POSITION & GUIDANCE DOCUMENTS OF ASHP

BEST PRACTICES

for Hospital & Health-System Pharmacy

2012-2013 Edition

American Society of Health-System Pharmacists®
Bethesda, Maryland

The ASHP policies in this book, positions and guidance documents, are intended to foster improvements in pharmacy practice and patient care. The content of individual positions and guidance documents should be assessed in the context of your own health system, its policies and procedures, as well as applicable federal and state laws and regulations.

Guidance documents, in particular, evolve because of advances in technology, new knowledge from research, and lessons from experience. Additionally, medication information is constantly evolving because of ongoing research and clinical experience, and it is often subject to interpretation and unique clinical situations. The American Society of Health-System Pharmacists (ASHP) endeavors to ensure the completeness and timeliness of the information presented. However, the reader is advised that the publisher, contributors, editors, and reviewers make no representations concerning the suitability of the information for any purpose, and are not responsible for the immediate currency of the information, for any errors or omissions, or for any consequences arising from the use of these materials. All decisions made within the context of pharmacy practice should be based on the independent judgment of the practitioner.

ASHP is the national professional organization whose nearly 40,000 members include pharmacists, pharmacy technicians, and pharmacy students who provide patient care services in hospitals, health systems, and ambulatory clinics. For 70 years, the Society has been on the forefront of efforts to improve medication use and enhance patient safety. For more information about the wide array of ASHP activities and the many ways in which pharmacists help people make the best use of medicines, visit ASHP's website, www.ashp.org, or its consumer website, www.safemedication.com.

Editor: Bruce Hawkins

Published by the American Society of Health-System Pharmacists, 7272 Wisconsin Avenue, Bethesda, MD 20814.

ASHP® is a service mark of the American Society of Health-System Pharmacists®, Inc.; registered in the U.S. Patent and Trademark Office.

ISBN: 978-1-58528-381-1

Contents

*Indicates content that has been added or revised since the 2011–2012 edition.

Ethics

Formulary Management (Medication-Use Policy Development)

*Indicates content that has been added or revised since the 2011–2012 edition.

Government, Law, and Regulation

Medication Misadventures

Medication Therapy and Patient Care

ORGANIZATION AND DELIVERY OF SERVICES

*Indicates content that has been added or revised since the 2011–2012 edition.

SPECIFIC PRACTICE AREAS

Pharmaceutical Industry

DRUG PRODUCTS, LABELING, AND PACKAGING

*Indicates content that has been added or revised since the 2011–2012 edition.

MARKETING

Pharmacy Management

COMPENSATION AND REIMBURSEMENT

HUMAN RESOURCES

Practice Settings

Research

*Indicates content that has been added or revised since the 2011–2012 edition.

ASHP Therapeutic Position Statements

ASHP Therapeutic Guidelines

Index

Page Locator for Guidance Documents by Type and Title

ASHP Statements

ASHP Guidelines

ASHP Report

ASHP Technical Assistance Bulletins

Acknowledgments

SHP gratefully acknowledges the following organizations and individuals for drafting and reviewing* the new and revised guidance documents in this edition.

ASHP Statement on the
Role of the Medication Safety Leader

Drafter: Lynn Eschenbacher, Pharm.D., M.B.A.

Reviewers: American Osteopathic Association (AOA)
 Emily Alexander, Pharm.D., BCPS
 Dean A. Bennett, CPHQ
 Toby Clark, M.Sc., FASHP
 Jorge Carrillo, Pharm.D., M.S.
 John B. Crosby, J.D. (AOA)
 Jean Douglas, Pharm.D.
 Michael S. Edwards, Pharm.D., M.B.A.,
 BCOP, FASHP
 Roy Guharoy, Pharm.D.
 Becky Harvey, Pharm.D.
 John Hertig, Pharm.D., M.S.
 James M. Hoffman, Pharm.D., M.S., BCPS
 Justin M. Julius, Pharm.D.
 Ambra King, Pharm.D.
 Joanne Kowiatek, M.P.M., FASHP
 Donna Luong, Pharm.D.
 Jeannell Mansur, Pharm.D., FASHP
 Elaine Mebel, Pharm.D., M.S.
 John F. Mitchell, Pharm.D., FASHP
 David B. Moore, M.P.A., CPh
 Ashley M. Overy, Pharm.D.
 Stephanie Peshek, Pharm.D., M.B.A.,
 FASHP
 James Ponto, M.S., FASHP
 Curt W. Quap, M.S., FASHP
 Marcus Ravnan, Pharm.D., FASHP, FCSHP
 Jennifer Schultz, Pharm.D., FASHP
 Nancy R. Smestad, M.S.
 Robert L. Stein, Pharm.D., J.D.
 Jody Jacobson Wedret, B.S.Pharm., FASHP,
 FCSHP

ASHP Statement on the
Pharmacist's Role in Medication Reconciliation

Drafter: Michelle M. Thoma, Pharm.D.

Reviewers: Academy of Managed Care Pharmacy
 (AMCP)
 Paul Barrett, Pharm.D., M.P.A., BCPS,
 FASHP
 Julie Cooper, Pharm.D., BCPS
 Michael S. Edwards, Pharm.D., M.B.A.,
 BCOP, FASHP
 Jean Douglas, Pharm.D.

 Kristine M. Gleason, B.S.Pharm.
 Kayla Hansen, Pharm.D., M.S.
 Becky Harvey, Pharm.D.
 John Hertig, Pharm.D., M.S.
 Justin Julius, Pharm.D.
 Nishaminy Kasbekar, Pharm.D., FASHP
 Carlo Lupano, B.S.Pharm., M.B.A., CCP
 Ashley M. Overy, Pharm.D.
 Fred J. Pane, B.S.Pharm., FASHP
 Barbara Petroff, M.S., FASHP
 James Ponto, M.S., FASHP
 Curt W. Quap, M.S., FASHP
 Elizabeth Sampsel, Pharm.D., M.B.A.,
 BCPS (AMCP)
 Jamie S. Sinclair, M.S., FASHP
 Richard L. Stambaugh, Pharm.D., M.S.,
 BCPS
 Robert L. Stein, Pharm.D., J.D.
 Jeffrey Stroup, Pharm.D., BCPS, AAHIVE

ASHP Statement on
Use of Social Media by Pharmacy Professionals

Drafter: Ashley M. Overy, Pharm.D.

Contributors: Kevin A. Clauson, Pharm.D.
 Brent I. Fox, Pharm.D., Ph.D.
 Karl F. Gumpper, BCNSP, BCPS, FASHP
 Arpit Mehta, Pharm.D.
 David R. Witmer, Pharm.D.

Reviewers: Academy of Managed Care Pharmacy
 (AMCP)
 Paul Barrett, Pharm.D., M.P.A., BCPS,
 FASHP
 Mark Brueckl, M.B.A. (AMCP)
 Jeff Cain, Ed.D., M.S.
 Michael S. Edwards, Pharm.D., M.B.A.,
 BCOP, FASHP
 Erin R. Fox, Pharm.D.
 Becky Harvey, Pharm.D.
 John Hertig, Pharm.D., M.S.
 Justin Julius, Pharm.D.
 Nishaminy Kasbekar, Pharm.D., FASHP
 Linda McElhiney, Pharm.D., FASHP, FIACP
 Sean Mirk, Pharm.D.
 John F. Mitchell, Pharm.D., FASHP
 David B. Moore, M.P.A., CPh
 Linda A. Nelson, Pharm.D.
 Agatha Nolen, Ph.D.
 James Ponto, M.S., FASHP

*Review does not imply endorsement.

Curt W. Quap, M.S., FASHP
Marcus Ravnan, Pharm.D.
Jamie S. Sinclair, M.S., FASHP
Kelly M. Smith, Pharm.D., BCPS, FASHP,
 FCCP
Jody Jacobson Wedret, B.S.Pharm., FASHP,
 FCSHP

*ASHP Guidelines: Minimum Standard
for Pharmacies in Hospitals*

Contributors: Thomas S. Brenner, B.S.Pharm., FASHP
Harold N. Godwin, M.S., FASHP, FAPhA
William A. Gouveia, M.S., FASHP
Brian D. Hodgkins, Pharm.D., FASHP,
 FCSHP
Stanley S. Kent, M.S., FASHP
Patricia C. Kienle, M.P.A., FASHP
Harold J. Kornfuhrer, B.S.Pharm., FASHP
Emory S. Martin III, Pharm.D., BCPS
J. Russell May, Pharm.D., FASHP
Gerald E. Meyer, Pharm.D., M.B.A., FASHP
Thomas E. O'Brien, Pharm.D., M.S.,
 FASHP
Sherri L. Ramsey, D.Ph., BCPS
Frank G. Saya, Pharm.D., FASHP, FCSHP
Donna L. Soflin, B.S.Pharm., FASHP
David K. Solomon, Pharm.D., FASHP
Kasey K. Thompson, Pharm.D., M.S.
Billy W. Woodward, B.S.Pharm.

Reviewers: American Nurses Association (ANA)
Institute for Safe Medication Practices
 (ISMP)
Rhode Island Society of Health-System
 Pharmacists (RISHP)
South Carolina Society of Health-system
 Pharmacists (SCSHP)
Wyoming Society of Health-Systems
 Pharmacy (WSHP)
Tuesday Adams, RN-C, WCC
John A. Armitstead, M.S., FASHP
Phil Ayers, Pharm.D., BCNSP
Ronald Barnes, M.S.
Paul J. Barrett, Pharm.D. BCPS
Carol J. Bickford, Ph.D., RN-BC, CPHIMS
 (ANA)
P. Justin Boyd, Pharm.D. BCPS, CDM
Tim Brown, Pharm.D., BCACP
Margaret Chrymko, Pharm.D.
Toby Clark, M.Sc., FASHP
Wayne F. Conrad, Pharm.D., FASHP
Gayle A. Cotchen, Pharm.D., M.B.A.
Debra Lynn Painter Cowan, Pharm.D.,
 FASHP
Arash Dabestani, Pharm.D., M.H.A.,
 FASHP, FABC
Denise F. Daly, Pharm.D., BCPS

Tina H. Denetclaw, Pharm.D., BCPS
Deanna Dossey, Pharm.D.
William L. Fritz, M.S., FASHP
Daphne Hsu Galang, RPhT, CPhT, B.S.,
 M.H.A.
Michael A. Gillette, Pharm.D., BCPS,
 BCACP
Kathleen M. Gura, Pharm.D., BCNSP,
 FASHP, FPPAG
Reginald L. Hain, B.S.Pharm.
Thomas G. Hall, Pharm.D.
George Hatfield, Pharm.D.
Jesse Hogue, Pharm.D.
Andrew Jarrell, Pharm.D.
Jack G. Kitrenos, Pharm.D., FASHP
Jamie Kuo, Pharm.D.
Jim Lile, Pharm.D.
Charles "Kurt" Mahan, Pharm.D., Ph.C.
Linda Gore Martin, Pharm.D., M.B.A.,
 BCPS (WSHP)
Justine Medina, M.S., RN
Dayna Mitchell, Pharm.D., BCPS
Holly Monatt, Pharm.D., BCPS
Selma Morrison
Robert J. Moura, M.S.
Jonathan M. Mundy, M.B.A. (RISHP)
Bruce A. Nelson, M.S.
Beth Norman, M.S., RN, CNS, ACNS-BC
Robert S. Oakley, M.S.
Fred J. Pane, B.S.Pharm., FASHP
Shreya Parekh, Pharm.D.
Jennifer Phillips, Pharm.D.
James Ponto, BCNP, FASHP
Curt W. Quap, M.S., FASHP
Todd Rowland, Pharm.D.
Renee B. Sager, Pharm.D.
Joseph Sceppa, M.S., M.B.A.
Nicole Shumiloff, Pharm.D.
Nancy R. Smestad, M.S.
Carolyn M. Smith, Pharm.D., M.B.A.,
 BCPS (SCHSP)
William E. Smith, Pharm.D., M.P.H., Ph.D.,
 FASHP
Richard L. Stambaugh, Pharm.D., M.S.,
 BCPS
Therese Staublin, Pharm.D.
Marc Stranz, Pharm.D.
Timothy P. Stratton, Ph.D.
Pamela Swarny, Pharm.D., J.D.
Jane Tennis, B.S.Pharm., M.B.A.
Sherry Umhoefer, M.B.A.
Allen J. Vaida, Pharm.D., FASHP (ISMP)
Jody Jacobson Wedret, B.S.Pharm., FASHP,
 FCSHP
Roger Woolf, Pharm.D.
Kevin Zak, Pharm.D.

ASHP Therapeutic Position Statement on the Institutional Use of 0.9% Sodium Chloride Injection to Maintain Patency of Peripheral Indwelling Intermittent Infusion Devices

Authors: Kim W. Benner, Pharm.D., BCPS, FASHP
 Amber J. Lucas, Pharm.D., BCPS, FASHP

Reviewers: Joseph M. Alessandrini, B.S.Pharm., FASHP
 Paul J. Barrett, Pharm.D., M.P.A., BCPS, FASHP
 Thomas Burnakis, Pharm.D.
 W. Duane Deaver, Pharm.D.

Brent R. Ekins, Pharm.D.
Randy Kuiper, Pharm.D., BCPS, FASHP
Marilyn Lee, Pharm.D., BCPS
Robert Long, B.S.Pharm.
Fred L. Meister, Pharm.D., FASHP
Edna Patatanian, Pharm.D.
James A. Ponto, M.S., BCNP, FASHP
Clyde Spence, Pharm.D., M.B.A.
Paul C. Walker, Pharm.D., FASHP
Jody Jacobson Wedret, B.S.Pharm., FASHP, FCSHP
William P. Yee, Pharm.D., FASHP, FCSHP

Introduction

The American Society of Health-System Pharmacists (ASHP) is the 35,000-member national professional association that represents pharmacists and pharmacy technicians who practice in inpatient, outpatient, home-care, and long-term-care settings, as well as pharmacy students. ASHP has extensive publishing and educational programs designed to help members improve their delivery of pharmaceutical care, and it is a national accrediting organization for pharmacy residency and pharmacy technician training programs.

The Compendium

ASHP, since its founding, has developed official professional policies in the form of policy positions and guidance documents about pharmacy practice, first for hospitals, and then for the continuum of practice settings in integrated health systems. Since 1984, these policies have been compiled annually in *Best Practices for Hospital & Health-System Pharmacy,* a compendium of ASHP policy positions, statements, guidelines, technical assistance bulletins, therapeutic position statements, therapeutic guidelines, and selected ASHP-endorsed documents. *Best Practices* reflects the intent of ASHP's professional policies to foster improvements in pharmacy practice and patient care.

The compendium is organized by topic to help readers quickly locate related documents. The table of contents is structured by topic, and under each topic the relevant ASHP policy positions, statements, guidelines, technical assistance bulletins, and endorsed documents are listed. The therapeutic documents are listed by type. Following the table of contents is a page locator for documents by type and title, and the index lists each document, to assist readers who are accustomed to searching for a specific document by its title.

Origins and Purposes of ASHP's Policy Positions and Guidance Documents

Policy positions generally originate with an ASHP council and are approved by the ASHP Board of Directors and ASHP House of Delegates. Some policy positions originate as House of Delegate resolutions. Statements, guidelines, and technical assistance bulletins originate with an ASHP council or commission. Statements are approved by the Board of Directors and the House of Delegates, because of their broad philosophical nature. Other types of documents are approved by the Board of Directors only. Therapeutic position statements and therapeutic guidelines originate with the ASHP Council on Therapeutics and are approved by the Board of Directors.

There is a gradation in detail among the guidance documents. Policy positions are short pronouncements, intended to address professional practice. Often, principles established in policy positions are elaborated on in statements and guidelines. Statements express basic philosophy, guidelines offer programmatic advice, and technical assistance bulletins offer more detailed programmatic advice. Of the two types of therapeutic documents, therapeutic guidelines are thorough discussions of drug use and thera-

peutic position statements are concise responses to specific therapeutic issues.

The guidance documents of ASHP represent a consensus of professional judgment, expert opinion, and documented evidence. They provide guidance and direction to ASHP members and pharmacy practitioners and to other audiences who affect pharmacy practice. Their use may help to comply with federal and state laws and regulations, to meet accreditation requirements, and to improve pharmacy practice and patient care. They are written to establish reasonable goals, to be progressive and challenging, yet attainable as "best practices" in applicable health-system settings. They generally do not represent minimum levels of practice, unless titled as such, and should not be viewed as ASHP requirements.

The use of ASHP's guidance documents by members and other practitioners is strictly voluntary. Their content should be assessed and adapted based on independent judgment to meet the needs of local health-system settings.

The need for authoritative guidance in pharmacy practice has grown with changes in health care and with the shifting influences from regulatory, accrediting, risk-management, financing, and other bodies. Because of the complex nature of ASHP guidance documents, ASHP does not typically undertake immediate development of new documents or expedited revisions to existing documents in response to environmental changes. Other ASHP activities and services, such as educational sessions at national meetings and *American Journal of Health-System Pharmacy (AJHP)* articles, provide more timely information that may be helpful, until sufficient experience is gained to serve as the basis for a document.

Definitions

The types of guidance documents included in this compendium are defined as follows:

ASHP Policy Position: A pronouncement on an issue related to pharmacy professional practice, as approved by the Board of Directors and House of Delegates.

ASHP Statement: A declaration and explanation of basic philosophy or principle, as approved by the Board of Directors and the House of Delegates.

ASHP Guideline: Advice on the implementation or operation of pharmacy practice programs, as approved by the Board of Directors.

ASHP Technical Assistance Bulletin: Specific, detailed advice on pharmacy programs or functions as developed by an ASHP staff division in consultation with experts, as approved by the Board of Directors.*

ASHP Therapeutic Guideline: Thorough, systematically developed advice for health-care professionals on appropriate use of medications for specific clinical circumstances, as approved by the Board of Directors.

ASHP Therapeutic Position Statement: Concise statements that respond to specific therapeutic issues of concern to health care consumers and pharmacists, as approved by the Board of Directors.

ASHP-Endorsed Document: Professional policy developed by another organization that offers guidance on some aspect of pharmacy practice or medication use, as approved by the Board of Directors.

**The ASHP Board of Directors voted in November 1997 to discontinue the title "Technical Assistance Bulletin" in ASHP guidance documents, assigning the title "Guidelines" in its place. Over time, the title "Guidelines" will replace the title "Technical Assistance Bulletin" on existing documents when they are revised.*

Development of Guidance Documents

The responsible ASHP council or commission recommends the development of a guidance document after considering whether the topic: a) has generated a need among practitioners for authoritative advice; b) has achieved some stability and there is sufficient experience upon which to base a statement or guideline; c) is relevant to the practice of a significant portion of ASHP's members; d) is within the purview of pharmacy practice in health systems; e) is without other sufficient guidance; and f) does not pose significant legal risks to ASHP. Another consideration is whether ASHP leadership believes that there is room for improvements in practice and that an ASHP document would foster that improvement. The Board of Directors must support the recommendations before developmental processes begin.

The processes used to draft and review new or revised documents vary depending on the body responsible for their development and on the type of document. These processes are described below. Once approved, the document draft becomes an official ASHP policy and is published in *AJHP*, added to ASHP's Web site, and incorporated into the next edition of *Best Practices for Hospital & Health-System Pharmacy.* Therapeutic documents are reviewed and revised as needed every three years, and policy positions and practice documents every five years.

ASHP Statements and Guidelines

Any of the ASHP policy-recommending bodies (councils and commissions) may initiate and oversee the development of ASHP statements and guidelines; however, most of them are initiated by the Council on Pharmacy Practice. The development of these documents generally includes the following steps:

1. A group of experts on a given topic volunteers to develop a preliminary draft. Drafters are selected based on demonstrated knowledge of the topic and their practice settings. Most often, the drafters are ASHP members.
2. The draft is sent by ASHP to reviewers who have interest and expertise in the given topic. Reviewers consist of members and selected individuals knowledgeable in the content area, representatives of various ASHP

bodies, and other professional organizations. A draft of particular interest to ASHP's membership may be published in *AJHP*, posted on ASHP's Web site, or discussed at an open hearing or in a network forum during an ASHP Summer or Midyear Clinical meeting to solicit comments.

3. Based on the comments, a revised draft is submitted to the appropriate ASHP policy-recommending body for action. When the draft meets the established criteria for content and quality, that body recommends that the Board of Directors approve the document.

ASHP Therapeutic Guidelines and Therapeutic Position Statements

The Council on Therapeutics (COT) has responsibility for the development of ASHP therapeutic guidelines and ASHP therapeutic position statements.

Therapeutic Guidelines—The development of these documents generally includes the following steps:

1. When the COT identifies a topic for therapeutic guidelines development, ASHP formally solicits proposals for a contractual arrangement with an individual, group, or organization to draft the guidelines document and coordinate its review. The contractor will work with a panel of 6–10 experts appointed by ASHP who have diverse backgrounds relevant to the topic.
2. A systematic analysis of the literature is performed, and scientific evidence is evaluated based on predetermined criteria. Recommendations in the document are based on scientific evidence or expert consensus. When expert judgment must be used, the document indicates the scientific reasoning that influenced the decision. Scientific evidence takes precedence over expert judgement. Each recommendation is accompanied by projections of the relevant health and cost outcomes that could result.
3. The expert panel and COT review each draft of the guidelines document and provide comments. This process is repeated until the expert panel and COT are satisfied with the content.
4. ASHP solicits multidisciplinary expert input on the draft. Reviewers consist of members and selected individuals knowledgeable in the content area, representatives of various ASHP bodies, and other professional organizations.
5. Once the above processes are completed, COT recommends that the ASHP Board of Directors approve it.

ASHP Therapeutic Position Statements (TPS)—The development of these documents generally includes the following steps:

1. One or more experts on a given topic are assigned to draft the TPS. Drafters are selected based on demonstrated knowledge of the topic and their practice setting. Most often, the drafters are ASHP members.
2. The proposed draft document is reviewed by COT, which may suggest modifications. This process is repeated until COT is satisfied with the content.

3. ASHP solicits multidisciplinary expert input on the draft. Reviewers consist of members and selected individuals knowledgeable in the content area, representatives of various ASHP bodies, and other professional organizations.

4. Once the above processes are completed, COT finalizes the draft and recommends that the ASHP Board of Directors approve it.

Access to ASHP Positions and Guidance Documents

Besides publishing in *AJHP* and *Best Practices for Hospital & Health-System Pharmacy,* policy positions and guidance documents are available through ASHP's Web site at **www.ashp.org.** They are located at the "Policy Positions & Guidelines" heading under "Policy and Practice" on the ASHP Web site (www.ashp.org/bestpractices), where a chronological compendium of policy positions (*ASHP Policy Positions 1982–2012*) is also available.

Opportunities to Be a Part of Guidance Document Development

ASHP members determine the needs for policy guidance documents. They write and review the drafts. And, as members of policy-recommending bodies, the Board of Directors, and House of Delegates, they approve the documents.

ASHP members are encouraged to take an active role in the development of documents by suggesting topic ideas for new documents or modifications to current ones, volunteering to be drafters or reviewers, and completing survey and evaluation forms. Members may comment on or express their interests in participating in the development of documents by contacting the editor at (301) 657-3000 or by e-mail at standards@ashp.org.

Mission Statement of the American Society of Health-System Pharmacists (ASHP)

ASHP believes that the **mission of pharmacists** is to help people make the best use of medications.

The **mission of ASHP** is to advance and support the professional practice of pharmacists in hospitals and health systems and serve as their collective voice on issues related to medication use and public health.

Approved by the ASHP House of Delegates, June 4, 2001.

The bibliographic citation for this document is as follows: American Society of Health-System Pharmacists. Mission statement of the American Society of Health-System Pharmacists (ASHP). *Am J Health-Syst Pharm.* 2001; 58:1524.

ASHP Vision Statement for Pharmacy Practice in Hospitals and Health Systems

ASHP dedicates itself to achieving a vision for pharmacy practice in hospitals and health systems in which pharmacists:

1. Will significantly enhance patients' health-related quality of life by exercising leadership in improving both the use of medications by individuals and the overall process of medication use.
2. Will manage patient medication therapy and provide related patient care and public health services.
3. Will be the primary individuals responsible for medication use and drug distribution systems.
4. Will be recognized as patient care providers and sought out by patients to help them achieve the most benefit from their therapy.
5. Will take a leadership role to continuously improve and redesign the medication-use process with the goal of achieving significant advances in (a) patient safety, (b) health-related outcomes, (c) prudent use of human resources, and (d) efficiency.
6. Will lead evidence-based medication-use programs to implement best practices.
7. Will have an image among patients, health professionals, administrators, and public policy makers as caring and compassionate medication-use experts.

Approved by the ASHP House of Delegates, June 4, 2001.

The bibliographic citation for this document is as follows: American Society of Health-System Pharmacists. ASHP vision statement for pharmacy practice in hospitals and health systems. *Am J Health-Syst Pharm.* 2001; 58:1524.

ASHP Policy Positions, Statements, Guidelines, and Technical Assistance Bulletins

Automation and Information Technology

Automation and Information Technology

Pharmacist's Role in Health Care Information Systems (1211)

Source: Council on Pharmacy Management

To strongly advocate key decision-making roles for pharmacists in the planning, selection, design, implementation, and maintenance of medication-use information systems, electronic health records, computerized provider order entry systems, and e-prescribing systems to facilitate clinical decision support, data analysis, and education of users for the purpose of ensuring the safe and effective use of medications; further,

To advocate for incentives to hospitals and health systems for the adoption of patient-care technologies; further,

To recognize that design and maintenance of medication-use information systems is an interdisciplinary process that requires ongoing collaboration among many disciplines; further,

To advocate that pharmacists must have accountability for strategic planning and direct operational aspects of the medication-use process, including the successful deployment of medication-use information systems.

This policy supersedes ASHP policy 0921.

Clinical Decision Support Systems (1212)

Source: Council on Pharmacy Management

To advocate for the development of clinical decision support (CDS) systems that are proven to improve medication-use outcomes and that include the following capabilities: (1) alerts, notifications, and summary data views provided to the appropriate people at the appropriate times in clinical workflows, based on (a) a rich set of patient-specific data, (b) standardized, evidence-based medication-use best practices, and (c) identifiable patterns in medication-use data in the electronic health record; (2) audit trails of all CDS alerts, notifications, and follow-up activity; (3) structured clinical documentation functionality linked to individual CDS alerts and notifications; and (4) highly accessible and detailed management reporting capabilities that facilitate assessment of the quality and completeness of CDS responses and the effects of CDS on patient outcomes.

Definition of Meaningful Use of Health Information Technology (1006)

Source: Council on Public Policy

To advocate to policymakers (public and private) that definitions of "meaningful use of health information technology" address interoperability of medication orders and prescriptions, medication decision support and continuous improvement, and quality reporting; further,

To advocate with respect to interoperability of medication orders and prescriptions that (1) a common medication vocabulary be mandated to promote the semantic interoperability of medication use across the continuum of care, because a common vocabulary is essential for comparative effectiveness research and for communicating medication information; and (2) communication of orders and electronic prescriptions must be demonstrated to be functional and semantically interoperable with pharmacy information systems; further,

To advocate with respect to medication decision support and continuous improvement that (1) medication decision support should include but not be limited to allergy, drug interaction (e.g., drug-lab or drug-disease interactions), duplicate therapy, and dose-range checking; and (2) that such a decision-support service must include an ongoing, continuous improvement process to attune the decision-support service to the needs of the providers who use it; further,

To advocate with respect to quality reporting that the ability to quantify improved patient safety, quality outcomes, and cost reductions in the medication-use process is essential, particularly in antimicrobial and adverse event surveillance.

Role of Pharmacists in Safe Technology Implementation (1020)

Source: Council on Pharmacy Practice

To affirm the essential role of the pharmacist in the evaluation, implementation, and ongoing assessment of all technology intended to ensure safety, effectiveness, and efficiency of the medication-use process.

Electronic Health and Business Technology and Services (0712)

Source: Council on Pharmacy Practice

To encourage pharmacists to assume a leadership role in their hospitals and health systems with respect to strategic planning for and implementation of electronic health and business technology and services; further,

To encourage hospital and health-system administrators to provide dedicated resources for pharmacy departments to design, implement, and maintain electronic health and business technology and services; further,

To advocate the inclusion of electronic health technology and telepharmacy issues and applications in college of pharmacy curricula.

This policy was reviewed in 2011 by the Council on Pharmacy Practice and by the Board of Directors and was found to still be appropriate.

Electronic Information Systems (0507)

Source: Council on Administrative Affairs

To advocate the use of electronic information systems, with appropriate security controls, that enable the integration of patient-specific data that is accessible in all components of a health system; further,

To support the use of technology that allows the transfer of patient information needed for appropriate medication management across the continuum of care; further,

To urge computer software vendors and pharmaceutical suppliers to provide standards for definition, collection, coding, and exchange of clinical data used in the medication-use process; further,

To pursue formal and informal liaisons with appropriate health care associations to ensure that the interests of patient care and safety in the medication-use process are fully represented in the standardization, integration, and implementation of electronic information systems; further,

To strongly encourage health-system administrators, regulatory bodies, and other appropriate groups to provide health-system pharmacists with full access to patient-specific clinical data.

This policy was reviewed in 2009 by the Council on Pharmacy Practice and by the Board of Directors and was found to still be appropriate.

Online Pharmacy and Internet Prescribing (0523)
Source: Council on Legal and Public Affairs
To support collaborative efforts of the Food and Drug Administration, the National Association of Boards of Pharmacy (NABP), and the Federation of State Medical Boards, as stated in the Principles of Understanding on the Sale of Drugs on the Internet, to regulate prescribing and dispensing of medications via the Internet; further,

To support legislation or regulation that requires pharmacy World Wide Web sites to list the states in which the pharmacy and pharmacists are licensed, and, if prescribing services are offered, requires that the sites (1) ensure that a legitimate patient-prescriber relationship exists (consistent with professional practice standards) and (2) list the states in which the prescribers are licensed; further,

To support mandatory accreditation by NABP of pharmacy Web sites and appropriate consumer education about the risks and benefits of using Internet pharmacies; further,

To support the principle that any medication distribution or drug therapy management system must provide timely access to, and interaction with, appropriate professional pharmacist patient-care services.

This policy was reviewed in 2009 by the Council on Pharmacy Practice and by the Board of Directors and was found to still be appropriate.

Computerized Prescriber Order Entry (0105)
Source: Council on Administrative Affairs
To advocate the use of computerized entry of medication orders or prescriptions by the prescriber when (1) it is planned, implemented, and managed with pharmacists' involvement, (2) such orders are part of a single, shared database that is fully integrated with the pharmacy information system and other key information system components, especially the patient's medication administration record, (3) such computerized order entry improves the safety, efficiency, and accuracy of the medication-use process, and (4) it includes provisions for the pharmacist to review and verify the order's appropriateness before medication administration, except in those instances when review would cause a medically unacceptable delay.

This policy was reviewed in 2010 by the Council on Pharmacy Management and by the Board of Directors and was found to still be appropriate.

Management of Blood Products and Derivatives (9919)
Source: Council on Legal and Public Affairs
To strongly encourage the computer software industry to provide data fields for lot number, expiration date, and other necessary and appropriate information for blood products and derivatives and biologicals, in order to facilitate compliance with regulatory requirements concerning the use of these products, particularly with respect to recalls or withdrawals.

This policy was reviewed in 2008 by the Council on Public Policy and by the Board of Directors and was found to still be appropriate.

Telepharmacy (9920)
Source: Council on Professional Affairs
To foster among health-system pharmacists and leaders of the telecommunications industry a common vision for the integration of telecommunication technology into the delivery of pharmaceutical care.

This policy was reviewed in 2008 by the Council on Pharmacy Practice and by the Board of Directors and was found to still be appropriate.

Regulation of Automated Drug Distribution Systems (9813)
Source: Council on Legal and Public Affairs
To work with the Drug Enforcement Administration and other agencies to seek regulatory and policy changes to accommodate automated drug distribution in health systems.

This policy was reviewed in 2007 by the Council on Public Policy and by the Board of Directors and was found to still be appropriate.

ASHP Statement on Bar-Code-Enabled Medication Administration Technology

Position

The American Society of Health-System Pharmacists (ASHP) encourages health systems to adopt bar-code-enabled medication administration (BCMA) technology to improve patient safety and the accuracy of medication administration and documentation. To support the goal of having all medications electronically verified before they are administered, BCMA systems should be used in all areas of health systems in which medications are used. Pharmacists must be involved in the interdisciplinary planning, development, implementation, and management of BCMA systems and must ultimately be responsible for developing and maintaining the infrastructure required to ensure BCMA success. Health systems deploying BCMA programs must provide the funding and staffing necessary to permit pharmacists to fulfill this role.

ASHP urges the Food and Drug Administration (FDA) and other regulatory agencies, standard-setting bodies, contracting entities, health systems, and others to mandate that pharmaceutical manufacturers use symbologies that are readily deciphered by commonly used scanning equipment to code for the National Drug Code (NDC), lot number, and expiration date on all unit dose, unit-of-use, and injectable drug packaging. Pharmaceutical manufacturers should also provide all medications used in health systems in unit dose packages. FDA, pharmaceutical manufacturers and packagers, and the manufacturers of BCMA systems should collaborate to minimize or eliminate the causes of false rejection of valid medication doses. Certain characteristics of the current NDC identification system contribute to the burden of implementing BCMA systems, and ASHP urges stakeholders to participate in efforts to develop a system that more reliably identifies the unique drug (or combination of drugs), strength, dosage form, and route of administration.

Although bar-coding systems are currently a widely used point-of-care technology, ASHP recognizes that other types of machine-readable coding (e.g., radio-frequency identification) may evolve. ASHP supports the use of new technologies that are as effective as or improve upon existing systems and believes the principles outlined in this statement apply to such systems. ASHP urges further research on such systems as well as research that will definitively determine the extent to which BCMA systems reduce preventable medication errors and provide a financial return on investment for health systems.

Background

Since the 1980s, health care practitioners and policymakers have recognized the potential benefits of using bar-coding technology in the medication dispensing and administration process.[1-5] Although there is a consensus of professional judgment and expert opinion on the advancement of BCMA technology, more studies are needed to definitively determine the impact of BCMA systems on medication errors and the finances of health systems. ASHP believes that optimally implemented BCMA systems have tremendous potential to improve patient safety. In addition, the reengineering of the medication-use process required to implement a BCMA system can provide opportunities for performance improvement in patient care and clinical documentation.

A 2005 ASHP survey estimated that only 13.2% of hospitals used a BCMA system.[6] Although this percentage is small, it represents an almost 10-fold increase since 2002.[7] The rapid adoption of BCMA systems presents challenges to health systems, and ASHP believes that pharmacists have a crucial role in responding to those challenges.

Role of the Pharmacist

Pharmacists should take the lead in ensuring that the implementation of BCMA systems and the reengineering of the medication-use system address the complexities of the process and that the goal of improving patient safety is achieved. Poor design and inadequate planning can compromise the effectiveness of a BCMA system and may even introduce new sources of error into the medication-use process.[8] Growing experience with BCMA systems has produced a body of knowledge that will aid hospitals and health systems in the adoption of BCMA systems.[9-12]

Pharmacy leadership needs to engage the chief information officer, chief nursing officer, and other key stakeholders in planning for BCMA systems as early as possible. Pharmacists and nurses should be involved with the preinstallation evaluation and selection of the BCMA system. Allowing end users to provide crucial advice about system design will increase acceptance and utility of the system.

Implementation of a BCMA system must be accompanied by the development of policies and procedures that ensure the system's safety. These policies and procedures should be developed by an interdisciplinary team that includes pharmacists.[10] Pharmacists and nurses should be involved with postinstallation evaluation and system improvement.

The role of nurses as end users of this technology should not be underestimated; nursing involvement is essential to successful system implementation and use. Processes for delivery and storage of medications (e.g., in medicine rooms or bedside storage spaces) should be examined by pharmacists and nurses to avoid workarounds or diversion.

Elements of a BCMA System

Although every hospital and health system will need to develop a BCMA system that meets its own needs, the following general principles should guide the implementation and use of such systems.

Use of the BCMA system should be universal within the health system. To the fullest extent feasible, every patient, care provider, and medication should receive a unique identifier, and that identifier should be used not only to verify care prescribed for a patient but also to document every significant step in the medication-use process.

A process should be in place to ensure simple, secure, and controllable placement and replacement of a patient identification tag. To ensure that there is only one active wristband per patient, this process should discourage the printing of multiple labels.[12] In addition to appropriate human-readable information, machine-readable patient wristbands should contain information (e.g., a photograph or the patient's medical record number) in order to uniquely identify the patient.

The BCMA system should have a secure user-identification system. Every care provider should be assigned and use a unique identifier. The care provider administering a medication should be able to use the BCMA system to verify that the medication to be administered is appropriate for the patient (i.e., confirming that the five rights of medication administration[13] are met). The BCMA system should document the information in the electronic medication administration record.

The pharmacy must be able to ensure that doses received in patient care areas can be scanned without inappropriate rejection and that those scans reliably indicate whether the medication is appropriate for a particular patient. For the implementation of a BCMA system to succeed, the health system must commit the pharmacy resources necessary to verify that each incoming medication is scannable and that the data encoded within its bar code accurately represent the product.

Every medication possible should be packaged in unit doses, and each unit dose package should be labeled with both human-readable medication identification information and a machine-readable code that includes the medication's unique identifier and, when feasible, its lot number and expiration date. Pharmacy information systems must be able to generate bar codes for multiple-component items. Pharmacy departments must develop a validation process for ensuring that every item has a bar code that can be scanned by all equipment supporting the BCMA system, including pharmacy automation systems, automated medication storage and distribution devices, and nursing BCMA scanning units.

An adequate number of scanners should be provided for each patient care area to facilitate scanning at peak times. Scanners should have the capacity to autodiscriminate the variety of symbologies encountered on pharmaceutical and pharmacy-prepared containers.

Finally, contingency plans should exist to ensure patient safety during system downtime. These policies should require that medications administered during downtime are retrospectively documented electronically in the medical record so that decision-support systems accurately reflect clinical trends associated with the patient, medication administration, and medication effects.

Conclusion

ASHP encourages health systems to adopt BCMA technology, with the goal of having all medications electronically verified before they are administered. Pharmacists must ultimately be responsible for developing and maintaining the infrastructure necessary to ensure BCMA success, and health systems deploying BCMA systems must provide the funding and staffing necessary to permit pharmacists to fulfill this role.

ASHP believes that pharmaceutical manufacturers should be required to place machine-readable coding that includes the NDC, lot number, and expiration date on all unit dose, unit-of-use, and injectable drug packaging, using symbologies that are readily deciphered by commonly used scanning equipment. ASHP also urges further research that will definitively determine the extent to which BCMA systems reduce preventable medication errors or provide a financial return on investment for health systems.

References

1. Hokanson JA, Keith MR, Guernsey BG et al. Potential use of barcodes to implement automated dispensing quality assurance programs. *Hosp Pharm.* 1985; 20:327–37.
2. Nold EG, Williams TC. Barcodes and their potential applications in hospital pharmacy. *Am J Hosp Pharm.* 1985; 42:2722–32.
3. Barry GA, Bass GE, Eddlemon JK et al. Bar-code technology for documenting administration of large-volume intravenous solutions. *Am J Hosp Pharm.* 1989; 46:282–7.
4. Lefkowitz S, Cheiken H, Barhart MR. A trial of the use of bar code technology to restructure a drug distribution and administration system. *Hosp Pharm.* 1991; 26:239–42.
5. Meyer GE, Brandell R, Smith JE et al. Use of bar codes in inpatient drug distribution. *Am J Hosp Pharm.* 1991; 48:953–66.
6. Pedersen CA, Schneider PJ, Scheckelhoff DJ. ASHP national survey of pharmacy practice in hospital settings: dispensing and administration—2005. *Am J Health-Syst Pharm.* 2006; 63:327–45.
7. Pedersen CA, Schneider PJ, Scheckelhoff DJ. ASHP national survey of pharmacy practice in hospital settings: dispensing and administration—2002. *Am J Health-Syst Pharm.* 2003; 60:52–68.
8. Patterson ES, Cook RI, Render ML. Improving patient safety by identifying side effects of introducing bar coding in medication administration. *J Am Med Inform Assoc.* 2002; 9:540–53.
9. Patterson E, Rogers M, Render M. Fifteen best practice recommendations for bar-code medication administration in the Veterans Health Administration. *Joint Comm J Qual Saf.* 2004; 30:355–65.
10. Neuenschwander M, Cohen MR, Vaida AJ et al. Practical guide to bar coding for patient medication safety. *Am J Health-Syst Pharm.* 2003; 60:768–79.
11. ASHP Research and Education Foundation Implementing a bar-coded medication safety program: a pharmacist's toolkit. www.ashpfoundation.org/MainMenuCategories/Education/SpecialPrograms/ImplementingaBarCodedMedSafetyProgram.aspx (accessed 2008 Dec 3).
12. Cummings J, Bush P, Smith D et al. Bar-coding medication administration overview and consensus recommendations. *Am J Health-Syst Pharm.* 2005; 62:2626–9.
13. 10 Golden rules for administering drugs safely. In: McGovern K. Preventing medication errors. Springhouse, PA: Springhouse; 1994:2–3.

Suggested Readings or Other Resources

ASHP guidelines on preventing medication errors in hospitals. *Am J Hosp Pharm.* 1993; 50:305–14.

Aspden P, Wolcott J, Bootman JL et al., eds. Preventing medication errors: quality chasm series. Washington, DC: National Academies Press; 2007.

Cohen MR, ed. Medication errors. Washington, DC: American Pharmaceutical Association; 1999.

Johnson CL, Carlson RA, Tucker CL et al. Using BCMA software to improve patient safety in Veterans Administration medical centers. *J Healthc Inf Manage.* 2002; 16:46–51.

Leape LL. Error in medicine. *JAMA.* 1994; 272:1851–7.

Poon EG, Cina JL, Churchill W et al. Medication dispensing errors and potential adverse drug events before and after implementing bar code technology in the pharmacy. *Ann Intern Med.* 2006; 145:426–34.

Puckett F. Medication management component of a point of care information system. *Am J Health-Syst Pharm.* 1995; 52:1305–9.

Developed through the ASHP Section of Pharmacy Informatics and Technology and approved by the ASHP Board of Directors on March 7, 2008, and by the ASHP House of Delegates on June 10, 2008. Supersedes ASHP policy position 0308.

Arash T. Dabestani, Pharm.D., M.H.A. and Alicia B. Perry, Pharm.D., are gratefully acknowledged for drafting versions of this statement.

The bibliographic citation for this document is as follows: American Society of Health-System Pharmacists. ASHP statement on barcode-enabled medication administration technology. *Am J Health-Syst Pharm.* 2009; 66:588–90.

ASHP Statement on Bar-Code Verification During Inventory, Preparation, and Dispensing of Medications

Position

The American Society of Health-System Pharmacists encourages hospital and health-system pharmacies to incorporate bar-code scanning into inventory management, dose preparation and packaging, and dispensing of medications. The purpose of such scanning is to ensure that drug products distributed, deployed to intermediate storage areas, or used in the preparation of patient doses are the correct products, are in-date, and have not been recalled. Such bar-code scanning should be employed in:

- Stocking of inventory both in the pharmacy and in other locations from which patient medications may be dispensed (e.g., an automated dispensing device),
- Manual packaging of oral solid and liquid medications,
- Compounding, repackaging, and labeling processes (e.g., scanning of source ingredients),
- Retrieving medications from automated dispensing devices, and
- Dispensing from the pharmacy to any location.

Prudent use of bar-coding technology in these processes will enhance patient safety and the quality of care by improving the accuracy of core pharmacy functions, closing potential gaps in the bar-code-assisted medication administration (BCMA) process, and allowing better allocation of pharmacists' knowledge and skills.

Background

Discussion of the role of technology in improving medication safety almost universally focuses on BCMA or computerized provider order entry (CPOE), despite evidence of medication errors that neither CPOE nor BCMA could prevent.[1,2] A number of activities in the medication-use process create opportunities for error outside of medication ordering and administration systems, such as:

- Receiving of inventory from suppliers and stocking of inventory locations from which patient medications may be dispensed (e.g., stocking unit-based automated dispensing devices with medications that may not be delivered to the bedside in their original packaging).
- Packaging of medications, which has become more prevalent as BCMA systems are more widely adopted by health systems and manufacturers have discontinued unit dose packaging of medications.
- Manual packaging of liquid medications in ready-to-administer form.
- The compounding of medications.
- The dispensing of patient-specific medications (e.g., 24-hour medication carts, nurse servers).

In addition, for BCMA to function, a vast majority of doses must be accurately bar coded, meaning there must be a highly reliable relationship between the information in the bar code and the contents of the dose. Additionally, the bar code must be readable by commercially-available scanners. Although doses delivered directly from manufacturer-labeled packages generally meet these conditions, there are numerous drug products that may not:

- Commercial products may lack a readily readable bar code, may have an irregular package shape that confounds the ability of scanning equipment to read the bar code, or may have a bar code in a symbology format that cannot be interpreted by the institution's bar-code scanning software.
- Nurse-prepared medications (e.g., insulin doses, heparin boluses, or syringes pre-drawn in the operating room) may be prepared at a location other than the patient's bedside, with the result that there is no labeling of any kind on the dose when it is administered.
- Compounded medications (e.g., sterile preparations) are often labeled by the pharmacy with a bar code that references a prescription or order number that describes the intended contents of the prescribed dose but provides no assurance that the prescribed contents were actually used in the product's preparation.

Benefits of Bar-Code Verification During Inventory, Preparation, and Dispensing

Initial estimates of the contribution of pharmacy dispensing errors to the overall medication errors were quite low.[3] However, recent reports have suggested that adding bar coding to the pharmacy dispensing process can significantly reduce opportunities for medication errors at the bedside and reduce the occurrence of potential adverse drug reactions.[4-6] Incorporating bar-code scanning in inventory management, dose preparation and packaging, and dispensing can improve patient safety in the following ways:

- Scanning during stocking in the pharmacy or patient-care locations (e.g., loading of an automated dispensing device) can help ensure that the product is placed in the correct location.
- Scanning during the retrieval of medications mitigates the hazards of erroneous medication stocking, which is especially important in the case of automated dispensing devices, where there is a potential risk that caregivers will override controls and remove medications for immediate use.
- Scanning of source ingredients during compounding, repackaging, or labeling processes can ensure that labeled doses contain the appropriate ingredients. Additionally, such scanning creates a reliable link be-

tween the information in the final package's bar code, its contents, and the National Drug Code (NDC) of the source container, which may be required to satisfy billing requirements (e.g., those of the Centers for Medicare & Medicaid Services).

- Scanning on dispensing can help prevent look-alike, sound-alike medication substitution errors that are difficult to visually detect, can identify and remove from distribution drug products whose bar codes are missing or unreadable, and prevent the distribution of expired or recalled products or facilitate retrieval in case of a recall.

- Scanning during any of these activities permits accumulation of an audit trail for each transaction in the inventory, preparation, and dispensing process. This information provides indications of the frequency of error encounter and detection, a record of the amount of time needed to perform selected functions, and evidence of success or failure of manual processes to deliver the correct medication.

Bar-code verification is optimized, and its potential negative impacts on productivity minimized, when the scanning system is configured to use bar codes on bulk packages (e.g., the bar code on an unopened case of unit-dose-packaged tablets) to confirm the contents of each item in the case, especially during batch processes. For patient-specific doses, each individual container used for the dose must be scanned.

The equipment and training costs for a pharmacy-based bar-code scanning implementation is quite small, especially when compared to those of BCMA systems.[7] Pharmacy-based bar-code scanning implementation may be considered a prerequisite for BCMA success, because unreadable bar codes are a significant cause of BCMA implementation failures.[8,9]

Limitations

As with BCMA, adoption of bar code scanning within distribution processes creates the necessity to ensure that the scanning system will recognize and appropriately respond to every bar code it scans. This verification activity is likely to create significant additional work for the pharmacy. Pharmacies planning on implementing such systems must plan for the resources needed to ensure that properly barcoded products are presented to, and readable by, the scanning system.

In addition, as with other bar-code technology implementations, pharmacy-based bar-code scanning systems will only be beneficial if appropriately deployed. For example, given the need to scan three vials of medication to prepare an IV admixture, such a system cannot distinguish between scanning each vial and scanning the same vial three times, although the latter defeats the purpose of the scanning. Any program of pharmacy-based bar-code scanning should be accompanied by appropriate training, policies, and procedures to promote and optimize safe use of the system, as well as a regular program of auditing to ensure that the program is being properly deployed by staff. Additionally, such programs require hospitals and health systems to compile and maintain a complete database of bar codes in use throughout the institution. The availability of such information in a timely fashion is a well-recognized problem.[10] An incomplete database or the absence of bar codes on drug products can undermine

the entire system, as the system cannot properly recognize and evaluate the drug products being scanned. Procedures should address such issues as the expected behavior while scanning occurs, specific prohibited acts, and the penalties associated with known at-risk behavior.[11]

In addition, this statement should not be interpreted to express a preference for bar-code scanning over other forms of automated identification of medications. Currently, bar coding is the least-expensive mechanism to introduce and deploy throughout the medication management cycle.[12] Should other technologies (e.g., radio-frequency identification) demonstrate similar or better capabilities, the principles articulated in this statement will continue to apply.

Validation

As with all such systems, bar coding on dispensing presumes that the scanning software, the scanning hardware, and the associated underlying database are accurate and complete. To ensure accuracy and completeness, organizations using a bar coding process will need to validate both that the software operates as expected and that the underlying database information is correct and reliable. A process will also need to be in place to immediately remediate problems if it is discovered that the hardware, software, or database are not operating properly.

Conclusion

Prudent use of bar-code scanning in inventory management, dose preparation and packaging, and dispensing of medications can enhance patient safety and the quality of care. Such scanning also provides the opportunity to accumulate and use statistics on the pharmacy distributive operation that can direct more appropriate staffing, identify sources of routine error, and generally permit better management of the drug distribution process.

References

1. Wolf R. Preventable medication error responsible for infant deaths. Injury Board.com. Available at: http://dallas.injuryboard.com/medical-malpractice/preventable-medication-error-responsible-for-infant-deaths.aspx?googleid=206592 (accessed 2010 Jan 11).
2. Institute for Safe Medication Practices. Failed check system for chemotherapy leads to pharmacist's no contest plea for involuntary manslaughter. www.ismp.org/Newsletters/acutecare/articles/20090423.asp (accessed 2010 Mar 4).
3. Bates DW, Cullen DJ, Laird N et al. Incidence of adverse drug events and potential adverse drug events. Implications for prevention. ADE Prevention Study Group. *JAMA.* 1995; 274:29-34.
4. Cina J, Fanikos J, Mitton P et al. Medication errors in a pharmacy-based bar-code-repackaging center. *Am J Health-Syst Pharm.* 2006; 63:165-8.
5. Poon EG, Cina JL, Churchill W et al. Medication dispensing errors and potential adverse drug events before and after implementing bar code technology in the pharmacy. *Ann Intern Med.* 2006;145:426-34.

6. Ragan R, Bond J, Major K et al. Improved control of medication use with an integrated bar-code-packaging and distribution system. *Am J Health-Syst Pharm.* 2005; 62:1075-9.

7. Maviglia SM, Yoo JY, Franz C et al. Cost-benefit analysis of a hospital pharmacy bar code solution. *Arch Intern Med.* 2007; 167:788-94.

8. Koppel R, Wetterneck T, Telles JL et al. Workarounds to barcode medication administration systems: their occurrences, causes and threats to patient safety. *J Am Med Inform Assoc.* 2008;15:408-23.

9. Young D. VA pursues bar code quality. *Am J Health-Syst Pharm.* 2004; 61:1312-4.

10. ASHP statement on bar-code-enabled medication administration technology. *Am J Health-Syst Pharm.* 2009; 66:588–90. www.ashp.org/DocLibrary/BestPractices/AutoITStBCMA.aspx. (accessed 2010 Mar 4).

11. ASHP policy position 0910: reporting medication errors. In: Hawkins B, ed. *Best practices for hospital and health-system pharmacy: positions and guidance documents of ASHP.* 2009-2010 ed. Bethesda, MD: American Society of Health-System Pharmacists; 2006:160. www.ashp.org/DocLibrary/BestPractices/MedMisPositions09.aspx (accessed 2010 Mar 08).

12. Cummings J, Bush P, Smith D et al. Bar-coding medication administration: overview and consensus recommendations. *Am J Health-Syst Pharm.* 2005; 62:2626-9.

Suggested Reading

Bates DW, Cullen JC, Laird N et al. Incidence of adverse drug events and potential adverse drug events. *JAMA.* 1995; 274:29-34.

Nold EG, Williams TC. Bar codes and their potential applications in hospital pharmacy. *Am J Hosp Pharm.* 1985; 42:2722-32.

Meyer GE, Brandell R, Smith JE et al. Use of bar codes in inpatient drug distribution. *Am J Hosp Pharm.* 1991; 48:953-66.

Santell JP, Hicks RW, McMeekin J et al. Medication errors: experience of the United States Pharmacopeia (USP) MEDMARX reporting system. *J Clin Pharmacol.* 2003; 43:760-7.

Ness JE, Sullivan SD, Stergachis A. Accuracy of technicians and pharmacists in identifying dispensing errors. *Am J Health-Syst Pharm.* 1994; 51:354-7.

Oswald S, Caldwell R. Dispensing error rate after implementation of an automated pharmacy carousel system. *Am J Health-Syst Pharm.* 2007; 64:1427-31.

Cina J, Fanikos J, Mitton P et al. Medication errors in a pharmacy-based bar-code-repackaging center. *Am J Health-Syst Pharm.* 2006; 63:165-8.

Ambrose PJ, Saya FG, Lovett LT et al. Evaluating the accuracy of technicians and pharmacists in checking unit dose medication cassettes. *Am J Health-Syst Pharm.* 2002; 59:1183-8.

Shane R. Current status of administration of medicines. *Am J Health-Syst Pharm.* 2009; 66:s42-s48.

Blair R. Medication transformation: pharmacists on the floor. A Midwest healthcare system takes bar code technology to new heights, as part of an enterprise initiative to optimize patient safety. *Health Manag Technol.* 2004; 25:26, 28, 30.

Nanji KC, Cina J, Patel N et al. Overcoming barriers to the implementation of a pharmacy bar code scanning system for medication dispensing: a case study. *J Am Med Inform Assoc.* 2009; 16:645-50.

Developed through the ASHP Section of Pharmacy Informatics and Technology and approved by the ASHP Board of Directors on April 15, 2010, and by the ASHP House of Delegates on June 6, 2010.

This statement was drafted by the ASHP Section of Pharmacy Informatics and Technology 2009–2010 Section Advisory Group on Pharmacy Operations Automation (Dennis A. Tribble, Pharm.D.; Ron Burnette, B.S.Pharm., M.B.A.; Dawn M. Biller; Leslie Brookins, M.S.; Richard Capps III, Pharm.D.; Marvin H. Choi; Kavish J. Choudhary, Pharm.D., M.S.; Seth Aaron Cohen, Pharm.D.; Thomas W. Cooley M.B.A.; Arash T. Dabestani, Pharm.D., M.H.A., FABC; Charles De la Torre, M.S., MIS; Doina Dumitru, Pharm.D., M.B.A.; Christopher Fortier, B.S.Pharm.; Barbara Giacomelli, Pharm.D., MBA, FASHP; Staci Hermann, M.S., Pharm.D.; Gary L. Johnson, Jr., Pharm.D., M.H.A.; Seth A. Kuiper, Pharm.D.; Denise Mckenzie, B.S.Pharm.; Rhonda B. McManus, Pharm.D.; Eric C. Nemec, II, Pharm.D.; Beth Prier, Pharm.D., M.S.; Brad Rognrud, M.S., R.Ph.; Kevin A. Scheckelhoff, M.B.A.; Paul M. Seelinger, B.S.Pharm.; Suzanne B. Shea, M.B.A.; David A. Tjhio, M.S., Pharm.D.; Christopher J. Urbanski, M.S.; Gwen Volpe, B.S.Pharm.; Rayburn Brian Vrabel, Pharm.D.; and Robynn P. Wolfschlag, M.B.A.).

ASHP gratefully acknowledges the following organizations and individuals for reviewing drafts of this statement (review does not imply endorsement): American Association of Critical Care Nurses (AACCN); American Nurses Association (ANA); Institute for Safe Medication Practices (ISMP); Rhode Island Society of Health System Pharmacists (RISHP); South Carolina Society of Health-System Pharmacists (SCSHP); Wyoming Society of Health-System Pharmacy (WSHP); Linda Annecchini, M.S.; James L. Besier, Ph.D., FASHP; Carol J. Bickford, Ph.D., RN-BC (ANA); Denny C. Briley, Pharm.D.; Mary E. Burkhardt, M.S., FASHP; Richard Capps, Pharm.D.; William W. Churchill, M.S.; Debra Cowan, Pharm.D.; Michele Danish, Pharm.D, FASHP; Brent I. Fox, Pharm.D., Ph.D.; Karl F. Gumpper, BCNSP, BCPS, FASHP; Kathleen M. Gura, Pharm.D., BCNSP, FASHP; J. Chad Hardy, Pharm.D., M.S.; Robi Hellman, RN, MSN, CNS (AACCN); Matthew R. Keith, B.S.Pharm., FASHP; Stan Kent, M.S.; Thomas E. Kirschling, Pharm.D., M.S.; Jim Lile, Pharm.D.; Jeff Little, Pharm.D., M.P.H.; Donald Lynx, M.B.A., FASHP; Leslie R. Mackowiak, M.S.; Linda Gore Martin, Pharm.D., M.B.A., BCPS (WSHP); Denise McKenzie, CPhT; Joel Melroy, Pharm.D., M.S., BCPS (SCSHP); Ian Orensky, Pharm.D., M.S.; Stephanie C. Peshek, Pharm.D., M.B.A., FASHP; Tommie Peterson, B.S.Pharm.; James Ponto, M.S., BCNP, FASHP; Brad Rognrud, M.S.; Martha J. Roberts, Pharm.D. (RISHP); Richard I. Sakai, Pharm.D., FASHP, FCSHP; Ronald Schneider, B.S.Pharm., M.H.A.; Paul Seelinger, B.S.Pharm.; Suzanne Shea, M.B.A.; Armen Simonian, Pharm.D.; Kirby K. Stiening, B.S.Pharm.; George Taniguchi, Pharm.D., M.P.H., M.A.; Greg Teale, Pharm.D.; Jennifer Thomas, Pharm.D.; Melanie J. Townsend, Pharm.D., BCPS; Dennis A. Tribble, Pharm.D.; Chris L. Tucker, B.S.Pharm.; Chris Urbanski, M.S.; Allen J. Vaida, Pharm.D., FASHP (ISMP); Rayburn B. Vrabel, Pharm.D.; Kelley A. Wasicek, B.S.Pharm.; and Jody Jacobson Wedret, FASHP, FCSHP.

The bibliographic citation for this document is as follows: American Society of Health-System Pharmacists. ASHP statement on bar-code verification during inventory, preparation, and dispensing of medications. *Am J Health-Syst Pharm.* 2011; 68:442-5.

ASHP Statement on the Pharmacist's Role in Informatics

Position

The American Society of Health-System Pharmacists (ASHP) believes that pharmacists have the unique knowledge, expertise, and responsibility to assume a significant role in medical informatics. As governments and the health care community develop strategic plans for the widespread adoption of health information technology, pharmacists must use their knowledge of information systems and the medication-use process to improve patient care by ensuring that new technologies lead to safer and more effective medication use.

ASHP has long recognized pharmacy informatics as a unique subset of medical informatics that focuses on the use of information technology and drug information to optimize medication use. The purpose of this statement is to reaffirm the responsibilities of the pharmacist and the pharmacy informaticist in medical informatics.

Background

Medical informatics was first defined during the 1960s.[1] Since then, the term informatics has been redefined several times, reflecting the dynamic nature of the health care information technology environment. The National Library of Medicine defines medical informatics as the "field of information science concerned with the analysis, use and dissemination of medical data and information through the application of computers to various aspects of health care and medicine."[2] The central purpose of medical informatics is the dissemination of two core types of information: (1) patient-specific information created in the care of patients and (2) knowledge-based information, which includes the scientific literature of health care.[3] Most researchers consider medical informatics an interdisciplinary or heterogeneous field, made of individuals with diverse backgrounds and levels of training with an inconsistently defined set of skills.[4] The broad definition of medical informatics and the number of disciplines potentially involved present an opportunity for the growth of subspecialties within the field. One of these subspecialties is pharmacy informatics, which can be defined as the use and integration of data, information, knowledge, technology, and automation in the medication-use process for the purpose of improving health outcomes.

The potential for medical informatics to improve health outcomes has prompted the health care industry, large health care purchasers, and state and federal governments to undertake sweeping health information technology initiatives that commonly include the following applications[5]:

- Computerized prescriber-order-entry systems integrated with electronic health records (EHRs) and pharmacy information systems,
- Clinical decision-support tools that bring best-practice information and guidelines to clinicians at the time they need them and rule-based systems for monitor-

ing, evaluating, responding, and reconciling medication-related events and information,
- Pharmacy information systems that allow electronic validation of medication orders in real time, provide the data flow needed to update both the medication administration record and order-driven medication dispensing systems, and support such operational activities as supply-chain management and revenue compliance,
- Automated dispensing cabinets and robotics integrated or interfaced with pharmacy information systems,
- Integrated medication administration management systems that enable the administration of bar-coded medications and use of "smart" infusion pumps, and
- Integrated medication surveillance applications for the reporting of medication incidents and adverse vents.

Development of these applications requires organizations to reengineer existing medication-use processes by introducing additional technologies and applications to support the end-to-end management of medications across the continuum of care. The drive to create a seamless environment for real-time sharing of medication- and patient-related information across all levels of care has highlighted the importance of medical and pharmacy informatics in health care. Traditional pharmacy systems that focus on the transcribing, preparation, and distribution phases of the medication-use process are often considered the foundation, or hub, for communicating meaningful information outside the pharmacy domain. The creation of such systems requires a unique blend of medication management and technology-related skills and draws new attention to the need for pharmacy informaticists.

Federal Initiatives

Reports issued by the Institute of Medicine[6,7] and subsequent research validating the importance of technology in health care led the federal government's launch of two important health care technology initiatives. In summer 2004, the Department of Health and Human Services released a 10-year plan entitled *The Decade of Health Information Technology: Delivering Consumer-Centric and Information-Rich Health Care*.[8] The plan was specifically designed to transform the delivery of health care by building a new health information infrastructure that links health care records nationwide. The plan describes the pressing need to achieve "always-current, always-available electronic health records for Americans." These EHR systems would allow physicians and other health professionals to share valuable health care information at the point of care. The report identified four major goals[8]:

1. *Inform clinical practice.* Bring information tools to the point of care, especially by investing in EHR systems in physicians' offices and hospitals.
2. *Interconnect clinicians.* Build an interoperable health information infrastructure so that records follow the

patient and clinicians have access to critical health care information when treatment decisions are being made.

3. *Personalize care.* Use health information technology to increase consumers' access to information and involvement in health care decisions.
4. *Improve population health.* Expand the capacity for monitoring public health, measuring quality of care, and accelerating implementation of research advances into medical practice.

The Centers for Medicare and Medicaid Services and the Department of Health and Human Services have published standards for an electronic prescription drug program under Title I of the Medicare Prescription Drug, Improvement, and Modernization Act of 2003 (MMA).[9] These standards are the first step in adopting final standards to address the MMA objectives of delivering cost-effective, efficient, safe, and high-quality patient care.

Electronic prescribing (e-prescribing) is the process of using a computer to enter, modify, review, and output or communicate prescriptions electronically to a patient's pharmacy.[10] E-prescribing with EHR systems further enhances the quality of care and patient safety by integrating the medication order into the overall process of medical care delivery.[8] Real-time access to patient information across the continuum of care and the provision of evidence-based clinical decision-support programs among stakeholders in the medication-use process offer opportunities to improve the quality of care, reduce errors, and improve workflow efficiency.

Pharmacists' Responsibilities

Pharmacists have unique, comprehensive knowledge about the safe and effective use of medications. More importantly, pharmacists understand core pharmacy operations and have developed expertise in end-to-end medication-use management, including communication with other information systems.[4] Pharmacists provide the expertise to effectively translate and seamlessly communicate the language of medication use across the continuum of care. They can interpret and implement requirements to ensure the safe and comprehensive communication of medication orders. An experienced pharmacist is skilled in the use of electronic medication-order-entry systems and has knowledge of human factor issues (e.g., interpretation of ambiguous clinical data) and the development of interfaces to disparate applications and systems.

Currently, there are many paths to becoming a pharmacy informaticist, with a growing number of training and residency programs focusing on this area. Although some pharmacy informaticists have formal academic or experiential training, the typical pharmacy informaticist is a pharmacist who has knowledge of computer systems, medication-use processes, safety issues, clinical management of medications, drug distribution, and administration and has developed extensive expertise in using technology to support these activities. Pharmacy informaticists are well suited to address the myriad issues involved with health care technology initiatives and provide leadership in the field of medical informatics. The pharmacy informaticist's responsibilities include active participation and leadership in all medical informatics activities that support medication use; education of pharmacy students, pharmacists, pharmacy technicians,

health care colleagues, and administrators; and research on the core areas of medical informatics.

Participation. The active participation of pharmacists in all aspects of medical informatics that support the medication-use process is imperative for safe and effective medication use. Such participation must be collaborative and comprehensive across the entire health care organization. It begins with system identification and vendor selection and includes identification of system requirements, as well as application design, development, implementation, and maintenance. Pharmacists must also be involved in the development and implementation of standards for medication-related vocabularies and terminologies to ensure safety and optimize deployment of activities related to clinical decision support.

Pharmacy informaticists are uniquely qualified to serve as liaisons between the pharmacy department and others involved in systems development, including vendors and other departments. The pharmacy informaticist's skills are needed to

* Work closely with information systems and pharmacy staff to develop system programming requirements while understanding system capabilities and limitations,
* Develop and oversee databases related to medication management systems,
* Identify, suggest solutions to, and resolve system or application problems,
* Assess medication-use systems for vulnerabilities to medication errors and implement medication-error prevention strategies,
* Actively participate in the development, prioritization, and determination of core clinical decision-support systems, and
* Assist in mining, aggregating, analyzing, and interpreting data from clinical information systems to improve patient outcomes.

The participation of pharmacy informaticists in the enhancement of the knowledge management infrastructure related to clinical decision support will make it possible for more providers to access high-quality references, rules, and guidelines that are comprehensive, usable, actionable, and configurable. Enhancing the vocabulary and terminology infrastructure will make broadly applicable research on the effectiveness of specific clinical decision-support methods possible.[11] Depending on the size of the organization and its scope of medication services, one or more pharmacists assigned and responsible for pharmacy informatics may provide the best means for attaining the level of participation required for safe and effective information systems.

Leadership. Pharmacists are responsible for patient safety throughout the medication-use process and need to take a leadership role in medical informatics at all levels of health care to ensure that health information technology supports safe medication use. Pharmacy informaticists must use their skills to

* Provide leadership to the institution's committees (e.g., practice, safety and quality, technology, pharmacy and therapeutics),
* Collaborate with other health care technology and clinical leaders to ensure that medication-related sys-

tems support interoperability and transportability of clinical information while maintaining patient safety and confidentiality,

- Attain key leadership roles within the health care technology industry, professional practice associations, and health care technology organizations, and
- Lead governmental and regulatory groups to sound conclusions regarding the use of technology in medication management, particularly as it relates to setting standards.

Education. Pharmacy informaticists need to develop a set of practical informatics competencies to manage medication-related data and information challenges across the continuum of health care.[12] Only a small percentage of U.S. pharmacy students currently receive the level of exposure to medical informatics needed to prepare for the dawning "decade of health information technology."[4] Pharmacy informaticists are responsible for providing strategic road maps for pharmacy educators that outline educational goals and objectives for training in medical informatics. Pharmacists actively involved in medical informatics within their own organizations are responsible for educating pharmacy staff and the institution's leadership about their role, particularly as it relates to using information technology to improve medication safety and quality of care. The education of leadership and staff must also include the inherent risks and negative aspects of implementing medication-use technologies. Their educational responsibilities include

- Supporting the continued growth of ASHP-accredited informatics residency training programs by serving as informatics residency program directors and preceptors,
- Coordination and implementation of staff development programs and curricula in pharmacy departments designed to teach fundamental concepts related to technology and outline those areas of medical informatics in which pharmacists are critical to the development process (e.g., electronic prescribing and ordering, clinical decision support, drug administration), and
- Training pharmacy technicians in the use of medication-related computer systems and technology in an effort to develop roles for credentialed pharmacy technicians to support pharmacy informaticists and other pharmacy staff.

Research. Pharmacy informaticists are responsible for performing research involving the core issues of medical informatics. Such research includes the study of standards, terminology, usability, and demonstrated value involving the economics, safety, and quality of health information technology.[3] Research efforts should be focused on designing and conducting research to expand informatics knowledge and its use in supporting patient care. The pharmacy informaticist, through qualitative and quantitative research, can assist in determining the balance of clinical informatics and health care system reengineering needed to optimize the medication-use process and improve patient safety and outcomes.

Conclusion

Pharmacists have the unique knowledge, expertise, and responsibility to assume a significant role in medical informat-

ics. As governments and the health care community develop strategic plans for the widespread adoption of health information technology, pharmacists must use their knowledge of information systems and the medication-use process to improve patient care by ensuring that new technologies lead to safer and more effective medication use.

References

1. Vanderbilt University Medical Center. What is biomedical informatics? www.mc.vanderbilt.edu/dbmi/informatics.html (accessed 2005 Dec 10).
2. National Library of Medicine. Collection development manual: medical informatics. www.nlm.nih.gov/tsd/acquisitions/cdm/subjects58.html (accessed 2005 Dec 10).
3. Hersh WR. Medical informatics: improving health care through information. *JAMA.* 2002; 288:1955–8.
4. Flynn AJ. The current state of pharmacy informatics education in professional programs at US colleges of pharmacy. *Am J Pharm Educ.* 2005; 69:490–4.
5. California HealthCare Foundation. Addressing medication errors in hospitals: a framework for developing a plan. www.chcf.org/documents/hospitals/addressing mederrorsframework.pdf (accessed 2006 Feb 9).
6. Committee on Quality of Health Care in America. Crossing the quality chasm: a new health system for the 21st century. Washington, DC: National Academy Press; 2001.
7. Kohn LT, Corrigan JM, Donaldson MS, eds. To err is human: building a safer health system. Washington, DC: National Academy Press; 1999.
8. Thompson TG, Brailer DJ. The decade of health information technology: delivering consumer-centric and information-rich health care. Framework for strategic action.www.hhs.gov/healthit/documents/hitframework.pdf (accessed 2006 Mar 10).
9. Centers for Medicare and Medicaid Services. Medicare program. Electronic prescription drug program; voluntary Medicare prescription drug benefit. *Fed Regist.* 2005; 70:67568–95.
10. eHealth Initiative. Executive summary—electronic prescribing: toward maximum value and rapid adoption. www.ehealthinitiative.org/initiatives/erx/document.aspx?Category=249&Document=269 (accessed 2006 Mar 10).
11. Teich JM, Osheroff JA, Pifer EA et al. Clinical decision support in electronic prescribing: recommendations and an action plan. Report of the Joint Clinical Decision Support Workgroup. www.amia.org/mbrcenter/pubs/docs/cdswhitepaperforhhs-final2005-03-08.pdf (accessed 2006 Feb 9).
12. Balen RM, Miller P, Malyuk D et al. Medical informatics: pharmacists' needs and applications in clinical practice. *J Inform Pharmacother.* 2000; 2:306–18.

Developed through the ASHP Section of Pharmacy Practice Managers and approved by the ASHP Board of Directors on March 28, 2006, and by the ASHP House of Delegates on June 27, 2006.

Mark H. Siska, B.S. is gratefully acknowledged for leading the drafting of this statement. ASHP also gratefully acknowledges the

following individuals for their participation in drafting this statement: Louis D. Barone, Pharm.D.; James L. Besier, B.S., M.S., Ph.D.; Toby Clark, M.S., FASHP; Kevin C. Marvin, B.S., M.S.; Scott R. McCreadie, Pharm.D., M.B.A.; Sandra H. Mitchell, M.S.I.S.; John C. Poikonen, Pharm.D.; Michael D. Schlesselman, Pharm.D.; Rita R. Shane, Pharm.D., FASHP; James G. Stevenson, Pharm.D., FASHP; Perry D. Taylor, Pharm.D.

The bibliographic citation for this document is as follows: American Society of Health-System Pharmacists. ASHP statement on the pharmacist's role in informatics. *Am J Health-Syst Pharm.* 2007; 64:200–3.

ASHP Statement on the Pharmacist's Role with Respect to Drug Delivery Systems and Administration Devices

Technological advances in drug delivery systems and administration devices frequently enable improved control of drug administration. Such advances may offer numerous potential benefits to patients, including improved therapeutic outcomes in disease management, improved patient compliance with drug regimens, and greater efficiency and economy in disease therapy. These advances constitute an important aspect of pharmaceutical knowledge and are routinely incorporated into pharmacy practice as they occur.

A drug delivery system is defined as one in which a drug (one component of the system) is integrated with another chemical, a drug administration device, or a drug administration process to control the rate of drug release, the tissue site of drug release, or both. A drug administration device is an apparatus that is used for introducing a drug to the body or controlling its rate of introduction. Drug delivery systems include (but are not limited to) osmotic pumps, thermal isolation, transdermal patches, liposomal encapsulation, iontophoresis, phonophoresis, magnetic migration, and implantation. Drug administration devices include (but are not limited to) mechanical (e.g., balloon-driven), gravity-driven, and electromechanical pumps. Some of the latter are portable, implantable, computer controlled, or patient controlled. Some enable the simultaneous infusion of multiple drugs. Drug administration control devices include plasma concentration monitoring and administration rate monitoring devices, which incorporate computers.

Pharmacists bear a substantial responsibility for ensuring optimal clinical outcomes from drug therapy and are suited by education, training, clinical expertise, and practice activities to assume responsibility for the professional supervision of drug delivery systems and administration devices. As a natural extension of efforts to optimize drug use, pharmacists should participate in organizational and clinical decisions with regard to these systems and devices. Some decisions and activities in which pharmacists should participate follow. Others may be appropriate as well.

1. Research and development of innovative drug delivery systems and administration devices.
2. Evaluation and research to determine the direct and comparative efficacy, safety, and cost-effectiveness of specific drug delivery systems and administration devices.
3. In conjunction with pharmacy and therapeutics committees (or other appropriate medical staff committees), decisions to choose or exclude particular drug delivery systems and administration devices for use in specific organizational settings.
4. Development of organization-specific policies and procedures regarding the acquisition, storage, distribution, use, maintenance, and ongoing product quality control of drug delivery systems and administration devices.
5. Choice of a particular drug delivery system or administration device for use in a specific patient's drug therapy.
6. Direct communication with patients to instruct them in the use of such systems and devices and to gather information necessary to monitor the outcome of their therapy.
7. Monitoring of the ongoing clinical effectiveness and suitability of specific drug delivery systems or administration devices with respect to specific patients and the communication of clinically relevant observations and recommendations to prescribers and other health professionals involved in the patients' care.

Failures or malfunctions of drug administration devices may lead to patient harm. Reports of such problems should be made in accordance with the provisions of the Safe Medical Devices Act of 1990 (PL 101–629).

Recommendations for Additional Reading

Acevedo ML. Electronic flow control. *NITA.* 1983; 6: 105–6.

Akers MJ. Current problems and innovations in intravenous drug delivery. Considerations in using the i.v. route for drug delivery. *Am J Hosp Pharm.* 1987; 44:2528–30.

Alexander MR. Current problems and innovations in intravenous drug delivery. Developing and implementing a contract for electronic infusion devices. *Am J Hosp Pharm.* 1987; 44:2553–6.

Anderson RW, Cohen JE, Cohen MR, et al. Hospital pharmacy symposium on new concepts in parenteral drug delivery. *Hosp Pharm.* 1986; 21:1033–55.

Baharloo M. Iontophoresis and phonophoresis: a role for the pharmacist. *Hosp Pharm.* 1987; 22:730–1.

Block LH, Shukla AJ. Drug delivery in the 1990s. *US Pharm.* 1986; 11(Oct):51–6, 58.

Boothe CD, Talley JR. Mechanical and electronic intravenous infusion devices. Part 1. *Infusion.* 1986; 10:6–8.

Chandrasekaran SK, Benson H, Urquhart J. Methods to achieve controlled drug delivery, the biomedical engineering approach. In: Robinson JR, ed. Sustained and controlled release drug delivery systems. New York: Marcel Dekker; 1978:557–93.

Colangelo A. Current problems and innovations in intravenous drug delivery. Drug preparation techniques for i.v. drug delivery systems. *Am J Hosp Pharm.* 1987; 44:2550–3.

Davis SR. Latest developments in drug delivery systems—abstracts. *Hosp Pharm.* 1987; 22:890–908.

Goodman MS, Wickham R. Venous access devices: oncology nurse overview. *Hosp Pharm.* 1985; 20:495–511.

Holm A, Campbell N. Role of institutional review boards in facilitating research, marketing of drugs and devices, and protecting human subjects. *Drug Dev Ind Pharm.* 1985; 11:1–12.

Juliano RL. Drug delivery systems. New York: Oxford University Press; 1980.

Kelly WN, Christensen LA. Selective patient criteria for the use of electronic infusion devices. *Am J IV Ther Clin Nutr.* 1983; 10(Mar):18, 19, 21, 25, 26, 29.

Kirschenbaum B, Klein S. Pharmacy-coordinated infusion device evaluation. *Am J Hosp Pharm.* 1984; 41:1181–3.

Leff RD. Current problems and innovations in intravenous drug delivery. Features of i.v. devices and equipment that affect i.v. drug delivery. *Am J Hosp Pharm.* 1987; 44:2530–3.

Longer MA, Robinson JR. Sustained-release drug delivery systems. In: Gennaro AR, ed. Remington's pharmaceutical sciences. Easton, PA: Mack Publishing Company; 1985:1644–61.

McFarlane AE. Role for pharmacists in the provision of medical devices. *Aust J Hosp Pharm.* 1986; 16:78.

Mutschler E. Now and future of drug delivery systems. *Pharm Tech.* 1983(Suppl); 7:13–5.

Nahata MC. Current problems and innovations in intravenous drug delivery. Effect of i.v. drug delivery systems on pharmacokinetic monitoring. *Am J Hosp Pharm.* 1987; 44:2538–42.

Piecoro JJ Jr. Current problems and innovations in intravenous drug delivery. Development of an institutional i.v. drug delivery policy. *Am J Hosp Pharm.* 1987; 44:2557–9.

Polack AE, Roberts MS. Drug delivery systems. *Med J Aust.* 1986; 144:311–4.

Rapp RP. Current problems and innovations in intravenous drug delivery. Considering product features and costs in selecting a system for intermittent i.v. drug delivery. *Am J Hosp Pharm.* 1987; 44:2533–8.

Reilly KM. Current problems and innovations in intravenous drug delivery. Problems in administration techniques and dose measurement that influence accuracy of i.v. drug delivery. *Am J Hosp Pharm.* 1987; 44:2545–50.

Reiss RE. Volumetric IV pumps. *Pharm Tech.* 1983(Suppl); 7:46–9.

Self TH, Brooks JB, Lieberman P, et al. The value of demonstration and role of the pharmacist in teaching the correct use of pressurized bronchodilators. *Can Med Assoc J.* 1983; 128:129–31.

Selton MV. Implantable pumps. *CRC Crit Rev Biomed Eng.* 1987; 14:201–40.

Smith KL. Developments in drug delivery systems. *Hosp Pharm.* 1987; 22:905–6.

Talley JR. Mechanical and electronic intravenous infusion devices. Part 2. *Infusion.* 1986; 10:31–4.

Talley JR. Mechanical and electronic intravenous infusion devices. Part 3. *Infusion.* 1986; 10:58–62.

Talsma H, Crommelin DJA. Liposomes as drug delivery systems, part I: preparation. *Pharm Tech.* 1992(Oct); 16:98, 100, 102, 104, 106.

Urquhart J. Implantable pumps in drug delivery. *Pharm Tech.* 1983(Suppl); 7:53–4.

Zenk KE. Current problems and innovations in intravenous drug delivery. Intravenous drug delivery in infants with limited i.v. access and fluid restriction. *Am J Hosp Pharm.* 1987; 44:2542–5.

This statement was reviewed in 1998 by the Council on Professional Affairs and by the ASHP Board of Directors and was found to still be appropriate.

Approved by the ASHP Board of Directors, November 18, 1992, and the ASHP House of Delegates, June 9, 1993. Revised by the ASHP Council on Professional Affairs. Supersedes a previous version approved by the ASHP House of Delegates on June 5, 1989, and the ASHP Board of Directors on November 16, 1988.

The bibliographic citation for this document is as follows: American Society of Hospital Pharmacists. ASHP statement on the pharmacist's role with respect to drug delivery systems and administration devices. *Am J Hosp Pharm.* 1993; 50:1724–5.

ASHP Statement on Use of Social Media by Pharmacy Professionals

Position

The American Society of Health-System Pharmacists (ASHP) encourages pharmacy professionals working in hospitals and health systems who use social media to do so in a professional, responsible, and respectful manner. Such use may complement and enhance their relationships with patients, caregivers, other members of the health care team, and the public. To achieve that goal, pharmacy professionals should

- thoroughly consider the purposes and potential outcomes of participation in social media and develop the strategies and skills required to effectively utilize social media to meet their goals, and
- exercise professional judgment and adhere to professional standards and legal requirements in both private and public social media communications, especially legal and ethical obligations to protect the privacy of personal health information.

Background

The term "social media" may be defined as online tools that allow interaction among individuals. Examples include professional networks such as ASHP Connect, career-building networks such as LinkedIn, and sites such as Facebook and Twitter that are primarily social but which may serve multiple purposes.[1-3] Informational sites regarding medical information that allow for commentary from users and medical professionals (e.g., PharmQD, The Pharmacist Society, Sermo) should also be considered collaborative social media.

Social media have transformed the way people communicate by reducing barriers to the exchange of information, increasing both the amount of communication and the number of people who can participate. Health care organizations (e.g., hospitals, health systems, professional societies, pharmaceutical companies, patient advocacy groups, and pharmacy benefit companies) have chosen to use social media for both communication and marketing.

Like other health care professionals, pharmacy professionals have adapted to advancing technology and are using social media to communicate with patients, caregivers, other health care professionals, and the public. Pharmacy professionals (including pharmacy students, as professionals in training) should continue to incorporate these new tools into the armamentarium of pharmacy practice and apply them with professional judgment to pursue the goal of helping people make the best use of medications. Social media provide pharmacy professionals with opportunities to educate patients and practitioners, seek advice from and provide advice to colleagues, optimize the medication use of individual patients and populations, promote the role of pharmacists in caring for patients, and engage in debate about issues in health care practice and policy, among other things.[1-5]

Participation in Social Media

Hospitals or health systems that choose to use social media or permit practice-related social media use by staff should have in place policies and procedures that

- balance the benefits social media provide with the obligations and liabilities they may create, and
- encourage the development and application of best practices by users of social media.

The details of such policies, procedures, and best practices are beyond the scope of this statement, which has as its purpose to briefly outline some of the considerations that should guide pharmacy professionals' participation in social media.

Pharmacy professionals should carefully consider the purposes and potential outcomes of their participation in social media and develop the strategies and skills required to achieve their goals. They need to be aware of and employ best practices when using social media, because health care practitioners, including pharmacy professionals, are held to a higher standard of professionalism within and outside the workplace than members of the public.[6] Pharmacy professionals who participate in social media should strive for a high degree of professionalism in their communications and ensure that patient privacy is not compromised.

Professionalism

ASHP has long advocated for the adoption of high professional aspirations for pharmacy practice. Pharmacists' responsibilities as professionals include "advancing the well-being and dignity of their patients, acting with integrity and conscience, [and] collaborating respectfully with health care colleagues."[7] The following recommendations for the use of social media represent high professional aspirations, and pharmacy professionals are encouraged to exercise their professional judgment in incorporating them into their practices.

Advancing the Well-Being and Dignity of Patients. The following recommendations can help pharmacy professionals who choose to participate in social media advance the well-being and dignity of patients.

1. Medical advice offered through social media should be provided in accordance with the professional standards of pharmacy practice. For example, pharmacy professionals should provide medical advice only with a complete understanding of the patient's medical conditions and only if they accept the associated liabilities, especially those regarding privacy and the requirements of pharmacy practice. Pharmacy professionals should be aware that providing medical advice may create a pharmacist–patient relationship, with all its attendant obligations and liabilities. All online relationships should conform to the ethical boundaries of an appropriate patient–pharmacist relationship.[8]

2. Pharmacy professionals should be cognizant of both the benefits and limitations of online communication. Social media may serve especially well as a point of initial contact or as a convenient way to maintain contact between patients and care providers, but professionals must recognize when a patient's health care needs would be better met through other means (e.g., phone consultation or an office visit).

3. Pharmacy professionals should view social media as a means to not only provide timely and accurate drug information but also to rebut inaccurate, misleading, or outdated information. While the purpose of specific social media content may not always be apparent, pharmacy professionals also need to be aware of and alert to the use of social media for marketing and sales purposes.

4. Complaining about or disparaging patients, even in general terms, does not advance the dignity of patients or the profession. Communications that contain patients' identifying information would violate privacy requirements, which are discussed in more detail below. Pharmacy professionals should keep in mind that simply avoiding the name of a patient may not be sufficient to avoid patient identification.

Acting with Integrity and Conscience. The following recommendations are intended to assist pharmacy professionals to act with integrity and conscience in their use of social media.

1. Pharmacy professionals should carefully distinguish between personal and professional information within social media and make conscientious decisions regarding who will have access to personal or professional information. Although some organizations recommend use of a strictly personal and a separate, strictly practice-related page,[9] professionals will quickly recognize the difficulty of making such distinctions. The higher standards of conduct expected of professionals, even in personal behavior, apply as well to their participation in social media.[6,10]

2. Pharmacy professionals must be conscious that content posted to social media may have consequences on reputations or careers for years to come, reflect poorly upon the pharmacy profession, or undermine patient confidence in the care provided. Postings on social media should be subject to the same professional standards and ethical considerations as other personal or public interactions.

3. The apparent anonymity provided by social media does not release pharmacy professionals from their ethical obligation to disclose potential conflicts of interest, especially when representing themselves as professionals. Some circumstances may require personal identification or disclosure of potential competing interests.[9]

4. Although all pharmacists should use social media in ways that set positive examples for pharmacy students and residents, preceptors and mentors have a special responsibility to model appropriate practices.[7,11]

Collaborating Respectfully with Health Care Colleagues. Although social media can and should be used to promote healthy debate about health care and pharmacy practice, such debate should be conducted in a respectful manner. Reasoned debate sometimes requires constructive criticism, but pharmacy professionals should not use social media to make ad hominem comments or needlessly denigrate specific care providers, institutions, or professions.

Patient Privacy

Health care professionals have long confronted the challenge of "communicat[ing] freely with each other while maintaining patient confidentiality and privacy."[12] Social media, by their very nature, present new issues of privacy and confidentiality by extending the reach of communications. The following recommendations may help pharmacy professionals protect patient privacy and confidentiality as they navigate this new terrain.

1. Pharmacy professionals should continue to adhere to all laws, regulations, standards, and other mandates intended to protect patient privacy and confidentiality in all environments, including social media.[8]

2. Pharmacy professionals should exercise professional judgment and employ established best practices to ensure compliance with privacy requirements when communicating with patients or about specific patient cases on social media.[9,13,14]

3. Pharmacy professionals should select privacy settings in social media accounts that provide the greatest degree of protection for personal information, keeping in mind that privacy settings are not perfect and that information posted online is likely permanent. Continuous self-monitoring of privacy settings is necessary, as social media sites change privacy policies.[10]

Conclusion

Social media are emerging as important modes of communication and are increasingly being used for personal, professional, and business communication, as well as for patient care. As medical professionals held to high standards of personal, professional, ethical, and moral conduct, pharmacy professionals have a responsibility to use social media appropriately.

References

1. Fox BI, Varadarajan R. Use of Twitter to encourage interaction in a multi-campus Pharmacy Management course. *Am J Pharm Educ.* 2011 Jun 10;75(5):88.

2. Estus E. Using Facebook within a geriatric pharmacotherapy course. *Am J Pharm Educ.* 2010 Oct 11;74(8):145.

3. Cain J, Fox BI. Web 2.0 and pharmacy education. *Am J Pharm Educ.* 2009 Nov 12;73(7):120.

4. Clauson KA, Seamon MJ, Fox BI. Pharmacists' duty to warn in the age of social media. *Am J Health Syst Pharm.* 2010 Aug 1; 67(15):1290–3.

5. Mattingly TJ, Cain J, Fink JL. Pharmacists on Facebook: Online social networking and the profession. *J Am Pharm Assoc.* 2010 May-Jun;50(3):424–7.

6. Williams J, Field C, James K. The effects of a social media policy on pharmacy students' Facebook secu-

rity settings. *Am J Pharm Educ.* 2011 Nov 10;75(9): 177.

7. American Society of Health-System Pharmacists [ASHP]. ASHP statement on professionalism. *Am J Health-Syst Pharm.* 2008 Jan 15; 65(2):172–4.

8. University of California, San Diego. Guidelines and best practices for online social media use by student pharmacists. http://pharmacy.ucsd.edu/current/pdf/Social_Media_Guidelines.pdf (accessed 01 Feb 2012).

9. Ohio State Medical Association. Social Networking and the medical practice: guidelines for physicians, office staff, and patients. www.osma.org/files/documents/tools-and-resources/running-a-practice/social-media-policy.pdf (accessed 01 Feb 2012).

10. American Medical Association [AMA]. AMA Policy: Professionalism in the Use of Social Media. www.ama-assn.org/ama/pub/meeting/professionalism-social-media.shtml (accessed 01 Feb 2012).

11. Kukreja P, Sheehan AH, Riggins J. Use of social media by pharmacy preceptors. *Am J Pharm Educ.* 2011 Nov 10; 75(9):176.

12. American Society of Health-System Pharmacists [ASHP]. ASHP statement on confidentiality of patient health care information. *Am J Health-Syst Pharm.* 2009 Feb 15; 66(4):411–2.

13. Dimov V. Case reports and HIPAA rules. http://casesblog.blogspot.com/2005/07/case-reports-and-hipaa-rules.html (accessed 01 Feb 2012).

14. Dimov V. How to write a medical blog and not get fired. http://casesblog.blogspot.com/2008/02/how-to-write-medical-blog-and-not-get.html (accessed 01 Feb 2012).

Approved by the ASHP Board of Directors on April 13, 2012, and by the ASHP House of Delegates on June 10, 2012. Developed through the ASHP Pharmacy Student Forum and the ASHP Section of Pharmacy Informatics and Technology.

Ashley M. Overy, Pharm.D., is gratefully acknowledged for drafting this statement. The following individuals are also gratefully acknowledged for their contributions to this statement: Kevin A. Clauson, Pharm.D.; Brent I. Fox, Pharm.D., Ph.D.; Karl F. Gumpper, BCNSP, BCPS, FASHP; Arpit Mehta, Pharm.D.; and David R. Witmer, Pharm.D.

Note: This statement had not been published in the *American Journal of Health-System Pharmacy* (*AJHP*) when *Best Practices for Hospital & Health-System Pharmacy 2012–2013* went to press. Some minor editorial differences may exist between this document and the official one that will eventually appear in *AJHP* and subsequent editions of this publication.

ASHP Guidelines on Pharmacy Planning for Implementation of Computerized Provider-Order-Entry Systems in Hospitals and Health Systems

Purpose and Scope

The purpose of these guidelines is to provide guidance to pharmacists in hospitals and health systems on planning for, implementing, and enhancing safe computerized provider-order-entry (CPOE) systems. To date, most CPOE guidelines have concentrated on the functionality required of a CPOE system, despite the fact that most CPOE system implementations occur using commercial systems whose functionality is largely pre-determined. These guidelines are intended to help pharmacy directors, managers, informaticists, and project managers successfully engage in this type of CPOE system implementation. CPOE is commonly part of a larger health information technology (IT) plan or system implementation. Though many health care technologies impact patient care and pharmacy practice, this guideline will focus on CPOE only. This document is the first of a planned series of ASHP guidelines on CPOE and related technologies and addresses the planning phase of a health-system CPOE implementation, primarily focusing on acute care and associated ambulatory care clinics. The guideline will focus on using CPOE in the medication-use process, though it is important to realize that CPOE includes all orders for patient care (laboratory, nursing, respiratory, and others). Topics covered in these guidelines include

- Developing an interdisciplinary planning and implementation team,
- Defining the vision, goals, and objectives of the CPOE system,
- Establishing essential metrics to measure the success of CPOE system implementation,
- Understanding current and future workflow in order to reengineer the medication-use process as part of CPOE system implementation,
- Planning for scope and depth of clinical decision support (CDS),
- Determining the functionality that ensures the safety of the CPOE system, and
- Educating and training health care providers to use the CPOE system.

Terms used in these guidelines are defined in the appended glossary. The recommendations presented in these guidelines can be used for strategic planning with the organization's decision-makers, drafting contract provisions, prospectively comparing CPOE systems, and creating an implementation plan. These guidelines should be used in conjunction with other literature on the topic and information from prospective or selected CPOE vendors. Pharmacists should exercise professional judgment in assessing their health system's needs regarding CPOE systems and in adapting these guidelines to meet those needs.

CPOE and the Electronic Health Record

In its 1999 report *To Err is Human,*[1] the Institute of Medicine (IOM) shocked the nation with its estimate of deaths due to medical errors. Two large studies, one conducted in New York[2,3] and the other in Utah and Colorado,[4] revealed adverse events occurring in 2.9% and 3.7% of hospitalizations, respectively. Over half of these adverse events were judged to be preventable. Based on these studies, IOM estimated that 44,000–98,000 Americans die each year due to medical errors in hospitals.[1] Many of these deaths are caused by medication errors or preventable adverse drug events (ADEs).[5,6]

When it was recognized that errors resulting in preventable ADEs involved a wide range of drug classes and most commonly occurred at the prescribing stage,[7] interest in CPOE systems grew. In a second report, *Crossing the Quality Chasm: A New Health System for the 21st Century,*[8] the IOM called for IT, including CPOE, to take a central role in the redesign of the health care system to improve quality, increase efficiency, and reduce errors. In addition to IOM, organizations such as the Leapfrog Group and the National Quality Forum have pushed for hospitals to adopt CPOE.[9,10] The American Recovery and Reinvestment Act of 2009 (Recovery Act) authorizes the Centers for Medicare and Medicaid Services (CMS) to provide reimbursement incentives for eligible professionals and hospitals who are successful in becoming "meaningful users" of certified electronic health record (EHR) technology. This law will likely increase the adoption of CPOE in hospitals and health systems.[11]

CPOE has the potential to affect the ordering of all medications, laboratory tests, medical imaging, nursing orders, and more. Even a basic CPOE system can eliminate illegible and incomplete orders and facilitate efficient order processing through instantaneous transmission of orders to hospital departments such as pharmacy and laboratory. Additionally, CPOE integrated with a pharmacy information system and the electronic medication administration record (eMAR) can nearly eliminate transcription errors, resulting in another potential 6% decrease in ADEs.[7] A homegrown CPOE system has been shown to decrease medication errors by 55–80%.[12,13] There are many reports of improvements in physician practices and patient outcomes with health IT related to ordering,[14-21] but in some reports it is difficult to distinguish whether the benefits were due to CPOE, CDS, the EHR, or a combination of all three. The synergy of the three of these will likely lead to the most significant improvements.[15,16] Although there are many reported benefits to CPOE, there is a growing body of research pointing to new problems introduced by CPOE. These new problems are collectively known as e-iatrogenesis, which is defined as patient harm caused at least in part by the application of health IT.[22] Though the systems themselves may contribute to these problems, design and implementation decisions play a role in the avoidance of these new errors.

More recently, attention has focused on the development of an integrated information system to support the coordination and integration of clinical and business processes. The terminology for such information systems is evolving, with *enterprise information system* sometimes used to describe the broader system that integrates clinical and business systems, and *EHR* used to describe the clinical information system, which may include a patient portal or the ability to link to a personal health record (PHR).[23] CPOE must be viewed in the context of the EHR, which would integrate CPOE, CDS, and departmental information systems and make patient-specific clinical information available to providers.

The EHR is a longitudinal electronic record of patient health information generated by one or more encounters in any care delivery setting.[24] It contains medical histories, medication histories, laboratory test results, diagnostic images, clinical documentation, progress notes, narrative summaries (such as operative reports or consultations), and other information related to patient encounters. EHRs provide the ability to manipulate, organize, and present data in ways that are clinically meaningful during the care planning, ordering, and care processes and allow broad clinician access to patient-specific clinical information, which is important to clinical quality and patient safety. When fully deployed within a facility through protected networks, the EHR serves as an information source and platform to coordinate patient care and communicate with the health care team. In addition, codified data can be used to trigger effective CDS as well as to provide data for continuous quality improvement.

For CPOE to be most useful it must be deployed as part of an EHR and not as a stand-alone module. CPOE is the process of health care providers entering orders and related information directly into the EHR. It places the provider at the center of patient care, allowing direct access and secure sharing of health information.

The EHR, including electronic clinician (e.g., physician, pharmacist, nurse) documentation with CPOE and CDS, is important to support the complex effort needed to improve hospital care.[15,16] The integration of CPOE and CDS within an EHR can create a platform upon which to build and improve the delivery of health care today and in the future. Many organizations implement these in a stepwise fashion because of the enormous work effort and the significant workflow changes required. Although there is no single solution that fits every circumstance, the literature offers many examples for others to follow or avoid.[25-28] Regardless of the vendor, organization size, or other factors that could potentially affect success, there are quite a number of implementation decisions that can increase the likelihood of a clinician-accepted CPOE installation that leads to quality and safety improvements.

Planning for the Transition to CPOE

A successful CPOE implementation starts with a well-organized, realistic plan. In planning for the transition to CPOE, initial tasks include assembling an interdisciplinary planning and implementation team; developing a vision, goals, and objectives for the CPOE system; establishing essential baseline and post-go-live metrics; mapping current physician, pharmacist, and nurse workflows as they relate to the medication-use process; defining the desired medication-use process; and planning for CDS. Project management and change management skills are vital for the conversion to CPOE. Because the enormous change in workflow will affect every clinician, standard project management and change management tools, such as a formal project charter, will help keep the implementation on track and manage expectations. Establishing a plan for communication is important from day 1.

Assembling an Interdisciplinary Planning and Implementation Team

The transition to CPOE is an immense cultural change that will affect every member of the health care team. No individual or department will be exempt from the impact of CPOE. Support for the project at the executive level is a prerequisite. Medical and administrative leadership/sponsorship are instrumental in the development of a clear vision for CPOE. An interdisciplinary team approach to planning and implementation is essential for a safe, well-designed, user-friendly, and successful CPOE system.

Physicians must be central players in the decision-making process, as prescriber buy-in and acceptance is crucial to CPOE success. Key departments (such as pharmacy, nursing, laboratory, radiology, admissions, dietary, and respiratory therapy) must dedicate resources and be involved in the initial effort, including workflow/process analysis and redesign, system analysis, integration between ancillary systems, review of organizational culture, and compliance with regulatory, legal, and reimbursement requirements.

The involvement of pharmacists in the development and implementation of CPOE is essential for several reasons. Pharmacists have the benefit of years of experience with electronic order entry systems. Pharmacists' experience with human factors issues related to the interaction between human and computer is invaluable, even though pharmacy systems may differ from CPOE systems in significant ways. In addition, the medication-order-entry aspect of CPOE systems leads to the most significant increase in patient safety and is likely the most complex part of the system.[21,29-32] The initial decision to purchase a completely integrated CPOE system or develop one that can interface with existing electronic systems (e.g., the pharmacy department's information system) is an important one that would benefit from the pharmacist's perspective. Although the number of successful implementations is increasing on a yearly basis,[33] the complexity of the systems should not be underestimated.

Collaboration among health care staff and the IT department is critical to the selection, implementation, and maintenance of CPOE systems. Although a CPOE system cannot be developed and implemented without IT expertise, the CPOE system is intended to serve the best interests of patients and clinicians. Clinicians and IT staff do not always talk the same language, and differences of opinion are not uncommon. Though difficult at times, these groups must work together for success. IT understands the technical aspects, but physicians, nurses, and pharmacists are best suited to determine how the CPOE system can be implemented to best serve the interests of patients and clinicians.

Recommendations for Team Structure. The organization should carefully consider the structure of the interdisciplin-

ary implementation team, which should include physicians, nurses, pharmacists, IT staff, the chief medical information officer, and staff from all ancillary departments (e.g., laboratory services, respiratory therapy). In addition to front-line practitioners, patient safety and quality improvement staff can help immensely with some of the workflow and design decisions. CPOE systems by definition require ownership by the medical staff. Therefore, prescribers (mainly physicians) must be actively solicited for system requirements and be involved in key decisions. CPOE system design, including the content, the user interface, and the flow of CDS, will be influenced by the vendor's product, but acceptance will ultimately reside with the medical staff.

The team structure for implementing CPOE must take into account the interests and expertise of the following types of individuals:

- *Clinical content experts.* Physicians, pharmacists, mid-level providers, nurses, and practitioners of other disciplines who have clinical knowledge and workflow experience that can help shape the CPOE system to be most useful in the local environment.
- *Medical record content experts.* Health care information management representatives who oversee the legal medical record.
- *Technical experts.* Typically, IT professionals who understand the capabilities of the system, write or configure the software, and test and troubleshoot problems.
- *Front-line users.* Physicians, nurses, pharmacists, and others who care for patients on a regular basis and who will understand the positive and negative implications of each proposal regarding CPOE. CPOE's effects on nurses cannot be overstated. The workflow of incoming information completely changes with the implementation of CPOE. The unit secretary will no longer be the gatekeeper and notifier of new orders. The development of an electronic means to notify nurses of new orders must be considered and incorporated into the nursing workflow to enhance patient care.
- *Project managers.* Individuals responsible for overseeing the completion of project tasks and managing timelines and resources. There may be both a facility project manager and a project manager for the vendor or outside contractor.
- *Workflow analysts.* Team members responsible for analyzing the workflow and processes of patient care, from admission through the entire hospitalization (including transfers, surgeries, and procedures) to discharge.
- *Project sponsors.* Clinician champions and organization leaders who can, with frequent reports from the CPOE team, help overcome the many real and imagined barriers to the CPOE transition and keep the implementation on track.
- *Others.* Ancillary staff whose roles or responsibilities may change with the implementation of CPOE.

Representatives from each of these areas of expertise should work together regularly, in a variety of committees and work group formats. The team should report to a key organizational committee (e.g., the pharmacy and therapeutics [P&T] committee) as well as medical staff or other governance-related bodies. Communication with many formal committees is

important as early as possible. The hospital should consider the merits of compensation for time spent away from clinical duties. The health system's existing committee structure may be utilized as oversight authority for CPOE initiatives before, during, and after the system goes live. However, it is highly recommended to create small work groups consisting of physicians, administrators, pharmacists, nurses, and IT personnel to make and approve design decisions and form specific task groups as needed when policy or process issues arise. Quick and timely action will be required during the implementation phase to keep the project moving forward on schedule and in an organized and cohesive manner. This interdisciplinary group should refer matters of policy to existing policy-making committees (e.g., P&T committee, medication safety committee, executive committee, practice guidelines committee, leadership council). The interdisciplinary CPOE committee is not a policymaking committee, but rather a tool to provide structure to existing policies. Some organizations may find it necessary to keep this new formal committee for ongoing oversight of clinical information systems and CDS decision-making.

Pharmacists are needed to provide oversight of medication-use process development. Pharmacist involvement should begin in the initial CPOE planning stages and continue throughout all phases of CPOE development and optimization. The pharmacists that serve on the interdisciplinary team would ideally be relieved of clinical duties to the extent possible in order to commit much of their time to the complex project. Those pharmacists could remain in the pharmacy or be physically relocated to whatever space the interdisciplinary team is allocated. Any pharmacist chosen to serve on the team should be

- A team player,
- Well-respected within and outside the pharmacy department,
- A good communicator,
- Knowledgeable about all facets of the medication-use system, especially the thought process prescribers use to determine a treatment or treatment plan,
- Well-versed in the regulatory and legal requirements of medication management,
- Current on patient safety initiatives and issues, both external and internal to the health system,
- Detail-oriented, with sharp analytical skills,
- Open to new ideas,
- Very interested in informatics,
- Capable of handling stressful situations and limited time lines, and
- Able to differentiate the requirements of an ordering system from those of a dispensing system and translate those requirements for others.

Outside Consultants. External consultants may be used in a variety of roles, including evaluation and vendor selection as well as project management and post-implementation assessments. Use of outside consultants may be warranted if there are insufficient resources, lack of on-site knowledge of the vendor's application, or a desire for a quicker implementation timeline. Consultants add a unique dimension to the team structure in that they have experienced how other hospitals have solved similar problems, can offer a variety of solutions based on their experience

from other facilities, and have a network of colleagues they can contact for advice. Having a consultant engaged early in the process can provide continuity to the development and implementation processes.

External consultants should work in conjunction with permanent members of the implementation team. It is important that the permanent members of the team know and understand how the system was designed, how its components fit together, and how each item was built by the consultants. Changes in one part of the system may have intended and unintended downstream effects. Modifications to the system are inevitable, and the on-site team must have the knowledge to understand and execute the necessary future changes. It is detrimental to have this knowledge leave with the consultant when the contract expires. Formal documentation and knowledge transfer meetings should be part of the consultant deliverables.

Allocating Resources. The resources required to manage the transition to a CPOE system will vary, based on a number of factors: the size and complexity of the institution, whether it is an academic or a community setting, types of patients served, current IT infrastructure, the scope of the CPOE project, commitment of implementation project team members, degree of system integration, and other circumstances. There are no general rules about the time, money, or number of employees required for such a transition. Vendors may perform an assessment to help determine the resources that will be required based on the institution's circumstances.

The resources needed should be identified and approved before the project begins, and monitoring of ongoing resource needs and allocation will be necessary. Planning often focuses on capital expenses, underestimating the personnel required to build, test, maintain, improve, and train staff on the use of the system.[29] Having these resources in place is critical to the success of an implementation. During planning and implementation, resource needs may vary, based on project activities. Following implementation, order sets and CDS are integral components of managing care, and the ongoing maintenance to keep the care components current and in line with practice requires ongoing resources. In addition, as the complexity of the system increases with enhancements and user requests, resources needed for ongoing management may increase. Understanding these needs before implementation can help in resource planning.

Developing a Vision for the CPOE System

A vision statement helps describe where the organization wants to be after CPOE implementation and helps define decision-making criteria and the framework for metrics. It is imperative that the CPOE vision align tightly with the vision of the organization as a whole. Large-scale projects should include a clear organizational vision, which might be as simple as increasing patient safety or improving provider access to information. Taking the time to develop these criteria will focus the team throughout the design and implementation processes, help the team communicate the rationale for the necessary change that front-line clinicians will have to make, and lay the groundwork for ongoing measurement.

CPOE is a vital component of the institution's overall patient safety and IT development plans. It is important to establish from the beginning that CPOE is a clinical interven-

tion and not an IT implementation. The implementation team should determine whether there are other issues that may influence CPOE implementation, such as new buildings or other system changes (e.g., pharmacy, bar-coding, or eMAR systems). The team should review and attempt to anticipate trends in regulation or best practices (e.g., from CMS, the Joint Commission, the Institute for Safe Medication Practices, or ASHP) and adopt practices from similar sites that have implemented CPOE. Finally, it should be remembered that CPOE is only one element of the hospital's IT infrastructure. Care should be taken to integrate these disparate systems, with the end result of a complete EHR.

Pharmacy involvement in CPOE development and implementation will be related mainly to medication use within the health system. Pharmacists often have experience with entry of medication orders into a computer system. This experience can be used to help providers adapt to the changes that come with CPOE, but pharmacists should be aware of the differences between ordering medications and verifying and dispensing them. Financial goals, hospital infrastructure, integration, and regulatory compliance also play an important role in the development of a vision for CPOE.

Developing a vision for medication orders in a CPOE system can be divided into three main tasks: defining the goals and objectives for the CPOE system, mapping the current and desired medication-use processes, and determining CPOE system performance requirements to reach those goals. An organization's physicians, nurses, pharmacists, other providers, and administrators can team up to prepare this vision. The vision might include describing how products should be named for easy identification or the configuration of special populations of orders. Consideration should also be given to how medication orders relate to other orders, laboratory test results, allergies, and other clinical information.

Defining Goals and Objectives for the CPOE System

Implementing CPOE is an immense cultural change that involves every part of an organization. After an overarching vision for the components of the CPOE system has been established, the implementation team should reach out to all areas of the institution to develop and explain the goals and objectives of the CPOE system. Widespread understanding and acceptance of these goals and objectives will facilitate development and implementation of the CPOE system. The central goals of a CPOE system typically include improving medication safety and the quality of health care processes.

Medication Safety. Improving the safety of the medication-ordering process should always be in the forefront of any design decision, programming modification, or enhancement to CPOE. The analysis of the existing medication-use process (see "Mapping the Current Medication-use Process" below) should identify any safety deficiencies that can be corrected with CPOE, as well as the strengths of the current processes. The addition of safety features to CPOE will be an ongoing endeavor, as acceptance of the system grows and clinicians realize how the system can improve their practices.

CPOE systems need to be monitored for unexpected safety failures. CPOE can introduce previously unknown safety failures through user interaction with the system, programming changes, or poor system design.[26] To prevent

the introduction of new medication errors, careful analysis, review, and testing needs to be conducted with initial implementation and subsequent additions, modifications, and enhancements. Constant surveillance for errors and unanticipated outcomes is an ongoing necessity.[29] This evaluation can also be used to develop the goals and objectives for implementation.

A major impetus behind CPOE is that the deployment of a well-designed CPOE system with effective CDS can reduce medication errors and ADEs. A systematic review of the effects of CPOE with CDS on medication errors and ADEs supports the successful use of CPOE in health care facilities.[18] Many hospitals will implement CPOE to improve patient care, while focusing less on research that explores its impact. Nevertheless, internal systems for tracking medication errors and ADEs should be continually used to assess the impact of CPOE. CPOE could potentially

- Reduce some forms of ADEs or medication errors,
- Qualitatively change some forms of ADEs or medication errors (e.g., an error of omission may become a wrong-time error), and
- Introduce new types of ADEs or medication errors (e.g., a physician may select the wrong drug or wrong patient from a list appearing on the computer screen or inappropriately select a default dose).

Quality of Health Care Processes. In addition to improving medication safety, the goals of CPOE implementation may include such things as decreasing drug or laboratory costs, reducing the time required for pharmacist medication order review, improving data collection, or increasing communication among health care team members. If efficiencies from the direct entry of medication orders by the physician result in time savings in the pharmacy, the pharmacy department could potentially direct more pharmacist resources to patient interaction or areas such as pharmacotherapy consultation, pharmacokinetics, anticoagulation monitoring, drug regimen review, antibiotic streamlining, or intravenous-to-oral (i.v.-to-p.o.) conversions. Such goals will be different for every organization, but it is important to establish them during the planning phase of the project. The transition to CPOE represents a major paradigm shift for most organizations. The organized, goal-oriented institution will benefit from creating concise, measurable goals and objectives.[19]

Establishing Baseline Data

In conjunction with the analysis of the current medication-use process, the interdisciplinary team should develop a clear and complete understanding of the institution's current medication safety data (e.g., medication errors, ADEs) as well as the resources devoted to the manual medication order system.[34,35] It is important to track data for at least three months in advance of implementation to assemble adequate baseline data. These data can then be compared with data from the CPOE system at designated intervals. Data should be tracked over time to assess the impact of the CPOE on the medication-use process. This information can help identify workflow bottlenecks or discrepancies in the CPOE system, providing opportunities for improvement. Examples of data that may change with the implementation of CPOE and CDS include errors related to known drug allergies, ADEs related

to drug–drug interactions, prescribing errors related to drug dose, and drugs withheld due to contraindications identified via CDS.

Establishing Post-Go-Live Metrics

Implementation metrics can be used to help measure achievement of organizational goals. Comparing baseline and post-go-live measures can identify which areas have improved and which need further review. Metrics are quantitative, measurable parameters, and may include

- Order entry time (e.g., average time it takes a provider to enter an order[36]),
- Compliance with established evidence-based order sets,
- Number of entered orders,
- Missing doses,
- Pharmacist interventions related to order entry problems,
- Changes to scheduled administration times in the system,
- First dose medication administration turnaround time,
- Assess possible financial indicators of success,
- Frequency of provider contact (e.g., pages for questions or errors on order entry), and
- Documented medication errors.

When reporting these data, the hospital should be careful not to overstate the impact of the CPOE system on patient outcomes. The measures listed above are process measures, not outcome measures. For example, although the CPOE system may have flagged a patient allergy and prevented administration of the medication, it is possible that even without the CPOE system the pharmacist or nurse would have identified the allergy and intervened before the drug was administered.

It is important to identify and report new errors or ADEs introduced by the CPOE system.[22,25,26,31,37-40] The hospital should actively engage clinicians at all levels in open dialogue and reporting of such issues. These reports should be used to make rapid changes in the design of the system in the spirit of continuous quality improvement.

Describing the Current Medication-Use Process And System Design

To ensure that the integrity, safety, and efficiency of the entire current medication process are maintained, if not enhanced, it is important to perform a complete analysis of the current medication-use process. This analysis should include the interdisciplinary workflows associated with medication use for multiple types of medications. The output can be represented in a variety of ways, including flow charts, narrative scenarios, analyzed issue/problem reports, and comparisons of current practices to known best practices.

The analysis of the current medication-use process should consider a variety of medication order types, based on frequency of use or potential impact on patient safety, in all different process settings (e.g., acute care, critical care, emergency department), procedural areas (e.g., diagnostic imaging), and patient populations (e.g., pediatric, geriatric, adult). The project team should consider a representa-

tive group of orders that includes the basic types of orders prescribers typically write. How orders are currently entered into the system may not necessarily be intuitive to a physician. Most importantly, the project team should consider how the prescriber currently orders medications and what would make the most sense to the prescriber when ordering electronically. CPOE systems should be designed from the prescribers' perspective, with an eye on how orders flow over the course of their existence, to encompass all facets of medication use, ensuring the process is complete from medication reconciliation through ordering, renewing, and discontinuing. Complex medication orders and/or protocols may need special attention because of current technology limitations or workflow differences. The types of medication orders that should be reviewed and included in the design, as well as the processes across which they should be considered, are listed in Figure 1.

The description of the current medication-use process should be developed from a number of sources: observation, paper order sets, discussion with clinicians, and the knowledge of those who have worked on the organization's previous process-improvement efforts. This process is an opportunity to engage staff pharmacists who service various areas of the organization. Pharmacists often have a broad view of the medication-use process, seeing it from end to end, both receiving orders from physicians and helping address complex administration scheduling issues. The project team should strive to understand the current state of the medication-use process in terms of the components listed in Table 1, which also lists the form best used to represent the component.

Developing the Future Medication-Use Process and System Design

Once the current state of the medication-use process is well understood, one or more instances of the future state (depending on the plan for phasing in the CPOE system) can be designed. This future state should be designed to meet or exceed the current levels of service and other important designated metrics and priorities (e.g. patient safety, first-dose delivery time) and address any desired improvements.

The CPOE system should be designed to support the hospital's ideal medication-use process as much as is possible. The system should be configured to support clinicians and promote improved patient care processes, rather than compromising these processes to accommodate system functionality. It will likely be necessary (and desirable) to change many of the key work processes to ensure that benefits (such as improved medication safety) are achieved. A description of the ideal medication-use process is beyond the scope of these guidelines, but key steps in a typical medication-use process are outlined in Figure 2.

A successful CPOE design is a combination of process, information systems, and supporting technologies that work together to allow the desired improvements to occur. Figures 3-6 list some of the process and technology enhancements that should be considered for incorporation into the new process/technology/system design.

The desired benefits of the CPOE implementation should be clearly identified, and the process and system design should make those benefits possible. The design should include the practices, work processes, and techno-

Figure 1. Types of medication orders and processes that should be reviewed and included in CPOE design.

Medication Order Types

Oral solids
Oral liquids
Topicals
High-risk medications (e.g., anticoagulants, heparin, insulin, or potassium chloride)
Compounded medications, such as triple mix or acetazolamide suspension (e.g., oral swish-and swallow or dermatological preparations made in the pharmacy)
Combination products (e.g., hydrocodone-acetaminophen, multi-drug inhalers)
Combination doses
Respiratory therapy
Total parenteral nutrition
I.V. medications
 Piggy-back i.v.'s
 Continuous infusion medications and titrations
Flushes

Medical staff protocols that include medications
Automated dispensing device overrides
Irrigations
Immunizations
Patient-controlled analgesia, including epidural analgesia
Sliding scale insulin and heparin
Chemotherapy standard and non-standard protocols
Conditional orders
Hemodialysis, peritoneal dialysis, and continuous renal replacement solutions
Investigational medications
Herbal medications
Ophthalmic or otic medications
Injectable medications (e.g., i.v. push, i.m.)
Medications used in operative and procedural areas
Linked or interdependent orders
Medications used for diagnostic imaging

Medication Order Processes

Ordering (physician or other clinician)
Electronic signature, signing of verbal orders
Medication reconciliation
Preparation and labeling
Medication order review
Dispensing and distribution (including interface to automated dispensing devices)
Administration and documentation

Medication schedule changes
Holding orders
Code medications
On-call to operating room or procedures
Future orders
Negative orders (e.g., do not give aspirin)
Charging
Transfer orders

Table 1.
Components of the Medication-use Process and Formats Best Suited to Representing Them

Component	Representation
Activities performed	Process flow chart
Strengths and weaknesses of the current process	Text/table
The person(s) performing the activities	Text
The information needed in order to perform the activitiy	Text
The tools and systems used to perform the activity	Flow chart
The outputs of the activity and where they are sent/recorded	Text
The time/effort used to perform the activities'	Text
The barriers, constraints, reductions in efficiency, and limitations on the activity	Text

logical components in an integrated fashion. General process design principles are listed in Figure 7.

The future state design should be an interdisciplinary effort that considers the entire medication-use process, even though parts of the process may not change or may not change much with CPOE implementation. It is important to maintain the continuity and integrity of the process by making sure that the design of the component activities is compatible and completely accounts for manual or previously automated processes.

The draft future state design is typically done with a small interdisciplinary group of clinicians (the "core team") who understand the current process and the capabilities and limitations of the CPOE system. This group should consist of clinicians who order (physicians, nurse practitioners, and pharmacists), dispense (pharmacists and pharmacy technicians), and administer (nurses and physicians) medications. This core team should have dedicated time for the project, or at least be relieved of their regular staff schedules for the time spent working on the project. The charge of this group is to weave into the system design the following factors:

- Existing work processes and systems,
- Best practices,
- New systems, with consideration for their capabilities and limitations,
- Physical limitations (e.g., space, facility issues, staffing limitations),
- Political issues (e.g., organizational priorities, limited physician cooperation or interest in CPOE),
- Desired benefits and performance improvements, and
- Compliance with regulatory, legal, and reimbursement requirements.

This redesign typically starts with a high-level process flow diagram that describes the activities performed by each member in the medication-use process, coupled with demonstrations of the system capabilities and flow. Through successive iterations, the workflow and system design is brought into increasing levels of detail and expanded to address the factors listed above.[34] Once the core team is satisfied with the design, practicing clinicians can be brought in to validate and improve the design. The clinicians involved in these process redesign sessions should be experienced and practicing clinicians who understand the current process and will likely find the potential issues with the new processes.

These process redesign sessions should be as practically focused as possible and should demonstrate prototypes of orders and output from the system. They should provide a forum to discuss what to do and how it will be done. The redesign will likely take at least three or four sessions to cover the necessary detail of all the affected processes. The information gathered from these sessions can then be used to complete the process and system design and build the policy and procedure and training documents.

Failure Mode and Effects Analysis. A safety analysis of the future state design should be done prior to implementation to identify unintended or unidentified consequences.[41] Failure mode and effects analysis (FMEA) is a useful tool to prospectively evaluate the potential risks associated with the new process and identify inconsistencies or omissions that may have the unwanted effect of increasing risk to patient safety rather than reducing it.[41-44]

Other Design Considerations. It should be determined whether there are required elements at provider order entry in order for the pharmacy to verify orders (e.g., patient allergies, weight). Integrated systems start to break down the silos in which physicians, nurses, and pharmacists sometimes practice. There should be one shared field for allergy and weight documentation, so any expected workflow changes need to be discussed prior to implementation. Though it is the right thing to do, this standardization often uncovers workflow issues that were previously hidden in the paper process. The current process for handling allergy conflicts or drug interactions should be examined and it should be determined how users will handle an alert in a critical or time-dependent area, such as the emergency room. It should also be determined whether there is a need for an additional set of elements for order processing (e.g., laboratory or other results).

Medication Use within the Context of CPOE and the EHR. Whether your organization implements CPOE alone or along with other parts of the EHR (such as the eMAR), other parts of the medication-use process will be affected. To meet the long-term goal of a complete EHR, all medication orders should be included in CPOE. Having disparate ordering systems (i.e., manual and electronic systems) causes confusion, creates additional work for health care professionals, and presents risks to patient safety. The hospital

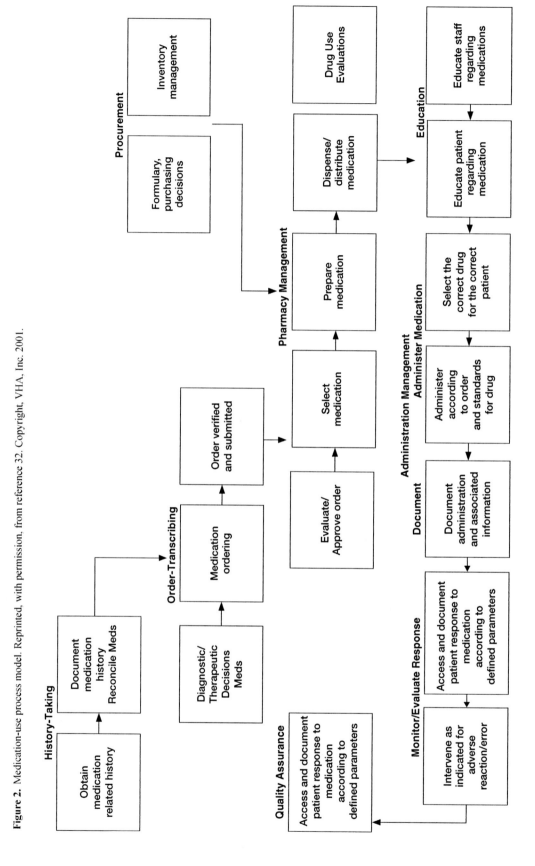

Figure 2. Medication-use process model. Reprinted, with permission, from reference 32. Copyright, VHA, Inc. 2001.

must recognize that CPOE may increase the amount of time the medical staff spends on prescribing medications, at least in the beginning.[45,46] Therefore, there must be considerable dialogue with the medical staff about their role in the overall medication-use process. It is important that they understand that CPOE is an effective way for them to communicate their orders and improve the timeliness, accuracy, and safety of patient care and that efficiency should improve over time.

Figure 3. Potential process and technology interventions in order writing and submission to improve medication safety. Reprinted, with permission, from reference 32. Copyright VHA, Inc. 2001.

Ordering: Order Writing and Submission

Process Interventions

Establish standards for abbreviations

Establish policies that do not accept incomplete or vague orders such as "continue previous medications"

Establish standard protocols for drug dosing and administration

Develop standard order sets to include drug order, time associated tests, and associated medicines

Provide routine staff education on common causes of error

Educate staff on back-up procedures for system down time

Establish policies for routine review and updating of current orders

Monitor the bypass of rules and alerts to complete order

Do not dispense drug prior to written order or verbal order verification unless critical

Minimize verbal order use

Technology Interventions

Implement tools to guide the user:

 Order entry (CPOE) with standard order sets and protocols

 Mandatory fields to complete an order

 Rules-based ordering to include dose adjustment, interaction checking, and accompanying orders

Provide formulary selections

Provide mobile charting devices to allow for ordering at the point of care

Adequate back-up procedures for system down

Updated Mar generated by CPOE or pharmacy sytem on routine basis (minimum every 24 hours)

Automated reminders or alerts for changes in patient status

Automated dispensing units do not dispense drug prior to order verification unless a critical medication

Figure 4. Potential process and technology interventions in medication history-taking and medication reconciliation to improve medication safety. Reprinted, with permission, from reference 32. Copyright VHA, Inc. 2001.

Medication History-Taking and Medication Reconciliation

Process Interventions

Establish procedures for obtaining admission history

Establish minimum data set to include medications, diagnoses, height, weight, and allergies

Establish accountability for obtaining minimum data set

Use standardized templates

Multi-disciplinary clinical documentation

Instruct patient/family on need to bring all current medications with them, including over-the-counter medications

Select and identify "record of truth"

Establish communication links with primary and extended care providers to support transitions in level of care

Replace free text with checklists when appropriate

Establish standard abbreviations for medication recording

Provide wallet cards or other forms to prompt patients to bring complete home medication information

Technology Interventions

Implement tools to guide the user

Clinical documentation with templates and checklists

Prompts for required fields to include minimum data set

Flags to highlight changes in minimum data set from previous data

Improve access to patient record through implementation of computer-based patient record/clinical data repository

Establish communication links with primary and extended care providers to support transitions in level of care

Provide mobile charting devices to allow for documentation at the point of care

Structured for computer-based clinical documentation

Technology adherence to standards

Figure 5. Potential process and technology interventions in pharmacy evaluation of orders to improve medication safety. Reprinted, with permission, from reference 32. Copyright VHA, Inc. 2001.

Pharmacy Evaluation of Orders

Process Interventions

Establish standards for abbreviations

Establish policies that do not accept incomplete or vague orders such as "continue previous medications"

Develop standard order sets to include drug order, associated tests and associated medications

Provide routine staff education on common causes of error

Do not dispense drug prior to order evaluation unless critical

Establish procedures for evaluation of orders and when to clarify

Establish procedures for pharmacy dosing

 Develop procedures for escalating an order that is on hold for clarification

Technology Interventions

Adequate back-up procedures for system downtime

Minimize system downtime

Automated reminders or alerts for patient changes in status

Pharmacy alerts and reminders based on change in lab value, drug-to-drug interaction, dose-checking, drug-to-diagnosis, drug-to-allergy checking

 Targeted alerts that vary by individual receiving them to reduce alert fatigue

Ability to view online clinical information to include: lab values, clinical documentation and orders

Interfaces to auto-populate pharmacy system with ADT, laboratory, clinical documentation

Access to drug knowledge base

Figure 6. Potential process and technology interventions in administering medications to improve medication safety. Reprinted, with permission, from reference 32. Copyright VHA, Inc. 2001. RFID = radio frequency identification.

Administering Medications

Process Interventions

Standardize medication administration times
Standardize equipment for IV infusion; minimize number
 of different kinds of devices
Provide tools that assist staff in calculating correct rate
 of infusion
Stock pre-mixed IV drugs
Establish standard dose packaging and labeling
Patients with multiple IV access lines have line clearly
 marked at distal end
Distal ports of non-IV tubing incompatible with
 medication oral syringe
Standard protocols for the physical assessment prior to
 administering a specific drug throughout the hospital

Technology Interventions

MAR with time based schedule
Electronic MAR
Automated drug distribution carts at the point of care
Smart infusion pumps
Alerts to caregiver to obtain and document clinical
 information prior to administering a drug
Bar code/RFID administration systems
Comprehensive wireless network coverage
Needleless administration system
Other medication delivery technologies

Figure 7. General CPOE process design principles.

CPOE Process Design Principles

Standardization of order entry and management information
 and workflows across the organization to the degree
 possible.
Simplifying processes.
Creating an effective interdisciplinary, team-based approach
 (i.e., improving communication).
Designing mechanisms for reporting and learning from
 errors.
Seeking redundancy through use of technology to support
 clinical decision making.
Avoiding reliance on memory.
Using constraints and forcing functions where appropriate.
Simulating planned and unplanned events for how people
 interact with each other and technology.
Planning for failure and designing for recovery.
Providing access to a core set of integrated clinical
 information at the time and point of decision-making.

The hospital should provide incentives for prescribers to utilize the system and disincentives for giving verbal orders or continuing to handwrite orders. To facilitate use of the system, prescribers should have access to the CPOE system from multiple venues, including their offices and homes and via wireless computers. If clinicians have the ability to enter orders from multiple locations such as home or office, a defined process should exist to easily reach the prescriber if there is a problem with the order (e.g., non-formulary, lack of availability).

All new orders should be verified by a pharmacist and reviewed by a nurse, and these actions should be documented in the EHR prior to medication administration. The nurse should work directly in the EHR for all clinical documentation, including medication administration. To comply with the "five rights" of medication administration,[47] a workstation must be available close to the patient's bedside with ready access to that patient's relevant information to facilitate resolution of any questions on the medications that arise. Figure 8 lists some design considerations for the workgroup as new workflows are designed for different clinical scenarios.

Computers (both wired and wireless) should be available in sufficient quantities so that no clinician has to wait to use one. It is critical that the technologies used for stationary and mobile computing be matched to the anticipated workflow. It is likely that stationary computers, handheld devices (e.g., personal digital assistants), and tablet and cart-mounted computers will all be needed for some part of medication ordering for various users. If they are not part of an integrated system, the CPOE, eMAR, and pharmacy information systems should be available on the same computer to facilitate switching between systems. Any other technologies that are used by providers (e.g., voice recognition) should not only be on the same computer but ideally available from these devices as well. Users should be able to easily switch between different applications if needed, and clinical data should freely flow between applications so that the pharmacist and other providers have real-time access to the same information.

Planning for CDS

CPOE is an important part of an organization's plan for improved safety and quality. The addition of CDS to the EHR and CPOE is essential for the prevention of adverse events and improvement in patient outcomes.[17,20,21] A full discussion of CDS is beyond the scope of this document. ASHP plans to cover the topic in future guidelines. The purpose of this section is to provide an overview of CDS that will allow incorporation of CDS to be addressed in planning.

CDS can be defined as providing the appropriate clinicians with clinical knowledge and/or patient information intelligently filtered and presented at appropriate times to enhance patient care.[48] CDS has many intervention types, including but not limited to the following[49]:

- Documentation forms/templates (structured guidance, required or restricted fields, checklists),
- Relevant data presentation (optimize decision making by ensuring all pertinent data are considered),
- Order/prescription creation facilitators (pick-lists, pre-completed order sentences and order sets),
- Protocol/pathway support (multistep care plans, link to evidence or protocol, pertinent reference information or institution-specific best practice guidance),

Figure 8. CPOE design considerations.

Design Considerations

How do orders post to the MAR, and what is the relationship between the MAR and intake/output flowsheets?

Are there other documentation flowsheets that are also used or needed (e.g., patient-controlled anesthesia, continuous renal replacement therapy)?

When do orders need to be approved by pharmacy before a nurse can chart or administer the first dose of the medication?

Can nursing staff easily tell when the order has been verified by pharmacy?

Is there a mechanism to have critically needed orders available on the eMAR before pharmacist review?

What medication information is displayed to the nurse for administration (i.e., both brand and generic names)?

How are orders sorted on the MAR (e.g., are as-needed orders separated from scheduled orders)?

Are administration instructions and notes required (e.g., do not administer oral ciprofloxacin with Maalox)? Will they be supplied from the CPOE system or from the pharmacy system?

Are nondrug items needed on the MAR (e.g., wet to dry dressings)? If so, how will these items be entered (i.e., are these orders that pharmacy must review and approve)? Can some type of treatment administration record be created for these items?

Is there a chart on removal from an automated dispensing cabinet or are auto-charting functions in use?

How will the health system develop a bar-coding system for medication administration?

Override rates of alerts by both pharmacists and providers to better set sensitivities for the warning.

Order verification times by pharmacists to determine turn-around times for different priorities of medication ordering.

Compliance to clinical practice guidelines and order sets.

If integration of the CPOE system is available with automated dispensing devices, then monitoring for overrides would be warranted.

Monitoring free-text orderables in the system, to better address the provider's needs and provide guidance for appropriate formulary build.

Does the software provide the ability to designate a medication and document "First Dose Effectiveness"?

How are enteral nutritional supplements and tube feeding supplements documented, ordered, etc?

Does the software provide "Query Tools"?

Will provider, pharmacist, nursing software "Hand Off" IT tools be needed?

Does the software handle "Look-A-Like, Sound-A-Like" medications and due to this aspect should generate medication nomenclature be utilized exclusively?

Does the software provide the functionality for "after hours" entry and how will the review be completed if pharmacy service is closed?

How will MAR/eMAR handle multi-component medication orders?

How will MAR/eMAR process fractional doses of medication package forms?

How will reporting needs be developed and integrated into the system for users? When?

How are co-signatures or verbal order sign-offs obtained?

- Alerts and reminders (drug–drug interactions, therapeutic duplication, drug–disease, allergy alerts, and others), and
- Automated ADE detection based on patient symptoms, labs, diagnostic results, and patient notes.

Because CDS has such a broad definition, the line between CDS and CPOE is not always clear. Basic forms of CDS, such as fully defined order sentences and order sets, are an important aspect of CPOE and can decrease errors while enhancing clinician acceptance of the system.[27,28] This type of basic CDS encourages clinicians to make proper choices initially rather than alerting them to potentially problematic choices after the fact and is an essential part of any CPOE implementation.

An organization must recognize that to realize the benefits of CDS, the CPOE system must be accepted by clinicians and used effectively. Poor design or too many alerts could lead to system rejection or, even worse, unanticipated outcomes such as increased errors or adverse events.[25,26,50-53]

Some CDS, including checks for allergies, drug–drug interactions, drug duplications, and dose ranges, are typically delivered via an interruptive alert to the user or displayed as a passive warning on an order entry screen. Such CDS should be considered before CPOE implementation, but designers should keep in mind that a high number of interruptive alerts may cause clinicians to ignore alerts alto-

gether and may even threaten clinician acceptance of CPOE. The way alerts are prioritized and presented to the user may be as important as which alerts are presented. Alerts for very serious clinical situations may be ignored when lost in a sea of less important ones.[54] Some vendor systems allow clients to change severity levels or even disable some alerts in an effort to bring alert interruptions to a better signal-to-noise ratio and thus decrease the potential for alert fatigue, particularly for physician recipients.[50-52] Ideally, there needs to be an alternative mechanism to provide CDS feedback to prescribers that is not intrusive but still allows the prescriber to know that there may be issues with an order. If ignored, these alerts can be acted upon by the pharmacist.

The strategy for prioritization of CDS should be defined as early as possible, and pharmacists should take a leading role in all medication-related CDS. It is likely that organizations will be eager to implement CDS along with CPOE. Pharmacists should ensure that the CPOE system is implemented with basic CDS, such as order sets and sentences, while using appropriate caution when implementing alerts.[27] Although vendor systems are continuously improving and may allow tiering of alerts, there is typically a significant amount of work necessary to vet any changes and carry out the technical work involved in the customization. The combination of pharmacists' clinical knowledge of drugs and their experience with the interruptive alerts that have been present in pharmacy information systems for

years provide pharmacists with a unique understanding of the many implications of implementing medication-related CDS. Pharmacists should work with medical leadership, either through the P&T, informatics, or another interdisciplinary committee, to decide how and when medication-related CDS will be added to CPOE. Pharmacists are well positioned to formulate local evidence criteria, collect information on medication therapy outcomes, and to bring together institutional health providers for the purpose of setting priorities and targeted outcomes where select IT interventions are made. The design, implementation, and optimization of CDS is an exciting area of opportunity for pharmacists now and in the years to come.

Elements of a Safe CPOE System

Minimum Features and Functions. The implementation group and key stakeholders should consider what features and functions of the CPOE system are desired both now and in the future. Starting with a pilot group of users allows experience with the system to build and permits users to work through some process issues before system usage is widespread. Any pilot should be brief, with plans for a roll-out shortly after addressing the major discoveries. A highly sophisticated system may take so long to develop that interest is lost, or it may be too sophisticated or rigid in its initial application to be well accepted.

An important consideration during CPOE implementation is the determination of which functionalities are required for go-live. CPOE will always be a work in progress, and there will be opportunities for modifications and enhancements. At a minimum, the project team should evaluate all existing manual medication ordering processes, including such complex orders as epidurals, patient-controlled analgesia, weight-based dosing, lab-result-dependent dosing, tapering medication doses, total parenteral nutrition, and chemotherapy, along with critical patient safety functionality driven from known internal or external sentinel events. An agreed-upon list of basic functionality should be established in order to ensure a timely yet successful go-live. If some complex or high-risk medication orders will be left on paper at the initial go-live (e.g., chemotherapy), be sure this is well communicated during training. As well, this principle applies to other identified yet unresolved design topics. The project team will to need re-visit these topics for completion in the post-go-live period.

General Features and Functions. The user interface is often a problematic aspect of CPOE. Users have been reported to enter orders for the wrong patient or to select the wrong item (or wrong feature of an order) unintentionally because they did not use selection lists properly or because it is very easy to select the wrong item from a drop-down list.[38] The CPOE user interface should incorporate appropriate human-factors engineering to avoid risk-prone workflows and controls (e.g., memorized mnemonic codes or function keys, long selection lists) that may produce order-entry errors. The order entry functionality should be independent of patient setting (e.g., inpatient, outpatient), and users should be able to combine data (e.g., order history) from all settings without a need for independent searches or screen selections. The system should include an online help function for system navigation and provide notification if another user modifies the patient record while an order session is ongoing, without losing the session. All displays should contain the patient name, patient location, user name, and function in consistent screen locations. The system should support third-party data entry for prescribers by simultaneous display of the same session in multiple locations and default fields where possible or helpful. The CPOE system should permit user definition of data elements and fields that can be attached to any portion of the database. The system should permit user-friendly, error-free medication order processing by providing the functionalities for the CPOE interface and order processing listed in Figure 9.

Levels of Access. The team will need to determine the levels of access or security permitted to staff throughout the hospital. The team may find it easier to begin with the current level of privileges for existing systems.

In general, pharmacists require a high level of access (full access to medication orders, and in some cases the ability place lab orders) because they cover multiple areas; place, alter, or discontinue orders; and may practice under protocols that require monitoring of laboratory test results. There may be different levels of access within the pharmacy department (e.g., actions by a pharmacy student, intern, or resident may need to be reviewed by a senior pharmacist; pharmacy technicians may require different levels of access, depending on duties). Staff may also need off-site or alternative site access.

In addition to pharmacy personnel access, the design team will need to determine levels of access for other staff members. This should include all categories of physicians that practice at the site (e.g., attendings, specialists, consultants, community clinicians with privileges, residents or other trainees, fellows, and medical students). The medical staff office, medical staff executive committees, or P&T committees may be able to make recommendations for appropriate access based on existing policies. Nursing will need to consider similar access issues and ensure compliance with provider practice acts. Ideally, these issues are addressed by existing policies that will only need to be reviewed and implemented. Other ancillary staff will need to be granted access, depending on their need for information and orders that will be built within CPOE and routed to the appropriate department for action.

User Levels and Co-Signatures. The CPOE system should permit restriction of medication orders by user type, individual order, or class of order. Each medication order should indicate the name and user level of the ordering party. The CPOE system should support the entry of unverified orders and the editing and verification of unverified orders, and this function should be role-based and restricted. The system should also support the creation of reminders or inbox messages for orders that require a co-signature. The pending prescriber co-signature name should default into the field from service, team, or coverage schedules, and there should be an option to override the name. The system should provide the ability to require that all orders be countersigned prior to placing a discharge order if the organization wishes to implement this.

Medication Order Status. Considerations regarding medication order status include the following:

Figure 9. Functionalities for CPOE interface and order processing.

CPOE Interface

- Multiple active sessions on one display (i.e., ability to put a current order session on hold and review other information, then return to the original work session without losing the work in progress).
- Side-by-side viewing of active order lists and any system-maintained order list (e.g., a standard order set, personal favorites list, or critical path order set).
- Alignment of orders by department while in side-by-side view.
- Switching between applications on the same display without exiting order functions.
- Utilization of all functions via either keyboard or mouse.
- Forward and backward navigation anywhere in the application.
- Access to the Internet from anywhere in the orders application.
- Access from multiple locations (e.g., sign-on, viewing, data entry, and verification at clinical or remote location).
- Order entry with minimal (<3) screen flips and user definition of defaulted fields.

CPOE Medication Order Processing

- Ability to return user to previous screen.
- Online access to error message documentation.
- Hospital-defined error messages.
- Ability to audit and track all errors and alerts.
- Robust search functionality available from all screens.
- Support for coding all diagnoses, tests, and procedures with institutional, departmental, and user-definable subsets of preferred terms (e.g., the appropriate edition of the International Classification of Diseases,[55] SnoMed CT,[56] or others).
- Ability to establish cross-references for tests or procedures, including:
 o Information regarding the name of a procedure or test (i.e., the ability to use alternate names for a procedure).
 o Information regarding indications for, execution of, cost of, and medical literature pertinent to a procedure.
 o Diagnosis codes that can be restricted based on type of exam or test.
 o Diagnosis code restrictions that staff can override by direct entry of the code or access to full table for lookup.
 o Ability to enter a diagnosis code along with reason for exam.
 o Ability to maintain orders online for the duration of the patient stay and to display the status of the orders (e.g., open, in process, completed, scheduled to expire, expired) during order inquiry.
 o Ability to store, display, and print patient test instructions as well as preparation instructions for the order.
- Ability to perform global set-up changes (i.e., changes to a master file table element can be optionally set to automatically populate all relevant items throughout the table).
- Ability to update patient service and physician(s).
- Ability to clearly note, flag and color-code order status.
- Option to have active orders remain visible on the same screen while writing new orders.
- Ability to view all orders, including stopped and interrupted (partially entered) orders.
- Automatic assignment of unique order identification numbers used in mapping to other systems, with the order identification number large enough, or based on an algorithm, so that such numbers are not repeated within 5 years.
- Ability to retain multiple order numbers or other unique identifiers from other systems.
- Option to manually update order status, with the ability to restrict such updates to specific order items or specific users or user classes.
- Ability to create user-defined order status.
- One-step cancel/reorder process.
- Discontinue, discontinue/renew, cancel occurrence, and hold order functions.
- Automatic calculations.
- Option to input order information using free text.
- Ability to search for, track, and audit free text orders.
- Ability to drill down for detail from every screen.
- Ability to drill down to the following during the order entry process:
 o Medication and doses, since initial orders include suspended and discontinued orders.
 o Termination date and time of current orders.
 o Allergies (coded).
 o Patient diagnoses (coded).
 o Demographic information.
 o Visit information (medical).
 o Physicians responsible for the patient (resident, attending, and consultant physicians, at a minimum).
 o Active and completed orders with dates and times.
 o Patient location and service.
- Modules with data specific to clinical specialties, including sets for reporting results, CDS, and order sets.

- Whether all orders must be reviewed by a pharmacist before they are active or posted to the MAR.
- If the answer to the above question is yes, the process in which the organization will handle urgent medications that are administered before pharmacist review.
- Should the CPOE system have some medications on override for urgent use? Are these medications always on override or are there alternative methods for ordering them?
- Does the pharmacy have sufficient staff to deal with the volume of orders? Pharmacy will potentially see all changes, i.v. fluid orders, discontinuation orders, and titration orders. Design considerations will need to address the disposition of the orders prior to implementation.
- If a prescriber enters and then changes an order, how are those two orders reconciled into one order?
- How does the system handle an order by a physician assistant or student that requires a co-signature before becoming active?
- Do hold orders need a defined duration to be accepted? Do these orders automatically discontinue if on hold for a certain amount of time?

Except in urgent situations as described by the Joint Commission,[57] a pharmacist should verify every medication order prior to drug dispensing and administration. Once verified by a pharmacist, the order should populate the pharmacy computer system, generate labels and other items necessary for dispensing, release the drug in the automated dispensing device (if applicable), and populate the eMAR as an active order. The order should be available to the eMAR as soon as it is placed, but it should be clear to the nurse whether the pharmacist has verified the order or not.

Order History. The CPOE system should permit viewing of orders from all previous patient encounters regardless of enterprise location, setting, or patient status. The system should be capable of storing and retrieving previous patient order lists and sorting, reporting, and printing patient order lists by date and date range, setting, patient status (e.g., discharge), service, department, and provider.

The system should allow pharmacists to maintain eMARs and permit online updates, provide online capability to automatically generate a hard copy of eMARs for downtime back-up, provide the ability to display and/or print patient medication profiles or eMARs on demand or at a specified time, and include the ability to have multiple formats that are definable by systems-level staff.

Documentation in the eMAR. The CPOE system should seamlessly build the eMAR from orders in real time. Some institutions may want medication administration time changes to be modifiable from the eMAR, and the eMAR may have a bi-directional interface to the pharmacy information system (if it is not an integrated system). The system should provide the ability to enable bar-code medication documentation. Pharmacist order validation should automatically update the eMAR. The pharmacy and nursing departments should work together to ensure that the eMAR is designed to be readable and user-friendly from the nurse's perspective. Pharmacists and nurses should have the ability to add or delete patient allergies, enter special instructions,

change administration times, and place medication orders on or remove them from hold or conditional status. Changes made to administration times in the eMAR should back-populate the CPOE and pharmacy information systems.

Medication Orderable Design and Build Considerations

The design and build of the medication orderables are key tasks in implementing the CPOE system. Care should be taken in designing and building the formulary or formularies, as well as the standard orders and order sets that are built from the formulary. The pharmacy department must have direct involvement in this task.

The CPOE formulary cannot be simply a copy of the pharmacy inventory. Prescribers need to have the orderables constructed to match how they order medications (therapeutic entity), rather than how the pharmacy maintains medication inventory (dosage form/product). In addition, care must be exercised when deciding on the default dose, frequency, and route values for items that will be displayed to the prescriber and in developing the construction of standard orders. Medication errors can result from a hurried prescriber accepting the default that he or she assumes must be correct.[25] The CPOE system should be able to generate formulary lists by generic name, trade name, and dosage form.

The CPOE system should allow routine online updating of the formulary and clinical checks of information without system functionality downtime. The system should provide authorized personnel the ability to maintain and display the formulary with pertinent data (e.g., formulary code, generic name, trade name, national drug code [NDC], or American Hospital Formulary Service [AHFS] number), while limiting access to certain formulary data by role. The CPOE system should include the ability to identify whether an i.v. with a medication additive is to be handled as a large-volume i.v. or as a small-volume i.v. for appropriate handling within the pharmacy department for compounding and dispensing. The system should allow the ability to make changes to the medication identifier (NDC or RxNorm identifier), communicate those changes to other systems, and receive changes from other systems.

Build Considerations

IT analysts design and build the system from documents or order sets reviewed and approved by the multidisciplinary group. Standard IT processes should be followed, beginning with the design phase. Once the design has been approved, IT staff should build the system in a test environment. A test environment protects from mishaps in the live (or "production") environment. It is important for the test environment to match the production environment so that testers get a true feel for how the build will work and interact. IT staff should meet with nursing and pharmacy throughout building and testing phases to resolve any issues that may arise.

After the builder is satisfied that the requested build or order set is complete, the builder should then develop a testing plan. The builder should work through the test plan initially and sign off when the build works as designed.

Next, pharmacy and nursing should perform testing. This testing should involve patient scenarios throughout

the patient's visit. Pharmacy is integral to this process and should ensure proper medication management and workflow. When the build passes pharmacy and nursing testing, physicians should review, test, and sign off.

When all aspects have been tested and fixed, and any necessary education is completed, the build may be moved to production. Follow-up is critical to ensure the build meets the needs of providers and is not adversely affecting ancillary staff. A mechanism to report issues quickly must be established, so that the implementation team can investigate and resolve them. The CPOE group should maintain reports of problems and review those lists for recurrent issues. Providing feedback and updates to the persons reporting problems is vital to progression of the project. Clinicians need to know they have been heard and resolution is being sought.

Dependent or Joined Orders. Support for dependent or joined orders is important in the case of i.v. medications and the diluent used for administration, two drugs to be taken together, or a drug and a measurement requirement (e.g., digoxin and pulse rate). The CPOE system needs to make it easy for the prescriber to order these types of formulary items. The system should be flexible enough for the prescriber to select the drug form and size or indicate the diluent for an i.v. piggy-back when ordering if so desired or to allow these choices to be made once the order reaches the pharmacy system.

Order Sets. Requiring providers to use a CPOE system requires a change in workflow, and many fear it may increase the time clinicians spend processing orders.[46] Configuring pre-constructed order sentences and order sets prior to implementing CPOE may increase speed, accuracy, and acceptability of CPOE.[27,28,58] Careful deliberation is needed prior to the creation of CPOE order sets, including consideration of how order sets are currently developed and revised (e.g., by department or by individual practitioners), what the process to propose and review order sets is, and what level of medical oversight is in place for order set development and use. It is also important to understand ordering patterns when developing order sets for use by clinicians. Many organizations use this opportunity to improve and standardize across important aspects of care, such as post-operative nausea and vomiting or pain management, as well as move to evidence-based order sets from their legacy order sets.[28]

The system should permit development of specific admission pathways (e.g., order sets capable of including any type of order and intervention) and integrate with data documented elsewhere in the EHR (e.g., medical histories, medication lists, laboratory results, diagnostic images, clinical documentation, progress notes, narrative summaries [such as operative reports or consultations]). Order set availability should be limitable by user, user role, location, service, or patient status or diagnosis. The system should permit an unlimited number of orders within an order set and an unlimited number of order sets within departments, across departments, and with user-definable time parameters. Order sets can include nursing orders, tests, and medications, and should include appropriate laboratory tests at appropriate intervals to assist in monitoring therapy. Though many systems allow users to create and save their own order sets in a favorites list, this flexibility needs to be weighed against the desire to standardize care by allowing hospital-based order

sets only.[28] Discontinuation of an order set should trigger the automatic ability to review, edit, or discontinue all linked orders.

Because the CPOE system may permit initiation of standard order sets with a single action (mouse click, keyboard stroke, etc.), order sets' ease of use may lead to inappropriate or excess medications being ordered. Order sets should be allowed to include linked orders, but orders grouped in a standard order set need not be linked. The institution should decide whether all orders in the set are going to be active once they are signed or if prescribers are required to actively check and click on each medication before signing.

The CPOE system should require designation of an owner (i.e., department, service, person, or role) for each order set. CPOE order sets should be reviewed on a periodic basis for therapy updates. Item and service maintenance should be performed at the departmental level, with updates in item or service definition flagged for review by the owner of the standard order set containing that item or service (i.e., the change triggers a report that the order set requires review). The CPOE system should support restriction of departmental or service standard order set creation or editing by role or individual.

The CPOE system should support standard order set maintenance and review by

- Grouping order sets by department/service,
- Dating the creation and review of order sets,
- Providing periodic (user-defined intervals or dates, or as-needed) reporting of standard order sets that require review by owner (department, service, person, or role), and
- Permitting global changes.

Critical Pathways and Protocol Order Sets. Critical pathways and paper-based order sets, a very basic form of CDS already widely used in hospitals, provide a starting point in efforts to standardize care and improve quality and safety through the CPOE system. With the implementation of evidence-based order sets, organizations can provide the prescriber with a direct link to the electronic literature supporting the recommended practice. The work of synthesizing and classifying the available evidence is done by organizations such as the National Guideline Clearinghouse[59] and the Cochrane Database of Systematic Reviews.[60] Organizations may incorporate these guidelines into electronic order sets and critical pathways, in addition to providing the link to give prescribers point-of-care access to the evidence-based literature at the time of order entry.

The CPOE system should support all functions listed under general order sets for critical pathways and protocol order sets. The system should provide a default set of protocols that are available by service and physician and a default set of protocols that are restricted by location. The CPOE system should include an alert system for orders not completed within user-defined time parameters or time parameters required by critical paths or research protocol.

Medication Order Linking. The CPOE system should include the ability to identify orders as linked and sequential or mutually exclusive or time off-set, and to specify intervals, as well as cascade changes in future orders to maintain sequence and timing. It should permit an order stop to automatically bring up any linked orders for re-verification, with

the default being to cancel unless re-verified. The system should provide automatic re-sequencing of future orders if any item identified as sequential is moved on the timeline, and it should permit linked orders (i.e., reflexive occurrences that trigger other procedures) that cascade through multiple levels.

Favorites Lists. The CPOE system should permit use of favorites lists by individual user that may include orders for multiple departments (e.g., laboratory, pharmacy, radiology). The system should provide default components of medication prescribing ("Sigs"), such as dose route frequency, and length of order, that are user-definable at the nursing unit level and that have discharge orders or discharge worksheet functionality. The system should provide default Sigs and permit users to save favorite Sigs in user favorites. Users should be able to create favorites lists that include orders from multiple departments on one list. Favorites lists should be fully editable on an ad hoc basis for an active order session, and user-specific favorites lists should be editable by the user. Users should be able to designate any order list as a favorite and may name or rename the list ad hoc (i.e., the save function automatically prompts for name, defaulting to the existing name if available). There should be an option to save an order list as a favorite, either as a new favorite or as a replacement for an existing favorite; that option should be available during any ordering session. Favorites lists should be allowed to contain ordering details that default into the order, and default details should be editable and replaceable during order entry. The CPOE system should support context-specific favorites lists by user, nursing unit, service, and diagnosis, and by combinations of user and diagnosis or by combinations of user, diagnosis, and setting (e.g., outpatient, inpatient). User favorites lists should be copied and shared easily, and the system should allow favorites lists to be built by opening and then editing standard order sets and saving as a favorite. Favorites lists may also include reminders. The system should permit review of favorites lists.

Pharmacy Department Considerations

The ideal CPOE system will have to be integrated with or have a fully functional bi-directional interface with the hospital's pharmacy computer system so that orders entered or modified in one system will populate fields in the other system, avoiding the need for dual order entry. The bi-directional feature of an interface is important because it prevents potentially dangerous discrepancies between data in the pharmacy and EHR systems and removes the transcription step of the medication-use process. In addition, if the distribution and administration components of medication management are not linked, then documentation and billing will not be either, causing more opportunities for error and audit problems.

In their day-to-day interaction with the CPOE system, pharmacists should be working primarily in the pharmacy system, which has all relevant patient information fully integrated with the EHR and CPOE module. The pharmacist's roles include verifying all orders, reviewing and responding to alerts, and clinical monitoring of the patient. The pharmacist should have security privileges to enter and modify orders under protocol (such as formulary or formulation changes).The pharmacist should see all orders within a particular group of orders so that they can see the con-

text in which each individual drug order was prescribed. Additionally, any functionality to help the pharmacist prioritize the review and approval of orders will improve the care of patients.

Pharmacists should receive and work with orders electronically in a queue. Patients with stat orders should appear at the top of the list and be clearly differentiated from less urgent orders. Pharmacists should have the ability to screen their view of orders based on the nursing units they are responsible for on a given shift. At no time should a pharmacist be able to view orders for more than one patient at the same time.

When working with paper orders, pharmacists often gain insight into the medication orders from the context of the surrounding patient care orders. CPOE systems should preserve that context so that pharmacists can view an order in terms of the other therapies, tests, nutrition, and nursing care surrounding it.

Communication Among Departments

The CPOE system should allow for notification of clinicians for pending orders needing signature via e-mail, pager, text message, or inbox message. Pharmacist order notification should be allowed via printout, work queue, e-mail message, system message, or pager. The default method for receiving notification of orders should be definable by the department or service, and the system should support special notification methods for specific services or items different from the departmental or service default, without affecting summary reporting by department. Users should be able to print orders to alternate locations and to send messages, orders, and alerts to additional departments (including information about scheduling and priority of orders) as a single order is being entered or completed. The CPOE system should have an option that order placement generates user-defined worklists. The system should also provide the ability to e-mail patient and preparation instructions and to reference on-call lists.

Education and Training of Health Care Providers

The rate of adoption of the new CPOE system may be directly linked to the extent of training provided to users prior to and during the implementation. One cannot spend too much time training users, as the change the new system entails will be overwhelming. This training can be in the form of formal classroom training, local expert training, or "at-the-elbow" support and training (the type of training typically most welcomed by physicians) during implementation. Organizations may find the most success in using a combination of all three. The more familiar the users are with the system at the time of implementation, the easier the transition will be.

The facility should train and employ a group of prescriber "super users." These users will support the go-live, help the institution refine the CPOE system to be as efficient as possible, and serve as liaisons and CPOE champions to the other members of the medical staff. There should be ongoing, open dialogue with leadership and medical staff members to continually improve the system.

Each training session should be geared toward the type of user, since utilization will differ by clinician type (e.g., physician, respiratory therapist, nurse, pharmacist, laboratory technician). The initial training of users is important, but ongoing training for new users, changes in programming, and functionality require that training be given a high priority after transition to the new system.

Overview of System. The initial introduction to the system should familiarize the user with the layout of the system. It should review toolbars and menus of each application. The first glimpse should include any definitions that are new or to which meanings may be different from the current process.

Accessing Data. This section of training should familiarize the user with the various methods for accessing data. It should provide information on sorting and filtering data. Because access to data will vary based upon the type of user, separating different user types for training purposes at this stage may be beneficial, and this is a good time to discuss security and privileges.

Documenting Information. This section should teach users how to document information pertinent to their practices. These tasks would include adding basic patient information and documentation onto flow sheets, as well as clinical progress notes.

Orders. The training sessions on medication orders will be the most comprehensive. Some users will be limited to ordering tests or procedures specific to their practices. Physicians, nurses, and pharmacists, however, will spend a large percentage of their time in the CPOE system working with orders. Time should be taken to demonstrate each type of order. After the demonstration, users should practice working with all types of orders that they may process in various scenarios. Though documented information may be sparse in test domains, practicing with realistic patient scenarios will provide the best training results and prepare the user for success when using the live CPOE system.

Pilot Project. A pilot with a defined scope is advisable at the beginning of the implementation phase. Organizers should consider the length of the pilot, which patients will be included, what the objectives of the pilot are (i.e., testing system performance, workflow, completeness of ordering), and what happens at the conclusion of the pilot (e.g., more programming, more testing, another pilot, or live rollout). Consideration should be given to type of prescriber/practitioner, order types and number of patient transfers into or out of pilot test area as well as flow of patient information to non-pilot areas. Because user feedback is a valuable objective of the pilot, organizers should develop and use a formal evaluation tool for the pilot clinicians. A time analysis should be performed, comparing how long it takes the pharmacy to process orders with the CPOE system versus their previous workflow. If the time analysis demonstrates a negative impact on workload, the facility may consider making appropriate staffing adjustments. These adjustments will vary, based on the percentage of orders directly entered by the prescriber, and should be continually assessed. True final measurement of process performance capabilities will

likely not be realized until implementation processes have been completed and stabilized. A time analysis should also be performed comparing how long it takes CPOE-trained nursing staff to administer and document medications in the CPOE system versus the manual system. This analysis should determine whether time is saved by eliminating manual transcription of orders and manual development and maintenance of MARs. If the time analysis demonstrates a negative impact on workload, the facility should make appropriate staffing adjustments. These adjustments will vary, based on the percentage of orders directly entered by the prescriber, and should be continually assessed.

Conclusion

These guidelines provide guidance to pharmacists in hospitals and health systems on planning for and implementing safe CPOE systems. Pharmacists should utilize their unique knowledge and skills as part of the interdisciplinary CPOE planning and implementation team. Participation by pharmacists is critical in defining the vision, goals, and objectives of the CPOE system; establishing essential metrics to measure the success of CPOE system implementation; re-engineering the medication-use process as part of CPOE system implementation; determining the functionality that ensures the safety of the CPOE system; planning for CDS; and educating and training health care providers to use the CPOE system. Finally, for optimal benefits to patients, organizations should realize that the implementation is merely the beginning and that pharmacists should continue to take a central role in ongoing system optimization and continued CDS implementation.

References

1. Kohn LT, Corrigan JM, Donaldson MS, eds. *To err is human—building a safer health system.* Washington, DC: National Academy Press; 1999.
2. Brennan TA, Leape LL, Laird NM et al. Incidence of adverse events and negligence in hospitalized patients. Results of the Harvard Medical Practice Study I. *N Engl J Med.* 1991; 324:370-6.
3. Leape LL, Brennan TA, Laird NM et al. The nature of adverse events in hospitalized patients: Results from the Harvard Medical Practice Study II. *N Engl J Med.* 1991; 324:377-84.
4. Thomas EJ, Studdert DM, Burstin HR et al. Incidence and types of adverse events and negligent care in Utah and Colorado. *Med Care.* 2000; 38:261-71.
5. Phillips DF, Christenfeld N, Glynn LM. Increase in U.S. medication-error deaths between 1983 and 1993. *Lancet.* 1998; 351:643-4.
6. Bates DW, Spell N, Cullen DJ et al. The costs of adverse drug events in hospitalized patients. *JAMA.* 1997; 277:307-11.
7. Bates DW, Cullen DJ, Laird N et al. Incidence of adverse drug events and potential adverse drug events. Implications for prevention. ADE Prevention Study Group. *JAMA.* 1995; 274:29-34.
8. Corrigan JM, Donaldson MD, Kohn LT et al. Crossing the quality chasm: a new health system for the 21st

century. Washington, DC: National Academy Press; 2001.

9. Birkmeyer JD, Dimick JB. The Leapfrog Group's Patient Safety Practices, 2003: The Potential Benefits of Universal Adoption. Leapfrog Group; February 2004. www.leapfroggroup.org/media/file/Leapfrog-Birkmeyer.pdf (accessed 2009 Jan 22).

10. National Quality Forum (NQF). Safe Practices for Better Healthcare–2009 Update: A Consensus Report. Washington, DC: NQF; 2009.

11. American Recovery and Reinvestment Act of 2009 [ARRA] (P.L. 111-5, 123 Stat. 115-521). http://edocket.access.gpo.gov/2010/E9-31217.htm (accessed 2010 May 19).

12. Bates DW, Teich JM, Lee J et al. The impact of computerized physician order entry on medication error prevention. *J Am Med Inform Assoc.* 1999; 6:313-21.

13. Bates DW, Leape LL, Cullen DJ et al. Effect of computerized physician order entry and a team intervention on prevention of serious medication errors. *JAMA.* 1998; 280:1311-6.

14. Hunt DL, Haynes RB, Hanna SE et al. Effects of computer-based clinical decision support systems on physician performance and patient outcomes: a systemic review. *JAMA.* 1998; 289:1330-46.

15. Amarasingham R, Plantinga L, Diener-West M et al. Clinical information technologies and inpatient outcomes: a multiple hospital study. *Arch Intern Med.* 2009; 169:108-11.

16. Bates DW. The effects of health information technology on inpatient care. *Arch Intern Med.* 2009; 169:105-7.

17. Wolfstadt JI, Gurwitz JH, Field TS et al. The effect of computerized physician order entry with clinical decisions support on the rates of adverse drug events: a systematic review. *J Gen Intern Med.* 2008; 23:451-8.

18. Ammenwerth E, Schnell-Inderst P, Machan C et al. The effect of electronic prescribing on medication errors and adverse drug events: a systematic review. *J Am Med Inform Assoc.* 2008; 15: 585-600.

19. Eslami S, de Keizer NF, Abu-Hanna A. The impact of computerized physician medication order entry in hospitalized patients—a systematic review. *Int J Med Informatics.* 2008; 77:365-76.

20. Teich JM, Merchia PR, Schmiz JL et al. Effects of computerized physician order entry on prescribing practices. *Arch Intern Med.* 2000; 160:2741-7.

21. Chaudry B, Wang J, Wu S et al. Systematic review: impact of health information technology on quality, efficiency and costs of medical care. *Ann Intern Med.* 2006; 144:E-12-22.

22. Weiner JP, Kfuri T, Chan K et al. "e-Iatrogenesis": the most critical unintended consequence of CPOE and other HIT. *J Am Med Inform Assoc.* 2007; 14:387-8.

23. Healthcare Information and Management Systems Society (HIMSS) Enterprise Information Systems Steering Committee. Clinical perspectives on enterprise information technology. www.himss.org/content/files/ClinicalPerspectives_whitepaper_052907.pdf (accessed 2009 Aug 26).

24. Healthcare Information and Management Systems Society (HIMSS). Electronic health record. www.himss.org/ASP/topics_ehr.asp (accessed 2009 Aug 26).

25. Koppel R, Metlay JP, Cohen A et al. Role of computerized physician order entry systems in facilitating medication errors. *JAMA.* 2005; 293:1197-203.

26. Han YY, Carcillo JA, Venkataraman ST et al. Unexpected increased mortality after implementation of a commercially sold computerized physician order entry system. *Pediatrics.* 2005; 116:1506-12.

27. Kuperman GJ, Bobb AM, Payne TH et al. Medication-related clinical decision support in computerized provider order entry systems: a review. *J Am Med Inform Assoc.* 2007; 14:29-40.

28. Bobb AM, Payne TH, Gross PA. Viewpoint: controversies surrounding use of order sets for clinical decision support in computerized provider order entry. *J Am Med Inform Assoc.* 2007; 14:41-7.

29. Bates DW. Computerized physician order entry and medication errors: finding a balance. *J Biomed Informatics.* 2005; 38:259-61.

30. Kaushal R, Shojania KG, Bates DW. Effects of computerized physician order entry and clinical decision support systems on medication safety: a systematic review. *Arch Intern Med.* 2003; 163:1409-16.

31. Bobb A, Gleason K, Husch M et al. The epidemiology of prescribing errors: the potential impact of computerized prescriber order entry. *Arch Intern Med.* 2004; 164:785-92.

32. Kilbridge PM, Classen DC. A process model of inpatient medication management and information technology interventions to improve patient safety. VHA Research Series, vol. 1. Irving, TX: VHA Inc.; 2001.

33. Pedersen CA, Gumpper KF. ASHP national survey on informatics: Assessment of the adoption and use of pharmacy informatics in U.S. hospitals—2007. *Am J Health-Syst Pharm.* 2008; 65:2244-64.

34. Khajouei R, Jaspers MW. The impact of CPOE medication systems' design aspects on usability, workflow and medication orders: a systematic review. *Methods Inf Med.* 2010; 49:3-19.

35. Niazkhani Z, Pirnejad H, Berg M et al. The impact of computerized provider order entry systems on inpatient clinical workflow: a literature review. *J Am Med Inform Assoc.* 2009; 16:539-49.

36. Wietholter J, Susan Sitterson S, Allison S. Effects of computerized prescriber order entry on pharmacy order-processing time. *Am J Health-Syst Pharm.* 2009; 66:1394-8.

37. Kaushal R, Jha AK, Franz C et al. Return on investment for a computerized physician order entry system. *J Am Med Inform Assoc.* 2006; 13:261-6.

38. Campbell EM, Sittig DF, Ash JS et al. Types of unintended consequences related to computerized provider order entry. *J Am Med Inform Assoc.* 2006; 13:547-56.

39. Campbell EM, Guappone KP, Sittig DF. Computerized provider order entry adoption: implications for clinical workflow. *J Gen Intern Med.* 2009; 24:21-6.

40. Singh H, Mani S, Espadas D et al. Prescription errors and outcomes related to inconsistent information transmitted through computerized order entry: a prospective study. *Arch Intern Med.* 2009; 169:982-9.

41. Bonnabry P, Despont-Gros C, Grauser D et al. A risk analysis method to evaluate the impact of a computerized provider order entry system on patient safety. *J Am Med Inform Assoc.* 2008; 15:453-60.

42. Kozakiewicz JM, Benis LJ, Fisher SM et al. Safe chemotherapy administration: using failure mode and effects analysis in computerized prescriber order entry. *Am J Health-Syst Pharm.* 2005; 62:1813-6.

43. Coles G, Fuller B, Nordquist K et al. Using failure mode effects and criticality analysis for high-risk processes at three community hospitals. *Jt Comm J Qual Patient Saf.* 2005; 31:132-40.

44. Beuscart-Zéphir MC, Pelayo S, Bernonville S. Example of a human factors engineering approach to a medication administration work system: potential impact on patient safety. *Int J Med Inform.* 2010; 79:e43-57.

45. Kuperman GJ, Gibson RF. Computer physician order entry: benefits, costs, and issues. *Ann Intern Med.* 2003; 139:31-9.

46. Bates DW, Boyle DL, Teich JM. Impact of computerized physician order entry on physician time. *Proc Annu Symp Comput Appl Med Care.* 1994:996.

47. McGovern K. 10 Golden rules for administering drugs safely. In: Preventing medication errors. Springhouse, PA: Springhouse; 1994:2-3.

48. Osheroff JA, Pifer EA, Teich JM et al. Improving outcomes with clinical decision support: an implementer's guide. Chicago: Healthcare Information and Management Systems Society; 2005.

49. Osheroff J, ed. Improving medication use and outcomes with clinical decision support: a step-by-step guide. Chicago: Healthcare Information and Management Systems Society; 2009.

50. Weingart SN, Toth M, Sands DZ et al. Physicians' decisions to override computerized drug alerts in primary care. *Arch Intern Med.* 2008; 163:2625-31.

51. Igboechi CA, Ng CL, Yang CS et al. Impact of computerized prescriber order entry on medication errors at an acute tertiary care hospital. *Hosp Pharm.* 2003; 38:227-31.

52. Hsieh TC, Kuperman GJ, Jaggi T et al. Characteristics and consequences of drug allergy alert overrides in a computerized physician order entry system. *J Am Med Inform Assoc.* 2004; 11:482-91.

53. Nebeker JR, Hoffman JM, Weir CR et al. High rates of adverse drug events in a highly computerized hospital. *Arch Intern Med.* 2005; 165:1111-6.

54. Paterno MD, Maviglia SM, Gorman PN et al. Tiering drug-drug interaction alerts by severity increases compliance rates. *J Am Med Inform Assoc.* 2009; 16:40-6.

55. International classification of diseases, ninth revision, clinical modification (ICD-9-CM). www.cdc.gov/nchs/about/otheract/icd9/abticd9.htm (accessed 2009 Jan 27).

56. SnoMed Clinical Terms (SnoMed CT). www.nlm.nih.gov/research/umls/Snomed/snomed_main.html (accessed 2009 Aug 28).

57. Medication Management Standard MM.4.10—preparing and dispensing. In: Comprehensive accreditation manual for hospitals. Oakbrook Terrace, IL: Joint Commission on the Accreditation of Healthcare Organizations: 2006:MM-10.

58. Payne TH, Hoey PJ, Nichol P et al. Preparation and use of preconstructed orders, order sets, and order menus in a computerized provider order entry system. *J Am Med Inform Assoc.* 2003; 10:322-9.

59. National Guideline Clearinghouse. www.guideline.gov (accessed 2009 Jan 22).

60. Cochrane Database of Systematic Reviews. www.cochrane.co.uk (accessed 2009 Jan 22).

Appendix—Glossary of Terms and Abbreviations

Adverse drug event (ADE): ASHP defines a significant ADE as any unexpected, unintended, undesired, or excessive response to a drug that
1. Requires discontinuing the drug (therapeutic or diagnostic),
2. Requires changing the drug therapy,
3. Requires modifying the dose (except for minor dosage adjustments),
4. Necessitates admission to a hospital,
5. Prolongs stay in a health care facility,
6. Necessitates supportive treatment,
7. Significantly complicates diagnosis,
8. Negatively affects prognosis, or
9. Results in temporary or permanent harm, disability, or death.

Bar-code-assisted medication administration (BCMA): A methodology involving the use of scanners and software to verify all medications electronically before they are administered to patients. These systems may also document the medication in the eMAR.

Clinical decision support (CDS): Clinical decision support systems are interactive computer programs or other tools, which are designed to assist physicians and other health professionals with decision making tasks usually at the point of care.

Computerized provider-order-entry; alternatively, computerized prescriber-order-entry (CPOE): An electronic system that health care professionals can use to enter drug, treatment, and test orders and transmit the orders directly to the department responsible for fulfilling the order.

e-iatrogenesis: Patient harm caused at least in part by the application of health information technology including but not limited to the systems and/or the design and implementation of the system.

Electronic health record (EHR): An electronic record of health-related information on an individual that conforms to nationally recognized interoperability standards and that can be created, managed, and consulted by authorized clinicians and staff across more than one health care organization.

Electronic medication administration record (eMAR): A version of the medication administration record viewable online and not printed.

Electronic medical record (EMR): An electronic record of health-related information on an individual that can be created, gathered, managed, and consulted by authorized clinicians and staff within one health care organization.

Enterprise information system: Broader system that integrates clinical systems such as an EHR and business systems such a scheduling and/or financial systems and quality reporting systems.

Leadership: Within a health-system, leadership may address three leadership groups: The governing body, the chief executive and other senior managers, and the leaders of the licensed independent practitioners.

Legal medical record (LMR): The legal health record is the documentation of health care services provided to an

individual during any aspect of health care delivery in any type of health care organization. It is consumer or patient-centric. The legal health record contains individually identifiable data, stored on any medium, and collected and directly used in documenting health care or health status.

National drug code (NDC): A universal 11-digit product identifier used in the United States for drugs intended for human use. The Drug Listing Act of 1972 requires registered drug establishments to provide the Food and Drug Administration (FDA) with a current list of all drugs manufactured, prepared, propagated, compounded, or processed by it for commercial distribution.

Orderable: An authoritative direction or instruction from a prescriber to perform a task (e.g., a radiology test or administer a medication or treatment).

Medication administration record (MAR): Medication administration record usually handwritten or printed from an electronic pharmacy information system.

Personal health record (PHR): An electronic record of health-related information on an individual that conforms to nationally recognized interoperability standards and that can be drawn from multiple sources while being managed, shared, and controlled by the individual.

RxNorm: RxNorm is a standardized nomenclature for clinical drugs and drug delivery devices and is produced by the National Library of Medicine.

Sponsorship: An identified executive or clinical leader who assumes responsibility for another person or a group during a period of project planning implementation follow-up.

Systematized nomenclature of medicine (SNOMed): A multiaxial, hierarchical classification system. As in any such system, a disease may be located in a body organ, which results in a code in a topography axis and may lead to morphological alterations represented by a morphology code.

Workflow: The flow or progress of work done by a company, industry, department, or person.

Developed through the ASHP Section of Pharmacy Informatics and Technology and approved by the ASHP Board of Directors on September 24, 2010.

A work group of the ASHP Section of Pharmacy Informatics and Technology Section Advisory Group on Clinical Information Systems is gratefully acknowledged for developing these guidelines: Anne M. Bobb, B.S.Pharm.; Jennifer Boehne, Pharm.D.; W. Lynn Ethridge, Pharm.D.; J. Chad Hardy, Pharm.D., M.S.; Randy Herring, B.S.Pharm.; Richard S. Jacobs, Pharm.D.; Michael A. Jones, Pharm.D.; Timothy W. Lynch, Pharm.D., M.S.; Leslie R. Mackowiak, M.S.; Tommy J. Mannino, B.S.; Jayson J. Przybyla, Pharm.D.; Brendan J. Reichert, M.S.; Ranee M. Runnebaum, Pharm.D.; Nancy R. Smestad, M.S.; David L. Troiano, M.B.A., MSIA; Laura L. Tyndall, Pharm.D.; and Lori Wright, Pharm.D.

ASHP also gratefully acknowledges the contributions of the following people: Bruce W. Chaffee, Pharm.D.; Toby Clark, M.Sc., FASHP; Kate Farthing, Pharm.D., BCPS; Burt W. Finkelstein, Pharm.D.; William L. Fritz, M.S., FASHP; Kimberly A. Galt, Pharm.D., FASHP; Barry R. Goldspiel, Pharm.D., FASHP; Frances M. Jordan, M.B.A., FASHP; Renee B. Marino, Pharm.D.; Kevin C. Marvin, M.S., FASHP; Steven Meisel, Pharm.D.; Alicia S. Miller, M.S.; Sandi Mitchell, M.S.I.S., FASHP; Kuldip R. Patel, Pharm.D.; Alicia B. Perry, Pharm.D.; John Poikonen, Pharm.D.; Mark H. Siska, B.S.Pharm.; and Mary Windle, Pharm.D.

ASHP also acknowledges the following organizations and individuals for reviewing drafts of these guidelines (review does not imply endorsement): American Academy of Family Physicians (AAFP); American Association of Critical Care Nurses (AACCN); American Health Information Management Association (AHIMA); American Hospital Association (AHA); California Society of Health-System Pharmacists (CSHP); Healthcare Information and Management Systems Society (HIMSS); Jeanine (Porter) Abrons, Pharm.D., M.S.; Christel Anderson (HIMSS); Dan Buffington; Peggy Brashear, B.S.Pharm.; Tim R. Brown, Pharm.D., FASHP; Dominick A. Caselnova III, M.H.A.; Thomas W. Cooley, M.B.A.; Debby Cowan, Pharm.D.; Michele Danish, Pharm.D., FASHP; Neil Davis; Charlie De la Torre; Robert DeChristoforo, M.S., FASHP; Jean Douglas, Pharm.D.; Brent R. Ekins, Pharm.D., DABA; Elizabeth Fang, Pharm.D.; Tim Lanese, M.B.A., FASHP, CPHIMS; Lisa Gunther Lum, Pharm.D., FASHP, FCSHP; Robi Hellman, RN, MSN, CNS (AACCN); James M. Hoffman, Pharm.D., M.S., BCPS; Carol J. Hope, Pharm.D., M.S.; Amey Hugg; Joan E. Kapusnik-Uner, Pharm.D., FCSHP; Linda L. Kloss, RHIA, FAHIMA (AHIMA); Ronald E. Lay, M.S.; Jeff Little, Pharm.D.; Bob Lobo, Pharm.D.; LTC Eric M. Maroyka, Pharm.D., BCPS; Greg Matsuura, Pharm.D., BCPS; Patrick J. McDonnell, Pharm.D.; Michael McGregory, Pharm.D., M.B.A., BCPS; Robert Moore, B.S.Pharm., BCPS; Susan J. Morikawa, Pharm.D., BCPS; Kevin Olsen, RN, BSN; Peg Panella-Spangler M.S.; Christine Pavlak, M.H.A., FASHP; Stephanie C. Peshek, Pharm.D., FASHP; Tommie Peterson; Minh James Pham, Pharm.D.; James A. Ponto, M.S., BCNP, FASHP; Donald W. Rucker, M.D.; Richard Sakai; Kevin Scheckelhoff; Thomas R. Schafer, Pharm.D., BCPS; Terry Seaton, Pharm.D.; Suzanne Shea; Pamela Shellner, M.A., RN (AACCN); Clyde Spence, Pharm.D., M.B.A.; Richard L. Stambaugh, Pharm.D., M.S., BCPS; Craig S. Stern, Pharm.D., M.B.A.; Scott H. Takahashi, Pharm.D., FCSHP (CSHP); Dennis A. Tribble, Pharm.D.; Jody Jacobson Wedret, FASHP, FCSHP; Rich Umbdenstock (AHA); Ray Vrabel, Pharm.D.; Steven E. Waldren, M.D., M.S. (AAFP); Eric Weber; Barbara White, M.S., PMP, FASHP.

The bibliographic citation for this document is as follows: American Society of Health-System Pharmacists. ASHP guidelines on pharmacy planning for implementation of computerized provider- order-entry systems in hospitals and health systems. *Am J Health-Syst Pharm.* 2011; 68:e9-31.

ASHP Guidelines on Remote Medication Order Processing

Purpose

Because of the complexity of the care that pharmacists provide patients, the American Society of Health-System Pharmacists (ASHP) advocates that patients have 24-hour access to the pharmacist responsible for their care and that the pharmacist be physically accessible to the patient when feasible. ASHP recognizes that such access is not always possible and encourages the development of remotely delivered pharmacist care as a supplement to onsite care.

Medication order review is one aspect of pharmacist patient care. All health-system pharmacies have an obligation to provide a review of medication orders that ensures safe medication use.[1] When onsite pharmacist review is not available, health systems may determine that remote pharmacist review of medication orders is a suitable alternative. The purpose of these guidelines is to describe the policies and procedures that must be in place to safely employ remote medication order processing (RMOP). Health-system policies and procedures regarding RMOP should address quality assurance and safety; access to drug information and hospital policy resources; training and orientation; minimum technical standards and specifications; confidentiality, privacy, and security; regulatory and accreditation standards; and communication and problem resolution. These guidelines also describe some general considerations for RMOP implementation, and Appendix A provides a checklist for assessing implementation readiness. Appendix B contains an outline of a model agreement for RMOP. A glossary of terms used in these guidelines appears in Appendix C.

Because of the rapid pace of change, differences in practice settings and RMOP models, and the complexities of health care organizational arrangements, aspects of these guidelines may not be applicable to all settings. These guidelines are not intended to describe best practices for the operational relationships between satellite and central pharmacies in acute care settings. Readers should also note that these guidelines do not attempt to address all aspects of remotely delivered pharmacist care and should interpret them as limited to the subject of RMOP. These guidelines address remote order verification only when medication order fulfillment occurs through automated medication storage and distribution devices. Remote end verification of the dispensed drug product (e.g., visual approval of the drug product by video camera or other means) is beyond the scope of these guidelines. Health-system administrators and pharmacy managers should therefore exercise their professional judgment in assessing and adapting these guidelines to meet the needs of their particular settings and to comply with the health care organization's policies and procedures.

Models of RMOP Services

The technologies used in RMOP are relatively new and rapidly changing, so different methods for RMOP have evolved, and further evolution should be encouraged. At least two models of RMOP are currently in use: contracted services and supplemental workload balancing, which includes network workload balancing and on-call assistance. Each of these models has unique characteristics that must be considered in planning for its use.

Contracted Services. In this model, a hospital pharmacy that is not continuously open contracts with a larger hospital or a service to provide RMOP when its pharmacy is closed. This model is typically applied when a hospital without 24-hour pharmacy services has sufficient automated dispensing cabinet capacity that RMOP allows nursing staff to keep functioning without having a pharmacist present,[2] although some institutions have developed models for remote verification by pharmacists of dispensing performed by pharmacy technicians at the client site.[3]

Supplemental Workload Balancing. Similar to the model described above, in this case a health system with a number of hospitals relies on the ones that have a 24-hour pharmacy department or on a service to provide RMOP for hospitals whose pharmacies are closed or that experience unanticipated peaks in order processing workload. For example, in an on-call model, a staff pharmacist from the client site or a contracted service is placed on call to help with managing workload. This pharmacist works remotely (sometimes from a home office, where allowed by state regulation) to help the client's pharmacy department manage unanticipated peaks in order processing workload (often on the second or third shift). In this model, the remote pharmacist is responsible for medication order entry and/or review, and medication order fulfillment occurs through the client-site pharmacy.

Quality Assurance and Safety

Medication-use management and safety in the RMOP environment require special efforts in the coordination of quality-assurance, quality-improvement, and patient safety practices between the client site and the remote site. Differences in local practice standards and organizational cultures, combined with unique human factors issues, have the potential to magnify the risk of errors. Quality, safety, and risk management strategies should be jointly examined and agreed on and should address the procedures and communication pathways unique to RMOP systems. These include critical workflow steps and handoffs involved in medication ordering, review, and verification; communication among prescriber, pharmacist, and nurse; and assessing the patient's response to drug therapy and achieving desired therapeutic outcomes.

Review of the Patient's Profile. The remote pharmacist must be able to review the patient's profile for

- Medication history and medication reconciliation reports,
- Diagnosis,
- Allergies and prior adverse drug reactions,

- Height, weight, age (measured versus estimated), and sex,
- Pregnancy status for women of childbearing potential,
- Duplications of drug therapies,
- Potential drug interactions,
- Pertinent laboratory data, and
- Other information as needed.

Clarification of Medication Orders. The remote pharmacist must have a process by which he or she can clarify the medication order with the prescriber. The remote pharmacist must alert other health care providers caring for the patient (e.g., the client nursing and pharmacy staff) of the need for additional review and clarification. There must be a mechanism for the remote pharmacist to readily communicate by phone or leave a note in the patient profile for other health care providers, including the client site pharmacy staff, to clarify the order or otherwise respond within an appropriate period of time. The remote pharmacy must have a mechanism for timely follow-up on medication orders that are pending clarification.

Quality-Assurance and Medication Error Reporting Systems. The remote pharmacy must participate in the client site's quality-assurance and medication error reporting systems. These systems should include the collection and reporting of medication errors and process variances as described below:

- The medication error reporting system should include potential adverse events that reach the patient (with or without harm) and potential adverse events that are intercepted before reaching the patient.
- Medication error reports related to RMOP procedures and communications should be tracked by outcome, type, cause, severity, preventability, and source.
- Corrective action plans should be directed toward the system failures that contributed to or caused the error, variance, or adverse event.
- Policies and procedures should ensure that quality-assurance data and medication error reports are jointly reviewed in a timely manner by pharmacy leadership and safety officers (if applicable) at both the client and remote sites and that relevant information is shared with relevant frontline practitioners at both sites, including remote pharmacists and client-site nursing and pharmacy staff.

The quality-assurance program should include indicators that measure important aspects of RMOP, including measures of (1) timeliness (e.g., elapsed time to receive and verify an order), (2) system performance (e.g., percentage of time information technology systems are not available for RMOP), (3) compliance with contractual requirements, (4) employee satisfaction at the client and remote sites, and (5) unanticipated problems (e.g., breaks in privacy standards, communication and handoff problems).

Handoff Communication. The remote site should have a documented process for handoff communication that meets the requirements of Joint Commission National Patient Safety Goals.[4]

Access to Drug Information and Hospital Policy Resources

Drug Information Resources. Drug information resources are essential tools for health care organizations. Drug information resources, specific to the needs and scope of patients served, are essential for practicing evidence-based medicine in a safe and efficient manner. In health care systems that use RMOP procedures, each institution needs point-of-care access to internal and external drug information systems. Internal drug information resources include the client's formulary, laboratory reference values, newsletters, and drug-use guidelines based on local standards. External drug information resources include commercially available electronic and print media that organize information into full-text and bibliographic retrieval systems.

Drug information resources available in the remote pharmacy should at a minimum meet the state board of pharmacy requirements for both the client and remote pharmacy sites and include the current edition of a drug information reference (hard copy or electronic). Other reference material (hard copy or electronic media) should be available, depending on the scope of care being provided. Recommended clinical and drug information reference materials available in the remote pharmacy include

- Two sources of pediatric dosing information (ideally, one of which is the same resource used by clinicians in the remote pharmacy),
- Internet access to online drug information resources, including the Food and Drug Administration,
- Drug compatibility and drug interaction resources,
- Poison information and poison control resources (at a minimum, the telephone number for a certified poison control center), and
- Drug information center contact number.

Drug information requirements, resources, and staff competencies in the use of drug information systems should be reviewed at least annually to ensure that patient care needs are met.

Hospital Policy and Procedures. The minimum information on client site hospital policies and procedures that the remote pharmacist should have available is

- Client site's pharmacy department's policies and procedures,
- Client site's formulary,
- Client site's relevant nursing department policies and procedures,
- Standard medication administration times,
- Standard drip concentrations or drug protocols,
- High-risk policies including the "Do Not Use" abbreviations list,
- Drug-specific clinical guidelines,
- Restrictions by indication or prescriber,
- Chemotherapy protocols, pain protocols, and anticoagulation protocols,
- Standing or protocol orders,

- Pre- and postoperative antibiotic selection and administration protocols, and other protocols as determined,
- Therapeutic interchange list,
- Client's policies and procedures for processing nonformulary medication orders,
- Client's policies and procedures for handling a clinical message order to alert nursing staff and pharmacy department of the need to address an issue at a future time, and
- Client's pharmacokinetic and renal dosing policies along with written medical staff approval to write orders in the patient's chart if required to comply with these policies.

The remote site must have a procedure that ensures the timely and complete communication of changes in client site hospital policies and procedures, including changes to formularies and medication protocols.

Training and Orientation

Pharmacists, through training and orientation, are competent to review and enter medication orders written by prescribers into a computerized database to maintain a complete patient profile. This patient profile can be used by nurses and other providers to access medications appropriate for their patients. This training and orientation are critical for pharmacists to accurately document and transcribe the appropriate information to maintain an accurate and up-to-date profile. Requirements for training and orientation include the following:

- All education and orientation are documented in a permanent record maintained in the pharmacy department of the remote site (if applicable) and shared with client sites or in the pharmacy department of the client site, as appropriate.
- All pharmacy personnel accessing the pharmacy information system are tested for competency prior to use of the system and annually thereafter.
- When upgrades or significant changes are made to the client site's computer system, the client site will communicate to the remote site the need for follow-up training.
- When significant changes are made to the client site's clinical policies or procedures, the client site will communicate to the remote site the need for follow-up training.
- The client and the remote site must have a process for documenting the remote pharmacist's competencies. If the remote site is responsible for the documentation of those competencies, the client and the remote site must have a system for reporting those competencies to the client.

Minimum Technical Standards and Specifications

The client and the remote site must ensure that the following minimum technical standards and specifications are met:

- The remote site must have access to the client's network or Internet, phone, and scan or fax access to the client.

- The remote site must have the ability to access the client facility via the client's Internet solution or via the client's computer network.
- The remote site must, to the extent possible, have redundant systems in place to ensure RMOP service availability (e.g., computer network and Internet connectivity, other information systems used to facilitate RMOP).
- The remote site must have the ability to operate remotely the client's order transmittal system.
- The systems used by the remote pharmacist to view the patient orders and other medical information must comply with the technical standards set by the Health Insurance Portability and Accountability Act of 1996 and ensure technical and physical safeguarding of patient health care information.

Confidentiality, Privacy, and Security

To ensure the confidentiality, privacy, and security of patient health care information, the following conditions must be met:

- Remote pharmacists must adhere to the client's confidentiality policy.
- The remote site, if a business entity, must have a signed business associate agreement with the client.
- The client must provide individual pharmacist-specific access to the client's hospital computer system.

Regulatory Considerations

State regulation of RMOP varies considerably. The client and the remote site should jointly analyze state regulations governing pharmacy practice at both sites to determine and meet applicable requirements. This analysis should be repeated on a routine basis, as regulations may change. To ensure regulatory compliance, at a minimum the following should be verified and approved by the client and the remote site before implementing RMOP:

- Remote site's approval to operate by the client's state board of pharmacy, if required,
- The policy and procedure manual for the RMOP operation, including but not limited to procedures for handling computer system or connectivity downtime, issue escalation, annual competency renewal verification, and communication between the client site and remote site personnel,
- Copies of all licensure required by the states in which the client and the remote site are located (some states require remote pharmacists to have a consultant license in addition to a state pharmacist license for each hospital for which the pharmacist performs RMOP services), and
- Copies of any hospital job-specific competency requirements for pharmacy personnel.

Communication and Problem Resolution

To ensure the safety of the RMOP service, the client and the remote site must establish effective communication chan-

nels between personnel at the two sites. Communication among prescriber, pharmacist, and nurse will be critical to assessing the patient's response to drug therapy and achieving desired therapeutic outcomes. The remote pharmacist must have the ability to immediately contact the prescriber or client site's nursing staff to discuss any concerns identified during review of the patient's information. The client must provide its nursing supervisor with a 24-hour telephone number to contact the remote site or remote pharmacist and encourage nurses to communicate with the remote pharmacist. In the event the nursing supervisor is unable to resolve a problem or concern, the client pharmacist on call is available for consultation and problem resolution if the problem cannot wait until the client pharmacist is on duty again. Patient profile information, including laboratory results, should be communicated to the remote site electronically; oral communication of laboratory results should be limited to exceptional circumstances, and such oral communications should be documented in the patient medical record as soon as possible. Downtime procedures should provide mechanisms for direct communication among the remote pharmacist, nurses, and the prescriber.

Considerations for Implementation

The success of RMOP implementation will depend on a host of specific factors. Below are some considerations that are generally applicable. Appendix A provides a brief checklist for implementation readiness.

- Terms of the contract or agreement should allow flexibility for the number of orders processed, since estimates prior to "go-live" may be inaccurate.
- Early and frequent communication between the client site and the remote site, especially in the first few weeks after go-live, is critical to the success of the implementation and ongoing operation.
- After-hours technical support at both the remote site and the client site will be essential to the success of the implementation and ongoing operation. Plan for information technology support in advance of go-live.
- Education will be required for all nurses at the client site, not just those whose shifts coincide with RMOP coverage. In particular, changes to the client site's override processes will need to be planned in collaboration with nurses.
- The client should implement a mechanism for communication between the remote site and nursing via the electronic medication administration record (eMAR) system. For example, if the remote pharmacist reviews the patient's home medication reconciliation list and identifies items not stocked by the pharmacy, it would be helpful to have a drug dictionary item (e.g., "Pharmacy Note to Nurse") whereby the remote pharmacist can make an entry in the eMAR that informs nurses that the remote pharmacist has reviewed the order but that some action at the client site is required.

Conclusion

ASHP believes that patients should have 24-hour access to the pharmacist responsible for their care and that the pharmacist should be physically accessible to the patient

when feasible. Because 24-hour pharmacy services are not achievable in all circumstances, health systems may employ remote pharmacist review and processing of medication orders. The purpose of these guidelines is to describe the policies and procedures that must be in place to safely employ RMOP. Health-system policies and procedures regarding RMOP should address quality assurance and safety; access to drug information and hospital policy resources; training and orientation; minimum technical standards and specifications; confidentiality, privacy, and security; regulatory and accreditation standards; and communication and problem resolution. Given the rapid pace of change in technology, differences in practice settings and RMOP models, and the complexities of health care organizational arrangements, health-system administrators and pharmacy managers should exercise their professional judgment in assessing and adapting these guidelines to their particular settings.

References

1. The Joint Commission. Elements of performance for medication management standard 4.10 (preparing and dispensing). Comprehensive accreditation manual for hospitals. Oakbrook Terrace, IL: The Joint Commission; 2007:MM-10.
2. Stratton TP, Worley MW, Schmidt M et al. Implementing after-hours pharmacy coverage for critical access hospitals in northeast Minnesota. *Am J Health-Syst Pharm.* 2008; 65:1727-34.
3. Clifton GD, Byer H, Heaton K et al. Provision of pharmacy services to underserved populations via remote dispensing and two-way videoconferencing. *Am J Health-Syst Pharm.* 2003; 60:2577-82.
4. The Joint Commission. 2009 National Patient Safety Goals: hospital program. www.jointcommission.org/PatientSafety/NationalPatientSafetyGoals/09_hap_npsgs.htm. (accessed 2009 Dec 28).

Appendix A—Checklist/Assessment for Implementation Readiness

1. All automation has been tested and is functional, including
 a. Communication of medication orders (fax machines or scanners)
 b. Computer systems maintaining patient profiles
 c. Connectivity to automated medication dispensing cabinets
 d. Electronic reference resources
 e. Remote connectivity
2. All personnel training for remote site and client site is completed and documented:
 a. Computer systems
 b. Clinical guidelines
 c. Client site pharmacy policies and procedures related to review, authorization, and entry of medication orders
 d. Communication procedures
3. Pre-go-live test of mock patients and scenarios has been performed for
 a. Fax/scan orders
 b. Admission, transfer, and discharge of patient

c. Medication order entry

d. Communication procedures

4. System downtime protocols have been well communicated to all applicable personnel at both the remote site and client site (e.g., pharmacy, nursing, information technology, and administrative personnel)

5. Go-live date and service level expectations have been well communicated to all applicable personnel at both the remote site and client site

6. Communication process that includes quality reporting, system changes/availability, and policy and procedure updates as well as shift change communication has been agreed on, established, and well communicated to all applicable personnel at both the remote site and client site

Appendix B—Outline for Model Agreement Between Remote Site and Client

The agreements between a remote site and the client must be approved by both contract office and risk management in both facilities (if applicable). The agreement should include

1. Services to be provided, including the roles of both parties:
 a. Hours of service
 b. Technology requirements
 c. Order processing services
 d. All clinical services provided
 e. Management services
 f. Quality measures
 g. Other services (e.g., vacation, emergency, or other hours of coverage)
 h. Qualification of pharmacy and pharmacists
 i. Security of information
 j. Limitations
 k. Access to records, including information required to review patient profiles
2. Terms and renewal of the agreement
3. Mutual indemnification and insurance
4. Termination of the agreement, including changes in laws or regulations
5. Confidentiality, including requirements set by the Health Insurance Portability and Accountability Act of 1996
6. Limitations of liability
7. No exclusion from federal health care programs
8. Dispute resolution
9. Fees and payment terms:
 a. Hourly rates
 b. Per-order rates
 c. Order volume
 d. Overpayment and underpayment exposure
 e. Penalty charges
 f. Addition of new services
10. Miscellaneous issues, including
 a. Independent contractors
 b. Notices
 c. Compliance with the terms
 d. Rights of the parties
 e. Conflict of laws

f. Compliance with laws, regulations, guidelines, and accrediting body standards (e.g., Joint Commission)

Appendix C—Glossary

Terms used to describe remote medication order processing (RMOP) practices are evolving and vary considerably. Readers should be alert to these inconsistencies and exercise caution in interpreting the literature. The following terms are used in these guidelines:

Client: The health care organization receiving the RMOP service.

Client Site: The site receiving the RMOP service (the site where the patient is receiving care).

RMOP: Medication order processing provided by a remote pharmacist; this term includes remote order entry and remote order review.

Remote Pharmacist: A licensed pharmacist processing the medication order from the remote site.

Remote Site: The site that is electronically linked to the client site via a computer system and/or a video or auditory communication system approved by the appropriate state board(s) of pharmacy. The remote site may be a licensed pharmacy or other location permitted by the appropriate state board(s) of pharmacy.

Developed through the ASHP Council on Pharmacy Management and approved by the ASHP Board of Directors on September 25, 2009.

ASHP gratefully acknowledges the expert panel that authored these guidelines. At the time of writing, members of the expert panel held the following positions. Bruce Thompson, M.S., was Director of Pharmacy Services, Hennepin County Medical Center, Minneapolis, MN; Greg Conrad was Director, Pharmacy, Willamette Falls Hospital, Oregon City, OR; Michael O. Gum was Pharmacy Director, Presbyterian Hospital, Charlotte, NC; John M. Kessler, Pharm.D., BCPS, was Founder and Chief Clinical Officer, SecondStory Health LLC, Carrboro, NC; Tim Larson was Pharmacy Director, Cardinal Rxe-source Center–Chicago region, Westmont, IL; Dallas Moore, M.S., was Pharmacy Director, American Fork Hospital–Intermountain Healthcare, American Fork, UT; Kelly Morrison was Director of Sales & Marketing, Rxe-source, Cardinal Health, Houston, TX; and Mickey Price was Vice President, Rxe-source, Cardinal Health, Dublin, OH.

The contributions of Stephen R. Novak, M.P.A., FASHP, to these guidelines are gratefully acknowledged. At the time of his contribution, Mr. Novak was Director, Pharmacy Services, Pardee Hospital, Hendersonville, NC. ASHP also acknowledges the following organizations and individuals for reviewing drafts of these guidelines (review does not imply endorsement): Accreditation Council for Pharmacy Education (ACPE); Healthcare Information and Management Systems Society (HIMSS) Pharmacy Informatics Task Force; Emily Alexander, Pharm.D., BCPS; David B. Archer, D.Ph.; David Aresco, B.S.Pharm., FASCP; John A. Armitstead, M.S., FASHP; Darrel W. Box, M.H.A.; Michael Brown, Pharm.D.; Kimberly K. Daugherty, Pharm.D., BCPS; Doug DeJong, M.B.A., FASHP; Mike Dudzik, M.H.A.; Francis J. Dunn, Jr., B.S.Pharm.; Jeanne Ezell, M.S., FASHP; Kelly Guhr, Pharm.D., BCPS; George Hill, M.B.A.; Linda Horton, Pharm.D.; Jody Jacobson Wedret, FASHP, FCSHP; Ken Kester, Pharm.D., J.D.; Patricia Kienle,

M.P.A., FASHP; Nancy Konieczny, M.B.A.; Donald H. Lynx, M.B.A., FASHP; Lynnae M. Mahaney, M.B.A.; Peter G. Mayberry; Roland Patry, Dr.P.H., FASHP; James A. Ponto, M.S., BCNP, FASHP; Cliff Richards, Pharm.D.; Mike Rouse, B.Pharm.(Hons), M.P.S. (ACPE); Terry Seaton, Pharm.D., FCCP, BCPS; Timothy P. Stratton, Ph.D., BCPS, FAPHA; Basil J. Thoppil, M.Sc., Pharm.D.; and Dennis A. Tribble, Pharm.D.

The bibliographic citation for this document is as follows: American Society of Health-System Pharmacists. ASHP guidelines on remote medication order processing. *Am J Health-Syst Pharm.* 2010; 67:672-7.

ASHP Guidelines on the Safe Use of Automated Compounding Devices for the Preparation of Parenteral Nutrition Admixtures

Purpose

Automated compounding devices are frequently used by pharmacists for the extemporaneous preparation of parenteral nutrition admixtures. This continuing shift from manual compounding procedures comes as a result of significant advances in automated technology, as well as in response to changing health care demands to provide admixture compounding in a safer, more efficient, and more accurate manner. Approximately 65% of the hospitals in the United States currently use automated compounding devices for parenteral nutrition admixtures on a daily basis.[a] Compounders are also used for other types of intravenous admixtures and in other settings, including home care and long-term-care facilities; therefore, the overall magnitude of their use may be substantial. As with other automated systems or devices, the benefits can be realized only when the technology is used appropriately. Significant patient harm may occur when safety and quality assurance measures are overlooked or circumvented.[1]

The purpose of these guidelines is to outline the key issues that should be considered to safely and cost-effectively incorporate this technology into the pharmacy operations of health care organizations. The guidelines focus on parenteral nutrition admixtures, but the safety issues are also applicable to the use of compounders for other types of i.v. admixtures. The term "health care organization" is used throughout the guidelines as a general descriptor and is intended to be inclusive of any of the practice settings and types of facilities in which compounders are used, including, for example, home infusion companies. These guidelines should be used in conjunction with the ASHP Guidelines on Quality Assurance for Pharmacy-Prepared Sterile Products and device manufacturers' instruction manuals and training materials. Pharmacists should use professional judgment in assessing their health care organization's needs for automated compounding devices and in adapting these guidelines to meet those needs.

Background

The act of extemporaneously compounding any parenteral formulation is complex and not without inherent risks; therefore, compounding tasks are best performed by personnel most qualified to do so. An incompatible, unstable, or contaminated i.v. infusion may induce significant patient morbidity and even mortality.[1] Pharmacists are specifically educated and legally responsible for performing these tasks safely. Pharmacists are also responsible for training other personnel to perform relatively simple tasks with the least risk possible.

The extemporaneous preparation of multiadditive products, such as parenteral nutrition admixture compounding, should be performed under the direct supervision of a pharmacist and in the appropriate environment.[2] The historical method of compounding these multicomponent admixtures has been to manually use gravity-driven transfers for large-volume additives, such as amino acids, dextrose, lipids, and sterile water. Small-volume additives, such as electrolytes, trace minerals, multivitamins, and drugs, have often been added manually and separately with a syringe. Thus, this compounding method is limited by the visual inspection of volumes transferred between stock containers, as well as by the precision of the calibrations marked on the stock containers or transfer devices.

The manual method of parenteral nutrition admixture compounding is labor-intensive and requires multiple manipulations of infusion containers, sets, syringes, needles, and so forth, which can lead to the extrinsic contamination of the final admixture with sterile and nonsterile contaminants. A sterile contaminant can be particulate matter from elastomeric vial enclosures (needle cores), and nonsterile contaminants can be bacteria and other infectious materials. Minimizing the number of extemporaneous manipulations of the parenteral infusion containers and supplies improves compounding efficiency and reduces the risk of extrinsic contamination and associated sequelae.[3]

The emergence of automated technology as an alternative approach to parenteral nutrition admixture compounding has led to potentially improved compounding accuracy with the use of fluid pump technology and software that controls the compounder pump. Fluid can be delivered from the source container to the final container by using either a volumetric or a gravimetric fluid pumping system. Volumetric systems transfer a specified volume of fluid from a source container to a final container via a rotary peristaltic pump. The tubing is stretched around a rotor and, as the rotor turns, solution is pulled from the source container and pushed toward the final container. Measurements are based on the theory that each rotor movement advances a constant amount of fluid through the system. The total volume delivered is calculated by the volume pulled into the tubing by each rotor movement multiplied by the number of movements. These systems usually incorporate a final check of the *actual* total bag weight by comparing it with a calculated *expected* weight.

In gravimetric systems, measurement of fluid volume delivered from the source container to the final container is determined by weighing the fluid transferred and dividing the weight by the solution's known specific gravity, thereby converting weight to volume. Two types of gravimetric pumps are available: additive and subtractive. With an additive pump, a single load cell is positioned to measure each fluid as it is delivered to the final container. With a subtractive pump, load cells are positioned beneath the source containers to measure each fluid as it is being pumped from its source container. Weight is determined by subtracting the posttransfer weight from the pretransfer weight of the container for each source solution. When all transfers are

completed, the system compares the *actual* total bag weight with a calculated *expected* weight.

In addition to the compounder, dedicated software may be used to electronically transfer information to the compounding device. Automated compounding software has additional features that can enhance the management of the parenteral nutrition program. Software issues and their integrity are additional critical components unique to compounder methods and require continuous monitoring to ensure that the operations are correct.[4]

Justification for the Use of Automated Compounding Devices

When is it appropriate to use compounders, and how will decisions affect others within and outside the pharmacy department? It is incumbent upon the pharmacist to ensure that the department is fully knowledgeable about the operation of the compounder and that a minimum acceptable standard of pharmacy practice is met. First, internal decisions need to be made to justify the expenses associated with this technology. Second, policies and procedures should be in place to assess workflow, establish training programs, and standardize compounder use in the specific pharmacy practice setting. Third, changing current compounder contracts may result in more cost than the savings that might appear in the new contracts. Specifically, the initial incorporation of an automated compounder into daily pharmacy practice is a labor-intensive effort, and such transitions can be disruptive and can even increase the risk of errors. This may be particularly true during staff orientation to new devices. Such changes must be carefully reviewed; if they are determined to be worthwhile, a well-coordinated transition plan should be devised beforehand. Whether transition costs (including the potential for unused sets and supplies) can be deferred to the new contract is another factor for consideration.

The principal emphasis associated with using automated compounding devices in health care organizations should be improving patient care and enhancing efficiency while remaining cost-effective. "Cost-effectiveness" is, therefore, a relative term with respect to personnel, as the labor saved is often redirected to other aspects of pharmaceutical care that could also improve patient safety. Time that was previously spent on operations associated with parenteral nutrition admixture compounding can now be aimed at other issues, such as optimization of drug and nutritional therapies, reorganization of product utilization, quality assurance programs, and augmentation of other core pharmaceutical services. Specific objectives related to cost justification of automated compounding devices may include the following:

1. Enhanced efficiency and worker safety during the parenteral nutrition compounding process and patient safety with parenteral use.
2. Reduction in labor associated with manually compounded parenteral nutrition admixtures. Assessment of the overall labor and material costs associated with the current manual compounding methods should include hidden costs such as pharmacists' time to perform calculations, quality assurance checks, and compounder set-up, as well as staff training (initial and on-going).
3. Reduction in waste through more efficient use of base solutions and additives. Inventory can often be reduced by consolidating source solutions to a few high-concentration, large-volume additives.

In some cases in which the cost of implementing automated compounding technology in one facility is prohibitive, health care organizations have opted to explore regional compounding centers or outsourcing to contractors.

Performance Requirements and Responsibilities

The use of automated devices for compounding parenteral nutrition admixtures should be clearly defined by the health care organization and the manufacturer. This includes the ongoing responsibilities of the pharmacy department and those of the manufacturer during and after implementation of the compounder in the pharmacy practice setting.

Three areas need to be clearly defined before choosing an automated compounding system: (1) the system's performance requirements, (2) the manufacturer's responsibilities, and (3) the pharmacy department's responsibilities. The performance requirements of the automated compounding system should ensure that

1. The compounder exceeds the level of accuracy achieved with manual compounding. The automated compounding device should be accurate to within 5% of the amount programmed, with verification of the amount pumped versus the programmed amount for each ingredient.
2. The automated compounding device has inherent safeguards, including the ability to detect inadvertent source-solution mixups; the ability to detect situations that could result in inaccurate deliveries, such as occluded transfer-set tubing and empty source containers; and the ability to keep incompatible source solutions separate.
3. The automated compounding software alerts the user when formulation issues arise.
4. The automated compounding software meets the standards of the American Society for Parenteral and Enteral Nutrition for parenteral nutrition label formats.[5]
5. The automated compounding software assists the pharmacist in producing physicochemically compatible parenteral nutrition formulations.
6. The automated compounding software provides useful clinical information.
7. The automated compounding software integrates with existing pharmacy programs wherever possible to optimize patient care and avoid therapeutic duplications.

The contractual agreement with the manufacturer should provide continuous support of the compounder and software, including information updates, problem solving, and emergency coverage. FDA considers all automated compounding devices class II devices,[6] and as such they must comply with federal regulations. The manufacturer's responsibilities are as follows:

1. The manufacturer should supply, and the pharmacist should verify, that the device is 510K cleared as evidence of compliance with regulatory requirements; that the device meets the fire and safety standards established by Underwriters Laboratories (i.e., is

UL-approved); that the operator's manual and other documentation support recommendations for use; and that accuracy statements and manufacturer claims are valid.

2. The manufacturer should provide 24-hour support for the compounder and its software throughout the life of the contract.

3. The manufacturer should routinely provide the latest version of the compounder software in a timely manner.

4. The manufacturer should ensure adequate availability of compounding supplies.

5. The manufacturer should provide detailed information and instructions on the appropriate use of the compounder and its software. References should be provided when appropriate.

6. The manufacturer should comply with FDA requirements for reporting adverse events.

Within the pharmacy department, specific policies and procedures should be developed that address responsibilities for compounder operations and maintenance, staff training, and monitoring compounder performance at all times. Before selecting and implementing an automated compounder, the pharmacy department should

1. Define and agree on automated compounding system needs and performance requirements.

2. Develop an implementation team with a lead person.

3. Develop a set of policies and procedures.

Control of the Automated Compounding Device in Daily Operations

The pharmacy department is responsible for the use, maintenance, and performance of the automated compounding device, including decisions about who has access to the compounder and its operations. Specific consideration should be given to the following:

1. Only designated pharmacy department personnel should have access to the compounder and its software. The level of access should correspond to the level of authority and expertise of the personnel.

2. Before being granted access to a compounder, pharmacy personnel should pass established competency-standard testing.

3. Access to and use of the compounder by pharmacy support personnel (i.e., pharmacy technicians, students, and other designated support staff) should be directly supervised by an authorized pharmacist.

4. The additive configuration or sequence of the compounder for compounding parenteral nutrition admixtures should not be altered from the established format without the authorization of a designated pharmacist.

5. The compounder should not be used for any purpose other than parenteral nutrition admixture compounding without authorization from a designated pharmacist. If the compounder is used for other extemporaneous drug preparation, this should be done separately from the schedule for parenteral nutrition admixtures. The use of the compounder in this manner will likely require the use of new compounding sets and admixture configurations.

Safety and Efficacy Features

The complexity of automated compounding device functions makes it imperative that the pharmacy department develop a specific plan for ensuring safe and efficacious use at all times. The safety and efficacy features should outline the core principles necessary for carrying out the complex tasks of parenteral nutrition compounding. The plan should identify the minimum standards that are routinely assessed through an established monitoring and surveillance program. Automated compounding devices on the market differ in hardware design, mechanisms of fluid transfer, and software applications. Consequently, sterility and quality assurance testing procedures and measures are also different, including routine assessments of accuracy in the delivery of correct amounts of nutrients. Consideration should be given to the following in accordance with the device manufacturer's specific instructions:

1. Establishing minimum competency standards for all personnel who have access to and operate the compounder. Competency standards should ensure that the compounder user has sufficient expertise to identify errors that may inadvertently bypass quality assurance systems. The competency standards should be reviewed and validated on a routine basis for all personnel operating the compounder.

2. Establishing specific procedures for the operation of the compounder that standardize its use, irrespective of the individual operator. Changes in compounder operations should occur only when authorized and should be communicated to all staff involved in compounding.

3. Including sterility and quality assurance measures to avoid extrinsic contamination and to ensure accurate delivery of parenteral nutrition additives.

4. Ensuring that compounder tubing changes occur at appropriate specified time intervals in accordance with the manufacturer's recommendations.

5. Devising methods for assessing and calibrating the accuracy of the compounder in delivering precise levels of substrates and additives.

6. Developing a contingency plan and a readily available backup system or method for providing uninterrupted parenteral nutrition therapy to patients in the event of compounder failure.

7. Ensuring that adequate amounts of solutions and supplies for automated compounding are on hand.

Quality Assurance Monitoring and Documentation

Automated compounding devices are intended to provide a higher margin of accuracy and to streamline the labor-intensive tasks associated with the manual extemporaneous preparation of large-volume, multiadditive parenteral nutrition admixtures and other admixtures. The compounders are not designed to replace oversight functions, which require the expertise of a pharmacist.

In theory, automated compounding devices provide compounding accuracy superior to that of traditional methods of manual compounding. However, the performance of compounders must be critically challenged by the pharmacist to ensure that their manufacturing specifications are

equal to the task. In the pharmaceutical industry, that process is called validation. Ongoing quality assurance measures specified by the device manufacturer for assessing the performance of the compounder, as well as corrective actions, should be clearly delineated in policies separate from those dedicated to operational tasks. "Ongoing" means daily, and whatever measures are determined to be essential should be performed each day because random checks may not detect a more insidious, intermittent flaw that could assume major clinical significance.[7,8]

The pharmacy department may work with other departments to assess the compounder's performance if such expertise is not available within the pharmacy department. For example, portions of parenteral nutrition admixtures may be sent to the health care organization's laboratory to determine dextrose content. However, laboratory methods are usually designed for biological rather than pharmaceutical systems and should be validated to meet USP requirements for the components being tested. If outside departments participate in the quality assurance program, their methods should be appropriately validated in accordance with USP specifications and the results documented within the pharmacy department records on the compounder's performance.

The pharmacy department should develop a monitoring and surveillance plan with output reports that encompasses the principles outlined under the section on safety and efficacy features. The plan should detail specific policies and procedures that will ensure the continuing operation of the automated compounding device at optimum performance levels at all times. The data generated by the monitoring procedures should be reported to the pharmacy director and other appropriate oversight personnel and kept as a permanent record of the compounder's operations. These reports should be regularly reviewed in the assessment of trends and other long-term measures of performance. Specific consideration should be given to

1. Establishing performance standards and continuous quality assurance measures for assessing the compounder's performance and product quality during setup and in-process (during compounding) and end-process testing.
2. Establishing quality assurance testing of user-defined software variables validating that the correct responses to user commands occur.
3. Validating all quality assurance testing before implementation.
4. Establishing a minimum performance standard for each quality assurance test. For example, deviations in the accuracy of delivering a single additive cannot exceed a predetermined percent error without immediate corrective actions.
5. Documenting all quality assurance data on a daily basis. A comprehensive review of the data and documentation of performance trends should be performed at scheduled intervals as necessitated by aseptic conditions. The compounder should have scheduled, routine cleaning and maintenance according to the manufacturer's recommendations to ensure proper operation.

Storage and Inventory

The pharmacy department is responsible for housing the automated compounding device, related disposable supplies,

and admixture ingredients. Other departments, such as materials management, may order and store additional supplies for the compounder yet defer to the pharmacy for the selection of the components necessary for proper compounder operation. Specific consideration should be given to

1. Maintaining an adequate inventory of supplies necessary for compounder operation and patient needs.
2. Procuring all large-volume parenteral nutrition components (amino acids, dextrose, and lipids) from one manufacturer unless such combinations have adequate physicochemical data that ensure the stability, compatibility, and safety of the final formulations commensurate with the data for single-source products.[5] Any proposed substitute products should be assessed for compatibility and approved by designated pharmacy personnel qualified to do so and possibly by the pharmacy and therapeutics committee if clinical issues are identified.
3. If a health care organization's contract requires a change in the brand of parenteral products, designated pharmacy personnel should verify that the new products are compatible. If a new product is approved, designated pharmacy personnel should verify that the new product is compatible, add it to the compounder formulary, and revise the admixture requirements and instructions relevant to the compounder's operations.

Education and Training

Pharmacists, by education and training, are competent to safely compound pharmaceuticals, including parenteral nutrition admixtures. Nevertheless, the introduction of automated compounding devices requires specific training of pharmacists as well as other pharmacy personnel in the operation, maintenance, and quality assurance of compounders. Specific consideration should be given to ensuring that

1. Pharmacy administration determines the individuals who will be responsible for education and training in the use of the compounders.
2. All education and training are documented in a permanent record maintained in the pharmacy department and in personnel files.
3. All pharmacy personnel using or supervising compounder operations are tested at regular intervals to ensure that individuals meet the department's minimum competency standards.
4. Retraining, competency assessment, and appropriate documentation accompany upgrades and new versions of the compounder to ensure the continued proficiency of personnel, safety of compounder operations, and adequacy of oversight.

Device Variability

Automated compounding devices are marketed by several manufacturers. Even though there are similarities among compounders, there may be significant differences in the design, accuracy, operation, maintenance, software, and manufacturing support, among other things. The safe operation and supervision of any given compounder depend on adherence to the manufacturer's specific instructions and

continuous quality assurance monitoring of compounder performance. The safe and efficient operation of an automated compounding system depends on defined responsibilities for the pharmacy and manufacturer, as well as on strict adherence to policies, procedures, and quality assurance programs.

References

1. Food and Drug Administration. Safety alert: hazards of precipitation associated with parenteral nutrition. *Am J Hosp Pharm.* 1994; 51:1427–8.

2. American Society of Hospital Pharmacists. ASHP technical assistance bulletin on quality assurance for pharmacy-prepared sterile products. *Am J Hosp Pharm.* 1993; 50:2386–98.

3. McClendon RR. A comparative evaluation of methods used to compound parenteral nutrition solutions. *Nutr Support Serv.* 1983; 3:46–9.

4. Driscoll DF. Clinical delivery of nutritional therapy: automated compounders and patient-specific feeding. *Nutrition.* 1996; 12:461–2. Editorial.

5. American Society for Parenteral and Enteral Nutrition National Advisory Group on Standards and Practice Guidelines for Parenteral Nutrition. Safe practices for parenteral nutrition formulations. *JPEN J Parenter Enteral Nutr.* 1998; 22:49–66.

6. Trautman KA. The FDA and worldwide quality system requirements guidebook for medical devices. Milwaukee, WI: ASQ Quality Press; 1997.

7. Driscoll DF. Delivery of nutritional therapy: quality assurance of automated compounding devices. *Nutrition.* 1996; 12:651–2. Editorial.

8. Fields HS. Establishing core performance requirements for automated TPN compounders. *Am J Health-Syst Pharm.* 1996; 53:1607. Letter.

[a] Mihalski T, Clintec Nutrition Division, Baxter Healthcare. Personal communication. 1999 Mar 15.

Approved by the ASHP Board of Directors on April 27, 2000. Developed through the ASHP Council on Professional Affairs.

The bibliographic citation for this document is as follows: American Society of Health-System Pharmacists. ASHP guidelines on the safe use of automated compounding devices for the preparation of parenteral nutrition admixtures. *Am J Health-Syst Pharm.* 2000; 57:1343–8.

ASHP Guidelines on the Safe Use of Automated Dispensing Devices

Purpose

The purposes of these guidelines are to (1) propose goals and objectives for the safe use of automated dispensing devices in the medication-use process, (2) provide guidance on the safe use of automated dispensing devices to pharmacists and others involved in the medication-use process, (3) advise vendors of automated dispensing devices about the safety needs of health care professionals who use their systems, and (4) recommend standardization for Health Level 7 (HL7) interfaces between pharmacy information systems and automated dispensing devices. The recommendations presented in these guidelines should be used in conjunction with other literature on the topic and information from prospective or selected automated dispensing device or system vendors, established guidelines, and state and federal regulations. Pharmacists should exercise professional judgment in assessing their health system's needs regarding automated dispensing devices and systems and in adapting these guidelines to meet those needs.

Automated pharmacy systems are designed for centralized filling of individual patient prescriptions and unit-dose medication orders, decentralized dispensing, and other purposes. These guidelines address primarily computer-controlled decentralized medication-dispensing cabinets, which will be referred to as "automated dispensing devices." Since many of the concepts discussed here may be applicable to related technologies, the term "automated pharmacy system" will be used generally and the term "automated dispensing device" will be used specifically. Automated dispensing devices are located in hospital patient care units, surgical suites, emergency rooms, long-term care facilities, physicians' offices, and other settings. Several manufacturers produce automated dispensing devices with a variety of configurations and software capabilities that may interface with the pharmacy or health care organization's information systems.[1,2]

Background

The appropriate, accurate, and timely distribution of medications to patients is a well-established responsibility of pharmacists. In acute care settings in particular, distribution systems have been developed that enable pharmacists to review patient-specific medication orders and oversee the preparation and packaging or selection of these medication doses, as well as the delivery of these medication doses to patient care units. Automation has evolved to ease fulfillment of pharmacists' distributive responsibilities, expand distribution system capabilities, and improve efficiency in distribution.

Automated dispensing devices are an increasingly prevalent component of the medication-use process in health care organizations today. The pharmacy profession's transition to an emphasis on direct patient care, changes in health care systems, and pressures to reduce costs have all created interest in the availability and use of automated dispensing devices. ASHP supports the use of automated dispensing devices when it frees pharmacists from labor-intensive distributive functions, helps improve patient care by both pharmacists and nurses, improves accountability and storage of medications, and improves the accuracy and timeliness of medication product availability. Experience with automated dispensing devices suggests that, when used appropriately, these benefits can be realized.[3-11] When automated dispensing devices are not used appropriately, their complexity, design and function variations, maintenance and education requirements, and other factors can have undesirable effects and compromise patient safety.[12,13] The National Association of Boards of Pharmacy (NABP) includes language on automation in the NABP Model State Pharmacy Act and Model Rules.[14,15] The NABP Model Act uses the term "automated pharmacy systems" and defines them to include, but not be limited to, "mechanical systems that perform operations or activities, other than Compounding or Administration, relative to the storage, packaging, Dispensing, or Distribution of medications, and which collect, control, and maintain all transaction information."[14] Data processing and bar code technologies, although incorporated as integral components of some of these systems, are not considered in the NABP Model Act definition as automated drug distribution technology. The NABP Model Rules suggest specific requirements and options for helping individual states determine which automated pharmacy systems are appropriate for use.[15] These ASHP guidelines reflect and expand on the requirements of the NABP Model Rules.

The use of automated dispensing devices continues to evolve. Some health care organizations deploy one or several devices in selected areas, such as emergency departments, that are floor-stock intensive and where lost charges can be substantial. Some devices are used for selected categories of medications, such as controlled substances, that have time-consuming tracking and documentation requirements. Some organizations deploy devices throughout patient care areas to cover nearly all medications used.

The rapid development of technology applications in health care, including automated dispensing devices, and pressures to expand their use have raised concerns about patient safety, access to medications, and possible legislative and regulatory barriers. While technologies can be designed to minimize opportunities for medication errors, that same design can create other, often unanticipated, opportunities for medication errors. Consideration of the use of automated dispensing devices, like consideration of any other technology, must include serious evaluation of existing and potential opportunities for error and the implementation of mitigating strategies to minimize or prevent such errors. Pharmacists have a professional responsibility to ensure that appropriate policies, procedures, and quality-assurance programs are in place to address the safety, accuracy, security, and patient confidentiality of automated pharmacy systems, including automated dispensing devices.

Goals and Objectives

Goals for the use of automated dispensing devices in the medication-use process should focus on improving patient

care and resource use. Specific objectives related to these goals may include the following:

- Information necessary for appropriate medication management and patient care is accurate, accessible, and timely.
- Appropriate medications are readily available and accessible to meet patient needs within safety and security controls.
- Vulnerabilities to medication errors are minimized, and those that remain are identified, documented, and mediated.
- Staff members involved in the medication-use process are safety conscious, accurate, and productive.
- Patients are satisfied with the quality and delivery of care.
- Medication distribution services are facilitated across the continuum of practice settings in the health care system.
- Resource management is improved by linking supply ordering channels to the medication distribution system.
- Billing accuracy is improved by allowing charges and credits to post when medications are dispensed from or returned to the automated dispensing device.

Requirements

Automated dispensing devices should be regarded by users as tools for improving the medication-use process rather than inherent solutions to problems in that process. Consideration should be given to how the technology can be adapted to meet the goals and objectives of the user rather than how the user's systems should be redesigned to fit the automated dispensing device. It is important to consider the recommended workflow for the automated dispensing device while simultaneously reviewing the facility's current workflow and practices to ultimately determine the best practices that will provide safe and efficient patient care while maximizing the safety and efficiency advantages offered by the automated dispensing device.

Before deciding to deploy automated dispensing devices in the medication-use process, an organization should assess its logistical, financial, and cultural circumstances; the safety, patient care, and resource benefits it hopes to gain; and how these benefits would be observed and measured. The organization should also determine if the automated dispensing devices in consideration are capable of producing the desired benefits. Specific consideration should be given to

- Incorporating the use of automated dispensing devices into the organization's strategic planning (i.e., ensuring that automation is compatible with the vision and mission of the organization).
- Assessing the use of automation from a complete systems perspective. Automated dispensing devices should integrate smoothly with other systems and processes, both manual and automated. Interfaces with overall patient care computer systems especially must be considered.
- Establishing performance standards for safety, accuracy, timeliness, and costs.[16]

- Determining the responsibilities of the automated dispensing device vendor and the organization for installation, validation, maintenance, education, operations, and troubleshooting.
- Assessing the impact of automation on organizational culture. Automation has a significant impact on employees, particularly pharmacy technicians and nurses. Optimal preparation and support should be considered.
- Ensuring effective education for the organization's employees who use the automated dispensing device or whose responsibilities are affected by its use.
- Developing an ongoing support plan.

Since the medication-use process involves multiple health care disciplines, selection of automated dispensing devices and establishment of policies and procedures for their use will require decisions that meet the needs of all disciplines involved. However, since pharmacists have a professional and legal responsibility for the safety and integrity of the entire medication-use process, they should provide leadership in the development and maintenance of policies and procedures for the safe use of automated pharmacy systems. Any system or device adopted for drug distribution and control, including automated dispensing devices, should meet the intent of established professional standards and guidelines regarding patient safety. The automated system or device should provide the following inherent safety features of unit-dose drug distribution systems:

- Medications are contained in, and administered from, single-unit or unit-dose packages.
- Medications are dispensed in ready-to-administer form to the extent possible.[17]
- Medications are available for administration to the patient only at the time at which they are to be administered, according to the institution's policy.
- An electronic patient medication profile is concurrently maintained in the pharmacy for each patient and made easily accessible to the pharmacist.
- Medications are accessible to different categories of health care professionals with the ability to limit access based on policy or law.

In addition, the automated systems or devices should ensure safe medication storage, distribution, access, and use wherever they are deployed, including meeting required environmental conditions for the storage and handling of medications. Plans for use of automated dispensing devices should include

- Sufficient quantity and appropriate location of devices to support intended use and efficient work processes,
- Selection of a location that minimizes distractions and interruptions during use,
- Consideration of surrounding work-space to allow efficient device operation and movement of staff,
- Ensuring appropriate ventilation and temperature control, including refrigeration for applicable medications,
- Ensuring adequate infection control policies and procedures are maintained when appropriate for the intended use and placement of the device,

- Ensuring appropriate and sufficient lighting to support the safe and accurate verification of medication orders, reading of medication labels, and administration documentation,
- Establishing proximity of the device to medication information and documentation systems,
- Selection of location or placement of the device that permits only the patient's caregivers access to protected health information, and
- Ensuring power and data connections essential to the operation of the device are included in the facility's emergency backup power and data management systems, so that support and information are provided in a reliable manner during power or data interruptions.

Finally, the automated system or device should comply with applicable federal and state consumer protection laws and regulations. State boards of pharmacy may have different requirements for the use of automated dispensing devices in various practice settings and for obtaining approval for their use.

Override Access to Medications Through Automated Dispensing Devices

All medication distribution systems have medication withdrawal functions that allow nurses and other caregivers limited access to certain medications before order review and approval by a pharmacist, especially in cases of patient emergencies. This function is typically referred to as an "override." Clearly stated organizational policies and criteria for system overrides should be developed that limit access to medications before orders have been reviewed and approved by a pharmacist.[16,18,19] Override access to medications should be limited to cases in which the drug product has been approved by a multidisciplinary committee of physicians, pharmacists, and nurses as having a clinically urgent need for the medication that outweighs the potential risk of medication error.

Subsequent order-based retrieval of the same medication should cause the user to be reminded that an override supply of medication was recently dispensed for the patient. Provision should be made for the retrospective review and reconciliation by a pharmacist of orders that were initiated without a pharmacist's review and approval. Override data (e.g., name of medication, quantity, location of the automated device, any associated adverse drug events) should be routinely reviewed to help evaluate and manage those medications approved for override access. Override data evaluation can aid an organization in improving the outcomes of automated dispensing device use by decreasing medication errors and potential adverse drug events[20] and should be considered part of the routine management process for automated dispensing devices.

Interfaces with Automated Pharmacy Systems

Proper planning should include the development of an interface strategy. Automated pharmacy systems interface with systems for pharmacy information, electronic medical records, admission/discharge/transfer, bar-coded medication administration (BCMA), and materials management for various purposes in support of the medication-use process, including the following:

- Commanding distribution of medications from a pharmacy location,
- Maintaining current data on patient population, including demographics and patient location, for the automated pharmacy system,
- Maintaining a current and accurate patient medication profile for each patient served by the automated pharmacy system,
- Maintaining current formulary information,
- Recording the addition, removal, or dispensing of medications from automated dispensing devices,
- Issuing charges for medications removed or dispensed from automated dispensing devices (if this is the charge method of choice), and
- Integrating with bedside point-of-care systems to assure accurate medication dispensing and patient administration.

Interfaces are effectively used to communicate patient demographic information, medication order information, formulary additions and updates, dispensing/charting information, and inventory management transactions between the automated dispensing device and the pharmacy information system (or pharmacy functionality in a hospital information system). Such interfaces may also pose challenges related to the complexity of their own deployment and maintenance. Their completeness and level of application may also impact the workflow associated with the use of automated dispensing devices. For these reasons, it is important to consider the impact that specific interfaces will have on the hospital and system users.

Interfaces between automated dispensing devices and pharmacy systems can be costly to create and maintain. Most vendors base these interfaces on HL7 standards[21] but do not necessarily interpret and apply the HL7 specifications in the same way. The result is that automated dispensing device interfaces should be easily customizable and thoroughly tested prior to implementation. Pharmacists should consult with other users of the same pharmacy system, automated dispensing device, and interface for advice on functionality and customization.

ASHP believes that the vendor community should work with the HL7 organization to identify one standard message set for communicating key transactions to and from automated dispensing devices to permit interfaces to be more easily implemented and supported. In addition, vendors should be prepared to support XML-based interfaces with the newer Web-based pharmacy applications.

Safety Checks

The pharmacy is responsible for ensuring that the automated pharmacy system operates as designed and is well maintained to prevent errors and system interruptions. All elements of the automated pharmacy system require periodic monitoring, including, as applicable, patient information and medication profiles, computer controls for access, operations of drawers and bins, and transaction records.

Any organization that uses an automated pharmacy system should have a written plan for the safe and effective

use of the system. The plan should be developed by the pharmacy and nursing staff, with input from respiratory therapy, medicine, and other disciplines that may be affected by the system.[22,23] The plan should address

- Conformance with industry and government standards as well as accepted practice standards,
- Potential sources of medication errors and the procedures to follow to avoid such errors,
- Limits on access to medications,[24]
- How medications will be packaged and labeled, including standardizing and limiting available concentrations,
- How medications will be safely and securely transported from the pharmacy to the automated dispensing device,
- The use of clinical alerts for high-risk medications,
- How medications will be transported from the automated dispensing device to the patient to reduce risk of administration to the wrong patient or at the wrong time,[16]
- How patient and medication information will be available and displayed while maintaining patient privacy,[16]
- How user privacy, security, and safety will be ensured,
- Procedures for ensuring the security of all stored medications, especially controlled substances, with a process in place to prevent and detect diversion,[25,26]
- Procedures for auditing all system transactions,
- Procedures for avoiding drug product cross-contamination (evident or trace amounts of a liquid or solid drug that may contaminate another drug or package),
- Procedures for identifying and removing medications prior to expiration, and
- Procedures for reporting malfunction or breakdown of the automated dispensing device.

The organization should have a written plan for ensuring the accuracy of (1) medications stored and accessed through an automated pharmacy system and (2) machine-readable identification on medication labels. This plan should provide

- A thorough review of the automated pharmacy system to identify potential sources of error that may be introduced by the system,
- Policies and procedures designed to preclude errors, and
- A quality-assurance program for reviewing override data and medication error data associated with the automated dispensing device and identifying opportunities for improvement, including a process for validating any medications that have been designated as high risk via machine-readable coding on removal.

Any organization that allows external suppliers to replenish medications in the automated pharmacy system should have a written plan for ensuring medication accuracy.[27] When possible, this plan should include the use of machine-readable identification to ensure placement of medications in the appropriate containers within automated dispensing devices, as well as recording that the proper filling was performed. To support this, processes must be in place to ensure that products do not reach the active inventory before confirmation that the product's bar code is accurately loaded into the appropriate cross-reference file. If possible, the machine-readable identification should also be used to ensure that medication supplies are not expired or in immediate danger of expiring.[28] If a hospital utilizes BCMA, all medications present in an automated dispensing device must be encoded with a bar code that will appropriately identify them in the BCMA system.

The organization should have a written contingency plan for maintaining timely medication distribution, security, and documentation when system interruptions occur.

A profile interface in which all medication order information is sent from the pharmacy information system to the automated dispensing device should be present whenever 24/7 pharmacy order entry is available. (For facilities that do not have 24/7 pharmacy order entry, a profile interface should be employed whenever feasible.) A profile interface is important for patient safety because it requires that a pharmacist review medication orders before the caregiver can access the medication from the automated dispensing device. Profiling functionality should include

- Transmission of all components of medication and i.v. orders, including drug, dose and/or infusion rate, route, frequency, dosing schedule, and order start/stop times,
- Ensuring that all patient care areas use the profiling functionality, including ambulatory and outpatient areas such as the emergency department, whenever possible,
- Limiting the variety and quantity of medications that are accessible without pharmacist review (override), and
- The option to require a double-check (witness) at the time of dispensing of an identified high-alert medication from automated devices, especially when pharmacist review and order entry have not occurred.[16]

The organization should include a process for comparing patient allergies with the current medication profile. Automated devices should receive coded allergy information from the pharmacy or hospital information system, which would allow an alert to be displayed when a medication to which a patient is allergic is dispensed.

Monitoring and Surveillance

Pharmacists are legally and organizationally responsible for ensuring that drug supplies are adequately controlled and that medication use is documented within the health care organization. Automated pharmacy systems usually provide options for tracking and accounting for medication use, which can be used to help monitor important data, such as the number of adverse drug events.[29,30] These options often include freestanding computer-controlled access and record keeping for each device, computer-controlled access and record keeping linked to the pharmacy information system, and computer linking among the pharmacy, patient record, and billing information systems. Appropriate interfaces with pharmacy and overall patient care computer systems are critical. Each of these options may require a different level of oversight.

The organization should have a written plan for the monitoring and surveillance of medications accessed through automated pharmacy systems. The plan should be developed by the pharmacy, with input from nursing staff and other clinicians, and communicated to staff members responsible for its implementation. The plan should include[18,25,26,31]

- Identification of the data to be captured and the reports to be generated for monitoring medication use, waste reconciliation, and discrepancies (data and reports may vary by drug categories and requirements for control and accountability),
- Assignment of responsibility for reviewing reports, scheduling the frequency of report reviews, and reporting discrepancies,
- Assignment of responsibility for resolving discrepancies, scheduling the resolution of discrepancies, following up on unresolved discrepancies, and taking action if the discrepancy is not resolved on schedule,
- A description of the process for investigating trends in discrepancies and assigning responsibility for conducting the investigation,
- Appropriate access by personnel, including timely removal of access when no longer employed or credentialed by the facility,
- Determination of frequency of narcotic counts, who will perform them, and who is responsible for verifying that the narcotic counts were completed,
- Examination of charge and credit flow to ensure billing accuracy, and
- Assignment of reviewing overrides to ensure the function is being used appropriately.

Compliance with the plan should be monitored through the organization's quality-assurance program.

Storage and Inventory

The drawer, bin, and pocket configurations of automated dispensing devices vary depending on device design and hospital preferences. Open matrix drawers, pockets that open or light up for a specific drug, and multiple open bins within a cabinet door are just a few of many different configurations available from various vendors. The pharmacy should develop criteria for determining the drug products and quantities that will be stored under different levels of access control in specific configurations of drawers, pockets, or bins. Patient safety should be the primary concern in establishing these criteria. The criteria should address

- The frequency and appropriateness of individual medication use,
- The effective use of reports related to the safe, accurate, and timely withdrawal of medications available through the automated pharmacy system,
- The party responsible for medication safety oversight and administrative control of drug availability in the automated pharmacy system (e.g., the pharmacy and therapeutics committee),[16]
- The identification of drug products that are considered inappropriate for inclusion in automated dispensing devices (e.g., products that have short expiration dates

or special preparation or storage requirements, present cross-contamination risks, or are hazardous),
- The need for ongoing monitoring and optimization of the contents of the automated dispensing device by a pharmacist, taking into consideration such matters as evolving therapeutic trends, the differing needs of individual patient care areas, and the capabilities and safety features of the automated pharmacy system,[17]
- Oversight of the positioning of look-alike and sound-alike drugs, high-alert drugs, and drugs with multiple strengths throughout the automated dispensing device as well as procedures to minimize the incorrect restocking of these medications (e.g., keeping these items as far apart as possible),
- Procedures to prevent and/or minimize the return of drugs directly to the automated dispensing device by nursing staff to decrease the potential for error,
- Specification of the individual(s) responsible for adding, modifying, or reviewing formulary items on a regular and ongoing basis to ensure they correctly display and interface map. Tall-man lettering, standardized concentration displays, and form designations are just a few of the many items that need to be maintained for safety,
- Procedures for keeping policies, procedures, and education current,
- Policies addressing drug product integrity, including
 - The importance of accuracy and integrity of product labels,
 - How to handle medications that are removed from an automated dispensing device but not used,
 - How medication waste is accounted for,
 - Checking products for expiration and beyond-use dates,
 - Identifying and following up on tampered products,
 - Storing products, and
 - Procedures for delivering medications to patient care units and individual patients.
- Controls that ensure accurate restocking of automated dispensing devices, such as
 - Access controls on drawers, bins, and pockets, including software restrictions and use of location lights and/or locking bin or pocket systems that support safe access,
 - Process redundancies to ensure correct restocking,[16]
 - Standardization of restocking procedures to limit process variation,[16] and
 - When the system permits, use of bar coding to restock the correct medication in the correct drawer, bin, or pocket, and
- Controlling access to medications to limit the potential for inadvertent selection of the wrong medication, and assuring that each drug has a unique and segregated location within the automated dispensing device so only the specific drug needed is accessible.[16]

Security and Responsibility

Among pharmacy's responsibilities for the medication-use process is preventing threats to patient and employee safety

and economic loss through medication misuse, pilferage, and diversion.

Any organization that uses an automated pharmacy system should have a written plan that assigns responsibility for and addresses issues of security. The plan should be developed by the pharmacy, with input from nursing, medicine, and other disciplines that may be affected by the system. The plan should clearly identify that the pharmacist in charge has general responsibility for the automated pharmacy system. The plan should specify who in the pharmacy and elsewhere in the organization has responsibility for computer interface issues; operational problems; the accuracy of medications contained in the system; maintenance of access codes, magnetic cards, and other positive identification methods; and education of users and the determination of skill levels those individuals must achieve.

The specific responsibilities and privileges of all personnel involved in operating or using the automated pharmacy system should be set forth in written policies and procedures. The policies and procedures should minimize the use of temporary user and patient identifications and should describe the circumstances in which these features may be used.

Downtime procedures in case of software or hardware malfunctions, power failures, or planned maintenance affecting normal operations should be developed to ensure medication security, accurate documentation of distribution and administration, and continued patient safety.[16]

Education

Automated pharmacy systems bring together information systems, machines, and humans in highly complex and interdependent relationships. Individuals involved in the use and operation of the system must possess the knowledge and skills required by their level of responsibility and understand the risks associated with the use and foreseeable misuse of automated pharmacy systems.[16] The organization should

- Have procedures in place for ensuring that all staff members who use the automated pharmacy system receive adequate education, both initially and on an ongoing basis,
- Ensure that adequate resources are provided for effective education,
- Ensure that the content of the education programs is continually updated,
- Evaluate staff members to ensure competency in the use of the automated pharmacy system and document the evaluations,
- Share with staff members the lessons learned from the evaluations and discuss medication errors related to the automated pharmacy system and near-miss reports,[16] and
- Include at least one higher-level user group capable of managing and supporting the system and its end users.

Support

When automated dispensing devices are utilized, alternative distribution systems need to be in place to deliver medications in case of failure. The organization must negotiate a service level agreement with the vendor that meets the organization's minimal acceptable downtime requirements.

The organization should define the level of support that will be provided internally and ensure that staff are sufficiently educated to deliver the defined level of internal support. The organization will need to negotiate with the vendor the purchase of spare parts needed to optimally recover from mechanical failures.

Conclusion

Automated dispensing devices are increasingly being used in health systems for centralized filling of individual patient prescriptions and unit-dose medication orders, decentralized dispensing, and other purposes. When such devices and the systems that support them are not used appropriately, their complexity, design and function variations, maintenance and education requirements, and other factors can compromise patient safety and have other harmful effects. ASHP supports the appropriate use of automated dispensing devices and has developed these guidelines to provide recommendations to pharmacists and others involved in their use.

References

1. Perini VJ, Vermeulen LC. Comparison of automated medication-management systems. *Am J Hosp Pharm.* 1994; 51:1883-91.
2. ECRI. Automated decentralized pharmacy dispensing systems. *Health Devices.* 1996; 25:436-73.
3. Ray MD, Aldrich LT, Lew PJ. Experience with an automated point-of-use drug distribution system. *Hosp Pharm.* 1995; 30: 18, 20-3, 27-30.
4. Borel JM, Karen LR. Effect of an automated, nursing unit-based drug-dispensing device on medication errors. *Am J Health-Syst Pharm.* 1995; 52:1875-9.
5. Guerrero RM, Nickman NA, Jorgenson JA. Work activities before and after implementation of an automated dispensing system. *Am J Health-Syst Pharm.* 1996; 53:548-54.
6. Schwarz HO, Brodowy BA. Implementation and evaluation of an automated dispensing system. *Am J Health-Syst Pharm.* 1995; 52:823-8.
7. Franklin BD, O'Grady K, Donyai P et al. The impact of a closed-loop electronic prescribing and administration system on prescribing errors, administration errors and staff time: a before-and-after study. *Qual Saf Health Care.* 2007; 16:279-84.
8. Gaunt MJ, Johnston J, Davis MM. Automated dispensing cabinets. Don't assume they're safe; correct design and use are crucial. *Am J Nurs.* 2007; 107:27-8.
9. Crane J, Crane FG. Preventing medication errors in hospitals through a systems approach and technological innovation: a prescription for 2010. *Hosp Top.* 2006; 84:3-8.
10. Chung K, Choi YB, Moon S. Toward efficient medication error reduction: error-reducing information management systems. *J Med Syst.* 2003; 27:553-60.
11. Oren E, Shaffer ER, Guglielmo BJ. Impact of emerging technologies on medication errors and adverse drug events. *Am J Health-Syst Pharm.* 2003; 60:1447-58.
12. Barker KN. Ensuring safety in the use of automated medication dispensing systems. *Am J Health-Syst Pharm.* 1995; 52:2445-7.

13. Tribble DA. How automated systems can (and do) fail. *Am J Health-Syst Pharm.* 1996; 53:2622-7.

14. National Association of Boards of Pharmacy. Model State Pharmacy Act. Article 1, section 105(h), p. 3. www.nabp.net/ftpfiles/NABP01/ModelActFINAL.doc (accessed 2009 Mar 18).

15. National Association of Boards of Pharmacy Model Rules for the Practice of Pharmacy. Section 3(p), pp. 94-95. www.nabp.net/ftpfiles/NABP01/ModelAct FINAL.doc (accessed 2009 Mar 18).

16. Institute for Safe Medication Practices (ISMP). ISMP guidance on the interdisciplinary safe use of automated dispensing cabinets. www.ismp.org/Tools/guidelines/ADC_Guidelines_Final.pdf (accessed 2009 Mar 19).

17. Fanikos J, Erickson A, Munz KE et al. Observations on the use of ready-to-use and point-of-care activated parenteral products in automated dispensing cabinets in U.S. hospitals. *Am J Health-Syst Pharm.* 2007; 64:2037-43.

18. Kowiatek JG, Weber RJ, Skledar SJ et al. Assessing and monitoring override medications in automated dispensing devices. *J Comm J Qual Patient Saf.* 2006; 32:309-17.

19. Kester K, Baxter J, Freudenthal K. Errors associated with medications removed from automated dispensing machines using override function. *Hosp Pharm.* 2006; 41:535-7.

20. Oren E, Griffiths L, Guglielmo J. Characteristics of antimicrobial overrides associated with automated dispensing machines. *Am J Health-Syst Pharm.* 2002; 59:1445-8.

21. Health Level 7 (HL7). HL7 standards. www.hl7.org/Library/standards.cfm (accessed 2009 Mar 19).

22. Novek J, Bettess S, Burke K et al. Nurses' perceptions of the reliability of an automated medication dispensing system. *J Nurs Care Qual.* 2000; 14:1-13.

23. Rebidas D, Smith ST, Denomme P. Redesigning medication distribution systems in the OR. *AORN J.* 1999; 69:184-6,188,190.

24. Botwin KJ, Chan J, Jacobs R et al. Restricted access to automated dispensing machines for surgical antimicrobial prophylaxis. *Am J Health-Syst Pharm.* 2001; 58:797-9.

25. Vigoda MM, Gencorelli FJ, Lubarsky DA. Discrepancies in medication entries between anesthetic and pharmacy records using electronic databases. *Anesth Analg.* 2007; 105:1061-5.

26. Epstein RH, Gratch DM, Grunwald Z. Development of a scheduled drug diversion surveillance system based on an analysis of atypical drug transactions. *Anesth Analg.* 2007; 105:1053-60.

27. Louie C, Brethauer B, Dong D et al. Use of a drug wholesaler to process refills for automated medication dispensing machines. *Hosp Pharm.* 1997; 32:367-75.

28. ASHP 2015 Initiative, Objective 5.1. www.ashp.org/s_ashp/docs/files/2015_Goals_Objectives_0508.pdf (accessed 2010 Jan 6).

29. Romero AV, Malone DC. Accuracy of adverse-drug-event reports collected using an automated dispensing system. *Am J Health-Syst Pharm.* 2005; 62:1375-80.

30. Institute for Safe Medication Practices, McIntosh ST, Petropoulos JB. Using data from automated dispensing units to identify adverse drug reactions. *Am J Health-Syst Pharm.* 2005; 62:2397-400.

31. Klibanov OM, Eckel SF. Effects of automated dispensing on inventory control, billing, workload, and potential for medication errors. *Am J Health-Syst Pharm.* 2003; 60:569-72.

Developed through the ASHP Section of Pharmacy Informatics and Technology and approved by the ASHP Board of Directors on July 21, 2009. These guidelines supersede the ASHP Guidelines on the Safe Use of Automated Medication Storage and Distribution Devices dated April 22, 1998.

A work group of the ASHP Section of Pharmacy Informatics and Technology 2008–2009 Section Advisory Group on Automation and Documentation (Leslie Brookins, M.S.; Ron Burnette, M.B.A.; Thomas W. Cooley, M.B.A.; Paul M. Seelinger, B.S.Pharm.; and Gwen Volpe, B.S.Pharm.) is gratefully acknowledged for revising these guidelines. Other members of the section advisory group included Christopher J. Urbanski, M.S., Chair; Arash T. Dabestani, Pharm.D., M.H.A., FABC, Vice Chair; Jim Besier, Ph.D., FASHP; Kimberly Dove, Pharm.D.; Craig P. Frost, M.B.A.; Rick K. Glabach, B.S.Pharm.; Gary L. Johnson, Jr., Pharm.D., M.H.A.; Denise Mckenzie; Brad Rognrud, M.S.; Charles De la Torre, M.S., M.I.S.; Rayburn Brian Vrabel, Pharm.D.; Matt Marshall, Pharm.D.; Marvin H. Choi (Student Member); Dennis A. Tribble, Pharm.D. (Executive Committee Liaison); and Karl Gumpper, Pharm.D., BCNSP, BCPS.

The bibliographic citation for this document is as follows: American Society of Health-System Pharmacists. ASHP guidelines on the safe use of automated dispensing devices. *Am J Health-Syst Pharm.* 2010; 67:483-90.

Drug Distribution and Control

Drug Distribution and Control

Redistribution of Unused Medications (0611)

Source: Council on Legal and Public Affairs

To advocate that any program for the return and reuse of medications comply with all federal and state laws (including laws regarding controlled substances); further,

To advocate that in order to ensure patient safety and provide an equal standard of care for all patients, such a program should include the following elements: (1) compliance with practice standards, accreditation standards, and laws related to prescription dispensing; (2) a requirement that these medications must not have been out of the possession of a licensed health care professional or his or her designee; (3) protection of the privacy of the patient for whom the prescription was originally dispensed; (4) inclusion of only those drug products that are in their original sealed packaging or in pharmacy-prepared unit-of-use packaging that is not expired and has been properly stored; (5) the presence of a system for identifying medications for the purpose of a drug recall or market withdrawal; (6) a definition of patient eligibility for participation in the program; and (7) adequate compensation of participating pharmacists for any associated costs.

This policy was reviewed in 2010 by the Council on Public Policy and by the Board of Directors and was found to still be appropriate.

Pharmaceutical Counterfeiting (0401)

Source: Council on Professional Affairs

To foster increased pharmacist and public awareness of drug product counterfeiting; further,

To encourage pharmacists to purchase and handle medications in ways that enhance the transparency and integrity of the drug product supply chain; further,

To encourage pharmacists to identify instances of drug product counterfeiting and to respond by assisting the patient in receiving appropriate treatment and monitoring, documenting patient outcomes, and notifying the patient, prescriber, and appropriate state and federal regulatory bodies (e.g., the Food and Drug Administration's MedWatch system); further,

To provide consumers and health professionals with information on how to avoid counterfeit drug products and how to recognize, respond to, and report encounters with suspicious drug products; further,

To foster research and education on the extent, methods, and impact of drug product counterfeiting and on strategies for preventing and responding to drug product counterfeiting.

This policy was reviewed in 2008 by the Council on Pharmacy Practice and by the Board of Directors and was found to still be appropriate.

Pharmacy Drug Theft (0303)

Source: House of Delegates Resolution

To support the development of policies and guidelines for health-system pharmacists designed to deter drug product theft and thereby enhance both the integrity of the drug distribution chain and the safety of the workplace; further,

To encourage the development of systems that limit the diversion and abuse potential of medications, including high-cost drugs and controlled substances, and thereby reduce the likelihood that these products will be targets of theft.

This policy was reviewed in 2007 by the Council on Pharmacy Management and by the Board of Directors and was found to still be appropriate.

Pharmacist's Role in Drug Procurement, Distribution, Surveillance, and Control (0232)

Source: Council on Professional Affairs

To affirm the pharmacist's expertise and responsibility in the procurement, distribution, surveillance, and control of all drugs used within health systems; further,

To encourage the Joint Commission on Accreditation of Healthcare Organizations, other accreditation bodies, and governmental entities to enhance patient safety by supporting the pharmacist's role in drug procurement, distribution, surveillance, and control.

(*Note:* For purposes of this policy, drugs include those used by inpatients and outpatients, large- and small-volume injectables, radiopharmaceuticals, diagnostic agents including radiopaque contrast media, anesthetic gases, blood-fraction drugs, dialysis fluids, respiratory therapy drugs, biotechnologically produced drugs, investigational drugs, drug samples, drugs brought to the setting by patients or family, and other chemicals and biological substances administered to patients to evoke or enhance pharmacologic responses.)

This policy was reviewed in 2011 by the Council on Pharmacy Practice and by the Board of Directors and was found to still be appropriate.

Optimizing the Medication-Use Process (9903)

Source: Council on Administrative Affairs

To urge health-system pharmacists to assume leadership, responsibility, and accountability for the quality, effectiveness, and efficiency of the entire medication-use process (including prescribing, dispensing, administration, monitoring, and education) across the continuum of care; further,

To urge health-system pharmacists to work in collaboration with patients, prescribers, nurses, and other health care providers in improving the medication-use process.

This policy was reviewed in 2008 by the Council on Pharmacy Management and by the Board of Directors and was found to still be appropriate.

ASHP Guidelines on Managing Drug Product Shortages in Hospitals and Health Systems

Purpose

Drug product shortages can adversely affect drug therapy, compromise or delay medical procedures, and result in medication errors.[1,2] Health care professionals are increasingly concerned about the clinical effect that shortages have on patients and the tremendous resources required to address shortages.[3-5] Adverse patient outcomes related to drug product shortages[1,2,6-9] have prompted aggressive management strategies by health care providers and gained the attention of the Joint Commission,[10] the government,[11,12] and the media.[13,14] Drug product shortages adversely affect health-system finances by increasing the cost of delivering patient care, largely through higher drug acquisition and personnel costs.[6] In addition, shortages create a high level of frustration for everyone involved, including purchasing agents, pharmacists, nurses, physicians, and patients.[7]

Managing drug product shortages is particularly complex for practitioners in hospitals and health systems (hereinafter, "health systems"), because these facilities routinely treat patients with acute or emergent conditions, use a significant number of medically necessary or single-source products, and use high-cost new drug technologies. These health care providers are challenged during drug product shortages to ensure the provision of seamless, safe, and therapeutically equivalent drug therapy, preferably at comparable costs. The pharmacy department must take a leadership role in efforts to develop and implement appropriate strategies and processes for informing practitioners of shortages and ensuring the safe and effective use of therapeutic alternatives. Strategic planning is required for managing drug product shortages, just as it is for disasters such as major weather events and mass-casualty incidents.

Because a thorough understanding of why drug product shortages occur is essential for their successful management, these guidelines begin with a description of factors that contribute to or exacerbate shortages. The guidelines then describe a three-phase approach to contingency planning for management of drug product shortages and include strategies for prevention. Given the differences and complexities in health-system organizational arrangements and practice settings, some aspects of these guidelines may not be applicable in all settings. Pharmacy managers should use their professional judgment in assessing and adapting these guidelines to meet their needs.

Contributing Factors

For the purpose of these guidelines, a drug product shortage is defined as a supply issue that affects how the pharmacy prepares or dispenses a drug product or influences patient care when prescribers must use an alternative agent. Shortages can be the result of one or a combination of factors throughout the supply chain. The supply chain includes sources of raw materials, manufacturers, regulators, wholesalers or distributors, prime vendors, group purchasing organizations, and end-user health care systems. The factors that follow contribute to disruptions in the availability of drug products.

Raw and Bulk Material Unavailability. Disruptions in the supply of raw or bulk materials are especially problematic when the primary or sole source experiences production difficulties or discontinues production, affecting multiple manufacturers. An estimated 80% of the raw materials used in pharmaceuticals comes from outside the United States.[4] Availability problems can arise when armed conflict or political upheaval disrupts trade, animal diseases contaminate tissue from which raw materials are extracted, climatic and other environmental conditions depress the growth of plants used to produce raw materials, or raw materials are degraded or contaminated during harvesting, storage, or transport.

Manufacturing Difficulties and Regulatory Issues. Drug product shortages can also occur when the primary or sole manufacturer of a drug product halts or delays production in response to a Food and Drug Administration (FDA) enforcement action concerning noncompliance with current good manufacturing practices (cGMPs). Contributing factors may include antiquated manufacturing equipment, a shift of resources from maintenance of equipment and facilities to research and development, loss of manufacturer personnel experienced in production and compliance issues as a result of company mergers or retirements, cGMP-related problems with subcontractors who supply products to multiple pharmaceutical manufacturers, and limited FDA resources for timely inspections of manufacturing sites.[4] Resolution of these issues is often a lengthy process and may include inspections to ascertain cGMP compliance, issuance of an injunction against the manufacturer, or seizure of products. In some instances, a manufacturer's decision to close a specific manufacturing facility results in unintended drug product shortages. Such was the case when the sole source for hyaluronidase production closed, leaving no supplier.[5]

FDA enforcement actions are intended to protect the public from potentially unsafe drug products. These actions are evaluated by FDA's Center for Drug Evaluation and Research (CDER) drug shortage coordinator to determine if the action might create a shortage of a medically necessary drug product.[12] (FDA's definition of a medically necessary product is discussed in the "Government intervention" section below.) In the event that a significant corrective action involves a medically necessary product, FDA will help the manufacturer return to compliance, consider qualifying additional manufacturing sites, or, in extreme circumstances, permit importation of the product from a foreign manufacturing source once the required quality controls are met.

Voluntary Recalls. Voluntary recalls, generally related to manufacturing problems, can cause shortages, especially when a sole manufacturer's drug product dominates the market supply. Voluntary recalls are generally temporary and occur as a result of a minor lapse in manufacturing procedures

that would not be subject to FDA legal action. Recalls usually affect specific lots and are conducted either because of a lack of assurance that the recalled product is safe or for reasons not related to safety, such as technical deficiencies in the drug's labeling. An ethical dilemma could arise when it is predictable that complying with the voluntary recall may cause a drug product shortage in a given health system.

Change in Product Formulation or Manufacturer. Changes in a product's formulation or manufacturer may also delay product availability. One example is the transition from albuterol metered-dose inhalers (MDIs) containing chlorofluorocarbons to MDIs containing hydro-fluoroalkanes in 2006.

Manufacturers' Production Decisions and Economics. Manufacturers' business decisions are based on a variety of factors, including availability of generic products, market size, patent expiration, drug-approval status, regulatory compliance requirements, and anticipated clinical demand. Occasionally, manufacturers temporarily or permanently reduce production quantities of certain drug products as they shift production efforts or reallocate resources to other products. A manufacturer's reasoned, sound business decision to discontinue production of a drug product because of insufficient financial return or a high cost to correct manufacturing issues can cause an unanticipated, serious shortage, especially in the instance of a sole-source or medically necessary product.[15] For example, a shortage of diphtheria and tetanus toxoids and acellular pertussis vaccine adsorbed was precipitated when one of the manufacturers, claiming low revenues, discontinued its product in 2000.[5] Manufacturers are not required to notify FDA of a drug discontinuation unless the product is a sole-source or medically necessary product.[16] For medically necessary drugs, FDA can encourage other manufacturers to produce the product or request that the manufacturer not suspend production until an alternative source is available. However, FDA does not have the authority to require a company to make any product, even if it is medically necessary. Even with advance notice, some agents, such as vaccines or antibiotics, are complex to manufacture, and shortages may result even if other manufacturers are willing and able to produce the product. Similarly, business decisions on the part of wholesale distributors and end-user health systems may contribute to drug product shortages.

Industry Consolidations. Manufacturer mergers often result in decisions to narrow the focus of product lines or move a production line to a new facility, resulting in the discontinuation or delayed availability of drug products. Mergers between two companies that manufacture similar product lines typically result in single-source products. As the number of manufacturers of a product decreases, resiliency in the supply chain also decreases, making product supplies more vulnerable. Many vaccines in the United States are single-source products, in part because of discontinuations and consolidations.

Restricted Drug Product Distribution And Allocation. Most hospitals and health systems obtain the majority of their drug products through wholesale distributors. Restricted distribution methods that bypass the normal supply chain can also create shortages. As the result of either market approval requirements or postmarketing surveillance, manufacturers

limit the availability of specific drug products. Only selected suppliers and end users who comply with manufacturer agreements can obtain the product. A manufacturer can also place restrictions on available limited supplies, requiring health systems to order directly from the manufacturer or through a specialty distributor to receive an allocation.

Inventory Practices. Communication and transportation efficiencies throughout the supply chain have allowed inventory reductions at all levels. Most manufacturers, distribution centers, and health systems use "just-in-time" inventory management to reduce the cost of inventory on hand and optimize cash flow. This strategy is recognized as sound business management for all stakeholders, but an unexpected shortage at any point in the supply chain can significantly affect the end user and patient. Some manufacturers and distributors use inventory management strategies that minimize end-of-quarter or end-of-year product inventories or limit shipments based on yearly quotas.

Poor ordering practices, stockpiling before price increases, hoarding caused by rumors of an impending shortage, and unexpected delivery delays may affect inventory levels in individual health systems. Hospitals in rural areas face additional inventory challenges caused by distant distribution centers and the inability to easily borrow an item from a nearby hospital. Drug product shortages may also occur when all hospitals in an area disproportionately use the same wholesaler. Some shortages are wholesaler dependent, as shortages of drugs can occur when contracts with suppliers are delayed.

Unexpected Increases in Demand and Shifts in Clinical Practice. Occasionally, the demand for a drug product unexpectedly increases or exceeds production capacity. This may occur when a new indication is approved for an existing drug product, when usage patterns change in response to new therapeutic guidelines, when a substantial disease outbreak occurs, or when unpredictable factors influence demand. Shortages may be prolonged when the raw materials are limited or manufacturing processes are complex or dependent on a long lead time. For example, when the Centers for Disease Control and Prevention (CDC) recommended annual influenza vaccination for children age 6–59 months in 2006, only one product had FDA-approved labeling for use in children 6–23 months old.[17,18]

Nontraditional Distributors. The increased frequency of drug product shortages has precipitated the development of nontraditional distributors, also known as open-market, graymarket, or alternative distributors. These specialty, licensed distributors or brokers obtain products in short supply for the purpose of reselling them to end users who are unable to obtain them through their normal suppliers. These distributors aggressively market the availability of these products to hospitals, specialty health systems, home care agencies, and physician practices, generally at substantially higher prices. Typically, these distributors have a limited quantity of product, often only enough for one or two patients. Many do not offer a return or refund on a product if it expires or is not used. Especially worrisome is the inability to ascertain the product's pedigree or ensure the reliability of the product's source, which could be outside the United States, and proper handling and storage throughout the chain of custody. The

extent to which the activities of such nontraditional distributors contribute to drug product shortages is unknown.

Compounding pharmacies have also pursued the production of drugs that are in short supply. Caution is warranted because preparations from these pharmacies may not meet applicable state or federal standards (e.g., United States Pharmacopeia chapter 797 or FDA labeling requirements). The sources of raw materials used by compounding pharmacies have been questioned, and apparent lapses in quality control have resulted in serious patient injury, including death.[13]

Natural Disasters. Natural disasters can have a profound effect on the availability of drug products. Damage to manufacturing facilities, particularly those that are the sole source of a drug product or category of products, is likely to cause long-term shortages. Damage to manufacturing facilities in Puerto Rico in 1998 from hurricane George caused shortages of several drug products. Fires, hurricanes, tornadoes, and floods are examples of natural disasters that may temporarily compromise drug product supplies. In some instances, these shortages may be exacerbated by an escalated need for certain classes of drug products to care for victims of the disaster. In 2005, areas affected by hurricanes Katrina and Rita were affected by both an increased need for medications and the inability to obtain them.

Phased Approach to Planning for Drug Product Shortages

The discovery of a shortage initiates a cascade of events surrounding drug procurement and therapeutic decision-making (Figure 1). Drug procurement considerations include validating the shortage and its anticipated duration, determining the availability of supplies from alternative sources, locating and procuring alternative supplies (if available), investigating the implications of compounding the product, and researching and providing education about alternative agents and the cost implications of all scenarios. The outcome of this process may prompt an evaluation of the shortage's potential effect on patient care and development of a strategy for effectively communicating the needed information to all professionals involved and to affected patients when warranted.

In an ideal world, there would be a system for warning providers in advance of impending drug product shortages; this would give them ample opportunity to proactively address and manage all aspects and implications of the shortage. In lieu of this ideal, pharmacists, when confronted with the unavailability of a drug product, want information on which to base decisions about meeting patient needs for the product. Segments of the supply chain, especially manufacturers and distributors, have been inconsistent in providing information and assistance to health systems. The difficulty in obtaining information is exacerbated by the many players, complexities, and uncertainties in the supply chain.

The pharmacy department must take a leadership role in managing shortages by developing and implementing appropriate strategies and processes for optimizing the safe

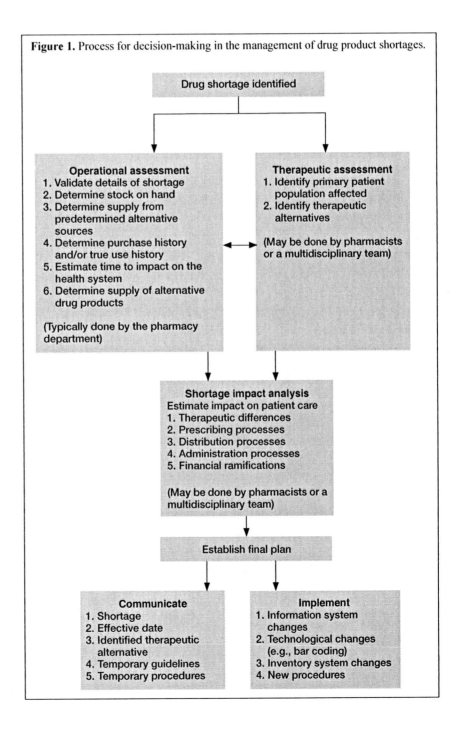

Figure 1. Process for decision-making in the management of drug product shortages.

and effective use of therapeutic alternatives. Health systems should develop a contingency planning strategy to prepare for the possibility of a prolonged drug product shortage.[19] Although it often is not possible to predict when shortages will occur, the process for dealing with them can be defined in advance. The health system should identify a point person to implement and monitor this process and establish an organizational approach to decision-making and communication. The institution should determine committee structures and responsibilities for decision-making during each phase of the process (e.g., pharmacy and therapeutics committee, medical executive committee).

Planning can be divided into three phases: identification and assessment, preparation, and contingency. Assessment requires a critical evaluation of the current situation and the potential effect of the shortage on the health system. An effective evaluation examines the reason for the shortage and estimates an end date; both internal and external supply availabilities are assessed.

The preparation phase consists of all activities that can be performed before the actual effects of the shortage are felt. Depending on the health system's inventory, when a back order or other notice is received, there is often lead-time before actual stock depletion. All patients whose treatment depends on the unavailable drug product and alternative therapies should be identified. Since many drug products have limited therapeutic alternatives, outages can have significant patient care and cost consequences. Health systems need to gauge the effect of those consequences on their institutions. Preparation should also include the development of methods for implementation and communication.

The contingency phase involves operations and circumstances for which preparation is limited because of incomplete information, financial constraints, or circumstances beyond the health system's control. For example, biological products are available only in increments and at a very high cost when no therapeutic alternatives are readily available or when shortages are longer than anticipated. Since direct control over availability is not possible, health systems must prepare for a product's unavailability.

Identification and Assessment Phase. The purchasing agent is often the person who identifies a shortage and may be the person responsible for managing drug product shortages. This person must be cognizant of aberrant fluctuations in the health system's supply chain that may indicate a potential shortage (e.g., partial orders filled, one strength difficult to obtain, most manufacturers have no more stock). If the purchasing agent is not a pharmacist, he or she must work with a designated pharmacist.

When a shortage is identified, the point person or his or her designee should conduct an assessment to evaluate its potential effect. A threat analysis using the shortage's expected duration and an assessment of the current inventory and usage patterns can be used to determine the potential consequences of the shortage.

Details and duration of shortage. Pharmacists can contact product manufacturers, distributors, FDA, CDC, and other sources to determine the reason for the shortage and its expected duration. This information may already be available on the ASHP Drug Shortage Resource Center Web site (www.ashp.org/shortages). If not, visitors to the site can report a shortage online. Predictions of when the product will be available help

determine the health system's ability to endure the shortage and guide its short- and long-term management strategies.

Although the end result is the same, the time to impact and the duration of effect vary according to the reason for the shortage and where in the supply chain problems occur—from raw materials to manufacturer, manufacturer to wholesaler, or wholesaler to health system. A lack of raw materials may affect several manufacturers of the finished drug product. A manufacturer's problems may affect only its product. Effects on distributors are dependent on their inventory levels.

Inventory on hand. Once a shortage is confirmed, the pharmacy should count the inventory on hand and estimate the time period it will cover. Available inventory includes all supplies of the drug product within the health system, including the pharmacies, inpatient units, ambulatory care clinics, automated medication storage and distribution devices, floor stock, resuscitation carts, and prepared trays.

Based on available quantities and historical usage, the pharmacy should estimate how long the health system can endure a shortage. Usage history can be obtained from procurement and issue records held by distributors, the purchasing department, and the pharmacy department. Billing and automated medication storage and dispensing device records can assist in determining actual usage within the system.

Inventory counts of all alternative drug products should be converted into common measurement units to augment estimates of use. Both current use rates and reduced rates after conservation measures are implemented should be included when assessing how long the available inventory of the shortage drug product and possible alternative products will last.

Threat to patient care and costs. A threat analysis evaluates all factors relevant to the shortage (e.g., duration, current inventory, medical necessity, alternative sources or therapies) to determine the shortage's potential effect on patient care and costs. Shortages affect safe medication practices throughout the medication distribution and administration process within a health system. When considering alternative dosage forms or therapies, pharmacists must consider changes in their procedures for look-alike and sound-alike medications, bar coding, distribution paths, and the effect on automation, contract compliance, and final product preparation.[20] The extent to which a health system will be affected by a given shortage depends on the health system's scope and level of services and its service population.

Preparation Phase. Once an imminent shortage is confirmed, the health system should take steps to prepare for known and potential problems in maintaining patient care and controlling costs.

Therapeutic alternatives. The first step in the preparation phase is to identify therapeutic alternatives to the unavailable drug product. A formal process for identifying and approving therapeutic alternatives for the health system should be established. The health system should make decisions about alternative agents in collaboration with medical, nursing, and pharmacy representatives and obtain approval of the appropriate medical committees. Therapeutic alternatives should be inventoried to ensure adequate supplies to meet new demand. In many cases, supplies of the best alternative agent may be affected by the current shortage.

Communication and patient safety. Information about the drug product shortage, alternative therapies, temporary

therapeutic guidelines, and implementation plans should be communicated to clinical staff by the most effective means available within the health system. Communication of this information is essential for ensuring patient safety and preventing medication errors caused by confusion over differences between drug products' dosages, onsets, durations, and other factors. Automated systems and order-entry systems must be updated with changes. Pharmacy department staff responsible for assisting prescribers with medication orders and aiding nursing staff with administration should be thoroughly informed about the alternative therapy decisions and implementation plans. Sustained communication is necessary to reach medical, nursing, and pharmacy staffs working varied shifts or services.

External relationships with other health systems. The preparation phase includes, when applicable, the establishment of collaborative arrangements with other institutions within a regional network or system. Available supplies of a potentially unavailable product and information about alternative therapies should be shared among the facilities. This option is limited for rural hospitals and for area hospitals served by a single wholesaler.

Patient prioritization. When a limited supply of a drug remains available and alternatives for specific patient groups are undesirable, a health system may prioritize the drug for specific patient groups. National organizations (e.g., CDC, medical organizations) may provide guidance on setting patient priorities. Medication-use evaluation data on prescribing and utilization trends, if available for the drug in question, may be useful in developing prioritization criteria to guide appropriate drug use. Such criteria are particularly helpful in dealing with long-term shortages such as with intravenous immunoglobulin. To limit product use for select patients or services in the health system, criteria should be developed by a multidisciplinary team. Communication is essential to ensure that adequate supplies are available to complete courses of therapy. Clear guidelines for prioritization must be provided to assist pharmacists in evaluating the appropriateness of medication orders.

Consultation with risk management and ethics staff members or committees may be useful when supplies are severely limited. For example, during the influenza vaccine shortage of 2004–05, many health systems did not have sufficient product to follow recommended CDC guidelines and further restricted use of the product to specific patient groups.

Stockpiling restraint. Inventory management is a challenge during a shortage. Despite pressure to do otherwise, stockpiling (hoarding) in advance of a feared shortage can occur; this can exacerbate the shortage and divert unneeded supplies away from other health systems with patients in need.[21] Health systems should refrain from stockpiling, which causes two distinct problems:

1. Stockpiling can cause artificial shortages when health systems drain the supply chain and exceed manufacturing capacities, and
2. Increased inventory is costly and may not be absorbed by normal usage if shortages do not occur as anticipated.

Speculative purchasing in response to a potential shortage has drawbacks, depending on the likely cause of the shortage and where it might occur in the supply chain. Problems may arise that pose threats to, but do not reach, end users. This happens when the supply chain, from raw material to finished product, contains several months' supply; the long lead-time allows corrections that avert a shortage.

During shortages, manufacturers and distributors often allocate a product on the basis of past usage. An initial stockpile order generally has no effect on increasing an allocation.

Contingency Phase. Health systems must establish clear guidelines for dealing with situations in which a product is available only from a compounding source or nontraditional source or when a critical drug is not available at all.

Risk management and liability. One potential complication of a shortage is litigation by patients who feel that they have received improper care or suffered unanticipated adverse drug events as a result of delays, prioritization, alternative therapy, or nontraditional drug product sources. This situation is most likely with agents for which no alternatives are available. Even though risk management and legal representatives may have participated in earlier phases of the process, they should be notified immediately when all options for obtaining either the drug product or acceptable alternatives have been exhausted.

Each health system must determine its philosophy on purchasing drugs from the gray-market or compounding pharmacies and on compounding agents inhouse. These decisions should be made before the pressure and emotion of a specific shortage occur. Each option and its potential effect on patient risk should be evaluated. Nontraditional drug product sources (e.g., secondary wholesalers) have extremely limited supplies, and the quality of these products may be questionable, as the provenance of the medication may be unknown. Compounding pharmacies may also present patient risks; several deaths have been associated with improperly sterilized compounded products.[9] Health systems may choose to compound products if they can meet the necessary guidelines; however, obtaining raw materials may be difficult in some cases.

Budget considerations. In the event that the drug product is available only from noncontracted manufacturers or through nontraditional distributors, the increased costs of using these sources should be estimated. Using alternative therapies may also increase costs. The financial implications should be presented through budget channels, with a request and justification for contingency funds. Additional expenditures caused by drug product shortages (e.g., overtime spent in locating product, extra or priority deliveries, inhouse compounding or packaging) must be documented to explain budget variances and to support future budget proposals.

Information coordination and communication. Clear communication with all affected clinicians about the status of a shortage is vital. Some health systems may designate a specific department to manage communications; others may find that a collaborative strategy involving various organizational departments and committees works best. Patients or family members should be counseled when a drug product shortage will delay or compromise care, especially when patients have been stabilized on the drug product and when alternatives may not be as effective (e.g., pain or blood pressure medications). The Joint Commission requires that prescribers potentially affected by drug product shortages be actively alerted.[10]

Strategies for Prevention

Communication with the media, national professional or patient organizations, and government agencies can raise awareness of the shortage and its potential consequences. Notifying ASHP or FDA about a drug product shortage can initiate these efforts. Drawing attention to the shortage may encourage production by other manufacturers, collaborative efforts to develop alternative therapies, and ad hoc training opportunities on the safe and effective use of alternatives.

Government Intervention

FDA is responsible for assisting with drug product shortages to the extent of its authority.[11] Its responsibilities are dispersed among several components of CDER. The extent of FDA's activities depends on whether a shortage meets "medical necessity" criteria. FDA will attempt to prevent or alleviate shortages of medically necessary products. A product is considered to be medically necessary or a medical necessity if it "is used to treat or prevent a serious disease or medical condition, and there is no other available source of that product or alternative drug that is judged by medical staff to be an adequate substitute."[12] Inconvenience to the patient and cost to the patient, institution, and manufacturer are insufficient reasons for classifying a product as a medical necessity.

A determination of medical necessity involves a risk–benefit evaluation of the compromising issue with the product versus the medical need. When FDA has determined that a shortage of a medically necessary product exists, the agency will act within its authority; actions may include discussions with pharmaceutical manufacturers to encourage additional sources, technical assistance to manufacturers experiencing cGMP difficulties, or expedited reviews of drug product marketing applications or cGMP-related improvements. FDA may take these actions whether the cause of the shortage involves business decisions to stop manufacturing the product, voluntary recalls, FDA enforcement actions, or other factors. Information on the availability of medically necessary drug products is posted on CDER's website, and information regarding the availability of blood and vaccine products regulated by FDA's Center for Biologics Evaluation and Research (CBER) is posted on CBER's website. FDA encourages consumers and health care professionals and organizations to report product shortages. Reports of drug product shortages can be made by e-mail via CDER's Drug Shortages website (www.fda.gov/cder/drug/shortages/default.htm), and reports on vaccine and blood product shortages via CBER's Biological Products Shortage website (www.fda.gov/cber/shortage/shortage.htm). FDA's shortage team will obtain information about availability and will work cooperatively with ASHP's drug product shortage team.

Conclusion

Drug product supply issues are becoming more frequent, whether they result from manufacturing difficulties or natural disasters that affect production, reductions in the supply of raw materials, voluntary recalls, manufacturer business decisions, FDA enforcement actions to ensure public safety, or stockpiling that leads to artificial shortages. Although it is impractical to prepare for every potential shortage, proper planning can minimize adverse effects on patient care and health-system costs and prevent problems from escalating into crises. The key to success will undoubtedly be found in the effectiveness of information gathering, teamwork to assess options, and communication with providers, patients, and administrators.

References

1. U.S. Pharmacopeia Center for the Advancement of Patient Safety. Section I: USP medication error analysis; drug shortages affect patient safety. www.usp.org/pdf/EN/patientSafety/capsLink2004-10-01.pdf (accessed 2008 Sep 17).
2. Institute for Safe Medication Practices. Safety briefs: drug shortage causes error. www.bfr06.com/ISMP_12_3.pdf (accessed 2009 Mar 23).
3. Schwartz MA. Prescription drugs in short supply: case histories. New York: Marcel Dekker; 1980.
4. Provisional observations on drug product shortages: effects, causes, and potential solutions. *Am J Health-Syst Pharm.* 2002; 59:2173–82.
5. Fox ER, Tyler LS. Managing drug shortages: seven years' experience at one health system. *Am J Health-Syst Pharm.* 2003; 60:245–53.
6. Baumer AM, Clark AM, Witmer DR et al. National survey of the impact of drug shortages in acute care hospitals. *Am J Health-Syst Pharm.* 2004; 61:2015–22.
7. Institute for Safe Medication Practices. National survey on drug shortages reveals high level of frustration, low regard for safety. www.ismp.org/Newsletters/acutecare/articles/20010321_2.asp (accessed 2009 Mar 23).
8. Institute for Safe Medication Practices. Recent national shortage of fentanyl products presents potential problems when substituting sufentanil. *ISMP Med Saf Alert.* 2001; 6(Feb 7):1.
9. Traynor K. Meningitis deaths linked to drug shortages. www.ashp.org/import/news/HealthSystemPharmacyNews/newsarticle.aspx?id=648 (accessed 2008 Sep 17).
10. Element of performance 7, medication management standard 2.10 (selection and procurement). In: Comprehensive accreditation manual for hospitals. Oakbrook Terrace, IL: Joint Commission; 2007:MM-7.
11. Jensen V, Kimzey LM, Goldberger MJ. FDA's role in responding to drug shortages. *Am J Health-Syst Pharm.* 2002; 59:1423–5.
12. CDER manual of policies and procedures (MAPP) 6003.1: drug shortage management. Rockville, MD: Food and Drug Administration; 2006.
13. Rubin AJ, Gosselin PG. Shortages of drugs threaten patients. http://articles.latimes.com/2001/may/06/news/mn-60196 (accessed 2009 Mar 23).
14. Szabo L. Shortages of pediatric cancer drugs are common. www.usatoday.com/news/health/2005-07-19-cancer-drugs_x.htm (accessed 2009 Mar 23).
15. Hensley S, Wysocki B. Shots in the dark. As industry profits elsewhere, U.S. lacks vaccines, antibiotics. *Wall St J.* 2005; Nov 8:A1.

16. Food and Drug Administration. Federal Food, Drug, and Cosmetic Act, Sec. 506C (21 U.S.C. 356c). Discontinuance of a life-saving product. www.fda.gov/opacom/laws/fdcact/fdcact5a3.htm#sec506c (accessed 2009 Mar 23).

17. Smith NM, Bresee JS, Shay DK et al. Prevention and control of influenza: recommendations of the Advisory Committee on Immunization Practices (ACIP). *MMWR Recomm Rep.* 2006; 55(RR-10):1–42. [Erratum, MMWR. 2006; 55:800.]

18. FluZone (influenza vaccine) package insert. Swiftwater, PA: Sanofi Pasteur; 2006.

19. Schrand LM, Troester TS, Ballas ZKet al. Preparing for drug shortages: one teaching hospital's approach to the IVIG shortage. *Formulary.* 2001; 36:52,56–9.

20. Pick AM, Massoomi F, Neff WJet al. A safety assessment tool for formulary candidates. *Am J Health-Syst Pharm.* 2006; 63:1269–72.

21. Myers CE. Artificial shortages of drug supplies. *Am J Health-Syst Pharm.* 1999; 56:727. Editorial.

Developed through the ASHP Council on Pharmacy Management and approved by the ASHP Board of Directors on January 15, 2009. These guidelines supersede the ASHP Guidelines on Managing Drug Product Shortages dated March 28, 2001.

ASHP gratefully acknowledges the expert panel that developed these guidelines: Erin R. Fox, Pharm.D.; Annette Birt, M.B.A., M.P.H.; Ken B. James, Pharm.D.; Heather Kokko, Pharm.D.; Sandra Salverson, Pharm.D., BCPS; and Donna L. Soflin, B.S.Pharm.

Erin R. Fox, Pharm.D., is Director, Drug Information Service, University of Utah Hospitals & Clinics, Salt Lake City. Annette Birt, M.B.A., M.P.H., is Pharmacy Communications Manager at Novation, Irving, TX. Ken B. James, Pharm.D., is Supervisor, Drug Information Services, Kaiser-Permanente Medical Center, Santa Clara, CA. Heather Kokko, Pharm.D., is Manager, Pharmacy Support Services, Department of Pharmacy Services, and Clinical Assistant Professor, Medical University of South Carolina. Sandra Salverson, Pharm.D., BCPS, is Drug Information/Infectious Disease Pharmacist, OSF Saint Francis Medical Center, Peoria, IL. Donna L. Soflin is Pharmacy Director, Tri-County Area Hospital, Lexington, NE.

The bibliographic citation for this document is as follows: American Society of Health-System Pharmacists. ASHP guidelines on managing drug product shortages in hospitals and health systems. *Am J Health-Syst Pharm.* 2009; 66:1399–406.

ASHP Guidelines for Selecting Pharmaceutical Manufacturers and Suppliers

Pharmacists are responsible for selecting, from hundreds of manufacturers and suppliers of drugs, those that will enable them to fulfill an important obligation: ensuring that patients receive pharmaceuticals and related supplies of the highest quality and at the lowest cost. These guidelines are offered as an aid to the pharmacist in achieving this goal.

Obligations of the Supplier

Pharmacists may purchase with confidence the products of those suppliers meeting the criteria presented here. Other factors such as credit policies, delivery times, and the breadth of a supplier's product line also must be considered when selecting a supplier.

Technical Considerations

1. On request of the pharmacist, the supplier should furnish
 a. Analytical control data.
 b. Sterility testing data.
 c. Bioavailability data.
 d. Bioequivalency data.
 e. Descriptions of testing procedures for raw materials and finished products.
 f. Any other information that may be indicative of the quality of a given finished drug product.
 Testing data developed by independent laboratories should be identified by the supplier. All information should be supplied at no charge.
2. There should be no history of recurring product recalls indicative of deficient quality control procedures.
3. The supplier should permit visits (during normal business hours) by the pharmacist to inspect its manufacturing and control procedures.
4. All drug products should conform to the requirements of *The United States Pharmacopeia—The National Formulary (USP—NF)* (the most recent edition) unless otherwise specified by the pharmacist. Items not recognized by *USP—NF* should meet the specifications set forth by the pharmacist.
5. To the extent possible, all products should be available in single unit or unit dose packages. These packages should conform to the "ASHP Technical Assistance Bulletin on Single Unit and Unit Dose Packages of Drugs."[1]
6. The name and address of the manufacturer of the final dosage form and the packager or distributor should be present on the product labeling.
7. Expiration dates should be clearly indicated on the package label and, unless stability properties warrant otherwise, should occur in January or July.
8. Therapeutic, biopharmaceutic, and toxicologic information should be available to the pharmacist on request. Toxicity information should be available around the clock.
9. Patient/staff educational materials that are important for proper use of the product should be routinely available.

10. On request, the supplier should furnish proof of any claims made with respect to the efficacy, safety, and superiority of its products.
11. On request, the supplier should furnish, at no charge, a reasonable quantity of its products to enable the pharmacist to evaluate the products' physical traits, including pharmaceutical elegance (appearance and absence of physical deterioration or flaws), packaging, and labeling.

Distribution Policies

1. Whenever possible, delivery of a drug product should be confined to a single lot number.
2. Unless otherwise specified or required by stability considerations, not less than a 12-month interval between a product's time of delivery and its expiration date should be present.
3. The supplier should accept for full credit (based on purchase price), without prior authorization, any unopened packages of goods returned within 12 months of the expiration date. Credits should be in cash or applied to the institution's account.
4. The supplier should ship all goods in a timely manner, freight prepaid, and enclose a packing list with each shipment. All items "out of stock" should be noted, and the anticipated availability of the item should be clearly indicated. There should be no extensive recurrence of back orders.
5. The supplier should warrant title to commodities supplied, warrant them to be free from defects and imperfections and fit for any rational use of the product, and indemnify and hold the purchaser harmless against any and all suits, claims, and expenses, includ-ing attorneys' fees, damages, and injuries or any claims by third parties relating to the products.

Marketing and Sales Policies

1. The supplier should not, without written consent, use the pharmacist's or his or her organization's name in any advertising or other promotional materials or activities.
2. The supplier should honor formulary decisions made by the organization's pharmacy and therapeutics committee, and the supplier's sales representatives should comply with the organization's regulations governing their activities.
3. The supplier should not offer cash, equipment, or merchandise to the organization or its staff as an inducement to purchase its products.
4. Discounts should be in cash or cash credit, not merchandise, and should be clearly indicated on invoices and bills rather than consisting of end-of-year rebates or similar discount practices.
5. In entering into a contract to supply goods, the supplier should guarantee to furnish, at the price specified, any minimum amount of products so stated. If the supplier

is unable to meet the supply commitment, the supplier should reimburse the organization for any excess costs incurred in obtaining the product from other sources. If, during the life of the contract, a price reduction occurs, the lower price should prevail.

6. All parties to the bidding process should respect the integrity of the process and the contracts awarded thereby.

Responsibilities of the Purchaser

It may be desirable to purchase drugs or other commodities on a competitive bid basis. The pharmacist should ensure that competitive bidding procedures conform to the guidelines below:

1. Invitations to bid should be mailed to the suppliers' home offices with copies to their local representatives (if any), unless suppliers specify otherwise.
2. Potential bidders should be given no less than 3 weeks to submit a bid.
3. The opening date for bids should be specified and honored by the purchaser.
4. The language of the invitation to bid should be clear and should indicate the person (and organization address and telephone number) the bidder should contact in the event of questions or problems. Specifications should be complete with respect to products, packagings, and quantities desired.
5. If bidding forms are used, they should contain adequate space for the bidder to enter the information requested.
6. The winning bidder should be notified in writing. Unsuccessful bidders may be informed of who won the award at what price, if they so request.

7. The quantities specified in the invitation to bid should be a reasonable estimate of requirements.
8. If the invitation to bid is offered on behalf of a group of purchasers, the individual members of the group should not engage in bidding procedures of their own and should purchase the goods in question from the winning bidder.

Reference

1. American Society of Hospital Pharmacists. ASHP technical assistance bulletin on single unit and unit dose packages of drugs. *Am J Hosp Pharm.* 1985; 42:378–9.

Approved by the ASHP Board of Directors, November 14, 1990. Revised by the ASHP Council on Professional Affairs. Supersedes previous versions approved November 17–*18, 1983,* and September 22, 1989.

The bibliographic citation for this document is as follows: American Society of Hospital Pharmacists. ASHP guidelines for selecting pharmaceutical manufacturers and suppliers. *Am J Hosp Pharm.* 1991; 48:523–4.

Preparation and Handling

Pharmaceutical Waste (0903)
Source: Council on Pharmacy Practice
To collaborate with regulatory bodies and appropriate organizations to develop standards for the disposal of pharmaceutical hazardous waste as defined in the Resource Conservation and Recovery Act (RCRA), for the purpose of simplifying the disposal of these substances by health systems; further,

To encourage pharmaceutical manufacturers and the Environmental Protection Agency (EPA) to provide guidance and assistance to hospitals and health systems in proper pharmaceutical waste disposal and destruction efforts; further,

To advocate that EPA update the list of hazardous substances under RCRA and establish a process for maintaining a current list; further,

To urge federal, state, and local governments to harmonize regulations regarding disposal of hazardous pharmaceutical waste; further,

To advocate that the Food and Drug Administration standardize labeling of drug products with information relating to appropriate disposal; further,

To promote awareness within hospitals and health systems of pharmaceutical waste regulations; further,

To encourage research on the environmental and public health impacts of drug products and metabolites excreted in human waste; further,

To encourage pharmaceutical manufacturers to streamline packaging of drug products to reduce waste materials.
This policy supersedes ASHP policy 0231.

Safe Disposal of Patients' Home Medications (0614)
Source: Council on Professional Affairs
To minimize the patient safety consequences and public health impact of inappropriate disposal of patients' home medications by working collaboratively with other interested organizations to (1) develop models for patient-oriented medication disposal programs that will minimize accidental poisoning, drug diversion, and potential environmental impact, (2) advocate that the pharmaceutical industry and regulatory bodies support the development and implementation of such models, and (3) educate health professionals, regulatory bodies, and the public regarding safe disposal of unused home medications.
This policy was reviewed in 2010 by the Council on Pharmacy Practice and by the Board of Directors and was found to still be appropriate.

Safe and Effective Extemporaneous Compounding (0616)
Source: Council on Professional Affairs
To affirm that extemporaneous compounding of medications, when done to meet immediate or anticipatory patient needs, is part of the practice of pharmacy and is not manufacturing; further,

To support the principle that medications should not be extemporaneously compounded when they are commercially and readily available in the form necessary to meet patient needs; further,

To encourage pharmacists who compound medications to use only drug substances that have been manufactured in Food and Drug Administration-approved facilities and that meet official United States Pharmacopeia (USP) compendial requirements where those exist; further,

To support the principle that pharmacists be adequately trained and have sufficient facilities and equipment that meet technical and professional standards to ensure the quality of compounded medications; further,

To encourage USP to develop drug monographs for commonly compounded preparations; further,

To educate prescribers and other health care professionals about the potential risks associated with the use of extemporaneously compounded preparations.
This policy was reviewed in 2010 by the Council on Pharmacy Practice and by the Board of Directors and was found to still be appropriate..

Accreditation of Compounding Facilities (0617)
Source: Council on Professional Affairs
To encourage unaccredited facilities where extemporaneous compounding of medications occurs to seek accreditation by a nationally credible accreditation body.
This policy was reviewed in 2010 by the Council on Pharmacy Practice and by the Board of Directors and was found to still be appropriate.

ASHP Guidelines on Handling Hazardous Drugs

In 1990, the American Society of Health-System Pharmacists (ASHP) published its revised technical assistance bulletin (TAB) on handling cytotoxic and hazardous drugs.[1] The information and recommendations contained in that document were current to June 1988. Continuing reports of workplace contamination and concerns for health care worker safety prompted the Occupational Safety and Health Administration (OSHA) to issue new guidelines on controlling occupational exposure to hazardous drugs in 1995.[2,3] In 2004, the National Institute for Occupational Safety and Health (NIOSH) issued the "NIOSH Alert: Preventing Occupational Exposure to Antineoplastic and Other Hazardous Drugs in Health Care Settings."[4] The following ASHP Guidelines on Handling Hazardous Drugs include information from these recommendations and are current to 2004.

Purpose

The purpose of these guidelines is to (1) update the reader on new and continuing concerns for health care workers handling hazardous drugs and (2) provide information on recommendations, including those regarding equipment, that have been developed since the publication of the previous TAB. Because studies have shown that contamination occurs in many settings, these guidelines should be implemented wherever hazardous drugs are received, stored, prepared, administered, or disposed.[2–7]

Comprehensive reviews of the literature covering anecdotal and case reports of surface contamination, worker contamination, and risk assessment are available from OSHA,[2,3] NIOSH,[4] and individual authors.[5–7] The primary goal of this document is to provide recommendations for the safe handling of hazardous drugs.

These guidelines represent the recommendations of many groups and individuals who have worked tirelessly over decades to reduce the potential harmful effects of hazardous drugs on health care workers. The research available to date, as well as the opinions of thought leaders in this area, is reflected in the guidelines. Where possible, recommendations are evidence based. In the absence of published data, professional judgment, experience, and common sense have been used.

Background

Workers may be exposed to a hazardous drug at many points during its manufacture, transport, distribution, receipt, storage, preparation, and administration, as well as during waste handling and equipment maintenance and repair. All workers involved in these activities have the potential for contact with uncontained drug.

Early concerns regarding the safety of workers handling potentially hazardous drugs focused on antineoplastic drugs when reports of second cancers in patients treated with these agents were coupled with the discovery of mutagenic substances in nurses who handled these drugs and cared for treated patients.[8,9] Exposure to these drugs in the workplace has been associated with acute and short-term reactions,

as well as long-term effects. Anecdotal and case reports in the literature range from skin-related and ocular effects to flu-like symptoms and headache.[4,5,10–17] Two controlled surveys have reported significant increases in a number of symptoms, including sore throat, chronic cough, infections, dizziness, eye irritation, and headaches, among nurses, pharmacists, and pharmacy technicians routinely exposed to hazardous drugs in the workplace.[18,19] Reproductive studies on health care workers have shown an increase in fetal abnormalities, fetal loss, and fertility impairment resulting from occupational exposure to these potent drugs.[20–23] Antineoplastic drugs and immunosuppressants are some of the types of drugs included on lists of known or suspected human carcinogens by the National Toxicology Program[24] and the International Agency for Research on Cancer.[25] Although the increased incidence of cancers for occupationally exposed groups has been investigated with varying results,[26,27] a formal risk assessment of occupationally exposed pharmacy workers by Sessink et al.[28] estimated that cyclophosphamide causes an additional 1.4–10 cases of cancer per million workers each year. This estimate, which considered workplace contamination and worker contamination and excretion in combination with animal and patient studies, was based on a conservative exposure level. Connor et al.[29] found greater surface contamination in a study of U.S. and Canadian clinical settings than had been reported in European studies conducted by Sessink and colleagues.[30–32] Ensslin et al.[33] reported an almost fivefold greater daily average excretion of cyclophosphamide in their study than that reported by Sessink. These later findings could add 7–50 additional cancer cases per year per million workers to Sessink's estimate. From these and other studies that show variations in work practices and engineering controls,[34,35] it may be assumed that such variations contribute to differences in surface and worker contamination.

Routes of Exposure. Numerous studies showed the presence of hazardous drugs in the urine of health care workers.[30–34,36–41] Hazardous drugs enter the body through inhalation, accidental injection, ingestion of contaminated foodstuffs or mouth contact with contaminated hands, and dermal absorption. While inhalation might be suspected as the primary route of exposure, air sampling studies of pharmacy and clinic environments have often demonstrated low levels of or no airborne contaminants.[30–32,40] Recent concerns about the efficacy of the sampling methods[42] and the possibility that at least one of the marker drugs may be volatile[42–45] and thus not captured on the standard sampling filter leave the matter of inhalational exposure unresolved. Surface contamination studies do, however, suggest that dermal contact and absorption may be a primary route of exposure.[31,46] While some hazardous drugs are dermally absorbed, a 1992 report showed no detectable skin absorption of doxorubicin, daunorubicin, vincristine, vinblastine, or melphalan.[47] An alternative to dermal absorption is that surface contamination transferred to hands may be ingested via the hand-to-mouth route.[48,49] One or more of these routes might be responsible for workers' exposure.

Hazard Assessment. The risk to health care personnel from handling hazardous drugs is the result of a combination of the inherent toxicity of the drugs and the extent to which workers are exposed to the drugs in the course of their daily job activities. Both hazard identification (the qualitative evaluation of the toxicity of a given drug) and an exposure assessment (the amount of worker contact with the drug) are required to complete a hazard assessment. As the hazard assessment is specific to the safety program and safety equipment in place at a work site, a formal hazard assessment may not be available for most practitioners. An alternative is a performance-based, observational approach. Observation of current work practices, equipment, and the physical layout of work areas where hazardous drugs are handled at any given site will serve as an initial assessment of appropriate and inappropriate practices.[4]

Hazardous Drugs as Sterile Preparations

Many hazardous drugs are designed for parenteral administration, requiring aseptic reconstitution or dilution to yield a final sterile preparation. As such, the compounding of these products is regulated as pharmaceutical compounding by the *United States Pharmacopeia (USP)*, chapter 797.[50] The intent of chapter 797 is to protect patients from improperly compounded sterile preparations by regulating facilities, equipment, and work practices to ensure the sterility of extemporaneously compounded sterile preparations. Chapter 797 addresses not only the sterility of a preparation but also the accuracy of its composition. Because many hazardous drugs are very potent, there is little margin for error in compounding.

The initial version of chapter 797, released in early 2004, provided only minimal guidance for the handling of hazardous drugs, limiting this issue to a short discussion of chemotoxic agents in the document's section on aseptic technique. The chapter referred to standards established by the International Organization for Standardization (ISO)[51] that address the acceptable air quality (as measured by particulate counts) in the critical environment but failed to discuss airflow, air exchanges per hour, or pressure gradients of the ISO standards for cleanrooms and associated environments for compounding sterile products. The chapter did not describe the containment procedures necessary for compounding sterile hazardous agents, leaving it to the practitioner to simultaneously comply with the need to maintain a critical environment for compounded sterile products for patient safety while ensuring a contained environment for worker safety. The use of positive-pressure isolators for compounding hazardous drugs or placement of a Class II biological-safety cabinet (BSC) for use with hazardous drugs in a positive-pressure environment may result in airborne contamination of adjacent areas. Engineering assessment of designs of areas where this may occur should be done to address concerns of contaminant dissemination. Because hazardous drugs are also compounded in areas adjacent to patients and their family members (e.g., in chemotherapy infusion centers), inappropriate environmental containment puts them, as well as health care workers, at risk. Because *USP* review is a dynamic and ongoing process, future revisions are likely to address these concerns. Practitioners are encouraged to monitor the process and participate when appropriate.

Definition of Hazardous Drugs

The federal hazard communication standard (HCS) defines a hazardous chemical as any chemical that is a physical or health hazard.[52,53] A health hazard is defined as a chemical for which there is statistically significant evidence, based on at least one study conducted in accordance with established scientific principles, that acute or chronic health effects may occur in exposed employees. The HCS further notes that the term *health hazard* includes chemicals that are carcinogens, toxic or highly toxic agents, reproductive toxins, irritants, corrosives, sensitizers, and agents that produce target organ effects.

A 1990 ASHP TAB proposed criteria to determine which drugs should be considered hazardous and handled within an established safety program.[1] OSHA adopted these criteria in its 1995 guidelines, which were posted on its Web site in 1999.[2,3] The TAB's definition of hazardous drugs was revised by the NIOSH Working Group on Hazardous Drugs for the 2004 alert.[4] These definitions are compared in Table 1.

Each facility should create its own list of hazardous drugs based on specific criteria. Appendix A of the NIOSH alert contains related guidance and a sample list.[4] When drugs are purchased for the first time, they must be evaluated to determine whether they should be included in the facility's list of hazardous drugs. As the use and number of hazardous drugs increase, so too do the opportunities for health care worker exposure. Investigational drugs must be evaluated according to the information provided to the principal investigator. If the information provided is deemed insufficient to make an informed decision, the investigational drug should be considered hazardous until more information is available.

Recommendations

Safety Program. Policies and procedures for the safe handling of hazardous drugs must be in place for all situations in which these drugs are used throughout a facility. A comprehensive safety program must be developed that deals with all aspects of the safe handling of hazardous drugs. This program must be a collaborative effort, with input from all affected departments, such as pharmacy, nursing, medical staff, housekeeping, transportation, maintenance, employee health, risk management, industrial hygiene, clinical laboratories, and safety. A key element of this safety program is the Material Safety Data Sheet (MSDS) mandated by the HCS.[52,53] Employers are required to have an MSDS available for all hazardous agents in the workplace. A comprehensive safety program must include a process for monitoring and updating the MSDS database. When a hazardous drug is purchased for the first time, an MSDS must be received from the manufacturer or distributor. The MSDS should define the appropriate handling precautions, including protective equipment, controls, and spill management associated with the drug. Many MSDSs are available online through the specific manufacturer or through safety-information services.

Drugs that have been identified as requiring safe handling precautions should be clearly labeled at all times during their transport and use. The HCS applies to all workers, including those handling hazardous drugs at the manufac-

Table 1.

Comparison of 2004 NIOSH and 1990 ASHP Definitions of Hazardous Drugs[a]

NIOSH[4]	ASHP[1]
Carcinogenicity	Carcinogenicity in animal models, in the patient population, or both as reported by the International Agency for Research on Cancer
Teratogenicity or developmental toxicity[b]	Teratogenicity in animal studies or in treated patients
Reproductive toxicity[b]	Fertility impairment in animal studies or in treated patients
Organ toxicity at low doses[b]	Evidence of serious organ or other toxicity at low doses in animal models or treated patients
Genotoxicity[c]	Genotoxicity (i.e., mutagenicity and clastogenicity in short-term test systems)
Structure and toxicity profile of new drugs that mimic existing drugs determined hazardous by the above criteria	

[a]NIOSH = National Institute for Occupational Safety and Health, ASHP = American Society of Health-System Pharmacists.

[b]NIOSH's definition contains the following explanation: "All drugs have toxic side effects, but some exhibit toxicity at low doses. The level of toxicity reflects a continuum from relatively nontoxic to production of toxic effects in patients at low doses (for example, a few milligrams or less). For example, a daily therapeutic dose of 10 mg/day or a dose of 1 mg/kg/day in laboratory animals that produces serious organ toxicity, developmental toxicity, or reproductive toxicity has been used by the pharmaceutical industry to develop occupational exposure limits (OELs) of less than 10 micrograms/meter3 after applying appropriate uncertainty factors. OELs in this range are typically established for potent or toxic drugs in the pharmaceutical industry. Under all circumstances, an evaluation of all available data should be conducted to protect health care workers."

[c]NIOSH's definition contains the following explanation: "In evaluating mutagenicity for potentially hazardous drugs, responses from multiple test systems are needed before precautions can be required for handling such agents. The EPA evaluations include the type of cells affected and *in vitro* versus *in vivo* testing."

turer and distributor levels. Employers are required to establish controls to ensure worker safety in all aspects of the distribution of these drugs.

The outside of the vials of many commercial drugs are contaminated by the time they are received in the pharmacy.[30,54,55] Although the possibility has not been studied, the contamination may extend to the inside of the packing cartons and onto the package inserts placed around the vial within the carton. Such contamination would present an exposure risk to anyone opening drug cartons or handling the vials, including workers receiving open or broken shipping cartons or selecting vials to be repackaged at a distribution point (e.g., a worker at the drug wholesaler selecting hazardous drugs for shipping containers or a pharmacy worker dividing a hazardous drug in a multidose container for repackaging into single-dose containers). These activities may present risks, especially for workers who too often receive inadequate safety training. Housekeepers and patient care assistants who handle drug waste and patient waste are also at risk and are not always included in the safe handling training required by safety programs. Safety programs must identify and include all workers who may be at risk of exposure.

The packaging (cartons, vials, ampuls) of hazardous drugs should be properly labeled by the manufacturer or distributor with a distinctive identifier that notifies personnel receiving them to wear appropriate personal protective equipment (PPE) during their handling. Sealing these drugs in plastic bags at the distributor level provides an additional level of safety for workers who are required to

unpack cartons. Visual examination of such cartons for outward signs of damage or breakage is an important first step in the receiving process. Policies and procedures must be in place for handling damaged cartons or containers of hazardous drugs (e.g., returning the damaged goods to the distributor using appropriate containment techniques). These procedures should include the use of PPE, which must be supplied by the employer. As there may be no ventilation protection in the area where damaged containers are handled, the use of complete PPE, including an NIOSH-certified respirator, is recommended.[56,57] As required by OSHA, a complete respiratory program, including proper training and fit testing, must be completed by all staff required to use respirators.[56] Surgical masks do not provide adequate protection from the harmful effects of these drugs.

Labeling and Packaging from Point of Receipt. Drug packages, bins, shelves, and storage areas for hazardous drugs must bear distinctive labels identifying those drugs as requiring special handling. Segregation of hazardous drug inventory from other drug inventory improves control and reduces the number of staff members potentially exposed to the danger. Hazardous drugs should be stored in an area with sufficient general exhaust ventilation to dilute and remove any airborne contaminants.[4] Hazardous drugs placed in inventory must be protected from potential breakage by storage in bins that have high fronts and on shelves that have guards to prevent accidental falling. The bins must also be appropriately sized to properly contain all stock. Care should be taken to separate hazardous drug inventory to reduce potential drug errors (e.g., pulling a look-alike vial from an adjacent drug bin). Because studies have shown that contamination on the drug vial itself is a consideration,[30,54,55] all staff members must wear double gloves when stocking and inventorying these drugs and selecting hazardous drug packages for further handling. All transport of hazardous drug packages must be done in a manner to reduce environmental contamination in the event of accidental dropping. Hazardous drug packages must be placed in sealed containers and labeled with a unique identifier. Carts or other transport devices must be designed with guards to protect against falling and breakage. All individuals transporting hazardous drugs must have safety training that includes spill control and have spill kits immediately accessible. Staff handling hazardous drugs or cleaning areas where hazardous drugs are stored or handled must be trained to recognize the unique identifying labels used to distinguish these drugs and areas. Warning labels and signs must be clear to non-English readers. All personnel

who work with or around hazardous drugs must be trained to appropriately perform their jobs using the established precautions and required PPE.[52]

Environment. Hazardous drugs should be compounded in a controlled area where access is limited to authorized personnel trained in handling requirements. Due to the hazardous nature of these preparations, a contained environment where air pressure is negative to the surrounding areas or that is protected by an airlock or anteroom is preferred. Positive-pressure environments for hazardous drug compounding should be avoided or augmented with an appropriately designed antechamber because of the potential spread of airborne contamination from contaminated packaging, poor handling technique, and spills.

Only individuals trained in the administration of hazardous drugs should do so. During administration, access to the administration area should be limited to patients receiving therapy and essential personnel. Eating, drinking, applying makeup, and the presence of foodstuffs should be avoided in patient care areas while hazardous drugs are administered. For inpatient therapy, where lengthy administration techniques may be required, hanging or removing hazardous drugs should be scheduled to reduce exposure of family members and ancillary staff and to avoid the potential contamination of dietary trays and personnel.

Because much of the compounding and administration of hazardous drugs throughout the United States is done in outpatient or clinic settings with patients and their family members near the compounding area, care must be taken to minimize environmental contamination and to maximize the effectiveness of cleaning (decontamination) activities. The design of such areas must include surfaces that are readily cleaned and decontaminated. Upholstered and carpeted surfaces should be avoided, as they are not readily cleaned. Several studies have shown floor contamination and the ineffectiveness of cleaning practices on both floors and surfaces.[29,30,46] Break rooms and refreshment areas for staff, patients, and others should be located away from areas of potential contamination to reduce unnecessary exposure to staff, visitors, and others.

Hazardous drugs may also be administered in nontraditional locations, such as the operating room, which present challenges to training and containment. Intracavitary administration of hazardous drugs (e.g., into the bladder, peritoneal cavity, or chest cavity) frequently requires equipment for which locking connections may not be readily available or even possible. All staff members who handle hazardous drugs should receive safety training that includes recognition of hazardous drugs and appropriate spill response. Hazardous drug spill kits, containment bags, and disposal containers must be available in all areas where hazardous drugs are handled. Techniques and ancillary devices that minimize the risk of open systems should be used when administering hazardous drugs through unusual routes or in nontraditional locations.

Ventilation Controls. Ventilation or engineering controls are devices designed to eliminate or reduce worker exposure to chemical, biological, radiological, ergonomic, and physical hazards. Ventilated cabinets are a type of ventilation or engineering control designed for the purpose of worker pro-

tection.[4] These devices minimize worker exposure by controlling the emission of airborne contaminants. Depending on the design, ventilated cabinets may also be used to provide the critical environment necessary to compound sterile preparations. When asepsis is not required, a Class I BSC or a containment isolator may be used to handle hazardous drugs. When sterile hazardous drugs are being compounded, a Class II or III BSC or an isolator intended for aseptic preparation and containment is required.[4] Recommendations for work practices specific to BSCs and isolators are discussed later in these guidelines.

Class II BSCs. In the early 1980s, the Class II BSC was determined to reduce the exposure of pharmacy compounding staff to hazardous preparations, as measured by the mutational response to the Ames test by urine of exposed subjects.[58,59] Studies in the 1990s, using analytical methods significantly more specific and sensitive than the Ames test, indicated that environmental and worker contamination occurs in workplace settings despite the use of controls recommended in published guidelines, including the use of Class II BSCs.[29–35,37–41,60,61] The exact cause of contamination has yet to be determined. Studies have shown that (1) there is contamination on the outside of vials received from manufacturers and distributors,[30,54,55] (2) work practices required to maximize the effectiveness of the Class II BSC are neglected or not taught,[32,46] and (3) the potential vaporization of hazardous drug solutions may reduce the effectiveness of the high-efficiency particulate air (HEPA) filter in providing containment.[42–45] Studies of surface contamination have discovered deposits of hazardous drugs on the floor in front of the Class II BSC, indicating that drug may have escaped through the open front of the BSC onto contaminated gloves or the final product or into the air.[29–32]

Workers must understand that the Class II BSC does not prevent the generation of contamination within the cabinet and that the effectiveness of such cabinets in containing hazardous drug contamination depends on operators' use of proper technique.

Some Class II BSCs recirculate airflow within the cabinet or exhaust contaminated air back into the work environment through HEPA filters.[62] The Class II BSC is designed with air plenums that are unreachable for surface decontamination; the plenum under the work tray collects room dirt and debris that mix with hazardous drug residue when the BSC is operational.[1] Drafts, supply-air louvers, and other laminar flow equipment placed near the BSC can interfere with the containment properties of the inflow air barrier, resulting in contamination of the work environment.[63] More information on the design and use of Class II BSCs is available from the NSF International (NSF)/American National Standards Institute (ANSI) standard 49-04.[62] Recommendations for use of Class II BSCs are listed in Appendix A.

Alternatives to Class II BSCs. Alternatives to the open-front Class II BSC include the Class III BSC, glove boxes, and isolators. By definition, a Class III BSC is a totally enclosed, ventilated cabinet of leak-tight construction.[64] Operations in the cabinet are conducted through fixed-glove access. The cabinet is maintained under negative air pressure. Supply air is drawn into the cabinet through HEPA filters. The exhaust air is treated by double HEPA filtration or by HEPA filtration and incineration. The Class III BSC is designed for use with highly toxic or infectious material. Because of the costs of

purchasing and operating a Class III BSC, it is seldom used for extemporaneous compounding of sterile products.

Less rigorous equipment with similar fixed-glove access include glove boxes and isolators. Although standardized definitions and criteria exist for glove boxes, these guidelines currently focus on applications in the nuclear industry and not on compounding hazardous drugs.[65] There are no standardized definitions or criteria for pharmaceutical compounding applications for this equipment and no performance standards determined by an independent organization to aid the purchaser in the selection process. NIOSH recommends that only ventilated engineering controls be used to compound hazardous drugs and that these controls be designed for containment.[4] NIOSH defines these controls and details their use and selection criteria as well as recommendations for airflow, exhaust, and maintenance. NIOSH further differentiates between ventilated engineering controls used for hazard containment that are intended for use with sterile products (aseptic containment) and those for use with nonsterile handling of hazardous drugs.[4]

An isolator may be considered a ventilated controlled environment that has fixed walls, floor, and ceiling. For aseptic use, supply air must be drawn through a high-efficiency (minimum HEPA) filter. Exhaust air must also be high-efficiency filtered and should be exhausted to the outside of the facility, not to the workroom. Workers access the isolator's work area, or main chamber, through gloves, sleeves, and air locks or pass-throughs. Currently available isolators have either unidirectional or turbulent airflow within the main chamber. For compounding sterile preparations, the filtered air and airflow must achieve an ISO class 5 (former FS-209E class 100) environment within the isolator.[50,51,66,67] Isolators for sterile compounding have become increasingly popular as a way to minimize the challenges of a traditional cleanroom and some of the disadvantages of the Class II BSC.[50,68–70] The totally enclosed design may reduce the escape of contamination during the compounding process. The isolator may be less sensitive to drafts and other laminar-airflow equipment, including positive-pressure environments. Issues unique to isolators include pressure changes when accessing the fixed-glove assembly, pressure changes in the main chamber when accessing the antechamber or pass-through, positive- versus negative-pressure isolators used to compound hazardous drugs, and ergonomic considerations associated with a fixed-glove assembly. Many isolators produce less heat and noise than Class II BSCs.[68] The Controlled Environment Testing Association has developed an applications guide for isolators in health care facilities.[71]

Isolators, like Class II BSCs, do not prevent the generation of contamination within the cabinet workspace, and their effectiveness in containing contamination depends on proper technique.[72] The potential for the spread of hazardous drug contamination from the pass-through and main chamber of the isolator to the workroom may be reduced by surface decontamination, but no wipe-down procedures have been studied. Surface decontamination may be more readily conducted in isolators than in Class II BSCs. (See *Decontamination, deactivation, and cleaning* for more information.)

Recirculating isolators depend on high-efficiency (HEPA or ultra-low penetrating air [ULPA]) filters. These filters may not sufficiently remove volatile hazardous drug contamination from the airflow. Isolators that discharge air into the workroom, even through high-efficiency filters,

present exposure concerns similar to those of unvented Class II BSCs if there is a possibility that the hazardous drugs handled in them may vaporize. Isolators used for compounding hazardous drugs should be at negative pressure or use a pressurized air lock to the surrounding areas to improve containment. Some isolators rely on a low-particulate environment rather than laminar-airflow technology to protect the sterility of the preparations. Recommendations for use of Class III BSCs and isolators are summarized in Appendix B.

Closed-system drug-transfer devices. Closed-system drug-transfer devices mechanically prevent the transfer of environmental contaminants into the system and the escape of drug or vapor out of the system.[4] ADD-Vantage and Duplex devices are closed-system drug-transfer devices currently available for injectable antibiotics. A similar system that may offer increased environmental protection for hazardous drugs is a proprietary, closed-system drug-transfer device known as PhaSeal. This multicomponent system uses a double membrane to enclose a specially cut injection cannula as it moves into a drug vial, Luer-Lok, or infusion-set connector.

Several studies have shown a reduction in environmental contamination with marker hazardous drugs during both compounding and administration when comparing standard techniques for handling hazardous drugs with the use of PhaSeal.[73–78] It should be noted, however, that PhaSeal components cannot be used to compound all hazardous drugs.

In 1984, Hoy and Stump[79] concluded that a commercial air-venting device reduced the release of drug aerosols during reconstitution of drugs packaged in vials. The testing was limited to visual analysis. The venting device does not lock onto the vial, which allows it to be transferred from one vial to another. This practice creates an opportunity for both environmental and product contamination. Many devices labeled as "chemo adjuncts" are currently available. Many feature a filtered, vented spike to facilitate reconstituting and removing hazardous drugs during the compounding process. However, none of these devices may be considered a closed-system drug-transfer device, and none has been formally studied with the results published in peer-reviewed journals. As other products become available, they should meet the definition of closed-system drug-transfer devices established by NIOSH[4] and should be required to demonstrate their effectiveness in independent studies. Closed-system drug-transfer devices (or any other ancillary devices) are not a substitute for using a ventilated cabinet.

Personal Protective Equipment. *Gloves.* Gloves are essential for handling hazardous drugs. Gloves must be worn at all times when handling drug packaging, cartons, and vials, including while performing inventory control procedures and when gathering hazardous drugs and supplies for compounding a batch or single dose. During compounding in a Class II BSC, gloves and gowns are required to prevent skin surfaces from coming into contact with these agents. Studies of gloves indicate that many latex and nonlatex materials are effective protection against penetration and permeation by most hazardous drugs.[80–84] Recent concerns about latex sensitivity have prompted testing of newer glove materials. Gloves made of nitrile or neoprene rubber and polyurethane have been successfully tested using a battery of antineoplastic drugs.[82–84] The American Society for Testing and Materials (ASTM) has developed testing standards for assessing the

resistance of medical gloves to permeation by chemotherapy drugs.[85] Gloves that meet this standard earn the designation of "chemotherapy gloves." Gloves selected for use with hazardous drugs should meet this ASTM standard.

Connor and Xiang[86] studied the effect of isopropyl alcohol on the permeability of latex and nitrile gloves exposed to antineoplastic agents. During the limited study period of 30 minutes, they found that the use of isopropyl alcohol during cleaning and decontaminating did not appear to affect the integrity of either material when challenged with six antineoplastic agents.

In most glove-testing systems, the glove material remains static, in contrast to the stressing and flexing that occur during actual use. In one study designed to examine glove permeability under static and flexed conditions, no significant difference in permeation was reported, except in thin latex examination gloves.[87] Another study, however, detected permeation of antineoplastic drugs through latex gloves during actual working conditions by using a cotton glove under the latex glove.[88] The breakthrough time for cyclophosphamide was only 10 minutes. The authors speculated that the cotton glove may have acted as a wick, drawing the hazardous drug through the outer glove. Nonetheless, under actual working conditions, double gloving and wearing gloves no longer than 30 minutes are prudent practices.

Permeability of gloves to hazardous drugs has been shown to be dependent on the drug, glove material and thickness, and exposure time. Powder-free gloves are preferred because powder particulates can contaminate the sterile processing area and absorb hazardous drug contaminants, which may increase the potential for dermal contact. Hands should be thoroughly washed before donning gloves and after removing them. Care must be taken when removing gloves in order to prevent the spreading of hazardous drug contaminants.

Several studies have indicated that contamination of the outside of gloves with hazardous drug is common after compounding and that this contamination may be spread to other surfaces during the compounding process.[30–33,39] Studies have also shown that hazardous drug contamination may lead to dermal absorption by workers not actively involved in the compounding and administration of hazardous drugs.[30,88] The use of two pairs of gloves is recommended when compounding these drugs. In an isolator, one additional pair of gloves must be worn within the fixed-glove assembly.[68]

Once compounding has been completed and the final preparation surface decontaminated, the outer glove should be removed and contained inside the BSC. The inner glove is worn to affix labels and place the preparation into a sealable containment bag for transport. This must be done within the BSC. In the isolator, the fixed gloves must be surface cleaned before wiping down the final preparation, placing the label onto the preparation, and placing it into the pass-through. The inner gloves should be worn to complete labeling and to place the final preparation into a transport bag in the pass-through. The inner gloves may then be removed and contained in a sealable bag within the pass-through. If the final check is conducted by a second staff member, fresh gloves must be donned before handling the completed preparation.

During batch compounding, gloves should be changed at least every 30 minutes. Gloves (at least the outer gloves) must be changed whenever it is necessary to exit and re-enter

the BSC. For aseptic protection of sterile preparations, the outer gloves must be sanitized with an appropriate disinfectant when reentering the BSC. Gloves must also be changed immediately if torn, punctured, or knowingly contaminated. When wearing two pairs of gloves in the BSC, one pair is worn under the gown cuff and the second pair placed over the cuff. When removing the gloves, the contaminated glove fingers must only touch the outer surface of the glove, never the inner surface. If the inner glove becomes contaminated, then both pairs of gloves must be changed. When removing any PPE, care must be taken to avoid introducing hazardous drug contamination into the environment. Both the inner and outer gloves should be considered contaminated, and glove surfaces must never touch the skin or any surface that may be touched by the unprotected skin of others. Gloves used to handle hazardous drugs should be placed in a sealable plastic bag for containment within the BSC or isolator pass-through before disposal as contaminated waste.

If an i.v. set is attached to the final preparation in the BSC or isolator, care must be taken to avoid contaminating the tubing with hazardous drug from the surface of the gloves, BSC, or isolator.

Class III BSCs and isolators are equipped with attached gloves or gauntlets. They should be considered contaminated once the BSC or isolator has been used for compounding hazardous drugs. For compounding sterile preparations, attached gloves or gauntlets must be routinely sanitized per the manufacturer's instructions to prevent microbial contamination. Hazardous drug contamination from the gloves or gauntlets may be transferred to the surfaces of all items within the cabinet. Glove and gauntlet surfaces must be cleaned after compounding is complete. All final preparations must be surface decontaminated by staff, wearing clean gloves to avoid spreading contamination.[68] Recommendations for use of gloves are summarized in Appendix C.

Gowns. Gowns or coveralls are worn during the compounding of sterile preparations to protect the preparation from the worker, to protect the worker from the preparation, or both. The selection of gowning materials depends on the goal of the process. Personal protective gowns are recommended during the handling of hazardous drug preparations to protect the worker from inadvertent exposure to extraneous drug particles on surfaces or generated during the compounding process.

Guidelines for the safe handling of hazardous drugs recommend the use of gowns for compounding in the BSC, administration, spill control, and waste management to protect the worker from contamination by fugitive drug generated during the handling process.[1–4,89,90] Early recommendations for barrier protective gowns required that they be disposable and made of a lint-free, low-permeability fabric with a closed front, long sleeves, and tight-fitting elastic or knit cuffs.[1] Washable garments (e.g., laboratory coats, scrubs, and cloth gowns) absorb fluids and provide no barrier against hazardous drug absorption and permeation. Studies into the effectiveness of disposable gowns in resisting permeation by hazardous drugs found variation in the protection provided by commercially available materials. In an evaluation of polypropylene-based gowns, Connor[91] found that polypropylene spun-bond nonwoven material alone and polypropylene–polyethylene copolymer spun-bond provided little protection against permeation by a battery of aqueous-

and nonaqueous- based hazardous drugs. Various constructions of polypropylene (e.g., spun-bond/melt-blown/spun-bond) result in materials that are completely impermeable or only slightly permeable to hazardous drugs. Connor[91] noted that these coated materials are similar in appearance to several other nonwoven materials but perform differently and that workers could expect to be protected from exposure for up to four hours when using the coated gowning materials. Harrison and Kloos[92] reported similar findings in a study of six disposable gowning materials and 15 hazardous drugs. Only gowns with polyethylene or vinyl coatings provided adequate splash protection and prevented drug permeation. In a subjective assessment of worker comfort, the more protective gowns were found to be warmer and thus less comfortable. These findings agree with an earlier study that found that the most protective gowning materials were the most uncomfortable to wear.[93] Resistance to the use of gowns, especially by nurses during administration of hazardous drugs, has been reported.[94] The lack of comfort could cause resistance to behavioral change.

Researchers have looked at gown contamination with fluorescent scans, high-performance liquid chromatography, and tandem mass spectrometry.[39,95] In one study, researchers scanned nurses and pharmacists wearing gowns during the compounding and administration of hazardous drugs.[95] Of a total of 18 contamination spots detected, 5 were present on the gowns of nurses after drug administration. No spots were discovered on the gowns of pharmacists after compounding. In contrast, researchers using a more sensitive assay placed pads in various body locations, both over and under the gowns used by the subjects during compounding and administration of cyclophosphamide and ifosfamide.[39] Workers wore short-sleeved nursing uniforms, disposable or cotton gowns, and vinyl or latex gloves. More contamination was found during compounding than administration. Contamination found on the pads placed on the arms of preparers is consistent with the design and typical work practices used in a Class II BSC, where the hands and arms are extended into the contaminated work area of the cabinet. Remarkably, one preparer had contamination on the back of the gown, possibly indicating touch contamination with the Class II BSC during removal of the final product. While early guidelines do not contain a maximum length of time that a gown should be worn, Connor's[91] work would support a two- to three-hour window for a coated gown. Contamination of gowns during glove changes must be a consideration. If the inner pair of gloves requires changing, a gown change should be considered. Gowns worn as barrier protection in the compounding of hazardous drugs must never be worn outside the immediate preparation area. Gowns worn during administration should be changed when leaving the patient care area and immediately if contaminated. Gowns should be removed carefully and properly disposed of as contaminated waste to avoid becoming a source of contamination to other staff and the environment.

Hazardous drug compounding in an enclosed environment, such as a Class III BSC or an isolator, may not require the operator to wear a gown. However, because the process of handling drug vials and final preparations, as well as accessing the isolator's pass-throughs, may present an opportunity for contamination, the donning of a gown is prudent. Coated gowns may not be necessary for this use if appropri-

ate gowning practices are established. Recommendations for use of gowns are summarized in Appendix D.

Additional PPE. Eye and face protection should be used whenever there is a possibility of exposure from splashing or uncontrolled aerosolization of hazardous drugs (e.g., when containing a spill or handling a damaged shipping carton). In these instances, a face shield, rather than safety glasses or goggles, is recommended because of the improved skin protection afforded by the shield.

Similar circumstances also warrant the use of a respirator. All workers who may use a respirator must be fit-tested and trained to use the appropriate respirator according to the OSHA Respiratory Protection Standard.[56,57] A respirator of correct size and appropriate to the aerosol size, physical state (i.e., particulate or vapor), and concentration of the airborne drug must be available at all times. Surgical masks do not provide respiratory protection. Shoe and hair coverings should be worn during the sterile compounding process to minimize particulate contamination of the critical work zone and the preparation.[50] With the potential for hazardous drug contamination on the floor in the compounding and administration areas, shoe coverings are recommended as contamination-control mechanisms. Shoe coverings must be removed with gloved hands when leaving the compounding area. Gloves should be worn and care must be taken when removing hair or shoe coverings to prevent contamination from spreading to clean areas. Hair and shoe coverings used in the hazardous drug handling areas must be contained, along with used gloves, and discarded as contaminated waste.

Work Practices. *Compounding sterile hazardous drugs.* Work practices for the compounding of sterile hazardous drugs differ somewhat with the use of a Class II BSC, a Class III BSC, or an isolator. Good organizational skills are essential to minimize contamination and maximize productivity. All activities not requiring a critical environment (e.g., checking labels, doing calculations) should be completed before accessing the BSC or isolator. All items needed for compounding must be gathered before beginning work. This practice should eliminate the need to exit the BSC or isolator once compounding has begun. Two pairs of gloves should be worn to gather hazardous drug vials and supplies. These gloves should be carefully removed and discarded. Fresh gloves must be donned and appropriately sanitized before aseptic manipulation.

Only supplies and drugs essential to compounding the dose or batch should be placed in the work area of the BSC or main chamber of the isolator. BSCs and isolators should not be overcrowded to avoid unnecessary hazardous drug contamination. Luer-Lok syringes and connections must be used whenever possible for manipulating hazardous drugs, as they are less likely to separate during compounding.

Spiking an i.v. set into a solution containing hazardous drugs or priming an i.v. set with hazardous drug solution in an uncontrolled environment must be avoided. One recommendation is to attach and prime the appropriate i.v. set to the final container in the BSC or isolator before adding the hazardous drug. Closed-system drug-transfer devices should achieve a dry connection between the administration set and the hazardous drug's final container. This connection allows the container to be spiked with a secondary i.v. set and the set to be primed by backflow from a primary nonhazardous solution. This process may be done outside the BSC or isolator, reducing the potential for surface contamination of the

i.v. set during the compounding process. A new i.v. set must be used with each dose of hazardous drug. Once attached, the i.v. set must never be removed from a hazardous drug dose, thereby preventing the residual fluid in the bag, bottle, or tubing from leaking and contaminating personnel and the environment.

Transport bags must never be placed in the BSC or in the isolator work chamber during compounding to avoid inadvertent contamination of the outer surface of the bag. Final preparations must be surface decontaminated after compounding is complete. In either the BSC or isolator, clean inner gloves must be worn when labeling and placing the final preparation into the transport bag. Handling final preparations and transport bags with gloves contaminated with hazardous drugs will result in the transfer of the contamination to other workers. Don fresh gloves whenever there is a doubt as to the cleanliness of the inner or outer gloves.

Working in BSCs or isolators. With or without ancillary devices, none of the available ventilation or engineering controls can provide 100% protection for the worker. Workers must recognize the limitations of the equipment and address them through appropriate work practices.[1] The effectiveness of Class II BSCs and isolators in containing contamination depends on proper technique.[72] Hazardous drug contamination from the work area of the isolator may be brought into the workroom environment through the pass-throughs or air locks and on the surfaces of items removed from the isolators (e.g., the final preparation). Surface decontamination of the preparation before removal from the isolator's main chamber should reduce the hazardous drug contamination that could be transferred to the workroom, but no wipe-down procedures have been studied. Surface decontamination may be accomplished using alcohol, sterile water, peroxide, or sodium hypochlorite solutions, provided the packaging is not permeable to the solution and the labels remain legible and intact. Recommendations for working in BSCs and isolators are summarized in Appendix E.

BSCs. Class II BSCs use vertical-flow, HEPA-filtered air (ISO class 5) as their controlled aseptic environment. Before beginning an operation in a Class II BSC, personnel should wash their hands, don an inner pair of appropriate gloves, and then don a coated gown followed by a second pair of gloves. The work surface should be cleaned of surface contamination with detergent, sodium hypochlorite, and neutralizer or disinfected with alcohol, depending on when it was last cleaned. For the Class II BSC, the front shield must be lowered to the proper level to protect the face and eyes. The operator should be seated so that his or her shoulders are at the level of the bottom of the front shield. All drugs and supplies needed to aseptically compound a dose or batch should be gathered and sanitized with 70% alcohol or appropriate disinfectant. Avoid exiting and reentering the work area. Being careful not to place any sterile objects below them, i.v. bags and bottles may be hung from the bar. All items must be placed well within the Class II BSC, away from the unfiltered air at the front barrier. By design, the intended work zone within the Class II BSC is the area between the front and rear air grilles. The containment characteristics of the Class II BSC are dependent on the airflow through both the front and back grilles; these grilles should never be obstructed. Due to the design of the Class II BSC, the quality of HEPA-filtered air is lowest at the sides of the

work zone, so manipulations should be performed at least six inches away from each sidewall in the horizontal plane. A small waste–sharps container may be placed along the sidewall toward the back of the BSC. One study has suggested that a plastic-backed absorbent preparation pad in a Class II BSC may interfere with airflow,[39] but another study determined that use of a flat firm pad that did not block the grilles of the cabinet had no effect on airflow.[96] The use of a large pad that might block the front or rear grilles must be avoided. In addition, because a pad may absorb small spills, it may become a source of hazardous drug contamination for anything placed upon it. Preparation pads are not readily decontaminated and must be replaced and discarded after preparation of each batch and frequently during extended batch compounding. More information on the design and use of Class II BSCs is available from the NSF/ANSI standard 49-04.[62]

Isolators. For work in an isolator, all drugs and supplies needed to aseptically compound a dose or batch should be gathered and sanitized with 70% alcohol or appropriate disinfectant and readied for placement in the pass-through. A technique described in the literature involves the use of a tray that will fit into the pass-through.[97] A large primary sealable bag is placed over the tray. Labels and a second sealable (transport) bag, which is used to contain the final preparation, are placed into the primary sealable bag on the tray surface. Vials, syringes, needles, and other disposables are placed on top of the sealed bag. The enclosed tray is then taken into the main chamber of the isolator, where the drug and supplies are used to compound the dose. The contaminated materials, including the primary sealable bag, are removed using the closed trash system of the isolator, if so equipped, or sealed into a second bag and removed via the pass-through for disposal as contaminated waste. The dose is then labeled and placed into the second sealable bag for transport.

This technique does not address contamination on the isolator gloves or gauntlets. Additional work practices may include cleaning off the gloves or gauntlets and final preparation after initial compounding and before handling the label and second sealable bag. Care must be taken when transferring products out of the pass-through and disposing of waste through the pass-through or trash chute to avoid accidental contamination.

Aseptic technique. Stringent aseptic technique, described by Wilson and Solimando[98] in 1981, remains the foundation of any procedure involving the use of needles and syringes in manipulating sterile dosage forms. This technique, when performed in conjunction with negative pressure technique, minimizes the escape of drug from vials and ampuls. Needleless devices have been developed to reduce the risk of blood-borne pathogen exposure through needle sticks. None of these devices has been tested for reduction of hazardous drug contamination. The appropriateness of these devices in the safe handling of hazardous drugs has not been determined.

In reconstituting hazardous drugs in vials, it is critical to avoid pressurizing the contents of the vial. Pressurization may cause the drug to spray out around the needle or through a needle hole or a loose seal, aerosolizing the drug into the work zone. Pressurization can be avoided by creating a slight negative pressure in the vial. Too much negative pressure, however, can cause leakage from the needle when it is with-

drawn from the vial. The safe handling of hazardous drug solutions in vials or ampuls requires the use of a syringe that is no more than three-fourths full when filled with the solution, which minimizes the risk of the plunger separating from the syringe barrel. Once the diluent is drawn up, the needle is inserted into the vial and the plunger is pulled back (to create a slight negative pressure inside the vial), so that air is drawn into the syringe. Small amounts of diluent should be transferred slowly as equal volumes of air are removed. The needle should be kept in the vial, and the contents should be swirled carefully until dissolved. With the vial inverted, the proper amount of drug solution should be gradually withdrawn while equal volumes of air are exchanged for solution. The exact volume needed must be measured while the needle is in the vial, and any excess drug should remain in the vial. With the vial in the upright position, the plunger should be withdrawn past the original starting point to again induce a slight negative pressure before removing the needle. The needle hub should be clear before the needle is removed.

If a hazardous drug is transferred to an i.v. bag, care must be taken to puncture only the septum of the injection port and avoid puncturing the sides of the port or bag. After the drug solution is injected into the i.v. bag, the i.v. port, container, and set (if attached by pharmacy in the BSC or isolator) should be surface decontaminated. The final preparation should be labeled, including an auxiliary warning, and the injection port covered with a protective shield. The final container should be placed, using clean gloves, into a sealable bag to contain any leakage.[1]

To withdraw hazardous drugs from an ampul, the neck or top portion should be gently tapped.[98] After the neck is wiped with alcohol, a 5-μm filter needle or straw should be attached to a syringe that is large enough that it will be not more than three-fourths full when holding the drug. The fluid should then be drawn through the filter needle or straw and cleared from the needle and hub. After this, the needle or straw is exchanged for a needle of similar gauge and length; any air and excess drug should be ejected into a sterile vial (leaving the desired volume in the syringe); aerosolization should be avoided. The drug may then be transferred to an i.v. bag or bottle. If the dose is to be dispensed in the syringe, the plunger should be drawn back to clear fluid from the needle and hub. The needle should be replaced with a locking cap, and the syringe should be surface decontaminated and labeled.

Training and demonstration of competence. All staff who will be compounding hazardous drugs must be trained in the stringent aseptic and negative-pressure techniques necessary for working with sterile hazardous drugs. Once trained, staff must demonstrate competence by an objective method, and competency must be reassessed on a regular basis.[99]

Preparation and handling of noninjectable hazardous drug dosage forms. Although noninjectable dosage forms of hazardous drugs contain varying proportions of drug to nondrug (nonhazardous) components, there is the potential for personnel exposure to and environmental contamination with the hazardous components if hazardous drugs are handled (e.g., packaged) by pharmacy staff. Although most hazardous drugs are not available in liquid formulations, such formulations are often prescribed for small children and adults with feeding tubes. Recipes for extemporane-

ously compounded oral liquids may start with the parenteral form, or they may require that tablets be crushed or capsules opened. Tablet trituration has been shown to cause fine dust formation and local environmental contamination.[100] Procedures for the preparation and the use of equipment (e.g., Class I BSCs or bench-top hoods with HEPA filters) must be developed to avoid the release of aerosolized powder or liquid into the environment during manipulation of hazardous drugs. Recommendations for preparation and handling of noninjectable hazardous drug dosage forms are summarized in Appendix F.

Decontamination, deactivation, and cleaning. Decontamination may be defined as cleaning or deactivating. Deactivating a hazardous substance is preferred, but no single process has been found to deactivate all currently available hazardous drugs. The use of alcohol for disinfecting the BSC or isolator will not deactivate any hazardous drugs and may result in the spread of contamination rather than any actual cleaning.[30,47]

Decontamination of BSCs and isolators should be conducted per manufacturer recommendations. The MSDSs for many hazardous drugs recommend sodium hypochlorite solution as an appropriate deactivating agent.[101] Researchers have shown that strong oxidizing agents, such as sodium hypochlorite, are effective deactivators of many hazardous drugs.[102,103] There is currently one commercially available product, SurfaceSafe (SuperGen, Dublin, CA), that provides a system for decontamination and deactivation using sodium hypochlorite, detergent, and thiosulfate neutralizer. A ventilated cabinet that runs continuously should be cleaned before the day's operations begin and at regular intervals or when the day's work is completed. For a 24-hour service, the cabinet should be cleaned two or three times daily. Cabinets used for aseptic compounding must be disinfected at the beginning of the workday, at the beginning of each subsequent shift (if compounding takes place over an extended period of time), and routinely during compounding.

Appropriate preparation of materials used in compounding before introduction into the Class II BSC or the pass-through of a Class III BSC or isolator, including spraying or wiping with 70% alcohol or appropriate disinfectant, is also necessary for aseptic compounding.

The Class II BSC has air plenums that handle contaminated air. These plenums are not designed to allow surface decontamination, and many of the contaminated surfaces (plenums) cannot be reached for surface cleaning. The area under the work tray should be cleaned at least monthly to reduce the contamination level in the Class II BSC (and in isolators, where appropriate).

Surface decontamination may be accomplished by the transfer of hazardous drug contamination from the surface of a nondisposable item to disposable ones (e.g., wipes, gauze, towels). Although the outer surface of vials containing hazardous drugs has been shown to be contaminated with hazardous drugs,[30,54,55] and hazardous drug contamination has been found on the outside of final preparations,[30] no wipe-down procedures have been studied. The amount of hazardous drug contamination placed into the BSC or isolator may be reduced by surface decontamination (i.e., wiping down) of hazardous drug vials. While no wipe-down procedures have been studied, the use of gauze moistened with alcohol, sterile water, peroxide, or sodium hypochlorite solutions

may be effective. The disposable item, once contaminated, must be contained and discarded as contaminated waste.

Administration of hazardous drugs. Policies and procedures governing the administration of hazardous drugs must be jointly developed by nursing and pharmacy for the mutual safety of health care workers. These policies should supplement policies designed to protect patient safety during administration of all drugs. All policies affecting multiple departments must be developed with input from managers and workers from the affected areas. Extensive nursing guidelines for the safe and appropriate administration of hazardous drugs have been developed by the Oncology Nursing Society[90,104] and OSHA.[2,3] Recommendations for reducing exposure to hazardous drugs during administration in all practice settings are listed in Appendix G.

Spill management. Policies and procedures must be developed to attempt to prevent spills and to govern cleanup of hazardous drug spills. Written procedures must specify who is responsible for spill management and must address the size and scope of the spill. Spills must be contained and cleaned up immediately by trained workers.

Spill kits containing all of the materials needed to clean up spills of hazardous drugs should be assembled or purchased (Appendix H). These kits should be readily available in all areas where hazardous drugs are routinely handled. A spill kit should accompany delivery of injectable hazardous drugs to patient care areas even though they are transported in a sealable plastic bag or container. If hazardous drugs are being prepared or administered in a nonroutine area (e.g., home setting, unusual patient care area), a spill kit and respirator must be obtained by the drug handler. Signs should be available to warn of restricted access to the spill area.

Only trained workers with appropriate PPE and respirators should attempt to manage a hazardous drug spill. All workers who may be required to clean up a spill of hazardous drugs must receive proper training in spill management and in the use of PPE and NIOSH-certified respirators.

The circumstances and handling of spills should be documented. Staff and nonemployees exposed to a hazardous drug spill should also complete an incident report or exposure form and report to the designated emergency service for initial evaluation.

All spill materials must be disposed of as hazardous waste.[105] Recommendations for spill cleanup procedure are summarized in Appendix I.

Worker contamination. Procedures must be in place to address worker contamination, and protocols for medical attention must be developed before the occurrence of any such incident. Emergency kits containing isotonic eyewash supplies (or emergency eyewashes, if available) and soap must be immediately available in areas where hazardous drugs are handled. Workers who are contaminated during the spill or spill cleanup or who have direct skin or eye contact with hazardous drugs require immediate treatment. OSHA-recommended steps for treatment are outlined in Appendix J.

Hazardous Waste Containment and Disposal. In 1976, the Resource Conservation and Recovery Act (RCRA) was enacted to provide a mechanism for tracking hazardous waste from its generation to disposal.[106] Regulations promulgated under RCRA are enforced by the Environmental Protection Agency and apply to pharmaceuticals and chemicals discarded by pharmacies, hospitals, clinics, and other commer-

cial entities. The RCRA outlines four "characteristics" of hazardous waste[107] and contains lists of agents that are to be considered hazardous waste when they are discarded.[108] Any discarded drug that is on one of the lists (a "listed" waste) or meets one of the criteria (a "characteristic" waste) is considered hazardous waste. The listed drugs include epinephrine, nicotine, and physostigmine, as well as nine chemotherapy drugs: arsenic trioxide, chlorambucil, cyclophosphamide, daunomycin, diethylstilbestrol, melphalan, mitomycin C, streptozocin, and uracil mustard. They require handling, containment, and disposal as RCRA hazardous waste.

The RCRA allows for the exemption of "empty containers" from hazardous waste regulations. Empty containers are defined as those that have held U-listed or characteristic wastes and from which all wastes have been removed that can be removed using the practices commonly employed to remove materials from that type of container and no more than 3% by weight of the total capacity of the container remains in the container.[109] Disposal guidelines developed by the National Institutes of Health (NIH) and published in 1984 coined the term "trace-contaminated" waste using the 3% rule.[110] Note that a container that has held an acute hazardous waste listed in §§261.31, 261.32, or 261.33(e), such as arsenic trioxide, is not considered empty by the 3% rule,[111] and that spill residues from cleanup of hazardous agents are considered hazardous waste.[105]

In addition, many states are authorized to implement their own hazardous waste programs, and requirements under these programs may be more stringent than those of the EPA. State and local regulations must be considered when establishing a hazardous waste policy for a specific facility.

General categories of hazardous waste found in health care settings would include trace-contaminated hazardous waste, bulk hazardous waste, hazardous drugs not listed as hazardous waste, and hazardous waste and mixed infectious–hazardous waste.

Trace-contaminated hazardous drug waste. By the NIH definition of trace chemotherapy waste,[110] "RCRA-empty" containers, needles, syringes, trace-contaminated gowns, gloves, pads, and empty i.v. sets may be collected and incinerated at a regulated medical waste incinerator. Sharps used in the preparation of hazardous drugs should not be placed in red sharps containers or needle boxes, since these are most frequently disinfected by autoclaving or microwaving, not by incineration, and pose a risk of aerosolization to waste-handling employees.

Bulk hazardous drug waste. While not official, the term *bulk hazardous drug waste* has been used to differentiate containers that have held either (1) RCRA-listed or characteristic hazardous waste or (2) any hazardous drugs that are not RCRA empty or any materials from hazardous drug spill cleanups. These wastes should be managed as hazardous waste.

Hazardous drugs not listed as hazardous waste. The federal RCRA regulations have not kept up with drug development, as there are over 100 hazardous drugs that are not listed as hazardous waste, including hormonal agents. In some states, such as Minnesota, these must be managed as hazardous waste. In other states, organizations should manage these drugs as hazardous waste as a best-management practice until federal regulations can be updated.

Hazardous waste and mixed infectious–hazardous waste. Most hazardous waste vendors are not permitted to

manage regulated medical waste or infectious waste; therefore, they cannot accept used needles and items contaminated with squeezable, flakable, or drippable blood. Organizations should check carefully with their hazardous waste vendors to ensure acceptance of all possible hazardous waste, including mixed infectious waste, if needed. Once hazardous waste has been identified, it must be collected and stored according to specific EPA and Department of Transportation requirements.[112] Properly labeled, leakproof, and spill-proof containers of nonreactive plastic are required for areas where hazardous waste is generated. Hazardous drug waste may be initially contained in thick, sealable plastic bags before being placed in approved satellite accumulation containers. Glass fragments should be contained in small, puncture-resistant containers to be placed into larger containers approved for temporary storage.

Waste contaminated with blood or other body fluids must not be mixed with hazardous waste. Transport of waste containers from satellite accumulation to storage sites must be done by individuals who have completed OSHA-mandated hazardous waste awareness training.[113,114] Hazardous waste must be properly manifested and transported by a federally permitted hazardous waste transporter to a federally permitted hazardous waste storage, treatment, or disposal facility.[115] A licensed contractor may be hired to manage the hazardous waste program. The waste generator, however, may be held liable for mismanagement of hazardous waste. Investigation of a contractor, including verification of possession and type of license, should be completed and documented before a contractor is engaged. More information on hazardous waste disposal is available at www. hercenter.org.

Alternative Duty and Medical Surveillance. A comprehensive safety program for controlling workplace exposure to hazardous drugs must include engineering controls, training, work practices, and PPE. Such safety programs must be able to identify potentially exposed workers and those who might be at higher risk of adverse health effects due to this exposure. Because reproductive risks have been associated with exposure to hazardous drugs, alternative duty should be offered to individuals who are pregnant, breast-feeding, or attempting to conceive or father a child. Employees' physicians should be involved in making these determinations.

All workers who handle hazardous drugs should be routinely monitored in a medical surveillance program.[2–4,90,104] Medical surveillance involves the collection and interpretation of data for the purpose of detecting changes in the health status of working populations. Medical surveillance programs involve assessment and documentation of symptom complaints, physical findings, and laboratory values (such as a blood count) to determine whether there is a deviation from the expected norms. Descriptions of medical surveillance programs for hazardous drug handlers are presented in the literature.[90,104] NIOSH encourages employees who handle hazardous drugs to participate in medical surveillance programs that are provided in the workplace.[4] Limited resources may preclude the implementation of a comprehensive medical surveillance program for health care workers who are exposed to hazardous drugs. In the absence of an institutional medical surveillance program, NIOSH encourages workers handling hazardous drugs to inform their personal health care providers of their occupation and possible hazardous drug exposure when obtaining routine medical care.[4]

Conclusion

These guidelines represent the recommendations of many groups and individuals who have worked tirelessly over decades to reduce the potential of harmful effects on health care workers exposed to hazardous drugs. No set of guidelines on this topic, however comprehensive, can address all the needs of every health care facility. Health care professionals are encouraged to rely on their professional judgment, experience, and common sense in applying these recommendations to their unique circumstances and to take into account evolving federal, state, and local regulations, as well as the requirements of appropriate accrediting institutions.

References

1. American Society of Hospital Pharmacists. ASHP technical assistance bulletin on handling cytotoxic and hazardous drugs. *Am J Hosp Pharm.* 1990; 47:1033–49.
2. Controlling occupational exposure to hazardous drugs. Chapter 21. In: OSHA technical manual (OSHA Instruction CPL 2-2.20B CH-4). Washington, DC: Directorate of Technical Support, Occupational Safety and Health Administration; 1995.
3. Occupational Safety and Health Administration. Controlling occupational exposure to hazardous drugs. OSHA technical manual, TED 1-0.15A. Section VI. Chapter 2. www.osha.gov/dts/osta/otm/otm_vi/otm_vi_2.html (accessed 2005 Feb 15).
4. National Institute for Occupational Safety and Health. NIOSH alert: preventing occupational exposure to anti-neoplastic and other hazardous drugs in health care settings. www.cdc.gov/niosh/docs/2004-165/ (accessed 2006 Mar 14).
5. Harrison BR. Risks of handling cytotoxic drugs. In: Perry MC, ed. The chemotherapy source book. 3rd ed. Philadelphia: Lippincott, Williams and Wilkins; 2001:566–82.
6. Baker ES, Connor TH. Monitoring occupational exposure to cancer chemotherapy drugs. *Am J Health-Syst Pharm.* 1996; 53:2713–23.
7. Sessink PJ, Bos RP. Drugs hazardous to healthcare workers: evaluation of methods for monitoring occupational exposure to cytostatic drugs. *Drug Saf.* 1999; 20:347–59.
8. Harris CC. The carcinogenicity of anticancer drugs: a hazard in man. *Cancer.* 1976; 37:1014–23.
9. Falck K, Grohn P, Sorsa M et al. Mutagenicity in urine of nurses handling cytostatic drugs. *Lancet.* 1979; 1:1250–1. Letter.
10. Ladik CF, Stoehr GP, Maurer MA. Precautionary measures in the preparation of antineoplastics. *Am J Hosp Pharm.* 1980; 37:1184,1186.
11. Crudi CB. A compounding dilemma: I've kept the drug sterile but have I contaminated myself? *NITA.* 1980; 3:77–8.

12. Crudi CB, Stephens BL, Maier P. Possible occupational hazards associated with the preparation/administration of antineoplastic agents. *NITA.* 1982; 5:264–6.

13. Reynolds RD, Ignoffo R, Lawrence J et al. Adverse reactions to AMSA in medical personnel. *Cancer Treat Rep.* 1982; 66:1885. Letter.

14. Knowles RS, Virden JE. Handling of injectable antineoplastic agents. *Br Med J.* 1980; 281:589–91.

15. McFarlane A. Ophthalmic problems in staff handling cytotoxic drugs. *Aust J Hosp Pharm.* 1986; 16:145. Letter.

16. Curran CF, Luce JK. Ocular adverse reactions associated with adriamycin (doxorubicin). *Am J Ophthalmol.* 1989; 108:709–11.

17. McLendon BF, Bron AJ. Corneal toxicity from vinblastine solution. *Br J Ophthalmol.* 1978; 62:97–9.

18. Valanis BG, Hertzberg V, Shortridge L. Antineoplastic drugs: handle with care. *AAOHN J.* 1987; 35:487–92.

19. Valanis BG, Vollmer WM, Labuhn KT et al. Association of antineoplastic drug handling with acute adverse effects in pharmacy personnel. *Am J Hosp Pharm.* 1993; 50:455–62.

20. Hemminki K, Kyyronen P, Lindholm ML. Spontaneous abortions and malformations in the offspring of nurses exposed to anaesthetic gases, cytostatic drugs, and other potential hazards, based on registered information of outcome. *J Epidemiol Community Health.* 1985; 39:141–7.

21. Selevan SG, Lindbohm ML, Hornung RW et al. A study of occupational exposure to antineoplastic drugs and fetal loss in nurses. *N Engl J Med.* 1985; 313:1173–8.

22. Valanis BG, Vollmer WM, Labuhn KT et al. Occupational exposure to antineoplastic agents and self-reported infertility among nurses and pharmacists. *J Occup Environ Med.* 1997; 39:574–80.

23. Valanis BG, Vollmer WM, Steele P. Occupational exposure to antineoplastic agents: self-reported miscarriages and stillbirths among nurses and pharmacists. *J Occup Environ Med.* 1999; 41:632–8.

24. National Toxicology Program. Report on carcinogens, 11th ed. http://ehis.niehs.nih.gov/roc/toc9.html (accessed 2005 Sep 15).

25. International Agency for Research on Cancer. Monographs database on carcinogenic risks to humans. www-cie.iarc.fr/ (accessed 2004 Nov 1).

26. Skov T, Lynge E, Maarup B et al. Risks for physicians handling antineoplastic drugs. *Lancet.* 1990; 336:1446. Letter.

27. Skov T, Maarup B, Olsen J et al. Leukaemia and reproductive outcome among nurses handling antineoplastic drugs. *Br J Ind Med.* 1992; 49:855–61.

28. Sessink PJ, Kroese ED, van Kranen HJ et al. Cancer risk assessment for health care workers occupationally exposed to cyclophosphamide. *Int Arch Occup Environ Health.* 1995; 67:317–23.

29. Connor TH, Anderson RW, Sessink PJ et al. Surface contamination with antineoplastic agents in six cancer treatment centers in Canada and the United States. *Am J Health-Syst Pharm.* 1999; 56:1427–32.

30. Sessink PJ, Boer KA, Scheefhals AP et al. Occupational exposure to antineoplastic agents at several departments in a hospital: environmental contamination and excretion of cyclophosphamide and ifosfamide in urine of exposed workers. *Int Arch Occup Environ Health.* 1992; 64:105–12.

31. Sessink PJ, Van de Kerkhof MC, Anzion RB et al. Environmental contamination and assessment of exposure to antineoplastic agents by determination of cyclophosphamide in urine of exposed pharmacy technicians: is skin absorption an important exposure route? *Arch Environ Health.* 1994; 49:165–9.

32. Sessink PJ, Wittenhorst BC, Anzion RB et al. Exposure of pharmacy technicians to antineoplastic agents: re-evaluation after additional protective measures. *Arch Environ Health.* 1997; 52:240–4.

33. Ensslin AS, Stoll Y, Pethran A et al. Biological monitoring of cyclophosphamide and ifosfamide in urine of hospital personnel occupationally exposed to cytostatic drugs. *Occup Environ Med.* 1994; 51:229–33.

34. Wick C, Slawson MH, Jorgenson JA et al. Using a closed-system protective device to reduce personnel exposure to antineoplastic agents. *Am J Health-Syst Pharm.* 2003; 60:2314–20.

35. Schmaus G, Schierl R, Funck S. Monitoring surface contamination by antineoplastic drugs using gas chromatography–mass spectrometry and voltammetry. *Am J Health-Syst Pharm.* 2002; 59:956–61.

36. Hirst M, Tse S, Mills DG et al. Occupational exposure to cyclophosphamide. *Lancet.* 1984; 1:186–8.

37. Ensslin AS, Pethran A, Schierl R et al. Urinary platinum in hospital personnel occupationally exposed to platinum-containing antineoplastic drugs. *Int Arch Occup Environ Health.* 1994; 65:339–42.

38. Ensslin AS, Huber R, Pethran A et al. Biological monitoring of hospital pharmacy personnel occupationally exposed to cytostatic drugs: urinary excretion and cytogenetics studies. *Int Arch Occup Environ Health.* 1997; 70:205–8.

39. Minoia C, Turci R, Sottani C et al. Application of high performance liquid chromatography/tandem mass spectrometry in the environmental and biological monitoring of health care personnel occupationally exposed to cyclophosphamide and ifosfamide. *Rapid Commun Mass Spectrom.* 1998; 12:1485–93.

40. Nygren O, Lundgren C. Determination of platinum in workroom air and in blood and urine from nursing staff attending patients receiving cisplatin chemotherapy. *Int Arch Occup Environ Health.* 1997; 70:209–14.

41. Pethran A, Schierl R, Hauff K et al. Uptake of antineoplastic agents in pharmacy and hospital personnel. Part I: monitoring of urinary concentrations. *Int Arch Occup Environ Health.* 2003; 76:5–10.

42. Larson RR, Khazaeli MB, Dillon HK. A new monitoring method using solid sorbent media for evaluation of airborne cyclophosphamide and other antineoplastic agents. *Appl Occup Environ Hyg.* 2003; 18:120–31.

43. Opiolka S, Schmidt KG, Kiffmeyer K et al. Determination of the vapor pressure of cytotoxic drugs and its effects on occupational safety. *J Oncol Pharm Practice.* 2000; 6:15. Abstract.

44. Kiffmeyer TK, Kube C, Opiolka S et al. Vapor pressures, evaporation behavior and airborne concentrations of hazardous drugs: implications for occupational safety. *Pharm J.* 2002; 268:331–7.

45. Connor TH, Shults M, Fraser MP. Determination of the vaporization of solutions of mutagenic antineoplastic agents at 23 and 36 °C using a dessicator technique. *Mutat Res.* 2000; 470:85–92.

46. Kromhout H, Hoek F, Uitterhoeve R et al. Postulating a dermal pathway for exposure to antineoplastic drugs among hospital workers. Applying a conceptual model to the results of three workplace surveys. *Ann Occup Hyg.* 2000; 44:551–60.

47. Dorr RT, Alberts DS. Topical absorption and inactivation of cytotoxic anticancer agents in vitro. *Cancer.* 1992; 70(4 suppl):983–7.

48. Bos RP, Leenaars AO, Theuws JL et al. Mutagenicity of urine from nurses handling cytostatic drugs, influence of smoking. *Int Arch Occup Environ Health.* 1982; 50:359–69.

49. Evelo CT, Bos RP, Peters JG et al. Urinary cyclophosphamide assay as a method for biological monitoring of occupational exposure to cyclophosphamide. *Int Arch Occup Environ Health.* 1986; 58:151–5.

50. Pharmaceutical compounding—sterile preparations (general information chapter 797). In: The United States pharmacopeia, 28th rev., and The national formulary, 23rd ed. Rockville, MD: United States Pharmacopeial Convention; 2004:2461–77.

51. Standard 14644-1. Cleanrooms and associated environments—part 1: classification of air cleanliness. 1st ed. Geneva, Switzerland: International Organization for Standardization; 1999.

52. 29 C.F.R. 1910-1200.

53. Occupational Safety and Health Administration. Hazard communication standard: hazard communication—final rule. 29 C.F.R. 1910. *Fed Regist.* 1987; 52:31852–86.

54. Kiffmeyer TK, Ing KG, Schoppe G. External contamination of cytotoxic drug packing: safe handling and cleaning procedures. *J Oncol Pharm Pract.* 2000; 6:13.

55. Connor TH, Sessink PJ, Harrison BR et al. Surface contamination of chemotherapy drug vials and evaluation of new vial-cleaning techniques: results of three studies. *Am J Health-Syst Pharm.* 2005; 62:475–84.

56. 29 C.F.R. 1910.134.

57. National Institute for Occupational Safety and Health. Summary for respirator users. www.cdc.gov/niosh/respsumm.html (accessed 2005 Sep 15).

58. Nguyen TV, Theiss JC, Matney TS. Exposure of pharmacy personnel to mutagenic antineoplastic drugs. *Cancer Res.* 1982; 42:4792–6.

59. Anderson RW, Puckett WH Jr, Dana WJ et al. Risk of handling injectable antineoplastic agents. *Am J Hosp Pharm.* 1982; 39:1881–7.

60. Rubino FM, Floridia L, Pietropaolo AM et al. Measurement of surface contamination by certain antineoplastic drugs using high-performance liquid chromatography: applications in occupational hygiene investigations in hospital environments. *Med Lav.* 1999; 90:572–83.

61. Sessink PJ, Anzion RB, Van den Broeck PH et al. Detection of contamination with antineoplastic agents in a hospital pharmacy department. *Pharm Weekbl Sci.* 1992; 14:16–22.

62. NSF/ANSI standard 49-04: class II (laminar flow) biosafety cabinetry. Ann Arbor, MI: NSF International; 2004.

63. Clark RP, Goff MR. The potassium iodide method for determining protection factors in open-fronted microbiological safety cabinets. *J Appl Bacteriol.* 1981; 51:439–60.

64. National Sanitation Foundation standard 49: Class II (laminar flow) biohazard cabinetry. Ann Arbor, MI: National Sanitation Foundation; 1987.

65. American Glovebox Society. Guidelines for gloveboxes. 2nd ed. Santa Rosa, CA: AGS; AGS-G001-1998.

66. General Services Administration. Federal standard 209e: clean room and work station requirements, controlled environments. Washington, DC: U.S. Government Printing Office; 1992.

67. Food and Drug Administration. Guidance for industry—sterile drug products produced by aseptic processing. Current good manufacturing practice. www.fda.gov/cder/guidance/5882fnl.pdf (accessed 2005 Sep 10).

68. Tillett L. Barrier isolators as an alternative to a cleanroom. *Am J Health-Syst Pharm.* 1999; 56:1433–6.

69. Mosko P, Rahe H. Barrier isolation technology: a labor-efficient alternative to cleanrooms. *Hosp Pharm.* 1999; 34:834–8.

70. Rahe H. Understanding the critical components of a successful cleanroom and barrier isolator project. *Am J Health-Syst Pharm.* 2000; 57:346–50.

71. Controlled Environment Testing Association. CETA applications guide for the use of barrier isolators in compounding sterile preparations in healthcare facilities. www.cetainternational.org/reference/isolator3.pdf (accessed 2005 Sep 10).

72. Mason HJ, Blair S, Sams C et al. Exposure to antineoplastic drugs in two UK hospital pharmacy units. *Ann Occup Hyg.* 2005; 49:603–10.

73. Nygren O, Gustavsson B, Strom L et al. Exposure to anti-cancer drugs during preparation and administration. Investigations of an open and a closed system. *J Environ Monit.* 2002; 4:739–42.

74. Sessink PJ, Rolf ME, Ryden NS. Evaluation of the PhaSeal hazardous drug containment system. *Hosp Pharm.* 1999; 34:1311–7.

75. Sessink PJ. How to work safely outside the biological safety cabinet. *J Oncol Pharm Pract.* 2000; 6:15. Abstract.

76. Connor TH, Anderson RW, Sessink PJ et al. Effectiveness of a closed-system device in containing surface contamination with cyclophosphamide and ifosfamide in an i.v. admixture area. *Am J Health-Syst Pharm.* 2002; 59:68–72.

77. Vandenbroucke J, Robays H. How to protect environment and employees against cytotoxic agents: the UZ Gent experience. *J Oncol Pharm Pract.* 2001; 6:146–52.

78. Spivey S, Connor TH. Determining sources of workplace contamination with antineoplastic drugs and comparing conventional IV drug preparation with a closed system. *Hosp Pharm.* 2003; 38:135–9.

79. Hoy RH, Stump LM. Effect of an air-venting filter device on aerosol production from vials. *Am J Hosp Pharm.* 1984; 41:324–6.
80. Connor TH. Permeability testing of glove materials for use with cancer chemotherapy drugs. *Oncology.* 1995; 52:256–9.
81. Singleton LC, Connor TH. An evaluation of the permeability of chemotherapy gloves to three cancer chemotherapy drugs. *Oncol Nurs Forum.* 1999; 26:1491–6.
82. Gross E, Groce DF. An evaluation of nitrile gloves as an alternative to natural rubber latex for handling chemotherapeutic agents. *J Oncol Pharm Pract.* 1998; 4:165–8.
83. Connor TH. Permeability of nitrile rubber, latex, polyurethane, and neoprene gloves to 18 antineoplastic drugs. *Am J Health-Syst Pharm.* 1999; 56:2450–3.
84. Klein M, Lambov N, Samev N et al. Permeation of cytotoxic formulations through swatches from selected medical gloves. *Am J Health-Syst Pharm.* 2003; 60:1006–11.
85. American Society for Testing and Materials D 6978-05 standard practice for assessment of resistance of medical gloves to permeation by chemotherapy drugs. West Conshohocken, PA: American Society for Testing and Materials; 2005.
86. Connor TH, Xiang Q. The effect of isopropyl alcohol on the permeation of gloves exposed to antineoplastic agents. *J Oncol Pharm Pract.* 2000; 6:109–14.
87. Colligan SA, Horstman SW. Permeation of cancer chemotherapeutic drugs through glove materials under static and flexed conditions. *Appl Occup Environ Hyg.* 1990; 5:848–52.
88. Sessink PJ, Cerna M, Rossner P et al. Urinary cyclophosphamide excretion and chromosomal aberrations in peripheral blood lymphocytes after occupational exposure to antineoplastic agents. *Mutat Res.* 1994; 309:193–9.
89. National Institutes of Health. Recommendations for the safe handling of cytotoxic drugs. www.nih.gov/od/ors/ds/pubs/cyto/index.htm (accessed 2004 Nov 1).
90. Polovich M, White JM, Kelleher LO, eds. Chemotherapy and biotherapy guidelines and recommendations for practice. 2nd ed. Pittsburgh: Oncology Nursing Society; 2005.
91. Connor TH. An evaluation of the permeability of disposable polypropylene-based protective gowns to a battery of cancer chemotherapy drugs. *Appl Occup Environ Hyg.* 1993; 8:785–9.
92. Harrison BR, Kloos MD. Penetration and splash protection of six disposable gown materials against fifteen antineoplastic drugs. *J Oncol Pharm Pract.* 1999; 5:61–6.
93. Laidlaw JL, Connor TH, Theiss JC et al. Permeability of four disposal protective-clothing materials to seven antineoplastic drugs. *Am J Hosp Pharm.* 1985; 42:2449–54.
94. Valanis B, Shortridge L. Self protective practices of nurses handling antineoplastic drugs. *Oncol Nurs Forum.* 1987; 14:23–7.
95. Labuhn K, Valanis B, Schoeny R et al. Nurses' and pharmacists' exposure to antineoplastic drugs: findings from industrial hygiene scans and urine mutagenicity tests. *Cancer Nurs.* 1998; 21:79–89.
96. NuAire. Containment capabilities of a Class II, type A2 BSC using a chemo pad on the worksurface. Technical bulletin. www.nuaire.com/tech_papers/Containment_Capabilities_using_Chemo_Pad.PDF (accessed 2006 Mar 23).
97. Farris J. Barrier isolators and the reduction of contamination in preparation of parenteral products. www.mic4.com/articles/parenteral-products.php (accessed 2006 Mar 23).
98. Wilson JP, Solimando DA. Aseptic technique as a safety precaution in the preparation of antineoplastic agents. *Hosp Pharm.* 1981; 15:575–81.
99. Harrison BR, Godefroid RJ, Kavanaugh EA. Quality-assurance testing of staff pharmacists handling cytotoxic agents. *Am J Health-Syst Pharm.* 1996; 53:402–7.
100. Shahsavarani S, Godefroid RJ, Harrison BR. Evaluation of occupational exposure to tablet trituration dust. Paper presented at ASHP Midyear Clinical Meeting. Atlanta, GA; 1993 Dec 6.
101. Johnson EG, Janosik JE. Manufacturers' recommendations for handling spilled antineoplastic agents. *Am J Hosp Pharm.* 1989; 46:318–9.
102. Benvenuto JA, Connor TH, Monteith DK et al. Degradation and inactivation of antitumor drugs. *J Pharm Sci.* 1993; 82:988–91.
103. Hansel S, Castegnaro M, Sportouch MH et al. Chemical degradation of wastes of antineoplastic agents: cyclophosphamide, ifosfamide, and melphalan. *Int Arch Occup Environ Health.* 1997; 69:109–14.
104. Polovich M, Belcher C, Glynn-Tucker EM et al. Safe handling of hazardous drugs. Pittsburgh: Oncology Nursing Society; 2003.
105. 40 C.F.R. 261.33.
106. Resource Conservation and Recovery Act of 1976. 42 U.S.C. 82 §6901-92.
107. 40 C.F.R. 261.20-24C.
108. 40 C.F.R. 261.3.38D.
109. 40 C.F.R. 261.7.
110. Vaccari PL, Tonat K, DeChristoforo R et al. Disposal of antineoplastic wastes at the National Institutes of Health. *Am J Hosp Pharm.* 1984; 41:87–93.
111. 40 C.F.R. 261.7(b)(1)-(3).
112. 49 C.F.R. 172.0-.123,173,178,179.
113. 29 C.F.R. 1910.120(e)(3)(i).
114. 29 C.F.R. 1910.120(q)(1-6).
115. 40 C.F.R. 260-8,270.

Appendix A—Recommendations for Use of Class II BSCs

1. The use of a Class II BSC must be accompanied by a stringent program of work practices, including training, demonstrated competence, contamination reduction, and decontamination.
2. Only a Class II BSC with outside exhaust should be used for compounding hazardous drugs; type B2 total exhaust is preferred. Total exhaust is required if the hazardous drug is known to be volatile.[4]
3. Without special design considerations, Class II BSCs are not recommended in traditional, positive-pressure cleanrooms, where contamination from hazardous drugs may result in airborne contamination that may spread from the open front to surrounding areas.
4. Consider using closed-system drug-transfer devices while compounding hazardous drugs in a Class II BSC; evidence documents a decrease in drug contaminants inside a Class II BSC when such devices are used.[4]
5. Reduce the hazardous drug contamination burden in the Class II BSC by wiping down hazardous drug vials before placing them in the BSC.

Appendix B—Recommendations for Use of Class III BSCs and Isolators

1. Only a ventilated cabinet appendix to protect workers and adjacent personnel from exposure and to provide an aseptic environment may be used to compound sterile hazardous drugs.
2. Only ventilated cabinets that are designed to contain aerosolized drug product within the cabinet should be used to compound hazardous drugs.
3. The use of a Class III BSC or isolator must be accompanied by a stringent program of work practices, including operator training and demonstrated competence, contamination reduction, and decontamination.
4. Decontamination of the Class III BSC or isolator must be done in a way that contains any hazardous drug surface contamination during the cleaning process.
5. Appropriate decontamination within the cabinet must be completed before the cabinet is accessed via pass-throughs or removable front panels.
6. Gloves or gauntlets must not be replaced before completion of appropriate decontamination within the cabinet.
7. Surface decontamination of final preparations must be done before labeling and placing into the pass-through.
8. Final preparations must be placed into a transport bag while in the pass-through for removal from the cabinet.

Appendix C—Recommendations for Use of Gloves

1. Wear double gloves for all activities involving hazardous drugs. Double gloves must be worn during any handling of hazardous drug shipping cartons or drug vials, compounding and administration of hazardous drugs, handling of hazardous drug waste or waste from patients recently treated with hazardous drugs, and cleanup of hazardous drug spills.
2. Select powder-free, high-quality gloves made of latex, nitrile, polyurethane, neoprene, or other materials that meet the ASTM standard for chemotherapy gloves.
3. Inspect gloves for visible defects.
4. Sanitize gloves with 70% alcohol or other appropriate disinfectant before performing any aseptic compounding activity.
5. Change gloves every 30 minutes during compounding or immediately when damaged or contaminated.
6. Remove outer gloves after wiping down final preparation but before labeling or removing the preparation from the BSC.
7. Outer gloves must be placed in a containment bag while in the BSC.
8. In an isolator, a second glove must be worn inside the fixed-glove assembly.
9. In an isolator, fixed gloves or appendix must be surface cleaned after compounding is completed to avoid spreading hazardous drug contamination to other surfaces.
10. Clean gloves (e.g., the clean inner gloves) should be used to surface decontaminate the final preparation, place the label onto the final preparation, and place it into the pass-through.
11. Don fresh gloves to complete the final check, place preparation into a clean transport bag, and remove the bag from the pass-through.
12. Wash hands before donning and after removing gloves.
13. Remove gloves with care to avoid contamination. Specific procedures for removal must be established and followed.
14. Gloves should be removed and contained inside the Class II BSC or isolator.
15. Change gloves after administering a dose of hazardous drugs or when leaving the immediate administration area.
16. Dispose of contaminated gloves as contaminated waste.

Appendix D—Recommendations for Use of Gowns

1. Gowns should be worn during compounding, during administration, when handling waste from patients recently treated with hazardous drugs, and when cleaning up spills of hazardous drugs.
2. Select disposable gowns of material tested to be protective against the hazardous drugs to be used.
3. Coated gowns must be worn no longer than three hours during compounding and changed immediately when damaged or contaminated.
4. Remove gowns with care to avoid spreading contamination. Specific procedures for removal must be established and followed.
5. Dispose of gowns immediately upon removal.
6. Contain and dispose of contaminated gowns as contaminated waste.
7. Wash hands after removing and disposing of gowns.

Appendix E—Recommendations for Working in BSCs and Isolators

1. The use of a Class II or III BSC or isolator must be accompanied by a stringent program of work practices, including operator training and demonstrated competence, contamination reduction, and decontamination.
2. Do not place unnecessary items in the work area of the cabinet or isolator where hazardous drug contamination from compounding may settle on them.
3. Do not overcrowd the BSC or isolator.
4. Gather all needed supplies before beginning compounding. Avoid exiting and reentering the work area of the BSC or isolator.
5. Appropriate handling of the preparation in the BSC or pass-through of the isolator, including spraying or wiping with 70% alcohol or another appropriate disinfectant, is necessary for aseptic compounding.
6. Reduce the hazardous drug contamination burden in the BSC or isolator by wiping down hazardous drug vials before placing them in the BSC or isolator.
7. Transport bags must never be placed in the BSC or the isolator work chamber during compounding to avoid inadvertent contamination of the outside surface of the bag.
8. Final preparations should be surface decontaminated within the BSC or isolator and placed into the transport bags in the BSC or in the isolator pass-through, taking care not to contaminate the outside of the transport bag.
9. Decontaminate the work surface of the BSC or isolator before and after compounding per the manufacturer's recommendations or with detergent, sodium hypochlorite solution, and neutralizer.
10. Decontaminate all surfaces of the BSC or isolator at the end of the batch, day, or shift, as appropriate to the workflow. Typically, a BSC or isolator in use 24 hours a day would require decontamination two or three times daily. Disinfect the BSC or isolator before compounding a dose or batch of sterile hazardous drugs.
11. Wipe down the outside of the Class II BSC front opening and the floor in front of the BSC with detergent, sodium hypochlorite solution, and neutralizer at least daily.
12. Seal and then decontaminate surfaces of waste and sharps containers before removing from the BSC or isolator.
13. Decontamination is required after any spill in the BSC or isolator during compounding.
14. Seal all contaminated materials (e.g., gauze, wipes, towels, wash or rinse water) in bags or plastic containers and discard as contaminated waste.
15. Decontamination of the Class III BSC or isolator must be done in a way that contains any hazardous drug surface contamination during the cleaning process.
16. Appropriate decontamination within the cabinet must be completed before the cabinet is accessed via the pass-throughs or removable front panels.
17. Gloves or gauntlets must not be replaced before completion of appropriate decontamination within the cabinet.
18. Surface decontamination of final preparations must be done before labeling and placing into the pass-through.
19. Final preparations must be placed into a transport bag while in the pass-through for removal from the cabinet.

Appendix F—Recommendations for Compounding and Handling Noninjectable Hazardous Drug Dosage Forms

1. Hazardous drugs should be labeled or otherwise identified as such to prevent improper handling.
2. Tablet and capsule forms of hazardous drugs should not be placed in automated counting machines, which subject them to stress and may introduce powdered contaminants into the work area.
3. During routine handling of noninjectable hazardous drugs and contaminated equipment, workers should wear two pairs of gloves that meet the ASTM standard for chemotherapy gloves.[85]
4. Counting and pouring of hazardous drugs should be done carefully, and clean equipment should be dedicated for use with these drugs.
5. Contaminated equipment should be cleaned initially with gauze saturated with sterile water; further cleaned with detergent, sodium hypochlorite solution, and neutralizer; and then rinsed. The gauze and rinse should be contained and disposed of as contaminated waste.
6. Crushing tablets or opening capsules should be avoided; liquid formulations should be used whenever possible.
7. During the compounding of hazardous drugs (e.g., crushing, dissolving, or preparing a solution or an ointment), workers should wear nonpermeable gowns and double gloves. Compounding should take place in a ventilated cabinet.
8. Compounding nonsterile forms of hazardous drugs in equipment designated for sterile products must be undertaken with care. Appropriate containment, deactivation, and disinfection techniques must be utilized.
9. Hazardous drugs should be dispensed in the final dose and form whenever possible. Unit-of-use containers for oral liquids have not been tested for containment properties. Most exhibit some spillage during preparation or use. Caution must be exercised when using these devices.
10. Bulk containers of liquid hazardous drugs, as well as specially packaged commercial hazardous drugs (e.g., Neoral [manufactured by Novartis]), must be handled carefully to avoid spills. These containers should be dispensed and maintained in sealable plastic bags to contain any inadvertent contamination.
11. Disposal of unused or unusable noninjectable dosage forms of hazardous drugs should be performed in the same manner as for hazardous injectable dosage forms and waste.

Appendix G—Recommendations for Reducing Exposure to Hazardous Drugs During Administration in All Practice Settings[104]

Intravenous administration

1. The use of gloves, gown, and face shield (as needed for splashing) is required.
2. Gather all necessary equipment and supplies, including PPE.
3. Use needleless systems whenever possible.
4. Use Luer-Lok fittings for all needleless systems, syringes, needles, infusion tubing, and pumps.
5. Needleless systems may result in droplets leaking at connection points; use gauze pads to catch leaks.
6. Designate a workplace for handling hazardous drugs.
7. Have a spill kit and hazardous drug waste container readily available.
8. Procedure for gowning and gloving: Wash hands, don first pair of gloves, don gown and face shield, and then don second pair of gloves. Gloves should extend beyond the elastic or knit cuff of the gown. Double-gloving requires one glove to be worn under the cuff of the gown and the second glove over the cuff.
9. Always work below eye level.
10. Visually examine hazardous drug dose while it is still contained in transport bag.
11. If hazardous drug dose appears intact, remove it from the transport bag.
12. Place a plastic-backed absorbent pad under the administration area to absorb leaks and prevent drug contact with the patient's skin.
13. If priming occurs at the administration site, prime i.v. tubing with an i.v. solution that does not contain hazardous drugs or by the backflow method.
14. Place a gauze pad under the connection at injection ports during administration to catch leaks.
15. Use the transport bag as a containment bag for materials contaminated with hazardous drugs, drug containers, and sets.
16. Discard hazardous drug containers with the administration sets attached; do not remove the set.
17. Wash surfaces that come into contact with hazardous drugs with detergent, sodium hypochlorite solution, and neutralizer, if appropriate.
18. Wearing gloves, contain and dispose of materials contaminated with hazardous drugs and remaining PPE as contaminated waste.
19. Hazardous drug waste container must be sufficiently large to hold all discarded material, including PPE.
20. Do not push or force materials contaminated with hazardous drugs into the hazardous drug waste container.
21. Carefully remove, contain, and discard gloves. Wash hands thoroughly after removing gloves.

Intramuscular or subcutaneous administration

1. The use of double gloves is required.
2. Gather all necessary equipment and supplies, including PPE.
3. Use Luer-Lok safety needles or retracting needles or shields.

4. Syringes should have Luer-Lok connections and be less than three-fourths full.
5. Designate a workplace for handling hazardous drugs.
6. Have a spill kit and hazardous drug waste container readily available.
7. Procedure for gloving: Wash hands; don double gloves.
8. Always work below eye level.
9. Visually examine hazardous drug dose while still contained in transport bag.
10. If hazardous drug dose appears intact, remove it from the transport bag.
11. Remove the syringe cap and connect appropriate safety needle.
12. Do not expel air from syringe or prime the safety needle.
13. After administration, discard hazardous drug syringes (with the safety needle attached) directly into a hazardous drug waste container.
14. Wearing gloves, contain and dispose of materials contaminated with hazardous drugs.
15. Do not push or force materials contaminated with hazardous drugs into the hazardous drug waste container.
16. Carefully remove, contain, and discard gloves.
17. Wash hands thoroughly after removing gloves.

Oral administration

1. Double gloves are required, as is a face shield if there is a potential for spraying, aerosolization, or splashing.
2. Workers should be aware that tablets or capsules may be coated with a dust of residual hazardous drug that could be inhaled, absorbed through the skin, ingested, or spread to other locations and that liquid formulations may be aerosolized or spilled.
3. No crushing or compounding of oral hazardous drugs may be done in an unprotected environment.
4. Gather all necessary equipment and supplies, including PPE.
5. Designate a workplace for handling hazardous drugs.
6. Have a spill kit and hazardous drug waste container readily available.
7. Procedure for gloving: Wash hands and don double gloves.
8. Always work below eye level.
9. Visually examine hazardous drug dose while it is still contained in transport bag.
10. If hazardous drug dose appears intact, remove it from the transport bag.
11. Place a plastic-backed absorbent pad on the work area, if necessary, to contain any spills.
12. After administration, wearing double gloves, contain and dispose of materials contaminated with hazardous drugs into the hazardous drug waste container.
13. Do not push or force materials contaminated with hazardous drugs into the hazardous drug waste container.
14. Carefully remove, contain, and discard gloves.
15. Wash hands thoroughly after removing gloves.

Appendix H—Recommended Contents of Hazardous Drug Spill Kit

1. Sufficient supplies to absorb a spill of about 1000 mL (volume of one i.v. bag or bottle).
2. Appropriate PPE to protect the worker during cleanup, including two pairs of disposable gloves (one outer pair of heavy utility gloves and one pair of inner gloves); nonpermeable, disposable protective garments (coveralls or gown and shoe covers); and face shield.
3. Absorbent, plastic-backed sheets or spill pads.
4. Disposable toweling.
5. At least two sealable, thick plastic hazardous waste disposal bags (prelabeled with an appropriate warning label).
6. One disposable scoop for collecting glass fragments.
7. One puncture-resistant container for glass fragments.

Appendix I—Recommendations for Spill Cleanup Procedure

General
1. Assess the size and scope of the spill. Call for trained help, if necessary.
2. Spills that cannot be contained by two spill kits may require outside assistance.
3. Post signs to limit access to spill area.
4. Obtain spill kit and respirator.
5. Don PPE, including inner and outer gloves and respirator.
6. Once fully garbed, contain spill using spill kit.
7. Carefully remove any broken glass fragments and place them in a puncture-resistant container.
8. Absorb liquids with spill pads.
9. Absorb powder with damp disposable pads or soft toweling.
10. Spill cleanup should proceed progressively from areas of lesser to greater contamination.
11. Completely remove and place all contaminated material in the disposal bags.
12. Rinse the area with water and then clean with detergent, sodium hypochlorite solution, and neutralizer.
13. Rinse the area several times and place all materials used for containment and cleanup in disposal bags. Seal bags and place them in the appropriate final container for disposal as hazardous waste.
14. Carefully remove all PPE using the inner gloves. Place all disposable PPE into disposal bags. Seal bags and place them into the appropriate final container.
15. Remove inner gloves; contain in a small, sealable bag; and then place into the appropriate final container for disposal as hazardous waste.
16. Wash hands thoroughly with soap and water.
17. Once a spill has been initially cleaned, have the area recleaned by housekeeping, janitorial staff, or environmental services.

Spills in a BSC or isolator
1. Spills occurring in a BSC or isolator should be cleaned up immediately.
2. Obtain a spill kit if the volume of the spill exceeds 30 mL or the contents of one drug vial or ampul.
3. Utility gloves (from spill kit) should be worn to remove broken glass in a BSC or an isolator. Care must be taken not to damage the fixed-glove assembly in the isolator.
4. Place glass fragments in the puncture-resistant hazardous drug waste container located in the BSC or discard into the appropriate waste receptacle of the isolator.
5. Thoroughly clean and decontaminate the BSC or isolator.
6. Clean and decontaminate the drain spillage trough located under the Class II BSC or similarly equipped Class III BSC or isolator.
7. If the spill results in liquid being introduced onto the HEPA filter or if powdered aerosol contaminates the "clean side" of the HEPA filter, use of the BSC or isolator should be suspended until the equipment has been decontaminated and the HEPA filter replaced.

Appendix J—OSHA-Recommended Steps for Immediate Treatment of Workers with Direct Skin or Eye Contact with Hazardous Drugs[3]

1. Call for help, if needed.
2. Immediately remove contaminated clothing.
3. Flood affected eye with water or isotonic eyewash for at least 15 minutes.
4. Clean affected skin with soap and water; rinse thoroughly.
5. Obtain medical attention.
6. Document exposure in employee's medical record and medical surveillance log.
7. Supplies for emergency treatment (e.g., soap, eyewash, sterile saline for irrigation) should be immediately located in any area where hazardous drugs are compounded or administered.

Glossary

Antineoplastic drug: A chemotherapeutic agent that controls or kills cancer cells. Drugs used in the treatment of cancer are cytotoxic but are generally more damaging to dividing cells than to resting cells.[4]

Aseptic: Free of living pathogenic organisms or infected materials.[4]

Biological-safety cabinet (BSC): A BSC may be one of several types.[4]

Class I BSC: A BSC that protects personnel and the work environment but does not protect the product. It is a negative-pressure, ventilated cabinet usually operated with an open front and a minimum face velocity at the work opening of at least 75 ft/min. A class I BSC is similar in design to a chemical fume hood except that all of the air from the cabinet is exhausted through a high-efficiency particulate air (HEPA) filter (either into the laboratory or to the outside).

Class II BSC: A ventilated BSC that protects personnel, the product, and the work environment. A Class II BSC has an open front with inward airflow for personnel protection, downward HEPA-filtered laminar airflow

for product protection, and HEPA-filtered exhausted air for environmental protection.

Type A1 (formerly type A): These Class II BSCs maintain a minimum inflow velocity of 75 ft/min, have HEPA-filtered down-flow air that is a portion of the mixed down-flow and inflow air from a common plenum, may exhaust HEPA-filtered air back into the laboratory or to the environment through an exhaust canopy, and may have positive-pressure contaminated ducts and plenums that are not surrounded by negative-pressure plenums. They are not suitable for use with volatile toxic chemicals and volatile radionucleotides.

Type A2 (formerly type B3): These Class II BSCs maintain a minimum inflow velocity of 100 ft/min, have HEPA-filtered down-flow air that is a portion of the mixed down-flow and inflow air from a common exhaust plenum, may exhaust HEPA-filtered air back into the laboratory or to the environment through an exhaust canopy, and have all contaminated ducts and plenums under negative pressure or surrounded by negative-pressure ducts and plenums. If these cabinets are used for minute quantities of volatile toxic chemicals and trace amounts of radionucleotides, they must be exhausted through properly functioning exhaust canopies.

Type B1: These Class II BSCs maintain a minimum inflow velocity of 100 ft/min, have HEPA-filtered down-flow air composed largely of uncontaminated, recirculated inflow air, exhaust most of the contaminated down-flow air through a dedicated duct exhausted to the at-mosphere after passing it through a HEPA filter, and have all contaminated ducts and plenums under negative pressure or surrounded by negative-pressure ducts and plenums. If these cabinets are used for work involving minute quantities of volatile toxic chemicals and trace amounts of radionucleotides, the work must be done in the directly exhausted portion of the cabinet.

Type B2 (total exhaust): These Class II BSCs maintain a minimum inflow velocity of 100 ft/min, have HEPA-filtered down-flow air drawn from the laboratory or the outside, exhaust all inflow and down-flow air to the atmosphere after filtration through a HEPA filter without recirculation inside the cabinet or return to the laboratory, and have all contaminated ducts and plenums under negative pressure or surrounded by directly exhausted negative-pressure ducts and plenums. These cabinets may be used with volatile toxic chemicals and radionucleotides.

Class III BSC: A BSC with a totally enclosed, ventilated cabinet of gastight construction in which operations are conducted through attached rubber gloves and observed through a nonopening view window. This BSC is maintained under negative pressure of at least 0.50 in of water gauge, and air is drawn into the cabinet through HEPA filters. The exhaust air is treated by double HEPA filtration or single HEPA filtration–incineration. Passage of materials in and out of the cabinet is generally performed through a dunk tank (accessible through the cabinet floor) or a double-door

pass-through box (such as an autoclave) that can be decontaminated between uses.

Chemotherapy drug: A chemical agent used to treat diseases. The term usually refers to a drug used to treat cancer.[4]

Chemotherapy glove: A medical glove that has been approved by FDA for use when handling antineoplastic drugs.[4]

Chemotherapy waste: Discarded items such as gowns, gloves, masks, i.v. tubing, empty bags, empty drug vials, needles, and syringes used while preparing and administering antineoplastic agents.[4]

Closed system: A device that does not exchange unfiltered air or contaminants with the adjacent environment.[4]

Closed-system drug-transfer device: A drug-transfer device that mechanically prohibits the transfer of environmental contaminants into the system and the escape of hazardous drug or vapor concentrations outside the system.[4]

Cytotoxic: A pharmacologic compound that is detrimental or destructive to cells within the body.[4]

Deactivation: Treating a chemical agent (such as a hazardous drug) with another chemical, heat, ultraviolet light, or another agent to create a less hazardous agent.[4]

Decontamination: Inactivation, neutralization, or removal of toxic agents, usually by chemical means.[4] Surface decontamination may be accomplished by the transfer of hazardous drug contamination from the surface of a nondisposable item to disposable ones (e.g., wipes, gauze, towels).

Disinfecting: Removal of viable organism from surfaces using 70% alcohol or other appropriate disinfectant prior to compounding of sterile hazardous drugs.

Engineering controls: Devices designed to eliminate or reduce worker exposures to chemical, biological, radiological, ergonomic, or physical hazards. Examples include laboratory fume hoods, glove bags, retracting syringe needles, sound-dampening materials to reduce noise levels, safety interlocks, and radiation shielding.[4]

Genotoxic: Capable of damaging DNA and leading to mutations.[4]

Glove box: A controlled environment work enclosure providing a primary barrier from the work area. Operations are performed through sealed gloved openings to protect the worker, the ambient environment, and/or the product.[4]

Hazardous drug: Any drug identified by at least one of the following six criteria: carcinogenicity, teratogenicity or developmental toxicity, reproductive toxicity in humans, organ toxicity at low doses in humans or animals, genotoxicity, and new drugs that mimic existing hazardous drugs in structure or toxicity.[4]

Hazardous waste: Any waste that is an RCRA-listed hazardous waste [40 C.F.R. 261.30-.33] or that meets an RCRA characteristic of ignitability, corrosivity, reactivity, or toxicity as defined in 40 C.F.R. 261.21-.24.[4]

Health care settings: All hospitals, medical clinics, outpatient facilities, physicians' offices, retail pharmacies, and similar facilities dedicated to the care of patients.[4]

Health care workers: All workers who are involved in the care of patients. These include pharmacists, pharmacy technicians, nurses (registered nurses, licensed practi-

cal nurses, nurses' aides, etc.), physicians, home health care workers, and environmental services workers (housekeeping, laundry, and waste disposal).[4]

HEPA filter: Filter rated 99.97% efficient in capturing particles 0.3-μm in diameter.[4]

Horizontal-laminar-airflow hood (horizontal-laminar-airflow clean bench): A device that protects the work product and the work area by supplying HEPA-filtered air to the rear of the cabinet and producing a horizontal flow across the work area and out toward the worker.[4]

Isolator: A device that is sealed or is supplied with air through a microbially retentive filtration system (HEPA minimum) and may be reproducibly decontaminated. When closed, an isolator uses only decontaminated interfaces (when necessary) or rapid transfer ports for materials transfer. When open, it allows for the ingress and egress of materials through defined openings that have been designed and validated to preclude the transfer of contaminants or unfiltered air to adjacent environments. An isolator can be used for aseptic processing, for containment of potent compounds, or for simultaneous asepsis and containment. Some isolator designs allow operations within the isolator to be conducted through a fixed-glove assembly without compromising asepsis or containment.[4]

Aseptic isolator: A ventilated isolator designed to exclude external contamination from entering the critical zone inside the isolator.[4]

Aseptic containment isolator: A ventilated isolator designed to meet the requirements of both an aseptic isolator and a containment isolator.[4]

Containment isolator: A ventilated isolator designed to prevent the toxic materials processed inside it from escaping to the surrounding environment.[4]

Laboratory coat: A disposable or reusable open-front coat, usually made of cloth or other permeable material.[4]

Material safety data sheet: Contains summaries provided by the manufacturer to describe the chemical properties and hazards of specific chemicals and ways in which workers can protect themselves from exposure to these chemicals.[4]

Mutagenic: Capable of increasing the spontaneous mutation rate by causing changes in DNA.[4]

Personal protective equipment (PPE): Items such as gloves, gowns, respirators, goggles, and face shields that protect individual workers from hazardous physical or chemical exposures.[4]

Respirator: A type of PPE that prevents harmful materials from entering the respiratory system, usually by filtering hazardous agents from workplace air. A surgical mask does not offer respiratory protection.[4]

Risk assessment: Characterization of potentially adverse health effects from human exposure to environmental or occupational hazards. Risk assessment can be divided into five major steps: hazard identification, dose–response assessment, exposure assessment, risk characterization, and risk communication.[4]

Surface decontamination: Transfer of hazardous drug contamination from the surface of nondisposable items to disposable ones (e.g., wipes, gauze, towels). No procedures have been studied for surface decontamination of hazardous drug contaminated surfaces. The use of gauze moistened with alcohol, sterile water, peroxide, or sodium hypochlorite solutions may be effective. The disposable item, once contaminated, must be contained and discarded as hazardous waste.

Ventilated cabinet: A type of engineering control designed for purposes of worker protection (as used in these guidelines). These devices are designed to minimize worker exposures by controlling emissions of airborne contaminants through (1) the full or partial enclosure of a potential contaminant source, (2) the use of airflow capture velocities to capture and remove airborne contaminants near their point of generation, and (3) the use of air pressure relationships that define the direction of airflow into the cabinet. Examples of ventilated cabinets include BSCs, containment isolators, and laboratory fume hoods.[4]

Developed through the ASHP Council on Professional Affairs and approved by the ASHP Board of Directors on January 12, 2006.

These guidelines supersede the ASHP technical assistance bulletin on handling cytotoxic and hazardous drugs (*Am J Hosp Pharm.* 1990; 47:1033–49).

Luci A. Power, M.S., is gratefully acknowledged for leading the revision of these guidelines. ASHP acknowledges the following individuals for their contributions to these guidelines: Thomas H. Connor, Ph.D., CAPT (ret.) Joseph H. Deffenbaugh Jr., M.P.H., CDR Bruce R. Harrison, M.S., BCOP, Dayna McCauley, Pharm.D., BCOP, Melissa A. McDiarmid, M.D., M.P.H., Kenneth R. Mead, M.S., PE, and Martha Polovich, M.N., RN, AOCN.

The bibliographic citation for this document is as follows: American Society of Health-System Pharmacists. ASHP guidelines on handling hazardous drugs. *Am J Health-Syst Pharm.* 2006; 63:1172–93.

ASHP Guidelines on
Pharmacy-Prepared Ophthalmic Products

Pharmacists are frequently called on to prepare sterile products intended for ophthalmic administration when a suitable sterile ophthalmic product is not available from a licensed manufacturer. These products may be administered topically or by subconjunctival or intraocular (e.g., intravitreal and intracameral) injection and may be in the form of solutions, suspensions, or ointments.

The sterility of these products, as well as accuracy in the calculation and preparation of doses, is of great importance. Ocular infections and loss of vision caused by contamination of extemporaneously prepared ophthalmic products have been reported.[1,2] Drugs administered by subconjunctival or intraocular injection often have narrow therapeutic indices. In practice, serious errors in technique have occurred in the preparation of intravitreal solutions, which resulted in concentrations up to double the intended amounts.[3] To ensure adequate stability, uniformity, and sterility, ophthalmic products from licensed manufacturers should be used whenever possible.

The following guidelines are intended to assist pharmacists when extemporaneous preparation of ophthalmic products is necessary. These guidelines do not apply to the manufacturing of sterile pharmaceuticals as defined in state and federal laws and regulations. Other guidelines on extemporaneous compounding of ophthalmic products also have been published.[4,5]

1. Before compounding any product for ophthalmic use, the pharmacist should review documentation that substantiates the safety and benefit of the product when administered into the eye. If no such documentation is available, the pharmacist must employ professional judgment in determining suitability of the product for ophthalmic administration.

2. Important factors to be considered in preparing an ophthalmic medication include the following:[6]
 a. Sterility.
 b. Tonicity.
 c. pH, buffering.
 d. Inherent toxicity of the drug.
 e. Need for a preservative.
 f. Solubility.
 g. Stability in an appropriate vehicle.
 h. Viscosity.
 i. Packaging and storage of the finished product.

3. A written procedure for each ophthalmic product compounded should be established and kept on file and should be easily retrievable. The procedure should specify appropriate steps in compounding, including aseptic methods, and whether microbiologic filtration or terminal sterilization (e.g., autoclaving) of the finished product is appropriate.

4. Before preparation of the product is begun, mathematical calculations should be reviewed by another person or by an alternative method of calculation in order to minimize error. This approach is especially important for products, such as intraocular injections, for which extremely small doses are frequently ordered, necessitating multiple dilutions. Decimal errors in the preparation of these products may have serious consequences.

5. Accuracy in compounding ophthalmic products is further enhanced by the use of larger volumes, which tends to diminish the effect of errors in measurement caused by the inherent inaccuracy of measuring devices. Larger volumes, however, also necessitate special attention to adequate mixing procedures, especially for ointments.

6. Strict adherence to aseptic technique and proper sterilization procedures are crucial in the preparation of ophthalmic products. All extemporaneous compounding of ophthalmic products should be performed in a certified laminar airflow hood (or, for preparing cytotoxic or hazardous agents, a biological safety cabinet).[5] Only personnel trained and proficient in the techniques and procedures should prepare ophthalmic products. Quality-assurance principles for compounding sterile products should be followed, and methods should be established to validate all procedures and processes related to sterile product preparation. In addition, the following should be considered:
 a. Ingredients should be mixed in sterile empty containers. Individual ingredients often can first be drawn into separate syringes and then injected into a larger syringe by insertion of the needles into the needle-free tip of the larger syringe. The larger syringe should be of sufficient size to allow for proper mixing of ingredients.
 b. To maximize measurement accuracy, the smallest syringe appropriate for measuring the required volume should be used. When the use of a single syringe would require estimation of the volume (e.g., measuring 4.5 ml in a 5-ml syringe with no mark at the 4.5-ml level), the use of two syringes of appropriate capacities (or two separate syringe "loads") should be considered in order to provide a more accurate measurement.
 c. A fresh disposable needle and syringe should be used at each step to avoid contamination and prevent error due to residual contents.
 d. When multiple dilutions are required, the containers of interim concentrations should be labeled to avoid confusion.
 e. In the preparation of an ophthalmic product from either (1) a sterile powder that has been reconstituted or (2) a liquid from a glass ampul, the ingredients should be filtered through a 5-μm filter to remove any particulate matter.

7. For ophthalmic preparations that must be sterilized, an appropriate and validated method of sterilization should be determined on the basis of the characteristics of the particular product and container. Filtration of the preparation through a 0.22-μm filter into a sterile final container is a commonly used method; however, this method is not suitable for sterilizing ophthalmic

suspensions and ointments.[7] When an ophthalmic preparation is compounded from a nonsterile ingredient, the final product must be sterilized before it is dispensed. Sterilization by autoclaving in the final container may be possible, provided that product stability is not adversely affected and appropriate quality control procedures are followed.[6]

8. Preservative-free ingredients should be used in the preparation of intraocular injections, since some preservatives are known to be toxic to many of the internal structures of the eye.[6]

9. In the preparation of ophthalmic products from cytotoxic or other hazardous agents, the pharmacist should adhere to established safety guidelines for handling such agents.[8,9]

10. The final container should be appropriate for the ophthalmic product and its intended use and should not interfere with the stability and efficacy of the preparation.[10] Many ophthalmic liquids can be packaged in sterile plastic bottles with self-contained dropper tips or in glass bottles with separate droppers. Ophthalmic ointments should be packaged in sterilized ophthalmic tubes. Injectables that are not for immediate use should be packaged in sterile vials rather than in syringes, and appropriate overfill should be included. All containers should be adequately sealed to prevent contamination.

11. The pharmacist should assign appropriate expiration dates to extemporaneously prepared ophthalmic products; these dates should be based on documented stability data as well as the potential for microbial contamination of the product.[11] The chemical stability of the active ingredient, the preservative, and packaging material should be considered in determining the overall stability of the final ophthalmic product.[12]

12. Ophthalmic products should be clearly and accurately labeled. In some cases, it may be appropriate to label the products with both the weight and concentration of active ingredients and preservatives. Labels should also specify storage and handling requirements and expiration dates. Extemporaneously prepared ophthalmic products dispensed for outpatient use should be labeled in accordance with applicable state regulations for prescription labeling.

References

1. Associated Press. Pittsburgh woman loses eye to tainted drugs; 12 hurt. *Baltimore Sun.* 1990; Nov 9:3A.

2. Associated Press. Eye drop injuries prompt an FDA warning. *N Y Times.* 1990; 140(Dec 9):391.

3. Jeglum EL, Rosenberg SB, Benson WE. Preparation of intravitreal drug doses. *Ophthalmic Surg.* 1981; 12:355–9.

4. Reynolds LA. Guidelines for preparation of sterile ophthalmic products. *Am J Hosp Pharm.* 1991; 48:2438–9.

5. Reynolds LA, Closson R. Ophthalmic drug formulations. A handbook of extemporaneous products. Vancouver, WA: Applied Therapeutics; (in press).

6. The United States Pharmacopeia, 22nd rev., and The National Formulary, 17th ed. Rockville, MD: The United States Pharmacopeial Convention; 1989:1692–3.

7. Allen LV. Indomethacin 1% ophthalmic suspension. *US Pharm.* 1991; 16(May):82–3.

8. American Society of Hospital Pharmacists. ASHP technical assistance bulletin on handling cytotoxic and hazardous drugs. *Am J Hosp Pharm.* 1990; 47:1033–49.

9. OSHA work-practice guidelines for personnel dealing with cytotoxic (antineoplastic) drugs. *Am J Hosp Pharm.* 1986; 43:1193–204.

10. Ansel HC, Popovich NG. Pharmaceutical dosage forms and drug delivery systems. 5th ed. Philadelphia: Lea & Febiger; 1990:354–7.

11. Stolar MH. Expiration dates of repackaged drug products. *Am J Hosp Pharm.* 1979; 36:170. Editorial.

12. Remington's pharmaceutical sciences. 19th ed. Gennaro AR, ed. Easton, PA: Mack Publishing; 1990:1581–959.

These guidelines were reviewed in 2008 by the Council on Pharmacy Practice and by the Board of Directors and were found to still be appropriate.

Approved by the ASHP Board of Directors, April 21, 1993. Developed by the ASHP Council on Professional Affairs.

The bibliographic citation for this document is as follows: American Society of Hospital Pharmacists. ASHP technical assistance bulletin on pharmacy-prepared ophthalmic products. *Am J Hosp Pharm.* 1993; 50:1462–3.

ASHP Guidelines on Quality Assurance for Pharmacy-Prepared Sterile Products

Patient morbidity and mortality have resulted from incorrectly prepared or contaminated pharmacy-prepared products.[1-7] Pharmacists seldom know that inaccurate or contaminated products are dispensed when pharmacy quality monitors are inadequate.[8-10] In contemporary health care organizations, more patients are receiving compounded sterile products that are stored for extended periods before use (allowing the growth of a pathological bioload of microorganisms[11]), more patients are seriously ill, and more patients are immunocompromised than ever before.

These ASHP guidelines are intended to help pharmacists and pharmacy technicians prepare sterile products of high quality.[a] The pharmacist is responsible for compounding and dispensing sterile products of correct ingredient identity, purity (freedom from physical contaminants, such as precipitates,[12] and chemical contaminants), strength (including stability[13] and compatibility), and sterility and for dispensing them in appropriate containers, labeled accurately and appropriately for the end user.

Other professional organizations have published useful guidelines on compounding and dispensing sterile products. The United States Pharmacopeia (USP) publishes the official compendium *The United States Pharmacopeia and The National Formulary (USP)* and its supplements, all of which may have legal implications for pharmacists.[14,15] The reader would especially benefit from studying the *USP* general information chapter on sterile drug products for home use,[13] which is referred to often in this ASHP guideline. The National Association of Boards of Pharmacy (NABP) has published less detailed model regulations for use by state boards of pharmacy.[16,17] The American Society for Parenteral and Enteral Nutrition (A.S.P.E.N.) recently published a special report on safe practices for parenteral nutrition formulations.[18]

Other governmental and accreditation sources are more general. The Joint Commission on Accreditation of Healthcare Organizations (JCAHO) publishes at least four sets of standards that mention pharmacy compounding. The hospital accreditation standards simply state that the organization adheres to laws, professional licensure, and practice standards governing the safe operation of pharmaceutical services.[19] The JCAHO home care standards require that medications be safely prepared, including "using appropriate techniques for preparing sterile and nonsterile medications and products." For example, the home care standards state that "appropriate quality-control techniques are used to check for preparation accuracy and absence of microbial contamination. Techniques for preparing sterile products follow guidelines established by the American Society of Health-System Pharmacists."[20] The JCAHO standards for long-term-care pharmacies list important conditions for product preparation, such as separate areas for sterile product preparation, use of a laminar-airflow workbench or class 100 cleanroom, and quality control systems to ensure the accuracy and sterility of final products.[21] The JCAHO standard for ambulatory care infusion centers states, among other things, several facility-related standards, for example the use of biological safety cabinets to protect personnel preparing cytotoxic or hazardous medications; work surfaces free of equipment, supplies, records, and labels unrelated to the medication being prepared; and a separate area for preparing sterile products that is constructed to minimize opportunities for particulate and microbial contamination.[22]

The Food and Drug Administration (FDA) publishes regulations on current good manufacturing practices that apply to sterile products made by pharmaceutical manufacturers for shipment in interstate commerce. Pursuant to the FDA Modernization Act of 1997 (FDAMA), Section 503A of the Food, Drug, and Cosmetic Act states that pharmacy compounding must comply with an applicable *USP* monograph, if one exists, and the *USP* chapter on pharmacy compounding[14] or be a component of an FDA-approved drug product; or, if neither of these apply to the ingredient being compounded, the substance must appear on a list of bulk drug substances developed by FDA and must be accompanied by a valid certificate of analysis and be manufactured in an FDA-registered establishment.[23] Inactive ingredients compounded by licensed pharmacies must comply with applicable *USP* monographs, if they exist, and the *USP* chapter on pharmacy compounding.[14] FDAMA prohibits pharmacists from compounding drug products that appear on a list of products that have been withdrawn or removed from the market because they have been found unsafe or ineffective. FDAMA also says that pharmacists may not compound, regularly or in inordinate amounts, drug products that are essentially copies of commercially available drug products; nor may they compound drug products identified by regulation as presenting demonstrable difficulties for compounding that reasonably demonstrate an adverse effect on safety or effectiveness.

The Centers for Disease Control and Prevention (CDC) has published guidelines for hand washing, prevention of intravascular infections, and hospital environmental control.[24,25]

The ASHP Guidelines on Quality Assurance for Pharmacy-Prepared Sterile Products are applicable to pharmaceutical services in various practice settings, including, but not limited to, hospitals, community pharmacies, nursing homes, ambulatory care infusion centers, and home care organizations. ASHP has also published practice standards on handling cytotoxic and hazardous drugs[26] and on pharmacy-prepared ophthalmic products.[27] These ASHP guidelines *do not* apply to the *manufacture* of sterile pharmaceuticals as defined in state and federal laws and regulations, *nor* do they apply to the preparation of medications by pharmacists, nurses, or physicians in emergency situations for *immediate* administration to patients (e.g., cardiopulmonary resuscitation). All guidelines may not be applicable to the preparation of radiopharmaceuticals.

These guidelines are referenced with supporting scientific data when such data exist. In the absence of published supporting data, guidelines are based on expert opinion or generally accepted pharmacy procedures. Pharmacists are urged to use professional judgment in interpreting these guidelines and applying them in practice. It is recognized that, in certain emergency situations, a pharmacist may be requested to compound products under conditions that do not meet these guidelines. In such situations, it is incumbent upon the pharmacist to employ professional judgment in

weighing the potential patient risks and benefits associated with the compounding procedure in question.

Objectives. The objectives of these guidelines are to provide

1. Information on quality assurance and quality control activities that should be applied to the preparation of sterile products in pharmacies and
2. A method to match quality assurance and quality control activities with the potential risks to patients posed by various types of products.

Multidisciplinary Input. Pharmacists are urged to participate in the quality or performance improvement, risk management, and infection control programs of their health care organizations, including developing optimal sterile product procedures.

Definitions. Definitions of selected terms, as used in this document, are provided in Appendix A. For brevity in this document, the term *quality assurance* will be used to refer to both quality assurance and quality control (as defined in Appendix A), as befits the circumstances.

Risk-Level Classification

In this document, sterile products are grouped into three levels of risk to the patient, increasing from least (level 1) to greatest (level 3) potential risk based on the danger of exposing multiple patients to inaccurate ingredients or pathogens and based on microbial growth factors influenced by product storage time, temperature and product ability to support microbial growth, surface and time exposure of critical sites, and microbial bioload in the environment. When circumstances make risk-level assignment unclear, guidelines for the higher risk level should prevail. Consideration should be given to factors that increase potential risk to the patient such as high-risk administration sites and immunocompromised status of the patient. A comparison of risk-level attributes appears in Appendix B.

Risk Level 1. Risk level 1 applies to compounded sterile products that exhibit characteristics 1, 2, *and* 3, stated below. All risk level 1 products should be prepared with sterile equipment (e.g., syringes and vials), sterile ingredients and solutions, and sterile contact surfaces for the final product. Risk level 1 includes the following:

1. Products
 a. Stored at room temperature (see Appendix A for temperature definitions) and completely administered within 28 hours after preparation or
 b. Stored under refrigeration for 7 days or less before complete administration to a patient over a period not to exceed 24 hours (Table 1) or
 c. Frozen for 30 days or less before complete administration to a patient over a period not to exceed 24 hours.
2. Unpreserved sterile products prepared for administration to one patient or batch-prepared products containing suitable preservatives prepared for administration to more than one patient.
3. Products prepared by closed-system aseptic transfer of sterile, nonpyrogenic, finished pharmaceuticals

(e.g., from vials or ampuls)[b] obtained from licensed manufacturers into sterile final containers (e.g., syringes, minibags, elastomeric containers, portable infusion-device cassettes) obtained from licensed manufacturers.

Examples of risk level 1 processes include transferring a sterile drug product from a vial into a commercially produced i.v. bag; compounding total parenteral nutrient (TPN) solutions by combining dextrose injection and amino acids injection via gravity transfer into a sterile empty container, with or without the subsequent addition of sterile drug products to the final container with a sterile needle and syringe; and transferring a sterile, preserved drug product into sterile syringes with the aid of a mechanical pump and appropriate sterile transfer tubing device.

Risk Level 2. Risk level 2 sterile products exhibit characteristic 1, 2, *or* 3, stated below. All risk level 2 products should be prepared with sterile equipment, sterile ingredients and solutions, and sterile contact surfaces for the final product and with closed-system transfer methods. Risk level 2 includes the following:

1. Products stored beyond 7 days under refrigeration, stored beyond 30 days frozen, or administered beyond 28 hours after preparation and storage at room temperature (Table 1).
2. Batch-prepared products *without preservatives* (e.g., epidural products) that are intended for use by more than one patient. (Note: Batch-prepared products without preservatives that will be administered to multiple patients carry a greater risk to the patients than products prepared for a single patient because of the potential effect of inaccurate ingredients or product contamination on the health and well-being of a larger patient group.)
3. Products compounded by complex or numerous manipulations of sterile ingredients obtained from licensed manufacturers in a sterile container or reservoir obtained from a licensed manufacturer by using closed-system aseptic transfer; for example, TPN solutions prepared with an automated compounder. (Note: So many risks have been associated with automated compounding of TPN solutions that its complexity requires risk level 2 procedures.[18])

Examples of risk level 2 processes include preparing portable-pump reservoirs for multiday (i.e., ambient temperature) administration; subdividing the contents of a bulk, sterile injectable (without preservatives) into single-dose syringes; and compounding TPN solutions with an automated compounding device involving repeated attachment of fluid containers to proximal openings of the compounder tubing set and of empty final containers to the distal opening, the process concluding with the transfer of additives into the filled final container from individual drug product containers or from a pooled additive solution.

Risk Level 3. Risk level 3 products exhibit either characteristic 1 *or* 2:

1. Products compounded from nonsterile ingredients or compounded with nonsterile components, containers, or equipment before terminal sterilization.

Table 1.
Assignment of Products to Risk Level 1 or 2 according to Time and Temperature before Completion of Administration

Risk Level	Room Temperature (15–30 °C)	No. Days Storage	
		Refrigerator (2–8 °C)	Freezer (–20 to –10°C)
1	Completely administered within 28 hr	≤7	≤30
2	Storage and administration exceed 28 hr	>7	>30

2. Products prepared by combining multiple ingredients—sterile or nonsterile—by using an open-system transfer or open reservoir before terminal sterilization.

Examples of risk level 3 products are calcium levulinate injection, estradiol in oil injection, and morphine sulfate 50-mg/mL injection.[32]

Quality Assurance for Risk Level 1

RL 1. 1: Policies and Procedures.[33] Up-to-date policies and procedures for compounding sterile products should be written and available to all personnel involved in these activities. When policies and procedures are changed they should be updated, as necessary, to reflect current standards of practice and quality. Additions, revisions, and deletions should be communicated to all personnel involved in sterile compounding and related activities. These policies and procedures should address personnel education and training requirements, competency evaluation, product acquisition, storage and handling of products and supplies, storage and delivery of final products, use and maintenance of facilities and equipment,[34] appropriate garb and conduct for personnel working in the controlled area, process validation, preparation technique,[35] labeling, documentation, and quality control.[36] Further, written policies and procedures should address personnel access and movement of materials into and near the controlled area. Policies and procedures for monitoring environmental conditions in the controlled area should take into consideration the amount of exposure of the product to the environment during compounding and the environmental control devices used to create the critical area. Sources of information include vendor-supplied inservice programs and multimedia training programs, such as videotapes and Internet-site information. Before compounding sterile products, all personnel involved should read the policies and procedures. Written policies and procedures are required for all environmental control devices used to create the critical area for manipulation of sterile products. Examples of such devices are laminar-airflow workstations, biological safety cabinets, class 100 cleanrooms, and barrier isolator workstations (see Appendix A).[c]

RL 1.2: Personnel Education, Training, and Evaluation. Training is the most important factor in ensuring the quality of sterile products. Pharmacy personnel preparing or dispensing sterile products must receive suitable didactic and experiential training and competency evaluation through demonstration, testing (written or practical), or both. Some aspects that should be included in training programs include aseptic technique; critical-area contamination factors; environmental monitoring; facilities, equipment, and supplies; sterile product calculations and terminology; sterile product compounding documentation; quality assurance procedures; aseptic preparation procedures; proper gowning and gloving

technique; and general conduct in the controlled area. In addition to knowledge of chemical, pharmaceutical, and clinical properties of drugs, pharmacists should be knowledgeable about the principles of pharmacy compounding.[14] Videotapes[37,38] and additional information on the essential components of a training, orientation, and evaluation program are described elsewhere.[39,40] All pharmacy and nonpharmacy personnel (e.g., environmental services staff) who work in the controlled area should receive documented training on cleaning, sanitizing, and maintaining equipment used in the controlled area. Training should be specific to the environmental control device and equipment present in the controlled area and should be based on current procedures.

The aseptic technique of each person preparing sterile products should be observed and evaluated as satisfactory during orientation and training and at least annually thereafter.[41] In addition to observation, methods of evaluating the knowledge of personnel include written or practical tests and process validation.[42,43]

RL 1.3: Storage and Handling within the Pharmacy.[44] Solutions, drugs, supplies, and equipment used to prepare or administer sterile products should be stored in accordance with manufacturer or *USP* requirements. Temperatures in refrigerators and freezers used to store ingredients and finished sterile preparations should be monitored and documented daily to ensure that compendial storage requirements are met. Warehouse and other pharmacy storage areas where ingredients are stored should be monitored to ensure that temperature, light, moisture, and ventilation remain within manufacturer and compendial requirements. To permit adequate floor cleaning, drugs, supplies, and compounding equipment should be stored on shelving, cabinets, and carts above the floor. Products that have exceeded their expiration dates should be removed from active storage areas. Before use, each drug, ingredient, and container should be visually inspected for damage, defects, and expiration date.[45]

Unnecessary personnel traffic in the controlled area should be minimized. Particle-generating activities, such as removal of intravenous solutions, drugs, and supplies from cardboard boxes, should not be performed in the controlled area. Products and supplies used in preparing sterile products should be removed from shipping containers outside the controlled area before aseptic processing is begun. Packaging materials and items generating unacceptable amounts of particles (e.g., cardboard boxes, paper towels [unless lint-free], reference books) should not be permitted in the controlled area or critical area. The removal of immediate packaging designed to retain the sterility or stability of a product (e.g., syringe packaging, light-resistant pouches) is an exception; obviously, this type of packaging should not be removed outside the controlled area. Disposal of packaging materials, used syringes, containers, and needles should be performed

at least daily, and more often if needed, to enhance sanitation and avoid accumulation in the controlled area. Trash cans should be below the level of the laminar-airflow workbench and should be removed from the controlled area before being emptied. Sharps containers should be safely placed into the waste stream, according to policies developed by the institution to comply with regulations of the Occupational Safety and Health Administration (OSHA).

In the event of a product recall, there should be a mechanism for tracking and retrieving affected products from specific patients to whom the products were dispensed.

RL 1.4: Facilities[46] and Equipment.[47]

The controlled area should be a limited-access area sufficiently separated from other pharmacy operations to minimize the potential for contamination that could result from the unnecessary flow of materials and personnel into and out of the area. The controlled area is a buffer from outside air that is needed because strong air currents from briefly opened doors, personnel walking past the laminar-airflow workbench, or the air stream from the heating, ventilating, and air conditioning system can easily exceed the velocity of air from the laminar-airflow workbench. Also, operators introducing supplies into the laminar-airflow workbench or reaching in with their arms can drag contaminants from the environment surrounding the workbench.[15] Cleanliness of the controlled area can be enhanced by (1) limiting access to those personnel assigned to work in the controlled area, (2) having those personnel wear the appropriate garb, (3) donning and removing garb outside the controlled area, (4) keeping doors to the controlled area closed, (5) limiting storage in the controlled area to items in constant use, (6) using low-particulate shelving, counters, and carts (e.g., stainless steel) in the controlled area, (7) not allowing cardboard and other particle-generating materials in the controlled area, (8) controlling the temperature and humidity inside the room, and (9) implementing a regular cleaning (e.g., nightly floor disinfection) and maintenance schedule.[48]

Barrier isolator workstations are closed systems and are not as sensitive to their external environment as laminar-airflow equipment. It is good practice to (1) place barrier isolator workstations in limited-access areas, (2) control the temperature and humidity of the surrounding area, and (3) clean and sanitize the surrounding area on a routine basis.[49]

Special precautions should be taken to clean equipment and compounding areas meticulously after preparing products that contain allergenic ingredients (e.g., sulfonamides and penicillins). Equipment should be of appropriate design and size for compounding and suitable for the intended uses. Equipment and accessories used in compounding should be inspected, maintained, and cleaned at appropriate intervals to ensure the accuracy and reliability of their performance.[14]

Computer entry, order processing, label generation, and record keeping should be performed outside the critical area. The controlled area should be well organized[50] and lighted[51] and of sufficient size to support sterile compounding activities. For hand washing, a sink with hot and cold running water should be in close proximity to but outside the controlled area. Refrigeration, freezing, ventilation, and room temperature control capabilities appropriate for storage of ingredients, supplies, and pharmacy-prepared sterile products in accordance with manufacturer, USP, and state or federal requirements should exist. The controlled area should be cleaned and disinfected at regular intervals with appropriate agents,

according to written policies and procedures.[52] Disinfectants should be alternated periodically to prevent development of resistant microorganisms.[d] The floors of the controlled area should be nonporous and washable to enable regular disinfection. Active work surfaces in the controlled area (e.g., carts, compounding devices, counter surfaces) should be disinfected, in accordance with written procedures. Refrigerators, freezers, shelves, and other areas where pharmacy-prepared sterile products are stored should be kept clean.

Sterile products must be prepared in a class 100 environment (i.e., the critical area).[29] Such an environment exists inside a certified horizontal- or vertical-laminar-airflow workbench, a class 100 cleanroom, or a barrier isolator.[53] Cytotoxic and other hazardous products should be prepared in a vented class II biological safety cabinet or a barrier isolator of appropriate design to meet the personnel exposure limits described in product material safety data sheets (MSDS).[54] Barrier isolators are gaining favor as clean environments, especially for cytotoxic drug compounding.[55–57] Properly maintained barrier isolators provide suitable environments for the preparation of risk level 1, 2, and 3 sterile products.[58]

Laminar-airflow workbenches are designed to be operated continuously. If a laminar-airflow workbench is turned off between aseptic processes, it should be operated long enough to allow complete purging of room air from the critical area (e.g., at least 30 minutes), then disinfected before use. Barrier isolators, because of their closed nature, require less start-up time. If the barrier isolator has been turned off for less than 24 hours, a two-minute start-up time is sufficient. For periods greater than 24 hours, the chamber should be sanitized and the isolator should not be used for a minimum of 10 minutes after application of the sanitizing agent. The critical-area work surface and all accessible interior surfaces of the workbench should be disinfected with an appropriate agent before work begins and periodically thereafter, in accordance with written policies and procedures.[52] The exterior surfaces of the laminar-airflow workbench should be cleaned periodically with a mild detergent or suitable disinfectant; 70% isopropyl alcohol may damage the workbench's clear plastic surfaces. The laminar-airflow workbench should be certified by a qualified contractor[59] every six months[53] or when it is relocated to ensure operational efficiency and integrity. Prefilters in the laminar-airflow workbench should be changed (or cleaned, if they are washable) periodically (e.g., monthly), in accordance with written policies and procedures.

A method should be established for calibrating and verifying the accuracy of automated compounding devices used in aseptic processing (e.g., routine reconstitution of bulk or individual vials, transferring of doses from a bulk container to a minibag, syringe, or other single-dose container).

RL 1.5: Garb.[60]

Procedures should require that personnel wear clean gowns or coveralls that generate few particles in the controlled area.[53] Scrub attire by itself is not acceptable (but can, like street clothes, be covered by a gown or coverall). Hand, finger, and wrist jewelry should be minimized or eliminated. Fingernails should be kept clean and trimmed. Head and facial hair should be covered. Masks are recommended because most personnel talk[61] or may cough or sneeze. Gloves are recommended. Personnel who have demonstrated sensitivity to latex should use either powder-free, low-latex protein gloves or, in the case of severe allergy, latex-free (synthetic) gloves.[62,63]

RL 1.6: Aseptic Technique[64,65] and Product Preparation.[66]
Sterile products must be prepared with aseptic technique in a class 100 environment. Personnel should scrub their hands and forearms for an appropriate length of time with a suitable antimicrobial skin cleanser at the beginning of each aseptic compounding process and when reentering the controlled area, in accordance with written procedures. Personnel should wear appropriate attire (see RL 1.5: Garb). Eating, drinking, and smoking are prohibited in the controlled area. Talking should be minimized in the critical area during aseptic preparation (even when masks are worn).

Ingredients used to compound sterile products should be determined to be stable, compatible, and appropriate for the product to be prepared, according to manufacturer or USP guidelines or appropriate scientific references. The ingredients of the preparation should be predetermined to result in a final product that meets physiological norms for solution osmolality and pH, as appropriate for the intended route of administration. Each ingredient and container should be inspected for defects, expiration date, and product integrity before use. Expired, inappropriately stored, or defective products must not be used in preparing sterile products. Defective products should be promptly reported to the FDA MedWatch Program.[67]

Only materials essential for preparing the sterile product should be placed in the laminar-airflow workbench or barrier isolator. The surfaces of ampuls, vials, and container closures (e.g., vial stoppers) should be disinfected by swabbing or spraying with an appropriate disinfectant solution (e.g., 70% isopropyl alcohol or 70% ethanol) before placement in the workbench. Materials used in aseptic preparation should be arranged in the critical area (within the laminar-airflow workbench or barrier isolator) in a manner that prevents interruption of the unidirectional airflow between the high-efficiency particulate air (HEPA) filter and critical sites of needles, vials, ampuls, containers, and transfer sets. All aseptic procedures should be performed at least 6 inches inside the front edge of the laminar-airflow workbench, in a clear path of unidirectional airflow between the HEPA filter and work materials (e.g., needles, closures). The number of personnel preparing sterile products in the workbench at one time should be minimized. Overcrowding of the critical work area may interfere with unidirectional airflow and increase the potential for compounding errors. Likewise, the number of units being prepared in the workbench at one time should allow unobstructed airflow over critical areas. Automated compounding devices and other equipment placed in or adjacent to the critical area should be cleaned, disinfected, and placed to avoid contamination or disruption of the unidirectional airflow between the HEPA filter and sterile surfaces. Closed systems like barrier isolators require less stringent placement of sterile units and equipment because the critical area encompasses the entire work surface. Hand and arm movements are not critical because the walls of the barrier isolator provide protection from the outside environment.[50]

Aseptic technique should be used to avoid touch contamination of sterile needles, syringe parts (e.g., plunger, syringe tip), and other critical sites. Solutions from ampuls should be properly filtered to remove particles. Solutions of reconstituted powders should be mixed carefully, ensuring complete dissolution of the drug with the appropriate diluent. Needle entry into vials should be performed in such a manner as to avoid coring of the vial closure. Some patients may require a latex-free admixture to avoid severe allergic reactions.[68] Latex-related policies and procedures should be developed by each institution, given the paucity of evidence that latex closures and syringe plungers are implicated in patient reactions to latex.[69,70] Before, during, and after the preparation of sterile products, the pharmacist should carefully check the identity and verify the amounts and sequence of the additives in sterile preparations against the original prescription, medication order, or other appropriate documentation (e.g., computerized patient profile, label generated from a pharmacist-verified order) before the product is released or dispensed.

RL 1.7: Process Validation.[71] Validation of aseptic processing procedures provides a mechanism for ensuring that processes consistently result in sterile products of acceptable quality.[10] In risk level 1, process validation (or process simulation) of compounding procedures is actually a method of assessing the adequacy of an operator's aseptic technique. Each individual involved in the preparation of sterile products should successfully complete a validation process on technique before being allowed to prepare sterile products. The validation process should follow written procedures.[42,43,45] Commercial kits are available for process validation; however, their ability to support microbial growth should be tested by challenging the intended kit with an indicator organism (e.g., *Bacillus stearothermophilus*) that can be purchased in known concentrations, is known not to be pathogenic, and grows only at relatively high temperatures.

Process simulation allows for the evaluation of opportunities for microbial contamination during all steps of sterile product preparation. The sterility of the final product is a cumulative function of all processes involved in its preparation and is ultimately determined by the processing step providing the lowest probability of sterility.[31] Process simulation testing is carried out in the same manner as normal production, except that an appropriate microbiological growth medium is used in place of the actual product used during sterile preparation. The same personnel, procedures, equipment, and materials are involved. Completed medium samples are incubated. If no microbial growth is detected, this provides evidence that adequate aseptic technique was used. If growth is detected, the entire sterile preparation process must be evaluated, corrective action taken, and the process simulation test performed again. No products intended for patient use should be prepared by an individual until the process simulation test indicates that the individual can competently perform aseptic procedures. It is recommended that personnel competency be revalidated at least annually, whenever the quality assurance program yields an unacceptable result, and whenever unacceptable techniques are observed; this revalidation should be documented.

RL 1.8: Expiration Dating.[72] All pharmacy-prepared sterile products should bear an appropriate expiration date. The expiration date assigned should be based on currently available drug stability information and sterility considerations. Sources of drug stability information include references (e.g., *AHFS Drug Information,*[73] *Extended Stability for Parenteral Drugs,*[74] *Handbook on Injectable Drugs,*[75] *King Guide to Parenteral Admixtures*[76]), manufacturer recommendations, and reliable, published research. When interpreting published drug stability information, the pharmacist should consider all aspects of the final sterile product being prepared (e.g., drug reservoir, drug concentration, storage conditions). Methods used for establishing expiration dates should be documented.

Appropriate inhouse (or contract service) stability testing may be used to determine expiration dates when drug stability data are not readily available. Home care pharmacies are often required to assign extended beyond-use dates to sterile products, so ASHP has published guidelines for home care pharmacies that address beyond-use dating.[74,77]

RL 1.9: Labeling.[78] Sterile products should be labeled with at least the following information:

1. For patient-specific products: the patient' name and any other appropriate patient identification (e.g., location, identification number); for batch-prepared products: control or lot number,
2. All solution and ingredient names, amounts, strengths, and concentrations (when applicable),
3. Expiration date and time, when applicable,
4. Prescribed administration regimen, when appropriate (including rate and route of administration),
5. Appropriate auxiliary labeling (including precautions),
6. Storage requirements,
7. Identification (e.g., initials) of the responsible pharmacist (and technician),
8. Device-specific instructions (when appropriate), and
9. Any additional information, in accordance with state or federal requirements; for example, a prescription number for products dispensed to ambulatory care, long-term-care, and home care patients.

The label should be legible and affixed to the final container in a manner enabling it to be read while the sterile product is being administered (when possible). Written policies and procedures should address proper placement of labels on containers.[79]

RL 1.10: End-Product Evaluation.[80] The final product should be inspected when preparation is completed and again when the product is dispensed. This inspection includes an evaluation for container leaks, container integrity, solution cloudiness or phase separation, particulates in the solution, appropriate solution color, and solution volume. The responsible pharmacist should verify that the product was compounded accurately with the correct ingredients, quantities of each ingredient, containers, and reservoirs; different methods may be used for end-product verification (e.g., observation, calculation checks, documented records). Refractive index measurement may also be used to verify the addition of dextrose, for example in parenteral nutrient solutions.[81]

RL 1.11: Handling of Sterile Products Outside the Pharmacy.[82] Pharmacists should participate in developing procedures for the safe use (e.g., stability, sterility) of sterile products once they are distributed outside the pharmacy. How the product is transported from the pharmacy, how it is stored outside the pharmacy, and methods for return, recycling, and disposal should be addressed in written policies and procedures.[15,83] Sterile products should be transported so as to be protected from extremes of temperature outside their range of stability and from light if they are photosensitive. Storage containers and packaging verified as suitable for protection during transport should be specified. Transit time and conditions should also be specified and controlled. Delivery personnel should be instructed on special handling procedures. Once

delivered to the end user, sterile products should be appropriately stored before use. Pharmacists should ascertain that the user has appropriate locations and equipment for storage (e.g., a refrigerator with a suitable thermometer). Special instructions for storage should be a part of the label or a separate information sheet (e.g., instructions for cleanliness, proper storage, interpretation of the expiration date and how to look for signs of product deterioration). The pharmacist should be notified if storage conditions do not remain suitable so that the pharmacist can give advice as to the disposition of the sterile products and remedies for storage problems. Pharmacists should participate in training end users on the proper care and storage of sterile products, either directly or through written instructional materials.

RL 1.12: Documentation.[84] The following should be documented and maintained on file for an adequate period of time, according to organizational policies and state regulatory requirements: (1) the training and competency evaluation of employees in sterile product procedures, (2) refrigerator and freezer temperatures, (3) certification of laminar-airflow workbenches, and (4) other facility quality control logs specific to the pharmacy's policies and procedures (e.g., cleaning logs for facilities and equipment). Pharmacists should also maintain appropriate dispensing records for sterile products, in accordance with state regulatory requirements.

Quality Assurance for Risk Level 2

Because the risks of inaccurate products are associated with more complex procedures and because instability and contamination are more likely with long-term storage and administration, more stringent requirements are appropriate for risk level 2 preparations. These requirements may be viewed as more important in circumstances where the medical need is *routine*. In circumstances where the medical need for a product is immediate (and there is not a suitable alternative) or when the preparation of such a product is rare, professional judgment should be applied to the extent to which some guidelines (e.g., cleanroom design and final product testing before product dispensing) must be applied.

RL 2.1: Policies and Procedures. In addition to all guidelines for risk level 1, a written quality assurance program should define and identify necessary environmental monitoring devices and techniques to be used to ensure an adequate environment for risk level 2 sterile product preparation. Examples include the use of airborne particle counters, air velocity and temperature meters, viable particle samplers (e.g., slit samplers), agar plates, and swab sampling of surfaces and potential contamination sites. All aspects of risk level 2 sterile product preparation, storage, and distribution, including such details as the choice of cleaning materials and disinfectants and the monitoring of equipment accuracy, should be addressed in written policies and procedures. Limits of acceptability (threshold or action levels) for environmental monitoring and process validation and actions to be implemented when thresholds are exceeded should be defined in written policies. For sterile batch compounding, written policies and procedures should be established for the use of master formulas and work sheets and for appropriate documentation. Policies and procedures should also address personnel attire in the controlled area, lot number determination and documentation, and any other quality assurance procedures unique to compounding risk level 2 sterile products.

RL 2.2: Personnel Education, Training, and Evaluation.
All guidelines for risk level 1 should be met. In addition to guidelines for risk level 1, assessment of the competency of personnel preparing risk level 2 sterile products should include appropriate process validation (as described in RL 1.7: Process validation). However, process simulation procedures for assessing the preparation of risk level 2 sterile products should be representative of all types of manipulations, products, and batch sizes personnel preparing risk level 2 products are likely to encounter.[15] Personnel should also be taught which products are to undergo end-product quantitative analysis (see RL 2.10).

RL 2.3: Storage and Handling. All storage and handling guidelines for risk level 1 should be met.

RL 2.4: Facilities and Equipment. In addition to all guidelines for risk level 1, the following guidelines should be followed for risk level 2 sterile product preparation:

1. The controlled area should meet the standards of a class 10,000 cleanroom,[e] as defined by Federal Standard 209E.[85,f] A positive air pressure relative to adjacent pharmacy areas is required, as are an appropriate number of air exchanges per hour and appropriate humidity and temperature levels.[86] For open-architecture cleanrooms, it is appropriate to measure the volume of air entering the cleanroom versus the volume of air entering adjacent rooms, so as to ensure a positive pressure gradient for the cleanroom. To allow proper cleaning and disinfection, walls, floors, and ceilings in the controlled area should be nonporous. To help reduce the number of particles in the controlled area, an adjacent support area (e.g., ante-room) should be provided. A properly maintained barrier isolator also provides an acceptable environment.[57] A barrier isolator provides a class 100 environment for product preparation; therefore, the isolator itself can be in a separate area of the pharmacy but need not actually be in a cleanroom.
2. Cleaning materials (e.g., mops, sponges, and germicidal disinfectants) for use in the cleanroom should be carefully selected. They should be made of materials that generate a low amount of particles. If reused, cleaning materials should be cleaned and disinfected between uses.
3. The critical-area work surfaces (e.g., interior of the laminar-airflow workbench) should be disinfected frequently and before and after each batch-preparation process with an appropriate agent, according to written policies and procedures. Floors should be disinfected at least daily. Carpet or porous floors, porous walls, and porous ceiling tiles are not suitable in the controlled area because these surfaces cannot be properly cleaned and disinfected. Exterior workbench surfaces and other hard surfaces in the controlled area, such as shelves, carts, tables, and stools, should be disinfected weekly and after any unanticipated event that could increase the risk of contamination. Walls should be cleaned at least monthly.
4. To ensure that an appropriate environment is maintained for risk level 2 sterile product preparation, an effective written environmental monitoring program is recommended.[87] Sampling of air and surfaces according to a written plan and schedule is recommended.[31] The plan and frequency should be adequate to document that the controlled area is suitable and that the laminar-airflow workbench or biological safety cabinet meets class 100 requirements. Limits of acceptability (thresholds or action levels) and appropriate actions to be taken in the event thresholds are exceeded should be specified. *USP* presents examples of environmental monitoring.[15] Settle plates or wipe samples can provide a simple but effective means of routinely monitoring airborne microbial contamination in controlled and critical areas.[45,88,89]
5. To help reduce the number of particles in the controlled area, an adjacent support area (e.g., anteroom) of high cleanliness, separated from the controlled area by a barrier (e.g., plastic curtain, partition, wall), is recommended. Appropriate activities for the support area include, but are not limited to, hand washing, gowning and gloving, removal of packaging and cardboard items, and cleaning and disinfecting hard-surface containers and supplies before placing these items into the controlled area.
6. Methods should be established for calibrating and verifying the accuracy and sterility of automated compounding methods used in aseptic processing.[90–96]

RL 2.5: Garb. All guidelines for risk level 1 should be met. Gloves, gowns, and masks are required for the preparation of all risk level 2 sterile products. Even when sterile gloves are used, they do not remain sterile during aseptic compounding; however, they do assist in containing bacteria, skin, and other particles that may be shed even from scrubbed hands. Clean gowns, coveralls, or closed jackets with sleeves having elastic binding at the cuff are recommended; these garments should be made of low-shedding materials. Shoe covers may be helpful in maintaining the cleanliness of the controlled area. Barrier isolators do not require the same level of gowning as laminar-airflow workstations as long as they operate as closed systems with HEPA filtration of air entering and leaving the barrier isolator and a separate area for entrance, such as an air lock for product transfers.

During sterile product preparation, gloves should be rinsed frequently with a suitable agent (e.g., 70% isopropyl alcohol) and changed when their integrity is compromised (i.e., when they are punctured or torn). Personnel should discard gloves upon leaving the cleanroom and don new gloves upon reentering the cleanroom.

RL 2.6: Aseptic Technique and Product Preparation.[97–99] All guidelines for risk level 1 sterile product preparation should be met. Relative to batch-prepared products, a master work sheet should be developed for a batch of each discrete identity and concentration of sterile product to be prepared. The master work sheet should consist of the formula, components, compounding directions or procedures, a sample label, and evaluation and testing requirements. Once the original master work sheet is approved by the designated pharmacist, a verified duplicate (e.g., a photocopy) of the master work sheet should be used as the preparation work sheet from which each batch is prepared and on which all documentation for each batch occurs. (For small-formula, frequently prepared batches, it may be more efficient to have multiple lines on the preparation work sheet for documenting more than one batch.) The preparation work sheet should be used to document the following:

1. Identity of all solutions and ingredients and their corresponding amounts, concentrations, or volumes,

2. Manufacturer lot number and expiration date for each component,
3. Component manufacturer or suitable manufacturer identification number,
4. Container specifications (e.g., syringe, pump cassette),
5. Lot or control number assigned to batch,
6. Expiration date of batch-prepared products,
7. Date of preparation,
8. Identity (e.g., initials, codes, signatures) of personnel involved in preparation,
9. End-product evaluation and testing specifications and results,
10. Storage requirements,
11. Specific equipment used during aseptic preparation (e.g., a specific automated compounding device), and
12. Comparison of actual yield with anticipated yield, when appropriate.

However documentation is done, a procedure should exist for easy retrieval of all records pertaining to a particular batch. Each batch of sterile products should bear a unique lot number. Identical lot numbers must never be assigned to different products or different batches of the same product. Lot numbers may be alphabetic, numeric, or alphanumeric.

The process of combining multiple sterile ingredients into a single sterile reservoir for subdivision into multiple units for dispensing may necessitate additional quality control procedures. A second pharmacist should verify calculations associated with this process, when possible; this verification should be documented. Because this process often involves making multiple entries into the intermediate sterile reservoir, the likelihood of contamination may be greater than that associated with the preparation of other risk level 2 sterile products.

For preparation involving automated compounding devices, a pharmacist should verify data entered into the compounding device before compounding begins. End-product checks should be performed to verify accuracy of ingredient delivery. These checks may include weighing and visually verifying the final product. For example, the expected weight (in grams) of the final product, based on the specific gravities of the ingredients and their respective volumes, can be documented on the compounding formula sheet, dated, and initialed by the responsible pharmacist. Once compounding is completed, each final product can be weighed and its weight compared with the expected weight. The product's actual weight should fall within a preestablished threshold for variance. Visual verification may be aided by marking the beginning level of each bulk container before starting the automated mixing process and checking each container after completing the mixing process to determine whether the final levels appear reasonable in comparison with expected volumes. The operator should also periodically observe the device during the mixing process to ensure that the device is operating properly (e.g., check to see that all stations are operating). If there are doubts whether a product or component has been properly prepared or stored, the product should not be used.

RL 2.7: Process Validation. Each individual involved in the preparation of risk level 2 sterile products should successfully complete a validation process, as recommended for risk level 1. Process simulation for compounding risk level 2 sterile products should be representative of all types of manipulations, products, and batch sizes that personnel preparing risk level 2 sterile products are likely to encounter.

RL 2.8: Expiration Dating. All guidelines for risk level 1 should be met.

RL 2.9: Labeling. All guidelines for risk level 1 should be met.

RL 2.10: End-Product Evaluation. All guidelines for risk level 1 should be met. For complex or toxic products, it is appropriate, when possible, to obtain quantitative testing of the accuracy of sterile additives, for example, the dextrose concentration in pediatric parenteral nutrient solutions or the potassium concentration in cardioplegia solutions.[g]

RL 2.11: Handling of Sterile Products Outside the Pharmacy. All guidelines for risk level 1 should be met.

RL 2.12: Documentation. All guidelines for risk level 1 should be met. Additionally, documentation of end-product sampling and batch-preparation records should be maintained for an adequate period, in accordance with organizational policies and procedures and state regulatory requirements.[100] Documentation for sterile batch-prepared products should include the

1. Master work sheet,
2. Preparation work sheet, and
3. End-product evaluation and testing results.

Quality Assurance for Risk Level 3

Risk level 3 addresses the preparation of products that pose the greatest potential risk to patients. The quality assurance activities described in this section are clearly more demanding—in terms of processes, facilities, and final product assessment—than for risk levels 1 and 2. Ideally, the activities described for risk level 3 would be used for all high-risk products. However, the activities may be viewed as most important in circumstances where the medical need for such high-risk products is *routine.* In circumstances where the medical need for such a product is immediate (and there is not a suitable alternative) or when the preparation of such a product is rare, professional judgment must be applied as to the extent to which some activities (e.g., strict facility design, quarantine, and final product testing before product dispensing) should be applied.

RL 3.1: Policies and Procedures. There should be written policies and procedures related to every aspect of preparation of risk level 3 sterile products. These policies and procedures should be detailed enough to ensure that all products have the identity, strength, quality, and purity purported for the product.[14,101] All policies and procedures should be reviewed and approved by the designated pharmacist. There should be a mechanism designed to ensure that policies and procedures are communicated, understood, and adhered to by personnel cleaning or working in the controlled area or support area. Written policies and procedures should define and identify the environmental monitoring activities necessary to ensure an adequate environment for risk level 3 sterile product preparation.

In addition to the policies and procedures required for risk levels 1 and 2, there should be written policies and procedures for the following:

1. Component selection, handling, and storage,
2. Any additional personnel qualifications commensurate with the preparation of risk level 3 sterile products,
3. Personnel responsibilities in the controlled area (e.g., sterilization, cleaning, maintenance, access to controlled area),
4. Equipment use, maintenance, calibration, and testing,
5. Sterilization and expiration dating,
6. Master formula and master work sheet development and use,
7. End-product evaluation and testing,
8. Appropriate documentation for preparation of risk level 3 sterile products,
9. Use, control, and monitoring of environmentally controlled areas and calibration of monitoring equipment,
10. Process simulation for each risk level 3 sterile product,
11. Quarantine of products and release from quarantine, if applicable,
12. A mechanism for recalling products from patients in the event that end-product testing procedures yield unacceptable results, and
13. Any other quality control procedures unique to the preparation of risk level 3 sterile products.

RL 3.2: Personnel Education, Training, and Evaluation.

Persons preparing sterile products at risk level 3 must have specific education, training, and experience to perform all functions required for the preparation of risk level 3 sterile products. However, final responsibility should lie with the pharmacist, who should be knowledgeable in pharmacy compounding practice[14] and proficient in quality assurance requirements, equipment used in the preparation of risk level 3 sterile products, and other aspects of sterile product preparation. The pharmacist should have sufficient education, training, experience, and demonstrated competency to ensure that all sterile products prepared from sterile or nonsterile components have the identity, strength, quality, and purity purported for the products.[101] In addition to the body of knowledge required for risk levels 1 and 2, the pharmacist should possess sufficient knowledge in the following areas:

1. Aseptic processing,
2. Quality control and quality assurance as related to environmental, component, and end-product testing,
3. Sterilization techniques,[98] and
4. Container, equipment, and closure system selection.

All pharmacy personnel involved in the cleaning and maintenance of the controlled area should be specially trained and thoroughly knowledgeable in the special requirements of class 100 critical-area technology and design. There should be documented, ongoing training for all employees to enable retention of expertise.

RL 3.3: Storage and Handling.

In addition to guidelines for risk levels 1 and 2, risk level 3 policies and procedures for storage and handling should include procurement, identification, storage, handling, testing, and recall of nonsterile components.[14,101]

Components and finished products ready to undergo end-product testing should be stored in a manner that prevents their use before release by a pharmacist, minimizes the risk of contamination, and enables identification. There should be identified storage areas that can be used to quarantine products, if necessary, before they are released.[15]

RL 3.4: Facilities and Equipment.

Preparation of risk level 3 sterile products should occur in a class 100 horizontal- or vertical-laminar-airflow workbench that is properly situated in a class 10,000 cleanroom *or* in a properly maintained and monitored class 100 cleanroom (without the workbench).[102] The cleanroom area should have a positive pressure differential relative to adjacent, less clean areas of at least 0.05 inch of water. A properly designed and maintained barrier isolator provides an aseptic environment for risk level 3 products.

To allow proper cleaning and disinfection, walls, floors, and ceilings in the controlled area should be nonporous. To help reduce the number of particles in the controlled area, an adjacent support area (e.g., anteroom) should be provided.

During the preparation of risk level 3 sterile products, access to the controlled area or cleanroom should be limited to those individuals who are required to be in the area and are properly attired. The environment of the main access areas directly adjacent to the controlled area (e.g., anteroom) should meet at least Federal Standard 209E class 100,000 requirements. To help maintain a class 100 critical-area environment during compounding, the adjacent support area (e.g., anteroom) should be separated from the controlled area by a barrier (e.g., plastic curtain, partition, wall). Written policies and procedures for monitoring the environment of the controlled area and adjacent areas should be developed.

No sterile products should be prepared in the controlled area if it fails to meet established criteria specified in the policies and procedures. A calibrated particle counter capable of measuring air particles 0.5 mm and larger should be used to monitor airborne particulate matter.[103] Before product preparation begins, the positive-pressure air status should meet or exceed the requirements. Air samples should be taken at several places in the controlled area with the appropriate environmental monitoring devices (e.g., nutrient agar plates). Surfaces on which work actually occurs, including laminar-airflow workbench surfaces and tabletops, should be monitored by using surface contact plates, the swab-rinse technique, or other appropriate methods.[104]

Test results should be reviewed and criteria should be preestablished to determine the point at which the preparation of risk level 3 sterile products will be disallowed until corrective measures are taken. When the environment does not meet the criteria specified in the policies and procedures, sterile product processing should immediately cease and corrective action should be taken. In the event that this occurs, written policies and procedures should delineate alternative methods of sterile product preparation to enable timely fulfillment of prescription orders.

Equipment should be adequate to prevent microbiological contamination. Methods should be established for the cleaning, preparation, sterilization, calibration, and documented use of all equipment.

Critical-area work surfaces should be disinfected with an appropriate agent before the preparation of each product. Floors in the controlled area should be disinfected at least daily. Exterior workbench surfaces and other hard surfaces in the controlled area, such as shelves, tables, and stools, should be disinfected weekly and after any unanticipated event that could increase the risk of contamination. Walls and ceilings in the controlled area or cleanroom should be disinfected at least weekly.

Large pieces of equipment, such as tanks, carts, and tables, used in the controlled area or cleanroom should be made of a material that can be easily cleaned and disinfected; stainless steel is recommended. Stools and chairs should be cleanroom

quality. Equipment that does not come in direct contact with the finished product should be properly cleaned, rinsed, and disinfected before being placed in the controlled area. All non-sterile equipment that will come in contact with the sterilized final product should be properly sterilized before introduction into the controlled area; this precaution includes such items as tubing, filters, containers, and other processing equipment. The sterilization process should be monitored and documented.[101]

RL 3.5: Garb. All guidelines for risk levels 1 and 2 should be met. Additionally, cleanroom garb should be worn inside the controlled area at all times during the preparation of risk level 3 sterile products. Attire should consist of a low-shedding coverall, head cover, face mask, and shoe covers. These garments may be either disposable or reusable. Head and facial hair should be covered. Before donning these garments over street clothes, personnel should thoroughly wash their hands and forearms with a suitable antimicrobial skin cleanser.[25] Sterile disposable gloves should be worn and rinsed frequently with an appropriate agent (e.g., 70% isopropyl alcohol) during processing. The gloves should be changed if their integrity is compromised. If persons leave the controlled area *or* support area during processing, they should regown with clean garments before reentering.

RL 3.6: Aseptic Technique and Product Preparation. All guidelines for risk levels 1 and 2 should be met. Methods should ensure that components and containers remain free from contamination and are easily identified as to the product, lot number, and expiration date. If components are not finished sterile pharmaceuticals obtained from licensed manufacturers, pharmacists should ensure that these components meet USP and FDA standards. Products prepared from nonsterile ingredients should be tested to ensure that they do not exceed specified endotoxin limits, unless the ingredient will denature all proteins (e.g., concentrated hydrochloric acid).[105] As each new lot of components and containers is received, the components should be quarantined until properly identified, tested, or verified by a pharmacist.[101]

The methods for preparing sterile products and using process controls should be designed to ensure that finished products have the identity, strength, quality, and purity they are intended to have. Any deviations from established methods should be documented and appropriately justified.

A master work sheet should be developed for the preparation of each risk level 3 sterile product. Once the pharmacist approves the master work sheet, a verified duplicate of the master work sheet should be used as the controlling document from which each sterile end product or batch of prepared products is compounded and on which all documentation for that product or batch occurs. The preparation work sheet should document all the requirements for risk level 2 plus the following:

1. Comparison of actual with anticipated yield,
2. Sterilization methods,[106,107]
3. Pyrogen testing,[108] and
4. Quarantine specifications.

The preparation work sheet should serve as the batch record for each time a risk level 3 sterile product is prepared. Each batch of pharmacy-prepared sterile products should bear a unique lot number, as described in risk level 2.

There should be documentation on the preparation work sheet of all additions of individual components plus the signatures or initials of those individuals involved in the measuring or weighing and addition of these components.

The selection of the final packaging system (including container and closure) for the sterile product is crucial to maintaining product integrity.[109] To the extent possible, presterilized containers obtained from licensed manufacturers should be used. If an aseptic filling operation is used, the container should be sterile at the time of the filling operation. If nonsterile containers are used, methods for sterilizing these containers should be established. Final containers selected should be capable of maintaining product integrity (i.e., identity, strength, quality, and purity) throughout the shelf life of the product.[110]

For products requiring sterilization, selection of an appropriate method of sterilization is of prime importance. Methods of product sterilization include sterile filtration, autoclaving, dry heat sterilization, chemical sterilization, and irradiation.[111,112] The pharmacist must ensure that the sterilization method used is appropriate for the product components and does not alter the pharmaceutical properties of the final product. A method of sterilization often used by pharmacists is sterile filtration.[113] In sterile filtration, the filter should be chosen to fit the chemical nature of the product, and the product should be filtered into presterilized containers under aseptic conditions. Sterilizing filters of 0.22-µm or smaller porosity should be used in this process. Colloidal or viscous products may require a 0.45-µm filter; however, extreme caution should be exercised in these circumstances, and more stringent end-product sterility testing is essential.[114]

To ensure that a bacteria-retentive filter did not rupture during filtration of a product, an integrity test should be performed on all filters immediately after filtration. This test may be accomplished by performing a bubble point test, in which pressurized gas (e.g., air in a syringe attached to the used filter) is applied to the upstream side of the filter with the downstream outlet immersed in water and the pressure at which a steady stream of bubbles begins to appear is noted.[98] The observed pressure is then compared with the manufacturer's specification for the filter. To compare the used filter with the manufacturer's specifications, which would be based on the filtration of water through the filter, it is necessary to first rinse the filter with sterile water for injection. An observed value lower than the manufacturer's specification indicates that the filter was defective or ruptured during the sterilization process. Methods should be established for handling, testing, and resterilizing any product processed with a filter that fails the integrity test.

RL 3.7: Process Validation. In addition to risk level 1 and 2 guidelines, written policies and procedures should be established to validate all processes involved in the preparation of risk level 3 sterile products (including all procedures, equipment, and techniques) from sterile or nonsterile components. In addition to evaluating personnel technique, process validation provides a mechanism for determining whether a particular process will, when performed by qualified personnel, consistently produce the intended results.[115]

RL 3.8: Expiration Dating. In addition to risk level 2 guidelines, there should be reliable methods for establishing all expiration dates, including laboratory testing of products for sterility, nonpyrogenicity, and chemical content, when

necessary. These tests should be conducted in a manner based on appropriate statistical criteria, and the results documented.

RL 3.9: Labeling. All guidelines for risk levels 1 and 2 should be met.

RL 3.10: End-Product Evaluation. For each preparation of a sterile product or a batch of sterile products, there should be appropriate laboratory determination of conformity (i.e., purity, accuracy, sterility, and nonpyrogenicity) to established written specifications and policies. Any reprocessed material should undergo complete final product testing. Additionally, process validation should be supplemented with a program of end-product sterility testing, according to a formal sampling plan.[116–127] Written policies and procedures should specify measurements and methods of testing. Policies and procedures should include a statistically valid sampling plan and acceptance criteria for the sampling and testing. The criteria should be statistically adequate to reasonably ensure that the entire batch meets all specifications. Products not meeting all specifications should be rejected and discarded. There should be a mechanism for recalling all products of a specific batch if end-product-testing procedures yield unacceptable results. On completion of final testing, products should be stored in a manner that ensures their identity, strength, quality, and purity.

It is advisable to quarantine sterile products compounded from nonsterile components, pending the results of end-product testing. If products prepared from nonsterile components must be dispensed before satisfactory completion of end-product testing, there must be a procedure to allow for immediate recall of the products from patients to whom they were dispensed.

RL 3.11: Handling of Sterile Products Outside the Pharmacy. All guidelines for risk levels 1 and 2 should be met.

RL 3.12: Documentation. In addition to the guidelines for risk levels 1 and 2, documentation for risk level 3 sterile products should include

1. Preparation work sheet,
2. Sterilization records of final products (if applicable),
3. Quarantine records (if applicable), and
4. End-product evaluation and testing results.

References

1. Hughes CF, Grant AF, Lick BD, et al. Cardioplegic solution: a contamination crisis. *J Thorac Cardiovasc Surg.* 1986; 91:296–302.
2. Pittsburgh woman loses eye to tainted drugs; 12 hurt. *Baltimore Sun.* 1990; Nov 9:3A.
3. ASHP gears up multistep action plan regarding sterile drug products. *Am J Hosp Pharm.* 1991; 48:386–90.
4. Dugleaux G, Coutour XL, Hecquard C, et al. Septicemia caused by contaminated parenteral nutrition pouches: the refrigerator as an unusual cause. *JPEN J Parenter Enteral Nutr.* 1991; 15:474–5.
5. Solomon SL, Khabbaz RF, Parker RH, et al. An outbreak of *Candida parapsilosis* bloodstream infections in patients receiving parenteral nutrition. *J Infect Dis.* 1984; 149:98–102.
6. Food and Drug Administration. Hazards of precipitation with parenteral nutrition. *Am J Hosp Pharm.* 1994; 51:427–8.
7. Pierce LR, Gaines A, Varricchio R, et al. Hemolysis and renal failure associated with use of sterile water for injection to dilute 25% human albumin solution. *Am J Health-Syst Pharm.* 1998; 55:1057,1062,1070.
8. Flynn EA, Pearson RE, Barker KN. Observational study of accuracy in compounding i.v. admixtures at five hospitals. *Am J Health-Syst Pharm.* 1997; 54:904–12.
9. Santell JP, Kamalich RF. National survey of quality assurance activities for pharmacy-prepared sterile products in hospitals and home infusion facilities—1995. *Am J Health-Syst Pharm.* 1996; 53:2591–605.
10. Kastango ES, Douglass K. Improving the management, operations and cost effectiveness of sterile-product compounding. *Int J Pharm Compd.* 1999; 3:253–8.
11. Guynn JB Jr, Poretz DM, Duma RJ. Growth of various bacteria in a variety of intravenous fluids. *Am J Hosp Pharm.* 1973; 30:321–5.
12. Hasegawa GR. Caring about stability and compatibility. *Am J Hosp Pharm.* 1994; 51:1533–4. Editorial.
13. Stability considerations in dispensing practice (general information chapter 1191). In: The United States pharmacopeia, 24th rev., and The national formulary, 19th ed. Rockville, MD: The United States Pharmacopeial Convention; 1999:2128–30.
14. Pharmacy compounding practices (general information chapter 1161). In: The United States pharmacopeia, 24th rev., and The national formulary, 19th ed. Rockville, MD: The United States Pharmacopeial Convention; 1999:2118–22.
15. Sterile drug products for home use (general information chapter 1206). In: The United States pharmacopeia, 24th rev., and The national formulary, 19th ed. Rockville, MD: The United States Pharmacopeial Convention; 1999:2130–43.
16. Good compounding practices applicable to state licensed pharmacies. *Natl Pharm Compliance News.* 1993; May:2–3, Oct:2–3.
17. Model rules for sterile pharmaceuticals. Chicago: National Association of Boards of Pharmacy; 1993:12.1–3.
18. National Advisory Group on Standards and Practice Guidelines for Parenteral Nutrition. Safe practices for parenteral nutrition formulations. *JPEN J Parenter Enteral Nutr.* 1998; 22:49–66.
19. Standard 3.3. Policies and procedures support safe medication prescription or ordering. In: 1999 Hospital accreditation standards. Chicago: Joint Commission on Accreditation of Healthcare Organizations; 1999:88.
20. Standard TX 5.1. Medications are prepared safely. In: 1999–2000 Comprehensive accreditation manual for home care. Chicago: Joint Commission on Accreditation of Healthcare Organizations; 1999:182.
21. Standard TX 2.3. The pharmacy organization maintains proper conditions of sanitation, temperature, light, moisture, ventilation, segregation, safety, and security for preparing medications. 1996–1998 Standards for long term care pharmacies. Chicago: Joint Commission on Accreditation of Healthcare Organizations; 1996:70–1.
22. Standard TX 3.3. Prescribing and ordering of medications follow established procedures. 1998–99 Comprehensive accreditation manual for ambulatory

care. Chicago: Joint Commission on Accreditation of Healthcare Organizations; 1998:211.

23. Food and Drug Modernization Act of 1997, Pub. L. No. 105–115, 111 Stat. 2296.

24. Centers for Disease Control. Guideline for prevention of intravascular infections. *Am J Infect Control.* 1983; 11(5):183–93.

25. Centers for Disease Control. Guideline for handwashing and hospital environmental control. *Am J Infect Control.* 1986; 4(8):110–29.

26. American Society of Hospital Pharmacists. ASHP technical assistance bulletin on handling cytotoxic and hazardous drugs. *Am J Hosp Pharm.* 1990; 47:1033–49.

27. American Society of Hospital Pharmacists. ASHP technical assistance bulletin on pharmacy-prepared ophthalmic products. *Am J Hosp Pharm.* 1993; 50:1462–3.

28. Cleanrooms and associated controlled environments—part 1: classification of air cleanliness. International standard ISO 14644-1. 1st ed. New York: American National Standards Institute; 1999.

29. Federal standard no. 209E. Airborne particulate cleanliness classes in cleanrooms and clean zones. Washington, DC: General Services Administration; 1992.

30. Microbiological evaluation of clean rooms and other controlled environments (general information chapter 1116). In: The United States Pharmacopeia, 24th rev., and The national formulary, 19th ed. Rockville, MD: The United States Pharmacopeial Convention; 1999:2009–106.

31. Validation of aseptic filling for solution drug products. Technical monograph no. 22. Philadelphia: Parenteral Drug Association; 1996.

32. Formulations: *Int J Pharm Compd.* 1999; 2:297–307.

33. Buchanan EC. Policies and procedures for sterile product preparation. In: Principles of sterile product preparation. Bethesda, MD: American Society of Health-System Pharmacists; 1995:133–8.

34. Standard operating procedure of a horizontal laminar air flow hood. *Int J Pharm Compd.* 1997(Sep/Oct); 1:344–5.

35. Standard operating procedure for general aseptic procedures carried out at a laminar air flow workbench. *Int J Pharm Compd.* 1998(May/Jun); 2:242.

36. Standard operating procedure for particulate testing for sterile products. *Int J Pharm Compd.* 1997(Jan/Feb); 2:78.

37. Quality assurance of pharmacy-prepared sterile products. Bethesda, MD: American Society of Hospital Pharmacists; 1994. Videotape and workbook.

38. Safe handling of cytotoxic and hazardous drugs. Bethesda, MD: American Society of Health-System Pharmacists; 1990. Videotape and study guide.

39. Schneider PJ, Buchanan EC. Personnel education, training and evaluation. In: Principles of sterile product preparation. Bethesda, MD: American Society of Health-System Pharmacists; 1995:9–15.

40. Hunt ML. Training manual for intravenous admixture personnel. 5th ed. Chicago: Precept; 1995.

41. Gallagher M. Home care pharmacist competency assessment program. *Am J Health-Syst Pharm.* 1999; 56:1549–53.

42. Dirks I, Smith FM, Furtado D, et al. Method for testing aseptic technique of intravenous admixture personnel. *Am J Hosp Pharm.* 1982; 39:457–9.

43. Brier KL. Evaluating aseptic technique of pharmacy personnel. *Am J Hosp Pharm.* 1983; 40:400–3.

44. McKinnon BT. Handling of sterile products within the pharmacy. In: Principles of sterile product preparation. Bethesda, MD: American Society of Health-System Pharmacists; 1995:111–6.

45. Morris BG, Avis KE. Quality-control plan for intravenous admixture programs. 1: Visual inspection of solutions and environmental testing. *Am J Hosp Pharm.* 1980; 37:189–95.

46. Buchanan EC. Sterile compounding facilities. In: Principles of sterile product preparation. Bethesda, MD: American Society of Health-System Pharmacists; 1995:25–35.

47. Schneider PJ. Equipment for sterile product preparation. In: Principles of sterile product preparation. Bethesda, MD: American Society of Health-System Pharmacists; 1995:37–43.

48. Lau D, Shane R, Yen J. Quality assurance for sterile products: simple changes can help. *Am J Hosp Pharm.* 1994; 51:1353. Letter.

49. Rahe H. Containment Technologies Group, Inc. Personal communication. 1999 Oct.

50. Hunt ML. Training manual for intravenous admixture personnel. 5th ed. Chicago: Precept; 1995:67–70.

51. Buchanan TL, Barker KN, Gibson JT, et al. Illumination and errors in dispensing. *Am J Hosp Pharm.* 1991; 48:2137–45.

52. Denny VF, Kopis EM, Marsik FJ. Elements for a successful disinfection program in the pharmaceutical environment. *PDA J Pharm Sci Technol.* 1999; 53:115–24.

53. Frieben WR. Control of the aseptic processing environment. *Am J Hosp Pharm.* 1983; 40:1928–35.

54. Scheckelhoff DJ. Handling, preparation and disposal of cytotoxic and hazardous agents. In: Principles of sterile product preparation. Bethesda, MD: American Society of Health-System Pharmacists; 1995:63–9.

55. Favier M, Hansel S, Bressole F. Preparing cytotoxic agents in an isolator. *Am J Hosp Pharm.* 1993; 50:2335–9.

56. Mosko P, Rahe H. Barrier isolation technology: a labor-efficient alternative to cleanrooms. *Hosp Pharm.* 1999; 34:834–8.

57. Pilong A, Moore M. Conversion to isolators in a sterile preparation area. *Am J Health-Syst Pharm.* 1999; 56:1978–80.

58. Tillett L. Barrier isolators as an alternative to a cleanroom. *Am J Health-Syst Pharm.* 1999; 56:1433–6.

59. Bryan D, Marback RC. Laminar air flow equipment certification: what the pharmacist needs to know. *Am J Hosp Pharm.* 1984; 41:1343–9.

60. McKinnon BT. Personnel behavior and garb use. In: Principles of sterile product preparation. Bethesda, MD: American Society of Health-System Pharmacists; 1995:57–62.

61. Coriell LL, McGarrity GJ, Horneff J. Medical applications of dust-free rooms: I. Elimination of airborne bacteria in a research laboratory. *Am J Public Health.* 1967; 57:1824–36.

62. NIOSH recommends steps for reducing work-related exposure to latex. *Am J Health-Syst Pharm.* 1997; 54:1688,1691.

63. Dasher G, Dasher T. The growing problem of latex allergies. *Infusion.* 1996; 2(Jan):23–7.

64. Hunt ML. Techniques used in preparing intravenous admixtures. In: Training manual for intravenous admixture personnel. Chicago: Precept; 1995:87–103.

65. Scheckelhoff DJ. Use of aseptic technique. In: Principles of sterile product preparation. Bethesda, MD: American Society of Health-System Pharmacists; 1995:49–56.

66. Buchanan EC. Sterile product formulation and compounding. In: Principles of sterile product preparation. Bethesda, MD: American Society of Health-System Pharmacists; 1995:17–24.

67. Kessler DA. MedWatch: The new FDA medical products reporting program. *Am J Hosp Pharm.* 1993; 50:1921–36.

68. Rice SP, Gutfeld MB. Preparation of latex-safe products. *Am J Health-Syst Pharm.* 1998; 55:1462–7.

69. Holzman RS. Latex allergy: an emerging operating room problem. *Anesth Analg.* 1993; 76:635–41.

70. McDermott JS, Gura KM. Procedures for preparing injectable medications for latex-sensitive patients. *Am J Health-Syst Pharm.* 1997; 54:2516–7.

71. Schneider PJ. Process validation. In: Principles of sterile product preparation. Bethesda, MD: American Society of Health-System Pharmacists; 1995:121–4.

72. McKinnon BT. Factors influencing expiration dates. In: Principles of sterile product preparation. Bethesda, MD: American Society of Health-System Pharmacists; 1995:95–103.

73. McEvoy GK, ed. AHFS drug information 99. Bethesda, MD: American Society of Health-System Pharmacists; 1999.

74. Bing C, ed. Extended stability for parenteral drugs. Bethesda, MD: American Society of Health-System Pharmacists; in press.

75. Trissel LA. Handbook on injectable drugs. 10th ed. Bethesda, MD: American Society of Health-System Pharmacists; 1998.

76. Catania PN, ed. King guide to parenteral admixtures. St. Louis, MO: King Guide; 1999.

77. American Society of Health-System Pharmacists. ASHP guidelines: minimum standard for home care pharmacies. *Am J Health-Syst Pharm.* 1999; 56:629–38.

78. Scheckelhoff DJ. Labeling of sterile products. In: Principles of sterile product preparation. Bethesda, MD: American Society of Health-System Pharmacists; 1995:105–9.

79. Davis NM. Optimal checking of pharmacy-prepared sterile products. *Hosp Pharm.* 1996; 31:102. Editorial.

80. Schneider PJ. End-product evaluation. In: Principles of sterile product preparation. Bethesda, MD: American Society of Health-System Pharmacists; 1995:125–8.

81. Meyer GE, Novielli KA, Smith JE. Use of refractive index measurement for quality assurance of pediatric parenteral nutrition solutions. *Am J Hosp Pharm.* 1987; 44:1617–20.

82. Scheckelhoff DJ. Handling of sterile products outside the pharmacy. In: Principles of sterile product preparation. Bethesda, MD: American Society of Health-System Pharmacists; 1995:117–20.

83. Chamallas SN, Fishwick JJ, Riesenberg M. Special delivery, keeping the product stable during shipping. *Infusion.* 1997; 4(3):30–2.

84. McKinnon BT. Documentation of sterile product preparations. In: Principles of sterile product preparation. Bethesda, MD: American Society of Health-System Pharmacists; 1995:129–31.

85. Schumock GT, Kafka PS, Tormo VJ. Design, construction, implementation, and cost of a hospital pharmacy cleanroom. *Am J Health-Syst Pharm.* 1998; 55:458–63.

86. Gianino RR. Misconceptions about cleanrooms. *Am J Hosp Pharm.* 1994; 51:239–40. Letter.

87. Fundamentals of a microbiological environmental monitoring program. Technical report no. 13. Philadelphia: Parenteral Drug Association; 1990.

88. Whyte W. In support of settle plates. *PDA J Pharm Sci Technol.* 1996; 50:201–4.

89. Hyde HA. Origin of bacteria in the clean room and their growth requirements. *PDA J Pharm Sci Technol.* 1998; 52:154–8.

90. American Society of Health-System Pharmacists. ASHP guidelines on the safe use of automated compounding devices for the preparation of parenteral nutrition admixtures. *Am J Health-Syst Pharm.* 2000; 57:1343–8.

91. Davis NM. Unprecedented procedural safeguards needed with the use of automated iv compounders. *Hosp Pharm.* 1992; 27:488. Editorial.

92. Murphy C. Ensuring accuracy in the use of automatic compounders. *Am J Hosp Pharm.* 1993; 50:60. Letter.

93. Dickson LB, Somani SM, Herrmann G, et al. Automated compounder for adding ingredients to parenteral nutrient base solutions. *Am J Hosp Pharm.* 1993; 50:678–82.

94. Fishwick JJ, Murphy CC, Riesenberg MC, et al. Weight-based accuracy of parenteral nutrient solutions prepared with an automated compounder. *Am J Health-Syst Pharm.* 1997; 54:678–9.

95. Johnson R, Coles BJ, Tribble DA. Accuracy of three automated compounding systems determined by end-product laboratory testing and comparison with manual preparation. *Am J Health-Syst Pharm.* 1998; 55:1503–7.

96. Combeau D, Rey JB, Rieutord A, et al. Accuracy of two filling systems for parenteral nutrient solutions. *Am J Health-Syst Pharm.* 1998; 55:1606–10.

97. Boylan JC. Essential elements of quality control. *Am J Hosp Pharm.* 1983; 40:1936–9.

98. McKinnon BT. Preparation and sterilization of batch compounds. In: Principles of sterile product preparation. Bethesda, MD: American Society of Health-System Pharmacists; 1995:71–7.

99. McKinnon BT. Batch preparation documentation. In: Principles of sterile product preparation. Bethesda, MD: American Society of Health-System Pharmacists; 1995:79–94.

100. Lima HA. Required documentation for home infusion pharmacies—compounding records. *Int J Pharm Compd.* 1998; 2:354–9.

101. Avis KE. Assuring the quality of pharmacy-prepared sterile products. *Pharmacopeial Forum.* 1997; 23:3567–76.

102. Fontan JE, Arnaud P, Brion F. Laminar-airflow ceiling in a hospital pharmacy cleanroom. *Am J Health-Syst Pharm.* 1998; 55:182–3. Letter.

103. Chandler SW, Trissel LA, Wamsley LM, et al. Evaluation of air quality in a sterile-drug preparation area with an electronic particle counter. *Am J Hosp Pharm.* 1993; 50:2330–4.

104. Schneider PJ. Environmental monitoring. In: Principles of sterile product preparation. Bethesda, MD: American Society of Health-System Pharmacists; 1995:45–8.

105. Bacterial endotoxins test (general tests and assays chapter 85). In: The United States pharmacopeia, 24th rev., and The national formulary, 19th ed. Rockville, MD: The United States Pharmacopeial Convention; 1999:1829-31.

106. Roberts JH, Wilson JD. Technical report no. 26: sterilizing filtration of liquids. *PDA J Pharm Sci Technol.* 1998; 52(suppl S1):1–31.

107. Akers MJ. Sterilization and depyrogenation: principles and methods. *Int J Pharm Compd.* 1999; 3:263–9.

108. Pyrogen test (general tests and assays chapter 151). In: The United States pharmacopeia, 24th rev., and The national formulary, 19th ed. Rockville, MD: The United States Pharmacopeial Convention; 1999:1850–1.

109. Aspects of container/closure integrity. Technical information bulletin no. 4. Philadelphia: Parenteral Drug Association; 1983.

110. Neidich RL. Selection of containers and closure systems for injectable products. *Am J Hosp Pharm.* 1983; 40:1924–7.

111. Validation of steam sterilization cycles. Technical information bulletin no. 1. Philadelphia: Parenteral Drug Association; 1978.

112. Turco S, ed. Sterile dosage forms: their preparation and clinical application. Philadelphia: Lea & Febiger; 1994:57–78.

113. McKinnon BT, Avis KE. Membrane filtration of pharmaceutical solutions. *Am J Hosp Pharm.* 1993; 50: 1921–36.

114. Eudailey WA. Membrane filters and membrane filtration processes for health care. *Am J Hosp Pharm.* 1983; 40:1921–3.

115. Wilson JD. Aseptic process monitoring—a better strategy. *PDA J Pharm Sci Technol.* 1999; 53:111–4.

116. Sterility tests (general tests and assays chapter 71). In: The United States pharmacopeia, 24th rev., and The national formulary, 19th ed. Rockville, MD: The United States Pharmacopeial Convention; 1999:1818–23.

117. Choy FN, Lamy PP, Burkhart VD, et al. Sterility-testing program for antibiotics and other intravenous admixtures. *Am J Hosp Pharm.* 1982; 39:452–6.

118. Doss HL, James JD, Killough DM, et al. Microbiologic quality assurance for intravenous admixtures in a small hospital. *Am J Hosp Pharm.* 1982; 39:832–5.

119. Posey LM, Nutt RE, Thompson PD. Comparison of two methods for detecting microbial contamination in intravenous fluids. *Am J Hosp Pharm.* 1981; 38:659–62.

120. Akers MJ. Progress toward a preferred method of monitoring the sterility of intravenous admixtures. *Am J Hosp Pharm.* 1982; 39:1297. Editorial.

121. Hoffman KH, Smith FM, Godwin HN, et al. Evaluation of three methods for detecting bacterial contamination in intravenous solutions. *Am J Hosp Pharm.* 1982; 39:1299–302.

122. Miller CM, Furtado D, Smith FM, et al. Evaluation of three methods for detecting low-level bacterial contamination in intravenous solutions. *Am J Hosp Pharm.* 1982; 39:1302–5.

123. DeChant RL, Furtado D, Smith FH, et al. Determining a time frame for sterility testing of intravenous admixtures. *Am J Hosp Pharm.* 1982; 39:1305–8.

124. Bronson MH, Stennett DJ, Egging PK. Sterility testing of home and inpatient parenteral nutrition solutions. *JPEN J Parenter Enteral Nutr.* 1988; 12:25–8.

125. Levchuk JW, Nolly RJ, Lander N. Method for testing the sterility of total nutrient admixtures. *Am J Hosp Pharm.* 1988; 45:1311–21.

126. Akers MJ, Wright GE, Carlson KA. Sterility testing of antimicrobial-containing injectable solutions prepared in the pharmacy. *Am J Hosp Pharm.* 1991; 48:2414-8.

127. Murray PR, Sandrock MJ. Sterility testing of a total nutrient admixture with a biphasic blood-culture system. *Am J Hosp Pharm.* 1991; 48:2419–21.

[a]Unless otherwise stated in this document, the term sterile products refers to sterile drugs or nutritional substances that are prepared (e.g., compounded or repackaged) by pharmacy personnel.

[b]Ampuls, swabbed and opened appropriately with contents filtered upon removal, should be considered part of a "closed" system.

[c]Isolator guidelines appear under risk level 1 sections because their greatest use is likely to be in the preparation of cytotoxic sterile products, most of which are risk level 1 processes.

[d]The need to alternate germicides is controversial. According to Akers and Moore (Microbiological monitoring of pharmaceutical cleanrooms: the need for pragmatism, *J Adv Appl Contam Control.* 1998; 1[1]:23-4,26,28,30), the data do not support alternating germicides. A literature search (Kopis EM. *Cleanrooms.* 1996; 10[10]:48-v50) found little evidence for periodic alternation of disinfectants; the search did find that alternating use of acidic and alkaline phenolic disinfectants reduces resistance arising in pseudomonads adhering to hard surfaces. If ethanol 70% or isopropyl alcohol 70% is used as the primary disinfectant, it should be sterile filtered through a 0.22-μm filter before use.

[e]According to Trissel and Chandler (*Am J Hosp Pharm.* 1993; 50:1858–61), pharmacy air is nearly class 10,000 cleanroom quality already. However, true cleanrooms add HEPA air filtering and designate room air changes and room air pressure differentials to ensure cleanliness (*Am J Hosp Pharm.* 1994; 51:239-40. Letter).

[f]Note that the International Organization for Sanitation (ISO) is preparing documents that should replace Federal Standard 209E. The ISO documents (numbered 14644-1 through 14644-7 and 14698-1 through 14698-3) are being prepared by a technical committee consisting of members from six countries, including the United States. Document 14644-1 is published in final form and classifies the air cleanliness of cleanrooms and associated controlled environments. In 14644-1 ISO cleanroom class 5 is equivalent to Federal Standard 209E class 100, and ISO class 7 is equivalent to Federal Standard 209E class 10,000.

[g]As in general information chapter 1206 in *USP*, which does not require sterility testing until the third risk level, this assumes that sterile components remain sterile throughout preparation. Many sterile products are prepared in batches too small or used too quickly after preparation to make sterility testing meaningful. Also, one of the purposes of process validation is to determine that personnel and processes can produce a sterile product.

Supersedes the ASHP Technical Assistance Bulletin on Quality Assurance for Pharmacy-Prepared Sterile Products, dated September 24, 1993.

Approved by the ASHP Board of Directors, on April 27, 2000 Developed through the ASHP Council on Professional Affairs.

The bibliographic citation for this document is as follows: American Society of Health-System Pharmacists. ASHP Guidelines on Quality

Assurance for Pharmacy-Prepared Sterile Products. *Am J Health-Syst Pharm*. 2000; 57:1150–69.

Appendix A—Glossary

Action Level: Established particulate or microbial counts or results that require corrective action when exceeded.

Aseptic Preparation or Aseptic Processing: The technique involving procedures designed to preclude contamination (of drugs, packaging, equipment, or supplies) by microorganisms during processing.

Batch Preparation: Compounding of multiple sterile product units, in a single discrete process, by the same individuals, carried out during one limited time period.

Cleanroom: A room (1) in which the concentration of airborne particles is controlled, (2) that is constructed and used in a manner to minimize the introduction, generation, and retention of particles inside the room, and (3) in which other relevant variables (e.g., temperature, humidity, and pressure) are controlled as necessary.[28] For example, the air particle count in a class 100 cleanroom cannot exceed a total of 100 particles 0.5 µm or larger per cubic foot of air.[29]

Clean Zone: Dedicated space (1) in which the concentration of airborne particles is controlled, (2) that is constructed and used in a manner that minimizes the introduction, generation, and retention of particles inside the zone, and (3) in which other relevant variables (e.g., temperature, humidity, and pressure) are controlled as necessary. This zone may be open or enclosed and may or may not be located within a cleanroom.[28] For example, an open-architecture controlled area should be a clean zone.

Closed-System Transfer: The movement of sterile products from one container to another in which the containers-closure system and transfer devices remain intact throughout the entire transfer process, compromised only by the penetration of a sterile, pyrogen-free needle or cannula through a designated closure or port to effect transfer, withdrawal, or delivery. Withdrawal of a sterile solution from an ampul through a particulate filter in a class 100 environment would generally be considered acceptable; however, the use of a flexible closure vial, when available, would be preferable.

Compounding: For purposes of these guidelines, compounding simply means the mixing of ingredients to prepare a medication for patient use. This activity would include dilution, admixture, repackaging, reconstitution, and other manipulations of sterile products.

Controlled Area: For purposes of these guidelines, a controlled area is the area designated for preparing sterile products. This is referred to as the buffer zone (i.e., the cleanroom in which the laminar-airflow workbench is located) by USP.[15]

Corrective Action: Action to be taken when the results of monitoring indicate a loss of control or when action levels are exceeded.

Critical Area: Any area in the controlled area where products or containers are exposed to the environment.

Critical Site: An opening providing a direct pathway between a sterile product and the environment or any surface coming into contact with the product or environment.

Critical Surface: Any surface that comes into contact with previously sterilized products or containers.

Designated Pharmacist: The pharmacist chosen by experience and training to be in charge of a sterile product preparation area or unit in a licensed pharmacy.

Expiration Date: The date (and time, when applicable) beyond which a product should not be used (i.e., the product should be discarded beyond this date and time). Expiration date and time should be assigned on the basis of both stability and risk level, whichever is the shorter period. **Note:** Circumstances may occur in which the expiration date and time arrive while an infusion is in progress. When this occurs, judgment should be applied in determining whether it is appropriate to discontinue that infusion and replace the product. Organizational policies on this should be clear.[15]

High-Efficiency Particulate Air (HEPA) Filter: A filter composed of pleats of filter medium separated by rigid sheets of corrugated paper or aluminum foil that direct the flow of air forced through the filter in a uniform parallel flow. HEPA filters remove 99.97% of all air particles 0.3 µm or larger. When HEPA filters are used as a component of a horizontal- or vertical-laminar-airflow workbench, an environment can be created consistent with standards for a class 100 cleanroom.

Isolator (or Barrier Isolator): A closed system made up of four solid walls, an air-handling system, and transfer and interaction devices. The walls are constructed so as to provide surfaces that are cleanable with coving between wall junctures. The air-handling system provides HEPA filtration of both inlet and exhaust air. Transfer of materials is accomplished through air locks, glove rings, or ports. Transfers are designed to minimize the entry of contamination. Manipulations can take place through either glove ports or half-suits.

Media Fill: See process validation or simulation.

Preservatives: For purposes of these guidelines, preservatives refer to any additive intended to extend the content, stability, or sterility of active ingredients (e.g., antioxidants, emulsifiers, bacteriocides).

Process Validation or Simulation: Microbiological simulation of an aseptic process with growth medium processed in a manner similar to the processing of the product and with the same container or closure system.[30] Process simulation tests are synonymous with medium fills, simulated product fills, broth trials, and broth fills.

Quality Assurance: For purposes of these guidelines, quality assurance is the set of activities used to ensure that the processes used in the preparation of sterile drug products lead to products that meet predetermined standards of quality.

Quality Control: For purposes of these guidelines, quality control is the set of testing activities used to determine that the ingredients, components (e.g., containers), and final sterile products prepared meet predetermined requirements with respect to identity, purity, nonpyrogenicity, and sterility.

Repackaging: The subdivision or transfer of a compounded product from one container or device to a different container or device, such as a syringe or an ophthalmic container.

Sterilization: A validated process used to render a product free of viable organisms.

Sterilizing Filter: A filter that, when challenged with a solution containing the microorganism *Pseudomonas diminuta* at a minimum concentration of 10^{12} organisms per square centimeter of filter surface, will produce a sterile effluent.

Temperatures (USP): Frozen means temperatures between −20 and −10 °C (−4 and 14 °F). Refrigerated means temperatures between 2 and 8°C (36 and 46 °F). Room temperature means temperatures between 15 and 30 °C (59 and 86 °F).

Validation: Documented evidence providing a high degree of assurance that a specific process will consistently produce a product meeting its predetermined specifications and quality attributes.

Worst Case: A set of conditions encompassing upper and lower processing limits and circumstances, including those within standard operating procedures, that pose the greatest chance of process or product failure when compared with ideal conditions. Such conditions do not necessarily induce product or process failure.[31]

Appendix B—Comparison of Risk-Level Attributes

This appendix does not show all details of the guidelines, nor does it tell whether an aspect of the sterile compounding process is "required" (must be) or "advisable" (should be). Regardless of the examples given, each compounding pharmacist must decide, according to the circumstances at the time, what conditions are appropriate for compounding a sterile product. In an emergency, it may be of more benefit to a patient to receive a sterile drug prepared under lower risk-level conditions. For the immunocompromised patient, even simple, single-patient admixtures may need to be compounded under higher risk-level conditions.

Definition of Products by Risk Level

Risk Level 1	Risk Level 2	Risk Level 3
Products that are (1) stored at room temperature and completely administered within 28 hours from preparation, (2) unpreserved and sterile and prepared for administration to one patient, or batch prepared for administration to more than one patient and contain suitable preservatives, and (3) prepared by closed-system aseptic transfer of sterile, nonpyrogenic, finished pharmaceuticals obtained from licensed manufacturers into sterile final containers obtained from licensed manufacturers.	Products that are (1) administered beyond 28 hours after preparation and storage at room temperature, (2) batch prepared without preservatives and intended for use by more than one patient, or (3) compounded by complex or numerous manipulations of sterile ingredients obtained from licensed manufacturers in a sterile container obtained from a licensed manufacturer by using closed-system, aseptic transfer.	Products that are (1) compounded from nonsterile ingredients or with nonsterile components, containers, or equipment before terminal sterilization or (2) prepared by combining multiple ingredients (sterile or nonsterile) by using an open-system transfer or open reservoir before terminal sterilization.

Examples of Sterile Products by Risk Level

Risk Level 1	Risk Level 2	Risk Level 3
Single-patient admixture Single-patient ophthalmic, preserved Single-patient syringes without preservatives used in 28 hours Batch-prefilled syringes with preservatives Total parenteral nutrient (TPN) solution made by gravity transfer of carbohydrate and amino acids into an empty container with the addition of sterile additives with a syringe and needle	Injections for use in portable pump or reservoir over multiple days Batch-reconstituted antibiotics without preservatives Batch-prefilled syringes without preservatives TPN solutions mixed with an automatic compounding device	Alum bladder irrigation Morphine injection made from powder or tablets TPN solutions made from dry amino acids TPN solutions sterilized by final filtration Autoclaved i.v. solutions

Policies and Procedures

Risk Level 1	Risk Level 2	Risk Level 3
Up-to-date policies and procedures for compounding sterile products should be available to all involved personnel. When policies are changed, they should be updated. Procedures should address personnel education and training, competency evaluation, product acquisition, storage and handling of products and supplies, storage and delivery of final products, use and maintenance of facilities and equipment, appropriate garb and conduct of personnel working in the controlled area, process validation, preparation technique, labeling, documentation, quality control, and material movement.	In addition to risk level 1 guidelines, procedures describe environmental monitoring devices and techniques, cleaning materials and disinfectants, equipment accuracy monitoring, limits of acceptability and corrective actions for environmental monitoring and process validation, master formula and work sheets, personnel garb, lot numbers, and other quality control methods.	Procedures cover every aspect of preparation of level 3 sterile products, so that all products have the identity, strength, quality, and purity purported for the product. Thirteen general policies and procedures, in addition to those in levels 1 and 2, are required.

Personnel Education, Training, and Evaluation

Risk Level 1	Risk Level 2	Risk Level 3
All pharmacy personnel preparing sterile products should receive suitable didactic and experiential training and competency evaluation through demonstration or testing (written or practical). In addition to the policies and procedures listed above, education includes chemical, pharmaceutical, and clinical properties of drugs and current good compounding practices.	In addition to guidelines in risk level 1, training includes assessment of competency in all types of risk level 2 procedures via process simulation. Personnel show competency in end-product testing as well.	Operators have specific education, training, and experience to prepare risk level 3 products. Pharmacist knows principles of good compounding practice for risk level 3 products, including aseptic processing; quality assurance of environmental, component, and end-product testing; sterilization; and selection and use of containers, equipment, and closures.

Storage and Handling in the Pharmacy

Risk Level 1	Risk Level 2	Risk Level 3
Solutions, drugs, supplies, and equipment must be stored according to manufacturer or USP requirements. Refrigerator and freezer temperatures should be documented daily. Other storage areas should be inspected regularly to ensure that temperature, light, moisture, and ventilation meet requirements. Drugs and supplies should be shelved above the floor. Expired products must be removed from active product storage areas. Personnel traffic in storage areas should be minimized. Removal of products from boxes should be done outside controlled areas. Disposal of used supplies should be done at least daily. Product-recall procedures must permit retrieving affected products from specific involved patients.	All guidelines for risk level 1 apply.	In addition to risk level 1 guidelines, procedures include procurement, identification, storage, handling, testing, and recall of components and finished products. Finished but untested products must be quarantined under minimal risk for contamination or loss of identity in an identified quarantine area.

Facilities and Equipment

Risk Level 1	Risk Level 2	Risk Level 3
The controlled area should be separated from other operations to minimize unnecessary flow of materials and personnel through the area. The controlled area must be clean, well lighted, and of sufficient size for sterile compounding. A sink with hot and cold water should be near, but not in, the controlled area. The controlled area and inside equipment must be cleaned and disinfected regularly. Sterile products must be prepared in a class 100 environment (the critical area), such as within a horizontal- or vertical-laminar-airflow workbench or barrier isolator. Computer entry, order processing, label generation, and record keeping should be performed outside the critical area. The critical area must be disinfected periodically. A workbench should be recertified every six months or when it is moved; prefilters should be changed periodically. Pumps should be recalibrated according to procedure.	In addition to risk level 1 guidelines, the following are recommended for risk level 2 products: controlled area must meet class 10,000 cleanroom standards; cleaning supplies should be selected to meet cleanroom standards; critical-area work surface must be cleaned between batches; floors should be disinfected daily, equipment surfaces weekly, and walls monthly; and there should be environmental monitoring of air and surfaces. An anteroom of high cleanliness is desirable. Automated compounding devices must be calibrated and verified as to accuracy, according to procedure.	Products must be prepared in a class 100 workbench in a class 10,000 cleanroom, in a class 100 cleanroom, or in a suitable barrier isolator. Access to the cleanroom must be limited to those preparing the products who are in appropriate garb. Methods are needed for cleaning, preparing, sterilizing, calibrating, and documenting the use of all equipment. Walls and ceilings should be disinfected weekly. All nonsterile equipment that is to come in contact with the sterilized final product should be sterilized before introduction into the cleanroom. An anteroom of high cleanliness (i.e., class 100,000) should be provided. Appropriate cleaning and disinfection of the environment and equipment are required.

Garb

Risk Level 1	Risk Level 2	Risk Level 3
In the controlled area, personnel wear low-particulate, clean clothing covers such as clean gowns or coverall with sleeves having elastic cuffs. Hand, finger, and wrist jewelry is minimized or eliminated. Nails are clean and trimmed. Gloves are recommended; those allergic to latex rubber must wear gloves made of a suitable alternative. Head and facial hair is covered. Masks are recommended during aseptic preparation. Personnel preparing sterile products scrub their hands and arms with an appropriate antimicrobial skin cleanser.	In addition to risk level 1 guidelines, gloves, gowns, and masks are required. During sterile preparation, gloves should be rinsed frequently with a suitable agent (e.g., 70% isopropyl alcohol) and changed when their integrity is compromised. Shoe covers are helpful in maintaining the cleanliness of the controlled area.	In addition to risk level 1 and 2 guidelines, cleanroom garb must be worn inside the controlled area at all times during the preparation of risk level 3 sterile products. Attire consists of a low-shedding coverall, head cover, face mask, and shoe covers. Before donning this garb, personnel must thoroughly wash their hands and arms. Upon return to the controlled area or support area during processing, personnel should regown with clean garb.

Aseptic Technique and Product Preparation

Risk Level 1	Risk Level 2	Risk Level 3
Sterile products must be prepared in a class 100 environment. Personnel scrub their hands and forearms for an appropriate period at the beginning of each aseptic compounding process. Eating, drinking, and smoking are prohibited in the controlled area. Talking is minimized to reduce airborne particles. Ingredients are determined to be stable, compatible, and appropriate for the product to be prepared, according to manufacturer, USP, or scientific references. Ingredients result in final products that meet physiological norms as to osmolality and pH for the intended route of administration. Ingredients and containers are inspected for defects, expiration, and integrity before use. Only materials essential for aseptic compounding are placed in the workbench. Surfaces of ampuls and vials are disinfected before placement in the workbench. Sterile components are arranged in the workbench to allow uninterrupted laminar airflow over critical surfaces of needles, vials, ampuls, etc. Usually only one person and one preparation are in the workbench at a time. Automated devices and equipment are cleaned, disinfected, and placed in the workbench to enable laminar airflow. Aseptic technique is used to avoid touch contamination of critical sites of containers and ingredients. Sterile powders are completely reconstituted. Particles are filtered from solutions. Needle cores are avoided. The pharmacist checks before, during, and after preparation to verify the identity and amount of ingredients before release.	In addition to risk level 1 guidelines, a master work sheet containing formula, components, procedures, sample label, final evaluation, and testing is made for each product batch. A separate work sheet and lot number are used for each batch. When combining multiple sterile ingredients, a second pharmacist should verify calculations. The pharmacist should verify data entered into an automatic compounder before processing and check the end product for accuracy.	In addition to risk level 1 and 2 guidelines, nonsterile components must meet USP standards for identity, purity, and endotoxin levels, as verified by a pharmacist. Batch master work sheets should also include comparisons of actual with anticipated yields, sterilization methods, and quarantine specifications. Presterilized containers should be used if feasible. Final containers must be sterile and capable of maintaining product integrity throughout shelf life. Sterilization method is based on properties of the product. Final filtration methods require attention to many elements of product, filter, and filter integrity.

Process Validation

Risk Level 1	Risk Level 2	Risk Level 3
All persons who prepare sterile products should pass a process validation of their aseptic technique before they prepare sterile products for patient use. Personnel competency should be reevaluated by process validation at least annually, whenever the quality assurance program yields an unacceptable result, and whenever unacceptable techniques are observed. If microbial growth is detected, the entire sterile process must be evaluated, corrective action taken, and the process simulation test performed again.	All risk level 1 guidelines apply, and process-simulation procedures should cover all types of manipulations, products, and batch sizes that are encountered in risk level 2.	In addition to risk level 1 and 2 guidelines, written policies should be made to validate all processes (including all procedures, components, equipment, and techniques) for each risk level 3 product.

Handling Sterile Products Outside the Pharmacy

Risk Level 1	Risk Level 2	Risk Level 3
Sterile products are transported so as to be protected from excesses of temperatures and light. Transit time and condition should be specified. Delivery personnel should be trained as appropriate. Pharmacists ascertain that the end user knows how to properly store products. End users notify pharmacists when storage conditions are exceeded or when products expire so that pharmacists can arrange safe disposal or return.	All guidelines for risk level 1 should be met.	All guidelines for risk level 1 should be met.

Documentation

Risk Level 1	Risk Level 2	Risk Level 3
The following must be documented according to policy, laws, and regulations: (1) training and competency evaluation of employees, (2) refrigerator and freezer temperature logs, (3) certification of workbenches, and (4) other facility quality control logs as appropriate. Pharmacists maintain appropriate records for the compounding and dispensing of sterile products.	In addition to the guidelines in risk level 1, documentation of end-product testing and batch-preparation records must be maintained according to policies, laws, and regulations.	In addition to the guidelines in risk levels 1 and 2, documentation for risk level 3 products must include (1) preparation work sheet, (2) sterilization records if applicable, (3) quarantine records if applicable, and (4) end-product evaluation and testing records.

Expiration Dating

Risk Level 1	Risk Level 2	Risk Level 3
All sterile products must bear an appropriate expiration date. Expiration dates are assigned based on current drug stability information and sterility considerations. The pharmacist considers all aspects of the final product, including drug reservoir, drug concentration, and storage conditions.	All guidelines for risk level 1 should be met.	In addition to risk level 1 and 2 guidelines, there must be a reliable method for establishing all expiration dates, including laboratory testing of product stability, pyrogenicity, and chemical content when necessary.

Labeling

Risk Level 1	Risk Level 2	Risk Level 3
Sterile products should be labeled with at least the following information: (1) for patient-specific product's, the patient's name and other appropriate patient identification; for batch-prepared products, control or lot numbers, (2) all solution and ingredient names, amounts, strengths, and concentrations, (3) expiration date (and time when applicable), (4) prescribed administration regimen, (5) appropriate auxiliary labeling, (6) storage requirements, (7) identification of the responsible pharmacist, (8) any device-specific instructions, and (9) any additional information, in accordance with state and federal regulations. A reference number for the prescription or order may also be helpful. The label should be legible and affixed to the product so that it can be read while being administered.	All guidelines for risk level 1 must be met.	All guidelines for risk levels 1 and 2 must be met.

End-Product Evaluation

Risk Level 1	Risk Level 2	Risk Level 3
The final product must be inspected for container leaks, integrity, solution cloudiness or phase separation, particulates in solution, appropriate solution color, and solution volume. The pharmacist must verify that the product was compounded accurately as to ingredients, quantities, containers, and reservoirs.	In addition to risk level 1 guidelines, toxic products, like concentrated glucose and potassium chloride, should be tested for accuracy of concentration.	In addition to risk level 1 and 2 guidelines, the medium-fill procedure should be supplemented with a program of end-product sterility testing according to a formal sampling plan. Samples should be statistically adequate to reasonably ensure that batches are sterile. A method for recalling batch products should be established if end-product testing yields unacceptable results. Each sterile preparation or batch must be laboratory tested for conformity to written specifications (e.g., concentration, pyrogenicity). It is advisable to quarantine sterile products compounded from nonsterile components pending the results of end-product testing.

ASHP Technical Assistance Bulletin on Compounding Nonsterile Products in Pharmacies

Introduction

Pharmacists are the only health care providers formally trained in the art and science of compounding medications.[1,2] Therefore pharmacists are expected, by the medical community and the public, to possess the knowledge and skills necessary to compound extemporaneous preparations. Pharmacists have a responsibility to provide compounding services for patients with unique drug product needs.

This Technical Assistance Bulletin is intended to assist pharmacists in the extemporaneous compounding of nonsterile drug products for individual patients. Included in this document is information on facilities and equipment, ingredient selection, training, documentation and record keeping, stability and beyond-use dating, packaging and labeling, and limited batch compounding. This document is not intended for manufacturers or licensed repackagers.

Facilities and Equipment

Facilities. It is not necessary that compounding activities be located in a separate facility; however, the compounding area should be located sufficiently away from routine dispensing and counseling functions and high traffic areas. The area should be isolated from potential interruptions, chemical contaminants, and sources of dust and particulate matter. To minimize chemical contaminants, the immediate area and work counter should be free of previously used drugs and chemicals. To minimize dust and particulate matter, cartons and boxes should not be stored or opened in the compounding area. The compounding area should not contain dust-collecting overhangs (e.g., ceiling utility pipes, hanging light fixtures) and ledges (e.g., windowsills). Additionally, at least one sink should be located in or near the compounding area for hand washing before compounding operations. Proper temperature and humidity control within the compounding area or facility is desirable.

Work areas should be well lighted, and work surfaces should be level and clean. The work surface should be smooth, impervious, free of cracks and crevices (preferably seamless), and nonshedding. Surfaces should be cleaned at both the beginning and the end of each distinct compounding operation with an appropriate cleaner or solvent. The entire compounding facility should be cleaned daily or weekly (as needed) but not during the actual process of compounding.

Equipment. The equipment needed to compound a drug product depends upon the particular dosage form requested. Although boards of pharmacy publish lists of required equipment and accessories, these lists are not intended to limit the equipment available to pharmacists for compounding.[2] Equipment should be maintained in good working order. Pharmacists are responsible for obtaining the required equipment and accessories and ensuring that equipment is properly maintained and maintenance is documented.

Weighing Equipment. In addition to a torsion balance, pharmacists who routinely compound may need to use a top-loading electronic balance that has a capacity of at least 300 g, a sensitivity of ±1 mg (or 0.1 mg), and 1-mg, 100-mg, 1-g, and 100-g weights for checking. Balances should be maintained in areas of low humidity and should be stored on flat, nonvibrating surfaces away from drafts. At least annually, the performance of balances should be checked according to the guidelines found in *Remington's Pharmaceutical Sciences,*[3] *USP XXII NF XVII: The United States Pharmacopeia–The National Formulary (USP–NF),*[4] or *USP DI Volume III: Approved Drug Products and Legal Requirements*[5] or the instructions of the balance manufacturer. Performance should be documented.

Weights should be stored in rigid, compartmentalized boxes and handled with metal, plastic, or plastic-tipped forceps—not fingers—to avoid scratching or soiling. Since most Class III prescription balances are only accurate to ±5 or 10 mg, Class P weights may be used for compounding purposes.[4] The *USP–NF* recommends that the class of weights used be chosen to limit the error to 0.1%. In practical terms this means that Class P weights can be used for weighing quantities greater than 100 mg.

The minimum weighable quantity must be determined for any balance being used for compounding. To avoid errors of 5% or more on a Class III balance with a sensitivity requirement of 6 mg, quantities of less than 120 mg of any substance should not be weighed. Smaller quantities may be weighed on more sensitive balances. If an amount is needed that is less than the minimum weighable quantity determined for a balance, an aliquot method of measurement should be used.

Measuring Equipment. The pharmacist should use judgment in selecting measuring equipment. The recommendations given in the *USP–NF* General Information section on volumetric apparatus should be followed. For maximum accuracy in measuring liquids, a pharmacist should select a graduate with a capacity equal to or slightly larger than the volume to be measured. The general rule is to measure no less than 20% of the capacity of a graduate. Calibrated syringes of the appropriate size may be preferred over graduated cylinders for measuring viscous liquids such as glycerin or mineral oil, since these liquids drain slowly and incompletely from graduated cylinders. Viscous liquids may also be weighed if this is more convenient, provided that the appropriate conversions from volume to weight are made by using the specific gravity of the liquid. Thick, opaque liquids should be weighed. For example, if a formulation specifies 1.5 mL of a liquid, it is better to use a 3-mL syringe with appropriate graduations to measure 1.5 mL than to use a 10-mL graduated cylinder, since quantities of less than 2.0 mL cannot be accurately measured in a 10-mL graduate. Also, if an opaque, viscous chemical, such as Coal Tar, USP, must be measured, it is more accurate to weigh the substance than to try to read a meniscus on a graduated cylinder or a fill line on a syringe.

For volumes smaller than 1 mL, micropipettes are recommended, in sizes to cover the range of volumes measured. Two or three variable pipettes can usually cover the range from about 50 µL to 1 mL.

Although conical graduates are convenient for mixing solutions, the error in reading the bottom of the meniscus increases as the sides flare toward the top of the graduate.

Therefore, for accurate measurements, cylindrical graduates are preferred. Conical graduates having a capacity of less than 25 mL should not be used in prescription compounding.[4]

Compounding Equipment. Pharmacists need at least two types of mortars and pestles—one glass and one Wedgwood or porcelain. The sizes of each will depend on the drug products being compounded. Glass mortars should be used for liquid preparations (solutions and suspensions) and for mixing chemicals that stain or are oily. Generally, glass mortars should be used for antineoplastic agents. Because of their rough surface, Wedgwood mortars are preferred for reducing the size of dry crystals and hard powder particles and for preparing emulsions. Porcelain mortars have a smoother surface than Wedgwood mortars and are ideal for blending powders and pulverizing soft aggregates or crystals. When Wedgwood mortars are used for small amounts of crystals or powders, the inside surface may first be lightly dusted with lactose to fill any crevices in which the crystals or powders might lodge. If the contact surfaces of the mortar and pestle become smooth with use, rubbing them with a small amount of sand or emery powder may adequately roughen them. Over extended use, a pestle and a mortar become shaped to each other's curvature. Thus, to ensure maximum contact between the surface of the head of each pestle and the interior of its corresponding mortar, pestles and mortars should not be interchanged.[3]

The compounding area should be stocked with appropriate supplies. Although supply selection depends on the types of products compounded, all areas should have weighing papers, weighing cups, or both to protect balance pans and spatulas. Glassine weighing papers (as opposed to bond weighing paper) should be used for products such as ointments, creams, and some dry chemicals. Disposable weighing dishes should also be stocked for substances like Coal Tar, USP.

Each compounding area should have stainless steel and plastic spatulas for mixing ointments and creams and handling dry chemicals. The pharmacist should exercise judgment in selecting the size and type of spatula. Small spatula blades (6 inches long or less) are preferred for handling dry chemicals, but larger spatula blades (>6 inches) are preferred for large amounts of ointments or creams and for preparing compactible powder blends for capsules. Plastic spatulas should be used for chemicals that may react with stainless steel blades. A variety of spatulas should be stocked in the compounding area, including 4-, 6-, and 8-inch stainless steel spatulas (one each) and 4- and 6-inch plastic spatulas (one each). Imprinted spatulas should not be used in compounding, since the imprinted ink on the spatula blade may contaminate the product.

The compounding area should contain an ointment slab, pill tile, or parchment ointment pad. Although parchment ointment pads are convenient and reduce cleanup time, parchment paper cannot be used for the preparation of creams because it will absorb water. Therefore, an ointment slab or pill tile is necessary. If suppositories are compounded, appropriate suppository molds, either reusable or disposable, should be available.

Other useful equipment and supplies may include funnels, filter paper, beakers, glass stirring rods, a source of heat (hot plate or microwave oven), a refrigerator, and a freezer—in some cases, an ultrafreezer capable of maintaining temperatures as low as –80 °C.

Ingredients

Ideally, only USP or NF chemicals manufactured by FDA-inspected manufacturers should be used for compounding. Although chemicals labeled USP or NF meet *USP–NF* standards for strength, quality, and purity for human drug products, the facilities in which the chemicals were manufactured may not meet FDA Good Manufacturing Practice (GMP) standards. In the event that a needed chemical is not available from an FDA-inspected facility, the pharmacist should, by next best preference, obtain a USP or NF product. If that is not available, the pharmacist should use professional judgment and may have to obtain the highest-grade chemical possible. Chemical grades that may be considered in this situation are ACS grade (meeting or exceeding specifications listed for reagent chemicals by the American Chemical Society) and FCC grade (meeting or exceeding requirements defined by the Food Chemicals Codex). Additional professional judgment is especially necessary in cases of chemical substances that have not been approved for *any* medical use. Particularly in these cases, but also in others as needed, the pharmacist, prescriber, and patient should be well informed of the risks involved.

Selection of ingredients may also depend on the dosage form to be compounded. In most cases, the prescriber specifies a particular dosage form, such as a topical ointment, oral solution or rectal suppository. Sometimes, however, the prescriber relies on the pharmacist to decide on an appropriate form. Irrespective of how the drug order is written, the pharmacist should evaluate the appropriateness of ingredients and the drug delivery system recommended. Factors to consider in selecting the dosage form include (1) physical and chemical characteristics of the active ingredient, (2) possible routes of administration that will produce the desired therapeutic effect (e.g., oral or topical), (3) patient characteristics (e.g., age, level of consciousness, ability to swallow a solid dosage form), (4) specific characteristics of the disease being treated, (5) comfort for the patient, and (6) ease or convenience of administration.

In checking the physical form of each ingredient, the pharmacist should not confuse drug substances that are available in more than one form. For example, coal tar is available as Coal Tar, USP, or Coal Tar Topical Solution, USP; phenol is available as Liquified Phenol, USP, or Phenol, USP; sulfur is available as Precipitated Sulfur, USP, or Sublimed Sulfur, USP. If ingredients are liquids, the pharmacist should consider compounding liquid dosage forms such as solutions, syrups, or elixirs for the final product. If ingredients are crystals or powders and the final dosage form is intended to be a dry dosage form, options such as divided powders (powder papers) or capsules should be considered. If ingredients are both liquids and dry forms, liquid formulations such as solutions, suspensions, elixirs, syrups, and emulsions should be considered.

Care must be exercised when using commercial drug products as a source of active ingredients. For example, extended-release or delayed-release products should not be crushed. Also, since chemicals such as preservatives and excipients in commercial products may affect the overall stability and bioavailability of the compounded product, their presence should not be ignored. Information on preservatives and excipients in specific commercial products can be found in

package inserts and also in the dosage form section of selected product monographs in *USP DI Volume I*.[6]

If an injectable drug product is a possible source of active ingredient, the pharmacist should check the salt form of the injectable product to make sure it is the same salt form ordered. If it is necessary to use a different salt because of physical or chemical compatibility considerations or product availability, the pharmacist should consult with the prescriber. Some injectable products contain active constituents in the form of prodrugs that may not be active when administered by other routes. For example, if an injectable solution is a possible source of active ingredient for an oral product, the pharmacist must consider the stability of the drug in gastric fluids, the first-pass effect, and palatability. Also, if injectable powders for reconstitution are used, expiration dating may have to be quite short.

Storage

All chemicals and drug products must be stored according to *USP–NF* and manufacturer specifications. Most chemicals and drug products marketed for compounding use are packaged by the manufacturer in tight, light-resistant containers. Chemicals intended for compounding should be purchased in small quantities and stored in the manufacturer's original container, which is labeled with product and storage information. This practice fosters the use of fresh chemicals and ensures that the manufacturer's label remains with the lot of chemical on hand. Certificates of purity for chemical ingredients should be filed for a period of time no less than the state's time requirement for retention of dispensing records.

The manufacturer's label instructions for storage should be followed explicitly to ensure the integrity of chemicals and drug products and to protect employees. Most chemicals and commercial drug products may be stored at controlled room temperature, between 15 and 30 °C (59 and 86 °F); however, the pharmacist should always check the manufacturer's label for any special storage requirements. Storage information provided for specific commercial drug products in *USP DI Volume I* and on product labels follows the definitions for storage temperatures found in the General Notices and Requirements section of *USP–NF*. An acceptable refrigerator maintains temperatures between 2 and 8 °C (36 and 46 °F); an acceptable freezer maintains temperatures between −20 and −10°C (−4 to +14 °F)

To protect pharmacy employees and property, hazardous products such as acetone and flexible collodion must be stored appropriately. Safety storage cabinets in various sizes are available from laboratory suppliers.

Personnel

Compounding personnel include pharmacists and supportive personnel engaged in any aspect of the compounding procedures.

Training. The pharmacist—who is responsible for ensuring that the best technical knowledge and skill, most careful and accurate procedures, and prudent professional judgment are consistently applied in the compounding of pharmaceuticals—must supervise all compounding activities and ensure that supportive personnel are adequately trained to perform assigned functions. Both pharmacists and the compounding personnel they supervise should participate in programs designed to enhance

and maintain competence in compounding. Training programs should include instruction in the following areas:

- Proper use of compounding equipment such as balances and measuring devices—including guidelines for selecting proper measuring devices, limitations of weighing equipment and measuring apparatus, and the importance of accuracy in measuring.
- Pharmaceutical techniques needed for preparing compounded dosage forms (e.g., levigation, trituration, methods to increase dissolution, geometric dilution).
- Properties of dosage forms (see Pharmaceutical Dosage Forms in *USP–NF*) to be compounded and related factors such as stability, storage considerations, and handling procedures.
- Literature in which information on stability, solubility, and related material can be found (see suggested references at the end of this document).
- Handling of nonhazardous and hazardous materials in the work area, including protective measures for avoiding exposure, emergency procedures to follow in the event of exposure, and the location of Material Safety Data Sheets (MSDSs) in the facility.[7–10]
- Use and interpretation of chemical and pharmaceutical symbols and abbreviations in medication orders and in product formulation directions.
- Pharmaceutical calculations.

Procedures should be established to verify the ability of staff to meet established competencies. These procedures may include observation, written tests, or quality control testing of finished products.

Attire. Personnel engaged in compounding should wear clean clothing appropriate for the duties they perform. Protective apparel, such as head, face hand, and arm coverings, should be worn as necessary to preclude contamination of products and to protect workers.

Generally, a clean laboratory jacket is considered appropriate attire for most personnel performing nonsterile compounding activities. Personnel involved in compounding hazardous materials should wear safety goggles, gloves, a mask or respirator, double gowns, and foot covers as required, depending on the substance being handled. To avoid microbial contamination of compounded drug products, written policies should be established that address appropriate precautions to be observed if an employee has an open lesion or an illness. Depending on the situation, an affected employee may be required to wear special protective apparel, such as a mask or gloves, or may be directed to avoid all contact with compounding procedures.

Reference Materials

Pharmacists and supportive personnel must have ready access to reference materials on all aspects of compounding (see suggested references at the end of this document). Earlier editions of some references, such as *Remington's Pharmaceutical Sciences,* provide more comprehensive compounding information than do the later editions. Information on compounding extemporaneous dosage forms from commercially available products can sometimes be obtained from the product's FDA-approved labeling (package insert), the manufacturer, a local pharmacy college, or a drug information center. It is essential

that the stability and proper storage conditions for extemporaneous products be thoroughly researched. Therefore, the availability of adequate references and appropriate training in the use of the references is important.

Documentation and Record Keeping

Each step of the compounding process should be documented. Pharmacists should maintain at least four sets of records in the compounding area: (1) compounding formulas and procedures, (2) a log of all compounded items, including batch records and sample batch labels (see section on packaging and labeling), (3) equipment-maintenance records, including documentation of checks of balances, refrigerators, and freezers, and (4) a record of ingredients purchased, including certificates of purity for chemicals (see section on ingredient selection) and MSDSs.

Compounding procedures should be documented in enough detail that preparations can be replicated and the history of each ingredient can be traced. Documentation should include a record of who prepared the product (if the compounder is not a pharmacist, the supervising pharmacist should also sign the compounding record); all names, lot numbers, and quantities of ingredients used; the order of mixing, including any interim procedures used (such as preparing a solution and using an aliquot); the assigned beyond-use date; and any special storage requirements (see section on stability and expiration dating). Compounding formulas and procedures should be written in a typeface that can be read easily. If formulas originate from published articles, copies of the articles should be attached to or filed with the written procedures.

Equipment maintenance and calibrations should be documented and the record maintained in an equipment-maintenance record file. Refrigerator and freezer thermometers should be checked and documented routinely, as should alarm systems indicating that temperatures are outside of acceptable limits.

Follow-up contact with patients who have received extemporaneously compounded products is recommended to ascertain that the product is physically stable and that no adverse effects have occurred from use of the product. Documentation of the contact and the findings is recommended.

Stability, Expiration, and Beyond-Use Dating

The *USP–NF*[4] defines stability as the extent to which a dosage form retains, within specified limits and throughout its period of storage and use, the same properties and characteristics that it possessed at the time of its preparation. The *USP–NF* lists the following five types of stability:

- Chemical
- Physical
- Microbiological
- Therapeutic
- Toxicological

Factors affecting stability include the properties of each ingredient, whether therapeutically active or inactive. Environmental factors such as temperature, radiation, light, humidity, and air can also affect stability. Similarly, such factors as particle size, pH, the properties of water and other solvents employed, the nature of the container, and the presence of other

substances resulting from contamination or from the intentional mixing of products can influence stability.[4]

Since compounded drug products are intended for consumption immediately or storage for a very limited time, stability evaluation and expiration dating are different for these products than for manufactured drug products. According to criteria for assigning dating in the *USP–NF*[4] General Notices and Requirements section and the Code of Federal Regulations,[11] the pharmacist labeling extemporaneously compounded drug products should be concerned with the beyond-use date as used by *USP–NF* or the expiration date as used by the Code of Federal Regulations. For uniformity, the term *beyond-use date* will be used in the remainder of this bulletin. The beyond-use date is defined as that date after which a dispensed product should no longer be used by a patient.

Determination of the period during which a compounded product may be usable after dispensing should be based on available stability information and reasonable patient needs with respect to the intended drug therapy. When a commercial drug product is used as a source of active ingredient, its expiration date can often be used as a factor in determining a beyond-use date. For stability or expiration information on commercial drug products, the pharmacist can refer to *USP DI Volume I*.[6] If no information is available, the manufacturer should be contacted. When the active ingredient is a USP or NF product, the pharmacist may be able to use the expiration dating of similar commercial products for guidance in assigning a beyond-use date. In addition, the pharmacist can often refer to published literature to obtain stability data on the same active ingredient under varying conditions and in different formulations.[12]

The pharmacist must assess the potential for instability that may result from the new environment for the active ingredients—from the combination of ingredients and the packaging materials. According to *USP–NF*,[4] hydrolysis, oxidation-reduction, and photolysis are the most common chemical reactions that cause instability. When the possibility of such reactions exists, the pharmacist should seek additional stability data or consider other approaches. These could, in extreme cases, include the preparation and dispensing of more than one compounded drug product or the use of alternative methods of dosing. For some drugs, the latter methods might include, for example, crushing a tablet or emptying the contents of a hard gelatin capsule into an appropriate food substance at each dosing time.

In assigning a beyond-use date for compounded drug products, the pharmacist should use all available stability information, plus education and experience in deciding how factors affecting product stability should be weighted. In the absence of stability data to the contrary or any indication of a stability problem, the following general criteria for assigning maximum beyond-use dates are recommended. It must be emphasized that these are *general* criteria. Professional judgment as discussed elsewhere in this section must be used in deciding when these general criteria may not be appropriate.

- When a manufactured final-dosage-form product is used as a source of active ingredient, use no more than 25% of the manufacturer's remaining expiration dating or six months, whichever is less;
- When a USP or NF chemical not from a manufactured final-dosage-form product is used, use no more than six months;

- In other cases, use the intended period of therapy or no more than 30 days, whichever is less.

All compounded products should be observed for signs of instability. Observations should be performed during preparation of the drug product and any storage period that may occur before the compounded drug product is dispensed. A list of observable indications of instability for solid, liquid, and semisolid dosage forms appears in *USP–NF*.

Packaging and Labeling

The packaging of extemporaneously compounded products for ambulatory patients should comply with regulations pertaining to the Poison Prevention Packaging Act of 1970. These regulations can be found in *USP–NF*.[4]

Containers for compounded products should be appropriate for the dosage form compounded. For example, to minimize administration errors, oral liquids should never be packaged in syringes intended to be used for injection.

The drug product container should not interact physically or chemically with the product so as to alter the strength, quality, or purity of the compounded product. Glass and plastic are commonly used in containers for compounded products. To ensure container inertness, visibility, strength, rigidity, moisture protection, ease of reclosure, and economy of packaging, glass containers have been the most widely used for compounded products.[3] Amber glass and some plastic containers may be used to protect light-sensitive products from degradation; however, glass that transmits ultraviolet or violet light rays (this includes green, blue, and clear ["flint"] glass) should not be used to protect light-sensitive products.

The use of plastic containers for compounded products has increased because plastic is less expensive and lighter in weight than glass. Since compounded products are intended for immediate use, most capsules, ointments, and creams should be stable in high-density plastic vials or ointment jars. Only plastic containers meeting *USP–NF* standards should be used.[4] Reclosable plastic bags may be acceptable for selected divided powders that are intended to be used within a short period of time.

Each compounded product should be appropriately labeled according to state and federal regulations. Labels should include the generic or chemical name of active ingredients, strength or quantity, pharmacy lot number, beyond-use date, and any special storage requirements. If a commercial product has been used as a source of drug, the generic name of the product should be used on the label. The trade name should not be used because, once the commercial drug product has been altered, it no longer exists as the approved commercial product. Listing the names and quantities of inactive ingredients on labels is also encouraged. The coining of short names for convenience (e.g., "Johnson's solution") is strongly discouraged; these names provide no assistance to others who may need to identify ingredients (e.g., in emergency circumstances).

Capsules should be labeled with the quantity (micrograms or milligrams) of active ingredient(s) per capsule. Oral liquids should be labeled with the strength or concentration per dose (e.g., 125 mg/5 mL or 10 meq/15 mL). If the quantity of an active ingredient is a whole number, the number should not be typed with a decimal point followed by a zero. For example, the strength of a capsule containing 25 mg of active ingredient should be labeled as 25 mg and not 25.0 mg. In cases where the dosage strength is less than a whole number, a zero should precede the decimal point (e.g., 0.25 µg).[3]

In expressing salt forms of chemicals on a label, it is permissible to use atomic abbreviations. For example, HCl may be used for hydrochloride, HBr for hydrobromide, Na for sodium, and K for potassium.

Vehicles should also be stated on labels, especially if similar products are prepared with different vehicles. For example, if a pharmacist prepares two potassium syrups, one using Syrup, USP, as the vehicle and one using a sugar-free syrup as the vehicle, the name of the vehicle should be included on the labels.

Liquids and semisolid concentrations may be expressed in terms of percentages. When the term "percent" or the symbol "%" is used without qualification for solids and semisolids, percent refers to weight in weight; for solutions or suspensions, percent refers to weight in volume; for solutions of liquids in liquids, percent refers to volume in volume.[4]

Labels for compounded products that are prepared in batches should include a pharmacy-assigned lot number. Assignment of a pharmacy lot number must enable the history of the compounded product to be traced, including the person compounding the product and the product's formula, ingredients, and procedures. Being able to trace the history of a batch is essential in cases of a drug product recall or withdrawal.

In the preparation of labels for batches of compounded products, all extra labels should be destroyed, since pharmacy lot numbers change with each batch. If computers, memory typewriters, or label machines are used to print batch labels, care must be taken to ensure that the memory and printing mechanism have been cleared and the correct information is programmed before any additional labels are made. It is a good practice to run a blank label between each batch of labels to ensure that the memory has been erased or cleared. To document the information printed on each set of labels, a sample label printed for the batch should be attached to the compounded-product log. If labels are sequentially prepared for different drug products, procedures should exist to minimize the risk of mislabeling the compounded products. These procedures should ensure, for example, that labels for one drug product are physically well separated from labels for any other drug product.

Auxiliary labels are convenient for conveying special storage or use information. Auxiliary labels should be attached conspicuously to containers, if possible. If the container is too small for both a general label and an auxiliary label, special storage and use instructions should appear on the label in a format that will emphasize the instructions.

Limited Batch Compounding

The purpose of extemporaneously compounding products is to provide individualized drug therapy for a particular patient. When a pharmacist is repeatedly asked to prepare identical compounded products, it may be reasonable and more efficient for the pharmacist to prepare small batches of the compounded product.

Batch sizes should be consistent with the volume of drug orders or prescriptions the pharmacist receives for the compounded product and the stability of the compounded product. The pharmacist should use judgment in deciding reasonable batch sizes. Product assays should be performed by a chemical analysis laboratory on a regular basis to ensure product

consistency among various lots, product uniformity, and stability. Analyses should be repeated every time an ingredient (active or inert) or procedure is changed. Documentation of assay findings should be filed for a period no less than the state's time requirement for the retention of dispensing records.

General Compounding Considerations

To provide the patient with the most stable drug product, the pharmacist should take the following steps upon receiving a prescription order that requires compounding.

First, the pharmacist should determine if a similar commercial product is available. A pharmacist can refer to various reference texts to check the availability of identical or similar products. Package inserts from commercially available products also contain information on inactive ingredients that can be compared with the requested formulation. If there is a commercially manufactured identical product, the local availability of the product should be determined.

When a similar product is commercially available, the pharmacist should determine which ingredients are different from the requested formulation to decide whether or not the commercial product can be used. At this stage, the pharmacist should seek answers to the following questions:

- Are all of the ingredients appropriate for the condition being treated?
- Are the concentrations of the ingredients in the drug order reasonable?
- Are the physical, chemical, and therapeutic properties of the individual ingredients consistent with the expected properties of the ordered drug product?

If the answers to these questions are positive, the pharmacist should consult the prescriber about the possibility of dispensing the commercial product. (In some states, pharmacists may not be required to obtain permission from the prescriber to dispense a commercial product if the formulation is identical to the drug order.) Dispensing a commercial product is preferable to extemporaneously compounding a drug product because commercial products carry the manufacturer's guarantee of labeled potency and stability.

If there is not a commercial product available with the same or similar formulation, the pharmacist should consider asking the prescriber the following questions:

- What is the purpose of the order? There may be another way to achieve the purpose without compounding a product.
- Where did the formula originate (article, meeting, colleague)?
- How will the drug product be used?
- Does the patient have other conditions that must be considered?
- For how long will the drug product be used?

If possible, the pharmacist should obtain a copy of the original formula to determine the extent to which the formulation has been tested for stability. When documentation is not available, the pharmacist should review the ingredients for appropriateness and reasonable concentrations.

For drug products that must be compounded, the pharmacist should closely observe the compounded drug product for any signs of instability. Such observations should be performed during preparation of the drug product and during any storage period that may occur before the compounded drug product is dispensed.

If specific packaging information is not available, a light-resistant, tight container, such as an amber vial or bottle, should be used to maximize stability (see section on packaging and labeling).

The pharmacist should label the compounded drug product, including an appropriate beyond-use date and storage instructions for the patient.

Specific Compounding Considerations

Accepted, proven compounding procedures for products including solutions, suspensions, creams, ointments, capsules, suppositories, troches, emulsions, and powders may be found in reference sources or the pharmacy literature. For additional information, pharmacists should check references cited in this document or consult colleagues or colleges of pharmacy with known expertise in compounding.

Glossary

For the purposes of this document, the following terms are used with the meanings shown.

Active Ingredient: Any chemical that is intended to furnish pharmacologic activity in the diagnosis, cure, mitigation, treatment, or prevention of disease or to affect the structure or function of the body of man or other animals.[4]

Batch: Multiple containers of a drug product or other material with uniform character and quality, within specified limits, that are prepared in anticipation of prescription drug orders based on routine, regularly observed prescribing patterns.

Cold: Any temperature not exceeding 8 °C (46 °F).[4]

Commercially Available Product: Any drug product manufactured by a producer registered with the Department of Health and Human Services as a pharmaceutical manufacturer.

Compounding: The mixing of substances to prepare a drug product.

Container: A device that holds a drug product and is or may be in direct contact with the product.[3]

Cool: Any temperature between 8 and 15 °C (46 and 59 °F).[4]

Drug Product: A finished dosage form that contains an active drug ingredient usually, but not necessarily (in the case of a placebo), in combination with inactive ingredients.[4]

Extemporaneous: Impromptu; prepared without a standard formula from an official compendium; prepared as required for a specific patient.

Inactive Ingredient: Any chemical other than the active ingredients in a drug product.[4]

Manufacturer: Anyone registered with the Department of Health and Human Services as a producer of drug products.[14]

Sensitivity Requirements: The maximal load that will cause one subdivision of change on the index plate in the position of rest of the indicator of the balance.[4]

Stability: The chemical and physical integrity of a drug product over time.[4]

Trituration: The reducing of substances to fine particles by rubbing them in a mortar with a pestle.[3]
Warm: Any temperature between 30 and 40 °C (86 and 104 °F).[4]

Suggested References

Product Availability
American Drug Index
Drug Facts & Comparisons
Physicians' Desk Reference
The Extra Pharmacopoeia (Martindale)
CHEMSOURCES
AHFS Drug Information

Compounding Techniques
Compounding Companion PC-Based Software
King's *Dispensing of Medications*
Remington's Pharmaceutical Sciences
Contemporary Compounding column in *U.S. Pharmacist*

Pharmaceutical Calculations
Stoklosa and Ansel's *Pharmaceutical Calculations*
Math—Use It or Lose It column in *Hospital Pharmacy*
Calculations in Pharmacy column in *U.S. Pharmacist*

Drug Stability and Compatibility
American Journal of Hospital Pharmacy
ASHP's *Handbook on Extemporaneous Formulations*
ASHP's *Handbook on Injectable Drugs*
International Pharmaceutical Abstracts
Journal of the Parenteral Drug Association (now *Journal of Pharmaceutical Science and Technology*)
Canadian Society of Hospital Pharmacists *Extemporaneous Oral Liquid Dosage Preparations*
Pediatric Drug Formulations
Physicians' Desk Reference
Contemporary Compounding column in *U.S. Pharmacist*
AHFS Drug Information
The Merck Index

References

1. Pancorbo SA, Campagna KD, Devenport JK, et al. Task force report of competency statements for pharmacy practice. *Am J Pharm Educ.* 1987; 51:196–206.
2. Allen LV Jr. Establishing and marketing your extemporaneous compounding service. *US Pharm.* 1990; 15(Dec):74–7.
3. Remington's pharmaceutical sciences. 18th ed. Gennaro AR, ed. Easton, PA: Mack Publishing; 1990; 1630–1, 1658, 1660.
4. The United States Pharmacopeia, 22nd rev., and The National Formulary, 17th ed. Rockville, MD: The United States Pharmacopeial Convention; 1989.
5. USP DI Volume III: Approved drug products and legal requirements. 14th ed. Rockville, MD: The United States Pharmacopeial Convention; 1994.
6. USP DI Volume I: Drug information for the health care professional. 14th ed. Rockville, MD: The United States Pharmacopeial Convention; 1994.
7. 29 §C.F.R. 1910. 1200(1990).
8. ASHP technical assistance bulletin on handling cytotoxic and hazardous drugs. *Am J Hosp Pharm.* 1990; 47:1033–49.
9. Feinberg JL. Complying with OSHA's Hazard Communication Standard. *Consult Pharm.* 1991; 6:444, 446, 448.
10. Myers CE. Applicability of OSHA Hazard Communication Standard to drug products. *Am J Hosp Pharm.* 1990; 47:1960–1.
11. 21 C.F.R. §211.137.
12. Connors KA, Amidon GL, Stella VJ. Chemical stability of pharmaceuticals: a handbook for pharmacists. 2nd ed. New York: Wiley; 1986.
13. American Society of Hospital Pharmacists. ASHP guidelines on preventing medication errors in hospitals. *Am J Hosp Pharm.* 1993; 50:305–14.
14. Fitzgerald WL Jr. The legal authority to compound in pharmacy practice. *Tenn Pharm.* 1990; 26(Mar):21–2.

Approved by the ASHP Board of Directors, April 27, 1994. Developed by the Council on Professional Affairs.

The bibliographic citation for this document is as follows: American Society of Hospital Pharmacists. ASHP technical assistance bulletin on compounding nonsterile products in pharmacies. *Am J Hosp Pharm.* 1994; 51:1441–8.

Distribution

Technician-Checking-Technician Programs (0310)
Source: Council on Administrative Affairs
To advocate technician-checking-technician programs (with appropriate quality control measures) in order to permit redirection of pharmacist resources to patient care activities; further,

To advocate state board of pharmacy approval of these programs.

This policy was reviewed in 2007 by the Council on Pharmacy Management and by the Board of Directors and was found to still be appropriate.

Dispensing by Nonpharmacists and Nonprescribers (0010)
Source: Council on Legal and Public Affairs
To reaffirm the position that all medication dispensing functions must be performed by, or under the supervision of, a pharmacist; further,

To reaffirm the position that any relationships that are established between a pharmacist and other individuals in order to carry out the dispensing function should preserve the role of the pharmacist in (a) maintaining appropriate patient protection and safety, (b) complying with regulatory and legal requirements, and (c) providing individualized patient care.

This policy was reviewed in 2009 by the Council on Public Policy and by the Board of Directors and was found to still be appropriate.

ASHP Statement on Pharmacist's Responsibility for Distribution and Control of Drug Products

A fundamental purpose of pharmaceutical services in any setting is to ensure the safe and appropriate use of drug products and drug-related devices. Fulfillment of this responsibility is enhanced through the pharmacist's involvement in all aspects of the use of drugs.[1]

This involvement should include decisions and actions with respect to the evaluation, procurement, storage, distribution, and administration of all drug products. The pharmacist is responsible for development, in consultation with appropriate other professionals, departments, and interdisciplinary committees in the setting, of all drug-use control policies. The pharmacist should be directly responsible for the control and distribution of all stocks of drugs.

The Federal Food, Drug, and Cosmetic Act defines the term *drug* as "(A) articles recognized in the official United States Pharmacopeia, official Homeopathic Pharmacopeia of the United States, or official National Formulary, or any supplement to any of them; and (B) articles intended for use in the diagnosis, cure, mitigation, treatment, or prevention of disease in man or other animals; and (C) articles (other than food) intended to affect the structure or any function of the body of man or other animals; and (D) articles intended for use as a component of any article specified in clauses (A), (B), or (C) of this paragraph; but does not include devices or their components, parts, or accessories."[2]

For purposes of this document, drugs include those used by inpatients and outpatients, large- and small-volume injections, radiopharmaceuticals, diagnostic agents including radiopaque contrast media, anesthetic gases, blood-fraction drugs, dialysis fluids, respiratory therapy drugs, biotechnologically produced drugs, investigational drugs, drug samples, drugs brought to the setting by patients or family, and other chemicals and biological substances administered to patients to evoke or enhance pharmacologic responses.

The pharmacist's responsibility for drug-use control extends throughout the setting served. This purview extends to all pharmacy satellite locations (inpatient and outpatient, including those serving the general public), emergency rooms, surgical and labor and delivery suites (and related areas such as recovery rooms), anesthesiology, nuclear medicine, radiology, dialysis areas, ambulatory care clinics and treatment (including surgery) areas, respiratory therapy areas, central sterile supply centers, blood banks, intensive care areas, cardiac catheterization suites,

research areas, and all other areas in which drugs are handled and used. The pharmacist should be responsible for drug-use policies and routine inspection of all drug stocks, even if direct custody and distribution are not possible.

The pharmacist also has an advocacy responsibility with respect to decisions and policies about the use of drug-related devices as they affect drug therapy. As appropriate, the pharmacist may also be assigned direct responsibility for control and distribution of drug-related devices.[3] Drug-related devices include electromechanical pumps, devices for administration of injectable drugs, devices for monitoring plasma drug concentration, and devices for monitoring drug administration rate.

References

1. American Society of Hospital Pharmacists. ASHP guidelines: minimum standard for pharmacies in institutions. *Am J Hosp Pharm.* 1985; 42:372–5.
2. 21 U.S.C. §321 (g) (1).
3. American Society of Hospital Pharmacists. ASHP statement on the pharmacist's role with respect to drug delivery systems and administration devices. *Am J Hosp Pharm.* 1989; 46:802–4.

This statement was reviewed in 2005 by the Council on Professional Affairs and by the Board of Directors and was found to still be appropriate.

Approved by the ASHP Board of Directors, November 16, 1994, and by the ASHP House of Delegates, June 5, 1995. Revised by the ASHP Council on Professional Affairs. Supersedes a previous version dated June 3, 1992.

The bibliographic citation for this document is as follows: ASHP statement on the pharmacist's responsibility for distribution and control of drug products. In: *Practice Standards of ASHP 1996–97.* Deffenbaugh JH, ed. Bethesda, MD: American Society of Health-System Pharmacists; 1996.

ASHP Statement on Unit Dose Drug Distribution

The unit dose system of medication distribution is a pharmacy-coordinated method of dispensing and controlling medications in organized health-care settings.

The unit dose system may differ in form, depending on the specific needs of the organization. However, the following distinctive elements are basic to all unit dose systems: medications are contained in single unit packages; they are dispensed in as ready-to-administer form as possible; and for most medications, not more than a 24-hour supply[a] of doses is delivered to or available at the patient-care area at any time.[1,2]

Numerous studies concerning unit dose drug distribution systems have been published over the past several decades. These studies indicate categorically that unit dose systems, with respect to other drug distribution methods, are (1) safer for the patient, (2) more efficient and economical for the organization, and (3) a more effective method of utilizing professional resources.

More specifically, the inherent advantages of unit dose systems over alternative distribution procedures are

1. A reduction in the incidence of medication errors.
2. A decrease in the total cost of medication-related activities.
3. A more efficient usage of pharmacy and nursing personnel, allowing for more direct patient-care involvement by pharmacists and nurses.
4. Improved overall drug control and drug use monitoring.
5. More accurate patient billings for drugs.
6. The elimination or minimization of drug credits.
7. Greater control by the pharmacist over pharmacy workload patterns and staff scheduling.
8. A reduction in the size of drug inventories located in patient-care areas.
9. Greater adaptability to computerized and automated procedures.

In view of these demonstrated benefits, the American Society of Hospital Pharmacists considers the unit dose system to be an essential part of drug distribution and control in organized health-care settings in which drug therapy is an integral component of health-care delivery.

References

1. Summerfield MR. Unit dose primer. Bethesda, MD: American Society of Hospital Pharmacists; 1983.
2. American Society of Hospital Pharmacists. ASHP technical assistance bulletin on hospital drug distribution and control. *Am J Hosp Pharm.* 1980; 37:1097–1103.

[a]In long-term care facilities, a larger supply of medication (e.g., 48 or 72 hours) may be acceptable.

Approved by the ASHP Board of Directors, November 16, 1988, and by the ASHP House of Delegates, June 5, 1989. Supersedes previous versions approved by the House of Delegates on June 8, 1981, and by the Board of Directors on April 19, 1975, and November 13–14, 1980.

The bibliographic citation for this document is as follows: American Society of Hospital Pharmacists. ASHP statement on unit dose drug distribution. *Am J Hosp Pharm.* 1989; 46:2346.

ASHP Technical Assistance Bulletin on Hospital Drug Distribution and Control

Drug control (of which drug distribution is an important part) is among the pharmacist's most important responsibilities. Therefore, adequate methods to assure that these responsibilities are met must be developed and implemented. These guidelines will assist the pharmacist in preparing drug control procedures for all medication-related activities. The guidelines are based on the premise that the pharmacy is responsible for the procurement, distribution, and control of *all* drugs used within the institution. In a sense, the entire hospital is the pharmacy, and the pharmacy service is simply a functional service extending throughout the institution's physical and organizational structures.

It should be noted that, although this document is directed toward hospitals, much of it is relevant to other types of health-care facilities.

Pharmacy Policies, Procedures, and Communications

Policy and Procedure Manuals.[1] The effectiveness of the drug control system depends on adherence to policies (broad, general statements of philosophy) and procedures (detailed guidelines for implementing policy). The importance of an up-to-date policy and procedure manual for drug control cannot be overestimated. All pharmacy staff must be familiar with the manual; it is an important part of orientation for new staff and crucial to the pharmacy's internal communication mechanism. In addition, preparing written policies and procedures requires a thorough analysis of control operations; this review might go undone otherwise.

Drug control begins with the setting of policy. The authority to enforce drug control policy and procedures must come from the administration of the institution, with the endorsement of the medical staff, via the pharmacy and therapeutics (P&T) committee and/or other appropriate committee(s). Because the drug control system interfaces with numerous departments and professions, the P&T committee should be the focal point for communications relating to drug control in the institution. The pharmacist, with the cooperation of the P&T committee, should develop media such as newsletters, bulletins, and seminars to communicate with persons functioning within the framework of the control system.

Inservice Training and Education. Intra- and interdepartmental education and training programs are important to the effective implementation of policies and procedures and the institution's drug control system in general. They are part of effective communication and help establish and maintain professional relationships among the pharmacy staff and between it and other hospital departments. Drug control policies and procedures should be included in the pharmacy's educational programs.

Standards, Laws, and Regulations

The pharmacist must be aware of and comply with the laws, regulations, and standards governing the profession. Many of these standards and regulations deal with aspects of drug control. Among the agencies and organizations affecting institutional pharmacy practice are those described below.

Regulatory Agencies and Organizations. The U.S. government, through its Food and Drug Administration (FDA), is responsible for implementing and enforcing the federal Food, Drug, and Cosmetic Act. The FDA is responsible for the control and prevention of misbranding and of adulteration of food, drugs, and cosmetics moving in interstate commerce. The FDA also sets label requirements for food, drugs, and cosmetics; sets standards for investigational drug studies and for marketing of new drug products; and compiles data on adverse drug reactions.

The U.S. Department of the Treasury influences pharmacy operation by regulating the use of tax-free alcohol through the Bureau of Alcohol, Tobacco and Firearms. The U.S. Department of Justice affects pharmacy practice through its Drug Enforcement Agency (DEA) by enforcing the Controlled Substances Act of 1970 and other federal laws and regulations for controlled drugs.

Another federal agency, the Health Care Financing Administration, has established Conditions of Participation for hospitals and skilled nursing facilities to assist these institutions to qualify for reimbursement under the health insurance program for the aged (Medicare) and for Medicaid.

The state board of pharmacy is the agency of state government responsible for regulating pharmacy practice within the state. Practitioners, institutions, and community pharmacies must obtain licenses from the board to practice pharmacy or provide pharmacy services in the state. State boards of pharmacy promulgate numerous regulations pertaining to drug dispensing and control. (In some states, the state board of health licenses the hospital pharmacy separately or through a license that includes all departments of the hospital.)

Standards and guidelines for pharmaceutical services have been established by the Joint Commission on Accreditation of Hospitals (JCAH)[2] and the American Society of Hospital Pharmacists (ASHP)[3]. The United States Pharmacopeial Convention also promulgates certain pharmacy practice procedures as well as official standards for drugs and drug testing. Professional practice guidelines and standards generally do not have the force of law but rather are intended to assist pharmacists in achieving the highest level of practice. They may, however, be employed in legal proceedings as evidence of what constitutes acceptable practice as determined by the profession itself.

In some instances, both federal and state laws may deal with a specific activity; in such cases, the more stringent law will apply.

The Medication System

Procurement: Drug Selection, Purchasing Authority, Responsibility, and Control.[4–6] The selection of pharmaceuticals is a basic and extremely important professional function of the hospital pharmacist who is charged with making decisions regarding products, quantities, product specifications, and

sources of supply. It is the pharmacist's obligation to establish and maintain standards assuring the quality, proper storage, control, and safe use of all pharmaceuticals and related supplies (e.g., fluid administration sets); this responsibility must not be delegated to another individual. Although the actual purchasing of drugs and supplies may be performed by a non-pharmacist, the setting of quality standards and specifications requires professional knowledge and judgment and must be performed only by the pharmacist.

Economic and therapeutic considerations make it necessary for hospitals to have a well-controlled, continuously updated formulary. It is the pharmacist's responsibility to develop and maintain adequate product specifications to aid in the purchase of drugs and related supplies under the formulary system. The *USP–NF* is a good base for drug product specifications; there also should be criteria to evaluate the acceptability of manufacturers and distributors. In establishing the formulary, the P&T committee recommends guidelines for drug selection. However, when his knowledge indicates, the pharmacist must have the authority to reject a particular drug product or supplier.

Although the pharmacist has the authority to select a brand or source of supply, he must make economic considerations subordinate to those of quality. Competitive bid purchasing is an important method for achieving a proper balance between quality and cost when two or more acceptable suppliers market a particular product meeting the pharmacist's specifications. In selecting a vendor, the pharmacist must consider price, terms, shipping times, dependability, quality of service, returned goods policy, and packaging; however, prime importance always must be placed on drug quality and the manufacturer's reputation. It should be noted that the pharmacist is responsible for the quality of all drugs dispensed by the pharmacy.

Records. The pharmacist must establish and maintain adequate recordkeeping systems. Various records must be retained (and be retrievable) by the pharmacy because of governmental regulations; some are advisable for legal protection, others are needed for JCAH accreditation, and still others are necessary for sound management (evaluation of productivity, workloads, and expenses and assessment of departmental growth and progress) of the pharmacy department. Records must be retained for at least the length of time prescribed by law (where such requirements apply).

It is important that the pharmacist study federal, state, and local laws to become familiar with their requirements for permits, tax stamps, storage of alcohol and controlled substances, records, and reports.

Among the records needed in the drug distribution and control system are

- Controlled substances inventory and dispensing records.
- Records of medication orders and their processing.
- Manufacturing and packaging production records.
- Pharmacy workload records.
- Purchase and inventory records.
- Records of equipment maintenance.
- Records of results and actions taken in quality-assurance and drug audit programs.

Receiving Drugs. Receiving control should be under the auspices of a responsible individual, and the pharmacist must ensure that records and forms provide proper control upon receipt of drugs. Complete accountability from purchase order initiation to drug administration must be provided.

Personnel involved in the purchase, receipt, and control of drugs should be well trained in their responsibilities and duties and must understand the serious nature of drugs. All nonprofessional personnel employed by the pharmacy should be selected and supervised by the pharmacist.

Delivery of drugs directly to the pharmacy or other pharmacy receiving area is highly desirable; it should be considered mandatory for controlled drugs. Orders for controlled substances must be checked against the official order blank (when applicable) and against hospital purchase order forms. All drugs should be placed into stock promptly upon receipt, and controlled substances must be directly transferred to safes or other secure areas.

Drug Storage and Inventory Control. Storage is an important aspect of the total drug control system. Proper environmental control (i.e., proper temperature, light, humidity, conditions of sanitation, ventilation, and segregation) must be maintained wherever drugs and supplies are stored in the institution. Storage areas must be secure; fixtures and equipment used to store drugs should be constructed so that drugs are accessible only to designated and authorized personnel. Such personnel must be carefully selected and supervised. Safety also is an important factor, and proper consideration should be given to the safe storage of poisons and flammable compounds. Externals should be stored separately from internal medications. Medications stored in a refrigerator containing items other than drugs should be kept in a secured, separate compartment.

Proper control is important wherever medications are kept, whether in general storage in the institution or the pharmacy or patient-care areas (including satellite pharmacies, nursing units, clinics, emergency rooms, operating rooms, recovery rooms, and treatment rooms). Expiration dates of perishable drugs must be considered in all of these locations, and stock must be rotated as required. A method to detect and properly dispose of outdated, deteriorated, recalled, or obsolete drugs and supplies should be established. This should include monthly audits of all medication storage areas in the institution. (The results of these audits should be documented in writing.)

Since the pharmacist must justify and account for the expenditure of pharmacy funds, he must maintain an adequate inventory management system. Such a system should enable the pharmacist to analyze and interpret prescribing trends and their economic impacts and appropriately minimize inventory levels. It is essential that a system to indicate subminimum inventory levels be developed to avoid "outages," along with procedures to procure emergency supplies of drugs when necessary.

In-House Manufacturing, Bulk Compounding, Packaging, and Labeling.[7,8] As with commercially marketed drug products, those produced by the pharmacy must be accurate in identity, strength, purity, and quality. Therefore, there must be adequate process and finished product controls for all manufacturing/bulk compounding and packaging operations. Written master formulas and batch records (including product test results) must be maintained. All technical personnel must be adequately trained and supervised.

Packaging and labeling operations must have controls sufficient to prevent product/package/label mixups. A lot number to identify each finished product with its production and control history must be assigned to each batch.

The Good Manufacturing Practices of the FDA is a useful model for developing a comprehensive control system.

The pharmacist is encouraged to prepare those drug dosage forms, strengths, and packagings that are needed for optimal drug therapy but that are commercially unavailable. Adequate attention must be given to the stability, palatability, packaging, and labeling requirements of these products.

Medication Distribution (Unit Dose System).[9-11] Medication distribution is the responsibility of the pharmacy. The pharmacist, with the assistance of the P&T committee and the department of nursing, must develop comprehensive policies and procedures that provide for the safe distribution of all medications and related supplies to inpatients and outpatients.

For reasons of safety and economy, the preferred method to distribute drugs in institutions is the *unit dose* system. Although the unit dose system may differ in form depending on the specific needs, resources, and characteristics of each institution, four elements are common to all: (1) medications are contained in, and administered from, single unit or unit dose packages; (2) medications are dispensed in ready-to-administer form to the extent possible; (3) for most medications, not more than a 24-hour supply of doses is provided to or available at the patient-care area at any time; and (4) a patient medication profile is concurrently maintained in the pharmacy for each patient. Floor stocks of drugs are minimized and limited to drugs for emergency use and routinely used "safe" items such as mouthwash and antiseptic solutions.

(1) Physician's drug order: writing the order. Medications should be given (with certain specified exceptions) only on the *written* order of a qualified physician or other authorized prescriber. Allowable exceptions to this rule (i.e., telephone or verbal orders) should be put in written form immediately and the prescriber should countersign the nurse's or pharmacist's signed record of these orders within 48 (preferably 24) hours. Only a pharmacist or registered nurse should accept such orders. Provision should be made to place physician's orders in the patient's chart, and a method for sending this information to the pharmacy should be developed.

Prescribers should specify the date and time medication orders are written.

Medication orders should be written legibly in ink and should include

- Patient's name and location (unless clearly indicated on the order sheet).
- Name (generic) of medication.
- Dosage expressed in the metric system, except in instances where dosage must be expressed otherwise (i.e., units, etc.).
- Frequency of administration.
- Route of administration.
- Signature of the physician.
- Date and hour the order was written.

Any abbreviations used in medication orders should be agreed to and jointly adopted by the medical, nursing, pharmacy, and medical records staff of the institution.

Any questions arising from a medication order, including the interpretation of an illegible order, should be referred to the ordering physician by the pharmacist. It is desirable for the pharmacist to make (appropriate) entries in the patient's medical chart pertinent to the patient's drug therapy. (Proper authorization for this must be obtained.[12]) Also, a duplicate record of the entry can be maintained in the pharmacy profile.

In computerized patient data systems, each prescriber should be assigned a unique identifier; this number should be included in all medication orders. Unauthorized personnel should not be able to gain access to the system.

(2) Physician's drug order: medication order sheets. The pharmacist (except in emergency situations) must receive the physician's original order or a direct copy of the order before the drug is dispensed. This permits the pharmacist to resolve questions or problems with drug orders before the drug is dispensed and administered. It also eliminates errors which may arise when drug orders are transcribed onto another form for use by the pharmacy. Several methods by which the pharmacy may receive physicians' original orders or direct copies are

1. Self-copying order forms. The physician's order form is designed to make a direct copy (carbon or NCR) which is sent to the pharmacy. This method provides the pharmacist with a duplicate copy of the order and does not require special equipment. There are two basic formats:
 a. Orders for medications included among treatment orders. Use of this form allows the physician to continue writing his orders on the chart as he has been accustomed in the past, leaving all other details to hospital personnel.
 b. Medication orders separated from other treatment orders on the order form. The separation of drug orders makes it easier for the pharmacist to review the order sheet.
2. Electromechanical. Copying machines or similar devices may be used to produce an exact copy of the physician's order. Provision should be made to transmit physicians' orders to the pharmacy in the event of mechanical failure.
3. Computerized. Computer systems, in which the physician enters orders into a computer which then stores and prints out the orders in the pharmacy or elsewhere, are used in some institutions. Any such system should provide for the pharmacist's verification of any drug orders entered into the system by anyone other than an authorized prescriber.

(3) Physician's drug order: time limits and changes. Medication orders should be reviewed automatically when the patient goes to the delivery room, operating room, or a different service. In addition, a method to protect patients from indefinite, open-ended drug orders must be provided. This may be accomplished through one or more of the following: (1) routine monitoring of patients' drug therapy by a pharmacist; (2) drug class-specific, automatic stop-order policies covering those drug orders not specifying a number of doses or duration of therapy; and (3) automatic cancellation of all drug orders after a predetermined (by the P&T committee) time interval unless rewritten by the prescriber. Whatever the method used, it must protect the patient, as well as provide for a timely notification to the prescriber that the order will be stopped *before* such action takes place.

(4) Physician's drug order: receipt of order and drug profiles. A pharmacist must review and interpret every medication order and resolve any problems or uncertainties with

it before the drug is entered into the dispensing system. This means that he must be satisfied that each questionable medication order is, in fact, acceptable. This may occur through study of the patient's medical record, research of the professional literature, or discussion with the prescriber or other medical, nursing, or pharmacy staff. Procedures to handle a drug order the pharmacist still believes is unacceptable (e.g., very high dose or a use beyond that contained in the package insert) should be prepared (and reviewed by the hospital's legal counsel). In general, the physician must be able to support the use of the drug in these situations. It is generally advisable for the pharmacist to document actions (e.g., verbal notice to the physician that a less toxic drug was available and should be used) relative to a questionable medication order on the pharmacy's patient medication profile form or other pharmacy document (not in the medical record).

Once the order has been approved, it is entered into the *patient's medication profile*. A medication profile must be maintained in the pharmacy for all inpatients and those outpatients routinely receiving care at the institution. (Note: Equivalent records also should be available at the patient-care unit.) This essential item, which is continuously updated, may be a written copy or computer maintained. It serves two purposes. First, it enables the pharmacist to become familiar with the patient's total drug regimen, enabling him to detect quickly potential interactions, unintended dosage changes, drug duplications and overlapping therapies, and drugs contraindicated because of patient allergies or other reasons. Second, it is required in unit dose systems in order for the individual medication doses to be scheduled, prepared, distributed, and administered on a timely basis. The profile information must be reviewed by the pharmacist *before* dispensing the patient's drug(s). (It also may be useful in retrospective review of drug use.)

Patient profile information should include

- Patient's full name, date hospitalized, age, sex, weight, hospital I.D. number, and provisional diagnosis or reason for admission (the format for this information will vary from one hospital to another).
- Laboratory test results.
- Other medical data relevant to the patient's drug therapy (e.g., information from drug history interviews).
- Sensitivities, allergies, and other significant contraindications.
- Drug products dispensed, dates of original orders, strengths, dosage forms, quantities, dosage frequency or directions, and automatic stop dates.
- Intravenous therapy data (this information may be kept on a separate profile form, but there should be a method for the pharmacist to review both concomitantly).
- Blood products administered.
- Pharmacist's or technician's initials.
- Number of doses or amounts dispensed.
- Items relevant or related to the patient's drug therapy (e.g., blood products) not provided by the pharmacy.

(5) Physician's drug order: records. Appropriate records of each medication order and its processing in the pharmacy must be maintained. Such records must be retained in accordance with applicable state laws and regulations. Any changes or clarifications in the order should be written in the chart. The signature(s) or initials of the person(s) verifying the transcription of medication orders into the medication profile should be noted. A way should be provided to determine, for all doses dispensed, who prepared the dose, its date of dispensing, the source of the drug, and the person who checked it. Other information, such as the time of receipt of the order and management data (number of orders per patient day and the like) should be kept as desired. Medication profiles also may be useful for retrospective drug use review studies.

(6) Physician's drug order: special orders.[5,6,13,14] Special orders (i.e., "stat" and emergency orders and those for nonformulary drugs, investigational drugs, restricted use drugs, or controlled substances) should be processed according to specific written procedures meeting all applicable regulations and requirements.

(7) Physician's drug order: other considerations. The pharmacy, nursing, and medical staffs, through the P&T committee, should develop a schedule of standard drug administration times. The nurse should notify the pharmacist whenever it is necessary to deviate from the standard medication schedule.

A mechanism to continually inform the pharmacy of patient admissions, discharges, and transfers should be established.

(8) Intravenous admixture services.[15] The preparation of sterile products (e.g., intravenous admixtures, "piggybacks," and irrigations) is an important part of the drug control system. The pharmacy is responsible for assuring that all such products used in the institution are (1) therapeutically and pharmaceutically appropriate (i.e., are rational and free of incompatibilities or similar problems) to the patient; (2) free from microbial and pyrogenic contaminants; (3) free from unacceptable levels of particulate and other toxic contaminants; (4) correctly prepared (i.e., contain the correct amounts of the correct drugs); and (5) properly labeled, stored, and distributed. Centralizing all sterile compounding procedures within the pharmacy department is the best way to achieve these goals.

Parenteral admixtures and related solutions are subject to the same considerations presented in the preceding sections on "physician's drug order." However, their special characteristics (e.g., complex preparation or need for sterility assurance) also mandate certain additional requirements concerning their preparation, labeling, handling, and quality control. These are described in Reference 15.

It is important that the pharmacy is notified of any problems that arise within the institution pertaining to the use of intravenous drugs and fluids (infections, phlebitis, and product defects).

(9) Medication containers, labeling, and dispensing: stock containers. The pharmacist is responsible for labeling medication containers. Medication labels should be typed or machine printed. Labeling with pen or pencil and the use of adhesive tape or china marking pencils should be prohibited. A label should not be superimposed on another label. The label should be legible and free from erasures and strikeovers. It should be firmly affixed to the container. The labels for stock containers should be protected from chemical action or abrasion and bear the name, address, and telephone number of the hospital. Medication containers and labels should not be altered by anyone other than pharmacy personnel. Prescription labels should not be distributed outside the pharmacy. Accessory labels and statements (shake well, may not be refilled, and the like) should be used as required. Any container to be used outside the institution should bear its name, address, and phone number.

Important labeling considerations are

1. The metric system should be given prominence on all labels when both metric and apothecary measurement units are given.
2. The names of all therapeutically active ingredients should be indicated in compound mixtures.
3. Labels for medications should indicate the amount of drug or drugs in each dosage unit (e.g., per 5 ml and per capsule).
4. rugs and chemicals in forms intended for dilution or reconstitution should carry appropriate directions.
5. he expiration date of the contents, as well as proper storage conditions, should be clearly indicated.
6. The acceptable route(s) of administration should be indicated for parenteral medications.
7. Labels for large volume sterile solutions should permit visual inspection of the container contents.
8. Numbers, letters, coined names, unofficial synonyms, and abbreviations should not be used to identify medications, with the exception of approved letter or number codes for investigational drugs (or drugs being used in blinded clinical studies).
9. Containers presenting difficulty in labeling, such as small tubes, should be labeled with no less than the prescription serial number, name of drug, strength, and name of the patient. The container should then be placed in a larger carton bearing a label with all necessary information.
10. The label should conform to all applicable federal, state, and local laws and regulations.
11. Medication labels of stock containers and repackaged or prepackaged drugs should carry codes to identify the source and lot number of medication.
12. Nonproprietary name(s) should be given prominence over proprietary names.
13. Amount dispensed (e.g., number of tablets) should be indicated.
14. Drug strengths, volumes, and amounts should be given as recommended in References 11 and 16.

(10) Medication containers, labeling, and dispensing: inpatient medications.[11,16] Drug products should be as ready for administration to the patient as the current status of pharmaceutical technology permits. Inpatient medication containers and packages should conform to applicable *USP* requirements and the guidelines in References 11 and 16.

Inpatient self-care and "discharge" medications should be labeled as outpatient prescriptions (see below).

(11) Medication containers, labeling, and dispensing: outpatient medications.[17] Outpatient medications must be labeled in accordance with state board of pharmacy and federal regulations. As noted, medications given to patients as "discharge medication" must be labeled in the pharmacy (not by nursing personnel) as outpatient prescriptions.

The source of the medication and initials of the dispenser should be noted on the prescription form at the time of dispensing. If feasible, the lot number also should be recorded.

An identifying check system to ensure proper identification of outpatients should be established.

Outpatient prescriptions should be packaged in accordance with the provisions of the Poison Prevention Packaging Act of 1970 and any regulations thereunder. They must also meet any applicable requirements of the *USP.*

Any special instructions to or procedures required of the patient relative to the drug's preparation, storage, and administration should be either a part of the label or accompany the medication container received by the patient. Counseling of the patient sufficient to ensure understanding and compliance (to the extent possible) with his medication regimen must be conducted. Nonprescription drugs, if used in the institution, should be labeled as any other medication.

(12) Delivery of medications. Couriers used to deliver medications should be reliable and carefully chosen.

Pneumatic tubes, dumbwaiters, medication carts, and the like should protect drug products from breakage and theft. In those institutions having automatic delivery equipment, such as a pneumatic tube system, provision must be made for an alternative delivery method in case of breakdown.

All parts of the transportation system must protect medications from pilferage. Locks and other security devices should be used where necessary. Procedures for the orderly transfer of medications to the nurse should be instituted; i.e., drug carts or pneumatic tube carriers should not arrive at the patient-care area without the nurse or her designee acknowledging their arrival.

Medications must always be properly secured. Storage areas and equipment should meet the requirements presented in other sections of these guidelines.

(13) Administration of medications. The institution should develop detailed written procedures governing medication administration. In doing so, the following guidelines should be considered:

1. All medications should be administered by appropriately trained and authorized personnel in accordance with the laws, regulations, and institutional policies governing drug administration. It is particularly important that there are written policies and procedures defining responsibility for starting parenteral infusions, administering all intravenous medications, and adding medications to flowing parenteral fluids. Procedures for drug administration by respiratory therapists and during emergency situations also should be established. Exceptions to any of these policies should be provided in writing.
2. ll medications should be administered directly from the medication cart (or equivalent) at the patient's room. The use of unit dose packaged drugs eliminates the need for medication cups and cards (and their associated trays), and they should not be used. A medication should not be removed from the unit dose package until it is to be administered.
3. Medications prepared for administration but not used must be returned to the pharmacy.
4. Medications should be given as near the specified time as possible.
5. The patient for whom the medication is intended should be positively identified by checking the patient's identification band or hospital number or by other means as specified by hospital policy.
6. The person administering the medication should stay with the patient until the dose has been taken. Exceptions to this rule are specific medications which may be left at the patient's bedside upon the physician's written order for self-administration.
7. Parenteral medications that are not to be mixed together in a syringe should be given in different injection sites on the patient or separately injected into the

administration site of the administration set of a compatible intravenous fluid.

8. The pharmacy should receive copies of all medication error reports or other medication-related incidents.
9. A system to assure that patients permitted to self-medicate do so correctly should be established.

(14) Return of unused medication. All medications that have not been administered to the patient must remain in the medication cart and be returned to the pharmacy. Only those medications returned in unopened sealed packages may be reissued. Medications returned by outpatients should not be reused. Procedures for crediting and returning drugs to stock should be instituted. A mechanism to reconcile doses not given with nursing and pharmacy records should be provided.

(15) Recording of medication administration. All administered, refused, or omitted medication doses should be recorded in the patient's medical record according to an established procedure. Disposition of doses should occur immediately after administering medications to each patient and before proceeding to the next patient. Information to be recorded should include the drug name, dose and route of administration, date and time of administration, and initials of the person administering the dose.

Drug Samples and Medical Sales Representatives.[18] The use of drug samples within the institution is strongly discouraged and should be eliminated to the extent possible. They should never be used for inpatients (unless, for some reason, no other source of supply is available to the pharmacy). Any samples used must be controlled and dispensed through the pharmacy.

Written regulations governing the activities of medical sales representatives within the institution should be established. Sales representatives should receive a copy of these rules and their activities should be monitored.

Investigational Drugs.[13] Policies and procedures governing the use and control of investigational drugs within the institution are necessary. Detailed procedural guidelines are given in Reference 13.

Radiopharmaceuticals. The basic principles of compounding, packaging, sterilizing, testing, and controlling drugs in institutions apply to radiopharmaceuticals. Therefore, even if the pharmacy department is not directly involved with the preparation and dispensing of these agents, the pharmacist must ensure that their use conforms to the drug control principles set forth in this document.

"Bring-In" Medications. The use of a patient's own medications within the hospital should be avoided to the extent possible. They should be used only if the drugs are not obtainable by the pharmacy. If they are used, the physician must write an appropriate order in the patient's medical chart. The drugs should be sent to the pharmacy for verification of their identity; if not identifiable, they must not be used. They should be dispensed as part of the unit dose system, not separate from it.

Drug Control in Operating and Recovery Rooms.[19] The institution's drug control system must extend to its operating room complex. The pharmacist should ensure that all drugs used within this area are properly ordered, stored, prepared, and accounted for.

Emergency Medication Supplies. A policy to supply emergency drugs when the pharmacist is off the premises or when there is insufficient time to get to the pharmacy should exist. Emergency drugs should be limited in number to include only those whose prompt use and immediate availability are generally regarded by physicians as essential in the proper treatment of sudden and unforeseen patient emergencies. The emergency drug supply should not be a source for normal "stat" or "p.r.n." drug orders. The medications included should be primarily for the treatment of cardiac arrest, circulatory collapse, allergic reactions, convulsions, and bronchospasm. The P&T committee should specify the drugs and supplies to be included in emergency stocks.

Emergency drug supplies should be inspected by pharmacy personnel on a routine basis to determine if contents have become outdated and are maintained at adequate levels. Emergency kits should have a seal which visually indicates when they have been opened. The expiration date of the kit should be clearly indicated.

Pharmacy Service When the Pharmacy Is Closed. Hospitals provide services to patients 24 hours a day. Pharmaceutical services are an integral part of the total care provided by the hospital, and the services of a pharmacist should be available at all times. Where around the clock operation of the pharmacy is not feasible, a pharmacist should be available on an "on call" basis. The use of "night cabinets" and drug dispensing by nonpharmacists should be minimized and eliminated wherever possible.

Drugs must not be dispensed to outpatients or hospital staff by anyone other than a pharmacist while the pharmacy is open. If it is necessary for nurses to obtain drugs when the pharmacy is closed and the pharmacist is unavailable, written procedures covering this practice should be developed. They generally should provide for a limited supply of the drugs most commonly needed in these situations; the drugs should be in proper single dose packages and a log should be kept of all doses removed. This log must contain the date and time the drugs were removed, a complete description of the drug product(s), name of the (authorized) nurse involved, and the patient's name.

Drugs should not be dispensed to emergency room patients by nonpharmacist personnel if the pharmacy is open. When no pharmacist is available, emergency room patients should receive drugs packaged, to the extent possible, in single unit packages; no more than a day's supply of doses should be dispensed. The use of an emergency room "formulary" is recommended.[20]

Adverse Drug Reactions. The medical, nursing, and pharmacy staffs must always be alert to the potential for, or presence of, adverse drug reactions. A written procedure to record clinically significant adverse drug reactions should be established. They should be reported to the FDA, the involved drug manufacturer, and the institution's P&T committee (or its equivalent). Adverse drug reaction reports should contain

- Patient's age, sex, and race.
- Description of the drug reaction and the suspected cause.
- Name of drug(s) suspected of causing the reaction.
- Administration route and dose.
- Name(s) of other drugs received by patient.
- Treatment of the reaction, if any.

These reports, along with other significant reports from the literature, should be reviewed and evaluated by the P&T committee. Steps necessary to minimize the incidence of adverse drug reactions in the facility should be taken.

Medication Errors. If a medication error is detected, the patient's physician must be informed immediately. A written report should be prepared describing any medication errors of clinical import observed in the prescribing, dispensing, or administration of a medication. This report, in accordance with hospital policy, should be prepared and sent to the appropriate hospital officials (including the pharmacy) within 24 hours.

These reports should be analyzed, and any necessary action taken, to minimize the possibility of recurrence of such errors. Properly utilized, these incident reports will help to assure optimum drug use control. Medication error reports should be reviewed periodically by the P&T committee. (It should be kept in mind that, in the absence of an organized, independent error detection system, most medication errors will go unnoticed.)

The following definitions of medication errors are suggested. A *medication error* is broadly defined as a dose of medication that deviates from the physician's order as written in the patient's chart or from standard hospital policy and procedures. Except for errors of omission, the medication dose must actually reach the patient; i.e., a wrong dose that is detected and corrected before administration to the patient is not a medication error. Prescribing errors (e.g., therapeutically inappropriate drugs or doses) are excluded from this definition.

Following are the nine categories of medication errors:

1. *Omission error:* the failure to administer an ordered dose. However, if the patient refuses to take the medication, no error has occurred. Likewise, if the dose is not administered because of recognized contraindications, no error has occurred.
2. *Unauthorized drug error:* administration to the patient of a medication dose not authorized for the patient. This category includes a dose given to the wrong patient, duplicate doses, administration of an unordered drug, and a dose given outside a stated set of clinical parameters (e.g., medication order to administer only if the patient's blood pressure falls below a predetermined level).
3. *Wrong dose error:* any dose that is the wrong number of preformed units (e.g., tablets) or any dose above or below the ordered dose by a predetermined amount (e.g., 20%). In the case of ointments, topical solutions, and sprays, an error occurs only if the medication order expresses the dosage quantitatively, e.g., 1 inch of ointment or two 1-second sprays.
4. *Wrong route error:* administration of a drug by a route other than that ordered by the physician. Also included are doses given via the correct route but at the wrong site (e.g., left eye instead of right).
5. *Wrong rate error:* administration of a drug at the wrong rate, the correct rate being that given in the physician's order or as established by hospital policy.
6. *Wrong dosage form error:* administration of a drug by the correct route but in a different dosage form than that specified or implied by the physician. Example of this error type include use of an ophthalmic ointment when a solution was ordered. Purposeful alteration (e.g., crushing of a tablet) or substitution (e.g.,

substituting liquid for a tablet) of an oral dosage form to facilitate administration is generally not an error.
7. *Wrong time error:* administration of a dose of drug greater than ± X hours from its scheduled administration time, X being as set by hospital policy.
8. *Wrong preparation of a dose:* incorrect preparation of the medication dose. Examples are incorrect dilution or reconstitution, not shaking a suspension, using an expired drug, not keeping a light-sensitive drug protected from light, and mixing drugs that are physically/chemically incompatible.
9. *Incorrect administration technique:* situations when the drug is given via the correct route, site, and so forth, but improper technique is used. Examples are not using Z-track injection technique when indicated for a drug, incorrect instillation of an ophthalmic ointment, and incorrect use of an administration device.

Special Considerations Contributing to Drug Control

Pharmacy Personnel and Management.[21–24] Adequate numbers of competent personnel and a well-managed pharmacy are the keys to an effective drug control system. References 21–24 provide guidance on the competencies required of the pharmacy staff and on administrative requirements of a well-run pharmacy department.

Assuring Rational Drug Therapy: Clinical Services.[21,25] Maximizing rational drug use is an important part of the drug control system. Although all pharmacy services contribute to this goal in a sense, the provision of drug information to the institution's patients and staff and the pharmacy's clinical services are those that most directly contribute to rational drug therapy. They are, in fact, institutional pharmacists' most important contributions to patient care.

Facilities. Space and equipment requirements relative to drug storage have been discussed previously. In addition to these considerations, space and equipment must be sufficient to provide for safe and efficient drug preparation and distribution, patient education and consultation, drug information services, and proper management of the department.

Hospital Committees Important to Drug Control.[26,27] Several hospital committees deal with matters of drug control, and the pharmacist must actively participate in their activities. Among these committees (whose names may vary among institutions) are the P&T committee, infection control committee, use review committee, product evaluation committee, patient care committee, and the committee for protection of human subjects. Of particular importance to the drug control system are the formulary and drug use review (DUR) functions of the P&T committee (although DUR in many institutions may be under a use review or quality-assurance committee).

Drug Use Review.[28] Review of how drugs are prescribed and used is an important part of institutional quality-assurance and drug control systems. DUR programs may be performed retrospectively or, preferably, concurrently or prospectively. They may utilize patient outcomes or therapeutic processes

as the basis for judgments about the appropriateness of drug prescribing and use. Depending on the review methodology, the pharmacist should be involved in

1. Preparing, in cooperation with the medical staff, drug use criteria and standards.
2. Obtaining quantitative data on drug use, i.e., information on the amounts and types of drugs used, prescribing patterns by medical service, type of patient, and so forth. These data will be useful in setting priorities for the review program. They also may serve as a measure of the effectiveness of DUR programs, assist in analyzing nosocomial infection and culture and sensitivity data, and help in preparing drug budgets.
3. Reviewing medication orders against the drug use criteria and standards.
4. Consulting with prescribers concerning the results of 3 above.
5. Participating in the followup activities of the review program, i.e., educational programs directed at prescribers, development of recommendations for the formulary, and changes in drug control procedures in response to the results of the review process.

It should be noted that the overall DUR program is a joint responsibility of the pharmacy and the organized medical staff; it is not unilaterally a pharmacy or medical staff function.

Quality Assurance for Pharmaceutical Services.[29] To ensure that the drug control system is functioning as intended, there should be a formalized method to (1) set precise objectives (in terms of outcome and process criteria and standards) for the system; (2) measure and verify the degree of compliance with these standards, i.e., the extent to which the objectives have been realized; and (3) eliminate any noncompliance situations. Such a *quality-assurance program* will be distinct from, though related to, the DUR activities of the department.

Drug Recalls. A written procedure to handle drug product recalls should be developed. Any such system should have the following elements:

1. Whenever feasible, notation of the drug manufacturer's name and drug lot number should appear on outpatient prescriptions, inpatient drug orders or profiles, packaging control records, and stock requisitions and their associated labels.
2. Review of these documents (prescriptions, drug orders, and so forth) to determine the recipients (patients and nursing stations) of the recalled lots. Optimally, this would be done by automated means.
3. In the case of product recalls of substantial clinical significance, a notice should go to the recipients that they have a recalled product. The course of action they should take should be included. In the case of outpatients, caution should be exercised not to cause undue alarm. The uninterrupted therapy of the patients must be assured; i.e., replacement of the recalled drugs generally will be required. The hospital's administration and nursing and medical staffs should be informed of any recalls having significant therapeutic implications. Some situations also may require notifying the physicians of patients receiving drugs that have been recalled.

4. Personal inspection of all patient-care areas should be made to determine if recalled products are present.
5. Quarantine of all recalled products obtained (marked "Quarantined—Do Not Use") until they are picked up by or returned to the manufacturer.
6. Maintenance of a written log of all recalls, the actions taken, and their results.

Computerization.[30] Many information handling tasks in the drug control system (e.g., collecting, recording, storing, retrieving, summarizing, transmitting, and displaying drug use information) may be done more efficiently by computers than by manual systems. Before the drug control system can be computerized, however, a comprehensive, thorough study of the existing manual system must be conducted. This study should identify the data flow within the system and define the functions to be done and their interrelationships. This information is then used as the basis to design or prospectively evaluate a computer system; any other considerations, such as those of the hospital accounting department, are subordinate.

The computer system must include adequate safeguards to maintain the confidentiality of patient records.

A backup system must be available to continue the computerized functions during equipment failure. All transactions occurring while the computer system is inoperable should be entered into the system as soon as possible.

Data on controlled substances must be readily retrievable in written form from the system.

Defective Drug Products, Equipment, and Supplies. The pharmacist should be notified of any defective drug products (or related supplies and equipment) encountered by the nursing or medical staffs. All drug product defects should be reported to the USP–FDA–ASHP Drug Product Defect Reporting Program.

Disposal of Hazardous Substances. Hazardous substances (e.g., toxic or flammable solvents and carcinogenic agents) must be disposed of properly in accordance with the requirements of the Environmental Protection Agency or other applicable regulations. The substances should not be poured indiscriminately down the drain or mixed in with the usual trash.

Unreconstituted vials or ampuls and unopened bottles of oral medications supplied by the National Cancer Institute (NCI) should be returned to the NCI's contract storage and distribution facility.

Other intact products should be returned to the original source for disposition.

Units of anticancer drugs no longer intact, such as reconstituted vials, opened ampuls, and bottles of oral medications, and any equipment (e.g., needles and syringes) used in their preparation require a degree of caution greater than with less toxic compounds to safeguard personnel from accidental exposure. The National Institutes of Health recommends that all such materials be segregated for special destruction procedures. The items should be kept in special containers marked *"Danger—Chemical Carcinogens."* Needles and syringes first should be rendered unusable and then placed in specially marked plastic bags. Care should be taken to prevent penetration and leakage of the bags. Excess liquids should be placed in sealed containers; the original vial is satisfactory. Disposal of all of the above materials should be by incineration to destroy organic material.

Alternate disposal for BCG vaccine products has been recommended by the Bureau of Biologics (BOB). The BOB suggests that all containers and equipment used with BCG vaccines be sterilized prior to disposal. Autoclaving at 121 ^{0}C for 30 minutes will sterilize the equipment.

At all steps in the handling of anticancer drugs and other hazardous substances, care should be taken to safeguard professional and support services personnel from accidental exposure to these agents.

References

1. Ginnow WK, King CM Jr. Revision and reorganization of a hospital pharmacy policy and procedure manual. *Am J Hosp Pharm.* 1978; 35:698–704.
2. Accreditation manual for hospitals 1980. Chicago: Joint Commission on Accreditation of Hospitals; 1979.
3. Publications, reprints and services. Washington, DC: American Society of Hospital Pharmacists; current edition.
4. American Society of Hospital Pharmacists. ASHP guidelines for selecting pharmaceutical manufacturers and distributors. *Am J Hosp Pharm.* 1976; 33:645–6.
5. American Society of Hospital Pharmacists. ASHP guidelines for hospital formularies. *Am J Hosp Pharm.* 1978; 35:326–8.
6. American Society of Hospital Pharmacists. ASHP statement of guiding principles on the operation of the hospital formulary system. *Am J Hosp Pharm.* 1964; 21:40–1.
7. American Society of Hospital Pharmacists. ASHP guidelines for repackaging oral solids and liquids in single unit and unit dose packages. *Am J Hosp Pharm.* 1979; 36:223–4.
8. 21 CFR Parts 210 and 211. Current good manufacturing practices in manufacturing, processing, packing or holding of drugs. April 1979.
9. Sourcebook on unit dose drug distribution systems. Washington, DC: American Society of Hospital Pharmacists; 1978.
10. American Society of Hospital Pharmacists. ASHP statement on unit dose drug distribution. *Am J Hosp Pharm.* 1975; 32:835.
11. American Society of Hospital Pharmacists. ASHP guidelines for single unit and unit dose packages of drugs. *Am J Hosp Pharm.* 1977; 34:613–4.
12. American Society of Hospital Pharmacists. ASHP guidelines for obtaining authorization for pharmacists' notations in the patient medical record. *Am J Hosp Pharm.* 1979; 36:222–3.
13. American Society of Hospital Pharmacists. ASHP guidelines for the use of investigational drugs in institutions. *Am J Hosp Pharm.* 1979; 36:221–2.
14. American Society of Hospital Pharmacists. ASHP guidelines for institutional use of controlled substances. *Am J Hosp Pharm.* 1974; 31:582–8.
15. Recommendations of the National Coordinating Committee on Large Volume Parenterals. Washington, DC: American Society of Hospital Pharmacists; 1980.
16. National Coordinating Committee on Large Volume Parenterals. Recommendations for the labeling of large volume parenterals. *Am J Hosp Pharm.* 1978; 35:49–51.
17. American Society of Hospital Pharmacists. ASHP guidelines on pharmacist-conducted patient counseling. *Am J Hosp Pharm.* 1976; 33:644–5.
18. Lipman AG, Mullen HF. Quality control of medical service representative activities in the hospital. *Am J Hosp Pharm.* 1974; 31:167–70.
19. Evans DM, Guenther AM, Keith TD, et al. Pharmacy practice in an operating room complex. *Am J Hosp Pharm.* 1979; 36:1342–7.
20. Mar DD, Hanan ZI, LaFontaine R. Improved emergency room medication distribution. *Am J Hosp Pharm.* 1978; 35:70–3.
21. American Society of Hospital Pharmacists. ASHP minimum standard for pharmacies in institutions. *Am J Hosp Pharm.* 1977; 34:1356–8.
22. American Society of Hospital Pharmacists. ASHP guidelines on the competencies required in institutional pharmacy practice. *Am J Hosp Pharm.* 1975; 32:917–9.
23. American Society of Hospital Pharmacists. ASHP training guidelines for hospital pharmacy supportive personnel. *Am J Hosp Pharm.* 1976; 33:646–8.
24. American Society of Hospital Pharmacists. ASHP competency standard for pharmacy supportive personnel in organized health care settings. *Am J Hosp Pharm.* 1978; 35:449–51.
25. American Society of Hospital Pharmacists. ASHP statement on clinical functions in institutional pharmacy practice. *Am J Hosp Pharm.* 1978; 35:813.
26. American Society of Hospital Pharmacists. ASHP statement on the pharmacy and therapeutics committee. *Am J Hosp Pharm.* 1978; 35:813–4.
27. American Society of Hospital Pharmacists. ASHP statement on the hospital pharmacist's role in infection control. *Am J Hosp Pharm.* 1978; 35:814–5.
28. Antibiotic use review and infection control: evaluating drug use through patient care audit. Chicago: InterQual, Inc.; 1978.
29. Model quality assurance program for hospital pharmacies, revised. Washington, DC: American Society of Hospital Pharmacists; 1980.
30. Sourcebook on computers in pharmacy. Washington, DC: American Society of Hospitals Pharmacists; 1978.

Developed by the ASHP Council on Professional Affairs. Approved by the ASHP Board of Directors, March 20, 1980. Revised November 1981.

This document contains numerous references to various official ASHP documents and other publications. Inclusion of the latter does not constitute endorsement of their content by the Society; they are, however, considered to be useful elaborations on certain subjects contained herein. To avoid redundancy with other ASHP documents, relevant references are cited in many sections of these guidelines. Most may be obtained from ASHP through its publications catalog

The bibliographic citation for this document is as follows: American Society of Hospital Pharmacists. ASHP technical assistance bulletin on hospital drug distribution and control. *Am J Hosp Pharm.* 1980; 37:1097–103.

ASHP Technical Assistance Bulletin on Repackaging Oral Solids and Liquids in Single Unit and Unit Dose Packages

To maximize the benefits of a unit dose drug distribution system, all drugs must be packaged in single unit or unit dose packages.[a] However, not all drugs are commercially available in single unit (or unit dose) packages. Therefore, the institutional pharmacist must often repackage drugs obtained in bulk containers (e.g., bottles of 500 tablets) into single unit packages so that they may be used in a unit dose system.

Certain precautions must be taken if the quality of drugs repackaged by the pharmacist is to be maintained. The guidelines presented herein will assist the pharmacist in developing procedures for repackaging drugs in a safe and acceptable manner:

1. The packaging operation should be isolated, to the extent possible, from other pharmacy activities.
2. Only one drug product at a time should be repackaged in a specific work area. No drug products other than the one being repackaged should be present in the immediate packaging area. Also, no labels other than those for the product being repackaged should be present in the area.
3. Upon completion of the packaging run, all unused stocks of drugs and all finished packages should be removed from the packaging area. The packaging machinery and related equipment should then be completely emptied, cleaned, and inspected before commencing the next packaging operation.
4. All unused labels (if separate labels are used) should be removed from the immediate packaging area. The operator should verify that none remains in the packaging machine(s). If labels are prepared as part of the packaging operation, the label plate (or analogous part of the printing apparatus) should be removed or adjusted to "blank" upon completion of the run. This will help assure that the correct label is printed during any subsequent run. There should be a procedure to reconcile the number of packages produced with the number of labels used (if any) and destroyed (if any) and the number of units or volume of drug set forth to be packaged.
5. Before beginning a packaging run, an organoleptic evaluation (color, odor, appearance, and markings) of the drug product being repackaged should be made. The bulk container should also be examined for evidence of water damage, contamination, or other deleterious effects.
6. All packaging equipment and systems should be operated and used in accordance with the manufacturer's or other established instructions. There should be valid justification and authorization by the supervisor for any deviation from those instructions on the part of the operator.
7. The pharmacist should obtain data on the characteristics of all packaging materials used. This information should include data on the chemical composition, light transmission, moisture permeability, size, thickness (alone or in laminate), recommended sealing temperature, and storage requirements.
8. Unit dose packages and labels should, to the extent possible, comply with the "ASHP Guidelines for Single Unit and Unit Dose Packages of Drugs."[1]
9. Whenever feasible, a responsible individual, other than the packaging operator, should verify that (a) the packaging system (drug, materials, and machines) is set up correctly and (b) all procedures have been performed properly. Ultimate responsibility for all packaging operations rests with the pharmacist.
10. Control records of all packaging runs must be kept. These records should include the following information: (1) complete description of the product, i.e., name, strength, dosage form, route of administration, etc.; (2) the product's manufacturer or supplier; (3) control number; (4) the pharmacy's control number if different from the manufacturer's; (5) expiration dates of the original container and the repackaged product; (6) number of units packaged and the date(s) they were packaged; (7) initials of the operator and checker (if any); (8) a sample of the label and, if feasible, a sample of the finished package, which should not be discarded until after the expiration date and which should be examined periodically for signs of deterioration; and (9) description (including lot number) of the packaging materials and equipment used.
11. It is the responsibility of the pharmacist to determine the expiration date to be placed on the package, taking into account the nature of the drug repackaged, the characteristics of the package, and the storage conditions to which the drug may be subjected. This date must not be beyond that of the original package.[b]
12. All drugs should be packaged and stored in a temperature- and humidity-controlled environment to minimize degradation caused by heat and moisture. A relative humidity of 75% at 23 °C should not be exceeded. Packaging materials should be stored in accordance with the manufacturer's instructions and any applicable regulations.
13. Written procedures (both general and product specific) governing repackaging operations should be prepared and updated as required. Any deviation from these procedures should be noted and explained on the control record. Operators must understand the procedures (and operation of all packaging equipment) before commencing the run.
14. Applicable FDA and USP requirements concerning the type of package required for specific drug products must be followed.
15. Drugs and chemicals with high vapor pressures should be stored separately from other products to minimize cross contamination.

References

1. American Society of Hospital Pharmacists. ASHP guidelines for single unit and unit dose packages of drugs. *Am J Hosp Pharm.* 1977; 34:613–4.
2. Stolar MH. Expiration dates of repackaged drug products. *Am J Hosp Pharm.* 1979; 36:170. Editorial.

[a]A *single unit* package is one which contains one discrete pharmaceutical dosage form, e.g., one tablet or one 5-ml volume of liquid. A *unit dose* package is one which contains the particular dose of drug ordered for the patient. A *single unit* package is a *unit dose (or single dose)* package if it contains that particular dose of drug ordered for the patient.

[b]For specific recommendations on expiration date policy, see Reference 2.

Revised by the ASHP Board of Directors, November 16–17, 1978.

Developed originally by a joint working group of the American Society of Hospital Pharmacists and the American Society of Consultant Pharmacists and representatives of the drug packaging industry. The original document subsequently was approved officially by the Boards of Directors of ASHP and ASCP. FDA reviewed the original document and commended ASHP and ASCP for developing the guidelines.

The bibliographic citation for this document is as follows: American Society of Hospital Pharmacists. ASHP technical assistance bulletin on repackaging oral solids and liquids in single unit and unit dose packages. *Am J Hosp Pharm.* 1983; 40:451–2.

ASHP Technical Assistance Bulletin on Single Unit and Unit Dose Packages of Drugs

Drug packages must fulfill four basic functions:

1. Identify their contents completely and precisely.
2. Protect their contents from deleterious environmental effects (e.g., photodecomposition).
3. Protect their contents from deterioration due to handling (e.g., breakage and contamination).
4. Permit their contents to be used quickly, easily, and safely.

Modern drug distribution systems use single unit packages to a great extent and, in fact, such packages are central to the operation of unit dose systems, intravenous admixture services, and other important aspects of pharmacy practice. These guidelines have been prepared to assist pharmaceutical manufacturers and pharmacists in the development and production of single unit and unit dose packages, the use of which has been shown to have substantial benefits.

A *single unit* package is one that contains one discrete pharmaceutical dosage form, i.e., one tablet, one 2-ml volume of liquid, one 2-g mass of ointment, etc. A *unit dose* package is one that contains the particular dose of the drug ordered for the patient. A single unit package is also a *unit dose* or *single dose* package if it contains the particular dose of the drug ordered for the patient. A unit dose package could, for example, contain two tablets of a drug product.

General Considerations

Packaging Materials. Packaging materials (and the package itself) must possess the physical characteristics required to protect the contents from (as required) light, moisture, temperature, air, and handling. The material should not deteriorate during the shelf life of the contents. Packages should be of lightweight, nonbulky materials that do not produce toxic fumes when incinerated. Materials that may be recycled or are biodegradable, or both, are to be preferred over those that are not. Packaging materials should not absorb, adsorb, or otherwise deleteriously affect their contents. Information should be available to practitioners indicating the stability and compatibility of drugs with various packaging materials.

Shape and Form. Packages should be constructed so that they do not deteriorate with normal handling. They should be easy to open and use, and their use should require little or no special training or experience. Unless the package contains a drug to be added to a parenteral fluid or otherwise used in compounding a finished dosage form, it should allow the contents to be administered directly to the patient (or IPPB apparatus or fluid administration set) without any need for repackaging into another container or device (except for ampuls).

Label Copy. Current federal labeling requirements must be adhered to, with attention also given to the items at right. The desired copy and format are as follows:

**Nonproprietary Name
(and proprietary name if to be shown)
Dosage Form (if special or other than oral)
Strength
Strength of Dose and Total Contents Delivered
(e.g., number of tablets and their total dose)
Special Notes (e.g., refrigerate)
Expiration Date
Control Number**

1. *Nonproprietary and proprietary names.* The nonproprietary name and the strength should be the most prominent part of the package label. It is not necessary to include the proprietary name, if any, on the package. The name of the manufacturer or distributor should appear on the package. In addition, the name of the manufacturer of the finished dosage form should be included in the product labeling. The style of type should be chosen to provide maximum legibility, contrast, and permanence.

2. *Dosage form.* Special characteristics of the dosage form should be a part of the label, e.g., extended release. Packages should be labeled as to the route of administration if other than oral, e.g., topical use. In a package containing an injection, the acceptable injectable route(s) of administration should be stated on both outer and inner packages, i.e., both on the syringe unit and carton (if any).

3. *Strength.* Strength should be stated in accordance with terminology in the *American Hospital Formulary Service*. The metric system should be used, with dosage forms formulated to provide the rounded-off figures in the *USP* table of approximate equivalents and expressed in the smallest whole number. Micrograms should be used through 999, then milligrams through 999, then grams. Thus, 300 mg, *not* 5 gr, nor 325 mg, nor 0.3 g; 60 mg, *not* 1 gr, nor 0.06 g, nor 64.5 mg, nor 65 mg; 400 mcg, *not* 1/150 gr, nor 0.4 mg, nor 0.0004 g; ml (milliliters) should be used instead of cc (cubic centimeters).

4. *Strength of dose and total contents delivered.* The total contents and total dose of the package should be indicated. Thus, a unit dose package containing a 600-mg dose as two 300-mg tablets should be labeled "600 mg (as two 300-mg tablets)." Likewise, a 500-mg dose of a drug in a liquid containing 100 mg/ml should be labeled "Delivers 500 mg (as 5 ml of 100 mg/ml)."

5. *Special notes.* Special notes such as conditions of storage (e.g., refrigerate), preparation (e.g., shake well or moisten), and administration (e.g., not to be chewed) that are not obvious from the dosage form designation are to be included on the label.

6. *Expiration date.* The expiration date should be prominently visible on the package. If the contents must be reconstituted prior to use, the shelf life of the final product should be indicated. Unless stability data warrant otherwise, expiration dates should fall during January and July to simplify recall procedures.

7. *Control number (lot number).* The control number should appear on the package.

Product Identification Codes. The use of product identification codes, appearing directly on the dosage form, is encouraged.

Evidence of Entry. The package should be so designed that it is evident, when the package is still intact, that it has never been entered or opened.

Specific Considerations

Oral Solids

1. *Blister package.* A blister package should
 a. Have an opaque and nonreflective backing (flat upper surface of package) for printing.
 b. Have a blister (dome or bubble) of a transparent material that is, preferably, flat bottomed.
 c. Be easily peelable.
 d. If it contains a controlled substance, be numbered sequentially for accountability purposes.
2. *Pouch package.* A pouch package should
 a. Have one side opaque and nonreflective for printing.
 b. Be easily deliverable, i.e., large tablets in large pouches, small tablets in small pouches.
 c. Tear from any point or from multiple locations.
 d. If it contains a controlled substance, be numbered sequentially for accountability purposes.
3. The packages should be such that contents can be delivered directly to the patient's mouth or hand.

Oral Liquids

1. The packages should be filled to deliver the labeled contents. It is recognized that overfilling will be necessary, depending on the shape of the container, the container material, and the formulation of the dosage form.
2. The label should state the contents as follows: Delivers ____mg (or g or mcg) in ____ml.
3. If reconstitution is required, the amount of vehicle to be added should be indicated. These directions may take the form of "fill to mark on container" in lieu of stating a specific volume.
4. Syringe-type containers for oral administration should not accept a needle and should be labeled "For Oral Use Only."
5. Containers should be designed to permit administration of contents directly from the package.

Injectables

1. The device should be appropriately calibrated in milliliters and scaled from the tip to the fill line. Calibrated space may be built into the device to permit addition of other drugs. The label should state the contents as follows: Delivers ____mg (or g or mcg) in ____ml.

2. An appropriate size needle may be an integral part of the device. The needle sheath should not be the plunger. The plunger should be mechanically stable in the barrel of the syringe.
3. The device should be of such a design that it is patient ready and assembly instructions are not necessary.
4. The sheath protecting the needle should be a nonpenetrable, preferably rigid material, to protect personnel from injury. The size of the needle should be indicated.
5. The device should be of such a design that easy and visible aspiration is possible. It should be as compact as possible and of such a size that it can be easily handled.

Parenteral Solutions and Additives

1. The approximate pH and osmolarity of parenteral solutions should be stated on the label. The amount of overfill also should be noted. Electrolyte solutions should be labeled in both mEq (or millimole) and mg concentrations. Solutions commonly labeled in terms of percent concentration, e.g., dextrose, should also be labeled in w/v terms.
2. Parenteral fluid container labels should be readable when hanging and when upright or in the normal manipulative position.
3. Drugs to be mixed with parenteral infusion solutions should be packaged into convenient sizes that minimize the need for solution transfers and other manipulations.
4. Partially filled piggyback-type containers should
 a. Be recappable with a tamperproof closure.
 b. Have a hanger.
 c. Have volume markings.
 d. Be designed to minimize the potential for contamination during use.
 e. Contain a partial vacuum for ease of reconstitution.
5. If an administration set is included with the container, it should be compatible with all large volume parenteral delivery systems.

Other Dosage Forms—Ophthalmics, Suppositories, Ointments, etc. Dosage forms other than those specifically discussed above should be adequately labeled to indicate their use and route of administration and should adhere to the above and other required package labeling and design criteria.

Approved by the ASHP Board of Directors, November 14–15, 1984. Revised by the ASHP Council on Clinical Affairs. Supersedes the previous version, which was approved on March 31–April 1, 1977.

The bibliographic citation for this document is as follows: American Society of Hospital Pharmacists. ASHP technical assistance bulletin on single unit and unit dose packages of drugs. *Am J Hosp Pharm.* 1985; 42:378–9.

Education and Training

Education and Training

Preceptor Skills and Abilities (1201)
Source: Council on Education and Workforce Development
To collaborate with pharmacy organizations on the development of standards to enhance the quality of experiential education and pharmacy residency precepting; further,

To provide tools, education, and other resources to develop preceptor skills.

Qualifications of Pharmacy Technicians in Advanced Roles (1203)
Source: Council on Education and Workforce Development
To recognize that highly trained and skilled pharmacy technicians working in advanced roles regularly perform complex and critical medication-use procedures, and that a safe and effective medication-use process depends significantly on the skills, knowledge, and competency of those pharmacy technicians to perform those tasks; further,

To reaffirm that all pharmacy technicians should complete an ASHP-accredited training program, be certified by the Pharmacy Technician Certification Board, and be licensed by state boards of pharmacy; further,

To advocate that beyond those requirements pharmacy technicians working in advanced roles should have additional training and should demonstrate ongoing competencies specific to the tasks to be performed; further,

To advocate that expansion of pharmacy technician duties into expanded, advanced roles should include consideration of potential risk to patients and that ongoing quality assurance metrics should be established to assure patient safety.

Role of Students in Pharmacy Practice Models (1204)
Source: Council on Education and Workforce Development
To encourage pharmacy practice leaders to incorporate students, including those in introductory and advanced pharmacy practice experiences and interns, into active, meaningful roles in new and evolving practice models.

Quality of Pharmacy Education and Expansion of Colleges of Pharmacy (1108)
Source: Council on Education and Workforce Development
To support the Accreditation Council for Pharmacy Education's continuing role of promulgating accreditation standards and guidelines and engaging in sound accreditation processes to ensure quality in the education provided by colleges of pharmacy; further,

To acknowledge that, in addition to a robust curriculum, access to quality experiential educational sites and the availability of qualified faculty (including preceptors and specialty-trained clinical faculty) are essential determinants of the ability to expand enrollment in existing or additional colleges of pharmacy; further,

To oppose expansion of enrollment in existing or new colleges of pharmacy unless well-designed projections demonstrate that such enrollment increases are necessary to maintain a viable pharmacist workforce.
This policy supersedes ASHP policy 0607.

Residency Equivalency (1109)
Source: Council on Education and Workforce Development
To acknowledge the distinct role of ASHP-accredited residency training in preparing pharmacists to be direct patient-care providers; further,

To recognize the importance of clinical experience in developing practitioner expertise; further,

To affirm that there are no objective means to convert or express clinical experience as equivalent to or a substitute for the successful completion of an ASHP-accredited residency.

Pharmacy Internships (1110)
Source: Council on Education and Workforce Development
To encourage the National Association of Boards of Pharmacy to develop standardized pharmacy internship hour requirements that would be used uniformly by all state boards of pharmacy; further,

To support structured requirements, goals, and objectives for pharmacy internship experiences, in alignment with requirements for introductory and advanced pharmacy practice experiences; further,

To promote and expand new staffing models that foster expanded roles for pharmacy interns, providing work experiences that build upon their knowledge and help them develop as future pharmacists.
This policy supersedes ASHP policy 0802.

State-Specific Requirements for Pharmacist Continuing Education (1111)
Source: Council on Education and Workforce Development
To support the standardization of state pharmacist continuing education requirements; further,

To advocate that state boards of pharmacy adopt continuing professional development (CPD) as the preferred model for maintaining pharmacist competence and structure continuing education requirements as a component of CPD.

Innovative Residency Models (1112)
Source: Council on Education and Workforce Development
To support the development of innovative residency models that meet ASHP accreditation requirements.

Employment Classification and Duty Hours of Pharmacy Residents (1008)
Source: Council on Public Policy
To advocate that pharmacy residents should be classified as exempt employees; further,

To advocate that pharmacy residents be subject to duty hour limits (similar to resident physicians) with respect to all clinical and academic activities during their training program in accordance with the Accreditation Council on Graduate Medical Education (ACGME) standards and ASHP accreditation standards for pharmacy residency programs.

Interprofessional Education and Training (1014)

Source: Council on Education and Workforce Development
To support interprofessional education as a component of didactic and experiential education in Doctor of Pharmacy degree programs; further,

To support interprofessional education as a part of professional development for pharmacy practitioners and to collaborate with other disciplines to facilitate and promote programs that support this goal; further,

To encourage and support pharmacists' collaboration with other health professionals and health care executives in the development of team-based, patient-centered care models; further,

To foster documentation and dissemination of outcomes achieved as a result of interprofessional education of health care professionals.

This policy supersedes ASHP policy 0608.

Pharmacy Student Experiences in Medically Underserved Areas (0913)

Source: Council on Education and Workforce Development
To encourage colleges of pharmacy to require student learning experiences in traditionally medically underserved areas and with diverse patient populations.

Education About Patient Safety in the Medication-Use Process (0914)

Source: Council on Education and Workforce Development
To encourage colleges of pharmacy to include instruction on patient safety throughout the medication-use process in the didactic curriculum and during experiential education.

Pharmacy Expertise in the Preparation and Handling of Injectable Medications (0915)

Source: Council on Education and Workforce Development
To encourage colleges of pharmacy to include sterile compounding and aseptic technique instruction in the didactic curriculum and during experiential education; further,

To support the development of postgraduate, curriculum-based sterile compounding training programs to foster an increase in the number of pharmacists with sterile compounding expertise.

Continuing Professional Development (0916)

Source: Council on Education and Workforce Development
To endorse and promote the concept of continuing professional development (CPD), which involves personal self-appraisal, educational plan development, plan implementation, documentation, and evaluation; further,

To continue the development of a variety of mechanisms and tools that pharmacists can use to assess their CPD needs; further,

To encourage individual pharmacists to embrace CPD as a means of maintaining their own professional competence; further,

To encourage pharmacy managers to promote CPD as the model for ensuring the competence of their staff; further,

To collaborate with other pharmacy organizations, state boards of pharmacy, accrediting bodies, and regulatory bodies in the development of effective methods for implementing CPD; further,

To strongly support objective assessment of the impact of CPD on pharmacist competence; further,

To endorse the efforts of colleges of pharmacy and ASHP-accredited pharmacy residency programs to teach the principles, concepts, and skills of CPD.

This policy supersedes ASHP policy 0408.

Pharmacy Residency Training (0917)

Source: Council on Education and Workforce Development
To continue efforts to increase the number of ASHP-accredited pharmacy residency training programs and positions available.

This policy supersedes ASHP policy 9911.

Standardized Pharmacy Technician Training as a Prerequisite for Certification (0803)

Source: Council on Education and Workforce Development
To advocate that completion of an ASHP-accredited pharmacy technician training program be a prerequisite for the Pharmacy Technician Certification Examination.

Collaboration Regarding Experiential Education (0804)

Source: Council on Education and Workforce Development
To promote collaboration of health-system teaching sites with the colleges of pharmacy (nationally or regionally), for the purpose of fostering preceptor development, standardization of experiential rotation schedule dates and evaluation tools, and other related matters.

Entry-Level Doctor of Pharmacy Degree (0805)

Source: Council on Education and Workforce Development
To be an active participant in the Accreditation Council for Pharmacy Education (ACPE) process for the revision of accreditation standards for entry-level education in pharmacy; further,

To actively monitor the long-range impact that the single entry-level degree will have on residency education, availability of experiential training sites, graduate education, and continuing education programs, and the resulting health-system pharmacist applicant pool.

This policy supersedes ASHP policy 9809.

Requirement for Residency (0701)

Source: House of Delegates Resolution
To support the position that by the year 2020, the completion of an ASHP-accredited postgraduate-year-one residency should be a requirement for all new college of pharmacy graduates who will be providing direct patient care.

This policy was reviewed in 2011 by the Council on Education and Workforce Development and by the Board of Directors and was found to still be appropriate.

Pharmacy Technician Training (0702)

Source: Council on Education and Workforce Development
To support the goal that pharmacy technicians entering the pharmacy workforce have completed an ASHP-accredited program of training; further,

To encourage expansion of ASHP-accredited pharmacy technician training programs.

This policy was reviewed in 2011 by the Council on Education and Workforce Development and by the Board of Directors and was found to still be appropriate.

Residency Programs (0704)
Source: Council on Education and Workforce Development
To strongly advocate that all pharmacy residency programs become ASHP-accredited as a means of ensuring and conveying program quality.
This policy supersedes ASHP policy 0216.

ASHP Guidelines, Statements, and Professional Policies as an Integral Part of the Educational Process (0705)
Source: Council on Education and Workforce Development
To encourage faculties in colleges of pharmacy and preceptors of ASHP-accredited residency training programs to use ASHP statements, guidelines, and professional policies as an integral part of training programs and courses.
This policy was reviewed in 2011 by the Council on Education and Workforce Development and by the Board of Directors and was found to still be appropriate.

Developing Leadership and Management Competencies (0509)
Source: Council on Educational Affairs
To work with health-system leadership to foster opportunities for pharmacy practitioners to move into pharmacy leadership roles; further,
To encourage current leaders to seek out and mentor practitioners in developing administrative, managerial, and leadership skills; further,
To encourage interested practitioners to obtain the skills necessary to pursue administrative, managerial, and leadership roles; further,
To encourage colleges of pharmacy and state affiliates to foster leadership skills in students through development and enhancement of curricula, leadership conferences, and other programs; further,
To encourage colleges of pharmacy to develop more opportunities for students to pursue combined degree programs; further,
To encourage colleges of pharmacy and health systems to develop more opportunities for students to pursue residency programs that develop administrative, management, and leadership skills; further,
To encourage residency programs to develop leadership skills by mentoring, training, and providing leadership opportunities; further,
To encourage residency programs to provide training for residents to develop administrative and management skills; further,
To foster leadership skills for pharmacists to use on a daily basis in their roles as leaders in medication safety and medication management in patient care.
This policy was reviewed in 2009 by the Council on Education and Workforce Development and by the Board of Directors and was found to still be appropriate.

Communication Among Health-System Pharmacy Practitioners, Patients, and Other Health Care Providers (0510)
Source: Council on Educational Affairs
To foster effective communication (with appropriate attention to patients' levels of general and health literacy) among health-system pharmacy practitioners, patients, and other health care providers; further,
To develop programs to enable pharmacy students, residents, and health-system pharmacy practitioners to self-assess their levels of health literacy and general communication skills; further,
To develop methods with which pharmacy students, residents, and health-system pharmacy practitioners can assess the level of general and health literacy of patients; further,
To disseminate information about resources for students, residents, and health-system pharmacy practitioners to use in working with patients and others having specific communication needs.
This policy was reviewed in 2009 by the Council on Education and Workforce Development and by the Board of Directors and was found to still be appropriate.

Patient-Centered Care (0313)
Source: Council on Educational Affairs
To encourage that the principles of patient-centered care be integrated throughout the college of pharmacy curriculum.
This policy was reviewed in 2007 by the Council on Education and Workforce Development and by the Board of Directors and was found to still be appropriate.

Cultural Competence (0314)
Source: Council on Educational Affairs
To foster cultural competence among pharmacy students, residents, and practitioners and within health systems for the purpose of achieving optimal therapeutic outcomes in diverse patient populations.
This policy was reviewed in 2007 by the Council on Education and Workforce Development and by the Board of Directors and was found to still be appropriate.

Practice Sites for Colleges of Pharmacy (0315)
Source: Council on Educational Affairs
To encourage practitioner input in pharmacy education; further,
To encourage that institutional and health-system environments be used as sites for experiential training of pharmacy students: further,
To encourage colleges of pharmacy and health systems to define and develop appropriate organizational relationships that permit a balance of patient care and service, as well as educational and research objectives, in a mutually beneficial manner: further,
To include the administrative interests of both the health system and the college of pharmacy in defining these organizational relationships to ensure compatibility of institutional (i.e., health system or university) and departmental (i.e., pharmacy department and department in the college) objectives; further,
To encourage pharmacists and pharmacy leaders to recognize that part of their professional responsibility is the development of new pharmacy practitioners.
This policy was reviewed in 2007 by the Council on Education and Workforce Development and by the Board of Directors and was found to still be appropriate.

Licensure for Pharmacy Graduates of Foreign Schools (0323)
Source: Council on Legal and Public Affairs
To support state licensure eligibility of a pharmacist who has graduated from a pharmacy program accredited by the Accreditation Council for Pharmacy Education (ACPE) or accredited by an ACPE-recognized accreditation program.

This policy was reviewed in 2007 by the Council on Public Policy and by the Board of Directors and was found to still be appropriate.

Public Funding for Pharmacy Residency Training (0325)
Source: Council on Legal and Public Affairs
To support legislation and regulation that ensures public funding for accredited pharmacy residency programs consistent with the needs of the public and the profession; further,

To oppose legislation or regulation involving reimbursement levels for graduate medical education that adversely affects pharmacy residencies at a rate disproportionate to other residency programs.

This policy was reviewed in 2007 by the Council on Public Policy and by the Board of Directors and was found to still be appropriate.

Residency Training for Pharmacists Who Provide Direct Patient Care (0005)
Source: Council on Educational Affairs
To recognize that optimal direct patient care by a pharmacist requires the development of clinical judgment, which can be acquired only through experience and reflection on that experience; further,

To establish as a goal that pharmacists who provide direct patient care should have completed an ASHP-accredited residency or have attained comparable skills through practice experience.

This policy was reviewed in 2009 by the Council on Education and Workforce Development and by the Board of Directors and was found to still be appropriate.

Fostering Pharmacy Leadership (9901)
Source: Council on Administrative Affairs
To encourage pharmacy managers to serve as mentors to their staff, pharmacy students, pharmacy residents, and peers in a manner that fosters the development of future pharmacy leaders.

This policy was reviewed in 2008 by the Council on Pharmacy Management and by the Board of Directors and was found to still be appropriate.

Career Counseling (8507)
Source: Council on Educational Affairs
To urge colleges of pharmacy to develop career counseling programs to make students aware of postgraduate career options, including residency training and career paths in various types of practice; further,

To urge that career counseling occur in a structured manner early in the curriculum and be continued throughout the curriculum; further,

To urge practitioners in various organized health care settings to make themselves available to colleges of pharmacy for participation in both structured and unstructured career counseling.

This policy was reviewed in 2011 by the Council on Education and Workforce Development and by the Board of Directors and was found to still be appropriate.

ASHP Statement on Continuing Education

Next to integrity, competence is the first and most fundamental moral responsibility of all the health professions....Each of our professions must insist that competence will be reinforced through the years of practice. After the degree is conferred, continuing education is society's only real guarantee of the optimal quality of health care.

—Edmund D. Pellegrino

In an era of rapidly accelerating change in health-care delivery, the roles of pharmacy practitioners are being constantly redefined. As roles change, competency requirements change; and as pharmacy practitioners assume the increased responsibilities demanded in these new roles, they must make a corresponding commitment to improve their professional competence. Continuing education is a means by which practitioners can gain the knowledge and skills necessary to develop, maintain, and improve their professional competence.

In keeping with the mission of the American Society of Health-System Pharmacists (ASHP), the purpose of continuing education for health professionals is the improvement of patient care and health maintenance and the enrichment of health careers. Every practitioner should assume personal responsibility for maintaining and improving professional competence through lifelong, self-directed education. Every pharmacist should set personal educational objectives based on individual needs and career goals. One way to achieve these objectives is through continuing education experiences judiciously selected from among area, regional, and national resources. It should be the role of ASHP to facilitate the efforts of the pharmacist in self-directed education.

Objectives

The objectives for the continuing education services of ASHP shall be

1. To help pharmacists develop a more complete understanding of the importance and methods of lifelong, self-directed education and to encourage and assist them toward this goal.
2. To help practitioners evaluate their professional performance, identify areas where improvement is needed, and set realistic and attainable educational goals.
3. To provide to practitioners information on available area, regional, and national educational resources which will help them achieve their personal educational objectives.
4. To assist pharmacists in selecting educational resources that most effectively fulfill their individual needs.
5. To provide to pharmacists continuing education resources in a variety of formats and media best suited for the

subject matter and needs of the greater number of learners.

Authority

Matters relating to continuing education services will be considered by the Council on Educational Affairs and will be submitted to the Board of Directors for review.

Guidelines

The following guidelines are used in the development and conduct of continuing education programs and activities of ASHP:

1. Continuing education programs will be planned and conducted in accordance with the Criteria for Quality of the Continuing Education Provider Approval Program of the Accreditation Council for Pharmacy Education.
2. ASHP will collaborate, when appropriate, with other professional organizations, agencies, and educational institutions in the planning and conduct of continuing education activities.
3. When appropriate, due consideration will be given to the curricular approach in the planning and implementation of continuing education activities.
4. ASHP may limit or restrict the enrollment for any continuing education program, depending on the nature and requirements of the particular program.
5. ASHP's overall continuing education activity is intended to be self-supporting; however, the benefit versus cost value to members of a specific educational program must also be considered.

This statement was reviewed in 2003 by the Council on Educational Affairs and by the ASHP Board of Directors and was found to still be appropriate.

Approved by the ASHP Board of Directors, November 15, 1989. Developed by the Council on Educational Affairs. Supersedes a previous version approved by the ASHP House of Delegates on May 15, 1978.

The bibliographic citation for this document is as follows: American Society of Hospital Pharmacists. ASHP statement on continuing education. *Am J Hosp Pharm.* 1990; 47:1855.

Definitions of Pharmacy Residencies and Fellowships

Pharmacy residencies (originally termed "internships") began in the early 1930s, primarily for the purpose of training pharmacists for the management of pharmacy services in hospitals. The first nonacademic residency program is believed to have been conducted by Harvey A. K. Whitney at the University of Michigan Hospital.[1] Approximately 10 years later, the first residency program combined with formal graduate studies was created.[2] Developments in these programs eventually led the American Society of Hospital Pharmacists to establish, in 1948, standards for pharmacy internships in hospitals.[3] Those standards defined an internship as "a period of organized training in an accredited hospital pharmacy under the direction and supervision of personnel qualified to offer such training."

Two types of internships were recognized, nonacademic and academic. The nonacademic internship consisted of a period of training in a hospital pharmacy. The academic internship consisted of training in a hospital pharmacy and study in an accredited graduate school associated with a college of pharmacy and leading to a Master of Science degree.

In 1962, following several revisions in the standards, ASHP established an accreditation process and accreditation standards for residencies in hospital pharmacy.[4,5] In this action, the term "internship" was replaced by "residency." A residency was defined as "a postgraduate program of organized training . . ." (and further detailed within the various standards). In 1985, the concept that a resident's training should be *directed* was incorporated into the definition.[6-9] It was also acknowledged that a residency is practice oriented and that it is possible for a residency to focus on a defined (specialized) area.

During the early 1970s, numerous residencies developed in *clinical* practice, leading to the establishment, in 1980, of accreditation standards for clinical pharmacy and specialized residency training.[10,11] In 1986, the American Pharmaceutical Association published a compilation of programmatic essentials for community pharmacy residencies.[12] In that same year, the American College of Apothecaries published specific guidelines for the accreditation of community pharmacy residencies.[13]

Paralleling these developments and fostered by a growing sophistication and clinical thrust in institutional pharmacy practice, postgraduate research-oriented programs (generally termed "fellowships") developed in the 1970s. These programs were conducted primarily in colleges of pharmacy and in academically based health centers to educate and train individuals to conduct pharmacy research. A 1981 survey of fellowship programs reported the existence of 58 fellowships in 19 topic areas.[14] Two-thirds of these fellowships had existed for 3 years or less. The oldest program had existed for less than 9 years. The ASHP Research and Education Foundation initiated clinical fellowships in 1978 and defined a pharmacy fellowship as "a directed, but highly individualized program [that] emphasizes research. The focus of a pharmacy fellowship is to develop the participant's (the fellow's) ability to conduct research in his or her area of specialization."[15,16]

ASHP publishes an annual directory of ASHP-accredited residency programs. In 1985, there were 184 accredited programs.[17] The American College of Clinical Pharmacy publishes an annual listing of residencies and fellowships conducted by its members. In 1985, ACCP reported the availability of 51 such residencies and 83 such fellowships.[18] Another source reported 115 known fellowships in 1986.[19] In that year, there were 12 clinical fellowships sponsored by the ASHP Research and Education Foundation in nine areas of specialization.

By 1986, a lack of conformity had arisen in the use of the terms "residency" and "fellowship," and considerable potential existed for program applicants to be misinformed or misled regarding program purposes and content. In 1986, at the recommendation of the ASHP Commission on Credentialing, ASHP invited six other national pharmacy organizations to discuss the issue and develop consensus definitions for the terms. The definitions and interpretations that follow resulted from that conference. These definitions and interpretations are viewed as accurate for current residencies and fellowships yet sufficiently broad and flexible to allow the development of new types of programs. Education, practice, and research developments may generate changes in residencies and fellowships and ultimately stimulate revisions in the definitions and interpretations.

Residency

Definition. A pharmacy residency is an organized, directed, postgraduate training program in a defined area of pharmacy practice.

Interpretation. Residencies exist primarily to train pharmacists in professional practice and management activities. Residencies provide experience in integrating pharmacy services with the comprehensive needs of individual practice settings and provide indepth experiences leading to advanced practice skills and knowledge. Residencies foster an ability to conceptualize new and improved pharmacy services. Within a given residency program, there is considerable consistency in content for each resident. In addition, accreditation standards and program guidelines produced by national pharmacy associations provide considerable program content detail and foster consistency among programs.

A residency is typically 12 months or longer in duration, and the resident's practice experiences are closely directed and evaluated by a qualified practitioner–preceptor. A residency may occur at any career point following an entry-level degree in pharmacy. Individuals planning practice-oriented careers are encouraged to complete all formal academic education before entry into a residency.

Fellowship

Definition. A pharmacy fellowship is a directed, highly individualized, postgraduate program designed to prepare the participant to become an independent researcher.

Interpretation. Fellowships exist primarily to develop competency in the scientific research process, including conceptualizing, planning, conducting, and reporting research. Under the close direction and instruction of a qualified researcher-

preceptor, the participant (the fellow) receives a highly individualized learning experience that utilizes research interests and knowledge needs as a focus for his or her education and training. A fellowship graduate should be capable of conducting collaborative research or functioning as a principal investigator.

Fellowships are typically offered through colleges of pharmacy, academic health centers, or specialized health-care institutions. Fellowships are usually offered for prede-termined, finite periods of time, often exceeding 12 or even 24 months. Individuals planning research-oriented careers should expect to complete formal education in research design and statistics either before or during a fellowship. A fellowship candidate is expected to possess basic practice skills relevant to the knowledge area of the fellowship. Such skills may be obtained through practice experience or through an appropriate residency and should be maintained during the program.

References

1. Niemeyer G. Ten years of the American Society of Hospital Pharmacists, 1942–1952: education and training. *Bull Am Soc Hosp Pharm.* 1952; 9:363–75.

2. American Society of Hospital Pharmacists. Approval program for internships in hospital pharmacy. *Bull Am Soc Hosp Pharm.* 1955; 12:309–13.

3. American Society of Hospital Pharmacists. Standards for internships in hospital pharmacies. *Bull Am Soc Hosp Pharm.* 1948; 5:233–4.

4. American Society of Hospital Pharmacists. Minimum standard for pharmacy internship in hospitals. *Bull Am Soc Hosp Pharm.* 1955; 12:288–90.

5. American Society of Hospital Pharmacists. Accreditation standard for residency in hospital pharmacy. *Am J Hosp Pharm.* 1963; 20:378–80.

6. American Society of Hospital Pharmacists. Accreditation standard for pharmacy residency in a hospital. *Am J Hosp Pharm.* 1971; 28:189–90.

7. American Society of Hospital Pharmacists. Accreditation standard for pharmacy residency in a hospital. *Am J Hosp Pharm.* 1973; 30:1129.

8. American Society of Hospital Pharmacists. ASHP accreditation standard for pharmacy residency in a hospital (with guide to interpretation). *Am J Hosp Pharm.* 1979; 36:74–80.

9. American Society of Hospital Pharmacists. ASHP accreditation standard for hospital pharmacy train-ing (with guide to interpretation). *Am J Hosp Pharm.* 1985; 42:2008–18.

10. American Society of Hospital Pharmacists. ASHP accreditation standard for residency training in clinical pharmacy (with guide to interpretation). *Am J Hosp Pharm.* 1980; 37:1223–8.

11. American Society of Hospital Pharmacists. ASHP accreditation standard for specialized residency train-ing (with guide to interpretation). *Am J Hosp Pharm.* 1980; 37:1229–32.

12. American Pharmaceutical Association, Academy of Pharmacy Practice. APhA community pharmacy resi-dency program: programmatic essentials. *Am Pharm.* 1986; NS26:35–43.

13. American College of Apothecaries. Guidelines for accreditation of community pharmacy residencies. Memphis, TN: American College of Apothecaries; 1986.

14. Kaul AF, Powell SH, Cyr DA. Postgraduate pharmacy fellowships. *Drug Intell Clin Pharm.* 1981; 15:981–5.

15. ASHP Commission on Credentialing. Statement of definition of pharmacy fellowships and resi-dency. Bethesda, MD: American Society of Hospital Pharmacists; 1981.

16. McConnell W. Fellowship program in critical care pharmacy. In: Majerus TC, Dasta JF, eds. Practice of critical care pharmacy. Rockville, MD: Aspen Systems; 1985:59–68.

17. American Society of Hospital Pharmacists. Residency directory. Accredited pharmacy residency programs and programs participating in the 1986 ASHP resident matching program. Bethesda, MD: American Society of Hospital Pharmacists; 1985.

18. American College of Clinical Pharmacy. Residency and fellowship programs offered by members of the American College of Clinical Pharmacy, 1986–87. Kansas City, MO: American College of Clinical Pharmacy; 1986.

19. Kaul AF, Janosik JE, Powell SH. Postgraduate phar-macy fellowships (1985–86). *Drug Intell Clin Pharm.* 1986; 20:203–8.

Developed by an ad hoc consortium made up of representatives from the American Association of Colleges of Pharmacy (AACP), the American College of Apothecaries (ACA), the American College of Clinical Pharmacy (ACCP), the American Pharmaceutical Association (APhA), the American Society of Consultant Pharmacists (ASCP), the American Society of Hospital Pharmacists (ASHP), and the National Association of Retail Druggists (NARD); the consortium was convened by ASHP and met on August 4, 1986. Approved by the ASHP Board of Directors, November 20, 1986, and subsequently approved by ACCP, APhA, ASCP, ACA, and AACP.

The bibliographic citation for this document is as follows: American Society of Hospital Pharmacists. Definitions of pharmacy residen-cies and fellowships. *Am J Hosp Pharm.* 1987; 44:1142-4.

Ethics

Ethics

Ethical Use of Placebos in Clinical Practice (1116)

Source: Council on Pharmacy Practice

To affirm that the use of placebos in clinical practice is ethically acceptable only when patients have been informed of and agree to such use as a component of treatment; further,

To encourage hospitals and health systems to develop policies and procedures to guide clinicians in making informed decisions regarding the use of placebos; further,

To oppose the use of pharmacologically active substances or medications as placebos.

This policy supersedes ASHP policy 0517.

Pharmacist's Right of Conscience and Patient's Right of Access to Therapy (0610)

Source: Council on Legal and Public Affairs

To recognize the right of pharmacists, as health care providers, and other pharmacy employees to decline to participate in therapies they consider to be morally, religiously, or ethically troubling; further,

To support the proactive establishment of timely and convenient systems by pharmacists and their employers that protect the patient's right to obtain legally prescribed and medically indicated treatments while reasonably accommodating in a nonpunitive manner the right of conscience; further,

To support the principle that a pharmacist exercising the right of conscience must be respectful of, and serve the legitimate health care needs and desires of, the patient, and shall provide a referral without any actions to persuade, coerce, or otherwise impose on the patient the pharmacist's values, beliefs, or objections.

This policy was reviewed in 2010 by the Council on Pharmacy Practice and by the Board of Directors and was found to still be appropriate.

Patient's Right to Choose (0013)

Source: Council on Legal and Public Affairs

To support the right of the patient or his or her representative as allowed under state law to develop, implement, and make informed decisions regarding his or her plan of care; further,

To acknowledge that the patient's rights include being informed of his or her health status, being involved in care planning and treatment, and being able to request or refuse treatment; further,

To support the right of the patient in accord with state law to (a) formulate advance directives and (b) have health care practitioners who comply with those directives.

This policy was reviewed in 2009 by the Council on Public Policy and by the Board of Directors and was found to still be appropriate.

ASHP Position on Assisted Suicide (9915)

Source: Council on Legal and Public Affairs

To remain neutral on the issue of health professional participation in assisted suicide of patients who are terminally ill; further,

To affirm that the decision to participate in the use of medications in assisted suicide is one of individual conscience; further,

To offer guidance to health-system pharmacists who practice in states in which assisted suicide is legal.

This policy was reviewed in 2008 by the Council on Pharmacy Practice and by the Board of Directors and was found to still be appropriate.

Nondiscriminatory Pharmaceutical Care (9006)

Source: Council on Professional Affairs

To adopt the following positions in regard to nondiscriminatory pharmaceutical care:

- All patients have the right to privacy, respect, confidentiality, and high-quality pharmaceutical care.
- No patient should be refused pharmaceutical care or denied these rights based solely on diagnosis.
- Pharmacists must always act in the best interest of individual patients while not placing society as a whole at risk.

This policy was reviewed in 2011 by the Council on Pharmacy Practice and by the Board of Directors and was found to still be appropriate.

Use of Drugs in Capital Punishment (8410)

Source: Council on Legal and Public Affairs

To support the following concepts:

1. The decision by a pharmacist to participate in the use of drugs in capital punishment is one of individual conscience.
2. Pharmacists, regardless of who employs them, should not be put at risk of any disciplinary action, including loss of their jobs, because of refusal to participate in capital punishment.

This policy was reviewed in 2008 by the Council on Pharmacy Practice and by the Board of Directors and was found to still be appropriate.

ASHP Statement on Leadership as a Professional Obligation

Position

The American Society of Health-System Pharmacists (ASHP) believes that all pharmacists have a professional obligation to serve as leaders in the safe and effective use of medications and encourages pharmacy practitioners, administrators, faculty members, preceptors, and students to advance patient care and strengthen the pharmacy profession by embracing the responsibility to exert leadership in their practices. ASHP urges all pharmacists to accept this responsibility, actively seek the development of leadership skills, and exercise leadership when working with others, including pharmacists, pharmacy technicians, pharmacy students and residents, administrators, other health care professionals, and patients.

ASHP encourages colleges of pharmacy to go beyond management coursework and integrate education on leadership as a practice philosophy throughout the pharmacy curriculum. All pharmacists share the responsibility to mentor pharmacy students, pharmacy residents, other pharmacists, and pharmacy technicians. Pharmacists in formal leadership roles have a specific responsibility to foster the development of leadership skills in pharmacists, facilitate the development of practice models that provide regular opportunities to exercise leadership, and encourage pharmacists to exercise leadership in practice. ASHP also encourages hospital and health-system executives to support the development of leadership skills of all health care professionals.

Leadership in Practice

The ASHP Statement on Professionalism includes leadership as 1 of 10 characteristics of a professional,[1] and the ASHP Statement on the Roles and Responsibilities of the Pharmacy Executive explains the formal leadership roles of the pharmacy executive.[2] Neither of these documents, however, describes the professional obligation every pharmacist has to serve as a leader in the safe and effective use of medications.

Definitions of leadership commonly focus on working toward goals and exerting influence.[3] For example, Nahata[4] stated that leadership "is about a vision, direction, strategies, motivating, and inspiring." The focus on goals and influence guides understanding of the inherent requirement for leadership in pharmacy. The success of current pharmacy practice models and the successful implementation of future models rest on the ability of members of the profession to influence others. In the complex and evolving health care environment, leadership from pharmacists is required to promote and advance the profession and our care for patients. Thus, leadership is not an option—it is a professional obligation.

The ASHP Research and Education Foundation convened a Student and New Practitioner Leadership Task Force that generated a report titled *Leadership as a Professional Obligation*.[5] This 2009 report addressed several issues regarding the current perceptions of leadership in the pharmacy profession, methods for training pharmacy

leaders, and the challenges presented by the leadership gap defined by White.[6] The Task Force report noted that leadership and management are different, stating that despite the synonymous use of "management" and "leadership" within the literature, hierarchy does not confer leadership, nor does leadership confer hierarchy. As Covey[7] wrote, "Management works in the system; leadership works on the system." He also further differentiated the concepts of leadership and management, saying, "Effective leadership is putting first things first. Effective management is discipline, carrying it out." Although the two terms are often used synonymously, leadership is a broader and more encompassing concept that extends to a wider array of situations, whereas management has a more specific focus.

The most successful organizations facilitate the development of routine leadership roles and encourage participation in those roles. Frontline pharmacists must exhibit themselves as leaders each time they step into the workplace. The practice of effectively influencing the behavior of physicians, nurses, pharmacy technicians, interns, support staff, and others to optimize medication safety and patient outcomes constitutes successful leadership. Innovative practice models can support the development of both clinical and leadership skills. ASHP encourages these types of practice models and their development.

The obligation to develop practitioners prepared for professional leadership requires colleges of pharmacy to adopt such values. Currently, leadership training is inconsistently present in both academic and practice settings. The Task Force report noted that pharmacy curricula commonly offer elective management courses without addressing fundamental leadership skills in a proactive or longitudinal manner and that the concept of using management training to teach leadership skills has led to further gaps in how new pharmacists perceive leadership.[5] The report emphasized the need for increased focus on leadership training in colleges of pharmacy and recommended that these institutions incorporate formalized leadership training throughout the curriculum in a formal, longitudinal manner and not exclusively through management course work.

White's[6] survey of student and new practitioners demonstrated that they are likely to be mentored by frontline pharmacists, supporting the critical need for expressions of leadership. All pharmacists should take personal responsibility for leadership of the medication-use process and for mentorship of students, residents, and colleagues. Although it is not the exclusive responsibility of formal pharmacy leaders such as pharmacy directors and managers, formal leaders must foster and support pharmacist leadership.

The report of the American Association of Colleges of Pharmacy Argus Commission, *Building a Sustainable System of Leadership Development for Pharmacy*, also argued that leadership is a responsibility for all pharmacists.[8] The report called for integration of leadership throughout pharmacy education and offered a number of specific recommendations. To support leadership development of students and practitioners, the report recommended greater focus on fostering leadership education in pharmacy curricula,

in residencies, and in practice sites. To cultivate high-quality candidates to fulfill the pharmacy leadership gap, the report also recommended expansion of didactic leadership training, distance learning programs, the use of social media for networking and mentorship, and an increased focus on the full spectrum of leadership. Colleges should also assess leadership potential during the application and selection process.

Pharmacists also have an obligation to exert leadership and participate in shaping the future of the profession. Participation in professional societies such as ASHP provides opportunities to shape the future of the profession and affords excellent opportunities for the development of leadership skills. Professional organizations such as ASHP also have an obligation to encourage the development of leadership skills and support their development among their memberships.

Conclusion

Leadership is a professional obligation of all pharmacists and not the exclusive responsibility of pharmacists who hold formal leadership roles or titles. All pharmacists should accept the obligation to develop and exert leadership skills to ensure the safe and effective use of medications. Pharmacy schools, professional organizations, and employers should encourage the development of these skills among students and practitioners and should provide both formal training and opportunities for pharmacists to develop leadership capacity.

References

1. American Society of Health-System Pharmacists. ASHP statement on professionalism. *Am J Health-Syst Pharm.* 2008; 65:172–4.
2. American Society of Health-System Pharmacists. ASHP statement on the roles and responsibilities of the pharmacy executive. *Am J Health-Syst Pharm.* 2009; 66:499–502.
3. Holdford DA. Leadership theories and their lessons for pharmacists. *Am J Health-Syst Pharm.* 2003; 60:1780–6.
4. Nahata MC. Balancing leadership and management. *Am J Pharm Educ.* 2001; 65:295–6.
5. American Society of Health-System Pharmacists Research and Education Foundation Center for Health-System Pharmacy Leadership Student and New Practitioner Leadership Task Force. Final report: leadership is a professional obligation (2009). www.ashpfoundation.org/MainMenuCategories/CenterforPharmacyLeadership/AbouttheCenter/StudentNewPractitionerLeadershipTaskForce/SNPFinalReport.aspx (accessed 2011 Mar 23).
6. White SJ. Will there be a pharmacy leadership crisis? An ASHP Foundation Scholar-in-Residence report. *Am J Health-Syst Pharm.* 2005; 62:845–55.
7. Covey SR. *The 7 habits of highly effective people.* New York: Free Press; 1989.
8. Kerr RA, Beck DE, Doss J, et al. Building a sustainable system of leadership development for pharmacy: report of the 2008–09 Argus Commission. *Am J Pharm Educ.* 2009; 73(suppl):S5.

Approved by the ASHP Board of Directors on April 14, 2011, and by the ASHP House of Delegates on June 12, 2011. Developed through the ASHP Council on Pharmacy Management.

Ashley L. Mains, Pharm.D., and David R. Witmer, Pharm.D., are gratefully acknowledged for drafting this statement.

The bibliographic citation for this document is as follows: American Society of Health-System Pharmacists. ASHP statement on leadership as a professional obligation. *Am J Health-Syst Pharm.* 2011; 68:2293–5.

ASHP Statement on Pharmacist's Decision-making on Assisted Suicide

Preamble

Consistent with the intent of the Code of Ethics for Pharmacists "to state publicly the principles that form the fundamental basis of the roles and responsibilities of pharmacists," the American Society of Health-System Pharmacists issues this Statement on Pharmacist Decision-making on Assisted Suicide. The practice of providing competent patients with pharmaceutical means of ending their lives raises issues of professional obligations to patients and to other professionals involved in patient care. We affirm the ASHP policy (9802) that supports the right of a pharmacist to participate or not in morally, religiously, or ethically troubling therapies.

This Statement establishes a framework for pharmacist participation in the legal and ethical debate about the appropriate care of patients at the end of life. This Statement will help pharmacists resolve the growing questions about the ethical obligations of health care professionals to provide care and alleviate suffering. It is hoped that this framework and its use by pharmacists will virtually eliminate a patient's request for assisted suicide.

When asked to evaluate and comment on legislative, regulatory, or judicial actions or on organizational policies of health systems regarding pharmaceutical care, pharmacists should use the principles expressed in this Statement in developing their responses.

Guiding Principles

Professional Tradition. The basic tenet of the profession is to provide care and affirm life. The pharmacy profession is founded on a tradition of patient trust. The trust developed between each patient and members of the health care team makes it important for each professional to examine the moral and ethical issues of patients' requests for assistance in dying. Pharmacists should serve as advocates for the patient throughout the continuum of care.

Respect for Patients. *Patient autonomy.* Pharmacists should ensure the rights of competent patients to know about all legally available treatment options while communicating to patients and their caregivers (including family members if appropriate) the overall duty of health care professionals to preserve life.

Confidentiality. Pharmacists should maintain the confidentiality of all patient information, regardless of whether they agree with the values underlying the patient's choice of treatment or decision to forgo any particular treatment.

Decision-making. Patients' ability to exercise their ethical and legal right to choose or decline treatment is dependent upon pharmacists informing patients and their health care providers about the nature of pharmaceutical options. Those options are constantly changing, given the dynamic aspect of the pharmaceutical marketplace and the evolving nature of hospice care and available palliative treatments.

Health Care Systems. *Collaboration.* Collaboration among members of the health care team must occur at both the patient care and the public policy levels. It is the pharmacist's responsibility to educate members of the health care team about the pharmacotherapeutic options available in treating the patient's condition. Health care team members include the patient, members of the patient's family, and caregivers.

Confidentiality. The patient's right of confidentiality and right to determine his or her therapy, including end-of-life decisions, shall be respected, included, and considered in the decision process in health care systems. Pharmacists should maintain the confidentiality of all patient information, regardless of whether they agree with the values underlying the patient's choice of treatment or decision to forgo any particular treatment.

Covenant with society. Health care is delivered in a system in which each profession makes a contribution on the patient's behalf. An act in one part of the system has consequences in other parts of that system. Each profession has a covenant with society, founded on a relationship of trust with the patient. The trust developed between each patient and members of the health care team makes it important for each professional to examine the moral and ethical issues of patients' requests for assistance in dying.

Barriers to care. Health care professionals must address the following barriers to adequate end-of-life care:

1. Inadequate knowledge and use of pain- and symptom-management therapies.
2. The paucity of published data related to the ingestion of lethal drugs and the outcomes thereof.
3. Insufficient education of health care professionals about end-of-life and palliative care issues.
4. Inadequate recognition that end-of-life care is the responsibility of the entire health care team.
5. Legal and regulatory issues that deter appropriate provision of pain and symptom management.

Professional Obligations. *Conscientious objection.* Pharmacists must retain their right to participate or not in morally, religiously, or ethically troubling therapies. Procedures should be in place to ensure that employers are able to provide care to the patient and provide adequate services to the patient and caregiver. The employer has specific responsibilities, and the employee cannot be a barrier to the employer's ability to fulfill those obligations. Employers must reasonably accommodate the employee pharmacist's right to not participate in morally, religiously, or ethically troubling therapies.

Obligation to the patient. Pharmacists should support appropriate drug therapy to ensure that palliative care and aggressive pain management are available for all patients in need. Pharmacists, as part of their professional responsibility, must offer to provide counseling services to the patient and caregivers and be prepared to provide pharmaceutical care to the patient until the end of life.

Obligation to team members. The pharmacist, as a member of a health care team responsible for the care of a patient, is accountable for providing the team members with detailed information concerning efficacious use of pharmaceutical and other therapies available that may affect the options open to the patient.

As active members of an interdisciplinary team caring for patients, pharmacists must be central participants in all decisions relating to medication management of the patient. Pharmacists should respect the opinions and specific areas of expertise of the other members of the health care team.

Pharmacist education. Pharmacists are often inadequately trained in the care of dying patients. Therefore, pharmacists' education at all levels (undergraduate, graduate, continuing education) should be sensitive to these issues and offer the development of skills and knowledge concerning care of the dying. Pharmacists should make a personal, professional commitment to learn more about end-of-life care.

Recommended Readings

Supreme Court Decisions

1. *Washington v. Glucksberg,* decided June 26, 1997.
2. *Vacco v. Quill,* decided June 26, 1977.
3. Angell M. The Supreme Court and physician-assisted suicide—the ultimate right. *N Engl J Med.* 1997; 336: 50–3.
4. Annas GJ. The bell tolls for a constitutional right to physician-assisted suicide. *N Engl J Med.* 1997; 337:1098–103.
5. Burt RA. The Supreme Court speaks: not assisted suicide but a constitutional right to palliative care. *N Engl J Med.* 1997; 337:1234–6.
6. Gostin LO. Deciding life and death in the courtroom: from *Quinlan to Cruzan, Glucksberg,* and *Vacco*—a brief history and analysis of constitutional protection of the "right to die" *JAMA* 1997; 278:1523–8.
7. Orentlicher D. The Supreme Court and physician-assisted suicide: rejecting assisted suicide but embracing euthanasia. *N Engl J Med.* 1997; 337:1236–9.
8. Palmer LI. Institutional analysis and physicians' rights after *Vacco v. Quill, Cornell J Law Public Policy.* 1998; 7:415–30.

Professional Organization Position Statements/Policies

1. American Bar Association house of delegates. Report of action taken at 1997 annual meeting.
2. American Pharmaceutical Association. Code of Ethics for Pharmacists.
3. American Pain Society. Treatment of pain at the end of life.
4. National League for Nursing. Life-terminating choices: a framework for nursing decision-making.
5. American Medical Association Policy on Physician-Assisted Suicide, 1996.
6. American Nurses Association. Position statement on assisted suicide.
7. American Geriatrics Society. Position statement on the care of dying patients.
8. National Hospice Organization.

Assisted Suicide

1. Dixon KM, Kier KL. Longing for mercy, requesting death: pharmaceutical care and pharmaceutically assisted death. *Am J Health-Syst Pharm.* 1998; 55:578–85.
2. Hamerly JP. Views on assisted suicide: perspectives of the AMA and the NHO. *Am J Health-Syst Pharm.* 1998; 55:543–7.
3. Lee BC. Views on assisted suicide: the aid-in-dying perspective. *Am J Health-Syst Pharm.* 1998; 55: 547–50.
4. Meier DE, Emmons CA, Wallenstein S et al. A national survey of physician-assisted suicide and euthanasia in the United States. *N Engl J Med.* 1998; 338: 1193–201.
5. Mullan K, Allen WL, Brushwood DB. Conscientious objection to assisted death: can pharmacy address this in a systematic fashion? *Ann Pharmacother.* 1996; 30:1185–91.
6. Rupp MT. Issues for pharmacists in assisted patient death. In: Battin MP, Lipman AG, eds. Drug use in assisted suicide and euthanasia. Binghamton, NY: Haworth; 1996.
7. Rupp MT. Physician-assisted suicide and the issues it raises for pharmacists. *Am J Health-syst Pharm.* 1995; 52:1455–60.
8. Rupp MT, Isenhower HL. Pharmacists' attitudes toward physician-assisted suicide. *Am J Hosp Pharm.* 1994; 51:69–74.
9. Stein GC. Assisted suicide: an issue for pharmacists. *Am J Health-Syst Pharm.* 1998; 55:539. Editorial.
10. Van der Maas PJ, van der Wal G, Haverkate I et al. Euthanasia, physician-assisted suicide, and other medical practices involving the end of life in the Netherlands, 1990–1995. *N Engl J Med.* 1996; 335:1699–705.
11. Van der Wal G, van der Maas PJ, Bosma JM et al. Evaluation of the notification procedure for physician-assisted death in the Netherlands. *N Engl J Med.* 1996; 335:1706–11.
12. Vaux KL. Views on assisted suicide: an ethicist's perspective. *Am J Health–Syst Pharm.* 1998; 55:551–3.

End-of-Life Care

1. Foley KM. Competent care for the dying instead of physician-assisted suicide. *N Engl J Med.* 1997; 336:54–8.
2. Quill TE, Lo B, Brock DW. Palliative options of last resort: a comparison of voluntarily stopping eating and drinking, terminal seda-tion, physician-assisted suicide, and voluntary active euthanasia. *JAMA.* 1997; 278:2099–104.
3. Suicide prevention: efforts to increase research and education in palliative care. Washington, DC: General Accounting Office, 1998 Apr; report HEHS-98-128.

Miscellaneous

1. Board of Directors report on the Council on Legal and Public Affairs, ASHP House of Delegates Session—1994.
2. Board of Directors report on the Council on Professional Affairs, ASHP House of Delegates Session—1998.

3. Board of Directors report on the Council on Legal and Public Affairs, ASHP House of Delegates Session—1998.
4. Statement of Attorney General Reno on Oregon's Death with Dignity Act. June 5, 1998.
5. Schnabel J, Schnabel G. Pharmacy information. In: Haley K, Lee M, eds. The Oregon Death With Dignity Act: A Guidebook for Health Care Providers. Portland: Oregon Health Sciences University, Center for Ethics in Health Care; 1998 Mar.

This statement was reviewed in 2008 by the Council on Pharmacy Practice and by the Board of Directors and was found to still be appropriate.

Approved by the ASHP Board of Directors, April 21, 1999, and by the ASHP House of Delegates, June 7, 1999. Developed by the Council on Legal and Professional Affairs.

Copyright © 1999, American Society of Health-System Pharmacists, Inc. All rights reserved.

The bibliographic citation for this document is as follows: American Society of Health-System Pharmacists. ASHP statement on pharmacist's decision-making on assisted suicide. *Am J Health-Syst. Pharm.* 1999; 56:1661–4.

Relevant ASHP Policies

Pharmacist Support for Dying Patients (0307)
Source: Council on Professional Affairs
To support the position that care for dying patients is part of the continuum of care that pharmacists should provide to patients; further,

To support the position that pharmacists have a professional obligation to work in a collaborative and compassionate manner with patients, family members, caregivers, and other professionals to help fulfill the patient care needs, especially the quality-of-life needs, of dying patients of all ages; further,

To support research on the needs of dying patients; further,

To provide education to pharmacists on caring for dying patients, including education on clinical, managerial, professional, and legal issues; further,

To urge the inclusion of such topics in the curricula of colleges of pharmacy.
This policy was reviewed in 2007 by the Council on Pharmacy Practice and by the Board of Directors and was found to still be appropriate.

Pharmacist's Right of Conscience and Patient's Right of Access to Therapy (0610)
Source: Council on Legal and Public Affairs
To recognize the right of pharmacists, as health care providers, and other pharmacy employees to decline to participate in therapies they consider to be morally, religiously, or ethically troubling; further,

To support the proactive establishment of timely and convenient systems by pharmacists and their employers that protect the patient's right to obtain legally prescribed and medically indicated treatments while reasonably accommodating in a nonpunitive manner the right of conscience; further,

To support the principle that a pharmacist exercising the right of conscience must be respectful of, and serve the legitimate health care needs and desires of, the patient, and shall provide a referral without any actions to persuade, coerce, or otherwise impose on the patient the pharmacist's values, beliefs, or objections.
This policy supersedes ASHP policy 9802.

Use of Drugs in Capital Punishment (8410)
To support the following concepts:

1. The decision by a pharmacist to participate in the use of drugs in capital punishment is one of individual conscience.
2. Pharmacists, regardless of who employs them, should not be put at risk of any disciplinary action, including loss of their jobs, because of refusal to participate in capital punishment.

This policy was reviewed in 2008 by the Council on Pharmacy Practice and by the Board of Directors and was found to still be appropriate.

ASHP Statement on Professionalism

Position

Pharmacy is a profession. Despite the challenges to professionalism presented by changes in health care, pharmacists must embrace the responsibilities that stem from their profession's guiding principles. Among those responsibilities are advancing the well-being and dignity of their patients, acting with integrity and conscience, collaborating respectfully with health care colleagues, and seeking justice in the distribution of health care resources.

The American Society of Health-System Pharmacists (ASHP) encourages pharmacy practitioners, administrators, faculty members, preceptors, and students to advance patient care and strengthen the pharmacy profession by promoting professionalism in everyday practice. ASHP urges pharmacists to dedicate themselves to serving the interests of their patients and to practicing with compassion and respect for patients and their families. Pharmacists should commit to working cooperatively with and with respect for other health care providers and to seeking to improve the quality of health care received by the communities in which they work and live. ASHP encourages pharmacists to serve as mentors to students, residents, and colleagues in a manner that fosters the adoption of high professional aspirations for pharmacy practice, high personal standards of integrity and competence, a commitment to serving humanity, habits of analytical thinking and ethical reasoning, and a commitment to lifelong learning.

Background

Between 1995 and 2005, the number of PubMed-indexed articles on professionalism quadrupled, from 50 to approximately 200 per year.[1] Professional associations from the American College of Physicians–American Society of Internal Medicine to the American College of Dentistry have convened task forces, developed white papers and charters, and initiated programs to increase the professionalism of their members.[2-6]

The rising interest in professionalism has been attributed to the perception that changes in health care delivery are eroding the professional standards of health care providers.[2] Among the changes confronting the pharmacy profession are managed care's continuing emphasis on cost containment[7]; increased demand for systems that ensure the safety of medication use[8]; technology-driven changes in pharmacy's core responsibilities, the most important of which is an expansion of the pharmacist's role in patient care[7,9,10]; and a prolonged shortage of pharmacists.[11] As such challenges mount, it is in the best interest of our profession and the public we serve to reaffirm our foundational principles. Hospital and health-system pharmacists must therefore define for themselves the principles that will guide them in their unique practice settings.

Guiding Principles and Responsibilities for Health-System Pharmacy

The use of the term "profession" to describe a group of individuals pursuing an occupation or career is based on the idea that these individuals profess a common purpose.[12] The common purpose of pharmacists is eloquently stated in the eight principles of the Code of Ethics for Pharmacists.[13]

Professing these principles creates responsibilities for pharmacists. Foremost among these responsibilities is the obligation to place the well-being of patients at the center of pharmacy practice. Many of the other principles flow from the covenantal relationship between the pharmacist and the patient. To provide the best possible care, pharmacists dedicate themselves to maintaining professional competence through lifelong learning and contemplation. Professional education and advancing standards of practice can only be achieved through a profession's collective efforts; pharmacists therefore commit themselves to serve not only their patients but also their profession. Finally, pharmacists commit themselves to improving health care institutions not simply for the well-being of individual patients but for the benefit of society as a whole.

Incorporating Professionalism into Practice

ASHP encourages practitioners, administrators, faculty members, preceptors, and pharmacy students to contemplate and to incorporate into their practices the guiding principles set forth in the Code of Ethics for Pharmacists[13] and the following 10 characteristics of a professional:

1. Knowledge and skills of the profession,
2. Commitment to self-improvement of skills and knowledge,
3. Service orientation,
4. Pride in and service to the profession,
5. Covenantal relationship with the patient,
6. Creativity and innovation,
7. Conscience and trustworthiness,
8. Accountability for his or her work,
9. Ethically sound decision-making, and
10. Leadership.[6]

Practicing and aspiring hospital and health-system pharmacists should develop a personal plan for professional development, encourage their colleagues to do the same, and share the results. Continuing education should be viewed as an opportunity to enhance one's practice rather than an obligation to be fulfilled in the most expedient manner.

Much could be done to make practice sites more conducive to professional behavior. Institutions can develop personnel recruitment, orientation, and evaluation systems that encourage professional development (e.g., by offering benefit packages that emphasize professional development rather than salary or by incorporating characteristics of professionalism into job descriptions).[14] Administrators and pharmacists can promote professionalism by improving the pharmacy practice area to reduce environmental barriers to professionalism (e.g., cluttered, isolated, outdated, or cramped working quarters).

One of the fundamental services of a professional is recruiting, nurturing, and securing new practitioners to that profession's ideals and mission.[15] For hospital and health-system pharmacists, professional socialization is especially important because the principles of institutional pharmacy practice are not emphasized in typical pharmacy curricula. Above all else, hospital and health-system pharmacists need to prevent "inconsistent socialization,"[16] in which the principles of professionalism instilled in pharmacy students are undermined by a lack of professionalism in the role models they encounter when they enter practice. Pharmacy departments can avoid inconsistent socialization by promoting a culture of professionalism in the workplace through personnel recruitment and evaluation systems that emphasize professional development.[16] Regardless of the level of support they receive, however, hospital and health-system pharmacists must commit themselves fully to their mentorship responsibilities.

ASHP urges practicing pharmacists to serve as mentors to students, residents, and colleagues in a manner that fosters the adoption of high professional aspirations for pharmacy practice, high personal standards of integrity and competence, a commitment to serve humanity, habits of analytical thinking and ethical reasoning, and a commitment to lifelong learning. Practice sites should designate preceptors, implement preceptor training programs, encourage preceptor adherence to the highest professional standards, solicit student feedback on preceptorship programs, and reward those who participate.[6] Hospitals and health systems should also explore other ways to promote mentorship relationships among staff. Hospital and health-system pharmacists and students can participate in ASHP's Virtual Mentoring Exchange.[17] ASHP encourages pharmacists, particularly new practitioners, to actively seek mentors.

Finally, hospital and health-system pharmacists can advance the cause of professionalism in health care by reinvigorating the mission development processes of their institutions, encouraging those institutions to revise their mission statements to describe how they will address such ethical issues as the treatment of patients, employees, and staff; institutions' responsibilities to their communities, to other institutions, and to their own futures; the need to honor founding traditions and sustaining principles; and the complex interactions of legal and ethical responsibilities and their obligations to meet legislatively and socially defined needs.[18]

In 1976, Anderson[15] called on hospital pharmacists to "create a code that reflects our relationships with all of the different people and conditions under which we practice." The time has come for hospital and health-system pharmacists to join forces with other health care providers and patients to engage what has been called "the new authorities of health care"[18] to attain the kind of health care system our patients deserve and our society demands.

Conclusion

The pharmacy profession's guiding principles are eloquently stated in the Code of Ethics for Pharmacists. Despite the challenges to professionalism presented by changes in health care, pharmacists must embrace the responsibilities that stem from their profession's guiding principles.

References

1. National Center for Biotechnology Information. PubMed online database. www.ncbi.nih.gov/entrez/query.fcgi (accessed 2006 Jun 16).
2. ABIM Foundation, ACP–ASIM Foundation, and European Federation of Internal Medicine. Medical professionalism in the new millennium: a physician charter. *Ann Intern Med.* 2002; 136:243–6.
3. Yeager AL. Dental ethics for the 21st century: learning from the Charter on Medical Professionalism. *J Am Coll Dent.* 2002; 69:53–60.
4. Popp RL, Smith SC Jr. Cardiovascular professionalism and ethics in the modern era. *J Am Coll Cardiol.* 2004; 44:1722–3.
5. American Society of Health-System Pharmacists. 2001 ASHP Leadership Conference on Pharmacy Practice Management Executive Summary. From management to leadership: the building blocks of professionalism. *Am J Health-Syst Pharm.* 2002; 59:661–5.
6. Adapted from: American Pharmaceutical Association Academy of Students of Pharmacy—American Association of Colleges of Pharmacy Council of Deans Task Force on Professionalism. White paper on pharmacy student professionalism. *J Am Pharm Assoc.* 2000; 40:96–102.
7. Zacker C, Mucha L. Institutional and contingency approaches to the reprofessionalization of pharmacy. *Am J Health-Syst Pharm.* 1998; 55:1302–5.
8. Pedersen CA, Schneider PJ, Scheckelhoff DJ. ASHP national survey of pharmacy practice in hospital settings: prescribing and transcribing—2004. *Am J Health-Syst Pharm.* 2005; 62:378–90.
9. Reeder CE, Dickson M, Kozma CM et al. ASHP national survey of pharmacy practice in acute care settings—1996. *Am J Health-Syst Pharm.* 1997; 54: 653–69.
10. Knapp KK, Okamoto MP, Black BL. ASHP survey of ambulatory care pharmacy practice in health systems—2004. *Am J Health-Syst Pharm.* 2005; 62: 274–84.
11. Knapp KK, Quist RM, Walton SM et al. Update on the pharmacist shortage: national and state data through 2003. *Am J Health-Syst Pharm.* 2005; 62:492–9.
12. Knowlton CH, Penna RP. Pharmaceutical care, 2nd ed. Bethesda, MD: American Society of Health-System Pharmacists; 2003:4.
13. Code of ethics for pharmacists. In: Hawkins BH, ed. Best practices for hospital and health-system pharmacy. Bethesda, MD: American Society of Health-System Pharmacists; 2005:103.
14. Hammer DP, Berger BA, Beardsley RS et al. Student professionalism. *Am J Pharm Educ.* 2003; 63:1-29.
15. Anderson RD. 1976 Harvey A.K. Whitney lecture: the peril of deprofessionalization. *Am J Hosp Pharm.* 1977; 34:133–9 [reprinted in *Am J Health-Syst Pharm.* 2004; 61:2373–9].
16. Manasse HR Jr, Stewart JE, Hall RH. Inconsistent socialization in pharmacy—a pattern in need of change. *J Am Pharm Assoc.* 1975; 15:616–21,658.
17. American Society of Health-System Pharmacists. ASHP virtual mentoring exchange. www.ashp.org/virtualmentoring/index.cfm (accessed 2005 Jun 16).

18. Reiser SJ, Banner RS. The Charter on Medical Professionalism and the limits of medical power. *Ann Intern Med.* 2003; 138:844–6.

Approved by the ASHP Board of Directors on January 12, 2007, and by the ASHP House of Delegates on June 26, 2007. Developed through the ASHP Council on Pharmacy Practice.

The bibliographic citation for this document is as follows: American Society of Health-System Pharmacists. ASHP statement on professionalism. *Am J Health-Syst Pharm.* 2008; 65:172–4.

ASHP Guidelines on Pharmacists' Relationships with Industry

In the practice of their profession, pharmacists should be guided only by the consideration of patient care. Pharmacists should neither accept nor retain anything of value that has the potential to affect materially their ability to exercise judgments solely in the interests of patients. A useful criterion in determining acceptable activities and relationships is this: Would the pharmacist be willing to have these relationships generally known? Notwithstanding this responsibility, pharmacists may benefit from guidance in their relationships with industry. To this end, the following suggestions are offered.

Gifts and Hospitality

Gifts, hospitality, or subsidies offered to pharmacists by industry should not be accepted if acceptance might influence, or appear to others to influence, the objectivity of clinical judgment or drug product selection and procurement.

Continuing Education

Providers of continuing education that accept industry funding for programs should develop and enforce policies to maintain complete control of program content.

Subsidies to underwrite the costs of continuing-education conferences, professional meetings, or staff development programs can contribute to the improvement of patient care and are permissible. Payments to defray the costs of a conference should not be accepted directly or indirectly from industry by pharmacists attending the conference or program. Contributions to special or educational funds for staff development are permissible as long as the selection of staff members who will receive the funds is made by the department of pharmacy.

It is appropriate for faculty at conferences or meetings to accept reasonable honoraria and reimbursement for reasonable travel, lodging, and meal expenses. However, direct subsidies from industry should not be accepted to pay the costs of travel, lodging, or other personal expenses of pharmacists attending conferences or meetings, nor should subsidies be accepted to compensate for the pharmacists' time.

Scholarships or other special funds to permit pharmacy students, residents, and fellows to attend carefully selected educational conferences may be permissible as long as the selection of students, residents, or fellows who will receive the funds is made by the academic or training institution.

Consultants and Advisory Arrangements

Consultants who provide genuine services for industry may receive reasonable compensation and accept reimbursement for travel, lodging, and meal expenses. Token consulting or advisory arrangements cannot be used to justify compensating pharmacists for their time, travel, lodging, and other out-of-pocket expenses.

Clinical Research

Pharmacists who participate in practice-based research of pharmaceuticals, devices, or other programs should conduct their activities in accord with basic precepts of accepted scientific methodology. Practice-based drug studies that are, in effect, promotional schemes to entice the use of a product or program are unacceptable.

Disclosure of Information

To avoid conflicts of interest or appearances of impropriety, pharmacists should disclose consultant or speaker arrangements or substantial personal financial holdings with companies under consideration for formulary inclusion or related decisions. To inform audiences fully, speakers and authors should disclose, when pertinent, consultant or speaker and research funding arrangements with companies.

Additional Issues

The advice in this document is noninclusive and is not intended to limit the legitimate exchange of prudent scientific information.

This guideline was reviewed in 2001 by the Council on Legal and Public Affairs and by the ASHP Board of Directors and was found to still be appropriate.

Approved by the ASHP Board of Directors, November 20, 1991. Developed by the ASHP Council on Legal and Public Affairs.

The language used in many of the guidance issues contained in this document was adapted, with permission, from documents developed by the American Medical Association (*JAMA.* 1991; 265:501) and the American College of Physicians (*Ann Intern Med.* 1990; 112:624–6).

The bibliographic citation for this document is as follows: American Society of Hospital Pharmacists. ASHP guidelines on pharmacists' relationships with industry. *Am J Hosp Pharm.* 1992; 49:154.

Code of Ethics for Pharmacists

Preamble

Pharmacists are health professionals who assist individuals in making the best use of medications. This Code, prepared and supported by pharmacists, is intended to state publicly the principles that form the fundamental basis of the roles and responsibilities of pharmacists. These principles, based on moral obligations and virtues, are established to guide pharmacists in relationships with patients, health professionals, and society.

Principles

I. *A pharmacist respects the covenantal relationship between the patient and pharmacist.*

 Interpretation: Considering the patient-pharmacist relationship as a covenant means that a pharmacist has moral obligations in response to the gift of trust received from society. In return for this gift, a pharmacist promises to help individuals achieve optimum benefit from their medications, to be committed to their welfare, and to maintain their trust.

II. *A pharmacist promotes the good of every patient in a caring, compassionate, and confidential manner.*

 Interpretation: A pharmacist places concern for the well-being of the patient at the center of professional practice. In doing so, a pharmacist considers needs stated by the patient as well as those defined by health science. A pharmacist is dedicated to protecting the dignity of the patient. With a caring attitude and a compassionate spirit, a pharmacist focuses on serving the patient in a private and confidential manner.

III. *A pharmacist respects the autonomy and dignity of each patient.*

 Interpretation: A pharmacist promotes the right of self-determination and recognizes individual self-worth by encouraging patients to participate in decisions about their health. A pharmacist communicates with patients in terms that are understandable. In all cases, a pharmacist respects personal and cultural differences among patients.

IV. *A pharmacist acts with honesty and integrity in professional relationships.*

 Interpretation: A pharmacist has a duty to tell the truth and to act with conviction of conscience. A pharmacist avoids discriminatory practices, behavior or work conditions that impair professional judgment, and actions that compromise dedication to the best interests of patients.

V. *A pharmacist maintains professional competence.*

 Interpretation: A pharmacist has a duty to maintain knowledge and abilities as new medications, devices, and technologies become available and as health information advances.

VI. *A pharmacist respects the values and abilities of colleagues and other health professionals.*

 Interpretation: When appropriate, a pharmacist asks for the consultation of colleagues or other health professionals or refers the patient. A pharmacist acknowledges that colleagues and other health professionals may differ in the beliefs and values they apply to the care of the patient.

VII. *A pharmacist serves individual, community, and societal needs.*

 Interpretation: The primary obligation of a pharmacist is to individual patients. However, the obligations of a pharmacist may at times extend beyond the individual to the community and society. In these situations, the pharmacist recognizes the responsibilities that accompany these obligations and acts accordingly.

VIII. *A pharmacist seeks justice in the distribution of health resources.*

 Interpretation: When health resources are allocated, a pharmacist is fair and equitable, balancing the needs of patients and society.

The endorsement of this document was reviewed in 2007 by the Council on Pharmacy Practice and by the Board of Directors and was found to still be appropriate.

Formulary Management

(Medication-Use Policy Development)

Formulary Management

Pharmacogenomics (1104)
Source: Council on Therapeutics
To advocate that pharmacists take a leadership role in the therapeutic applications of pharmacogenomics, which is essential to individualized drug therapy; further,

To support research to validate and standardize genetic markers and genetic testing for drug therapy and to support research and other efforts that guide and accelerate the application of pharmacogenomics to clinical practice; further,

To advocate for the inclusion of pharmacogenomic test results in medical and pharmacy records in a format that clearly states the implications of the results for drug therapy and facilitates availability of the genetic information throughout the continuum of care and over a patient's lifetime; further,

To encourage pharmacists to educate prescribers and patients about the use of pharmacogenomic tests and their appropriate application to drug therapy management; further,

To encourage pharmacist education on the use of pharmacogenomics and advocate for the inclusion of pharmacogenomics and its application to therapeutic decision-making in college of pharmacy curricula.
This policy supersedes ASHP policy 0016.

Medications Derived from Biologic Sources (0809)
Source: Council on Pharmacy Practice
To encourage pharmacists to take a leadership role in their health systems for all aspects of the proper use of medications derived from biologic sources, including preparation, storage, control, distribution, administration procedures, safe handling, and therapeutic applications; further,

To facilitate education of pharmacists about the proper use of medications derived from biologic sources.

(*Note:* Section 351(a) of the Public Health Service Act [42 U.S.C. 262(a)] defines *biological product* as follows: a virus, therapeutic serum, toxin, antitoxin, vaccine, blood, blood component or derivative, allergenic product, or analogous product, or arsphenamine or derivative of arsphenamine [or any other trivalent organic arsenic compound], applicable to the prevention, treatment, or cure of a disease or condition of human beings.)
This policy supersedes ASHP policy 0316.

Generic Substitution of Narrow Therapeutic Index Drugs (0817)
Source: Council on Therapeutics
To support the current processes used by the Food and Drug Administration (FDA) to determine bioequivalence of generic drug products, including those with a narrow therapeutic index, and to recognize the authority of the FDA to decide if additional studies are necessary to determine equivalence; further,

To oppose a blanket restriction on generic substitution for any medication or medication class without evidence from well-designed, independent studies that demonstrate inferior efficacy or safety of the generic drug product.

Expression of Therapeutic Purpose of Prescribing (0305)
Source: Council on Professional Affairs
To advocate that the prescriber provide or pharmacists have immediate access to the intended therapeutic purpose of prescribed medications in order to ensure safe and effective medication use.
This policy was reviewed in 2007 by the Council on Pharmacy Practice and by the Board of Directors and was found to still be appropriate.

Appropriate Dosing of Medications in Patient Populations with Unique Needs (0228)
Source: Council on Professional Affairs
To advocate reforms in medication-use systems, including electronic systems, and health care provider education and training that facilitate optimal patient-specific dosing in populations of patients (e.g., pediatrics, geriatrics) with altered pharmacokinetics and pharmacodynamics.
This policy was reviewed in 2011 by the Council on Pharmacy Practice and by the Board of Directors and was found to still be appropriate.

Medication Formulary System Management (0102)
Source: Council on Administrative Affairs
To declare that decisions on the management of a medication formulary system (1) should be based on clinical, ethical, legal, social, philosophical, quality-of-life, safety, and pharmacoeconomic factors that result in optimal patient care, and (2) must include the active and direct involvement of physicians, pharmacists, and other appropriate health care professionals; further,

To declare that decisions on the management of a medication formulary system should not be based solely on economic factors.
This policy was reviewed in 2010 by the Council on Pharmacy Management and by the Board of Directors and was found to still be appropriate.

Gene Therapy (0103)
Source: Council on Administrative Affairs
To declare that health-system decisions on the selection, use, and management of gene therapy agents should be based on the same principles as a medication formulary system in that (1) decisions are based on clinical, ethical, legal, social, philosophical, quality-of-life, safety, and pharmacoeconomic factors that result in optimal patient care and (2) such decisions must include the active and direct involvement of physicians, pharmacists, and other appropriate health care professionals.
This policy was reviewed in 2010 by the Council on Pharmacy Management and by the Board of Directors and was found to still be appropriate.

Role of Pharmacists and Business Leaders in Health Care Services and Policies (9819)
Source: Council on Professional Affairs
To support the principle that business leaders and health professionals must share responsibility and accountability for providing optimal health care services to patients; further,

To support the principle that business leaders should expect practicing pharmacists to formulate policies that affect the prerogative of pharmacists to make optimal care decisions on behalf of patients.

This policy was reviewed in 2008 by the Council on Pharmacy Practice and by the Board of Directors and was found to still be appropriate.

Standardization of Drug Medication Formulary Systems (9601)

Source: Council on Administrative Affairs

To support the concept of a standardized medication formulary system among components of integrated health systems when standardization leads to improved patient outcomes; further,

To include in the formulary-standardization process the direct involvement of the health system's physicians, pharmacists, and other appropriate health care professionals.

This policy was reviewed in 2009 by the Council on Pharmacy Practice and by the Board of Directors and was found to still be appropriate.

Medical Devices (9106)

Source: Council on Legal and Public Affairs

To support public and private initiatives to clarify and define the relationship among drugs, devices, and new technologies in order to promote safety and effectiveness as well as better delivery of patient care.

This policy was reviewed in 2012 by the House of Delegates and by the Board of Directors and was found to still be appropriate.

Therapeutic Interchange (8708)

Source: Council on Legal and Public Affairs

To support the concept of therapeutic interchange of various drug products by pharmacists under arrangements where pharmacists and authorized prescribers interrelate on the behalf of patient care.

This policy was reviewed in 2008 by the Council on Pharmacy Practice and by the Board of Directors and was found to still be appropriate.

ASHP Statement on the Pharmacy and Therapeutics Committee and the Formulary System

Position

American Society of Health-System Pharmacists (ASHP) believes that health systems should develop, organize, and administer a formulary system that follows the principles below in order to optimize patient care by ensuring access to clinically appropriate, safe, and cost-effective medications.

Background

A formulary is a continually updated list of medications and related information, representing the clinical judgment of pharmacists, physicians, and other experts in the diagnosis and treatment of disease and promotion of health.[1] A formulary includes, but is not limited to, a list of medications and medication-associated products or devices, medication-use policies, important ancillary drug information, decision-support tools, and organizational guidelines. The multiplicity of medications available, the complexities surrounding their safe and effective use, and differences in their relative value make it necessary for health systems to have medication-use policies that promote rational, evidence-based, clinically appropriate, safe, and cost-effective medication therapy. The formulary system is the ongoing process through which a health care organization establishes policies on the use of drugs, therapies, and drug-related products and identifies those that are most medically appropriate and cost-effective to best serve the health interests of a given patient population.

Pharmacy and Therapeutics Committee

To be effective, medication-use policies must have the concurrence of individuals involved in the medication-use process. Such consensus is achieved by developing medication-use policies through a properly organized and representative pharmacy and therapeutics (P&T) committee or equivalent body and ensuring that those policies are approved by the organized medical staff.

The P&T committee is composed of actively participating physicians, other prescribers, pharmacists, nurses, administrators, quality-improvement managers, and other health care professionals and staff who participate in the medication-use process. Customarily, P&T member appointments are based on guidance from the medical staff. The P&T committee should serve in an evaluative, educational, and advisory capacity to the medical staff and organizational administration in all matters that pertain to the use of medications (including investigational medications). The P&T committee is a policy-recommending body to the medical staff and the administration of the organization on matters related to the safe and therapeutic use of medications. The P&T committee is responsible to the medical staff as a whole, and its recommendations are subject to approval by the organized medical staff as well as the administrative approval process. The basic policies and procedures that govern the P&T committee's administration of the formulary system should be incorporated, as appropriate, in the health system's medical staff bylaws, medical staff rules and regulations, and other organizational policies.

The overarching purposes of the P&T committee are policy development, communication and education, and formulary management.

Policy Development

The P&T committee formulates policies regarding evaluation, selection, diagnostic and therapeutic use, and monitoring of medications and medication-associated products and devices. The P&T committee should establish and assist in programs and procedures that ensure safe and effective medication therapy (e.g., clinical care plans, treatment guidelines, critical pathways, disease management protocols). Members of the P&T committee, or their representatives from appropriate specialties (including pharmacists), should participate in or direct the development and review of such programs or procedures, which should be kept current.

The P&T committee should participate in performance improvement activities related to procurement, prescribing, dispensing, administering, monitoring, and overall use of medications. The P&T committee should advise the institution, including the pharmacy department, in the implementation of effective medication distribution and control procedures, incorporating technological advances when appropriate. The P&T committee should initiate, direct, and review the results of medication-use evaluation programs to optimize medication use and routinely monitor outcomes (economic, clinical, and humanistic) of formulary decisions. Medication-use evaluation should result in performance-improvement initiatives to improve the medication-use process.

The P&T committee should take actions to prevent, monitor, and evaluate adverse drug reactions and medication errors in the health care setting, including those occurring with biological products and vaccines. Information from these activities should be disseminated to the appropriate health care personnel for informational and educational purposes (e.g., newsletters, memoranda) and, when appropriate, to the Food and Drug Administration (FDA).

The P&T committee should establish clearly defined policies and procedures related to manufacturer sales representatives' activities within the organization.

Communication and Education

The P&T committee ensures that mechanisms are in place to communicate with health care professionals, patients, and payers about all aspects of the formulary system, including changes made to the formulary or policies and how formulary system decisions are made. The P&T committee also recommends or assists in the formulation of educational programs designed to meet the needs of professional staff, patients, families, and caregivers on matters related to medications and medication use. The P&T committee should establish or plan suitable educational programs on matters related to medication use for staff involved in the care of patients and the use of medications.

Formulary Management

Health systems should develop, organize, and administer a formulary system that follows the principles below in order to optimize patient care by ensuring access to clinically appropriate, safe, and cost-effective medications.

Formulary System. The P&T committee is responsible for administering the formulary system. Although the basic organization of each health care setting and its medical staff may influence the specific functions and scope of the P&T committee, key elements of a formulary system that should also be included are the evaluation of the clinical use of medications (including outcomes), the development of policies and quality assurance activities for medication use and administration, and the evaluation and monitoring of adverse drug reactions and medication errors. The formulary system shall be endorsed by the medical staff based on the recommendations of the P&T committee. The medical staff should adapt the principles of the system to fit the needs of the particular organization and affiliated institutions and ambulatory care settings. The organization, often through the pharmacy department, should make certain that all personnel involved in the care of patients and the use of medications in all health-system components are informed about the existence of the formulary system, how to access the formulary, the procedures governing its operation, any changes in those procedures, and other necessary information (e.g., changes in drug product availability). This information may be further disseminated to other interested entities (e.g., affiliated managed care organizations).

Formulary. The P&T committee develops an evidence-based formulary of medications and medication-associated products accepted for use in the organization. The committee also provides timely revision and maintenance for the formulary and promotes the rational, clinically appropriate, safe, and cost-effective use of medications via guidelines, protocols, and other mechanisms. The P&T committee, on an ongoing basis, objectively appraises, evaluates, and selects medications for addition to or deletion from the formulary. The formulary is based on the best clinical evidence available and reflects the current clinical judgment of the medical staff, pharmacists, and other health care experts. The selection of items to be included in the formulary should be based on objective evaluation of their relative economic, clinical, and humanistic outcomes. The decisions should not be based solely on economic factors. The committee should identify potential safety concerns for each medication considered for inclusion in the formulary and should ensure those safety concerns are addressed if the medication is added to the formulary or used in the health system.

The committee should minimize unnecessary duplication of the same basic drug type, drug entity, or drug product. Optimizing the number of drug entities and products available from the pharmacy can produce substantial patient care and financial benefits. These benefits are greatly increased through the use of generic equivalents (drug products considered identical or equivalent by FDA) and therapeutic equivalents (drug products differing in composition or basic drug entity that are considered to have similar pharmacologic and therapeutic activities).[2] The P&T committee must set forth policies and procedures that govern the dispensing of generics and therapeutic equivalents.

The P&T committee, when considering formulary options, should evaluate coordination issues with local health care plans and other organizations' formularies. At a minimum, appropriateness of therapeutic interchange should be evaluated for any formulary decisions that may conflict with known managed care or other health plan formularies.

The formulary should be published and updated regularly. It should also be readily available and accessible at all times, either manually or electronically, to all personnel involved in the care of patients and the use of medications. Medications should be identified in the formulary by their generic names, and prescribers should be strongly encouraged to order medications by their generic names.

The P&T committee should clearly define terminology related to formulary status of medications (e.g., formulary, nonformulary, not stocked at a given site, restricted by criteria specific to a given site), especially in multihospital organizations, and disseminate this information to health care professionals involved in the medication-use process. The P&T committee should establish a procedure for appraisal and use by the medical staff of medications not included in the formulary (i.e., nonformulary medication use).

The pharmacist shall be responsible for specifications for the quality, quantity, and source of supply of all medications, chemicals, biologicals, and pharmaceutical preparations used in the diagnosis and treatment of patients.

Conclusion

ASHP believes that medication-use policies should be developed and implemented in organized health-care systems to promote the rational, evidence-based, clinically appropriate, safe, and cost-effective use of medications. The P&T committee of a health system should develop, organize, and administer a formulary system that follows the principles set forth in this statement in order to optimize patient care.

References

1. Principles of a sound drug formulary system [consensus statement]. In: Hawkins B, ed. Best practices for hospital & health-system pharmacy: positions and guidance documents of ASHP. Bethesda, MD: American Society of Health-System Pharmacists; 2006:110–3.
2. U.S. Department of Health and Human Services. Electronic orange book: approved drug products with therapeutic equivalence evaluations. www.fda.gov/cder/ob/ (accessed 2008 Sep 24).

Approved by the ASHP Board of Directors on January 23, 2008 and by the ASHP House of Delegates on June 10, 2008. Developed through the ASHP Council on Pharmacy Practice. This statement supersedes the ASHP Statement on Pharmacy and Therapeutics Committee dated November 20, 1991, and the ASHP Statement on the Formulary System dated November 18, 1982.

Linda S. Tyler, Pharm.D., FASHP; Mirta Millares, Pharm.D., FCSHP, FASHP; Andrew L. Wilson, Pharm.D., FASHP; Lee C. Vermeulen, Jr., B.S.Pharm., M.S.; J. Russell (Rusty) May, Pharm.D., FASHP; Michael A. Valentino, M.H.S.A.; and Sabrina W. Cole, Pharm.D., are gratefully acknowledged for drafting this statement. The drafters have declared no potential conflicts of interest.

ASHP also acknowledges the following organizations and individuals for reviewing drafts of this statement: Academy of Managed Care Pharmacy (AMCP); American Nurses Association (ANA); American Society for Clinical Pharmacology and Therapeutics (ASCPT); American Society of Consultant Pharmacists (ASCP); Institute for Safe Medication Practices (ISMP); Pharmacy Compounding Accreditation Board (PCAB); Daniel T. Abazia, Pharm.D.; Philip Anderson, Pharm.D., FASHP; Lilian M. Azzopardi, B.Pharm., M.Phil., Ph.D.; Kenneth R. Baker, J.D. (PCAB); James L. Besier, Ph.D., FASHP; J. Lyle Bootman, Ph.D., Sc.D.; David G. Bowyer, B.S.; Maureen Brady, Pharm.D.; Margaret Chrymko, Pharm.D., FASHP; Joseph W. Cranston, Ph.D.; Steven Dzierba, M.S., FASHP; Michael Gaunt, Pharm.D. (ISMP); Pamela C. Hagan, M.S.N., R.N. (ANA); Raymond W. Hammond, Pharm.D., BCPS, FCCP; Eric T. Hola, M.S.; Patricia Kienle, B.S.Pharm., M.P.A., FASHP; Katharine Kiser, Pharm.D.; Thomas L. Kurt, M.D., M.P.H., FACPM, FACMMT, FAACT, FCP, FACE (ASCPT); Timothy R. Lanese, M.B.A., FASHP, FACHE; Rosario (Russ) J. Lazzaro, M.S.; Melvin E. Liter, M.S., Pharm.D.; Patrick M. Malone, Pharm.D., FASHP; Candis M. Morello, Pharm.D., CDE, FCSHP; Richard O'Brocta, Pharm.D., BCPS; Folakemi T. Odedina, Ph.D.; James A. Ponto, M.S., BCNP, FASHP; Curt W. Quap, M.S.; Mike Rouse, B.Pharm., M.P.S.; Marissa Schlaifer, M.S. (AMCP); Shelley Hoppe Schliesser, Pharm.D.; Michele F. Shepherd, Pharm.D., M.S., BCPS, FASHP; Jonalan Smith, Pharm.D. (ASCP); Allen J. Vaida, Pharm.D., FASHP (ISMP); William E. Wade, Pharm.D., FASHP, FCCP; Tom W. Woller, M.S., FASHP; and John L. Woon, Pharm.D., FASHP. (Review does not imply endorsement.)

The bibliographic citation for this document is as follows: American Society of Health-System Pharmacists. ASHP statement on the pharmacy and therapeutics committee and the formulary system. *Am J Health-Syst Pharm.* 2008; 65:2384–6.

ASHP Statement on the Use of Medications for Unlabeled Uses

The freedom and responsibility to make drug therapy decisions that are consistent with patient-care needs is a fundamental precept supported by ASHP. This activity is a professional duty of pharmacists not limited by language in Food and Drug Administration (FDA)-approved product labeling.

The prescribing, dispensing, and administration of FDA-approved drugs for uses, treatment regimens, or patient populations that are not reflected in FDA-approved product labeling often represent a therapeutic approach that has been extensively studied and reported in medical literature. Such uses are *not* indicative of inappropriate usage. Health-care professionals should appreciate the critical need for freedom in making drug therapy decisions and understand the implications of unlabeled uses. ASHP supports third-party reimbursement for FDA-approved drug products appropriately prescribed for unlabeled uses.

Definition of Unlabeled Use

The FDA approves drug products for marketing in the United States. Such a product approved for marketing is often termed an "FDA-approved drug." FDA also approves each drug product's labeling (container label, package insert, and certain advertising); the term "FDA-approved labeling" applies here. Drug uses that are not included in the indications or dosage regimens listed in the FDA-approved labeling are defined as "unlabeled uses." For purposes of this document, unlabeled use includes the use of a drug product in (1) doses, (2) patient populations, (3) indications, or (4) routes of administration that are not reflected in FDA-approved product labeling.

It is important to recognize that FDA cannot approve or disapprove physician prescribing practices of legally marketed drugs. FDA does regulate what manufacturers may recommend about uses in their products' labeling and what manufacturers can include in advertising and promotion.

The sometimes-used term "unapproved use" is a misnomer, implying that FDA regulates prescribing and dispensing activities. This term should be avoided.[1] Other terminology that is sometimes used to describe unlabeled use includes "off-label use," "out-of-label use," and "usage outside of labeling."

According to FDA, unlabeled use encompasses a range of situations that extend from inadequate to carefully conceived investigations, from hazardous to salutary uses, and from infrequent to widespread medical practice. Accepted medical practice often involves drug use that is not reflected in FDA-approved drug-product labeling.[2]

Health-Care Issues Related to Unlabeled Use

Access to Drug Therapies. The prescribing and dispensing of drugs for unlabeled uses are increasing.[3,4] In many clinical situations, unlabeled use represents the most appropriate therapy for patients. Failure to recognize this or, more importantly, regarding such use as "unapproved" or "experimental" may restrict access to necessary drug therapies.

Lack of Practice Standards. Well-defined medical practice standards that differentiate between experimental therapies and established practice will probably always be somewhat lacking, owing to the advancement of medical science and the dynamic nature of medical practice. Standards of practice for certain drug therapies, particularly biotechnologically produced drugs, cancer chemotherapy, and AIDS treatments, are continually evolving. The dynamic nature of these drug therapies makes it difficult for professional societies to review scientific data expediently and to develop standards that remain absolutely current.

Failure of Package Insert and FDA-Approved Labeling to Reflect Current Practice. For FDA-approved product labeling to be modified, scientific data must be submitted by a product's manufacturer to FDA to support any additional indication(s) and dosage regimen(s). Once they are submitted, FDA must review the data and make a decision to permit alteration of the package insert.

Knowing that unlabeled uses are permitted, and knowing that the accumulation and submission of scientific data to FDA to modify labeling is a time-consuming and often expensive process, some pharmaceutical manufacturers elect not to pursue labeling changes. Therefore, a product's labeling sometimes fails to represent the most current therapeutic information for a drug, and situations naturally occur when it is appropriate to prescribe drugs for unlabeled uses.

Pharmacist's Role

ASHP believes that pharmacists in organized health-care settings bear a significant responsibility for ensuring optimal outcomes from all drug therapy. With respect to unlabeled uses, the role of the pharmacist should be to

1. Fulfill the roles of patient advocate and drug information specialist.
2. Develop policies and procedures for evaluating drug orders (prescriptions) and dispensing drugs for unlabeled uses in their own work settings. Such policies and procedures might address the documentation of scientific support, adherence to accepted medical practice standards, or a description of medical necessity.
3. Develop proactive approaches to promote informed decisionmaking by third-party payers for health-care services.

Role of Drug Information Compendia

The Medicare Catastrophic Coverage Act of 1988 (now repealed) included the statements that "in carrying out the legislation, the Secretary [of Health and Human Services] shall establish standards for drug coverage. In establishing such standards, which are based on accepted medical practice, the Secretary shall incorporate standards from such current authoritative compendia as the Secretary may select."[5] Specific compendia recommended were the *AHFS Drug Information,*

AMA Drug Evaluations, and *USP Dispensing Information, Volume I.* Despite the repeal of the Act, some third-party payers have adopted guidelines that endorse these three compendia as authoritative information sources with respect to unlabeled uses for drug products.

Positions on Unlabeled Use

FDA Position. A statement entitled "Use of Approved Drugs for Unlabeled Indications" was published in the *FDA Drug Bulletin* in April 1982 to address the issues of appropriateness and legality of prescribing approved drugs for uses not included in FDA's approved labeling. This statement included the following:

> The Food, Drug and Cosmetic Act does not limit the manner in which a physician may use an approved drug. Once a product has been approved for marketing, a physician may prescribe it for uses or in treatment regimens or patient populations that are not included in approved labeling. Such "unapproved" or, more precisely, "unlabeled" uses may be appropriate and rational in certain circumstances, and may, in fact, reflect approaches to drug therapy that have been extensively reported in medical literature.[1]

Other Organizations. Other organizations that have published positions on the issue of unlabeled uses of drug products are the Health Care Financing Administration (HCFA),[6] the Blue Cross and Blue Shield Association of America (BC/BS),[7] and the Health Insurance Association of America (HIAA).[8]

The American Medical Association, American Society of Clinical Oncology, Association of American Cancer Institutes, Association of Community Cancer Centers, Candlelighters Childhood Cancer Foundation, Memorial Sloan Kettering Cancer Center, National Cancer Institute, and the National Institute of Allergy and Infectious Diseases jointly developed a consensus statement and recommendations regarding use and reimbursement of unlabeled uses of drug products.[9]

These statements are consistent with the ASHP position.

Reimbursement Issues

As a cost-containment measure, most third-party payers exclude coverage for experimental therapies. Drug therapy coverage decisions are complicated, because often it is difficult to differentiate among an accepted standard of practice, an evolving standard of practice, and investigational therapies. Data demonstrating medical necessity and improved patient outcome are often difficult to retrieve. Consequently, insurance carriers and managed care providers

have sometimes elected to cover only those indications included in FDA-approved drug-product labeling and have frequently denied coverage for unlabeled uses of drug products.

ASHP believes that such coverage denials restrict patients from receiving medically necessary therapies that represent the best available treatment options. A growing number of insurance carriers are following the BC/BS and HIAA guidelines that encourage the use of the three authoritative drug compendia, peer-reviewed literature, and consultation with experts in research and clinical practice to make specific coverage decisions. ASHP supports informed decisionmaking that promotes third-party reimbursement for FDA-approved drug products appropriately prescribed for unlabeled uses.

References

1. Use of approved drugs for unlabeled indications. *FDA Drug Bull.* 1982; 12:4–5.
2. Nightingale SL. Use of drugs for unlabeled indications. *FDA Q Rep.* 1986(Sep); 269.
3. Mortenson LE. Audit indicates many uses of combination therapy are unlabeled. *J Cancer Program Manage.* 1988; 3:21–5.
4. Off-label drugs: initial results of a national survey. Washington, DC: U.S. General Accounting Office. 1991:1–27.
5. PL 100-360, 1988.
6. Health Care Financing Administration. Medicare carriers' manual. Section 2050.5. Washington, DC: U.S. Department of Health and Human Services; 1987 Aug.
7. Statement on coverage recommendation for FDA-approved drugs. Chicago: Blue Cross and Blue Shield Association; 1989 Oct 25.
8. Statement of the Health Insurance Association of America (HIAA) on coverage for unapproved drugs and drug-related costs. Presented to the National Committee to Review Current Procedures for Approval of New Drugs for Cancer and AIDS. 1989 Oct 25.
9. Cancer economics. *Cancer Lett.* 1989; Suppl(Jun):2–3.

Approved by the ASHP Board of Directors, November 20, 1991, and by the ASHP House of Delegates, June 1, 1992. Developed by the Council on Professional Affairs.

The bibliographic citation for this document is as follows: American Society of Hospital Pharmacists. ASHP statement on the use of medications for unlabeled uses. *Am J Hosp Pharm.* 1992; 49:2006–8.

ASHP Guidelines on Medication-Use Evaluation

Medication-use evaluation (MUE) is a performance improvement method that focuses on evaluating and improving medication-use processes with the goal of optimal patient outcomes. MUE may be applied to a medication or therapeutic class, disease state or condition, a medication-use process (prescribing, preparing and dispensing, administering, and monitoring), or specific outcomes.[1] Further, it may be applied in and among the various practice settings of organized health systems.

MUE encompasses the goals and objectives of drug-use evaluation (DUE) in its broadest application, with an emphasis on improving patient outcomes. Use of "MUE," rather than "DUE,"[2] emphasizes the need for a more multifaceted approach to improving medication use. MUE has a common goal with the pharmaceutical care it supports: to improve an individual patient's quality of life through achievement of predefined, medication-related therapeutic outcomes.[3,4] Through its focus on the system of medication use, the MUE process helps to identify actual and potential medication-related problems, resolve actual medication-related problems, and prevent potential medication-related problems that could interfere with achieving optimum outcomes from medication therapy.

In organized health systems, MUE must be conducted as an organizationally authorized program or process that is proactive, criteria based, designed and managed by an interdisciplinary team, and systematically carried out. It is conducted as a collaborative effort of prescribers, pharmacists, nurses, administrators, and other health care professionals on behalf of their patients.

MUE Objectives

Some typical objectives of MUE include

- Promoting optimal medication therapy.
- Preventing medication-related problems.
- Evaluating the effectiveness of medication therapy.
- Improving patient safety.
- Establishing interdisciplinary consensus on medication-use processes.
- Stimulating improvements in medication-use processes.
- Stimulating standardization in medication-use processes.
- Enhancing opportunities, through standardization, to assess the value of innovative medication-use practices from both patient-outcome and resource-utilization perspectives.
- Minimizing procedural variations that contribute to suboptimal outcomes of medication use.
- Identifying areas in which further information and education for health care professionals may be needed.
- Minimizing costs of medication therapy. These costs may be only partly related to the direct cost of medications themselves. When medications are selected and managed optimally from the outset, the costs of complications and wasted resources are minimized, and overall costs are decreased.
- Meeting or exceeding internal and external quality standards (e.g., professional practice standards, accreditation standards, or government laws and regulations).

Steps of the MUE Process

While the specific approach varies with the practice setting and patient population being served, the following common steps occur in the ongoing MUE process:

- Establish organizational authority for the MUE process and identify responsible individuals and groups.
- Develop screening mechanisms (indicators) for comprehensive surveillance of the medication-use system.
- Set priorities for in-depth analysis of important aspects of medication use.
- Inform health care professionals (and others as necessary) in the practice setting(s) about the objectives and expected benefits of the MUE process.
- Establish criteria, guidelines, treatment protocols, and standards of care for specific medications and medication-use processes. These should be based on sound scientific evidence from the medical and pharmaceutical literature.
- Educate health care professionals to promote the use of criteria, guidelines, treatment protocols, and standards of care.
- Establish mechanisms for timely communication among health care professionals.
- Initiate the use of MUE criteria, guidelines, treatment protocols, and standards of care in the medication-use process.
- Collect data and evaluate care.
- Develop and implement plans for improvement of the medication-use process based on MUE findings (if indicated).
- Assess the effectiveness of actions taken, and document improvements.
- Incorporate improvements into criteria, guidelines, treatment protocols, and standards of care, when indicated.
- Repeat the cycle of planning, evaluating, and taking action for ongoing improvement in medication-use processes.
- Regularly assess the effectiveness of the MUE process itself and make needed improvements.

Selecting Medications and Medication-Use Processes for Evaluation

Medications or medication-use processes should be selected for evaluation for one or more of the following reasons:

1. The medication is known or suspected to cause adverse reactions, or it interacts with another medication, food, or diagnostic procedure in a way that presents a significant health risk.
2. The medication is used in the treatment of patients who may be at high risk for adverse reactions.
3. The medication-use process affects a large number of patients or the medication is frequently prescribed.
4. The medication or medication-use process is a critical component of care for a specific disease, condition, or procedure.

5. The medication is potentially toxic or causes discomfort at normal doses.
6. The medication is most effective when used in a specific way.
7. The medication is under consideration for formulary retention, addition, or deletion.
8. The medication or medication-use process is one for which suboptimal use would have a negative effect on patient outcomes or system costs.
9. Use of the medication is expensive.

Indicators Suggesting a Need for MUE Analysis

Certain events (indicators) serve as "flags" of potential opportunities to improve medication use. Some are

- Adverse medication events, including medication errors, preventable adverse drug reactions, and toxicity.
- Signs of treatment failures, such as unexpected readmissions and bacterial resistance to anti-infective therapy.
- Pharmacist interventions to improve medication therapy, categorized by medication and type of intervention.
- Nonformulary medications used or requested.
- Patient dissatisfaction or deterioration in quality of life.

Roles and Responsibilities in the MUE Process

The roles of individual health care professionals in MUE may vary according to practice setting, organizational goals, and available resources. The organizational body (e.g., quality management committee, pharmacy and therapeutics committee) responsible for the MUE process should have, at a minimum, prescriber, pharmacist, nurse, and administrator representation. Other health care professionals should contribute their unique perspectives when the evaluation and improvement process addresses their areas of expertise and responsibility. Temporary working groups may be used for specific improvement efforts.

Pharmacist's Responsibilities in MUE

Pharmacists, by virtue of their expertise and their mission of ensuring proper medication use, should exert leadership and work collaboratively with other members of the health care team in the ongoing process of medication-use evaluation and improvement.[5] Responsibilities of pharmacists in the MUE process include

- Developing an operational plan for MUE programs and processes that are consistent with the health system's overall goals and resource capabilities.
- Working collaboratively with prescribers and others to develop criteria for specific medications and to design effective medication-use processes.
- Reviewing individual medication orders against medication-use criteria and consulting with prescribers and others in the process as needed.
- Managing MUE programs and processes.

- Collecting, analyzing, and evaluating patient-specific data to identify, resolve, and prevent medication-related problems.
- Interpreting and reporting MUE findings and recommending changes in medication-use processes.
- Providing information and education based on MUE findings.

Resources

Some resources helpful in designing and managing an MUE process are listed here.

- The primary professional literature and up-to-date reference texts are key resources necessary for the development of MUE criteria. In general, local consensus should be based on medical and pharmaceutical literature recommendations.
- Published criteria, such as found in *AJHP* and ASHP's *Criteria for Drug Use Evaluation* (volumes 1–4), provide medication-specific criteria that may be adapted for local use.
- Computer software programs, including proprietary programs designed specifically for MUE functions, may be helpful in managing data and reporting.
- External standards-setting bodies, such as the Joint Commission on Accreditation of Healthcare Organizations, publish medication-use indicators that can help to identify portions of the medication-use system that require improvement.

Follow-up Actions in an MUE Process

The MUE process itself should be reviewed regularly to identify opportunities for its improvement. The success of an MUE process should be assessed in terms of improved patient outcomes. Medication-use system changes that evolve from MUE findings should be developed by the departments and medical services with responsibility for providing care, rather than solely through a committee having oversight for MUE (e.g., a pharmacy and therapeutics committee). Typical follow-up actions based on MUE findings include contact with individual prescribers and other health care professionals, information and education (newsletters, seminars, clinical care guidelines) for health care professionals, changes in medication-use systems, and changes in medication-therapy monitoring processes. MUE should be conducted as an ongoing interdisciplinary and collaborative improvement process. Punitive reactions to quality concerns are often counterproductive. It is important to communicate and commend positive achievements (care that meets or exceeds expectations) and improvements.

Pitfalls

Some common pitfalls to avoid in performing MUE activities include the following:[6]

1. Lack of authority. An MUE process that does not involve the medical staff is likely to be ineffective. Authoritative medical staff support and formal organizational recognition of the MUE process are necessary.

2. Lack of organization. Without a clear definition of the roles and responsibilities of individuals involved (e.g., who will develop criteria, who will communicate with other departments, who will collect and summarize data, and who will evaluate data), an MUE process may not succeed.

3. Poor communication. Everyone affected by the MUE process should understand its importance to the health system, its goals, and its procedures. The pharmacist should manage the MUE process and have the responsibility and authority to ensure timely communication among all professionals involved in the medication-use process. Criteria for medication use should be communicated to all affected professionals prior to the evaluation of care. MUE activity should be a standing agenda item for appropriate quality-of-care committees responsible for aspects of medication use.

4. Poor documentation. MUE activities should be well documented, including summaries of MUE actions with respect to individual medication orders and the findings and conclusions from collective evaluations. Documentation should address recommendations made and follow-up actions.

5. Lack of involvement. The MUE process is not a one-person task, nor is it the responsibility of a single department or professional group. Medication-use criteria should be developed through an interdisciplinary consensus process. Lack of administrative support can severely limit the effectiveness of MUE. The benefits of MUE should be conveyed in terms of improving patient outcomes and minimizing health-system costs.

6. Lack of follow-through. A one-time study or evaluation independent of the overall MUE process will have limited success in improving patient outcomes. The effectiveness of initial actions must be assessed and the action plan adjusted if necessary. It is important not to lose sight of the improvement goals.

7. Evaluation methodology that impedes patient care. Data collection should not consume so much time that patient care activities suffer. Interventions that can improve care for an individual patient should not be withheld because of the sampling technique or evaluation methodology.

8. Lack of readily retrievable data and information management. Existing data capabilities need to be assessed and maximum benefit obtained from available computerized information management resources. Deficiencies in information gathering and analysis should be identified and priorities for upgrading information support established.

References

1. Nadzam DM. Development of medication-use indicators by the Joint Commission on Accreditation of Healthcare Organizations. *Am J Hosp Pharm.* 1991; 48:1925–30.

2. American Society of Hospital Pharmacists. ASHP guidelines on the pharmacist's role in drug-use evaluation. *Am J Hosp Pharm.* 1988; 45:385–6.

3. Hepler CD, Strand LM. Opportunities and responsibilities in pharmaceutical care. *Am J Hosp Pharm.* 1990; 47:533–43.

4. American Society of Hospital Pharmacists. ASHP statement on pharmaceutical care. *Am J Hosp Pharm.* 1993; 50:1720–3.

5. Angaran DM. Quality assurance to quality improvement: measuring and monitoring pharmaceutical care. *Am J Hosp Pharm.* 1991; 48:1901–7.

6. Todd MW. Drug use evaluation. In: Brown TR, ed. Handbook of institutional pharmacy practice. 3rd ed. Bethesda, MD: American Society of Hospital Pharmacists; 1992.

Approved by the ASHP Board of Directors, April 24, 1996. Developed by the ASHP Council on Professional Affairs. Supersedes the ASHP Guidelines on the Pharmacist's Role in Drug-Use Evaluation, dated November 19, 1987.

The bibliographic citation for this document is as follows: American Society of Health-System Pharmacists. ASHP guidelines on medication-use evaluation. *Am J Health-Syst Pharm.* 1996; 53:1953–5.

ASHP Guidelines on the Pharmacy and Therapeutics Committee and the Formulary System

Purpose

These guidelines outline the recommended processes and techniques for formulary system management and describe the pharmacist's responsibilities and roles in managing the formulary system in partnership with other health care professionals. These guidelines also provide assistance to pharmacists in the organization and operation of the pharmacy and therapeutics (P&T) committee or equivalent body, evaluation of medications for formularies, and development and implementation of strategies to manage medication use through the formulary system. A glossary of terms is provided in the appendix.

Formulary and Formulary System

A *formulary* is a continually updated list of medications and related information, representing the clinical judgment of physicians, pharmacists, and other experts in the diagnosis, prophylaxis, or treatment of disease and promotion of health. A formulary includes, but is not limited to, a list of medications and medication-associated products or devices, medication-use policies, important ancillary drug information, decision-support tools, and organizational guidelines. A *formulary system* is the ongoing process through which a health care organization establishes policies regarding the use of drugs, therapies, and drug-related products and identifies those that are most medically appropriate and cost-effective to best serve the health interests of a given patient population.[1] Formulary systems are used in many different settings, including hospitals, acute care facilities, home care settings, and long-term-care facilities, as well as by payers such as Medicare, Medicaid, insurance companies, and managed care organizations. Many organizations have policy statements on the use of formularies.[2–8] This document focuses on the use of formulary systems in hospitals and health systems.

Evolution of Formularies

Formulary systems have evolved over time. Modern formularies began as rudimentary drug lists developed by the military in the 1940s and came into more widespread use during the 1950s. Pharmacists, in conjunction with their organizations, developed policies to dispense generic equivalent drugs when a specific brand-name drug was prescribed. Protests from the National Pharmaceutical Council and the American Medical Association (AMA) resulted in state laws prohibiting this activity. Community pharmacies complied, but hospital pharmacies resisted. In the late 1950s, the ASHP minimum standard for pharmacies in hospitals called for the implementation of a formulary system.[9]

During the 1960s, the concept of a hospital formulary continued to grow. Hospitals developed policies that authorized pharmacists to make generic interchanges in an institutional formulary system based on prior consent from physicians.[10] ASHP and the American Hospital Association

(AHA) issued joint statements on the legality of formularies.[11,12] AMA and the American Pharmaceutical (later Pharmacists) Association subsequently joined with ASHP and AHA to revise the statements.[13] In 1965, two significant events occurred: (1) Medicare listed formularies as a reimbursement eligibility requirement[14] and (2) the Joint Commission on the Accreditation of Hospitals (now known as the Joint Commission) included an active P&T committee in its accreditation requirements.[15] Even with these actions, formularies were typically no more than lists of drugs stocked by the pharmacy.

By the 1980s, literature describing the clinical and economic value of well-designed formularies had emerged. Evidence from the hospital setting was published first, soon followed by evidence from the ambulatory care environment.[10] This literature led to more widespread acceptance of formularies. In 1986, the Pharmaceutical Research and Manufacturers Association officially accepted the concept of therapeutic interchange in hospitals and opposed its use in other settings.[10] As more evidence emerged, AMA's views on formularies for inpatient and outpatient settings became more closely aligned with those of ASHP. AMA's official policy on drug formularies and therapeutic interchange was first published in 1994[16] and has since been updated several times.[5]

Today, formulary systems are considered an essential tool for health care organizations. Formularies have grown from simple drug lists to comprehensive systems of medication-use policies intended to ensure safe, appropriate, and cost-effective use of pharmaceuticals in patient care.

P&T Committee

The P&T committee is responsible for managing the formulary system. It is composed of actively practicing physicians, other prescribers, pharmacists, nurses, administrators, quality-improvement managers, and other health care professionals and staff who participate in the medication-use process. Customarily, P&T committee member appointments are based on guidance from the medical staff. The P&T committee should serve in an evaluative, educational, and advisory capacity to the medical staff and organizational administration in all matters pertaining to the use of medications (including investigational medications). The P&T committee should be responsible for overseeing policies and procedures related to all aspects of medication use within an institution. The P&T committee is responsible to the medical staff as a whole, and its recommendations are subject to approval by the organized medical staff as well as the administrative approval process. The P&T committee's organization and authority should be outlined in the organization's medical staff bylaws, medical staff rules and regulations, and other organizational policies as appropriate.

Other responsibilities of the P&T committee include medication-use evaluation (MUE), adverse-drug-event monitoring and reporting, medication-error prevention, and development of clinical care plans and guidelines. Information about these activities is available in ASHP guidelines on the topics.[17–20]

P&T committees have been credited with increasing practitioners' knowledge about drug therapy, improving the safety of drug therapy, and improving therapeutic outcomes.[21]

Consideration of patient care and unbiased reviews of the biomedical literature are the cornerstone principles of formulary decision-making. A conflict of interest (COI), financial or otherwise, may interfere with professionals' ability to make evidence-based decisions,[22] and even the appearance of a potential COI can undermine a formulary decision. The P&T committee has a responsibility to its patients and its organization to identify and address COI issues in its decision-making processes. Professionals participating in the P&T committee should disclose financial relationships with pharmaceutical manufacturers, medical supply vendors, other health care provider organizations, and other commercial interests. Some health care organizations exclude heath care professionals with COIs from P&T committee membership, whereas others allow participation in committee discussions but prohibit voting on particular items. Practitioners requesting additions or changes to the formulary should disclose financial relationships with pharmaceutical companies and other potential COIs to the P&T committee.

Finally, the role of pharmaceutical company representatives and medical science liaisons in a health care organization should be carefully considered. Organizational guidelines should define appropriate relationships and interactions with such individuals. At a minimum, these guidelines should address the provision of pharmaceutical samples, indirect or direct funding support, and educational programming regarding formulary and nonformulary medications. Applications for formulary additions should be initiated and completed independently by the requesting health care provider and not by an industry representative or vendor. Refer to ASHP's "Guidelines on Pharmacists' Relationships with Industry" for more information on appropriate interactions with industry.[23]

Managing the Formulary System

Health systems should develop, maintain, and implement a formulary management process. Decisions on the management of a formulary system should be founded on the evidence-based clinical, ethical, legal, social, philosophical, quality-of-life, safety, and economic factors that result in optimal patient care.[24,25] The process must include the active and direct involvement of physicians, pharmacists, and other appropriate health care professionals. This evidence-based process should not be based solely on economic factors. The formulary system should be standardized among components of integrated health systems when standardization leads to improved patient outcomes and safety.

Management of a formulary system is a significant component of a health care organization's ongoing medication-use policy development process. A comprehensive, well-maintained formulary that is tailored to the organization's patient care needs, policy framework, and medication-use systems ensures that the six critical processes identified by the Joint Commission (selection and procurement, storage, ordering and transcribing, preparing and dispensing, administration, and monitoring) work in concert to ensure optimal outcomes.[26] A well-managed formulary system ensures a close relationship among the organization's medication-use policies, the therapies offered by the organization, and the medications routinely stocked in the pharmacy. A formulary also identifies those medications that are most medically appropriate and cost-effective to best serve the health interests of the health system's patient population. The P&T committee should interpret the term *medication* broadly in the context of care delivery to include alternative remedies (herbals and supplements), nonprescription drugs, blood derivatives, contrast media, and other diagnostic and treatment agents.[26]

The formulary system should include review and approval of all policies related to the medication-use process. All medication-use policies, regardless of their origination, should flow through the P&T committee. The organization's medical staff leadership (i.e., the body to which the P&T committee reports) should complete the final policy approval. Policy review and revision should occur as new information becomes available and at regularly established intervals (e.g., annually). Specific medication-use policies should address

- How medications are requested for addition to or deletion from the formulary,
- How medications are reviewed for addition to or deletion from the formulary, including who performs the reviews,
- The process for developing, implementing, and monitoring medication-use guidelines,
- Methods for ensuring the safe prescribing, distribution, administration, and monitoring of medications,
- Methods for selection of suitable manufacturers for specific medications (a pharmacist shall be responsible for specifications for the quality, quantity, and source of supply of all medications, chemicals, biologicals, and pharmaceutical preparations used in the diagnosis and treatment of patients),[27]
- The process for using nonformulary agents within the institution,
- The process for managing drug product shortages,
- The process for developing an organization-specific MUE plan,
- Policies regarding specific medication-use processes (e.g., procurement, prescribing, distribution, administration, monitoring), and
- The process for disseminating medication-use policies and how users will be educated regarding the process.

A formal process to review medication-use policies should be in place. This process may include the use of expert panels or subcommittees of the P&T committee. Expert panels should serve in an advisory role to the P&T committee, and their membership should include recognized experts in their areas of practice. Such panels can be helpful in applying clinical study results to specific patient populations, and panel members can help educate groups of physicians, who ultimately drive prescribing behaviors, about significant formulary changes. User groups, representing those primarily affected by the policy, may also be helpful. The P&T committee may also find subcommittees that address specific therapeutic areas to be beneficial (e.g., antimicrobial, cancer chemotherapy, cardiovascular, adverse-drug-reaction, or biotechnology subcommittees).

The P&T committee should have formal interactions (i.e., communication lines) with other committees whose functions may affect the medication-use process. These

committees would include those responsible for developing tools to facilitate medication use (e.g., forms or order set review committee, computerized prescriber-order-entry committee), those concerned with safety or performance improvement (e.g., quality-improvement or patient safety committees), those involved in developing patient care policies (e.g., medical and nursing committees), those involved with investigational medications (e.g., investigational review boards), and other committees whose actions may affect medication use (e.g., nutrition, equipment and supply, or finance committees). Recommendations from other committees, subcommittees of P&T, expert panels, and others should be submitted to the P&T committee for review. P&T committee decisions on recommendations should be communicated to the recommending group in a timely fashion.

Evaluating Medications for Inclusion in the Formulary

The P&T committee should use a structured, evidence-based process in the evaluation of medications for formulary consideration. The P&T committee should be provided with information that reflects a thorough, accurate, and unbiased review and analysis of the evidence available in the scientific literature. The evaluation process should encourage objective consideration of clinical and care delivery information, facilitate communication, foster positive patient outcomes, and support safe and effective medication ordering, dispensing, administration, and monitoring. Decisions made by the P&T committee should support improved patient care outcomes across the continuum of care.

Evidence-Based Evaluation. Inclusion of a medication on a health system's formulary should reflect that an evidence-based evaluation of the relative merits and risks of the medication has been performed and that the institution's P&T committee, with input from appropriate experts, has determined that the medication is appropriate for routine use in the management of the patient population at that institution.

Evidence-based medicine is a systematic approach to the evaluation of biomedical literature and application to clinical practice and should be applied to formulary decision-making for medication product selection.[24] Evidence-based decision-making standardizes and improves the quality of patient care and promotes cost-effective prescribing.[24,25] To practice evidence-based medicine, practitioners must be proficient in retrieving, evaluating, and applying the biomedical literature to clinical practice.

Evidence-based decision-making incorporates the systematic approach to reviewing, evaluating, and applying the biomedical literature to guide formulary decisions. Various types and strengths of evidence (e.g., meta-analyses, randomized clinical trials, case reports, association consensus statements) may be useful in the decision-making process. Although different types of evidence are available for application, those with stronger evidence should be used to drive formulary decisions (e.g., meta-analyses, randomized controlled trials). Other types of evidence have a role in the decision-making process, however, and may be appropriate when stronger evidence is not available. Observational studies (i.e., case–control and cohort studies), case reports, and consensus opinions may be valuable even when stronger evidence is available. Some organizations find it useful to

grade evidence when evaluating formulary requests; several tools are available for this purpose.[28–32]

Published evidence and expert opinion are not the only resources available to aid in the formulary decision-making process. Internal data and prescribing and outcomes information may be helpful in formulary decision-making. When published data are not available, it may be appropriate to incorporate expert opinion into the review process. Experts in practice areas sometimes have access to unpublished data or reports that may offer insight into difficult formulary decisions.

The P&T committee should use formulary packets and dossiers prepared by pharmaceutical manufacturers with the utmost caution, since the objectivity of these documents may be challenged. The formulary decision-making process should instead be guided by an independent review of evidence published in the biomedical literature, application of expert opinion, and use of internal data and benchmarking programs.

The information should be provided to the P&T committee in a written document with a standard format (e.g., a drug monograph, drug review, drug-evaluation document). All information provided in the drug-evaluation document should be referenced to the evidence or identified as a conclusion supported by evidence. Any areas of consensus recommendations or opinion should be clearly identified.

Types of Drug Reviews. There are four major types of drug reviews: new drug monographs, reevaluations of previous formulary decisions, therapeutic class reviews, and expedited reviews of newly approved medications. Because of the expertise and training of pharmacists (drug information specialists in particular), pharmacists should play an integral part in the preparation and presentation of the drug review document to the P&T committee.

New drug monographs. When the Food and Drug Administration (FDA) approves a new drug for marketing that is relevant to the health system, a drug monograph should be prepared for formulary consideration by the P&T committee. New chemical entities warrant a thorough evaluation and a written drug monograph. A short (e.g., one-page) summary could be provided along with the full monograph.[33] Some organizations use an executive summary format. A new drug that is significantly similar to other available therapeutic alternatives may be presented in a more abbreviated manner (e.g., an abbreviated monograph) provided that the P&T committee or experts agree that the drug is therapeutically equivalent to agents already available on the formulary.

Addenda to original monographs used to reevaluate previous formulary decisions. Formulary decisions may need to be reassessed based on relevant new information or in light of newly marketed drugs or dosage forms. New data on safety, efficacy, stability, methods of administration, cost, or pharmacoeconomics may warrant a reevaluation of the drug or dosage strengths or formulations stocked by the health system. An addendum to the original monograph summarizing the new information should be developed for evaluation by the P&T committee. The P&T committee may want to establish reassessment dates at the time of formulary review so that the committee can reassess the effect of a formulary decision on quality or cost of care.

Therapeutic class reviews. Review of an entire therapeutic class of drugs should be performed at regular intervals, which may be determined by the P&T committee or

influenced by regulatory agencies. A therapeutic class review should include all formulary and nonformulary medications within the class and may include institutional utilization or outcomes data and newly published information. Therapeutic class reviews may lead to formulary removal of therapeutically equivalent drugs or a change in restriction or guideline status for a drug.

Expedited reviews. A process should be available for the P&T committee to conduct an expedited review of a new drug, new indication for a drug, or reevaluation of a previous formulary decision. Criteria should be in place to describe when an expedited review is warranted. For example, approval of a new chemical entity for a disease with no therapeutic alternative may warrant an expedited review to ensure availability of the drug for patients who need it. Likewise, a significant new safety concern may warrant an expedited review for addition of restrictions or removal from the formulary.

Elements of a Drug-Evaluation Document. The drug-evaluation document should present the evidence in a manner that is thorough, is consistent from medication to medication, and provides all necessary facts and analysis to the P&T committee to allow for an informed formulary decision. Document structure may vary, depending on the needs of the specific health system and P&T committee, but the following elements are essential to all such documents:

- Brand and generic names and synonyms,
- FDA approval information, including date and FDA rating,
- Pharmacology and mechanism of action,
- FDA-approved indications,
- Potential non-FDA-approved (off-label) uses,
- Dosage forms and storage,
- Recommended dosage regimens,
- Pharmacokinetic considerations,
- Use in special populations (e.g., children, elderly, patients with renal or liver failure),
- Pregnancy category and use during breast-feeding,
- Comparisons of the drug's efficacy, safety, convenience, and costs with those of therapeutic alternatives (with evidence tables when feasible),
- If information on comparative efficacy is minimal or lacking, data on absolute efficacy (i.e., efficacy versus placebo),
- Clinical trial analysis and critique,
- Medication safety assessment and recommendations (adverse drug reactions; drug–drug and drug–food interactions; specific therapy monitoring requirements; unusual administration, storage, or stability issues; and potential for medication errors, such as look-alike or sound-alike issues), and
- Financial analysis, including pharmacoeconomic assessments.

Formulary status recommendations (e.g., from drug information services or expert groups) may be included in the drug evaluation document. In some organizations, recommendations are not provided in the written document in order to promote an unbiased discussion by the P&T committee. Recommendations should consider the formulary status (addition or rejection) of a medication, as well as the need for restrictions, educational efforts, or policies and procedures to ensure safe and appropriate use within the health system.

Pharmacoeconomic Assessments. Rigorous pharmacoeconomic evaluations can and should be conducted in some cases when reviewing new medications. These evaluations should explicitly state the perspective of the analysis (e.g., patient, health care provider, payer) and should include consideration of all costs and consequences relevant to that perspective. When new medications being considered are found to be therapeutically equivalent to existing alternatives (having equivalent efficacy and safety), then the cost-minimization approach is appropriate. In these circumstances, it is important to consider costs associated with the medication and nonmedication-related costs (e.g., costs of administration, monitoring, prolonged hospital stay, and laboratory test monitoring; costs to patients and providers).

While cost-effectiveness analysis (evaluating the incremental difference in investment necessary to produce an incremental difference in clinical outcome) is another potentially useful analytic approach, it is not often used for formulary decision-making because of its complexity and need for strong evidence or data. The academic value of this approach lies in its ability to show how little (or how much) must be spent to achieve a particular margin of clinical advantage when comparing an alternative that is more expensive but safer or more efficacious. No standards currently exist to determine how much money is reasonable to spend for any given improvement in out-come; however, it is unreasonable to recommend alternatives of lower quality simply to achieve cost savings. This approach can be used to demonstrate how a decrease in clinical outcomes associated with the use of a less expensive agent can be offset by investing the savings achieved in other interventions that produce even greater total benefits.

Cost-utility evaluations (evaluating the incremental difference in investment necessary to produce an incremental difference in quality-of-life-adjusted clinical outcome [e.g., incremental cost per quality-adjusted life years gained for one medication versus another]) may also be beneficial by serving to reflect patient preference in formulary decision-making. However, the same concerns related to the use of cost-effectiveness evaluations apply to this approach.[34–36]

Decision analysis models incorporating local data can be employed when published pharmacoeconomic data are limited or unavailable. Probabilities for each outcome can be extracted from the published literature or drawn from local data sources, which would provide a more relevant local perspective on outcomes. Costs associated with medications and outcomes should reflect those of the health care system.

Pharmacoeconomic analyses published in the medical literature or provided in the manufacturer's formulary dossier should be analyzed carefully before being included as part of the review process. Particular attention should be paid to the assumptions made in these studies. In many situations, assumptions made to simplify economic studies are not valid in particular institutions. Institution-specific costs are often different from the costs used in published studies, and local data should be used when incorporating their results into medication reviews.[37,38]

Even if a formal pharmacoeconomic evaluation is not included in a drug review document, a financial evaluation must be conducted, including consideration of nonmedication-related costs and financial consequences to the pharmacy and to the organization as a whole.

Formulary Exceptions. Exclusion of a medication from a formulary may affect coverage of and access to the medication. In a closed formulary system, for example, only medications listed on the formulary are covered under the patient's drug benefit. Regardless of health-system setting, the formulary system should include an exception process that provides prescribers and patients with timely access to medications that are not on the formulary but are medically necessary for the care of the patient. The underlying principle for such a process is that unique patient needs may not be satisfied by use of the formulary medications. The formulary exception process should generate information on nonformulary medication use that will enable the P&T committee to evaluate trends in such use. Criteria for approval of nonformulary medications should be developed (e.g., allergy to or therapeutic failure of formulary alternative, condition not treatable by formulary medications).

Subformularies. Depending on state regulations, subformularies may be developed and maintained, using the same evidence-based process, to provide lists of appropriate and approved medications for furnishing by nonphysician providers or to specific patient subsets, such as Medicare patients. Health systems must follow specific rules and regulations provided under the U.S. Medicare Modernization Act of 2003 in their evaluation and inclusion of medications in a Medicare formulary for those medications to be covered.[39]

Strategies for Managing Medication Use

Common strategies for managing medication use via the formulary include use of generic drugs, therapeutic interchange, guided-use policies, clinical practice guidelines, and policies for off-label prescribing and the use of research pharmaceuticals. MUE is also important in managing medication use.

Generic Drugs. Optimizing the number of medication entities and products available from the pharmacy can produce substantial patient care and financial benefits. These benefits are greatly increased through the use of generic equivalents (drugs considered bioequivalent by FDA [i.e., AB-rated drug products[40]] and therapeutic equivalents (drug products differing in composition or in their basic drug entity that are considered to have very similar pharmacologic and therapeutic activities). The use of high-quality generic equivalents is encouraged in order to provide the best possible care at an affordable cost. Use of generic drugs that have been deemed bioequivalent by FDA does not require review or approval by the P&T committee, although a review of all new medications for key safety issues (e.g., look-alike, sound-alike concerns) should be conducted to prevent medication errors. For some drug categories, such as those with a narrow therapeutic range, a more thorough evaluation of the bioequivalency data and approval of experts or the P&T committee should be considered before implementing a generic substitution.

The P&T committee must establish policies and procedures governing the dispensing of generic equivalents. These policies and procedures should include the following points:

- The pharmacist is responsible for selecting from available generic equivalents those drugs to be dispensed pursuant to a prescriber's order for a particular medication.

- The prescriber has the option, at the time of prescribing, to specify the brand or supplier of the drug to be dispensed for that particular medication order if considered clinically justified.
- The prescriber's decision should be based on pharmacologic or therapeutic considerations (or both) relative to that patient.

Therapeutic Interchange. Therapeutic interchange is the authorized exchange of therapeutic alternatives in accordance with previously established and approved written guidelines, policies, or protocols within a formulary system.[1] Therapeutic interchange provides pharmacists with the authorization to use a formulary therapeutic alternative in place of a nonformulary medication or a non-preferred formulary medication without having to contact the prescriber. Drugs appropriate for therapeutic interchange are drug products with different chemical structures that are expected to have similar therapeutic effects and safety profiles when administered to patients in therapeutically equivalent doses. The authorization of a therapeutic interchange and notification of the prescriber should occur according to the organization's policy. In some organizations, prescribers agree to the therapeutic interchange process as part of their overall agreement to follow the organization's policies when they are granted prescribing privileges. Other organizations require that the prescriber be notified each time a medication is interchanged. A process should be established for when the prescriber wishes to opt out of the interchange. Adequate educational initiatives should be undertaken to ensure that everyone affected (prescribers, patients, pharmacists, nurses, and other health care professionals) is notified of the therapeutic interchange. Guidelines on therapeutic interchange are available elsewhere.[41]

Guided-Use Strategies. Medications may be added to the formulary with additional processes in place to guide the use of the medications to improve therapeutic outcomes, prevent adverse events, or reduce costs. Examples of strategies to help guide the use of medications in addition to therapeutic interchange may include the following.

Established-use criteria. Patients must meet the established criteria before the medication is dispensed. A process should be developed to cover situations in which the patient does not meet the established criteria, but the medication is nevertheless determined to be medically necessary. This strategy may also be useful when medications are in short supply.

Restricting drug use to a service. A specific service must approve the use of the drug before dispensing. This strategy can be used when inappropriate use or severe adverse effects may occur, and it can also be employed for antimicrobial agents when inappropriate use or overuse can result in resistant organisms and pose a danger to the general patient population or the public.

Limiting use of the drug to specially trained individuals. This strategy may be appropriate when the drug is inherently dangerous and should only be used by individuals with specific training (e.g., restricting use of chemotherapy agents to oncologists).

Designating medications for use in specific areas. Such policies can be helpful when administration of a medication requires special equipment or staff with particular skills to use the medication safely (e.g., limiting neuromuscular blockers to operating rooms and critical care areas).

Approval of medical director (or designee) before drug use. This strategy is particularly appropriate when the P&T committee has reviewed a high-cost medication and determined that the drug has little or no role in the care of patients at that organization but a prescriber would like to use the medication on a nonformulary basis.

Clinical Practice Guidelines. The implementation of medication-use policy decisions is a complicated process that, when properly conducted, can decrease variability in practice and improve patient outcomes, including clinical and economic consequences of care. Many tools are used to reduce practice variability, reduce cost, and improve quality, including order sets, clinical pathways, treatment algorithms, and clinical practice guidelines. While active intervention tools, such as order sets, directly influence prescribing for individual patients, clinical practice guidelines influence prescriber behavior in a passive manner, primarily through education. Like the medication formulary, clinical practice guidelines should reflect current biomedical evidence, although they may also include expert opinion of prescribers within a practice seting. Clinical practice guidelines are developed and disseminated by national and international organizations, but they can also be developed locally. Not all guidelines are equally valuable, however. Policymakers should not assume that guidelines, even those endorsed by respected organizations, are necessarily evidence based and should carefully review guidelines to ensure that they are truly evidence driven and current. Regardless of the source of the synthesis of biomedical evidence that forms the framework for an individual guideline, a locally conducted consensus development process, incorporating local expertise, must be performed if a guideline is to be accepted and followed.

Whether the medication formulary is a reflection of existing clinical practice guidelines in a particular organization or vice versa, it is critical that the guidelines and formulary are consistent. If a specific medication is recommended by a clinical practice guideline, it should in the majority of cases be on the formulary. As formulary changes are made, agents may need to be removed from or replaced in existing guidelines. Guidelines should avoid recommending use of nonformulary medications, and they can be useful in discouraging nonformulary medication use and guiding the appropriate use of nonformulary products when necessary.

Guidelines are frequently developed to address complex or particularly expensive medication therapies. However, complicated specialty therapies that will affect the care of very few patients may not justify the time and resources necessary to develop and maintain a guideline. Guidelines may be medication specific or disease oriented and may overlap in their scope of coverage.

The development of a clinical practice guideline should begin with the synthesis of all available biomedical evidence addressing the guideline topic. In many cases, guidelines from other organizations, both national and local, can be used as a starting point for development. The national guideline clearinghouse sponsored by the Agency for Healthcare Research and Quality is a useful source of previously developed guidelines (www.guideline.gov). The subsequent consensus process, eliciting feedback and input from local stakeholders, is critical. Stakeholders may not reach unanimous agreement about all dimensions of the guideline, but their involvement in its development increases their awareness of it and may create a sense of investment in its goals. Process-of-care and outcomes data from the organization's MUE activities (or, in some organizations, from such sources as the electronic medical records and computerized prescriber-order-entry systems) can also be used to make informed decisions during the consensus process. After the consensus process is completed, the guideline should be reviewed and approved by the P&T committee.

The dissemination and implementation of guidelines in the practice environment must also be carefully executed. Unlike active intervention tools that directly influence behavior, guidelines change behavior only when they are accessed, read, accepted, and put into practice. Exhaustive communication about the availability of guidelines is necessary. The dissemination of guidelines in hardcopy format is common, but electronic distribution (often in the form of a library of guidelines available via the Internet) is more efficient. Given the dynamic nature of the biomedical evidence and the quickening pace of changes in practice, maintaining current practice guidelines is an important challenge. Every guideline should include a time frame for future review and revision. If resources are not available to properly update and revise an older guideline, the guideline should be retired and removed from circulation.

Off-Label Use. The use of a drug prescribed for an indication not specifically approved by FDA is often referred to as off-label use. Off-label use can include the use of pharmaceuticals outside of specified populations, for different diseases or stages of diseases, or by different routes of administration. Other types of off-label use involve changes to dosing or dosing schedules or in chronology or sequence of use.

Before considering off-label use, supporting safety and efficacy evidence must be carefully evaluated and a risk-benefit determination made, especially when alternatives with FDA-approved labeling are available for the intended off-label use.[42] When considering or reviewing off-label use, the P&T committee should use an evidence-based process. The approach to evaluating evidence and benefit developed by the U.S. Preventive Services Task Force is an example.[43,44]

The following principles should guide the off-label use of medications:

1. Off-label pharmaceutical prescribing should be based on published evidence, and patient safety should be the primary consideration.
2. When the off-label use of an agent is expected to occur frequently, the P&T committee should establish protocols guiding that use. The P&T committee should be considered the arbiter of off-label use and should rely on the scientific evidence to guide its decisions.
3. The ultimate responsibility for the safety and efficacy of off-label use resides with the prescriber, who should be familiar with the evidence before considering off-label use, be aware of local protocols for use of the agent, and, when necessary, consult with an appropriately knowledgeable pharmacist.
4. Proper assessment of evidence for off-label use should involve as comprehensive and balanced a review as possible. Selective use of studies to support a position is strongly discouraged and, in the event of a negative

outcome, may not withstand the rigor of a thorough peer review.

Research Pharmaceuticals (Investigational Drugs). An investigational drug is defined as a chemical or biological used in a clinical investigation and can include prescription and nonprescription drugs, nutritional supplements, and herbal preparations. Investigational drug study procedures must be consistent with all applicable laws and regulations. Efforts should be made to ensure that the prescribing and distribution of investigational drugs benefit from the safe medication management systems used for other medications. More information on the management of investigational drugs can be found in other ASHP guidelines.[45,46]

MUE Process. Although distinctions have historically been made among the terms *drug-use evaluation*, *drug-use review*, and *medication-use evaluation*, they all refer to the systematic evaluation of medication use employing standard, observational quality-improvement methods (e.g., traditional "plan–do–check–act" approach). MUE is a quality-improvement activity, but it can also be considered a formulary system management technique.

MUE methods have traditionally involved establishing evidence-based criteria for medication use and applying those criteria retrospectively to determine the degree to which a particular medication was used in discordance with established criteria. Interventions could then be used to improve prescribing based on those data. As electronic medical records have become increasingly important and more widely available, MUE activities have matured from simple paper-based medical record reviews to sophisticated analyses drawing on multiple sources of data regarding medication use. A more expansive approach to MUE has been described in which not only the use of individual medications but the entire process of care for disease states is examined.[47] The use of quasiexperimental research methods may provide more meaningful information for quality-improvement purposes (e.g., economic, clinical, and humanistic outcomes of greater relevance than arbitrarily set appropriateness criteria).

MUE can be simply informative (collecting data to guide decision-making) or be used to measure the effect of interventions, such as the addition of a new agent to the formulary or the implementation of a new medication-use policy. MUE activities can focus on any dimension of the medication-use process (from medication acquisition to patient monitoring) that presents an opportunity for improvement. While MUE often focuses on problem-prone, high-risk, or high-cost medications, MUE can be used to examine any aspect of medication use that is problematic to the institution conducting the evaluation.

A systematic plan to monitor, evaluate, and improve medication use should be established within the organization.[17] Such a plan is an accreditation requirement for many organizations (e.g., Joint Commission[26]). MUE should be a part of the organization's overall quality-improvement program. MUE activities should be conducted to examine the effect of medication-use policy decisions (particularly those made in the absence of convincing evidence from the biomedical literature) but can also be conducted to inform decision-making (again, particularly when making policy decisions under conditions of uncertainty). Specific projects to evaluate medication use can either involve assessing how an individual medication is used or evaluate medication management of a given disease state. All steps of the medication-use process should be evaluated over time. The P&T committee, or its equivalent, should be involved in the MUE process.

Concurrent evaluation (collecting data during care delivery and sometimes as a component of the care process) is usually preferred over retrospective methods because it allows organizations to select relevant outcomes for collection rather than rely on out-comes routinely documented in patient medical records. For example, quality-of-life measures remain an infrequently documented measure in medical records. Only through concurrent evaluation can that outcome measure be reliably captured. Medications recently added to the formulary should be evaluated, especially if there is the potential for inappropriate use or adverse effects of concern. This review should occur 6–12 months after their addition to the formulary. High-cost, high-use, and problem-prone medications are also good candidates for evaluation.

Incorporating Patient Safety Issues in the Decision-Making Process

P&T committees have always addressed medication safety issues. However, as medication errors have received increased scrutiny and more is understood about the process failures that contribute to such errors, P&T committees have more opportunities to address patient safety issues. The P&T committee should systematically address patient safety as part of its deliberations. Opportunities for including patient safety in P&T committee deliberations include the following:

1. When evaluating a medication for inclusion on the formulary, the P&T committee should consider adverse effects, issues in preparation, sound-alike or look-alike potential, and dosing or administration issues. Assessments should be conducted to identify potential safety concerns posed by use of the medication. The P&T committee should make recommendations for managing identified risks.
2. Organizations, in collaboration with the appropriate committees, should undertake projects to proactively assess risk in medication-use processes. The use of high-risk medications or major system changes (e.g., a new computer system, new equipment) offer opportunities to perform proactive risk assessments. Failure mode and effects analysis (FMEA) can be used to structure these assessments. The Joint Commission, Institute for Healthcare Improvement, and National Center on Patient Safety provide information about conducting and examples of FMEA projects on their websites (www.jointcommission.org/, www.ihi.org/, and www.patientsafety.gov).
3. The P&T committee should consistently review medication-event data, including data on near misses, and make recommendations to prevent future events.
4. The P&T committee should conduct targeted quality-improvement projects to improve the safety of specific medications or to evaluate the processes involved.
5. When reviewing policies, the P&T committee should ensure that the policies adequately address the potential risk issues.

6. The P&T committee should champion evidence-based fail-safe techniques (e.g., bar-coding) to prevent medication events.

7. The P&T committee should review information available on patient safety or events reported by other organizations to identify ways to prevent medication events and disseminate the information to health care providers and, when appropriate, patients.

Resources on medication safety should be routinely reviewed to identify potential issues an organization could address. Examples of resources include the Institute for Safe Medication Practices (www.ismp.org), Medwatch (www.fda.gov/medwatch), FDA Patient Safety News (www.accessdata.fda.gov/scripts/cdrh/cfdocs/psn/), and the U.S. Pharmacopeia Patient Safety Program (www.usp.org/hqi/patientSafety/).

Drug Product Shortages

Health systems frequently need to address drug product shortages. Drug product shortages disrupt patient care and the processing of medication orders, increasing the risks presented by all aspects of the medication-use system, including purchasing, storage, pharmacy computer and automation systems, ordering, preparation, administration, and monitoring.

During a drug product shortage, the P&T committee plays an important role in setting organizational priorities. The P&T committee needs to develop strategies to address shortages in a timely manner, including designating appropriate alternatives, identifying strategies for rationing available drug product, establishing use restrictions, and implementing evidence-based review procedures. Therapeutic interchange can be useful in dealing with critical drug product shortages. When necessary, the P&T committee should work collaboratively with other committees and departments, such as risk management or specific medical departments affected by the shortage, to develop effective management plans for addressing shortages. Many organizations include a drug shortage update as a regular agenda item for the P&T committee. Communication with patients and staff is crucial to effectively manage shortages.

More information about managing drug product shortages can be found in the ASHP Guidelines on Managing Drug Product Shortages.[48]

Implementing Medication-Use Policies

Various tools can be used to implement medication-use policies. The policy should be integrated directly into the therapeutic decision-making processes that guide the use of a medication as the health care professional orders it or incorporated into a preprinted order form. Other specific ways of communicating information about a medication-use policy may include the use of

- Inservice education,
- Grand rounds,
- Interactions between pharmacists and prescribers at the time of prescribing or dispensing,
- Staff meetings,
- e-mail,
- Newsletters,
- Mailings,
- Prescriber detailing, and
- Pharmacy or institutional websites.

Pilot or demonstration projects may be beneficial in illustrating the value of a new medication-use policy and may generate data that could justify a decision or help communicate why a specific policy is necessary.

Conclusion

A formulary system is the multidisciplinary, evidence-based process employed by an organization to select and use medications that offer the best therapeutic outcomes while minimizing potential risks and costs for patients. Organizations employ the MUE process to continually improve how medications are used within the organization at all steps in the medication-use process. Medication use is an inherently complex and dangerous process that requires constant evaluation. Organizations need to implement tools and processes necessary to meet the goals of using medications effectively and safely. Professionals involved in the medication-use process need to know and understand how the organization's medication-use policies and processes can be incorporated into their daily work so that medications are used appropriately and safely. Technology offers many opportunities to make those processes more effective. Communicating the actions related to medication use is a constant challenge that organizations need to address.

References

1. Principles of a sound drug formulary system. In: Hawkins B, ed. Best practices for hospital and health-system pharmacy: positions and guidance documents of ASHP. Bethesda, MD: American Society of Health-System Pharmacists; 2006:110–3.

2. American Society of Consultant Pharmacists. ASCP statement on medication formulary principles for older adults. www.ascp.com/resources/policy/upload/Sta01-Formulary%20Older%20Adults.pdf (accessed 2008 Mar 27).

3. American Society of Consultant Pharmacists. ASCP statement on formularies in nursing facilities. www.ascp.com/resources/policy/upload/Sta96-Formularies.pdf (accessed 2008 Mar 27).

4. Laing R, Tisocki K. How to develop a national formulary based on the WHO model formulary. http://whqlibdoc.who.int/hq/2004/WHO_EDM_PAR_2004.8.pdf (accessed 2008 Apr 24).

5. American Medical Association. Policy H-125.991: drug formularies and therapeutic interchange. www.ama-assn.org/apps/pf_new/pf_online?f_n=resultLink&doc=policyfiles/HnE/H-125.991.HTM (accessed 2008 Mar 27).

6. American Medical Association. Policy H-285.965: managed care cost containment involving prescription drugs. www.ama-assn.org/apps/pf_new/pf_online?f_n=resultLink&doc=policyfiles/HnE/H-285.965.HTM (accessed 2008 Mar 27).

7. Academy of Managed Care Pharmacy. AMCP format for formulary submissions, version 2.1. www.fmcpnet.org/cfr/waSys/f.cfc?method=getListFile&id=A2D0F502 (accessed 2008 Mar 27).

8. American Academy of Family Physicians. Patient-centered formularies. www.aafp.org/online/en/home/policy/policies/p/patientcenteredformularies.html (accessed Mar 27).

9. American Society of Hospital Pharmacists. Minimum standard for pharmacies in hospitals. *Am J Hosp Pharm.* 1958; 15:992–4.

10. May JR. Formulary systems. In: DiPiro JT, ed. Encyclopedia of clinical pharmacy. New York: Marcel Dekker; 2002.

11. Willcox AM. The legal basis of the formulary system. *Am J Hosp Pharm.* 1960; 17:603–8.

12. American Society of Hospital Pharmacists, American Hospital Association. Statement of guiding principles on the operation of hospital formularies. *Am J Hosp Pharm.* 1960; 17:609–10.

13. American Society of Hospital Pharmacists, American Hospital Association, American Pharmaceutical Association et al. Statement of guiding principles on the operation of hospital formularies. *Am J Hosp Pharm.* 1964; 21:40–1.

14. Social Security Administration. Conditions of participation for hospitals. *Am J Hosp Pharm.* 1966; 23:179–80.

15. Lammy PP, Flack HL. Pharmacy and therapeutics committee, consent, and the hospital formulary. *Am J Hosp Pharm.* 1966; 23:662–72.

16. American Medical Association. AMA policy on drug formularies and therapeutic interchange in inpatient and ambulatory patient care settings. *Am J Hosp Pharm.* 1994; 51:1808–10.

17. American Society of Health-System Pharmacists. ASHP guidelines on medication-use evaluation. *Am J Health-Syst Pharm.* 1996; 53:1953–5.

18. American Society of Health-System Pharmacists. ASHP guidelines on adverse drug reaction monitoring and reporting. *Am J Health-Syst Pharm.* 1995; 52:417–9.

19. American Society of Hospital Pharmacists. ASHP guidelines on preventing medication errors in hospitals. *Am J Hosp Pharm.* 1993; 50:305–14.

20. American Society of Health-System Pharmacists. ASHP guidelines on the pharmacist's role in the development, implementation, and assessment of critical pathways. *Am J Health-Syst Pharm.* 2004; 61:939–45.

21. Nair KV, Ascione FJ. Evaluation of P&T committee performance: an exploratory study. *Formulary.* 2001; 36:136–46.

22. Brennan TA, Rothman DJ, Blank L et al. Health industry practices that create conflicts of interest: a policy proposal for academic medical centers. *JAMA.* 2006; 295:429–33.

23. American Society of Hospital Pharmacists. ASHP guidelines on pharmacists' relationships with industry. *Am J Hosp Pharm.* 1992; 49:154.

24. Nakahiro S. Contemporary issues in formulary management. In: Millares M, ed. Applied drug information: strategies for information management. Vancouver: Applied Therapeutics Inc.; 1998:8.1–8.43.

25. Nakahiro RK, Ho SS, Okamoto MP. Concepts of pharmacoeconomics. In: Millares M, ed. Applied drug information: strategies for information management. Vancouver: Applied Therapeutics Inc.; 1998:7.1–7.37.

26. Comprehensive accreditation manual for accreditation of hospitals. Joint Commission on Accreditation of Healthcare Organizations. Oakbrook Terrace, IL; 2006.

27. ASHP guidelines for selecting pharmaceutical manufacturers and suppliers. *Am J Hosp Pharm.* 1991; 48:523–4.

28. Briss PA, Zaza S, Pappaioanou M et al. Developing an evidence-based guide to community preventive services—methods. *Am J Prev Med.* 2000; 18(suppl 1):35–43.

29. Atkins D, Best D, Briss PA et al. Grading quality of evidence and strength of recommendations. *BMJ.* 2004; 328:1490–8.

30. Guyatt G, Gutterman D, Baumann MH et al. Grading strength of evidence of recommendations and quality of evidence in clinical guidelines: report from an American College of Chest Physicians task force. *Chest.* 2006; 129:174–81.

31. Harbour R, Miller J. A new system for grading recommendations in evidence based guidelines. *BMJ.* 2001; 323:334–6.

32. Corman SL, Skledar SJ, Culley CM. Evaluation of conflicting literature and application to formulary decisions. *Am J Health-Syst Pharm.* 2007; 64:182–5.

33. Sterné SC, Uchida KM, Iteen SA. Improving the presentation of drug information to pharmacy and therapeutics committees for formulary decisions. *Am J Health-Syst Pharm.* 1996; 53:1162–4.

34. Reeder CE. Overview of pharmacoeconomics and pharmaceutical outcomes evaluations. *Am J Health-Syst Pharm.* 1995; 52(19, suppl 4):S5–8.

35. Drummond MF, Sculpher MJ, Torrance GW et al. Methods for the economic evaluation of health care programmes. 3rd ed. Oxford, England: Oxford Univ. Press; 2005:137–89.

36. Gold MR, Siegel JE, Russell LB et al., eds. Cost-effectiveness in health and medicine. New York: Oxford Univ. Press; 1996:176–213.

37. Sanchez LA. Applied pharmacoeconomics: evaluation and use of pharmacoeconomic data from the literature. *Am J Health-Syst Pharm.* 1999; 56:1630–8.

38. Ofman JJ, Sullivan SD, Neumann PJ et al. Examining the value and quality of health economic analyses: implications of utilizing the QHES. *J Manag Care Pharm.* 2003; 9:53–61.

39. U.S. Medicare Prescription Drug, Improvement, and Modernization Act of 2003. Pub. L. No. 108–173.

40. Food and Drug Administration. Electronic orange book: approved drug products with therapeutic equivalence evaluations. www.fda.gov/cder/ob/ (accessed 2008 Mar 27).

41. Gray T, Bertch K, Galt K et al. Guidelines for therapeutic interchange—2004. *Pharmacotherapy.* 2005; 25:1666–80.

42. American Society of Hospital Pharmacists. ASHP statement on the use of medications for unlabeled uses. *Am J Hosp Pharm.* 1992; 49:2006–8.

43. U.S. Preventive Services Task Force. Strength of recommendations rating guide. www.ahrq.gov/clinic/3rduspstf/ratings.htm (accessed 2008 Mar 27).

44. U.S. Preventive Services Task Force. Current methods of the U.S. Preventive Services Task Force: a review of the process.www.ahrq.gov/clinic/ajpmsuppl/harris2.htm#assessing (accessed 2008 Mar 27).

45. American Society of Hospital Pharmacists. ASHP guidelines for pharmaceutical research in organized health-care settings. *Am J Hosp Pharm.* 1989; 46:129–30.

46. American Society of Health-System Pharmacists. ASHP guidelines on clinical drug research. *Am J Health-Syst Pharm.* 1998; 55:369–76.

47. Vermeulen LC, Beis SJ, Cano SB. Applying outcomes research in improving the medication-use process. *Am J Health-Syst Pharm.* 2000; 57:2277–82.

48. American Society of Health-System Pharmacists. ASHP guidelines on managing drug product shortages. *Am J Health-Syst Pharm.* 2001; 58:1445–50.

Appendix—Glossary of Terms

Formulary: A continually updated list of medications and related information, representing the clinical judgment of physicians, pharmacists, and other experts in the diagnosis, prophylaxis, or treatment of disease and promotion of health.

Formulary System: An ongoing process whereby a health care organization, through its physicians, pharmacists, and other health care professionals, establishes policies on the use of drug products and therapies and identifies drug products and therapies that are the most medically appropriate and cost-effective to best serve the health interests of a given patient population.[1]

Generic Substitution: The substitution of drug products that contain the same active ingredient or ingredients and are chemically identical in strength, concentration, dosage form, and route of administration to the drug product prescribed.[1]

Medication: Any prescription medications, herbal remedies, vitamins, nutraceuticals, nonprescription drugs, vaccines, or diagnostic and contrast agents used to diagnose, treat, or prevent disease and other abnormal conditions and radioactive medications, respiratory therapy treatments, parenteral nutrition, blood derivatives, intravenous solutions (plain or with electrolytes or drugs), or any product designated by the Food and Drug Administration as a drug (including investigational drugs).[26]

Medication-Use Evaluation: A performance-improvement method that focuses on evaluating and improving medication-use processes with the goal of optimal patient outcomes.[17]

Pharmacy and Therapeutics (P&T) Committee: An advisory committee that is responsible for developing, managing, updating, and administering a formulary system.[1]

Therapeutic Alternatives: Drug products with different chemical structures but of the same pharmacologic or therapeutic class and usually have similar therapeutic effects and adverse-reaction profiles when administered to patients in therapeutically equivalent doses.[1]

Therapeutic Interchange: Authorized exchange of therapeutic alternatives in accordance with previously established and approved written guidelines or protocols within a formulary system.[1,41]

Therapeutic Substitution: The act of dispensing a therapeutic alternative for the drug product prescribed without prior authorization of the prescriber. This is an illegal act because only the prescriber may authorize an exchange of therapeutic alternatives.[1]

Approved by the ASHP Board of Directors on January 28, 2008. These guidelines supersede the ASHP Guidelines on Formulary System Management dated November 20, 1991, the ASHP Technical Assistance Bulletin on Drug Formularies dated November 14, 1990, and the ASHP Technical Assistance Bulletin on the Evaluation of Drugs for Formularies dated November 19, 1987. Developed through the ASHP Council on Pharmacy Practice.

ASHP gratefully acknowledges the expert panel that developed these guidelines: Linda S. Tyler, Pharm.D., FASHP; Mirta Millares, Pharm.D., FCSHP, FASHP; Andrew L. Wilson, Pharm.D., FASHP; Lee C. Vermeulen, Jr., B.S.Pharm., M.S.; J. Russell (Rusty) May, Pharm.D., FASHP; Michael A. Valentino, R.Ph. MHSA; and Sabrina W. Cole, Pharm.D.

The bibliographic citation for this document is as follows: American Society of Health-System Pharmacists. ASHP guidelines on the pharmacy and therapeutics committee and the formulary system. *Am J Health-Syst Pharm.* 2008; 65:1272–83.

Principles of a Sound Drug Formulary System

These principles have been endorsed by the following organizations:

- Academy of Managed Care Pharmacy
- Alliance of Community Health Plans
- American Medical Association
- American Society of Health-System Pharmacists
- Department of Veterans Affairs, Pharmacy Benefits Management Strategic Healthcare Group
- National Business Coalition on Health
- U.S. Pharmacopeia

Preamble

A coalition of national organizations representing health care professionals, government, and business leaders formed a working group (see Appendix III) to develop a set of principles specifying the essential components that contribute to a sound drug formulary system. The Coalition was formed in September 1999 in response to the widespread use of drug formularies in both inpatient and outpatient settings and the lack of understanding about formularies among the public. Also, proposed federal legislation that would provide a prescription drug benefit for Medicare beneficiaries has brought increased attention to the appropriate role and management of drug formulary systems within drug benefit programs.

The formulary system, when properly designed and implemented, can promote rational, clinically appropriate, safe, and cost-effective drug therapy. The Coalition has enumerated these principles, however, because it recognizes that patient care may be compromised if a formulary system is not optimally developed, organized, and administered. This document contains "Guiding Principles" that the Coalition believes must be present for a drug formulary system to appropriately serve the patients it covers. The absence of one or more of these "Guiding Principles" should be cause for careful scrutiny of a formulary system. A glossary (see Appendix I) and bibliography (see Appendix II) are included with the "Guiding Principles" to clarify terminology and to provide additional resources, respectively.

The Coalition believes that the presence of consensus-based Formulary System Principles can assist decision-makers who must balance the health care quality and cost equation. Further, the Guiding Principles will be a valuable educational tool for national, state, and local public policy makers, health care system administrators, purchasers and third-party payers, practitioners, and consumers and patient advocates. These parties all have an interest in designing formulary systems that ensure patients have access to rational, clinically appropriate, safe, and cost-effective therapy and which supports an affordable and sustainable drug benefit program.

Definitions

Drug Formulary System. An ongoing process whereby a health care organization, through its physicians, pharmacists, and other health care professionals, establishes policies on the use of drug products and therapies, and identifies drug products and therapies that are the most medically appropriate and cost-effective to best serve the health interests of a given patient population.

Drug Formulary. A continually updated list of medications and related information, representing the clinical judgement of physicians, pharmacists, and other experts in the diagnosis and/or treatment of disease and promotion of health.

Guiding Principles

Formulary system decisions are based on scientific and economic considerations that achieve appropriate, safe, and cost-effective drug therapy.

- Clinical decisions are based on the strength of scientific evidence and standards of practice that include, but are not limited, to the following:
 - Assessing peer-reviewed medical literature, including randomized clinical trials (especially drug comparison studies), pharmacoeconomic studies, and outcomes research data.
 - Employing published practice guidelines, developed by an acceptable evidence-based process.
 - Comparing the efficacy as well as the type and frequency of side effects and potential drug interactions among alternative drug products.
 - Assessing the likely impact of a drug product on patient compliance when compared to alternative products.
 - Basing formulary system decisions on a thorough evaluation of the benefits, risks, and potential outcomes for patients; risks encompass adverse drug events (adverse drug reactions and medication errors, such as those caused by confusing product names or labels).
- Economic considerations include, but are not limited, to the following:
 - Basing formulary system decisions on cost factors only after the safety, efficacy, and therapeutic need have been established.
 - Evaluating drug products and therapies in terms of their impact on total health care costs.
 - Permitting financial incentives only when they promote cost management as part of the delivery of quality medical care. Financial incentives or pressures on practitioners that may interfere with the delivery of medically necessary care are unacceptable.

The formulary system encompasses drug selection, drug utilization review, and other tools to foster best practices in prescribing, dispensing, administration, and monitoring of outcomes.

- The formulary system:
 - Provides drug product selection and formulary maintenance (see above).
 - Provides drug use evaluation (also called drug utilization review) to enhance quality of care for patients by assuring appropriate drug therapy.

- Provides for the periodic evaluation and analysis of treatment protocols and procedures to ensure that they are up-to-date and are consistent with optimum therapeutics.
- Provides for the monitoring, reporting, and analysis of adverse results of drug therapy (e.g., adverse drug reactions, medication errors) to continuously improve the quality of care.

The Pharmacy and Therapeutics (P&T) Committee, or equivalent body, comprised of actively practicing physicians, pharmacists, and other health care professionals, is the mechanism for administering the formulary system, which includes developing and maintaining the formulary and establishing and implementing policies on the use of drug products.

- The Pharmacy and Therapeutics Committee:
 - Objectively appraises, evaluates, and selects drugs for the formulary.
 - Meets as frequently as is necessary to review and update the appropriateness of the formulary system in light of new drugs and new indications, uses, or warnings affecting existing drugs.
 - Establishes policies and procedures to educate and inform health care providers about drug products, usage, and committee decisions.
 - Oversees quality improvement programs that employ drug use evaluation.
 - Implements generic substitution and therapeutic interchange programs that authorize exchange of therapeutic alternatives based upon written guidelines or protocols within a formulary system. (Note: Therapeutic substitution, the dispensing of therapeutic alternates without the prescriber's approval, is illegal and should not be allowed—see Glossary.)
 - Develops protocols and procedures for the use of and access to non-formulary drug products.

Physicians, pharmacists, and other health care professionals provide oversight of the formulary system.

- Health care organization policies should ensure appropriate oversight of the P&T Committee and its decisions by the medical staff or equivalent body.

The formulary system must have its own policies, or adhere to other organizational policies, that address conflicts of interest and disclosure by P&T committee members.

- Formulary system policies should:
 - Require P&T committee members to reveal, by signing a conflict of interest statement, economic and other relationships with pharmaceutical entities that could influence Committee decisions.
 - Exclude product sponsor representatives from P&T committee membership and from attending P&T committee meetings.
 - Require P&T committee members to adhere to the formulary system's policy on disclosure and participation in discussion as it relates to conflict of interest.

The formulary system should include educational programs for payers, practitioners, and patients concerning their roles and responsibilities.

- The formulary system should:
 - Inform physicians, pharmacists, other health care professionals, patients, and payers about the factors that affect formulary system decisions, including cost containment measures; the procedures for obtaining non-formulary drugs; and the importance of formulary compliance to improving quality of care and restraining health care costs.
 - Proactively inform practitioners about changes to the formulary or to other pharmaceutical management procedures.
 - Provide patient education programs that explain how formulary decisions are made and the roles and responsibilities of the patient, especially the importance of patient compliance with drug therapy to assure the success of that therapy.
 - Disclose the existence of formularies and have copies of the formulary readily available and accessible.
 - Provide rationale for specific formulary decisions when requested.

The formulary system should include a well-defined process for the physician or other prescriber to use a non-formulary drug when medically indicated.

- The formulary system should:
 - Enable individual patient needs to be met with non-formulary drug products when demonstrated to be clinically justified by the physician or other prescriber.
 - Institute an efficient process for the timely procurement of non-formulary drug products and impose minimal administrative burdens.
 - Provide access to a formal appeal process if a request for a non-formulary drug is denied.
 - Include policies that state that practitioners should not be penalized for prescribing non-formulary drug products that are medically necessary.

Appendix I—Glossary

Drug Formulary System: An ongoing process whereby a health care organization, through its physicians, pharmacists, and other health care professionals, establishes policies on the use of drug products and therapies, and identifies drug products and therapies that are the most medically appropriate and cost effective to best serve the health interests of a given patient population.

Drug Formulary: A continually updated list of medications and related information, representing the clinical judgement of physicians, pharmacists, and other experts in the diagnosis and/or treatment of disease and promotion of health.

Pharmacy & Therapeutics (P&T) Committee: An advisory committee that is responsible for developing, managing, updating, and administering the drug formulary system.

Generic Substitution: The substitution of drug products that contain the same active ingredient(s) and are chemically identical in strength, concentration, dosage form, and route of administration to the drug product prescribed.

Therapeutic Alternates: Drug products with different chemical structures but which are of the same

pharmacological and/or therapeutic class, and usually can be expected to have similar therapeutic effects and adverse reaction profiles when administered to patients in therapeutically equivalent doses.

Therapeutic Interchange: Authorized exchange of therapeutic alternates in accordance with previously established and approved written guidelines or protocols within a formulary system.

Therapeutic Substitution: The act of dispensing a therapeutic alternate for the drug product prescribed without prior authorization of the prescriber. This is an illegal act because only the prescriber may authorize an exchange of therapeutic alternates.

Drug Utilization Review (Drug Use Review, DUR, and Drug Use Evaluation): Process used to assess the appropriateness of drug therapy by engaging in the evaluation of data on drug use in a given health care environment against predetermined criteria and standards.

Appendix II—Bibliography

1. Academy of Managed Care Pharmacy, Concepts in Managed Care Pharmacy Series—Formulary Management (Alexandria, VA: 1998).

2. American Medical Association. Board of Trustees Report PPP, Principles of Drug Utilization Review. In, American Medical Association House of Delegates Proceedings, 140th Annual Meeting. Chicago: American Medical Association; June 1991; 225–7.

3. American Medical Association. Board of Trustees Report 45, Drug Formularies and Therapeutic Interchange. In, American Medical Association House of Delegates Proceedings, 47th Interim Meeting. New Orleans: American Medical Association; December 1993; 155–8.

4. American Medical Association. Council on Ethical and Judicial Affairs Report 2, Managed Care Cost Containment Involving Prescription Drugs. In, American Medical Association House of Delegates Proceedings, 144th Annual Meeting. Chicago: American Medical Association; June 1995; 207–13.

5. American Medical Association. Board of Trustees Report 9, Pharmaceutical Benefits Management Companies. In, American Medical Association House of Delegates Proceedings, 51st Interim Meeting. Dallas: American Medical Association; December 1997; 33–44.

6. American Society of Consultant Pharmacists. Guidelines for the Development of Formulary Systems in Nursing Facilities; July 1996.

7. American Society of Hospital Pharmacists. ASHP Statement on the Formulary System. *Am J Hosp Pharm.* 1983; 40:1384–5.

8. American Society of Hospital Pharmacists. ASHP Guidelines on Formulary System Management. *Am J Hosp Pharm.* 1992; 49:648–52.

9. American Society of Hospital Pharmacists. ASHP Statement on the Pharmacy and Therapeutics Committee. *Am J Hosp Pharm.* 1992; 49:2008–9.

10. American Society of Health-System Pharmacists. ASHP Guidelines on Medication-Use Evaluation. *Am J Health-syst Pharm.* 1996; 53:1953–5.

11. American Society of Hospital Pharmacists. ASHP Technical Assistance Bulletin on Drug Formularies. *Am J Hosp Pharm.* 1991; 48:791–3.

12. American Society of Hospital Pharmacists. ASHP Technical Assistance Bulletin on the Evaluation of Drugs for Formularies. *Am J Hosp Pharm.* 1988; 45:386–7.

13. Covington TR and Thornton JL. The formulary system: A cornerstone of drug benefit management, in A Pharmacist's Guide to Principles and Practices of Managed Care Pharmacy. Ito S and Blackburn S, eds. Foundation for Managed Care Pharmacy, Alexandria VA. 1995:35–49.

14. Dillon MJ. Drug Formulary Management, in Managed Care Pharmacy Practice. Navarro RP ed. Aspen Publishers, Inc., Gaithersburg, MD. 1999:145–65.

15. Hejna CS and Shepherd MD. Pharmacy and therapeutics committee and formulary development, in A Pharmacist's Guide to Principles and Practices of Managed Care Pharmacy. Ito S and Blackburn S, eds. Foundation for Managed Care Pharmacy, Alexandria VA. 1995:27–34.

16. National Committee for Quality Assurance. UM 10 procedures for pharmaceutical management. 2000 Standards for Accreditation of MCOs. 1999:58–60.

17. National Committee for Quality Assurance. UM 10 procedures for pharmaceutical management. 2000 Surveyor Guidelines for the Accreditation of MCOs. 1999:173–82.

18. PCMA Response to American Medical Association Report, I-97, "Pharmaceutical Benefits Management Companies." September 1998.

19. Rucker TD and Schiff GD. Drug formularies: myths-information. *Medical Care.* 1990; 28:928–42. Reprinted in *Hospital Pharmacy,* 1991; 26:507–14.

Appendix III—Coalition Working Group

Public Comment Requested

To ensure that knowledgeable and interested parties beyond the Coalition Working Group had an opportunity to contribute to the Principles development process, a preliminary set of principles was distributed for public comment to 50-plus organizations in February 2000. Comments received were thoroughly reviewed and considered by the Coalition Working Group.

These principles were endorsed by the ASHP Board of Directors on June 4, 2000.

The endorsement of this document was reviewed in 2011 by the Council on Pharmacy Practice and by the Board of Directors and was found to still be appropriate.

Government, Law, and Regulation

Government, Law, and Regulation

Pharmacy Technicians (1216)

Source: Council on Public Policy

To advocate that pharmacy move toward the following model with respect to the evolving pharmacy technician workforce as the optimal approach to protecting public health and safety: (1) development and adoption of uniform state laws and regulations regarding pharmacy technicians, (2) mandatory completion of an ASHP-accredited program of education and training as a prerequisite to pharmacy technician certification, (3) mandatory certification by the Pharmacy Technician Certification Board as a prerequisite to licensure by the state board of pharmacy, and (4) licensure of pharmacy technicians by state boards of pharmacy granting the technician permission to engage in the full scope of responsibilities authorized by the state; further,

To advocate, with respect to certification, as an interim measure until the optimal model is fully implemented, that individuals be required either (1) to have completed an ASHP-accredited program of education and training or (2) to have at least one year of full-time equivalent experience as pharmacy technicians before they are eligible to become certified; further,

To advocate that all pharmacy functions be performed under the general supervision of a licensed pharmacist and that licensed pharmacists and technicians be held accountable for the quality of pharmacy services provided.

(*Note:* Licensure is the process by which an agency of government grants permission to an individual to engage in a given occupation upon finding that the applicant has attained the minimal degree of competency necessary to ensure that the public health, safety, and welfare will be reasonably well protected. Certification is the process by which a nongovernmental agency or association grants recognition to an individual who has met certain predetermined qualifications specified by that agency or association.)

This policy supersedes ASHP policy 0815.

Approval of Biosimilar Medications (1218)

Source: Council on Public Policy

To encourage the development of safe and effective biosimilar medications in order to make such medications more affordable and accessible; further,

To encourage research on the safety, effectiveness, and interchangeability of biosimilar medications; further,

To support legislation and regulation to allow Food and Drug Administration (FDA) approval of biosimilar medications; further,

To support legislation and regulation to allow FDA approval of biosimilar medications that are also determined by the FDA to be interchangeable and therefore may be substituted for the reference product without the intervention of the prescriber; further,

To require postmarketing surveillance for all biosimilar medications to ensure their continued safety, effectiveness, purity, quality, identity, and strength; further,

To advocate for adequate reimbursement for biosimilar medications that are deemed interchangeable; further,

To promote and develop ASHP-directed education of pharmacists about biosimilar medications and their appropriate use within hospitals and health systems; further,

To advocate and encourage pharmacist evaluation and the application of the formulary system before biosimilar medications are used in hospitals and health systems.

This policy supersedes ASHP policy 0906.

Stable Funding for HRSA Office of Pharmacy Affairs (1219)

Source: Council on Public Policy

To advocate for a sustainable level of funding, including appropriations, sufficient to support the public health mission of the Health Resources and Services Administration (HRSA) Office of Pharmacy Affairs; further,

To support initiatives of the Office of Pharmacy Affairs, including the 340B Drug Pricing Program and innovative pharmacy service models in HRSA-funded programs; further,

To encourage research on the potential impact of any proposed fees or alternative funding sources for the Office of Pharmacy Affairs.

This policy supersedes ASHP policy 0911.

Standardized Immunization Authority to Improve Public Health (1220)

Source: Council on Public Policy

To advocate that, to improve public health and patient access to immunizations, states grant pharmacists the authority to initiate and administer all adult and child immunizations through a universal protocol developed by state health authorities; further,

To advocate that only pharmacists who have completed a training and certification program acceptable to state boards of pharmacy and meeting the standards established by the Centers for Disease Control and Prevention may provide such immunizations; further,

To advocate that state health authorities establish a centralized database for documenting administration of immunizations that is accessible to all health care providers.

Globalization of Clinical Trials (1223)

Source: Council on Therapeutics

To encourage the Food and Drug Administration (FDA) to use its existing authority to increase monitoring and inspection of foreign clinical trials to ensure the integrity and quality of those studies; further,

To advocate that the FDA expand its oversight of clinical trials conducted abroad by continuing to pursue innovative strategies, such as increased collaboration with foreign regulatory agencies and changes in domestic regulatory processes that support timely submission of foreign clinical trial information; further,

To encourage the FDA to establish a standardized electronic format and reporting standards that would be required for submission of data from foreign clinical trials; further,

To support the ethical treatment of patients in foreign clinical trials in accordance with international standards designed to protect human subjects; further,

To encourage public and private research to study the impact of the globalization of clinical trials on patient care.

Medical Marijuana (1101)
Source: Council on Therapeutics

To oppose state legislation that authorizes the use of medical marijuana until there is sufficient evidence to support its safety and effectiveness and a standardized product that would be subject to the same regulations as a prescription drug product; further,

To encourage research to define the therapeutically active components, effectiveness, safety, and clinical use of medical marijuana; further,

To advocate for the development of processes that would ensure standardized formulations, potency, and quality of medical marijuana products to facilitate research; further,

To encourage the Drug Enforcement Administration to eliminate barriers to medical marijuana research, including review of medical marijuana's status as a Schedule I controlled substance, and its reclassification, if necessary to facilitate research; further,

To oppose the procurement, storage, preparation, or distribution of medical marijuana by licensed pharmacies or health care facilities for purposes other than research; further,

To oppose the smoking of marijuana in settings where smoking is prohibited; further,

To encourage continuing education that prepares pharmacists to respond to patient and clinician questions about the therapeutic and legal issues surrounding medical marijuana use.

(*Note:* As defined by the Congressional Research Service, the term *medical marijuana* refers to uses of botanical marijuana that qualify for a medical use exception under the laws of certain states and under the federal Investigational New Drug Compassionate Access Program. Botanical marijuana includes the whole or parts of the natural marijuana plant and therapeutic products derived therefrom, as opposed to drugs produced synthetically in the laboratory that replicate molecules found in the marijuana plant.)

Agricultural Use of Hormone and Prohormone Therapies (1102)
Source: Council on Therapeutics

To advocate that the Food and Drug Administration and United States Department of Agriculture re-evaluate the agricultural use of hormone and prohormone therapies for purposes of animal growth promotion based on evidence demonstrating potential adverse effects on human health; further,

To encourage additional research to better define the public health impact of using hormone therapies for agricultural purposes.

Direct-to-Consumer Clinical Genetic Tests (1103)
Source: Council on Therapeutics

To support research to validate and standardize genetic markers used in direct-to-consumer clinical genetic tests and guide the application of test results to clinical practice; further,

To encourage the Food and Drug Administration to use existing authority to regulate these tests as medical devices and to work with the National Institutes of Health to expedite establishment of a process to evaluate and approve direct-to-consumer clinical genetic tests; further,

To advocate that direct-to-consumer clinical genetic tests to support disease diagnosis or management of drug therapy be provided to consumers only through the services of appropriate health care professionals that order tests from laboratories that are certified under the Clinical Laboratories Improvement Amendments of 1988 (CLIA); further,

To oppose advertising of direct-to-consumer clinical genetic tests unless such testing includes the established patient-health care provider relationship as a mechanism to provide information and interpretation of test results; further,

To oppose advertising of direct-to-consumer clinical genetic tests unless the following requirements are met: (1) that the relationship between the genetic marker and the disease or condition being assessed is clearly presented, (2) that the benefits and risks of testing are discussed, and (3) that such advertising is provided in an understandable format, at a level of health literacy that allows the intended audience to make informed decisions, and includes a description of the established patient-health care provider relationship as a critical source for information about the test and interpretation of test results; further,

To encourage pharmacists to educate consumers and clinicians on the appropriate use of direct-to-consumer clinical genetic tests for disease diagnosis and drug therapy management.

Drug Product Shortages (1118)
Source: Council on Public Policy

To advocate that the Food and Drug Administration (FDA) have the authority to require manufacturers to report drug product shortages and the reason(s) for the shortage, and to make that information available to the public; further,

To strongly encourage the FDA to consider, in its definition of "medically necessary" drug products, the patient safety risks created by use of alternate drug products during a shortage; further,

To support government-sponsored incentives for manufacturers to maintain an adequate supply of medically necessary drug products; further,

To advocate laws and regulations that would (1) require pharmaceutical manufacturers to notify the appropriate government body at least 12 months in advance of voluntarily discontinuing a drug product, (2) provide effective sanctions for manufacturers that do not comply with this mandate, and (3) require prompt public disclosure of a notification to voluntarily discontinue a drug product; further,

To encourage the appropriate government body to seek the cooperation of manufacturers in maintaining the supply of a drug product after being informed of a voluntary decision to discontinue that product.

This policy supersedes ASHP policy 0319.

Poison Control Center Funding (1121)
Source: Council on Public Policy

To advocate that poison control centers be considered an essential emergency service; further,

To advocate for new and stable funding mechanisms for poison control centers to continue to provide these essential and valuable services; further,

To support the integration and coordination of poison control center services where appropriate.

State Prescription Drug Monitoring Programs (1122)
Source: Council on Public Policy
To advocate for uniform state prescription drug monitoring programs that collect standard information about controlled substances prescriptions; further,

To advocate that the design of these programs should balance the need for appropriate therapeutic management with safeguards against fraud, misuse, abuse, and diversion; further,

To advocate that such programs be structured as part of electronic health records and exchanges to allow prescribers, pharmacists, and other practitioners to proactively monitor data for appropriate assessment; further,

To advocate for interstate integration to allow for access by prescribers, pharmacists, and other practitioners across state lines; further,

To advocate for federal and state funding to establish and administer these programs.

Health Insurance Coverage for U.S. Residents (1001)
Source: Council on Public Policy
To advocate health insurance for all residents of the United States, including coverage of medications and related pharmacist patient-care services; further,

To advocate that the full range of available methods be used to (1) ensure the provision of appropriate, safe, and cost-effective health care services; (2) optimize treatment outcomes; and (3) minimize overall costs without compromising quality; further,

To advocate that health insurers seek to optimize continuity of care in their design of benefit plans.
This policy supersedes ASHP policy 0512.

Risk Evaluation and Mitigation Strategies (1002)
Source: Council on Public Policy
To advocate for research on the impact of the Food and Drug Administration's Risk Evaluation and Mitigation Strategies (REMS) on patient safety, cost effectiveness, and pharmacy workflow; further,

To advocate pharmacist involvement in the development and implementation of REMS; further,

To urge computer software vendors to assist pharmacists in the identification of and compliance with REMS; further,

To advocate that any REMS that include constraint on traditional drug distribution systems be consistent with ASHP policy on restricted drug distribution.

FDA Authority on Recalls (1003)
Source: Council on Public Policy
To strongly encourage the Food and Drug Administration (FDA) to develop a standard recall notification process and format to be used by all manufacturers to facilitate the timely removal of recalled drugs; further,

To advocate that such notification should (1) come from a single source, (2) clearly identify the recalled product, (3) explain why the product is being recalled, (4) provide a way to report having the recalled product, (5) give instructions on what to do with the recalled product, and (6) be provided concurrently to all entities in the supply chain; further,

To advocate that the FDA be given the authority to order mandatory recalls of medications; further,

To urge the FDA to require drug manufacturers and the computer software industry to provide bar codes and data fields for lot number, expiration date, and other necessary and appropriate information on all medication packaging, including unit dose, unit-of-use, and injectable drug packaging, in order to facilitate compliance with recalls or withdrawals and to prevent the administration of recalled products to patients; further,

To urge the FDA to encourage postmarketing reporting of adverse events and product quality issues to enhance the recall system.

Postmarketing Comparative Clinical and Pharmacoeconomic Studies (1004)
Source: Council on Public Policy
To advocate expansion of comparative clinical and pharmacoeconomic studies on the effectiveness, safety, and cost comparison of marketed medications in order to improve therapeutic outcomes and promote cost-effective medication use; further,

To advocate that such studies compare a particular medication with (as appropriate) other medications, medical devices, or procedures used to treat specific diseases; further,

To advocate adequate funding for the Agency for Healthcare Research and Quality and other federal agencies to carry out such studies; further,

To encourage impartial private-sector entities to also conduct such studies.
This policy supersedes ASHP policy 0513.

Regulation of Home Medical Equipment Medication Products and Devices (1007)
Source: Council on Public Policy
To advocate for consistent regulatory oversight of all home medical equipment, with the goals of continuity of care, patient safety, and appropriate pharmacist involvement whenever equipment is used for medication administration; further,

To monitor the impact of the Centers for Medicare & Medicaid Services quality standards on the accreditation of suppliers of medication-related durable medical equipment and supplies.

Preservation of Antimicrobials for Medical Treatment (1009)
Source: Council on Therapeutics
To advocate that the Food and Drug Administration (FDA) eliminate future approval of antimicrobials for nontherapeutic uses in agricultural animals that represent a safety risk by contributing to antibiotic resistance; further,

To encourage efforts to phase out and eliminate the nontherapeutic uses of antimicrobials previously approved by the FDA; further,

To support the therapeutic use of antimicrobials in animals only under the supervision of a veterinarian; further,

To encourage the FDA, Centers for Disease Control and Prevention, and other stakeholders to monitor and limit, when effective alternatives are available, the therapeutic use of antimicrobials that are essential to the treatment of critically ill human patients; further,

To advocate for the inclusion of pharmacists in antimicrobial surveillance and related public health efforts based on pharmacists' knowledge of antimicrobial drug products and antimicrobial resistance.

Use of Surrogate Endpoints for FDA Approval of Drug Uses (1011)

Source: Council on Therapeutics

To support the continued use of qualified surrogate endpoints by the Food and Drug Administration (FDA) as a mechanism to evaluate the effectiveness and safety of new drugs and new indications for existing therapies, when measurement of definitive clinical outcomes is not feasible; further,

To support efforts by the FDA and other stakeholders to qualify surrogate endpoints; further,

To advocate that the FDA consistently enforce existing requirements that drug product manufacturers complete postmarketing studies for drugs approved based on qualified surrogate endpoints in order to confirm that the expected improvement in outcomes occurs, and to require that these studies be completed in a timely manner.

Quality Consumer Medication Information (1012)

Source: Council on Therapeutics

To support efforts by the Food and Drug Administration (FDA) and other stakeholders to improve the quality, consistency, and simplicity of written consumer medication information (CMI); further,

To encourage the FDA to work in collaboration with patient advocates and other stakeholders to create evidence-based models and standards, including establishment of a universal literacy level, for CMI; further,

To advocate that research be conducted to validate these models in actual-use studies in pertinent patient populations; further,

To advocate that state boards of pharmacy require that pharmacies comply with FDA-established standards for content, format, and distribution of CMI.

Automatic Stop Orders (0904)

Source: Council on Pharmacy Practice

To advocate that the Centers for Medicare & Medicaid Services (1) revise the requirement in the Hospital Conditions of Participation that all medication orders automatically stop after an arbitrarily assigned period to include other options to protect patients from indefinite, open-ended medication orders, and (2) revise the remainder of the medication management regulations and interpretive guidelines to be consistent with this practice.

Pharmaceutical Product and Supply Chain Integrity (0907)

Source: Council on Public Policy

To encourage the Food and Drug Administration (FDA) and relevant state authorities to take the steps necessary to ensure that (1) all drug products entering the supply chain are thoroughly inspected and tested to establish that they have not been adulterated or misbranded and (2) patients will not receive improperly labeled and packaged, deteriorated, outdated, counterfeit, adulterated, or unapproved drug products; further,

To encourage FDA and relevant state authorities to develop and implement regulations to (1) restrict or prohibit licensed drug distributors (drug wholesalers, repackagers, and manufacturers) from purchasing legend drugs from unlicensed entities and (2) ensure accurate documentation at any point in the distribution chain of the original source of drug products and chain of custody from the manufacturer to the pharmacy; further,

To advocate the establishment of meaningful penalties for companies that violate current good manufacturing practices (cGMPs) intended to ensure the quality, identity, strength, and purity of their marketed drug product(s) and raw materials; further,

To urge Congress and state legislatures to provide adequate funding, or authority to impose user fees, to accomplish these objectives.

This policy supersedes ASHP policy 0722.

Regulation of Interstate Pharmacy Practice (0909)

Source: Council on Public Policy

To advocate that state governments, including legislatures and boards of pharmacy, adopt laws and regulations that harmonize the practice of pharmacy across state lines in order to provide a consistent, transparent, safe, and accountable framework for pharmacy practice.

Regulation of Dietary Supplements (0811)

Source: Council on Public Policy

To advocate that Congress grant authority to the Food and Drug Administration (FDA) to (1) require that dietary supplements undergo FDA approval for evidence of safety and efficacy; (2) mandate FDA-approved dietary supplement labeling that includes disclosure of excipients; (3) mandate FDA-approved patient information materials that describe safe use in a clear, standardized format, including the potential for interaction with medications and cautions for special populations; and (4) establish and maintain an adverse-event reporting system specifically for dietary supplements, and require dietary supplement manufacturers to report suspected adverse reactions to the FDA; further,

To oppose direct-to-consumer advertising of dietary supplements unless the following criteria are met: (1) federal laws are amended to include all the requirements described above to ensure that dietary supplements are safe and effective; (2) evidence-based information regarding safety and efficacy is provided in a format that allows for informed decision-making by the consumer; (3) the advertising includes a recommendation to consult with a health care professional before initiating use; (4) any known warnings or precautions regarding dietary supplement–medication interactions or dietary supplement-disease interactions are provided as part of the advertising; and (5) the advertising is educational in nature and includes pharmacists as a source of information.

(*Note: Dietary supplement* as used in this policy is defined by the Dietary Supplement Health and Education Act of 1994, as amended; 21 U.S.C. 321.)

This policy supersedes ASHP policy 0718.

Medicare Prescription Drug Benefit (0813)

Source: Council on Public Policy

To strongly advocate a fully funded prescription drug program for eligible Medicare beneficiaries that maintains continuity of care and ensures the best use of medications; further,

To advocate that essential requirements in the program include (1) appropriate product reimbursement; (2) affordability for patients, including elimination of coverage gaps; (3) payment for indirect costs and practice expenses related to the provision of pharmacist services, based on a study of those costs; (4) appropriate coverage and payment for pa-

tient care services provided by pharmacists; (5) open access to the pharmacy provider of the patient's choice; (6) formularies with sufficient flexibility to allow access to medically necessary drugs; and (7) well-publicized, unbiased resources to assist beneficiaries in enrolling in the most appropriate plan for their medication needs.

(*Note: Fully funded* means the federal government will make adequate funds available to fully cover the Medicare program's share of prescription drug program costs; *eligible means* the federal government may establish criteria by which Medicare beneficiaries qualify for the prescription drug program.)

This policy supersedes ASHP policy 0721.

Federal Review of Anticompetitive Practices by Drug Product Manufacturers (0814)
Source: Council on Public Policy
To strongly oppose anticompetitive practices by manufacturers that adversely affect drug product availability and price; further,

To encourage appropriate federal review of these practices.

This policy supersedes ASHP policy 0520.

Regulation of Telepharmacy Services (0716)
Source: Council on Public Policy
To advocate that boards of pharmacy adopt regulations that enable the use of United States-based telepharmacy services for all practice settings; further,

To advocate that boards of pharmacy consider the following when drafting regulations for telepharmacy services: (1) education and training of participating pharmacists and technicians; (2) information system requirements; (3) remote order entry, remote prospective order review, remote double-checking of the completed medication order before dispensing, actual dispensing, and patient counseling and education; (4) licensure (including reciprocity) of participating pharmacies and pharmacists; (5) service arrangements that cross state borders; (6) service arrangements within the same corporate entity or between different corporate entities; (7) service arrangements for workload relief in the point-of-care pharmacy during peak periods; and (8) pharmacist access to minimum required elements of patient information; further,

To acknowledge the need to explore and resolve additional legal and professional issues in the provision of international telepharmacy services from sites not located in the United States.

This policy was reviewed in 2011 by the Council on Public Policy and by the Board of Directors and was found to still be appropriate.

FDA Authority to Prohibit Reuse of Brand Names (0719)
Source: Council on Public Policy
To advocate for Food and Drug Administration authority to prohibit reuse of brand names of prescription and nonprescription drugs when any active component of the product is changed or after any other changes are made in the product that may affect its safe use.

This policy was reviewed in 2011 by the Council on Public Policy and by the Board of Directors and was found to still be appropriate.

Minimum Effective Doses (0602)
Source: Commission on Therapeutics
To advocate that the Food and Drug Administration require manufacturers to identify minimum effective doses for medications and make this information available to health care providers.

This policy was reviewed in 2010 by the Council on Therapeutics and by the Board of Directors and was found to still be appropriate.

Streamlined Licensure Reciprocity (0612)
Source: Council on Legal and Public Affairs
To advocate that state boards of pharmacy grant temporary licensure to pharmacists who are relocating from another state in which they hold a license in good standing, permitting them to engage in practice while their application for licensure reciprocity is being processed; further,

To advocate that the National Association of Boards of Pharmacy collaborate with state boards of pharmacy to streamline the licensure reciprocity process.

This policy was reviewed in 2010 by the Council on Public Policy and by the Board of Directors and was found to still be appropriate.

Accessibility and Affordability of Pharmaceuticals (0506)
Source: Council on Administrative Affairs
To advocate legislation or regulation that would expand eligibility for federal discount drug-pricing programs (e.g., the 340B program) to inpatient drugs for disproportionate-share hospitals; further,

To advocate administrative simplification of existing and any future federal discount drug-pricing programs with respect to qualification and implementation.

This policy was reviewed in 2009 by the Council on Pharmacy Practice and by the Board of Directors and was found to still be appropriate.

Premarketing Comparative Clinical Studies (0514)
Source: Council on Legal and Public Affairs
To advocate that the Food and Drug Administration (FDA) have the flexibility to decrease the requirement for placebo-controlled studies, and correspondingly impose a requirement for comparative clinical trials, as more new drug applications are filed for products in the same drug class.

This policy was reviewed in 2009 by the Council on Public Policy and by the Board of Directors and was found to still be appropriate.

Postmarketing Safety Studies (0515)
Source: Council on Legal and Public Affairs
To advocate that Congress grant the Food and Drug Administration (FDA) authority to require the manufacturer of an approved drug product or licensed biologic product to conduct postmarketing studies on the safety of the product when the agency deems it to be in the public interest; further,

To advocate that Congress grant FDA broader authority to require additional labeling or withdrawal of the product on the basis of a review of postmarketing studies; further,

To advocate that Congress provide adequate funding to FDA to fulfill this expanded mission related to postmarketing surveillance.

This policy was reviewed in 2009 by the Council on Public Policy and by the Board of Directors and was found to still be appropriate.

Mandatory Registry of Clinical Trials (0516)
Source: Council on Legal and Public Affairs
To advocate disclosure of the most complete information on the safety and efficacy of drug products; further,

To advocate that the Department of Health and Human Services establish a mandatory registry for all Phase II, III, and IV clinical trials that are conducted on drugs intended for use in the United States; further,

To advocate that each clinical trial have a unique identifier; further,

To advocate that all data from registered clinical trials be posted electronically with unrestricted access, and that such posting occur (1) after Food and Drug Administration approval of the related new product but before marketing begins and (2) as soon as possible for trials completed after initial marketing.

This policy was reviewed in 2009 by the Council on Public Policy and by the Board of Directors and was found to still be appropriate.

Funding, Expertise, and Oversight of State Boards of Pharmacy (0518)
Source: Council on Legal and Public Affairs
To advocate appropriate oversight of pharmacy practice (including nontraditional practice) and the pharmaceutical supply chain by state boards of pharmacy and other state agencies whose mission it is to protect the public health; further,

To advocate adequate representation on state boards of pharmacy and related agencies by pharmacists who are knowledgeable about hospitals and health systems to ensure appropriate oversight of hospital and health-system pharmacy practice; further,

To advocate adequate funding for state boards of pharmacy and related agencies to ensure the effective oversight and regulation of pharmacy practice and the pharmaceutical supply chain.

This policy was reviewed in 2009 by the Council on Public Policy and by the Board of Directors and was found to still be appropriate.

Compounding by Health Professionals (0411)
Source: Council on Legal and Public Affairs
To advocate the adoption, in all applicable state laws and regulations governing health care practice, of the intent of the requirements and the outcomes for patient safety as described in *United States Pharmacopeia* Chapter 797 ("Pharmaceutical Compounding—Sterile Preparations").

This policy was reviewed in 2008 by the Council on Public Policy and by the Board of Directors and was found to still be appropriate.

Importation of Pharmaceuticals (0413)
Source: Council on Legal and Public Affairs
To advocate for the continuation and application of laws and regulations enforced by the Food and Drug Administration and state boards of pharmacy with respect to the importation of pharmaceuticals in order to (1) maintain the integrity of the pharmaceutical supply chain and avoid the introduction of counterfeit products into the United States; (2) provide for continued patient access to pharmacist review of all medications and preserve the patient-pharmacist-prescriber relationship; and

(3) provide adequate patient counseling and education, particularly to patients taking multiple high-risk medications; further,

To urge the FDA and state boards of pharmacy to vigorously enforce federal and state laws in relation to importation of pharmaceuticals by individuals, distributors (including wholesalers), and pharmacies that bypass a safe and secure regulatory framework.

This policy was reviewed in 2008 by the Council on Public Policy and by the Board of Directors and was found to still be appropriate.

Intermediate Category of Drugs (0220)
Source: Council on Legal and Public Affairs
To support, with appropriate changes in federal statutes and regulations, the establishment of an intermediate category of drug products that do not require a prescription but are available only from pharmacists and licensed health care professionals who are authorized to prescribe medications; further,

To base such support on the following facts:

1. Some drug products that are potential candidates for switching from prescription-only to nonprescription status raise concerns about patient safety as nonprescription products; these products could be better controlled, monitored, and evaluated by making them available only from pharmacists and licensed health care professionals who are authorized to prescribe medications; and
2. Pharmacists have the education, training, and expertise to help patients make appropriate therapeutic decisions associated with the use of such drug products; further,

To support that the regulatory system for this intermediate category of drug products contain the following features:

1. Drug products appropriate for this intermediate category would be identified through the advice of pharmacists, physicians, and other licensed health professionals who are authorized to prescribe medications, on the basis of the medical conditions to be treated and potential adverse effects (as indicated in FDA-approved labeling);
2. Pharmacists would be able to provide drugs in this intermediate category directly to patients without a prescription, on the basis of appropriate assessment and professional consultation;
3. Licensed health professionals who currently have prescribing authority would continue to have the ability to prescribe medications in this intermediate category; and
4. Data from postmarketing surveillance, epidemiologic studies, and adverse-drug-reaction reporting would be collected to help determine a drug product's eventual movement to nonprescription status, return to prescription-only status, or continuation in the intermediate category.

This policy was reviewed in 2011 by the Council on Public Policy and by the Board of Directors and was found to still be appropriate.

Greater Access to Less Expensive Generic Drugs (0222)
Source: Council on Legal and Public Affairs
To support legislation and regulations that promote greater patient access to less expensive generic drug products.

This policy was reviewed in 2011 by the Council on Public Policy and by the Board of Directors and was found to still be appropriate.

FDA's Public Health Mission (0012)
Source: Council on Legal and Public Affairs
To support the Food and Drug Administration's public health mission of ensuring the safety and effectiveness of drugs, biologics, and medical devices through risk assessment, appropriate product approval, labeling approval, manufacturing oversight, and consultation with health professionals, while deferring to state regulation and professional self-regulation on matters related to the use of drugs, biologics, and medical devices; further,

To support the allocation of sufficient federal resources to allow FDA to meet its defined public health mission; further,

To support the appointment of practicing pharmacists to FDA advisory committees as one mechanism of ensuring that decisions made by the agency incorporate the unique knowledge of the profession of pharmacy for the further benefit of the patient; further,

To support an ongoing dialogue between FDA and ASHP for the purpose of exploring ways to advocate the best use of FDA-regulated products by consumers and health care professionals.

This policy was reviewed in 2009 by the Council on Public Policy and by the Board of Directors and was found to still be appropriate.

Generic Pharmaceutical Testing (9010)
Source: House of Delegates Resolution
To support and foster legislative and regulatory initiatives designed to improve and restore public and professional confidence in the drug approval and regulatory process in which all relevant data are subject to public scrutiny.

This policy was reviewed in 2010 by the Council on Public Policy and by the Board of Directors and was found to still be appropriate.

ASHP Statement on Criteria for an Intermediate Category of Drug Products

Position

The American Society of Health-System Pharmacists (ASHP) supports the establishment of an intermediate category of drug products that would not require a prescription but would be available from a pharmacist after appropriate patient assessment and professional consultation.[1] These drug products would continue to be available by prescription from licensed health care professionals who are authorized to prescribe medications. Drug products appropriate for this intermediate category should have proven public health benefits and be identified by processes that include the input and advice of experts, such as pharmacists, physicians, and other licensed health care professionals. Identification of drug products for inclusion in the intermediate category should be based on the medical condition to be treated and potential adverse effects of the drug. Concerns that patients may not be able to fulfill a substantial self-care role associated with these drug products will be alleviated by taking into consideration the benefits of pharmacist oversight of these drug regimens. Data from postmarketing surveillance, epidemiologic studies, and adverse-drug-reaction reports should be collected and analyzed to evaluate the ongoing safety and effectiveness of drug products placed in this category. This information would be used to determine whether the product would remain in the intermediate category, return to prescription-only status, or move to nonprescription status.

Background

Rationale for Establishing an Intermediate Drug Category. Reclassification of prescription drug products to nonprescription status (e.g., antifungal products used for the treatment of vaginitis, nonsedating antihistamines) has been associated with improvements in patient autonomy, health care knowledge, and self-care behavior.[2-4] However, proposals to reclassify some prescription drug products to nonprescription status have been denied because of concerns about safety and whether patients would be capable of determining if they were suitable candidates for treatment. In 2008, for example, the Food and Drug Administration (FDA) ruled a third time against making lovastatin, a hydroxymethylglutaryl-coenzyme A reductase inhibitor (or statin), available without a prescription,[5] although the predicted public health benefit of increasing the availability of statins was estimated to range between 23,000 and 33,000 coronary heart disease events prevented per 1 million treated for 10 years.[6] ASHP supports inclusion of statins in an intermediate category of drug products that provides the benefit of pharmacist oversight.[7] Other drug products that should be considered for the intermediate category include injectable epinephrine to treat anaphylaxis; inhaled corticosteroids, leukotriene modifiers, and inhaled ß-agonists used in the treatment of asthma; select therapies for osteoporosis and hypertension; and vaccines.

ASHP and other pharmacy organizations have long proposed the creation of an intermediate category of drug products that would bridge the large gap between prescription and nonprescription status.[1,8,9] An intermediate drug category could improve patient access to medications that offer substantial public health benefit but present challenges for safety or effectiveness if used under existing models for nonprescription drug dispensing. Two concerns regarding the use of existing models are that (1) a product's labeling information may be beyond most consumers' capacity to understand (or may be subject to misinterpretation) and (2) monitoring procedures are not readily accessible to patients. Pharmacists' expertise, licensure, and education, which includes instruction on physiology, pharmacology, disease management, and physical assessment, make pharmacists well qualified to help patients make appropriate therapeutic decisions about the use of these drug products.

The terms "behind-the-counter (BTC) drugs" and "pharmacist-only drugs" have also been used to describe the proposed intermediate category of drug products. While an FDA-established BTC category does not currently exist, the term BTC has been used to refer to drug products such as pseudoephedrine and levonorgestrel (marketed as Plan B) that are available for purchase only at the pharmacy counter.[10,11] Implementation of that restriction has largely been a policing action (e.g., to restrict the amount of drug a patient can obtain or to confirm the patient's age). In some instances, these functions are completed by pharmacy support staff under the supervision of a pharmacist. ASHP recommends the use of the terminology intermediate category of drugs to describe drug products appropriate for this category that would be used by patients in conjunction with clinical assessment and consultation provided by pharmacists. Distribution of the aforementioned nonprescription products via an intermediate category model of dispensing could improve appropriate use of those products.

The purpose of this statement is to describe the criteria that should be used to identify drug products for inclusion in an intermediate category. While the practice implications of an intermediate drug category are briefly described, that discussion is beyond the scope of this statement. Pharmacoeconomic analyses should be conducted to assess the overall impact and costs of an intermediate category of drug products on patients, health systems, and health insurers, and new models of reimbursement for pharmacists' services should be developed. It should be noted that a few studies have demonstrated that overall costs to the health system decrease when the cost of these medications is not transferred solely to the patient.[12,13] Alternative reimbursement models, such as insurance coverage for these products, would be necessary to optimize the use of the intermediate category of drug products.

Criteria for an Intermediate Category of Drug Products

Appropriate identification of drug products for inclusion in the intermediate category should address the concerns associated with a substantial self-care role for patients by

providing the benefits of pharmacist oversight of these drug therapy regimens (e.g., assessing for appropriate indications, contraindications, precautions, adverse drug events, drug interactions, and therapeutic response). ASHP believes drug products proposed for inclusion in the intermediate category should

- Meet many of the criteria currently used to reclassify prescription drugs to nonprescription status (e.g., the drug product has a well-established benefit:risk ratio and a wide safety margin),
- Have been marketed as a prescription product for a length of time and been used by a number of patients deemed sufficient by FDA to detect serious adverse effects. Likewise, a product could be marketed as a nonprescription product but would benefit from pharmacist oversight because safety and effectiveness concerns have arisen with its nonprescription use,
- Have evidence of effectiveness and safety for the dosage and regimen recommended for the formulation intended for intermediate classification, and
- Be used to prevent or treat a disease, symptom, or condition that can be readily detected by the patient or identified by the pharmacist or other health care provider.

Further, if the drug is used for a condition that requires laboratory or other medical monitoring, the pharmacy should be able to offer testing or have access to the results of that monitoring. Signs and symptoms of deterioration in health and the need for medical attention should be identifiable by the pharmacist or patient, as should signs demonstrating the effectiveness of the drug therapy. If the drug has the potential to rarely cause serious toxicity that can result in death or serious harm, there should be reliable early warning signs that can be readily detected and interpreted by the pharmacist or patient.

Antiinfective agents (systemic or other formulations) for which the emergence of resistance is a concern would not be appropriate for the intermediate category.

In applying these criteria, an independent decision should be made about each individual chemical entity, dosage form, and drug product because differences among various members of a drug class and dosage forms prevent using therapeutic class as a basis for classifying groups of related drug products.

Because drug information is continually evolving, drug products in the intermediate category may be reclassified as prescription or nonprescription medications as new effectiveness and safety information becomes available. Similarly, products could be permanently classified in the intermediate category if ongoing evidence documents the necessity of pharmacist intervention to ensure safe and effective use. The postmarketing surveillance of these medications through the collaboration of FDA and product manufacturers should be supported, in part, by information reported by pharmacists and patients to an established surveillance system, such as MedWatch, or similar reporting mechanisms.

Practice Implications

Implementation of the intermediate drug category would require that an ongoing relationship be established and maintained between the pharmacist and the patient and that documentation of the care provided be available to the patient's other health care providers, upon approval of the patient to provide such information. The exact nature and duration of the patient–pharmacist relationship would depend on the condition being treated and the drug therapy selected. A practice model that includes collaboration among the patient, the pharmacist, and the patient's physician (or other primary care provider) would enhance the use of these drug products and result in improved patient outcomes.

Increased pharmacist time for patient assessment, counseling, and documentation of services provided with these drug products would require reimbursement for these cognitive services. In addition, other conditions and procedures would be necessary to ensure the safety and effectiveness of these therapies, including the following:

- If the drug is to be used in conjunction with other therapies, such as diet and exercise, information about those adjunct therapies should be readily available to the patient from the pharmacist or through recommendation of the pharmacist or other health care provider.
- Patient care services provided by the pharmacist should be documented in the pharmacy record and available for sharing with other health care providers.
- Pharmacists and patients should provide information on actual or suspected adverse effects or drug interactions to programs such as MedWatch for the purposes of drug safety surveillance.
- Pharmacies should adopt standardized processes for the use of medications in the intermediate category that would guide patient triage, treatment, and referral to a physician when necessary. The expertise offered by clinical practice guidelines and professional associations should serve as the basis for these protocols, with appropriate modifications based on the unique characteristics of the patient population at the practice site.
- Pharmacies should adhere to quality measures that would be developed to assess the care provided (similar to those offered by the Pharmacy Quality Alliance) and engage in ongoing quality-improvement activities to assess and improve the quality of services provided.

A detailed discussion of these topics is addressed by other ASHP position and guidance documents, including the ASHP Statement on the Pharmacist's Role in Primary Care[14]; the ASHP Guidelines on Pharmacist-Conducted Patient Education and Counseling[15]; the ASHP Guidelines on the Pharmacist's Role in the Development, Implementation, and Assessment of Critical Pathways[16]; the ASHP Guidelines on Documenting Pharmaceutical Care in Patient Medical Records[17]; and the ASHP Guidelines on Adverse Drug Reaction Monitoring and Reporting.[18]

Conclusion

An intermediate category of drug products would increase patient access to and benefit from drug products that would otherwise be available only by prescription. The use of appropriate criteria for classifying drug products in an inter-

mediate drug category—in conjunction with pharmacist oversight of patient assessment, counseling, and monitoring—would improve public health without compromising patient safety.

References

1. American Society of Health-System Pharmacists. ASHP policy position 0220: intermediate category of drugs. www.ashp.org/DocLibrary/BestPractices/DistributionPositions.aspx (accessed 2008 Dec 3).

2. Brass EP. Implications of a switch from prescription to over-the-counter status for allergy drugs. *Curr Allergy Asthma Rep.* 2004; 4:245–50.

3. Lipsky MS, Waters T. The "prescription-to-OTC switch" movement. Its effects on antifungal vaginitis preparations. *Arch Fam Med.* 1999; 8:297–300.

4. Gurwitz JH, McLaughlin TJ, Fish LS. The effect of an Rx-to-OTC switch on medication prescribing patterns and utilization of physician services: the case of vaginal antifungal products. *Health Serv Res.* 1995; 30:672–85.

5. Merck and Company. Merck receives not approvable letter from FDA for OTC Mevacor (lovastatin) 20 mg. www.merck.com/newsroom/press_releases/product/2008_0125a.html (accessed 2008 Feb 14).

6. Brass EP, Allen SE, Melin JM. Potential impact on cardiovascular public health of over-the-counter statin availability. *Am J Cardiol.* 2006; 97:851–6.

7. American Society of Health-System Pharmacists. ASHP statement on the over-the-counter availability of statins. *Am J Health-Syst Pharm.* 2005; 62:2420–2.

8. National Association of Boards of Pharmacy. Groups advocate various Plan B classifications as FDA delays decision on OTC application. www.nabp.net/ftpfiles/newsletters/NABP/nabp022006.pdf (accessed 2008 Dec 3).

9. American Pharmacists Association. Report of the APhA 2005 House of Delegates. Transition class of drugs. *J Am Pharm Assoc.* 2005; 45:557.

10. Food and Drug Administration. Legal requirements for the sale and purchase of drug products containing pseudoephedrine, ephedrine, and phenylpropanolamine. www.fda.gov/cder/news/methamphetamine.htm (accessed 2008 Dec 3).

11. Food and Drug Administration. Plan B: questions and answers. www.fda.gov/cder/drug/infopage/planB/planBQandA20060824.htm (accessed 2008 Dec 3).

12. West DS, Johnson JT, Hone SH. A 30-month evaluation of the effects on the cost and utilization of proton pump inhibitors from adding OTC to drug benefit coverage in a state employee health plan. *J Manag Care Pharm.* 2006; 12:25–32.

13. Trygstad TK, Hansen RA, Wegner SE. Evaluation of product switching after a state Medicaid program began covering loratadine OTC one year after market availability. *J Manag Care Pharm.* 2006; 12:108–20.

14. American Society of Health-System Pharmacists. ASHP statement on the pharmacist's role in primary care. *Am J Health-Syst Pharm.* 1999; 56:1665–7.

15. American Society of Health-System Pharmacists. ASHP guidelines on pharmacist-conducted patient education and counseling. *Am J Health-Syst Pharm.* 1997; 54:431–4.

16. American Society of Health-System Pharmacists. ASHP guidelines on the pharmacist's role in the development, implementation, and assessment of critical pathways. *Am J Health-Syst Pharm.* 2004; 61:939–45.

17. American Society of Health-System Pharmacists. ASHP guidelines on documenting pharmaceutical care in patient medical records. *Am J Health-Syst Pharm.* 2003; 60:705–7.

18. American Society of Health-System Pharmacists. ASHP guidelines on adverse drug reaction monitoring and reporting. *Am J Health-Syst Pharm.* 1995; 52:417–9.

Developed through the ASHP Council on Therapeutics and approved by the ASHP Board of Directors on March 7, 2008, and by the ASHP House of Delegates on June 10, 2008.

The assistance of Susan R. Dombrowski, B.S.Pharm., M.S., in drafting this statement is gratefully acknowledged.

The bibliographic citation for this document is as follows: American Society of Health-System Pharmacists. ASHP statement on criteria for an intermediate category of drug products. *Am J Health-Syst Pharm.* 2009; 66:502–9.

ASHP Statement on
the Over-the-Counter Availability of Statins

The American Society of Health-System Pharmacists (ASHP) believes that existing models for over-the-counter (OTC) dispensing do not provide the safeguards required to ensure the safe and effective use of 3-hydroxy-3-methylglutaryl coenzyme A (HMG-CoA) reductase inhibitors ("statins") as part of a multimodal approach to preventing coronary heart disease (CHD). ASHP supports the goal of more widespread use of CHD-preventive therapies, including statin therapy, and encourages consideration of alternative nonprescription dispensing models for statins that would advance CHD prevention.

Since 1985, ASHP has called for changes in federal statutes and regulations to establish an intermediate category of drug products that do not require a prescription but are available only from pharmacists and other licensed health care professionals authorized to prescribe medications.[1] ASHP believes consideration of OTC reclassification for statins presents an opportunity to explore the creation of such a category of drugs. ASHP has suggested that the regulatory system for such an intermediate category of drug products would allow pharmacists to provide drugs in this intermediate category directly to patients without a prescription, on the basis of appropriate assessment and professional consultation, while ensuring that licensed health professionals who currently have prescribing authority would continue to have the ability to prescribe such medications. ASHP believes that under such a regulatory system, data from postmarketing surveillance, epidemiologic studies, and adverse-drug-reaction reporting should be collected to help determine a drug product's eventual movement to nonprescription status, return to prescription-only status, or continuation in the intermediate category.[1] ASHP believes statins are an ideal candidate for dispensing under such a model.

Background

ASHP supports the use of statins to lower cholesterol and reduce morbidity and mortality in patients at risk for cardiovascular events.[2] Elevated cholesterol, specifically low-density lipoprotein cholesterol (LDL-C), is an important risk factor for the development of CHD. ASHP has recommended that evaluation and management of lipid disorders be guided by the recommendations of the National Cholesterol Education Program (NCEP), the latest of which are contained in the Adult Treatment Panel III (ATP III) guidelines.[3,4] Statins are considered the drug of choice for most patients with dyslipidemia who require lipid-lowering therapy. They are effective in lowering elevated LDL-C, and studies have demonstrated that statins reduce the risk of cardiovascular events in patients without known CHD (primary prevention). In addition, statins have been shown to reduce cardiovascular events and mortality in patients with CHD (secondary prevention). Cardiovascular disease is the leading cause of death for both men and women in the United States, and CHD is responsible for nearly 75% of all deaths from cardiovascular disease.[5] Individuals with multiple cardiovascular risk factors and a low LDL-C derive

an absolute benefit in reducing risk of CHD for a given milligram-per-deciliter lowering of LDL-C. However, for individuals with lower LDL-C levels and fewer risk factors for CHD, the benefits of lowering LDL-C level are less dramatic.[6]

Nonprescription Dispensing Models

The efficacy of statins in reducing LDL-C has prompted calls for more widespread use, including suggestions for a reclassification of statins as an OTC medication. Although ASHP does not support reclassification to OTC status as that status is currently constructed, alternative nonprescription models for dispensing these valuable medications should be explored.

To approve a reclassification to OTC status, FDA reviewers must find that (1) a drug is safe and effective in its proposed use(s), (2) the benefits of the drug outweigh its risks, and (3) consumers will be able to use the drug's labeling (e.g., its package insert) to safely use the medication in an OTC setting.[7] ASHP believes a decision to approve nonprescription dispensing models for statins should be based on evidence that, under the proposed model, the target population would receive a clinical benefit in primary prevention of CHD from the medication and patients can safely use the medication to achieve that clinical benefit. To achieve the goal of safe and effective use, any nonprescription dispensing model for statins should

- Identify candidates for appropriate therapeutic interventions, including statin therapy, on the basis of cholesterol levels, other risk factors for CHD events, and the patient's medical and family histories;
- Allow patients and health care providers to monitor response to treatment, including adverse reactions; and
- Maximize the effectiveness of treatment by encouraging adherence to therapy and appropriate interactions with health care professionals.

ASHP believes that before a patient begins statin therapy, a cardiac risk assessment should be performed by a competent health care professional in order to

- Determine the patient's LDL-C value, which can be used as a baseline value if the patient is a candidate for treatment;
- Assess the individual for other cardiovascular risk factors such as smoking, diabetes, hypertension, diet, weight, amount of exercise, and family history of cardiovascular disease; and
- Develop the optimal treatment plan based on ATP III guidelines and the assessment above.

Individuals with two or more risk factors or a family history of cardiovascular disease who have never been evaluated should have a complete medical assessment and appropriate interventions by a physician. If statins are

an appropriate therapeutic option, they should be part of a multimodal approach to reducing the overall CHD risk, which would include managing and treating modifiable risk factors such as hypertension, smoking, obesity, diet, and lack of exercise. Diet and exercise therapy should be a fundamental part of all cholesterol-lowering regimens.

Current OTC Model

Statins are not suitable for OTC status as that class is currently regulated. One study has examined the use of statins in a simulated OTC setting. The CUSTOM study[8] was an open-label study designed to observe consumers' initial and continued use of a statin to lower LDL-C. Although the results may indicate that some individuals in the study sample were able to use an OTC statin as directed, the study was, by the investigators' own admission, not designed to evaluate clinical outcomes and therefore not able to demonstrate efficacy. The study certainly did not prove that the existing OTC model would provide the level of counseling required to reduce cardiovascular risk factors other than LDL-C levels.

However encouraging these results might seem, caution should be exercised in extrapolating such information to a larger population, especially information regarding safety. Adverse drug effects should always be assessed, especially if the medications that cause them are easily available to the public. A system that relies on the voluntary reporting of adverse drug effects by patients may be inadequate to protect the public or detect subtle signals. It is imperative that the decision to reclassify a statin to a nonprescription status include a wide margin of safety. After statin therapy starts, ongoing evaluations should assess the patient's response, reassess risk factors, and monitor for and report adverse events. The existing model for OTC medications would place the entire burden for performing this evaluation and reassessment on the patient. Most patients are likely to be unfamiliar with the system used to report an adverse event, if the adverse event is even recognized. Although adverse events from prescription statins are rare, particularly at lower doses, they can occur months or years after therapy is initiated. Since OTC status would encourage wider use of statins, these drugs might be used by individuals with multiple disease states or those taking potentially interacting medications (e.g., cyclosporine, diltiazem, verapamil, macrolide antibiotics, azole antifungals, or protease inhibitors). Because statins are a chronic therapy, new risks may be introduced as the patient's health varies, requiring vigilance on the part of the patient as well as health care providers.

ASHP believes, for these reasons, that reclassification of statins to OTC status as currently constructed is not advisable but that alternative nonprescription models for dispensing these valuable medications should be explored.

Alternative Nonprescription Models

ASHP believes that there are alternatives to prescription-only status that would allow expanded use of statins to reduce cardiovascular events in primary prevention patients. Since 1985, ASHP has had a policy urging changes in federal statutes and regulations to create an intermediate category of drug products that do not require a prescription but are available only from pharmacists and other licensed health care professionals.[1] ASHP believes the regulatory system for this intermediate category of drug products should have the following features:

1. Drug products appropriate for this intermediate category would be identified through the advice of pharmacists, physicians, and other licensed health professionals who are authorized to prescribe medications, on the basis of the medical conditions to be treated and potential adverse effects (as indicated in FDA-approved labeling);
2. Pharmacists would be able to provide drugs in this intermediate category directly to patients without a prescription, on the basis of appropriate assessment and professional consultation;
3. Licensed health professionals who currently have prescribing authority would continue to have the ability to prescribe medications in this intermediate category; and
4. Data from postmarketing surveillance, epidemiologic studies, and adverse-drug-reaction reporting would be collected to help determine a drug product's eventual movement to nonprescription status, return to prescription-only status, or continuation in the intermediate category.[1]

Drugs that would raise safety and efficacy concerns if used as nonprescription products could be better controlled, monitored, and evaluated if they were available only from pharmacists and licensed health care professionals who are authorized to prescribe medications. Pharmacists have the education, training, and expertise to help patients make appropriate therapeutic decisions about the use of such products. ASHP believes statins are a good candidate for dispensing under such a model, much as is done in Great Britain, where simvastatin was approved for "counterprescribing" in May 2004.[9]

Conclusion

ASHP supports nonprescription dispensing models for statins that ensure their safe and effective use as part of a multimodal approach to CHD prevention. Given the complexities of therapies to prevent CHD, ASHP encourages consideration of alternatives to the current model of OTC distribution for statins.

References

1. Policy Position 0220: Intermediate Category of Drugs. In: Best practices for hospital and health-system pharmacy 2004–2005. Positions and practice documents of ASHP. Bethesda, MD: American Society of Health-System Pharmacists; 2004:89.
2. ASHP Therapeutic Position Statement on the Use of Statins in the Prevention of Atherosclerotic Disease in Adults. *Am J Health Syst Pharm.* 2003; 60:593-8.
3. Expert Panel on Detection, Evaluation, and Treatment of High Blood Cholesterol in Adults. Executive summary of the Third Report of the National Cholesterol Education Program (NCEP) Expert Panel on Detection, Evaluation, and Treatment of High Blood Cholesterol in Adults (Adult Treatment Panel III). *JAMA.* 2001; 285:2486-97.

4. National Cholesterol Education Program (NCEP) Expert Panel on Detection, Evaluation, and Treatment of High Blood Cholesterol in Adults (Adult Treatment Panel III). Third Report of the National Cholesterol Education Program (NCEP) Expert Panel on Detection, Evaluation, and Treatment of High Blood Cholesterol in Adults (Adult Treatment Panel III) final report. *Circulation.* 2002; 106:3143-421.

5. American Heart Association. 2002 heart and stroke statistical update. Available at: www.americanheart.org/presenter (accessed 2002 May 14).

6. Grundy SM, Cleeman JI, Merz CN et al. Implications of recent clinical trials for the National Cholesterol Education Program Adult Treatment Panel III Guidelines. *Circulation.* 2004; 110:227-39.

7. Food and Drug Administration, Center for Drug Evaluation and Research, Endocrinologic and Metabolic Drugs Advisory Committee, Questions to the Committee (joint meeting of January 13–14, 2005, to consider new drug application 21-213). Available at: http://www.fda.gov/ohrms/dockets/ac/05/questions/2005-4086S2_02_FDA-Questions.htm (accessed January 26, 2005).

8. Melin JM, Struble WE, Tipping RW et al. A consumer use study of over-the-counter lovastatin (CUSTOM). *Am J Cardiol.* 2004; 94:1243-8.

9. Royal Pharmaceutical Society of Great Britain. Concise version of practice guidance on the sale of OTC simvastatin. July 2004. Available at: http://www.rpsgb.org. uk/pdfs/otcsimvastatincardguid.pdf (accessed January 4, 2005).

This statement was reviewed in 2009 by the Council on Therapeutics and by the Board of Directors and was found to still be appropriate.

Approved by the ASHP Board of Directors on January 6, 2005, and by the ASHP House of Delegates on June 14, 2005. Developed through the ASHP Commission on Therapeutics.

The bibliographic citation for this document is as follows: American Society of Health-System Pharmacists. ASHP statement on the over-the-counter availability of statins. *Am J Health-Syst Pharm.* 2005; 62:2420–2.

ASHP Statement on Principles for Including Medications and Pharmaceutical Care in Health Care Systems

Introduction

The United States government, individual state governments, and private health care systems are moving toward reforming the way that they provide health care to their citizens or beneficiaries. As they do so, policy makers must improve their medication-use systems to address problems of access, quality, and cost of medicines and pharmaceutical care services. This document offers principles for achieving maximum value from the services of the nation's pharmacists.

Although pharmaceuticals and pharmaceutical care are among the most cost-effective methods of health care available, there is evidence that the public is not currently realizing the full potential benefit from these resources. Illnesses related to improper medication use are costing the health care systems in the United States billions of dollars per year in patient morbidity and mortality. Pharmacists are prepared and eager to help other health providers and patients prevent and resolve medication-related problems, and health care systems should facilitate and take advantage of pharmacists' expertise.

These principles are offered to guide health policy makers in their deliberations concerning the inclusion of medications and pharmacists' services in health care systems.

Principles

Principle I. Health care systems must make medications available to patients and provide for pharmaceutical care, which encompasses pharmacists' health care services and health promotional activities that ensure that medications are used safely, effectively, and efficiently for optimal patient outcomes.

Principle II. Careful distinction must be made between policies that affect pharmacist reimbursement and policies that affect pharmacist compensation. Health care systems must reimburse pharmacists for the medications they provide patients (including the costs of drug products, the costs associated with dispensing, and related administrative costs). Health care systems also must compensate pharmacists for the services and care that they provide to patients, which result in improved medication use and which may not necessarily be associated with dispensing.

Principle III. Patients differ in their needs for pharmaceutical care services. The method of compensating pharmacists for their services must recognize the value of the different levels and types of services that pharmacists provide to patients based on pharmacists' professional assessments of patients' needs.

Principle IV. Pharmacists must be enabled and encouraged to use their professional expertise in making medication-related judgments in collaboration with patients and health care colleagues. Health care systems must not erect barriers to pharmacists' exercising professional judgments; nor should health care systems prescribe specific services or therapies for defined types of patients.

Principle V. Pharmacists should have access to relevant patient information to support their professional judgments and activities. Pharmacists should be encouraged and permitted to make additions to medical records for the purpose of adding their findings, conclusions, and recommendations. Pharmacists will respect the confidential nature of all patient information.

Principle VI. Health care systems must be designed to enable, foster, and facilitate communication and collaboration among pharmacists and other care providers to ensure proper coordination of patients' medication therapies.

Principle VII. Quality assessment and assurance programs related to individual patient care should be implemented at local levels through collaborative efforts of health care practitioners rather than through centralized bureaucracies. Quality assessment and assurance procedures for medication use (such as pharmacy and therapeutics committees, formulary systems, drug-use evaluation programs, and patient outcomes analyses) are most effective when the professionals who care for covered patients are involved in the design and implementation of the procedures. Moreover, such programs must recognize local variations in epidemiology, demography, and practice standards. Information related to quality assessment and assurance activities must be held in confidence by all parties.

Principle VIII. Demonstration projects and evaluation studies in the delivery of pharmaceutical care must be enabled, fostered, and implemented. New services, quality assessment and assurance techniques, and innovative medication delivery systems are needed to improve the access to and quality of medication therapy and pharmaceutical care while containing costs.

Principle IX. Health care policies that are intended to influence practices of those associated with pharmacy, such as the pharmaceutical industry or prescribers, should address those audiences directly rather than through policies that affect reimbursement, compensation, or other activities of pharmacists.

This statement was reviewed in 2007 by the Council on Public Policy and by the Board of Directors and was found to still be appropriate.

Approved by the ASHP Board of Directors, November 18, 1992, and by the ASHP House of Delegates, June 7, 1993. Developed by a committee of the Joint Commission of Pharmacy Practitioners and subsequently reviewed and approved by the ASHP Council on Legal and Public Affairs.

The bibliographic citation for this document is as follows: American Society of Hospital Pharmacists. ASHP statement on principles for including medications and pharmaceutical care in health care systems. *Am J Hosp Pharm.* 1993; 50:756–7.

Medication Misadventures

Medication Misadventures

Just Culture (1115)
Source: Council on Pharmacy Practice
To recognize that the principles of *just culture* promote an environment in health care organizations in which safety is valued, reporting of safety risks is encouraged, and a fair process is used to hold staff and leaders accountable; further,

To encourage hospitals and health systems to include *just culture* as a component in organizational safety culture surveys and quality improvement initiatives.

Standardization of Device Connections to Avoid Wrong-Route Errors (1018)
Source: Council on Pharmacy Practice
To advocate for development and use of medication administration device connectors and fittings that are designed to prevent misconnections and wrong-route errors; further,

To support the use of oral syringes that are readily distinguishable from injectable syringes and connect only to oral or enteral adapters and fittings; further,

To oppose the use of injectable syringes for other than injectable routes of administration; further,

To identify and promote the implementation of best practices for preventing wrong-route errors.

Medication Safety Officer Role (1019)
Source: Council on Pharmacy Practice
To advocate that accountability for development and maintenance of a medication safety program in hospitals and health systems be assigned to a qualified individual (i.e., a medication safety officer or leader of a medication safety team); further,

To advocate that individuals in these roles have the authority and autonomy to establish priorities for medication-use safety and make the necessary changes as authorized by the medical staff committee responsible for medication-use policy; further,

To affirm that pharmacists are uniquely prepared by education, experience, and knowledge to assume the role of medication safety officer or other leadership role in all activities that ensure the safety, effectiveness, and efficiency of the medication-use process; further,

To support all pharmacists in their leadership roles in organizational medication-use safety, reflecting their authority over and accountability for the performance of the medication-use process.

Just Culture and Reporting Medication Errors (1021)
Source: Council on Pharmacy Practice
To encourage pharmacists to exert leadership in establishing a just culture in their workplaces and a nonpunitive systems approach to addressing medication errors while supporting a nonthreatening reporting environment to encourage pharmacy staff and others to report actual and potential medication errors in a timely manner; further,

To provide leadership in supporting a single, comprehensive, hospital- or health-system-specific medication error reporting program that (1) fosters a confidential, nonthreat-

ening, and nonpunitive environment for the submission of medication error reports; (2) receives and analyzes these confidential reports to identify system-based causes of medication errors or potential errors; and (3) recommends and disseminates error prevention strategies; further,

To provide leadership in encouraging the participation of all stakeholders in the reporting of medication errors to this program.

(*Note:* A just culture is one that has a clear and transparent process for evaluating errors and separating events arising from flawed system design or inadvertent human error from those caused by reckless behavior, defined as a behavioral choice to consciously disregard what is known to be a substantial or unjustifiable risk.)

This policy supersedes ASHP policy 0910.

Minimizing the Use of Abbreviations (0604)
Source: Council on Administrative Affairs
To support efforts to minimize the use of abbreviations in health care; further,

To collaborate with others in the development of a lexicon of a limited number of standard drug name abbreviations that can be safely used in patient care.

This policy was reviewed in 2010 by the Council on Pharmacy Management and by the Board of Directors and was found to still be appropriate.

Statutory Protection for Medication-Error Reporting (0011)
Source: Council on Legal and Public Affairs
To collaborate with other health care providers, professions, and stakeholders to advocate and support federal legislative and regulatory initiatives that provide liability protection for the reporting of actual and potential medication errors by individuals and health care providers; further,

To seek federal liability protection for medication-error reporting that is similar in concept to that which applies to reporting safety incidents and accidents in the aviation industry.

This policy was reviewed in 2009 by the Council on Public Policy and by the Board of Directors and was found to still be appropriate.

Drug Names, Labeling, and Packaging Associated with Medication Errors (0020)
Source: Council on Professional Affairs
To urge drug manufacturers and FDA to involve practicing pharmacists, nurses, and physicians in decisions about drug names, labeling, and packaging to help eliminate (a) look-alike and sound-alike drug names, and (b) labeling and packaging characteristics that contribute to medication errors; further,

To inform pharmacists and others, as appropriate, about specific drug names, labeling, and packaging that have documented association with medication errors.

This policy was reviewed in 2009 by the Council on Pharmacy Practice and by the Board of Directors and was found to still be appropriate.

Medication Errors and Risk Management (0021)

Source: Council on Professional Affairs

To urge that pharmacists be included in health care organizations' risk management processes for the purpose of (a) assessing medication-use systems for vulnerabilities to medication errors, (b) implementing medication-error prevention strategies, and (c) reviewing occurrences of medication errors and developing corrective actions.

This policy was reviewed in 2009 by the Council on Pharmacy Practice and by the Board of Directors and was found to still be appropriate.

Medication Misadventures (9805)

Source: Council on Administrative Affairs

To affirm that pharmacists must assume a leadership role in preventing, investigating, and eliminating medication misadventures across the continuum of care.

This policy was reviewed in 2007 by the Council on Pharmacy Management and by the Board of Directors and was found to still be appropriate.

Human Factors Concepts (9609)

Source: Council on Professional Affairs

To encourage pharmacists to apply human factors concepts (human errors related to inadequate systems or environment) in the prevention, analysis, and reporting of medication errors; further,

To encourage research (in conjunction with other groups, as appropriate) to identify human factors causes of medication errors and opportunities for their prevention.

This policy was reviewed in 2009 by the Council on Pharmacy Practice and by the Board of Directors and was found to still be appropriate.

ASHP Statement on Reporting Medical Errors

Position

The incidence of death and serious harm caused by mistakes and accidents in health care is unacceptable.[1] This serious public health problem merits top-priority national attention. Addressing this issue will require major reforms and sizable investment of resources throughout the health care system, including the medication use process, which is a particular focus of the American Society of Health-System Pharmacists (ASHP).

ASHP believes that the following steps should be taken as part of a comprehensive national solution to the problem: (1) The establishment of a standardized, uniform nationwide system (with the characteristics noted below) of mandatory reporting of adverse medical events that cause death or serious harm, (2) continued development and strengthening of systems for voluntary reporting of medical errors, and (3) strengthening efforts to implement process changes that reduce the risk of future errors and improve patient care.

The fundamental purpose of reporting systems for medical errors is to learn how to improve the health care delivery process to prevent these errors. Reporting of medical errors must become culturally accepted throughout health care. A major investment of resources will be required in the health care system to apply the lessons derived from the reporting of medical errors. Marshaling those resources is an urgent issue for the governing boards of health care institutions, health care administrators, health professionals, purchasers of health care (including federal and state governments), third party payers, public policy makers, credentialing organizations, the legal profession, and consumers.

Requirements

The primary goal of *mandatory reporting* of adverse medical events that cause death or serious harm should be to foster accountability for health care delivery process changes to prevent errors or adverse medical events. If a patient dies or is seriously harmed because of a mistake or accident in the health care system, the practitioner or institution responsible for the patient's care should report the incident to a designated state health body. Further, states should be obligated to share information based on these reports promptly with a national coordinating body and with national programs that are designed to improve the quality and enhance the safety of patient care.

ASHP's support of a mandatory reporting system is contingent upon the system having the following characteristics:

1. An overall focus on improving the processes used in health care, with the proper application of technical expertise to analyze and learn from reports,
2. Legal protection of confidentiality of patients, health care workers, and the information submitted to the extent feasible while preserving the interest of public accountability,
3. Nonpunitive in the sense that the submission of a report, per se, does not engender a penalty on the reporting institution or practitioner or others involved in the incident,
4. A definition of "serious harm" that concentrates on long-term or irreversible patient harm, so as not to overburden the reporting system,
5. National coordination and strong federal efforts to ensure compliance with standardized methods of reporting, analysis, and follow up, that emphasize process improvement and avoid a culture of blame,
6. Adequate resources devoted to report analysis, timely dissemination of advisories based on report analysis, and development of appropriate quality improvement efforts, and
7. Periodic assessment of the system to ensure that it is meeting its intent and not having serious undesired consequences.

Experience associated with current mandatory state reporting of adverse medical events and mandatory public health reporting of certain infectious diseases should be assessed, and the best practices of such programs should be applied to the new system of mandatory reporting of adverse medical events that cause death or serious harm.

The primary goals of *voluntary reporting* of medical errors should be quality improvement and enhancement of patient safety. Reports by frontline practitioners of errors and "near misses" are a strength of such programs when report analysis and communication lead to prevention of similar occurrences. The public interest will be served if protection is granted to individuals who submit reports to voluntary reporting programs. The Medication Errors Reporting Program operated by the United States Pharmacopeia in cooperation with the Institute for Safe Medication Practices is an important initiative that merits strengthening; this program may be a model for voluntary reporting of other types of medical error.

Reference

1. Institute of Medicine Division of Health Care Services Committee on Quality of Health Care in America. To err is human: building a safer health system. Washington, DC: National Academy Press; 1999.

This statement was reviewed in 2005 by the Council on Professional Affairs and by the Board of Directors and was found to still be appropriate.

Approved by the ASHP House of Delegates, June 5, 2000.

The bibliographic citation for this document is as follows: American Society of Health-System Pharmacists. ASHP statement on reporting medical errors. *Am J Health-Syst Pharm.* 2000; 57:1531–2.

ASHP Statement on the Role
of the Medication Safety Leader

Position

The American Society of Health-System Pharmacists (ASHP) believes that medication safety is a fundamental responsibility of all members of the profession of pharmacy. For a medication safety program to succeed, however, it is essential that there be an innovative leader to set a vision and direction, identify opportunities to improve the medication-use system, and lead implementation of error-prevention strategies. The medication safety leader's role includes responsibility for leadership, medication safety expertise, influencing practice change, research, and education. ASHP believes that because of their training, knowledge of the medication-use process, skills, and abilities, pharmacists are uniquely qualified to fill the roles and meet the responsibilities of the medication safety leader in hospitals and health systems.

Background

Hospital and health-system pharmacists have improved pharmacy systems over the past 60 years to reduce the risk that medications could harm patients. Medication safety was at the heart of such historic innovations in pharmacy services as unit-dose systems, decentralized clinical pharmacy services, and intravenous admixture services. The crucial leadership role of pharmacists in medication safety has been summarized as follows:

Pharmacy leadership is the core of a successful medication safety program. Pharmacy leaders can play an enormously important role in performance improvement. They can be part of the senior leadership team's DNA because their impact and view go far beyond the walls of the pharmacy.... Pharmacists can play an important role as leaders to reduce patient safety risks, optimize the safe function of medication management systems, and align pharmacy services with national initiatives that measure and reward quality performance.[1]

The landmark Institute of Medicine (IOM) report *To Err is Human: Building a Safer Health System*[2] generated major patient safety initiatives by government agencies, regulatory and accrediting bodies, professional and organizational associations, and health care organizations. The Joint Commission (TJC) National Patient Safety Goals (NPSGs)[3] are an example of a response to the original IOM report. The Pharmacy Practice Model Initiative (PPMI)[4] and the National Quality Forum (NQF) Safe Practice 18[5] incorporate medication safety principles to ensure optimal patient safety and outcomes.

The medication safety leader (also referred to as a medication safety officer, medication safety manager, or medication safety coordinator, among other titles) is a clinical practitioner designated by an organization to serve as the authoritative expert in safe medication use. Traditionally, the medication safety leader has been a clinical pharmacist

or manager within the department of pharmacy, although the position is sometimes filled by a nurse or physician. The medication safety leader may report to the organization's risk management department, its office of quality, or to a senior administrator (e.g., hospital vice president, chief medical officer, or chief executive officer). Reporting outside the pharmacy department may foster interdisciplinary approaches to medication safety. Medication safety leadership may encompass a single hospital or a group of organizations (e.g., spanning a health system or at a corporate level of a larger organization). Regardless of organization size, it is critical that the fundamentals of medication safety are the central component of the medication safety leader's job function. Although medication safety leaders may have other responsibilities in smaller institutions, medication safety should remain their core responsibility, and they must be strategically positioned and empowered to lead efforts to reduce the risks of medication use.

The characteristics of a medication safety leader include:

1. A strong understanding of the facility's internal systems and processes developed through firsthand experience, observations, medication-use evaluations, interviews, and data analysis for a spectrum of patient populations (e.g., pediatric, geriatric, cardiac, oncology).
2. Clinical expertise and a broad understanding of health care systems and processes to facilitate accurate interpretation of clinical events.
3. Knowledge of and experience with all aspects of the medication-use system, including procurement, prescribing, transcribing, preparation, distribution, administration, documentation, and monitoring.
4. Strong analytical skills and an understanding of statistics, population data, and the concepts of risk and prioritization.
5. Knowledge of performance improvement methodology and tools, including root cause analysis (RCA), failure mode and effects analysis (FMEA), cause-and-effect diagramming, process-flow mapping, and methods for monitoring projects and measuring the progress of performance improvement initiatives.
6. Three or more years of post-training health-system practice experience.
7. Demonstrated leadership skills.
8. Excellent small and large group presentation skills.
9. Excellent verbal communication skills, especially the ability to communicate to all types of health care providers, as individuals as well as in small and large groups.
10. Excellent writing and editing skills.
11. Strong personal belief that resolving the problem of medication errors is a systems issue and not an individual health care provider issue.
12. Ability to function proactively rather than reactively.

13. Strong personal belief in the concept of a "just culture"[6] that enhances transparency, opens participation to all health care professionals, and fosters a "lessons learned" environment in an organization's medication-error reporting system.

14. Understanding of concepts and application of safety principles, continuous quality improvement, and human factors engineering.

15. Appropriate assertiveness.

16. A passion for medication safety and improving patient outcomes.

17. Proven success in working with interdisciplinary teams and engaging diverse groups.

18. Strong personal belief in engaging patients as part of the health care team.

19. Eagerness to learn from events outside one's own facility (e.g., through external sources of information) to apply learning about what went wrong in order to identify and remedy possible system weaknesses to prevent patient harm.[7]

The scope of a medication safety leader's responsibilities reaches into every corner of the health care system and encompasses many roles, such as educator, preceptor, mentor, detective, compliance officer, risk manager, engineer, accountant, statistician, computer analyst, and counselor. A typical day may include attending safety rounds, precepting pharmacy students and residents, writing policies, reviewing adverse drug reactions and medication error reports, developing error-prevention strategies, leading process improvement teams, implementing action items, reviewing smart pump libraries, ensuring safe use of automated medication dispensing systems, assessing the safety of replacement drug products during drug shortages, orienting new professional staff, assisting with medication reconciliation, conducting tracers to ensure compliance with accreditation standards (e.g., TJC medication management standards and NPSGs), working with practitioners to resolve acute events, attending medical staff meetings, or educating the corporate board on the culture of safety. Most medication safety leaders quickly find themselves involved in many projects and committees as well as serving as the contact person when nursing, pharmacy, or medical staff have questions or problems. The medication safety leader needs a solid understanding of patient safety principles and must have the ability to prioritize work activities to have a positive impact on the safety of patient care. The medication safety leader should strive to acquire additional skills crucial to success, such as presentation and communications skills, as well as expertise in process improvement methodologies such as Six Sigma and Lean. Formalized training in medication safety can be achieved through residency, fellowship, certificate programs, and other methods of continuing education. ASHP supports the expansion of pharmacy education and postgraduate residency training to include an emphasis on medication safety.[8]

Responsibilities of Medication Safety Leaders

Medication safety leaders must collaborate with all types of health care professionals, support staff, and management, and consider all components of the medication-use process in both inpatient and clinic settings in order to improve medication safety. The medication safety leader's role includes responsibility for leadership, medication safety expertise, influencing practice change, research, and education.

Leadership. To provide leadership, the medication safety leader will:

1. Develop a vision of an ideal safe medication-use system for the organization.

2. Oversee the planning, creation, review, and refinement of a medication safety plan.

3. Proactively develop and lead implementation of error-prevention strategies based on practice standards, literature review, medication safety tools, and analysis of the organization's medication safety data.

4. Participate in the planning, design, and implementation of the organization's medication-use technology and automation systems.

5. Build a culture of safety through "lesson learned" education and communication across the entire organization.

6. Oversee processes to collect information on the organization's medication errors and system failures to ensure that they are captured and barriers to reporting are addressed.

7. Ensure compliance with state and federal regulatory and legal requirements relating to medication safety, and assist in the accreditation process by ensuring that the organization's medication-use processes meet applicable medication management standards and NPSGs.

Medication Safety Expertise. In the role of medication safety expert, the medication safety leader will:

1. Serve as an authoritative resource on medication safety for the organization.

2. Contribute the medication safety perspective for technology initiatives.

3. Contribute the medication safety perspective to internal and external emergency preparedness planning.

4. Serve as an internal consultant to investigate medication safety events or issues and develop recommendations for action.

5. Serve as the chair of the Medication Safety Committee, whose duties may include setting the agenda, reviewing general and specific error reports, and examining the progress of projects and initiatives assigned to the medication safety team.

6. Be knowledgeable in the application and use of a variety of quality improvement methodologies and tools (e.g., FOCUS-PDCA or Lean methodologies, root cause analysis, failure mode and effects analysis).

7. Collect, review, and analyze, as the leader of review teams, the organization's medication-use, medication error, adverse drug reaction, and continuous quality improvement data (e.g., markers of adverse drug events, smart pump event data, triggers and surveillance information, and automated dispensing system and bedside barcode scanning reports) and use appropriate data analysis techniques to identify needed im-

provements and develop high-leverage error-reduction strategies.

8. Predict and prepare to manage medication safety issues caused by potential or actual drug product shortages and the use of replacement drug products.
9. Maintain knowledge of trends and developments in the patient safety field through continuous professional development; reading articles, journals, and related material; attending appropriate seminars, conferences, or educational programs; and utilization of information from the Institute of Safe Medication Practices (ISMP) National Medication Error Reporting Program, the Food and Drug Administration (FDA) MedWatch program, and similar programs.
10. Participate at a local and national level in patient safety and medication safety organizations and initiatives.

Influencing Practice Change. To influence practice change, the medication safety leader will:

1. Collaborate with other departments (e.g., pharmacy, risk management, and patient safety), hospital or health-system senior leadership, frontline staff, and nursing and medical staff leadership to identify and prioritize safety issues and develop risk-reduction strategies using the methods listed above to identify opportunities to improve medication safety.
2. Manage changes in the medication-use system to enhance medication safety, ensure that appropriate measures are taken to address and resolve medication safety issues, and see that hospital staff and faculty are supported in providing safe care for patients.
3. Work closely with others (e.g., the patient safety officer) to integrate medication safety into the overall strategic plan for patient safety and coordinate medication safety initiatives with organizational patient safety initiatives.
4. Participate in or lead multidisciplinary hospital and health-system committees concerned with medication errors, adverse drug events and reactions, near misses, policy review, safe medication use, new product review, and patient safety to identify risk points and prioritize system improvements to reduce the potential for medication error and patient harm.
5. Consult with and advise specific clinical teams and the hospital and health system generally on opportunities and strategies to improve patient care.
6. Encourage organization-wide medication error reporting through an established and accepted error reporting system that utilizes appropriate error detection methods (e.g., trigger tools) and through other appropriate avenues such as the Pharmacy & Therapeutics Committee, Medication Safety Committee, or Patient Safety Committee.
7. Develop effective methods for spreading best medication-use practices throughout the organization.
8. Use continuous quality improvement principles to assess and report on the status of efforts to improve medication safety.
9. Periodically review and update clinical decision support tools to alert staff to high-risk situations and educate staff as needed.

Research and Education. To further research and education regarding medication safety, the medication safety leader will:

1. Design and assist in the implementation of education and orientation programs in safe medication use, including:

 - development of competency assessment for staff tasks related to medication safety (e.g., use of smart pumps and automated medication dispensing systems);
 - education of health care providers, other pertinent staff, and (as possible) patients to ensure they are competent in safe medication-use practices; and
 - provision of effective ongoing programs and presentations related to safe medication use to diverse audiences (e.g., nursing, pharmacy, respiratory care, and medical staff).

2. Share information about actual or potential medication errors or harm with safety organizations such as the Institute for Safe Medication Practices (ISMP), the FDA, drug or product manufacturers, and state error reporting programs.
3. Conduct medication-use safety research through well-designed, externally validated studies, and implement evidence-based practices for medication safety.
4. Contribute to the literature on medication safety.
5. Provide medication safety education to pharmacy colleagues, students, and residents, as well as other health care professionals.
6. Integrate medication safety into orientation and training for all health care providers who participate in the medication-use process.

Conclusion

ASHP believes that pharmacists, as experts on medication use, are uniquely qualified to serve as medication safety leaders. Medication safety leaders articulate the vision and direction for improving the safety of the medication-use system to prevent patient harm. The medication safety leader's role includes responsibility for leadership through direction and prioritization, medication safety expertise, influencing practice change, research, and education. Through analysis of the organization's medication safety data and literature review, the medication safety leader will lead development and implementation of proactive error-prevention strategies and build a culture of safety across the organization.

References

1. Burgess LH, Cohen MR, Denham CR. A new leadership role for pharmacists: a prescription for change. *J Patient Saf.* 2010; 6:31–7.
2. Kohn KT, Corrigan JM, Donaldson MS. To Err Is Human: Building a Safer Health System. Washington, DC: National Academy Press; 1999.

3. The Joint Commission. Facts about the National Patient Safety Goals. www.jointcommission.org/facts_about_the_national_patient_safety_goals/ (accessed 03 Nov 2012).

4. The consensus of the Pharmacy Practice Model Summit. *Am J Health-Syst Pharm.* 2011; 68:1148–52.

5. National Quality Forum. Safe Practices for Better Healthcare 2009 Update: A Consensus Report. Washington, DC: The National Quality Forum; 2009. Available at: www.qualityforum.org/publications/reports/safe_practices_2009.aspx (accessed 31 Jan 2012).

6. Marx D. Patient safety and the "just culture": a primer for health care executives. New York: Columbia University Press; 2001.

7. Adapted from: ASHP. Desired entry characteristics for those to be trained for medication-use safety coordinator positions. www.ashp.org/DocLibrary/Accreditation/Regulations-Standards/RTPEntryCharactMedUseSafety.aspx (accessed 28 Nov 2011).

8. American Society of Health-System Pharmacists. Required Educational Outcomes, Goals, and Objectives for Postgraduate Year Two (PGY2) Pharmacy Residencies in Medication-Use Safety. www.ashp.org/DocLibrary/Accreditation/Regulations-Standards/RTPObjMedicationSafety032608.aspx (accessed 03 Feb 2012).

Suggested Readings

1. Cohen MR (Ed.). Medication errors. Washington, DC: American Pharmacists Association; 2007.

2. Manasse HR, Thompson KK (Eds.). Medication safety: a guide for health care facilities. Bethesda, MD: American Society of Health-System Pharmacists; 2005.

3. Hepler CD, Segal R. Preventing medication errors and improving drug therapy outcomes: a management systems approach. Boca Raton, FL: CRC Press; 2003.

4. Joint Commission Resources. Medication use: a systems approach to reducing errors, 2nd ed. Oakbrook Terrace, IL: Joint Commission Resources; 2008.

5. Kohn LT, Corrigan JM, Donaldson MS (Eds.). To err is human: building a safer health system. Washington, DC: National Academy Press; 1999.

6. Committee on Quality of Health Care in America, Institute of Medicine. Crossing the quality chasm: a new health system for the 21st Century. Washington, DC: National Academy Press; 2001.

7. Committee on Data Standards for Patient Safety, Institute of Medicine. Patient safety: achieving a new standard for care. Washington, DC: National Academy Press; 2004.

8. Committee on the Work Environment for Nurses and Patient Safety, Board on Health Care Services, Institute of Medicine. Page A (Ed.). Keeping patients safe: transforming the work environment of nurses. Washington, DC: National Academy Press; 2004.

9. Committee on Identifying and Preventing Medication Errors, Board on Health Care Services, Institute of Medicine. Aspden P, Wolcott JA, Bootman JL, et al. (Eds.). Preventing medication errors. Washington, DC: National Academy Press; 2007.

Web Resources

www.ashp.org
www.ismp.org
www.safemedication.com
www.asmso.org
www.ahrq.gov
http://www.fda.gov/cder/drugSafety.htm
www.ihi.org
http://www.jointcommission.org/standards_information/npsgs.aspx
http://www.leapfroggroup.org/
www.qualityforum.org
www.nccmerp.org
www.usp.org
http://www.patientsafety.gov/

Approved by the ASHP Board of Directors on April 13, 2012, and by the ASHP House of Delegates on June 10, 2012. Developed through the ASHP Section of Inpatient Care Practitioners Section Advisory Group on Medication Safety and approved by the ASHP Council on Education and Workforce Development on February 21, 2012.

Lynn Eschenbacher, Pharm.D., M.B.A., is gratefully acknowledged for drafting this statement.

Note: This statement had not been published in the *American Journal of Health-System Pharmacy* (*AJHP*) when *Best Practices for Hospital & Health-System Pharmacy 2012–2013* went to press. Some minor editorial differences may exist between this document and the official one that will eventually appear in *AJHP* and subsequent editions of this publication.

ASHP Guidelines on Adverse Drug Reaction Monitoring and Reporting

Pharmacists in organized health care systems should develop comprehensive, ongoing programs for monitoring and reporting adverse drug reactions (ADRs).[1] It is the pharmacist's responsibility and professional obligation to report any suspected ADRs. ADR-monitoring and reporting programs encourage ADR surveillance, facilitate ADR documentation, promote the reporting of ADRs, provide a mechanism for monitoring the safety of drug use in high-risk patient populations, and stimulate the education of health professionals regarding potential ADRs. A comprehensive, ongoing ADR program should include mechanisms for monitoring, detecting, evaluating, documenting, and reporting ADRs as well as intervening and providing educational feedback to prescribers, other health care professionals, and patients. Additionally, ADR programs should focus on identifying problems leading to ADRs, planning for positive changes, and measuring the results of these changes. Positive outcomes resulting from an ADR program should be emphasized to support program growth and development.

ASHP does not suggest that there is a predictable rate of incidence or severity of ADRs. The number and severity of ADRs reported in a given organization or setting would vary with the organization's size, type, patient mix, drugs used, and the ADR definition used.

Definitions

ASHP defines a significant ADR as any unexpected, unintended, undesired, or excessive response to a drug that

1. Requires discontinuing the drug (therapeutic or diagnostic),
2. Requires changing the drug therapy,
3. Requires modifying the dose (except for minor dosage adjustments),
4. Necessitates admission to a hospital,
5. Prolongs stay in a health care facility,
6. Necessitates supportive treatment,
7. Significantly complicates diagnosis,
8. Negatively affects prognosis, or
9. Results in temporary or permanent harm, disability, or death.

Consistent with this definition, an *allergic reaction* (an immunologic hypersensitivity, occurring as the result of unusual sensitivity to a drug) and an *idiosyncratic reaction* (an abnormal susceptibility to a drug that is peculiar to the individual) are also considered ADRs.

Several other definitions of ADRs exist, including those of the World Health Organization (WHO),[2] Karch and Lasagna,[3] and the Food and Drug Administration (FDA).[4]

WHO: "Any response to a drug which is noxious and unintended, and which occurs at doses normally used in man for prophylaxis, diagnosis, or therapy of disease, or for the modification of physiological function."

Karch and Lasagna: "Any response to a drug that is noxious and unintended, and that occurs at doses used in humans for prophylaxis, diagnosis, or therapy, excluding failure to accomplish the intended purpose."

FDA: For reporting purposes, FDA categorizes a *serious adverse event* (events relating to drugs or devices) as one in which "the patient outcome is death, life-threatening (real risk of dying), hospitalization (initial or prolonged), disability (significant, persistent, or permanent), congenital anomaly, or required intervention to prevent permanent impairment or damage."

For perspective, it may be helpful to note events that are not classified as ADRs. A *side effect* is defined by ASHP as an expected, well-known reaction resulting in little or no change in patient management (e.g., drowsiness or dry mouth due to administration of certain antihistamines or nausea associated with the use of antineoplastics). ASHP further defines a side effect as an effect with a predictable frequency and an effect whose intensity and occurrence are related to the size of the dose. Additionally, drug withdrawal, drug-abuse syndromes, accidental poisoning, and drug-overdose complications should not be defined as ADRs.

While individual health care organizations may need to apply ADR surveillance to different degrees for different groups of patients, ASHP believes it would be greatly beneficial if a common definition of ADRs were used in all settings to facilitate reporting, collective surveillance, and ADR-trend research.

Program Features

A comprehensive ADR-monitoring and reporting program should be an integral part of an organization's overall drug-use system. An ADR-monitoring and reporting program should include the following features:

1. The program should establish
 a. An ongoing and concurrent (during drug therapy) surveillance system based on the reporting of suspected ADRs by pharmacists, physicians, nurses, or patients.[5]
 b. A prospective (before drug therapy) surveillance system for high-risk drugs or patients with a high risk for ADRs.
 c. A concurrent surveillance system for monitoring alerting orders. Alerting orders include the use of "tracer" drugs that are used to treat common ADRs (e.g., orders for immediate doses of antihistamines, epinephrine, and corticosteroids), abrupt discontinuation or decreases in dosage of a drug, or stat orders for laboratory assessment of therapeutic drug levels.[6,7]
2. Prescribers, caregivers, and patients should be notified regarding suspected ADRs.
3. Information regarding suspected ADRs should be reported to the pharmacy for complete data collection

and analysis, including the patient's name, the patient's medical and medication history, a description of the suspected ADR, the temporal sequence of the event, any remedial treatment required, and sequelae.

4. High-risk patients should be identified and monitored. High-risk patients include but are not limited to pediatric patients, geriatric patients, patients with organ failure (e.g., hepatic or renal failure), and patients receiving multiple drugs.[6]

5. Drugs likely to cause ADRs ("high-risk" drugs) should be identified, and their use should be monitored. Examples of drugs that may be considered as high risk include aminoglycosides, amphotericin, antineoplastics, corticosteroids, digoxin, heparin, lidocaine, phenytoin, theophylline, thrombolytic agents, and warfarin.[6]

6. The cause(s) of each suspected ADR should be evaluated on the basis of the patient's medical and medication history, the circumstances of the adverse event, the results of dechallenge and rechallenge (if any), alternative etiologies, and a literature review.

7. A method for assigning the probability of a reported or suspected ADR (e.g., confirmed or definite, likely, possible, and unlikely) should be developed to categorize each ADR. Algorithms[8–10] may be useful in establishing the causes of suspected ADRs. Subjective questions and the professional judgment of a pharmacist can be used as additional tools to determine the probability of an ADR. Questions might include the following:
 a. Was there a temporal relationship between the onset of drug therapy and the adverse reaction?
 b. Was there a dechallenge; i.e., did the signs and symptoms of the adverse reaction subside when the drug was withdrawn?
 c. Can signs and symptoms of the adverse reaction be explained by the patient's disease state?
 d. Were there any laboratory tests that provide evidence for the reaction being an ADR?
 e. What was the patient's previous general experience with the drug?
 f. Did symptoms return when the agent was readministered?

8. A method for ranking ADRs by severity should be established.[11]

9. A description of each suspected ADR and the outcomes from the event should be documented in the patient's medical record.

10. Serious or unexpected ADRs should be reported to the Food and Drug Administration (FDA) or the drug's manufacturer (or both).[a]

11. All ADR reports should be reviewed and evaluated by a designated multidisciplinary committee (e.g., a pharmacy and therapeutics committee).

12. ADR-report information should be disseminated to health care professional staff members for educational purposes. Good topics for medical staff education include preventing ADRs and appropriate and effective care for patients who experience ADRs. Educational programs can be conducted as morning "report" discussions, newsletters, "grand rounds" presentations, algorithms for treatment, and multidisciplinary reviews of drug-use evaluations. Patient confidentiality should be preserved.

13. In settings where it is possible, a pharmacy-coordinated ADR team or committee, consisting of a physician, nurse, quality improvement leader, an administrator, and a pharmacist is recommended.[12–15] The team should be charged with adopting a definition for the organization, promoting awareness of the consequences of ADRs, establishing mechanisms for identifying and reporting ADRs, reviewing ADR patterns or trends, and developing preventive and corrective interventions.

14. Continuous monitoring of patient outcomes and patterns of ADRs is imperative. Findings from an ADR-monitoring and reporting program should be incorporated into the organization's ongoing quality improvement activities. The process should include the following:
 a. Feedback to all appropriate health care staff,
 b. Continuous monitoring for trends, clusters, or significant individual ADRs,
 c. Educational efforts for prevention of ADRs, and
 d. Evaluation of prescribing patterns, patient monitoring practices, patient outcomes, and the ADR program's effect on overall and individual patient outcomes.

An overall goal of the ADR process should be the achievement of positive patient outcomes.

Benefits

An ongoing ADR-monitoring and reporting program can provide benefits to the organization, pharmacists, other health care professionals, and patients. These benefits include (but are not limited to) the following:

1. Providing an indirect measure of the quality of pharmaceutical care through identification of preventable ADRs and anticipatory surveillance for high-risk drugs or patients.

2. Complementing organizational risk-management activities and efforts to minimize liability.

3. Assessing the safety of drug therapies, especially recently approved drugs.

4. Measuring ADR incidence.

5. Educating health care professionals and patients about drug effects and increasing their level of awareness regarding ADRs.

6. Providing quality-assurance screening findings for use in drug-use evaluation programs.

7. Measuring the economic impact of ADR prevention as manifested through reduced hospitalization, optimal and economical drug use, and minimized organizational liability.

Role of the Pharmacist

Pharmacists should exert leadership in the development, maintenance, and ongoing evaluation of ADR programs. They should obtain formal endorsement or approval of such programs through appropriate committees (e.g., a pharmacy and therapeutics committee and the executive committee of the medical staff) and the organization's administration. In settings where applicable, input into the design of the pro-

gram should be obtained from the medical staff, nursing staff, quality improvement staff, medical records department, and risk managers.[8,16–18] The pharmacist should facilitate

1. Analysis of each reported ADR,
2. Identification of drugs and patients at high risk for being involved in ADRs,
3. The development of policies and procedures for the ADR-monitoring and reporting program,
4. A description of the responsibilities and interactions of pharmacists, physicians, nurses, risk managers, and other health professionals in the ADR program,
5. Use of the ADR program for educational purposes,
6. Development, maintenance, and evaluation of ADR records within the organization,
7. The organizational dissemination and use of information obtained through the ADR program,
8. Reporting of serious ADRs to the FDA or the manufacturer (or both), and
9. Publication and presentation of important ADRs to the medical community.

Direct patient care roles for pharmacists should include patient counseling on ADRs, identification and documentation in the patient's medical record of high-risk patients, monitoring to ensure that serum drug concentrations remain within acceptable therapeutic ranges, and adjusting doses in appropriate patients (e.g., patients with impaired renal or hepatic function).

References

1. American Society of Hospital Pharmacists. ASHP technical assistance bulletin on hospital drug distribution and control. *Am J Hosp Pharm.* 1980; 37:1097–103.
2. Requirements for adverse reaction reporting. Geneva, Switzerland: World Health Organization; 1975.
3. Karch FE, Lasagna L. Adverse drug reactions—a critical review. *JAMA.* 1975; 234:1236–41.
4. Kessler DA. Introducing MedWatch, using FDA form 3500, a new approach to reporting medication and device adverse effects and product problems. *JAMA.* 1993; 269:2765–8.
5. Prosser TR, Kamysz PL. Multidisciplinary adverse drug reaction surveillance program. *Am J Hosp Pharm.* 1990; 47:1334–9.
6. Koch KE. Adverse drug reactions. In: Brown TR, ed. Handbook of institutional pharmacy practice. 3rd ed. Bethesda, MD: American Society of Hospital Pharmacists; 1992.
7. Koch KE. Use of standard screening procedures to identify adverse drug reactions. *Am J Hosp Pharm.* 1990; 47:1314–20.
8. Karch FE, Lasagna L. Toward the operational identification of adverse drug reactions. *Clin Pharmacol Ther.* 1977; 21:247–54.
9. Kramer MS, Leventhal JM, Hutchinson TA, et al. An algorithm for the operational assessment of adverse drug reactions. I. Background, description, and instructions for use. *JAMA.* 1979; 242:623–32.
10. Naranjo CA, Busto U, Sellers EM, et al. A method for estimating the probability of adverse drug reactions. *Clin Pharmacol Ther.* 1981; 30:239–45.
11. Hartwig SC, Siegel J, Schneider PJ. Preventability and severity assessment in reporting adverse drug reactions. *Am J Hosp Pharm.* 1992; 49:2229–32.
12. Accreditation Manual for Hospitals. Chicago: Joint Commission on Accreditation of Healthcare Organizations; 1989:121, 180.
13. Keith MR, Bellanger-McCleery RA, Fuchs JE. Multidisciplinary program for detecting and evaluating adverse drug reactions. *Am J Hosp Pharm.* 1989; 46:1809–12.
14. Kimelblatt BJ, Young SH, Heywood PM, et al. Improved reporting of adverse drug reactions. *Am J Hosp Pharm.* 1988; 45:1086–9.
15. Nelson RW, Shane R. Developing an adverse drug reaction reporting program. *Am J Hosp Pharm.* 1983; 40:445–6.
16. Swanson KM, Landry JP, Anderson RP. Pharmacy-coordinated, multidisciplinary adverse drug reaction program. *Top Hosp Pharm Manage.* 1992; 12(Jul):49–59.
17. Flowers P, Dzierba S, Baker O. A continuous quality improvement team approach to adverse drug reaction reporting. *Top Hosp Pharm Manage.* 1992; 12(Jul): 60–7.
18. Guharoy SR. A pharmacy-coordinated, multidisciplinary approach for successful implementation of an adverse drug reaction reporting program. *Top Hosp Pharm Manage.* 1992; 12(Jul):68–74.

[a]To report an adverse drug event to the FDA, use the MedWatch program. Reports can be mailed (MedWatch, 5600 Fishers Lane, Rockville, MD 20852–9787), faxed (800-FDA-0178), called in (800-FDA-1088), or reported by modem (800-FDA-7737). An easy-to-use FDA form 3500 can be used. This form should be available from a pharmacy.

Approved by the ASHP Board of Directors, November 16, 1994. Revised by the ASHP Council on Professional Affairs. Supersedes a previous version dated November 16, 1988.

The bibliographic citation for this document is as follows: American Society of Health-System Pharmacists. ASHP guidelines on adverse drug reaction monitoring and reporting. *Am J Health-Syst Pharm.* 1995; 52:417–9.

ASHP Guidelines on Preventing Medication Errors in Hospitals

The goal of drug therapy is the achievement of defined therapeutic outcomes that improve a patient's quality of life while minimizing patient risk.[1] There are inherent risks, both known and unknown, associated with the therapeutic use of drugs (prescription and nonprescription) and drug administration devices. The incidents or hazards that result from such risk have been defined as drug misadventuring, which includes both adverse drug reactions (ADRs) and medication errors.[2] This document addresses medication errors—episodes in drug misadventuring that should be preventable through effective systems controls involving pharmacists, physicians and other prescribers, nurses, risk management personnel, legal counsel, administrators, patients, and others in the organizational setting, as well as regulatory agencies and the pharmaceutical industry.

This document suggests medication error prevention approaches that should be considered in the development of organizational systems and discusses methods of managing medication errors once they have occurred. These guidelines are primarily intended to apply to the inpatient hospital setting because of the special collaborative processes established in the setting [e.g., formulary system, pharmacy and therapeutics (P&T) committee, and opportunity for increased interaction among health-care providers].

Recommendations for practice settings other than hospitals are beyond the scope of this document, although many of the ideas and principles may be applicable.

Medication errors compromise patient confidence in the health-care system and increase health-care costs. The problems and sources of medication errors are multidisciplinary and multifactorial. Errors occur from lack of knowledge, substandard performance and mental lapses, or defects or failures in systems.[3,4] Medication errors may be committed by both experienced and inexperienced staff, including pharmacists, physicians, nurses, supportive personnel (e.g., pharmacy technicians), students, clerical staff (e.g., ward clerks), administrators, pharmaceutical manufacturers, patients and their caregivers, and others. The incidence of medication errors is indeterminate; valid comparisons of different studies on medication errors are extremely difficult because of differences in variables, measurements, populations, and methods.[2]

Many medication errors are probably undetected. The outcome(s) or clinical significance of many medication errors may be minimal, with few or no consequences that adversely affect a patient. Tragically, however, some medication errors result in serious patient morbidity or mortality.[3] Thus, medication errors must not be taken lightly, and effective systems for ordering, dispensing, and administering medications should be established with safeguards to prevent the occurrence of errors. These systems should involve adequately trained and supervised personnel, adequate communications, reasonable workloads, effective drug handling systems, multiple procedural and final product checks by separate individuals, quality management, and adequate facilities, equipment, and supplies.

The pharmacist's mission is to help ensure that patients make the best use of medications.[5] This applies to all drugs used by inpatients or ambulatory patients, including oral or injectable products, radiopharmaceuticals, radiopaque contrast media, anesthetic gases, blood-fraction drugs, dialysis fluids, respiratory therapy agents, investigational drugs, drug samples, drugs brought into the hospital setting by patients, and other chemical or biological substances administered to patients to evoke a pharmacological response.[6]

Through a systems-oriented approach, the pharmacist should lead collaborative, multidisciplinary efforts to prevent, detect, and resolve drug-related problems that can result in patient harm.[1] An understanding of the risk factors associated with medication errors should enable improved monitoring of patients and medications associated with increased risk for serious errors and should enable the development of organizational systems designed to minimize risk.[7] The pharmacist should participate in appropriate organizational committees and work with physicians, nurses, administrators, and others to examine and improve systems to ensure that medication processes are safe.

Types of Medication Errors

Medication errors include prescribing errors, dispensing errors, medication administration errors, and patient compliance errors. Specific types of medication errors are categorized in Table 1, based on a compilation of the literature.[3,7–18]

A *potential error* is a mistake in prescribing, dispensing, or planned medication administration that is detected and corrected through intervention (by another health-care provider or patient) before actual medication administration. Potential errors should be reviewed and tabulated as separate events from errors of occurrence (errors that actually reach patients) to identify opportunities to correct problems in the medication use system even before they occur. Detection of potential errors should be a component of the hospital's routine quality improvement process. Documentation of instances in which an individual has prevented the occurrence of a medication error will help identify system weaknesses and will reinforce the importance of multiple checks in the medication use system.

Recommendations for Preventing Medication Errors

Organizational systems for ordering, dispensing, and administering medications should be designed to minimize error. Medication errors may involve process breakdowns in more than one aspect of a system. This section provides recommendations to the management staff (general and departmental) of hospitals, as well as to individual prescribers, pharmacists, nurses, patients, pharmaceutical manufacturers, and others.

Organizational and Departmental Recommendations. Organizational policies and procedures should be established to prevent medication errors. Development of the policies and procedures should involve multiple departments, including pharmacy, medicine, nursing, risk management, legal counsel, and organizational administration. The following recommendations are offered for organizational management and clinical staff:[3,8,11–14,16,19–29]

Table 1.
Types of Medication Errors[3,7–18,a]

Type	Definition
Prescribing error	Incorrect drug selection (based on indications, contraindications, known allergies, existing drug therapy, and other factors), dose, dosage form, quantity, route, concentration, rate of administration, or instructions for use of a drug product ordered or authorized by physician (or other legitimate prescriber); illegible prescriptions or medication orders that lead to errors that reach the patient
Omission error[b]	The failure to administer an ordered dose to a patient before the next scheduled dose, if any
Wrong time error	Administration of medication outside a predefined time interval from its scheduled administration time (this interval should be established by each individual health care facility)
Unauthorized drug error[c]	Administration to the patient of medication not authorized by a legitimate prescriber for the patient
Improper dose error[d]	Administration to the patient of a dose that is greater than or less than the amount ordered by the prescriber or administration of duplicate doses to the patient, i.e., one or more dosage units in addition to those that were ordered
Wrong dosage-form error[e]	Administration to the patient of a drug product in a different dosage form than ordered by the prescriber
Wrong drug-preparation error[f]	Drug product incorrectly formulated or manipulated before administration
Wrong administration-technique error[g]	Inappropriate procedure or improper technique in the administration of a drug
Deteriorated drug error[h]	Administration of a drug that has expired or for which the physical or chemical dosage-form integrity has been compromised
Monitoring error	Failure to review a prescribed regimen for appropriateness and detection of problems, or failure to use appropriate clinical or laboratory data for adequate assessment of patient response to prescribed therapy
Compliance error	Inappropriate patient behavior regarding adherence to a prescribed medication regimen
Other medication error	Any medication error that does not fall into one of above predefined categories

[a] The categories may not be mutually exclusive because of the multidisciplinary and multifactorial nature of medication errors.

[b] Assumes no prescribing error. Excluded would be (1) a patient's refusal to take the medication or (2) a decision not to administer the dose because of recognized contraindications. If an explanation for the omission is apparent (e.g., patient was away from nursing unit for tests or medication was not available), that reason should be documented in the appropriate records.

[c] This would include, for example, a wrong drug, a dose given to the wrong patient, unordered drugs, and doses given outside a stated set of clinical guidelines or protocols.

[d] Excluded would be (1) allowable deviations based on preset ranges established by individual health care organizations in consideration of measuring devices routinely provided to those who administer drugs to patients (e.g., not administering a dose based on a patient's measured temperature or blood glucose level) or other factors such as conversion of doses expressed in the apothecary system to the metric system and (2) topical dosage forms for which medication orders are not expressed quantitatively.

[e] Excluded would be accepted protocols (established by the pharmacy and therapeutics committee or its equivalent) that authorize pharmacists to dispense alternate dosage forms for patients with special needs (e.g., liquid formulations for patients with nasogastric tubes or those who have difficulty swallowing), as allowed by state regulations.

[f] This would include, for example, incorrect dilution or reconstitution, mixing drugs that are physically or chemically incompatible, and inadequate product packaging.

[g] This would include doses administered (1) via the wrong route (different from the route prescribed), (2) via the correct route but at the wrong site (e.g., left eye instead of right), and (3) at the wrong rate of administration.

[h] This would include, for example, administration of expired drugs and improperly stored drugs.

1. Using the principles of the formulary system, the P&T committee (or its equivalent)—composed of pharmacists, physicians, nurses, and other health professionals—should be responsible for formulating policies regarding the evaluation, selection, and therapeutic use of drugs in organized health-care settings.

2. Care and consideration must be given in hiring and assigning personnel involved in medication ordering, preparation, dispensing, administration, and patient education. Policies and procedures should be developed that ensure adequate personnel selection, training, supervision, and evaluation. This would include the need to ensure proper interviewing, orientation, evaluation of competency, supervision, and opportunities for continuing professional and technical education.

3. Sufficient personnel must be available to perform tasks adequately. Policies and procedures should ensure that reasonable workload levels and working hours are established and rarely exceeded.

4. Suitable work environments should exist for the preparation of drug products. Potential error sources within the work environment, such as frequent interruptions, should be identified and minimized.

5. Lines of authority and areas of responsibility within the hospital should be clearly defined for medication ordering, dispensing, and administration. The system should ensure adequate written and oral communications among personnel involved in the medication use process to optimize therapeutic appropriateness and to enable medications to be prescribed, dispensed, and administered in a timely fashion. All systems should provide for review and verification of the prescriber's original order (except in emergency situations) before a drug product is dispensed by a pharmacist. Any necessary clarifications or changes in a medication order must be resolved with the prescriber before a medication is administered to the patient. Written documentation of such consultations should be made in the patient's medical record or other appropriate record. Nursing staff should be informed of any changes made in the medication order. Changes required to correct incorrect orders should be regarded as potential errors, assuming the changes occurred in time to prevent the error from reaching the patient.

6. There should be an ongoing, systematic program of quality improvement and peer review with respect to the safe use of medications. A formal drug use evaluation (DUE) program, developed and conducted through collaborative efforts among medicine, pharmacy, and nursing, should be integrated and coordinated with the overall hospital quality improvement program. To prevent medication errors, a portion of the DUE program should focus on monitoring

the appropriate use of any drugs associated with a high frequency of adverse events, including specific drug classes (such as antimicrobials, antineoplastic agents, and cardiovascular drugs) and injectable dosage forms (e.g., potassium products, narcotic substances, heparin, lidocaine, procainamide, magnesium sulfate, and insulin). The quality improvement program should include a system for monitoring, reviewing, and reporting medication errors to assist in identifying and eliminating causes of errors (system breakdowns) and preventing their recurrence. Table 2 lists common causes of medication errors, i.e., areas where there may be system breakdowns.

7. Pharmacists and others responsible for processing drug orders should have routine access to appropriate clinical information about patients (including medication, allergy, and hypersensitivity profiles; diagnoses; pregnancy status; and laboratory values) to help evaluate the appropriateness of medication orders.

8. Pharmacists should maintain medication profiles for all patients, both inpatients and ambulatory patients, who receive care at the hospital. This profile should include adequate information to allow monitoring of medication histories, allergies, diagnoses, potential drug interactions and ADRs, duplicate drug therapies, pertinent laboratory data, and other information.

9. The pharmacy department must be responsible for the procurement, distribution, and control of all drugs used within the organization. Adequate hours for the provision of pharmaceutical services must be maintained; 24-hour pharmaceutical service is strongly recommended in hospital settings. In the absence of 24-hour pharmaceutical service, access to a limited supply of medications should be available to authorized nonpharmacists for use in initiating urgent medication orders. The list of medications to be supplied and the policies and procedures to be used (including subsequent review of all activity by a pharmacist) should be developed by the P&T committee (or its equivalent). Items should be chosen with safety in mind, limiting wherever possible medications, quantities, dosage forms, and container sizes that might endanger patients. The use of well-designed night cabinets, after-hours drug carts, and other methods would preclude the need for non-pharmacists to enter the pharmacy. Access to the pharmacy by nonpharmacists (e.g., nurses) for removal of doses is strongly discouraged; this practice should be minimized and eliminated to the fullest extent

Table 2.
Common Causes of Medication Errors

Ambiguous strength designation on labels or in packaging
Drug product nomenclature (look-alike or sound-alike names, use of lettered or numbered prefixes and suffixes in drug names)
Equipment failure or malfunction
Illegible handwriting
Improper transcription
Inaccurate dosage calculation
Inadequately trained personnel
Inappropriate abbreviations used in prescribing
Labeling errors
Excessive workload
Lapses in individual performance
Medication unavailable

possible. When 24-hour pharmacy service is not feasible, a pharmacist must be available on an "on-call" basis.

10. The pharmacy manager (or designee), with the assistance of the P&T committee (or its equivalent) and the department of nursing, should develop comprehensive policies and procedures that provide for efficient and safe distribution of all medications and related supplies to patients. For safety, the recommended method of distribution within the organized health-care setting is the unit dose drug distribution and control system.

11. Except in emergency situations, all sterile and nonsterile drug products should be dispensed from the pharmacy department for individual patients. The storage of non-emergency floor stock medications on the nursing units or in patient-care areas should be minimized. Particular caution should be exercised with respect to drug products that have commonly been involved in serious medication errors or whose margin of safety is narrow, such as concentrated forms of drug products that are intended to be diluted into larger volumes (e.g., concentrated lidocaine and potassium chloride for injection concentrate). All drug storage areas should be routinely inspected by pharmacy personnel to ensure adequate product integrity and appropriate packaging, labeling, and storage. It is important that drug products and other products for external use be stored separately from drug products for internal use.

12. The pharmacy director and staff must ensure that all drug products used in the organizational setting are of high quality and integrity. This would include, for example, (1) selecting multisource products supported by adequate bioavailability data and adequate product packaging and labeling, (2) maintaining an unexpired product inventory, and (3) keeping abreast of compendial requirements.

13. The use of a patient's own or "home" medications should be avoided to the fullest extent possible. Use of such medications should be allowed only if there is a need for the patient to receive the therapy, the drug product is not obtainable by the pharmacy, and no alternative therapy can be prescribed. If such medications are used, the prescribing physician must write an appropriate order in the patient's medical record. Before use, a pharmacist should inspect and identify the medication. If there are any unresolved questions with respect to product identity or integrity, the medication must not be used.

14. All discontinued or unused drugs should be returned to the department of pharmacy immediately on discontinuation or at patient discharge. Discharged patients must not be given unlabeled drug products to take home, unless they are labeled for outpatient use by the pharmacy in accordance with state and federal regulations. Discharged patients should be counseled about use of any medications to be used after discharge.

15. It is recommended that there be computerized pharmacy systems in place that enable automated checking for doses, duplicate therapies, allergies, drug interactions, and other aspects of use. Where possible, the use of technological innovations such as bar coding is recommended to help identify patients, products, and care providers. Pharmacy-generated medication administra-

tion records or labels are recommended to assist nurses in interpreting and documenting medication activities.

16. Adequate drug information resources should be available for all health-care providers involved in the drug use process.

17. Standard drug administration times should be established for the hospital by the P&T committee (or its equivalent), with input from the departments of nursing and pharmacy. Policies and procedures should allow for deviations from the standard times when necessary. Further, standard drug concentrations and dosage charts should be developed to minimize the need for dosage calculations by staff.

18. The P&T committee (or its equivalent) should develop a list of standard abbreviations approved for use in medication ordering. There should be efforts to prohibit or discourage the use of other abbreviations in medication ordering.

19. A review mechanism should be established through the P&T committee specifying those responsible for data collection and evaluation of medication error reports. The review group should investigate causes of errors and develop programs for decreasing their occurrence. The review group should be composed of representatives from pharmacy, nursing, medicine, quality assurance, staff education, risk management, and legal counsel.

20. The pharmacy department, in conjunction with nursing, risk management, and the medical staff, should conduct ongoing educational programs to discuss medication errors, their causes, and methods to prevent their occurrence. Such programs might involve seminars, newsletters, or other methods of information dissemination.

Recommendations for Prescribers. Prescribing is an early point at which medication errors can arise. It has been estimated that 1% of hospitalized patients suffer adverse events as the result of medical mismanagement[30] and that drug-related complications are the most common type of adverse event.[7] The following recommendations for preventing medication errors are suggested for physicians and other prescribers[3,7,11–16,31]:

1. To determine appropriate drug therapy, prescribers should stay abreast of the current state of knowledge through literature review, consultation with pharmacists, consultation with other physicians, participation in continuing professional education programs, and other means. It is especially crucial to seek information when prescribing for conditions and diseases not typically experienced in the prescriber's practice.

2. Prescribers should evaluate the patient's total status and review all existing drug therapy before prescribing new or additional medications to ascertain possible antagonistic or complementary drug interactions. To evaluate and optimize patient response to prescribed drug therapy, appropriate monitoring of clinical signs and symptoms and of relevant laboratory data is necessary.

3. In hospitals, prescribers should be familiar with the medication ordering system (e.g., the formulary system, participation in DUE programs, allowable delegation of authority, procedures to alert nurses and others to new drug orders that need to be processed, standard medication administration times, and approved abbreviations).

4. Drug orders should be complete. They should include patient name, generic drug name, trademarked name (if a specific product is required), route and site of administration, dosage form, dose, strength, quantity, frequency of administration, and prescriber's name. In some cases, a dilution, rate, and time of administration should be specified. The desired therapeutic outcome for each drug should be expressed when the drug is prescribed. Prescribers should review all drug orders for accuracy and legibility immediately after they have prescribed them.

5. Care should be taken to ensure that the intent of medication orders is clear and unambiguous. Prescribers should

 a. Write out instructions rather than using nonstandard or ambiguous abbreviations. For example, write "daily" rather than "q.d.," which could be misinterpreted as q.i.d. (causing a drug to be given four times a day instead of once) or as o.d. (for right eye).

 b. Do not use vague instructions, such as "take as directed," because specific instructions can help differentiate among intended drugs.

 c. Specify exact dosage strengths (such as milligrams) rather than dosage form units (such as one tablet or one vial). An exception would be combination drug products, for which the number of dosage form units should be specified.

 d. Prescribe by standard nomenclature, using the drug's generic name (United States Adopted Name or USAN), official name, or trademarked name (if deemed medically necessary). Avoid the following: locally coined names (e.g., Dr. Doe's syrup); chemical names [e.g., 6-mercaptopurine (instead of mercaptopurine) could result in a six-fold overdose if misinterpreted]; unestablished abbreviated drug names (e.g., "AZT" could stand for zidovudine, azathioprine, or aztreonam); acronyms; and apothecary or chemical symbols.

 e. Always use a leading zero before a decimal expression of less than one (e.g., 0.5 ml). Conversely, a terminal zero should never be used (e.g., 5.0 ml), since failure to see the decimal could result in a 10-fold overdose. When possible, avoid the use of decimals (e.g., prescribe 500 mg instead of 0.5 g).

 f. Spell out the word "units" (e.g., 10 units regular insulin) rather than writing "u," which could be misinterpreted as a zero.

 g. Use the metric system.

6. Written drug or prescription orders (including signatures) should be legible. Prescribers with poor handwriting should print or type medication or prescription orders if direct order entry capabilities for computerized systems are unavailable. A handwritten order should be completely readable (not merely recognizable through familiarity). An illegible handwritten order should be regarded as a potential error. If it leads to an error of occurrence (that is, the error actually reaches the patient), it should be regarded as a prescribing error.

7. Verbal drug or prescription orders (that is, orders that are orally communicated) should be reserved only for those situations in which it is impossible or impractical for the prescriber to write the order or enter it in the computer. The prescriber should dictate verbal orders slowly, clearly, and articulately to avoid confusion. Special caution is urged in the prescribing of drug dosages in the teens (e.g., a 15-mEq dose of potassium chloride could be misheard as a 50-mEq dose). The order should be read back to the prescriber by the recipient (i.e., the nurse or pharmacist, according to institutional policies). When read back, the drug name should be spelled to the prescriber and, when directions are repeated, no abbreviations should be used (e.g., say "three times daily" rather than "t.i.d."). A written copy of the verbal order should be placed in the patient's medical record and later confirmed by the prescriber in accordance with applicable state regulations and hospital policies.

8. When possible, drugs should be prescribed for administration by the oral route rather than by injection.

9. When possible, the prescriber should talk with the patient or caregiver to explain the medication prescribed and any special precautions or observations that might be indicated, including any allergic or hypersensitivity reactions that might occur.

10. Prescribers should follow up and periodically evaluate the need for continued drug therapy for individual patients.

11. Instructions with respect to "hold" orders for medications should be clear.

Recommendations for Pharmacists. The pharmacist is expected to play a pivotal role in preventing medication misuse. The value of pharmacists' interventions to prevent medication errors that would have resulted from inappropriate prescribing has been documented.[7,32,33] Ideally, the pharmacist should collaborate with the prescriber in developing, implementing, and monitoring a therapeutic plan to produce defined therapeutic outcomes for the patient.[1] It is also vital that the pharmacist devote careful attention to dispensing processes to ensure that errors are not introduced at that point in the medication process. The following recommendations are suggested for pharmacists[3,4,8–10,14,16,18–20,28,29]:

1. Pharmacists should participate in drug therapy monitoring (including the following, when indicated: the assessment of therapeutic appropriateness, medication administration appropriateness, and possible duplicate therapies; review for possible interactions; and evaluation of pertinent clinical and laboratory data) and DUE activities to help achieve safe, effective, and rational use of drugs.

2. To recommend and recognize appropriate drug therapy, pharmacists should stay abreast of the current state of knowledge through familiarity with literature, consultation with colleagues and other health-care providers, participation in continuing professional education programs, and other means.

3. Pharmacists should make themselves available to prescribers and nurses to offer information and advice about therapeutic drug regimens and the correct use of medications.

4. Pharmacists should be familiar with the medication ordering system and drug distribution policies and procedures established for the organizational setting to provide for the safe distribution of all medications and related supplies to inpatients and ambulatory patients. In particular, pharmacists should be familiar with all elements that are designed into the system to prevent or detect errors. Actions by any staff that would (even unintentionally) defeat or compromise those elements should serve as "alerts" to the pharmacist that safety may be affected. Any necessary followup action (e.g., education or reeducation of staff) should ensue promptly. Policies and procedures to be followed for "hold" orders should be clear and understood by pharmacy, medical, and nursing staffs.

5. Pharmacists should never assume or guess the intent of confusing medication orders. If there are any questions, the prescriber should be contacted prior to dispensing.

6. When preparing drugs, pharmacists should maintain orderliness and cleanliness in the work area and perform one procedure at a time with as few interruptions as possible.

7. Before dispensing a medication in nonemergency situations, the pharmacist should review an original copy of the written medication order. The pharmacist should ensure that all work performed by supportive personnel or through the use of automated devices is checked by manual or technological means. All processes must conform with applicable state and federal laws and regulations. Pharmacists should participate in, at a minimum, a self-checking process in reading prescriptions, labeling (drug or ingredients and pharmacist-generated labeling), and dosage calculations. For high risk drug products, when possible, all work should be checked by a second individual (preferably, another pharmacist). Pharmacists must make certain that the following are accurate: drug, labeling, packaging, quantity, dose, and instructions.

8. Pharmacists should dispense medications in ready-to-administer dosage forms whenever possible. The unit dose system is strongly recommended as the preferred method of drug distribution. The need for nurses to manipulate drugs (e.g., measure, repackage, and calculate) prior to their administration should be minimized.

9. Pharmacists should review the use of auxiliary labels and use the labels prudently when it is clear that such use may prevent errors (e.g., "shake well," "for external use only," and "not for injection").

10. Pharmacists should ensure that medications are delivered to the patient-care area in a timely fashion after receipt of orders, according to hospital policies and procedures. If medication doses are not delivered or if therapy is delayed for any reason pending resolution of a detected problem (e.g., allergy or contraindications), the pharmacist should notify the nursing staff of the delay and the reason.

11. Pharmacists should observe how medications are actually being used in patient-care areas to ensure that dispensing and storage procedures are followed and to assist nurses in optimizing patient safety.

12. Pharmacy staff should review medications that are returned to the department. Such review processes may reveal system breakdowns or problems that resulted in medication errors (e.g., omitted doses and unauthorized drugs).

13. When dispensing medications to ambulatory patients (e.g., at discharge), pharmacists should counsel patients or caregivers and verify that they understand why a medication was prescribed and dispensed, its intended use, any special precautions that might be observed, and other needed information. For inpatients, pharmacists should make their services available to counsel patients, families, or other caregivers when appropriate.
14. Pharmacists should preview and provide advice on the content and design of preprinted medication order forms or sheets if they are used.
15. Pharmacists should maintain records sufficient to enable identification of patients receiving an erroneous product.

Recommendations for Nurses. By virtue of their direct patient-care activities and administration of medications to patients, nurses—perhaps more than any other health-care providers—are in an excellent position to detect and report medication errors. Nurses often serve as the final point in the checks-and-balances triad (physicians and other prescribers, pharmacists, and nurses) for the medication use process; thus, they play an important role in risk reduction. The following recommendations for preventing medication administration errors are suggested[3,14,16,17,34]:

1. Nurses who practice in organized health-care settings should be familiar with the medication ordering and use system (e.g., participation in DUE activities, order processing, and standard medication administration times).
2. Nurses should review patients' medications with respect to desired patient outcomes, therapeutic duplications, and possible drug interactions. Adequate drug information (including information on medication administration and product compatibilities) should be obtained from pharmacists, nurses, other health-care providers, the literature, and other means when there are questions. There should be appropriate followup communication with the prescriber when this is indicated.
3. All drug orders should be verified before medication administration. Nurses should carefully review original medication orders before administration of the first dose and compare them with medications dispensed. Transcriptions of orders should be avoided to the extent possible and should be recognized as prime opportunities for errors. Doses should not be administered unless the meaning of the original order is clear and unambiguous and there are no questions with respect to the correctness of the prescribed regimen. Nurses should check the identity and integrity (e.g., expiration date and general appearance) of the medications dispensed before administering them. When there are discrepancies, the nurse should contact the pharmacy department and determine the appropriate action.
4. Patient identity should be verified before the administration of each prescribed dose. When appropriate, the patient should be observed after administration of the drug product to ensure that the doses were administered as prescribed and have the intended effect.
5. All doses should be administered at scheduled times unless there are questions or problems to be resolved. Medication doses should not be removed from packaging or labeling until immediately before administra-

tion. The administration of medication should be documented as soon as it is completed.
6. When standard drug concentrations or dosage charts are not available, dosage calculations, flow rates, and other mathematical calculations should be checked by a second individual (e.g., another nurse or a pharmacist).
7. The drug distribution system should not be circumvented by "borrowing" medications from one patient (or another hospital area) to give to a different patient or by stockpiling unused medications. If there are apparent missing doses, it is important that the pharmacy be contacted for explanation or correction. There may be an important reason why the dose was not sent to the patient-care area (e.g., allergy, contraindication, and questionable dose), and resolution of the potential question or problem may be pending.
8. If there are questions when a large volume or number of dosage units (e.g., more than two tablets, capsules, vials, or ampuls) is needed for a single patient dose, the medication order should be verified. Consult with the pharmacist and prescriber as appropriate.
9. All personnel using medication administration devices (e.g., infusion pumps) should understand their operation and the opportunities for error that might occur with the use of such devices.
10. Nurses should talk with patients or caregivers to ascertain that they understand the use of their medications and any special precautions or observations that might be indicated. Any counseling needed should be provided before the first dose is administered, when possible.
11. When a patient objects to or questions whether a particular drug should be administered, the nurse should listen, answer questions, and (if appropriate) double check the medication order and product dispensed before administering it to ensure that no preventable error is made (e.g., wrong patient, wrong route, and dose already administered). If a patient refuses to take a prescribed medication, that decision should be documented in the appropriate patient records.

Recommendations for Patients and Personal Caregivers. Patients (or their authorized caregivers or designees) have the right to know about all aspects of their care, including drug therapy. When patient status allows, health-care providers should encourage patients to take an active role in their drug use by questioning and learning about their treatment regimens. Generally, if patients are more knowledgeable, anxieties about the uncertainty of treatments can be alleviated and errors in treatment may be prevented. The following suggestions are offered to help patients whose health status allows, and their caregivers, make the best use of medications[3]:

1. Patients should inform appropriate direct health-care providers (e.g., physicians, nurses, and pharmacists) about all known symptoms, allergies, sensitivities, and current medication use. Patients should communicate their actual self-medication practices, even if they differ from the prescribed directions.
2. Patients should feel free to ask questions about any procedures and treatments received.
3. atients should learn the names of the drug products that are prescribed and administered to them, as well as dosage strengths and schedules. It is suggested that

patients keep a personal list of all drug therapy, including prescribed drugs, nonprescription drugs, home remedies, and medical foods. Patients should also maintain lists of medications that they cannot take and the reasons why. This information should be shared with health-care providers. Patients should be assertive in communicating with health-care providers when anything seems incorrect or different from the norm.

4. After counseling from an authorized health-care provider about the appropriateness of the medication, patients should take all medications as directed.

Recommendations for Pharmaceutical Manufacturers and Approval Organizations. Poor designs with respect to drug product packaging and labeling, as well as selection of inappropriate or confusing nomenclature, have been identified as factors that contribute to serious medication errors by practitioners.[4,35–37] Pharmaceutical manufacturers and approval agencies should be responsive to efforts of practitioners to minimize errors. The following guidelines are recommended for the pharmaceutical industry and regulatory authorities[3,4,16,38]:

1. Drug manufacturers and the Food and Drug Administration are urged to involve pharmacists, nurses, and physicians in decisions about drug names, labeling, and packaging.
2. Look-alike or sound-alike trademarked names and generic names should be avoided.
3. Similar proprietary appearances of packaging and labeling should be avoided, because look-alike products contribute to medication errors.
4. The use of lettered or numbered prefixes and suffixes in trademarked names is generally discouraged. Lettered prefixes or suffixes could be mistaken for instructions or strength. Commonly used medical abbreviations should never be used in trademarked names (e.g., "HS" could stand for half-strength or a bedtime dose). Numbers as part of trademarked names could be mistaken for quantities to be administered. Coined abbreviations that could be misinterpreted (e.g., MTX, U, and HCTZ) should not be used in trademarked names.
5. Special instructions should be highlighted on labeling, such as the need for dilution before administration.
6. The most prominent items on the product label should be information in the best interest of safety (e.g., product name and strength). Less prominence should be given to company names or logos.
7. Drug manufacturers are encouraged to make dosage forms available commercially in unit dose and unit-of-dispensing containers, as well as bulk packaging, to facilitate their appropriate use in all practice settings.
8. Drug manufacturers must communicate with health-care providers (i.e., pharmacists, physicians, and nurses) when changes are made in product formulations or dosage forms.

Monitoring and Managing Medication Errors

Monitoring Medication Errors. Ongoing quality improvement programs for monitoring medication errors are needed. The difficulty in detecting errors has long been recognized as one of the barriers to studying the problem effectively.[39] Medication errors should be identified and documented and their causes studied in order to develop systems that minimize recurrence.[3,4,7,10,11,14,16,22,40] Several error monitoring techniques exist (e.g., anonymous self-reports, incident reports, critical incident technique, and disguised observation technique) and may be applied as appropriate to determine the rates of errors.[9,40,41] There are differences in the validity of data obtained by the various error monitoring techniques or combined techniques. Program managers should determine the best method for use in their organizations in consideration of utility, feasibility, and cost. Monitoring programs for medication errors should consider the following risk factors[6,10,11,22,40,41]:

1. Work shift (higher error rates typically occur during the day shift).
2. Inexperienced and inadequately trained staff.
3. Medical service (e.g., special needs for certain patient populations, including geriatrics, pediatrics, and oncology).
4. Increased number or quantity of medications per patient.
5. Environmental factors (lighting, noise, and frequent interruptions).
6. Staff workload and fatigue.
7. Poor communication among health-care providers.
8. Dosage form (e.g., injectable drugs are associated with more serious errors).
9. Type of distribution system (unit dose distribution is preferred; floor stock should be minimized).
10. Improper drug storage.
11. Extent of measurements or calculations required.
12. Confusing drug product nomenclature, packaging, or labeling.
13. Drug category (e.g., antimicrobials).
14. Poor handwriting.
15. Verbal (orally communicated) orders.
16. Lack of effective policies and procedures.
17. Poorly functioning oversight committees.

Managing Medication Errors. Medication errors result from problematic processes, but the outcomes of medication errors could range from minimal (or no) patient risk to life-threatening risk. Classification of the potential seriousness and clinical significance of detected medication errors should be based on predefined criteria established by the P&T committee (or its equivalent). The error classification should be based on the original order, standard medication dispensing and administration procedures, dosage forms available, acceptable deviation ranges, potential for adverse consequences and patient harm, and other factors.[6,32,41]

Classification of medication errors should allow for better management of followup activities upon medication error detection. A simple classification of medication errors is the following: (1) clinically significant (includes potentially fatal or severe, potentially serious, and potentially significant errors) or (2) minor.[7,33] Hartwig, Denger, and Schneider defined seven medication error severity levels, as follows[41]:

Level 0—Nonmedication error occurred (potential errors would be classified here).
Level 1—An error occurred that did not result in patient harm.
Level 2—An error occurred that resulted in the need for increased patient monitoring but no change in vital signs and no patient harm.

Level 3—An error occurred that resulted in the need for increased patient monitoring with a change in vital signs but no ultimate patient harm, or any error that resulted in the need for increased laboratory monitoring.

Level 4—An error occurred that resulted in the need for treatment with another drug or an increased length of stay or that affected patient participation in an investigational drug study.[a]

Level 5—An error occurred that resulted in permanent patient harm.

Level 6—An error occurred that resulted in patient death.

Medication error classifications could also be based on probability and severity scales analogous to those used in ADR reporting programs.[42,43]

Determination of the causes of medication errors should be coupled with assessment of the severity of the error. While quality management processes should include programs to decrease the incidence of all medication errors, effort should be concentrated on eliminating the causes of errors associated with greater levels of severity. There should be established mechanisms for tracking drugs or drug classes that are involved in medication errors. Correlations between errors and the method of drug distribution should also be reviewed (e.g., unit dose, floor stock, or bulk medications; premixed or extemporaneously compounded products; and oral or injectable products). These processes will help identify system problems and stimulate changes to minimize the recurrence of errors.

Quality improvement programs should provide guidance for patient support, staff counseling and education, and risk management processes when a medication error is detected. Incident reporting policies and procedures and appropriate counseling, education, and intervention programs should be established in all hospitals. Risk management processes for medication errors should include pharmacists, physicians, and nurses, in addition to risk management specialists, legal counsel, and others as appropriate. The following actions are recommended upon error detection[3,7,10,11,16,17,27,43]:

1. Any necessary corrective and supportive therapy should be provided to the patient.
2. The error should be documented and reported immediately after discovery, in accordance with written procedures. For clinically significant errors, an immediate oral notice should be provided to physicians, nurses, and pharmacy managers. A written medication error report should follow promptly.
3. For clinically significant errors, fact gathering and investigation should be initiated immediately. Facts that should be determined and documented include what happened, where the incident occurred, why the incident occurred, how the incident occurred, and who was involved. Appropriate product evidence (e.g., packaging and labeling) should be retrieved and retained for future reference until causative factors are eliminated or resolved.
4. Reports of clinically significant errors and the associated corrective activities should be reviewed by the supervisor and department head of the area(s) involved, the appropriate organizational administrator, the organizational safety committee (or its equivalent), and legal counsel (as appropriate).
5. When appropriate, the supervisor and the staff members who were involved in the error should confer on how the error occurred and how its recurrence can be prevented. Medication errors often result from problems in systems rather than exclusively from staff performance or environmental factors[2,3,44]; thus, error reports should not be used for punitive purposes but to achieve correction or change.
6. Information gained from medication error reports and other means that demonstrates continued failure of individual professionals to avoid preventable medication errors should serve as an effective management and educational tool in staff development or, if necessary, modification of job functions or staff disciplinary action.
7. Supervisors, department managers, and appropriate committees should periodically review error reports and determine causes of errors and develop actions to prevent their recurrence (e.g., conduct organizational staff education, alter staff levels, revise policies and procedures, or change facilities, equipment, or supplies).
8. Medication errors should be reported to a national monitoring program so that the shared experiences of pharmacists, nurses, physicians, and patients can contribute to improved patient safety and to the development of valuable educational services for the prevention of future errors. Reports of medication errors can be made by telephone to the United States Pharmacopeial Convention, Inc. (USP) Medication Errors Reporting Program (1-800-23ERROR). Reports can be submitted to USP on a confidential basis if the reporter so chooses. Other reporting programs may also be in existence or under development. Reporting programs are intended to track trends and inform practitioners, regulators, and the pharmaceutical industry of potential product and system hazards that have a documented association with medication errors.

References

1. Hepler CD, Strand LM. Opportunities and responsibilities in pharmaceutical care. *Am J Hosp Pharm.* 1990; 47:533–43.
2. Manasse HR Jr. Medication use in an imperfect world: drug misadventuring as an issue of public policy, part 1. *Am J Hosp Pharm.* 1989; 46:929–44.
3. Davis NM, Cohen MR. Medication errors: causes and prevention. Huntingdon Valley, PA: Neil M. Davis Associates; 1981.
4. Zellmer WA. Preventing medication errors. *Am J Hosp Pharm.* 1990; 47:1755–6. Editorial.
5. Zellmer WA. ASHP plans for the future. *Am J Hosp Pharm.* 1986; 43:1921. Editorial.
6. American Society of Hospital Pharmacists. ASHP statement on the pharmacist's responsibility for distribution and control of drugs. *Am J Hosp Pharm.* 1991; 48:1782.
7. Lesar RS, Briceland LL, Delcoure K, et al. Medication prescribing errors in a teaching hospital. *JAMA.* 1990; 263:2329–34.
8. American Society of Hospital Pharmacists. ASHP technical assistance bulletin on hospital drug distribution and control. *Am J Hosp Pharm.* 1980; 37:1097–103.
9. Allan EL, Barker KN. Fundamentals of medication error research. *Am J Hosp Pharm.* 1990; 47:555–71.

10. Betz RP, Levy HB. An interdisciplinary method of classifying and monitoring medication errors. *Am J Hosp Pharm.* 1985; 42:1724–32.

11. Leape LL, Brennan TA, Laird N, et al. The nature of adverse events in hospitalized patients—results of the Harvard medical practice study II. *N Engl J Med.* 1991; 324:377–84.

12. Ingrim NB, Hokanson JA, Guernsey BG, et al. Physician noncompliance with prescription-writing requirements. *Am J Hosp Pharm.* 1983; 40:414–7.

13. Anderson RD. The physician's contribution to hospital medication errors. *Am J Hosp Pharm.* 1971; 28:18–25.

14. Cooper JW. Consulting to long-term care patients. In: Brown TR, Smith MC, eds. Handbook of institutional pharmacy practice. 2nd ed. Baltimore, MD: Williams & Wilkins; 1986:649–61.

15. Bedell SE, Dertz DC, Leeman D, et al. Incidence and characteristics of preventable iatrogenic cardiac arrest. *JAMA.* 1991; 265:2815–20.

16. Fuqua RA, Stevens KR. What we know about medication errors: a literature review. *J Nurs Qual Assur.* 1988; 3:1–17.

17. Intravenous Nurses Society. Intravenous nursing standards of practice. *J Intraven Nurs.* 1990; 13(Apr): Suppl.

18. American Society of Hospital Pharmacists. ASHP statement on the pharmacist's clinical role in organized health care settings. *Am J Hosp Pharm.* 1989; 46:2345–6.

19. American Society of Hospital Pharmacists. ASHP guidelines on the pharmacist's role in drug-use evaluation. *Am J Hosp Pharm.* 1988; 45:385–6.

20. American Society of Hospital Pharmacists. ASHP guidelines: minimum standard for pharmacies in institutions. *Am J Hosp Pharm.* 1985; 42:372–5.

21. American Society of Hospital Pharmacists. ASHP guidelines for obtaining authorization for documenting pharmaceutical care in patient medical records. *Am J Hosp Pharm.* 1989; 46:338–9.

22. Barker KN, Pearson RE. Medication distribution systems. In: Brown TR, Smith MC, eds. Handbook of institutional pharmacy practice. 2nd ed. Baltimore, MD: Williams & Wilkins; 1986:325–51.

23. Cohen MR, Davis NM. Assuring safe use of parenteral dosage forms in hospitals. *Hosp Pharm.* 1990; 25:913–5. Editorial.

24. American Society of Hospital Pharmacists. ASHP statement on the pharmacy and therapeutics committee. *Am J Hosp Pharm.* 1992; 49:2008–9.

25. Barker KN, Pearson RE, Hepler CD, et al. Effect of an automated bedside dispensing machine on medication errors. *Am J Hosp Pharm.* 1984; 41:1352–8.

26. American Society of Hospital Pharmacists. ASHP guidelines for selecting pharmaceutical manufacturers and suppliers. *Am J Hosp Pharm.* 1991; 48:523–4.

27. Joint Commission on Accreditation of Healthcare Organizations. 1992 Accreditation manual for hospitals, vol. 1: standards. Oakbrook Terrace, IL: Joint Commission on Accreditation of Healthcare Organizations; 1991.

28. American Society of Hospital Pharmacists. ASHP guidelines on pharmacist-conducted patient counseling. *Am J Hosp Pharm.* 1984; 41:331.

29. American Society of Hospital Pharmacists. ASHP statement on unit dose drug distribution. *Am J Hosp Pharm.* 1989; 46:2346.

30. Brennan TA, Leape LL, Laird NM, et al. Incidence of adverse events and negligence in hospitalized patients—results of the Harvard medical practice study I. *N Engl J Med.* 1991; 324:370–6.

31. American Society of Hospital Pharmacists. Medication errors: a closer look (videocassette). Bethesda, MD: American Society of Hospital Pharmacists; 1988. 20 min.

32. Folli HL, Poole RL, Benitz WE, et al. Medication error prevention by clinical pharmacists in two children's hospitals. *Pediatrics.* 1987; 19:718–22.

33. Blum KV, Abel SA, Urbanski CJ, et al. Medication error prevention by pharmacists. *Am J Hosp Pharm.* 1988; 45:1902–3.

34. American Society of Hospital Pharmacists and American Nurses Association. ASHP and ANA guidelines for collaboration of pharmacists and nurses in institutional care settings. *Am J Hosp Pharm.* 1980; 37:253–4.

35. Derewicz HJ. Color-coded packaging and medication errors. *Am J Hosp Pharm.* 1978; 35:1344–6. Letter.

36. Myers CE. Color-coding of drug product labels and packages. *Am J Hosp Pharm.* 1988; 45:1660.

37. Clifton GD, Record KE. Color coding of multisource products should be standardized or eliminated. *Am J Hosp Pharm.* 1988; 45:1066. Letter.

38. Proceedings of the 41st annual session of the ASHP House of Delegates. Report of the House of Delegates. *Am J Hosp Pharm.* 1990; 47:1807–17.

39. Barker KN, McConnell WE. The problems of detecting medication errors in hospitals. *Am J Hosp Pharm.* 1962; 19:361–9.

40. McClure ML. Human error—a professional dilemma. *J Prof Nurs.* 1991; 7:207.

41. Hartwig SC, Denger SD, Schneider PJ. A severity-indexed, incident-report based medication-error reporting program. *Am J Hosp Pharm.* 1991; 48:2611–6.

42. Maliekal J, Thornton J. A description of a successful computerized adverse drug reaction tracking program. *Hosp Formul.* 1990; 25:436–42.

43. Miwa LJ, Fandall RJ. Adverse drug reaction program using pharmacist and nurse monitors. *Hosp Formul.* 1986:1140–6.

44. Anderson ER Jr. Disciplinary action after a serious medication error. *Am J Hosp Pharm.* 1987; 44:2690, 2692.

[a]The mention of investigational drugs in the definition of level 4 errors (and nowhere else in the levels) may lead some to believe that any error involving an investigational drug should automatically be classified as a level 4 error. However, in discussing this issue at its September 1992 meeting, the ASHP Council on Professional Affairs noted that it is the effect on the patient (for a medication of any type) that really should determine what level of error is involved. Approved by the ASHP Board of Directors, June 23, 1993, reaffirming the version approved November 18, 1992. Developed by the ASHP Council on Professional Affairs.

The bibliographic citation for this document is as follows: American Society of Hospital Pharmacists. ASHP guidelines on preventing medication errors in hospitals. *Am J Hosp Pharm.* 1993; 50:305–14.

ASHP Guidelines on Preventing Medication Errors with Antineoplastic Agents

Purpose

The purpose of these guidelines is to assist practitioners in improving their antineoplastic medication-use system and error-prevention programs. They supplement ASHP's Guidelines on Preventing Medication Errors in Hospitals and address error prevention within diverse health care settings.[1] Further, these guidelines provide updated general guidance to include a standard definition of a "medication error" and applicable aspects of recommendations from the National Coordinating Council on Medication Error Reporting and Prevention (NCCMERP).

NCCMERP's definition of a medication error is "any preventable event that may cause or lead to inappropriate medication use or patient harm while the medication is in the control of the health care provider, patient, or consumer. Such events may be related to professional practice, health care products, procedures, and systems, including prescribing; order communication; product labeling, packaging, and nomenclature; compounding; dispensing; distribution; administration; education; monitoring; and use."[2]

Comprehensive recommendations are provided in these guidelines for preventing errors with antineoplastic agents in health care organizations, with an emphasis on hospitals and ambulatory care clinics that offer direct pharmacy services. Nevertheless, it is strongly recommended that the guidance also be adopted by other settings, including physician office practices and home care. The recommendations cover known procedural, technical, and behavioral elements that could systematically reduce a health care organization's vulnerabilities to errors. However, strict adherence to good practice recommendations is not sufficient. Since the complexities of antineoplastic therapy afford unlimited opportunities for system failures, continuous diligence to verify accuracy is critical by all persons responsible for medication-use functions.

These guidelines focus on the medication-use responsibilities shared by and unique to specific professional health care disciplines, progressing from general to specific applications. The structure of the guidelines, by necessity, includes the repetition of some material, repeated and enhanced in specific sections and recommendations for different health care disciplines.

The guidelines contain the following major sections:

1. Recommendations for health care organizations,
2. Recommendations for multidisciplinary monitoring of medication use and verification,
3. Recommendations for prescribing systems and prescribers,
4. Recommendations for medication preparation and dispensing systems and roles for pharmacists,
5. Recommendations for medication administration systems and roles for nurses,
6. Recommendations for patients,
7. Recommendations for manufacturers and regulatory agencies, and
8. Managing medication errors.

Because of the complexity of and differences in practice settings and organizational arrangements, aspects of these guidelines may be more applicable to some practice settings than others. Pharmacists, physicians, nurses, and other health care providers should use their professional judgment in assessing and adapting the guidance to their own setting. These guidelines address a specific aspect of the medication-use process and should be augmented as appropriate by other ASHP practice statements and guidelines.

Background

The prevalence of medication errors associated with antineoplastic agents, as with other drug categories, is not precisely known, but it may be surmised that incorrect use of antineoplastic agents consistently produces serious adverse effects in patients. Antineoplastics are drug products that cause serious toxicities at FDA-approved dosages and with FDA-approved administration schedules. Extra precautions are therefore necessary to prevent antineoplastic-related medication errors. Advocates for safe medication use and oncology pharmacy specialists have recommended that health care organizations improve their medication-use systems specifically to prevent medication errors with antineoplastics.[3-6] Antineoplastic-related medication-error prevention has become a priority, especially in hospitals. However, many antineoplastic therapies are also administered outside the inpatient setting. An increasing number of patients receive treatment for cancer in ambulatory care settings. Thus, error-prevention strategies should be applicable to the diverse settings in which antineoplastic agents are used.

Recommendations for Health Care Organizations

Optimal and comprehensive patient care, especially for patients receiving antineoplastic agents, requires the participation of multiple health care disciplines. Systems are necessary to coordinate the functions throughout the medication-use process of prescribing, preparing, dispensing, and administering drugs, and to educate and counsel patients.

Health care organizations in which multiple disciplines are represented should establish committees with representatives from each discipline to develop policies and procedures for the medication-use process and to oversee its operation. These should include educational and competency requirements for persons with medication-use responsibilities, general system requirements that minimize vulnerabilities to errors, and periodic auditing of physicians', pharmacists', and nurses' proficiency with the system. Further, near misses and errors should be analyzed, and problems in the procedures that place patients and staff at risk should be resolved.

Education, Competency, and Credentialing. All practice settings should establish policies and procedures ensuring that health care providers who prescribe, prepare, dispense, and administer antineoplastic medications and monitor

patients receiving those medications are competent to perform those functions. For pharmacists and nurses, specific education and experience or board certification in a practice specialty may be included in the credentialing process.

Employers should evaluate prospective employees' training and previous practice experiences for knowledge and mastery of the skills that are essential prerequisites for the new position. Prerequisites for employment should include discipline-appropriate training in how to safely handle antineoplastic drug products. Deficiencies in applicants' training and experience must be identified and remedied before new employees assume patient care responsibilities. Training for new and current employees should emphasize collaboration among health care providers to ensure optimal patient care and outcomes and worker safety.

All health care providers who prescribe, prepare, dispense, and administer antineoplastic medications and monitor patients receiving those medications should be oriented in their practice setting before commencing patient care responsibilities. Orientation should introduce to new employees all of the departments, service providers, and functions that affect patient care. Each provider's roles and responsibilities should be identified, and it should be clarified how health care providers from different disciplines are expected to interact.

Further, health care organizations should require that all personnel who prescribe, prepare, dispense, administer, and handle hazardous drugs and materials that are contaminated with hazardous drugs and that all persons who may be exposed to hazardous-drug-contaminated materials during their job performance complete job-appropriate training and evaluation. They should demonstrate competence, knowledge, and proficiency in techniques and procedures for safely handling (preventing exposure to oneself, other persons, and the environment, and managing accidental exposure) hazardous drugs. Those competencies should be reassessed annually or more frequently if performance problems occur. It is the responsibility of medication-use system administrators and supervisory personnel to know the current government restrictions that limit or prohibit some health care providers from preparing and administering antineoplastic medications.

Health care providers who participate in an antineoplastic medication-use process and those who monitor patients receiving antineoplastics should be knowledgeable and have current information available about each of the following factors on the antineoplastic drug products used in their practice setting:

1. Names of antineoplastic drug formulations,
2. Indications and whether those indications comply with the FDA-approved labeling or are part of an investigational protocol,
3. Routes of administration,
4. Administration schedules,
5. Appropriate dosages and, when applicable, constraints for the maximum dose of medication that can be safely given during a single administration,
6. Appropriate handling conditions,
7. Potential adverse effects, and
8. Potential drug interactions.

Every practice setting where cancer patients receive antineoplastic therapy should provide opportunities for continuing professional and technical education related to

antineoplastic drug use. A portion of the annual continuing-education programs for health care providers specializing in oncology should be related to antineoplastic agents and their uses.

Providers who use drug-delivery devices, such as i.v. pumps and infusion controllers, to administer antineoplastic medications should be required to demonstrate competencies related to the clinical application, function (general use, operational limits, alarms), and care of these devices; problems that may occur with the devices; and troubleshooting.

Communication and Access to Information. Many errors occurring in the medication-use process are caused or promulgated by inadequate patient-specific information. Patients' medical records should be organized and made readily accessible for use by all providers who prescribe, dispense, and administer antineoplastic medications to enable independent confirmation that all prerequisite criteria have been met before commencing antineoplastic treatment. In some cases, individual disciplines may keep additional patient records that supplement the patient's primary medical record. For example, it has historically been the responsibility of pharmacists and pharmacies to maintain patient-specific medication profiles, records of medications that were prescribed and dispensed for each patient.

Providers who practice at sites where pharmacists do not participate in patient care also should document and maintain medication profiles for their patients. Medication profiles for antineoplastic therapies should include at least the following information:

1. Patient's name and a unique identifying code or number,
2. A brief medical history that identifies a patient's cancer diagnosis,
3. Known drug-related adverse events, allergies, and medication-, nutrient-, and food-related sensitivities,
4. Vital statistics that may affect treatment intensity, particularly those needed to calculate medication doses, including height, weight, body surface area (BSA), age, sex, and pertinent laboratory values (e.g., serum creatinine, creatinine clearance, liver transaminases),
5. Data about all medications used by a patient, including the date the medications were prescribed if it differs from the date they were prepared and administered, the date the medications were prepared and dispensed if it differs from the date the medications were administered, drug identity, drug dosage, total drug dosage administered per unit interval (e.g., day, week, treatment cycle), administration route, administration schedule as a function of the treatment plan (e.g., every three hours; days 1, 8, and 15), rate of administration (when relevant), prescribed duration of use (e.g., number of doses to administer; number of treatment hours, days, or weeks), and the product manufacturer's identity and product lot numbers and expiration dates for drugs dispensed from that facility,
6. Additional ingredients and diluting agents and the amounts used in extemporaneously compounded medications,
7. Primary references that describe the treatment regimen, and
8. An up-to-date treatment history, including the treatment cycle or course number for each treatment repetition, the dates on which a patient last received treatment,

how previous treatment was tolerated, and the cumulative amount of drug previously administered for medications with established absolute cumulative dosage limits (e.g., anthracyclines, bleomycin) or constraints against repeated administration as a function of time.

Ambulatory care, home care, and managed care organizations are vulnerable to the same communication and interpretation errors that occur in hospitals. These settings and organizational arrangements, however, introduce additional opportunities for errors of omission and duplication when treatments and other services are provided at multiple locations and by more than one participating provider or group of providers. In hospitals and integrated health systems, patient-specific medical information has traditionally been communicated through a single comprehensive medical record. In contrast, providers in private practice, home care, and managed care organizations generally cannot rely on the availability of a comprehensive medical record, because medication prescribing, preparing, and administering may occur at geographically separate facilities.

Local policies should be developed to ensure that orders for a patient's antineoplastic medications are transmitted accurately and completely, simultaneously protecting patient confidentiality. Electronic means of communication are recommended to transmit up-to-date, accurate, and comprehensive patient-specific medical information among providers. Thus, data entered into this electronic system by any one provider are immediately available to all. Until a single unifying network becomes available for all health care providers, portable printed and electronic records that ensure patient safety and confidentiality must be devised.

Schedule Coordination. Since oncology patients often receive care from more than one health care provider, their primary provider should coordinate patient care with other providers and facilities. Efficient organizational systems should have someone to coordinate a patient's health care needs with the providers' schedules. Administrative coordinators are an interface between a patient's primary provider and other providers and services. They plan and document scheduling for patients' treatments, laboratory tests, follow-up visits, consultations, supportive care, and assistance from home health care contractors, hospice facilities, and social services.

Standardize Medication Ordering. To the extent possible, medication prescribing, preparation, dispensing, and administration should be standardized. Patient care facilities should develop and use standardized preprinted medication-order forms or forms that are retrievable from a computerized database for requesting frequently used antineoplastic treatments and treatment-related services. Well-designed standardized medication-order forms decrease potential errors by organizing treatment information in a clear, consistent, and uniform format.

Standardized forms should be developed collaboratively with all local health care providers who prescribe, prepare, and administer antineoplastic medications. Forms should be preprinted with treatment-specific information, such as generic drug names, specifications for drug dosage and dosage modifications as a function of patient-specific variables, and administration routes and schedules. They should also include space for prescribers to note laboratory test results that affect dosages, administration rates, and treatment duration. These forms may also permit prescribers to schedule laboratory tests and request other services for comprehensive patient care.

Standardized medication-order forms simplify and expedite ordering medications by requiring prescribers to supply only patient-specific information, such as

1. Patient's name and unique identifying code or number,
2. Date the order was generated,
3. Time and date treatments are to be administered,
4. Patient-specific laboratory values (e.g., height, body weight, BSA, pertinent laboratory values) from which dosages and administration rates are calculated,
5. Planned medication dosages and administration rates as a function of patient-specific factors and the calculated doses and rates to be administered,
6. Patient's allergies and medication and nutrient sensitivities,
7. Prescriber's name and signature, and
8. Prescriber's telephone, pager, or fax number (or another means to communicate with the prescriber).

Preprinted forms should specify, by protocol number or publication reference, the treatment that is to be administered.[3,7]

For investigational antineoplastic treatments, standardized forms should also include the study name and protocol number. Color-coded forms, for example, may be used to designate different types of treatment, such as commercially marketed antineoplastic and investigational medications.

Standardized order forms eliminate many of the problems related to misinterpreting medication orders that are commonly associated with nonstandardized orders; however, health care providers must be aware that interpretation errors may still result from illegible handwriting. Multipurpose preprinted forms that list antineoplastic medications alphabetically may also contribute to prescribing errors when two similar drug names appear in close proximity. Since lined paper can obscure the details of a prescriber's orders, preprinted forms should be printed on unlined paper.

Self-replicating forms (e.g., carbon copies, no-carbon-required paper) can produce copies that are difficult to read. Providers who prepare and administer medications on the basis of a copy of a prescriber's order should be wary of ambiguous notations, artifact markings, and omissions on the copy. Each facility should restrict antineoplastic ordering (e.g., access to medication-order forms) to providers with the appropriate clinical privileges. Health care organizations that depend on standardized forms must also ensure that only the most current versions of standardized forms are available and that obsolete forms are recalled and destroyed.

Computerized Prescriber Order Entry. Computerized prescriber order-entry (CPOE) systems provide many of the same safety and convenience features as preprinted order forms with several important advantages, including an efficient means for simultaneously disseminating orders to various providers. CPOE simplifies prescribing and eliminates the potential for introducing errors into a medication-use system when intermediaries are required to accurately interpret and transcribe orders into a manual database.

CPOE can also provide online information about drug dosages and administration schedules, both of which can be updated from a central location. Computer software can also provide additional safety and convenience features, such as

automated scheduling of multiple-day treatments, repeated treatment cycles, and laboratory tests and automated calculation of mathematically derived patient-specific data (e.g., BSA, lean body weight, drug dosages). In addition, software can decrease the likelihood of errors by incorporating features that detect drug dosages and administration schedules greater than and less than predetermined limits and by alerting system users when potentially interacting medications are prescribed.[8]

Safeguards are also required for CPOE systems. Access privileges should be limited to authorized health care providers. The system should electronically record when users enter, change, and discontinue orders. Providers should review and verify orders before treatment is started.

Oral Orders for Antineoplastic Medications. Except for discontinuing treatment, medication-use systems should not permit health care providers to transmit or accept orders to commence or modify antineoplastic medication that are communicated orally.[3,4,9] Oral orders for medications, spoken face-to-face or by telephone, circumvent an essential checkpoint in the order-verification process, whether they are communicated directly to persons who prepare medications or received and reported by one or more intermediaries.[10]

Stat Orders for Antineoplastic Medications. It is rarely necessary to begin antineoplastic treatment as quickly as possible. In general, Stat orders for antineoplastic medications potentially compromise essential order-verification safeguards and are almost never appropriate. Except for urgently required treatments, antineoplastic medication preparation and administration should be scheduled when staffing is adequate to ensure that appropriate safety checks are performed and to implement treatment. It is essential that patient care is not compromised under any circumstances. Persons who design medication-use systems are challenged to incorporate antineoplastic medication-order-verification systems that cannot be circumvented and do not introduce unnecessary delays in processing the orders.

Standardize Dosage Calculation. Medication-use systems should establish whether drug dosages should be routinely calculated as a function of actual or ideal (lean) body weight and develop standardized criteria that direct dosage calculation as a function of this weight. Treatment plans and medication orders should indicate whether patients' actual or ideal body weight was used in calculating drug dosages and identify the equation from which dosages were calculated.

Methods should be standardized for calculating BSA and ideal body weight, rounding calculated results (e.g., drug dosages and administration rates), and changing dosages and administration rates in response to changes in patients' weight and stature. For dosage and administration rates calculated from pharmacokinetic data, the mathematical equations that describe how calculated values were derived should appear in the treatment plans and medication orders.

Standardize Medication Orders. Standards should be established for the content of an acceptable medication order, requirements for patient-specific measurements, and data that must be included on medication-order forms.[11,12] The following standards are recommended:

1. All orders for patient care services should be clearly dated;

2. When ordering antineoplastic medications, the generic drug name should be used; use generic drug names approved by the United States Adopted Names (USAN) program. Brand names are not acceptable unless they aid in identifying combination drug products or a particular drug formulation (e.g., to distinguish between liposomal and nonliposomal product formulations);

3. Specify the dosage form;

4. Orders for medications should include the patient-specific data from which drug doses are calculated (height, weight, BSA, laboratory test results). When drug dosages and schedules are modified for current or anticipated pathologies, treatment plans and medication orders should explicitly identify the factors on which treatment modifications are based;

5. Drug dosages and calculated doses should be expressed in metric notation whenever possible. The word *units* should never be abbreviated in medication orders where drug dosages and administration rates are expressed in biological activity units (e.g., aldesleukin, asparaginase, bleomycin);

6. Medication orders should specify the drug dosage, calculated dose, and append the total cycle or course dosage;

7. Administration vehicle solutions and volumes should be specified, unless standard solutions and volumes have been established;

8. Specify the administration route;

9. Specify the administration rate;

10. Specify the administration schedule and the duration of treatment. Treatment plans and medication orders should specify the interval between repeated doses, the days on which each dose is to be given within a treatment cycle or course, and the total length of a treatment cycle or course;

11. Specify the dates and times when drug administration is to commence, or identify the temporal sequence in which each medication is to be administered. When 1200 is written as 12 a.m. or 12 p.m., it may be incorrectly interpreted. Directions indicating events for 1200 should be written as 12:00 noon, or 12:00 midnight, or expressed in the 24-hour system.

A medication order that complies with these recommendations would appear as follows for a patient with a BSA of 2 m²: Azorhubarb injection 100 mg/m²/dose = 200 mg in 100 mL 5% dextrose injection/dose, administer by continuous intravenous infusion over 24 hours, every 48 hours for three doses days 1, 3, and 5. Start at 8:00 a.m. on April 1, 2001 (total dose/cycle = 600 mg).

Although health care providers have traditionally used abbreviations, acronyms, and nicknames to describe antineoplastic medications and treatment regimens (e.g., ADR [doxorubicin], MTX [methotrexate], VBL [vinblastine], "platinum" [carboplatin or cisplatin], ICE [ifosfamide, carboplatin, and etoposide], MOPP [mechlorethamine, vincristine, procarbazine, and prednisone], ProMACE [prednisone, methotrexate, doxorubicin, cyclophosphamide, and epipodophyllotoxicin], and Cy-TBI [cyclophosphamide and total body irradiation]), the practice is potentially dangerous and should be avoided. Abbreviations for drug names, scheduling information, and directions for medication use should be prohibited in medication orders. Nonstandard abbreviations, Latin abbreviations, and apothecaries' weights and measures should not be used

in orders for antineoplastic medications. Whenever possible, measurement units should be expressed in metric notation.

Establish Dosage Limits and Acceptable Routes of Administration. Medication-use systems should include utilization limits for antineoplastic medications. Constraints should be developed to limit maximum antineoplastic drug dosages and administration routes and schedules. Multidisciplinary peer review should be completed before established drug administration limits are exceeded.[3,4] These constraints should include the maximum amount of an antineoplastic drug that may be administered as a single dose, the maximum amount that may be administered during a defined time interval (including maximum administration rates for parenterally administered medications), and the routes by which each drug should be administered.

Constraints for dosage and administration rate may be defined by treatment regimens and protocols and may vary among protocols. In contrast, the types of treatments administered in some practice settings may be consistently similar, permitting the establishment of absolute maximum dose limits within that practice setting.

Limits should also be established for the maximum amount of an antineoplastic drug that may be administered during one treatment course or cycle and, when appropriate, the maximum amount of drug that may be administered to a single patient within his or her lifetime.[3] In addition, dosage limits should be established for antineoplastic medications used in specific combination regimens (defined for each drug) in which clinical toxicities may be exacerbated by combining agents with overlapping adverse-effect profiles.

Antineoplastic drug-use limits should appear prominently in printed treatment descriptions (e.g., protocol summaries, "care maps,"; schematic treatment diagrams) and on printed medication-order forms and computer-based medication-order templates. Computer software that alerts health care providers whenever an order for antineoplastic medications exceeds defined limits would be ideal.[13] For patients who receive antineoplastic medications for which cumulative dosage limits have been established, cumulative dosage data should be constantly updated in their permanent medical records and in any supplementary records. Patients' cumulative dosage data should be audited and independently confirmed by health care providers when verifying orders for antineoplastic medications.[3,14]

In each health care organization, the medication-use system should include a multidisciplinary committee that oversees matters related to medication-use limits. The committee should proactively develop and establish policies and procedures for resolving disagreements related to patient treatment among providers; whether medications should be prepared, dispensed, and administered if a discrepancy cannot be resolved; and how medication-use-related disputes are to be resolved. Committee membership should comprise all providers who have responsibilities in the medication-use process in the organization.[3]

Investigational Antineoplastic Medications. Cancer patients often receive investigational (i.e., experimental) anticancer treatments at facilities participating in clinical trials. Consideration must be given to ensure that the same safety precautions and checks that are used for FDA-approved antineoplastic therapies apply similarly to prescribing, preparing, dispensing, and administering investigational medications and monitoring patients who receive those therapies.

Facility administrators should ensure that adequate staff is maintained to support an investigational drug program.[10] Ideally, nurses and pharmacists should be involved early in the process of developing clinical protocols involving the use of commercially marketed and investigational antineoplastic medications.[15] This helps to ensure that investigational medications are prepared and administered in accordance with local policies and procedures. Nurses and pharmacists should be voting members on regulatory and review committees that evaluate the scientific and ethical treatment of patients receiving antineoplastic medications and monitor investigational therapies (e.g., institutional review boards).[3]

Because a protocol governs and supplies the rules for drug use in clinical trials, an up-to-date copy of the study protocol should be available for review at all sites where medications are prepared and administered. All staff should be informed through inservice education programs before new protocols are implemented. Inservice programs and study-related information should be provided by persons associated with the investigational study (e.g., principal investigator, associate investigators, protocol chairperson, study-coordinating personnel). If an investigational protocol is to be conducted at more than one site within a health care system, procedures should be developed to ensure that up-to-date information is available at all study sites where patients receive protocol-directed care.

Procedures for supplying health care providers with information about patients' dose assignments, drug dosage, and schedule modifications should also be devised. A separate procedure should be established allowing independent dose-checking activity among all disciplines involved in the medication-use process for investigational drugs.

Recommendations for Multidisciplinary Monitoring of Medication Use and Verification

Independent medication-order verification is an essential safeguard that ensures the accuracy and appropriateness of medical treatment. It is imperative that health care providers resolve any questions related to medication orders before treatment commences. Providers should recognize that medication-order verification and other system safeguards ensure patients' safety.[3,7,14]

Lack of information about patients and their medications has been described as the most frequent cause of medication errors.[9,16] In order to independently verify prescribers' orders for medications, all persons who prepare and administer antineoplastic medications and those who monitor patients who have received antineoplastics should also have access to complete, up-to-date copies of treatment protocols and patient-specific data.[3,9,14] Drug information and reference materials should be readily available to all persons who provide patient care.

Each health care provider has a responsibility to share information with other providers and consultants to ensure patient safety and an optimal treatment outcome. Policies that regulate treatment verification standards should describe how prescribers, medically responsible and senior authorizing physicians, pharmacists and pharmacy technicians, persons responsible for administering medications, and other persons who are responsible for transcribing and transmitting medication orders should interact.

Providers who prescribe, prepare, dispense, and administer antineoplastic medications should perform as many independent manual checks as possible. Treatment-verification systems may incorporate computerized medication-order safety checks but should also include as many independent manual checks as possible.[3,10] Ideally, computerized systems are used to calculate and verify dosages and the rate and route of administration for antineoplastic drug orders and to screen medication orders for compliance with dosage limits. In addition to facilitating chemotherapy-order processing, computer software can also serve as a double check on prescribers' orders. Systems requiring pharmacists to transcribe prescribers' medication orders into a computerized or manual drug-ordering system should have a second pharmacist recheck all order-processing documents and product labeling before a drug product is dispensed.

Providing medications to patients includes four discreet steps: prescribing, preparation, dispensing, and administration. The ideal verification system has nine established checkpoints to ensure that an antineoplastic drug is accurately prescribed, prepared, dispensed, and administered to the patient for whom it was intended (Figure 1). Different individuals should complete each check so that no single person bears responsibility for checking his or her own work.

Prescribing antineoplastic medications (checkpoint 1). Health care providers who prescribe, prepare, and administer antineoplastic drugs should be familiar with the entire treatment regimen. A prescriber should complete as many orders as possible comprising a patient's antineoplastic treatment regimen and include orders for preparative and supportive care medications. This practice ensures that orders can be checked for completeness and accuracy and compliance with planned treatment.

When orders for antineoplastic drugs must be countersigned by a second medically responsible individual, the person who countersigns the medication orders should critically evaluate each order for an antineoplastic treatment. This is checkpoint 1. The orders should be compared with patient-specific data and verified against original reference sources that describe the treatment regimen (e.g., a published article, validated standard reference text, investigational protocol).

Preparing antineoplastic medications (checkpoints 2–4). Checkpoint 2 requires persons receiving a prescriber's order for antineoplastic medications to review the original written medication orders and independently verify them against published standards (e.g., product package labeling, reports published in professional journals, treatment protocols, standard reference textbooks).

Because erroneous information sometimes appears in published information, orders for noninvestigational antineoplastic medications should be verified against the primary reference in which the specific treatment was described (e.g., published reports, study protocols, meeting proceedings). If a primary reference is not available, the treatment regimen should be confirmed with a resource that previously had been validated as accurately describing the planned treatment (locally compiled handbooks, guides, and compendia) or at least two alternative publications, including reviews and reference textbooks.[3,12] Investigational drug doses and administration schedules must be verified against a study protocol that was approved by all relevant regulatory agencies and study sponsors (e.g., institutional review board, National Cancer Institute, FDA).

Although preprinted order forms preclude the necessity of repeatedly verifying drug names, dosages, routes, and schedules each time a preprinted form is used, all medication orders should be evaluated for completeness, compliance with the planned regimen, and, during repeated courses, deviations from previous treatments by following these requirements:

1. Measurements from which a patient's medication dosage and administration rate are calculated should be confirmed (e.g., height, weight, BSA);
2. The date a patient was last treated and the next planned treatment date should be compared to ensure that an appropriate interval has elapsed since treatment was last administered;
3. Patient-specific data (e.g., height, weight, BSA) should be remeasured and, when applicable, recalculated to determine whether changes from previous measurements indicate corresponding changes in dosage or administration rates;
4. Appropriate laboratory test and physical assessment values should be evaluated, and primary treatment references should be consulted to determine whether they are within acceptable ranges or if treatment modifications are indicated; and
5. A patient's allergy, drug sensitivity, and adverse drug effect histories and his or her current medication profile should be evaluated for potential drug interactions with planned antineoplastic treatment.

Orders prescribed by physicians-in-training and nonphysician health care providers with prescribing privileges (e.g., nurse practitioners, physician assistants) should be verified with at least

Figure 1. Medication-order verification system. These nine established checkpoints ensure that an antineoplastic drug is accurately prescribed, prepared, dispensed, and administered to the patient for whom it was intended.

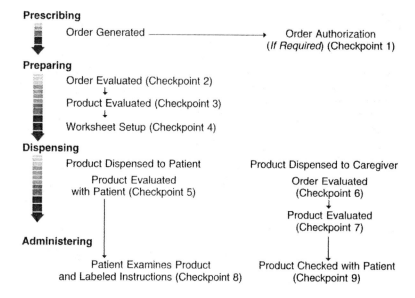

one medically responsible person, other than the prescriber, who is knowledgeable about medical oncology. Verification includes confirming correct treatment before commencing the initial cycle, dosage and administration schedule modifications, and deviations from planned or expected treatment.

For patients who receive treatment in clinical studies in which more than one primary or ancillary treatments are prescribed (e.g., dose-and-duration-escalating studies), treatment assignment and dosage and administration schedule modifications should be confirmed with at least one person directly associated with the clinical trial, other than the prescriber (e.g., the principal investigator, an associate investigator, research nurses or pharmacists, a study coordinator or chairperson). Consult with the prescriber when expected treatment modifications were not ordered or when nonstandard modifications were prescribed.

Instructions for diluents, drug administration sequence and duration, number of doses, and starting date and time should be checked. Review and confirm that appropriate ancillary and supportive medications that facilitate antineoplastic drug delivery and those required by protocol have been prescribed and are complete and accurate (e.g., premedications, hydration, cytoprotectant and "rescue" medications, antiemetics, hematopoietic growth factors). Discrepancies between prescribed medications and planned treatment should be brought to the prescriber's attention and resolved before medication preparation proceeds.

At checkpoint 3, after treatment orders have been verified, all work related to medication-order processing and preparation accuracy should be routinely documented in a standardized format. Drug preparation work sheets (sometimes referred to as work cards or admixture or compounding logs, sheets, and cards) identify the drug products prepared for each patient and the persons who prepared and checked the medications. Although layout and design may vary among work sheets, and data may be organized as a continuous log in which each drug product appears on separate consecutive lines or as a separate record for each patient, all work sheets should detail the techniques used in preparing the drug products. They should also identify special preparation and dispensing information, such as the indication of special product containers, requirements for filtration, the need for special diluents, intermediate dilution steps, and how and when administration sets should be attached to the drug product container. Order processing, drug preparation, and processing records should be confirmed by a second individual (preferably a pharmacist).[3,4] The calculations written on preparation work sheets should be independently verified by a second health care provider who did not prepare the work sheet. Independent verification should include checking the work sheet for completeness and accuracy of content, with particular attention given to special preparation instructions. A checklist identifying the necessary elements in a drug preparation work sheet may be helpful for this step (Figure 2).[3]

At checkpoint 4, drug products should be checked, after preparation, against both the preparation work sheet and the original order by an individual who was not involved in preparing the work sheet. Checklists may also be helpful for this step.[3]

Dispensing antineoplastic medications (checkpoint 5). Checkpoint 5 requires persons dispensing medications to patients or caregivers for outpatient use to verify a patient's identity when a medication is dispensed. Patients who self-administer their medications or personal caregivers should visually examine the medication, confirm whether its appearance meets their expectations, and compare its instructions with information they received from their health care providers (e.g., a chemotherapy calendar).

Dispensing and administering antineoplastic medications (checkpoints 6–9). At checkpoint 6, before starting treatment, each antineoplastic medication should be checked against the prescriber's orders by at least two individuals who are trained and competent to administer antineoplastic medications. All dosage- and administration rate-related calculations should be independently confirmed. Health care providers should routinely confirm that the medication will be administered to the intended patient by comparing a patient's name and unique identifying code or number with medication labels (e.g., alpha–numeric characters or bar codes) and that a drug product's identity, ancillary components (e.g., additional medications, diluent, and vehicle solutions), route of administration, and schedule are correct.

At checkpoint 7, health care providers should examine the medication container and note whether the content's general appearance is what was expected. Many chemotherapeutic parenteral products have distinctive colors, and product coloration should be confirmed before administration.

At checkpoint 8, patients who self-administer their medications (or receive it from personal caregivers) should carefully read the container's label to confirm the product's identity and review its instructions for use each time they take a medication.

At checkpoint 9, patients should be encouraged to ask questions about their treatment before its administration and compare its appearance and medication label with information they received about the treatment.

In ambulatory care practice, it is common for patients to receive parenteral antineoplastic medications in a setting where a physician and a nurse complete all tasks related to prescribing, preparing, administering, and monitoring treatment without a pharmacist's participation. Under these circumstances, the two health care providers involved should check the other's work. Both providers should be involved in the entire process. The person preparing antineoplastic medications should work from written orders.

Recommendations for Prescribing Systems and Prescribers

Antineoplastic prescribing is complicated by numerous medical publications that report indications, dosages, and administration schedules inconsistent with FDA-approved product labeling. Antineoplastic treatments are frequently based on preliminary reports, meta-analyses, and promising, albeit anecdotal, information. Prescribers must exercise great care in correctly interpreting this information and clearly communicating orders for antineoplastic medications with other health care providers.

System administrators should weigh the merits of requiring orders for all antineoplastic medications and other high-risk drugs prescribed by physicians-in-training to be countersigned by a senior physician with expertise in the specialty to safeguard against errors in interpretation and prescribing.

Health care providers with privileges of prescribing antineoplastic drugs should complete an orientation of local policies and procedures related to prescribing antineoplastics before they are permitted to order them for patient care.

Figure 2. Antineoplastic drug preparation checklists.

Checklist for Initial Setup of Antineoplastic Drug Work Card

This form should be completed by the pharmacist checking the work card. Place check mark (or N/A) in each space after each check is completed. Your check marks and initials at the bottom of this work sheet are your personal assurance that you checked all these items for accuracy in the setup and transcription of information onto the work card. Each drug requires a separate checklist.

Patient _____ Drug _____

Start date _____

Administration time _____

Stop date _____

Duration _____

Correct drug name _____

Number of doses _____

Dose _____

Drug concentration _____

Drug volume _____

Diluent _____

Volume of diluent _____Overfill _____Drug in overfill ____

Expiration time _____

Special delivery devices (tubing, cassette, container, etc.)

Correct route of administration _____

Correct mixing instructions (special directions, e.g., "Do Not Filter") _____

Auxiliary label information (e.g., "Do Not Refrigerate," "Use In-line Filter," "For Intrathecal Use Only") _____

Correct total volume _____

Pharmacist's initials _____ Date _____

This record should remain with the work card for the duration of the order and be saved for the supervisor for review after discontinuation of the order.

Supervisor's initials _____ Date _____

Checklist for Preparing and Labeling Antineoplastic Drugs

For each order you check, verify that each element is correct with a check mark.

Patient _____ Drug _____

Date _____

Label check

Patient name is same as on front of work card _____

Drug name on label matches drug name written on back of work card _____

Dose on label matches dose written on back of work card_____

Diluent on label matches diluent written on back of work card _____

Volume of diluent on label matches volume of diluent on back of work card _____

Correct date to prepare _____

Expiration date and time _____

Correct time (expiration date not greater than administration time) _____

For each drug/additive

Correct drug used _____Proper protocol supply ____

Drug concentration in each vial _____

Additives, such as sodium bicarbonate solution, for which large stock bottles are used (which remain in hood) are visually checked, lot number is verified, and technician is asked to verify volume used

Syringe plunger is pulled back to volume required for dose

Drug lot number on each vial matches lot number written on work card _____

Calculations are checked _____

Drug has not expired _____

For each diluent

Correct diluent _____Volume of diluent _____

Diluent has not expired _____

Special instructions followed

Air purged from bag ____

Tubing affixed/primed to end of line _____

Diluent for reconstitution _____

Correct container _____Proper overfill ___Drug in overfill ___

Final miscellaneous steps

Chemotherapy work card checklist is in card pocket _____

Solution is inspected for impurities/floaters_____

Label is initialed (on left-hand side of label just below last additive or drug) **after** being affixed to correct admixture _____

Total volume to be infused _____Red chemo i.v. seal _____

"Caution chemo" label _____Other auxiliary labeling ____

Zip-lock bag _____

Work card is initialed _____

Pharmacist's initials _____ Date _____
Supervisor's initials _____ Date _____

Health care providers should locally develop standardized dosage and administration schedule modifications for each antineoplastic medication. Treatment modifications may be appropriate for patients with the following characteristics: (1) preexisting pathologies and whose health may be compromised by treatment with particular antineoplastics (e.g., withholding or decreasing bleomycin dosages in patients with preexisting pulmonary dysfunction or cardiotoxic agents in patients with congestive heart failure), (2) a history of severe, prolonged, or cumulative adverse effects after previous antineoplastic treatments, (3) impaired physiological function that predisposes patients to altered pharmacodynamic responses (e.g., renal or hepatic impairment), and (4) low or decreased performance status.

Health care providers should also establish standardized guidelines for prescribing drugs that are routinely administered concomitantly with antineoplastic medications. Medication-use guidelines for supportive care and ancillary agents (e.g., antiemetics, hydration, chemoprotec-

tants) should be made accessible to all health care providers who prescribe, prepare, and administer antineoplastic drugs and for persons who perform clinical monitoring.

When generating medication orders in a setting where preprinted ordering forms, CPOE, and other electronic

and mechanical means (e.g., a typewriter) are not available, prescribers should legibly print the names of medications, dosages, routes of administration, and administration schedules in plain block letters and Arabic numerals. Unless it is considered inappropriate by the prescriber, handwritten medication orders should include the indications for which they are prescribed (e.g., for sore mouth, for nausea, for chronic lymphocytic leukemia).

When antineoplastic treatment (ordering, preparing, and administering) is coordinated at a single location, it is the prescriber's responsibility, or in the conduct of clinical trials, it is the principal investigator's responsibility, to provide information about the treatment (e.g., protocols, publication reprints) to those who prepare and administer medications and monitor patient outcomes. It remains the prescriber's responsibility to answer questions and provide information to other health care providers when treatment is implemented in a place that is geographically separate from the prescriber's location. Prescribers, clinical investigators, and medically responsible staff are strongly urged to provide to healthcare providers who prepare and administer antineoplastic medications a complete printed (or electronically reproduced) copy of the treatment regimen.

General Guidelines for Prescribing Antineoplastic Medications.[3,5,7,17] The following are general guidelines for prescribing antineoplastic drugs:

1. Instructions for medication regimens should be explicit, complete, clear, and easy to follow. Treatment regimens should be described accurately and consistently in all written and published materials in which antineoplastic medication use is described;
2. Medication-use systems should require health care providers to use standardized vocabulary and nomenclature for describing treatment with antineoplastic medications;
3. Use uniform and consistent notations to express quantifiable amounts (dosage, concentration, volume, and time);
4. Never trail a whole number with a decimal point followed by a zero (e.g., write "5 mg," not "5.0 mg");
5. When writing amounts less than one, the expression should be written with a leading zero, which precedes the decimal point (e.g., "0.125 mg");
6. In all treatment plans and medication orders, identify the dosage, the calculated dose, and, parenthetically, the total dosage (the amount of drug as a function of body weight, BSA, or other factors) that patients are to receive during a treatment cycle; and
7. When treatment day enumeration is arbitrary, day 1 typically describes the day treatment commences. In contrast, hematopoietic progenitor-cell transplantation regimens of ten include day 0, and significant treatment-related events both before and after a progenitor-cell graft is administered are distinguished by negative (minus) and positive (plus) prefixes, respectively.

Specific Recommendations for Parenterally Administered Medications.[7] Health care providers should adhere to the following guidelines for parenteral antineoplastic drugs:

1. In treatment plans and orders, doses should be expressed as the total amount of medication to be administered from a single container (i.e., the total amount of medication per syringe, bag, or other container);

2. For medication admixtures that can be prepared in more than one way, practitioners should institute a priori, standard, and consistent methods directing how each medication will be prepared and administered; and
3. For drug products with extended stability and when a medication is administered from a single container for more than 24 hours, a prescriber's order for treatment should specify the amount of medication to be administered during each 24-hour interval.[7] A drug order for a patient with a BSA of 2 m² should read: "Drug XYZ" (8 mg/m²/day × 3 days) 48 mg in 150 mL 0.9% sodium chloride injection by continuous intravenous infusion over 72 hours, days 1–3. Start on 04/01/2001 at 0800 (total dose/cycle = 48 mg).

Specific Recommendations for Orally Administered Medications.[7] Health care providers should adhere to the following guidelines when oral medications are the prescribed antineoplastic treatment:

1. In treatment plans and medication orders, describe drug doses and schedules as the amount of medication to be taken per dose, not as a total daily dose that is to be taken in divided doses;
2. In treatment plans, medication orders, and instructions to a patient, identify the number of doses to be administered or taken;
3. When doses for a solid orally administered dosage form are greater or less than available dose strengths, specify whether and how doses are to be rounded to the nearest capsule or tablet strength (e.g., Should tablet formulations be broken to deliver a calculated dose? Should high and low doses be administered on alternating days to deliver an average dose?);
4. Whenever possible, include instructions about how medications are to be taken with respect to food ingestion and whether particular types of food may affect medication activity; and
5. Explicitly identify essential ancillary medications and supportive care that should accompany an antineoplastic treatment regimen.

Recommendations for Medication Preparation and Dispensing Systems and Roles for Pharmacists

For each practice setting, persons representing the various health care disciplines that prescribe, prepare, and administer antineoplastic medications should participate in planning and managing local medication-use systems.

Standardize Medication Preparation Guidelines. Health care providers should establish standardized guidelines for reconstituting, diluting, admixing, packaging, and labeling commonly used antineoplastics and other medications that are routinely administered with antineoplastics. Each practice facility should also establish a standardized method for labeling multidose vials and reconstituted drug products. Standardized medication preparation guidelines should be prominently displayed (e.g., as a chart) for easy accessibility in areas where orders are processed and medications prepared.

Policies and procedures should be developed for situations in which medications are prepared at facilities that are geographically removed from where treatment is administered. Procedural protocols should describe requirements for medication packaging, storage conditions during transportation, duration of transport, and handling after delivery. Medication couriers should receive training in organizational policies for handling medications and should immediately report when conditions and handling practices deviate from procedural standards. In addition, handling procedures should ensure patient confidentiality and provide guidelines for emergency situations, such as hazardous-drug spills.

Persons who prepare and dispense antineoplastic medications should ensure timely drug delivery to patients and patient care areas after receiving written orders. If dispensing is delayed for any reason, health care providers awaiting the medications should be notified.[3]

Quality Assurance. In collaboration with health care providers who prescribe and administer medications, pharmacists and persons who prepare and dispense medications should take the initiative in developing and managing quality-assurance programs for their medication-use systems. These programs should preeminently include surveillance and reporting systems that track potential and actual medication errors and evaluate the proximal causes of errors among processes and systems and preventive measures.[3,18] The major advantage of multidisciplinary participation is that each discipline's perspectives and methods for conceptualizing system flaws and solutions can be incorporated in designing strategies for preventing medication errors. Confidential reporting is essential to the success of a medication-error surveillance and reporting system. Only by understanding what causes and contributes to errors can the number of errors be reduced. In designing a medication-error surveillance and reporting system, strategic emphasis should be placed on understanding why errors occur and not on blaming or censuring personnel.[19]

Orientation on Medication-Error Reduction. Pharmacy supervisors and managers should develop an orientation program about medication errors commonly associated with antineoplastic drugs to train pharmacy personnel who prepare and dispense antineoplastic medications. Pharmacists should develop ongoing interdisciplinary educational programs that focus awareness on potential medication errors with antineoplastic medications, strategies for preventing errors, and local and national medication-error reporting and evaluation systems for all practitioners who have direct patient contact.

Pharmacists should engage the support of medical and nursing administrators and supervisors to encourage their staff (particularly those in professional training programs) to complete antineoplastic medication-error awareness programs.[9] Educational programs should be discipline specific. Program content should include medication-error case scenarios and discussion about the effects that medication errors have on patients' quality of life and the health system.[3,10]

Standardize Drug Procurement and Storage. Pharmacists who select and procure drugs should strive to minimize or eliminate look-alike drug product containers and limit the availability of different vial sizes for parenteral medications whenever possible.[4] Frequent additions to the variety of available drug products and changes among alternative

manufacturers' drug products can contribute to medication-use errors and should be avoided. When practicable, drug products with similar names and packaging should not be stored next to each other. Medication-use systems that involve a formulary should separate nonformulary products from those that are on the formulary. Health care providers should familiarize themselves with antineoplastic drugs that are not on their formulary before prescribing, preparing, and administering them.

Standardize Medication Preparation and Dispensing. Antineoplastic medications should be dispensed in ready-to-administer dosage forms whenever possible. Generally, antineoplastics for intermittent parenteral administration should be prepared so that each medication container has only one dose. The risk of incorrect medication use is increased when the amount of drug dispensed in a single container exceeds the amount to be administered during a 24-hour period. It is essential that individuals and committees responsible for developing and overseeing medication-use systems establish guidelines on whether prescribers may order antineoplastic preparations to be administered from a single container for more than 24 hours. In all practices where parenteral drugs with extended stability (more than 24 hours) are sanctioned, it is imperative that the duration of their use is clearly labeled and that health care providers are trained to correctly prescribe, prepare, and administer them.[7]

When preparing an antineoplastic admixture, a quantity of medication that most closely approximates the prescribed dose should be segregated from other drug supplies. For treatment regimens that include two or more drugs, especially when medications are to be administered by different routes, the medications should be physically segregated during preparation and when administered. Compounded medications should be prepared one at a time, using standardized techniques whenever possible. When measuring diluent solutions used to reconstitute medications and drugs to be added to a secondary container, a person other than the individual who measured the volume should visually confirm the measurement before the solutions are transferred from the measuring device to the secondary container. This may be accomplished by visual inspection or by weighing syringes, other transfer devices, and intermediate product containers before fluid transfer is completed. Alternatively, post hoc methods for checking medication preparation include "pulling back" syringe plungers and marking syringe barrels to demonstrate the volume of fluid that was injected into the secondary container. In any medication-checking system, the person who confirms the technical accuracy of the person who prepares the admixture should examine all containers used during preparation.

Antineoplastic agents are administered parenterally by many routes other than the intravenous route (e.g., intrathecally, intrahepatically, intrapleurally, intraarterially). Inadvertent administration by the wrong route (e.g., giving vincristine intrathecally) can result in serious or fatal consequences. Medication-use systems should include policies and procedures that distinguish medications administered by the intravenous route from those intended for administration by other routes.

Standardize Medication Labeling. Strict procedures should be established for standardizing medication labeling. A uniform, systematic labeling method should be used, especially when multiple drugs are prepared for a single patient. Medication labels should be mechanically printed (not handwritten). Extemporaneously

compounded antineoplastic medications should be labeled immediately after preparation. Oral medications should also be sealed with childproof or poisoning-prevention closures. Auxiliary labels may facilitate distinguishing among medications that are administered by particular delivery methods.

Labels for oral dosage forms, rectal suppositories, and topically applied unit-dose products should include all of the following information:

1. Patient's name and unique identifying code or number and patient's location within a treatment facility (when applicable),
2. Date (with or without specifying time) the medication was dispensed,
3. Generic drug name,
4. Dosage form and strength,
5. Amount of medication per dose (when the container dispensed holds more than one dose),
6. Administration route,
7. Detailed instructions to the patient for self-administering the medication,
8. Supplemental administration instructions, such as the starting and completion dates and times, number of doses to administer, cautionary information about when medications are to be taken in relation to food ingestion and other medications, and instructions and warnings regarding administration route, storage conditions, and container closures, and
9. The number of drug product units dispensed within each container (the number of tablets, capsules, or suppositories, packaged in a single container).

Labels for injectable dosage form containers should include all of the following information:

1. Patient's name and unique identifying code or number and patient's location within a treatment facility (when applicable);
2. Generic drug name;
3. The amount of medication per container and the amount of medication per dose when a product container holds more than one dose, as drug product containers may hold more medication than is intended for a single administration (e.g., multiple doses for intermittent administration). Identify how much overfill is added to a container when excess medication and fluid volumes are added to displace air from the tubing lumen ("dead space") in administration sets;
4. Route of administration; for example, medications prescribed for administration other than by the intravenous route—especially those for intrathecal administration—should bear ancillary labels that distinctively identify the intended administration route;
5. The name and either the amount or concentration of all drug additives in a drug product;
6. Diluent (vehicle fluid) name;
7. The volume of fluid to be administered. Volume to be administered should be specified, especially when it differs from the total volume within a medication container (i.e., when the product contains an amount of fluid in excess of the volume to be delivered);
8. Administration rate and duration. Ideally, both administration rate and duration should be specified. Because administration rates can be calculated from the volume to be administered and duration of administration, duration is the essential component;
9. Supplemental administration instructions, such as starting and completion dates and times, prohibitions about when medications are not to be administered in relation to other medications, instructions and warnings regarding administration route, handling, and storage conditions (e.g., information about special requirements for administration sets including inline filtration, warnings to avoid intrathecal administration with vinca alkaloid drugs, and hazardous-drug warning labels);
10. When it is necessary to prepare more than one medication intended for sequential administration, the container labels should be numbered. Indicate the sequence in which each container is to be used plus the total number of containers (e.g., bag 1 of 3, bottle 3 of 7);
11. Date (with or without specifying time) the medication was ordered or prepared. Investigational compounds, in particular, should be labeled with the date and time they were prepared;
12. Date (with or without specifying time) after which a medication should no longer be used (expiration information);
13. Cautionary warnings as required for hazardous-drug products;[20]
14. Storage specifications; and
15. The name (with or without specifying location or telephone number) of the institution, pharmacy, or practice from which a medication was dispensed and the prescriber's identity.

Credentialing Pharmacists for Antineoplastic Medication-Use Programs. Pharmacy managers and supervisors should require pharmacist employees to complete training and demonstrate competencies related to antineoplastic medication use, evaluating medication orders, preparing antineoplastic medications, safe handling procedures, error surveillance and reporting programs, and local policies as a prerequisite to pharmacist credentialing. Health care organizations should periodically reassess pharmacist employees' competencies related to their responsibilities, increasing the frequency of reassessment if performance problems occur.[6]

Roles for Pharmacists. Among primary health care providers, pharmacists generally are best positioned to ensure that medications are used rationally and safely and increase others' awareness about medication errors and how to prevent them. Pharmacists should participate in all aspects of patient care related to antineoplastic treatment, including developing rational policies for safe and appropriate medication use and other services consistent with pharmaceutical care.[3,9] Pharmacists should participate with other primary health care providers in multidisciplinary groups that develop, implement, and periodically reevaluate practice-specific procedures and processes for verifying antineoplastic medication orders, resolving procedural questions related to confirming and processing medication orders, and evaluating and resolving disputes among health care providers.

Each organization should establish a minimum acceptable level of pharmacist participation in the error-prevention elements of patient care, such as proactively reviewing medication orders, screening laboratory results, providing drug

information and patient counseling, and reviewing drug storage conditions.[3,21]

The following areas are recommended for pharmacist participation:

1. Educate health care providers about medication errors,
2. Independently verify medication dosages, routes of administration, and schedules,
3. Participate in multidisciplinary efforts to establish drug-specific utilization constraints that limit maximum doses, administration rates, and administration schedules for antineoplastic medications,
4. Participate in multidisciplinary efforts to standardize the prescribing vocabulary,
5. Participate in multidisciplinary efforts to educate patients, their families, and personal caregivers,
6. Improve communication among health care providers and among health care providers, patients, and caregivers, and
7. Work with drug manufacturers.

Drug information resources and education for providers. Pharmacists should help ensure the availability of up-to-date references on the appropriate use of antineoplastic drugs for all health care providers involved in medication use.[3,10] Drug information resources should provide information about drug products' FDA-approved labeling and investigational uses. Information should be developed or selected, including drug-specific precautionary warnings and information about adverse effects, particularly dosage- and schedule-limiting effects; potential interactions with other drugs, disease states, and foods; administration methods, including drug admixture stability and compatibility data; usual adult and pediatric dosages; dosage recommendations for single- and multiple-treatment courses; treatment modifications for persons with concurrent pathologies or end-organ impairment; and pharmacokinetically based dosing and monitoring guidelines.

Pharmacists should develop and provide discipline-specific educational materials about antineoplastic medication use to health care providers who prescribe, prepare, and administer antineoplastic medications. The instructional tools developed for each professional health care discipline should complement the materials developed for the other disciplines.[3] Whenever new antineoplastics, treatment regimens, and treatment protocols are introduced into their practice setting, pharmacists should assume a continuous, proactive leadership role in developing educational programs and materials for health care providers, patients, and caregivers.[3,10]

For patients whose care is transferred from oncologists to nonspecialist practitioners, oncology pharmacy specialists should develop and provide drug monographs, medication-use summaries, and other treatment-related materials describing how antineoplastic medications and treatment regimens are to be accomplished.[4,9] The need is especially acute among organizations and practitioners who provide local care for patients enrolled in clinical trials or receiving investigational antineoplastic treatments.

Treatment protocols. Oncology pharmacy specialists should participate in developing treatment protocols for standard treatments and clinical investigations. In practice settings where antineoplastic agents and treatment regimens are used routinely, pharmacists should initiate the development of tools that standardize the way medications are ordered,

thereby facilitating accurate and appropriate prescribing, order interpretation and verification, and medication processing and dispensing.[10,22] Pharmacists should lead initiatives to standardize drug preparation procedures, including reconstitution, dilution, and drug admixture methods for commonly used parenteral antineoplastic medications.[4]

CPOE. When circumstances and resources permit, pharmacists should work with information systems personnel, computer programmers, and software vendors to develop CPOE systems. System requirements should include mechanisms for standardizing medication orders, decreasing opportunities for error by minimizing data entry, and screening orders for medication doses and administration schedules that exceed established limits. Pharmacists should advocate for and participate in establishing maximum safe antineoplastic dosage and scheduling limits with physicians, nurses, and other primary health care providers.

Vocabulary and nomenclature. Pharmacists are uniquely qualified to lead multidisciplinary efforts toward developing and implementing clear, detailed, standardized vocabulary and nomenclature for antineoplastic treatment regimens, medication orders, and administration instructions. Pharmacists should participate in the early stages of protocol development for standard treatments and clinical investigations to ensure that pharmacotherapeutic regimens are clearly described, easily understood, and incorporate standardized language, content, abbreviations, and units of measure.[3,7,9]

Patient education and counseling. When meeting or interviewing patients, their family members, or other home-based caregivers (e.g., completing medication-use and allergy histories, screening blood pressure, performing ongoing treatment response assessment, dispensing medications), pharmacists should provide medication education and counseling. They should verify that patients and their caregivers understand the following:

1. The purpose of the medication and its intended use,
2. The appropriate use and safe handling of medications and administration devices,
3. Appropriate temperature and safe storage conditions,
4. Special precautions to prevent exposure to hazardous materials that may be present in patients' clothing, linens, body fluids, and excreta during and after treatment,
5. The potential interactions with other medications and foods,
6. Common and possible adverse effects associated with the medication,
7. Methods for preventing and managing adverse effects, and
8. What to do if potentially serious adverse effects occur.[3,13]

Pharmacists should provide educational materials to patients and suggest supplemental and alternative information resources, such as the National Cancer Institute information services department (1-800-4-CANCER or 1-800-422-6237 and www.nci.nih.gov), the American Cancer Society, libraries, and bookstores.[3]

Advocates for patients' rights. Pharmacists should encourage patients and their caregivers to participate in their own care and advise patients how to protect themselves from medication errors. Pharmacists should advise patients that they are entitled to satisfactory answers from their health care providers. Pharmacists should encourage patients to double-check the details of their treatment, including drug names and dosages, and to request

dosage recalculation if their biological measurements change. Pharmacists who participate in developing treatment plans and protocols should ensure that consent-for-treatment forms truly secure patients' informed consent. Pharmacists should help to prepare treatment consent forms; provide patients with an accurate and detailed description of their treatment plan in clear, unambiguous, and easily understood language and answers to their questions about the treatment and alternative treatment options; and assess patients' understanding of expected and possible outcomes. Pharmacists should also describe their role as primary care providers and the care they provide.[3,4]

Clinical intervention, analysis, and performance improvement. In addition to dispensing medications, pharmacists in various settings can provide a vital service toward improving the quality of patient care by implementing a proactive clinical intervention program and documenting health care providers' deviations from planned antineoplastic treatments. Longitudinal data collection, analysis, and reporting can reveal system flaws that failed to prevent or facilitated prescribing errors, suggest targets for quality improvement, and validate pharmacists' interventions.

Pharmacists should proactively work with other primary care providers to establish medication-use reporting and surveillance programs. Committees established for this purpose should comprise representatives from medical, nursing, pharmacy, and risk-management disciplines. Programs should continually evaluate local medication-use systems to identify potential problems and solutions related to medication use and prevent medication errors.[3,18] Such programs in institutions should seek endorsement from appropriate local multidisciplinary committees (e.g., pharmacy and therapeutics, medical executive, and clinical practice committees).

Feedback for pharmaceutical manufacturers and regulators. Pharmacists should work with pharmaceutical manufacturers and FDA to eliminate ambiguous, confusing, and potentially misleading drug product and treatment information from published resources (e.g., product packaging, package inserts, official compendia, and promotional information). Pharmacists working in the pharmaceutical manufacturing industry should proactively identify preventable causes of product-user errors and adverse effects associated with product labeling, packaging, and promotion.[23] Pharmacists' voluntary participation in national reporting programs can increase the awareness of medication errors and promote error prevention throughout the nation's health care system. These aggregate data promote changes in product identity, packaging, labeling, commercial information, and marketing practices that are subject to manufacturers' control and governmental regulation.[3,17]

Recommendations for Medication Administration Systems and Roles for Nurses

Nurses are often the last link in the chain of health care providers who provide treatment with antineoplastic medications. To safeguard patients from mistakes that have potentially lethal consequences, elaborate systems have evolved that include

- Requirements for credentialing persons who administer antineoplastic medications,
- Tools and methods to facilitate documentation and identification of correct medication use,
- Independent verification of medication orders,

- Accurate documentation of medication use and effects and patient care,
- Strict compliance with regulations and practice standards, and
- Patient education regarding medication safety.

Credentialing Nurses for Antineoplastic Medication-Use Programs. Nursing managers and supervisors should require nurse employees to complete training and demonstrate nursing care-related competencies, such as administering antineoplastic medications, caring for patients who have received antineoplastic medications, and knowing about local policies. Specialty certification is encouraged. Nurses may be required to complete additional training and competency assessments before they are permitted to administer experimental medications. Training usually combines didactic and supervised practical instruction. Didactic instruction generally includes training about specific antineoplastic agents, appropriate dosages and dosage ranges, adverse effects and clinical toxicities, administration techniques, and safe handling. Technical experience in administering antineoplastic medications commonly starts with role-playing exercises and practicing technical skills on nonhuman models and proceeds through clinical interactions under the supervision of an experienced mentor. Performance evaluations test trainees for satisfactory cognitive and motor competencies. Health care organizations should periodically (annually or more frequently if performance problems occur) reassess nurses' competencies related to their responsibilities.

Standardized Tools for Recording Medication Administration. Nurses with a variety of experiences have devised and contributed to designing tools to facilitate the prevention of drug administration errors, such as standardized work sheets used to calculate medication dosages and administration rates and checklists of pertinent laboratory results and physiological measurements. Treatment flow sheets provide easily interpretable information about when a patient's previous treatments were administered, whether dosages and medication delivery deviated from planned treatment, and the cumulative amount of medication administered. Thoughtfully designed treatment flow sheets may become part of a patient's permanent medical record and can be an invaluable resource for patient care.

Checking Orders and Equipment for Administering Antineoplastic Medications. Medication orders for antineoplastics are commonly checked by two nurses working independently. As has been discussed previously, double checks by two licensed health care providers help to ensure that medications are prescribed and administered appropriately. In addition, nurses should evaluate and confirm the functional integrity of vascular access devices (and devices for other administration routes), medication pumps, and other devices that control medication delivery. For adjustable and programmable mechanical and electronic devices, mechanical adjustments or electronic programming for delivering the correct dose at the appropriate rate should be verified with another health care provider who is knowledgeable about the delivery device before it is used to administer medications. Another individual who checks adjustments and programming should independently examine the adjustments made to the device and review the programming.

Recording and Tracking Antineoplastic Use. After medications have been administered, it is a nurse's responsibility to manually

or electronically record the activity. The documentation should include the patient's name, the names of all medications administered, dosages, administration routes, rates of administration, the date and time administration began, the duration of administration or time that treatment was completed, and whether adverse effects were observed or reported by the patient during or after administration. Communications with patients, other health care providers, and personal caregivers should be documented in an objective, chronological narrative style, reporting the dates and times the events occurred, the names of involved persons, and how questions and problems were resolved.

Nurses and other personnel should immediately report to medically responsible personnel and their supervisors any instance in which medications were used incorrectly and the events attributable to the error. In response to discovering a medication-use error, a provider's primary responsibility is to ensure the patient's safety. Subsequently, the error and related circumstances should be recorded as is indicated by specific policies and procedures. Medication-use error reports (also called occurrence or incident reports) should be written in an objective, chronological, narrative style without editorial remarks and speculative comments. Comprehensive incident reports are useful in discovering and evaluating system flaws and may provide the impetus for improving medication-use systems.

To prevent medication errors, nurses and other personnel who administer antineoplastic medications must comply with policies and procedures that define standards of practice. It is important, however, to periodically reevaluate practice standards in order to assess how well a medication-use system functions, make appropriate changes, and, ultimately, improve patient safety and the quality of care.

Health care providers administering antineoplastic medications should not deviate from previously stated guidelines for ordering, preparing, and administering antineoplastic agents. Examples of inappropriate practice include borrowing medications from a patient's drug supply to give to another patient and preparing agents without the proper facilities or staff. Medication administration schedules should be followed as closely as possible; providers and caregivers should strive to comply with treatment plans. Drug administration should be documented promptly after it is completed, and providers administering antineoplastic medications should rigorously comply with local requirements for documenting treatment. To prevent the inadvertent duplication of treatment, it is recommended that one individual assumes the primary responsibility for each patient during a work period (shift or tour of duty).

Nurses and Patient Education. Nurses and other personnel who administer antineoplastic medications should encourage patients and their personal caregivers to ask questions about their treatment. Patient education guidelines may be included in treatment maps and clinical care plans.

Recommendations for Patient Education

Well-informed patients (and their authorized caregivers) are the vital last link in the safety chain to prevent errors related to antineoplastic medications. Patients are entitled to know all pertinent facts about the medications they receive during their treatment. Health care providers have an obligation to encourage patients to ask questions and to provide answers.

The following suggestions are offered to help patients and their caregivers ensure optimal outcomes from the cancer therapy medications.

Multifocal Medication Education. Patients need multifocal education about the purpose, adverse effects, schedules, routes of administration, and descriptions (e.g., colors, shapes) for all the medications they will receive during their treatment. This includes the primary antineoplastic regimen and all ancillary and supportive medications, such as anti-emetics and medications that hasten bone marrow recovery. When patients are well informed and the information they receive is reinforced by nurses, pharmacists, and other caregivers, they are better prepared to detect a misinterpreted medication order and assertively question conflicting information.[24] Health care professionals should be sensitive to the emotional aspects of patients with cancer when planning medication education. Education should take place at a time when a patient is able to listen and understand. Medication education should not be attempted when patients are sedated or confused as a result of medications or immediately after receiving their cancer diagnosis.

Patients should participate in their care by asking questions about their cancer treatment and related medications and by confirming the regimen with their nurse before receiving treatment. Health care providers should make educational materials available in counseling and treatment areas to encourage patients to learn more about their cancer therapies.

Health-System Procedures Education. Patients should understand the health system's plan for antineoplastic medication-error prevention. They should become familiar with their providers' routine procedures for checking medication orders so that they can understand the safeguards that have been established and why delays may occur before their treatment can be started. For example, patients can remind the person administering chemotherapy to compare medication labels with a patient's identity and can verify their height and weight each time they are measured.

Patient Participation in a Medication-Use System. Patients (or their caregivers) should be knowledgeable about their medications and the ways in which the medications are to be administered according to their treatment plan. In some circumstances, patients should be encouraged to take responsibility for some of their care to help improve their quality of life. Examples include self-administering medications, maintaining the patency of vascular access devices, giving themselves a subcutaneous injection, and troubleshooting a problem with the portable infusion pump. Patients should demonstrate their abilities to perform these functions if they are included in the therapy plan.

Patients should be given a detailed treatment calendar that identifies all of the medication events that are expected to occur throughout their treatment. Patients should be encouraged to keep their calendar with them to compare the expected treatment with what is being dispensed and administered.

Patients' Responsibilities. Patients should be taught to detect and to seek help in managing adverse effects that may occur during their cancer treatment. Patients should promptly inform their health care providers about adverse effects experienced during a chemotherapy cycle before the next cycle commences. Patients should keep a list of the medications that they self-administered to treat these adverse effects.

It is important for health care providers to be able to determine a potential for interactions between a patient's non-antineoplastic medications and the chemotherapy they are to receive. Therefore, patients should provide to their providers a list of all medications they are using, including over-the-counter preparations, natural products and dietary supplements, and other complementary and alternative medicines.

Recommendations for Manufacturers and Regulatory Agencies

Pharmaceutical manufacturers have a responsibility to exercise care in designing product packaging and labeling and in promoting their products, as these features may contribute to errors in prescription, product selection, preparation, and administration. Companies that market antineoplastic agents should develop and support educational programs that encourage safe and accurate prescribing, preparation, administration, and handling of their products. The following guidelines address some of the major areas.

Product Naming, Packaging, and Labeling. Companies should avoid trademarking drug names that look or sound similar to those of other drug products. Proprietary drug names for new products and product formulations should be dissimilar from other generic and proprietary names. Manufacturers should avoid appending letters and numbers to drug names as this practice can result in potential confusion with dosage strengths, medication quantities, and the amount of medication to be administered.

Product packaging and labeling should provide clear, easily distinguished features to identify a drug and the amount of drug per dosage unit (e.g., tablet, capsule, wafer) and within a product container (e.g., vials, bags, bottles, prefilled syringes). It is particularly important that a drug product's USAN-approved generic name appear more prominently than other information on the product label. Drug names should be printed on both the front and back of the containers and packaging of parenteral drugs; "TALL man" characters should be used to distinguish between similar drug names. Container labels for drugs that are in solution and for those that require reconstitution or dilution before they are used should identify the total drug content in mass units (or biological activity units) rather than concentration.[24] Product packaging and labeling that include both mass and concentration values should be designed to display mass units more prominently.

Labels should be unique and well designed. Distinguishing colors and contrasting hues facilitate identifying and distinguishing drug products and products in different strengths and concentrations. Warnings and special or unique instructions should be prominently displayed on product packaging and labeling. Unique labeling and packaging techniques should be used to prevent product misidentification and to warn about dosing errors and unique characteristics that predispose medication users to potentially serious or life-threatening toxicities. Examples include the unique way that the Platinol-AQ brand of cisplatin injection (Bristol-Myers Squibb, Princeton, NJ) is packaged to prevent misidentification with carboplatin and the cautionary statements on vials containing vincristine sulfate injection that warn against using the entire contents of a vial for a single patient (on bulk packages) and that intrathecal administration may be fatal.

A statement that declares a drug's approved routes of administration is optional and may or may not appear on product packaging. If the agent is approved for administration by only one route, it must be clearly indicated.

Appropriate storage temperatures or conditions should be clearly visible on drug labeling and packaging.

Drug labeling and packaging must identify the manufacturer's product lot or control number.

Drugs that must be reconstituted and diluted before clinical use should include reconstitution instructions that identify appropriate diluents and volumes.

A manufacturer's drug product preparation date (for experimental drugs) or an expiration date should be clearly visible on the product label.

Special instructions, such as "Shake Well," "Do Not Shake," "Albumin Required," and instructions for dilution, should appear on product labeling. In cases where important information will not fit on a product label, a package insert may be required as part of the labeling and packaging.

Product changes should be widely communicated to prescribers, pharmacists, nurses, and other health care providers involved in drug prescribing, preparation, and administration.

Package inserts and product information that describe medical indications, medication doses, administration schedules, and product use should not include abbreviations. This is especially important for drugs used in complex treatment regimens.

Educational Materials and Programs. Pharmaceutical manufacturers and drug product sponsors should be encouraged to provide educational materials and programs that promote and encourage safe use of their drug products. Programs should clearly explain the indications appearing on FDA-approved labeling, dosages, methods for preparation, and administration routes and schedules. Treatment descriptions should be standardized and consistent with guidelines designed to prevent medication-use errors.[7] Medication names and administration information should not be abbreviated in educational and promotional materials.

Regulatory Oversight. Regulatory agencies have a responsibility to review product packaging, labeling, and advertising to ensure that their content accurately reflects safety and efficacy data and conforms with language that has been approved by the FDA. A key component in those reviews should be that the product packaging and labeling facilitate safe and appropriate use and prevent users from making errors in selecting, preparing, and administering a drug product. Pharmacists should be consulted in screening proprietary drug names, product packaging, and labeling before drug products are approved for commercial use.

Managing Medication Errors

Medication-use errors with antineoplastics are distinguished from errors with other types of drugs in two important ways, both of which relate to antineoplastics' inherent toxicity. Individually and categorically, the therapeutic index for antineoplastic drugs is less than that for any other class of drugs. Adverse effects are an expected pharmacodynamic consequence attendant with antineoplastic use, and clinical toxicities may occur and persist at substantially lower dosages and schedules than are therapeutically used. The second characteristic distinguishing between antineoplastics and other types of drugs is that with the latter,

subtherapeutic doses may not produce adverse effects that delay retreatment. In contrast, antineoplastic medications given in error at subtherapeutic doses (or underdoses) may not provide a therapeutic benefit, but they may compromise patients' ultimate response to therapy by delaying effective treatment until adverse effects are resolved. Underdoses may also cause or contribute to cumulative long-term patient harm as a result of adverse effects, delayed treatment, or both. It should be noted that antineoplastic treatments are almost always repeated, and the effect of a medication-use error may not be apparent until long after the error occurred. Consequently, if treatment plans and medication orders are not verified during each treatment cycle, errors may be compounded during repeated cycles and go undetected throughout an entire treatment course.

In addition to the actions already set forth in the "ASHP Guidelines on Preventing Medication Errors in Hospitals,"[1] the following are recommended after detecting a medication error[6]:

1. Implement monitoring and interventions for controlling injurious effects and ensuring patient safety;
2. Determine if an error could have previously occurred during prior treatment in the same patient and in other patients. Medication preparation work sheets or logs and drug administration records should be evaluated. Unexpected toxicities and an apparent or unaccountable lack of therapeutic and adverse effects should be investigated when it is suspected that a medication error occurred;
3. Seek the advice of health care professionals from various disciplines. The perspective of providers in other disciplines may facilitate discovering and understanding the circumstances that allowed a medication error to occur;
4. Determine whether an immediate temporizing or "stopgap" change in policy or procedure is necessary to prevent recurrence of an error while the proximal cause is being analyzed;
5. Provide immediate professional counseling and support for employees implicated in causing or contributing to an error resulting in serious patient harm. Counseling and support should be offered to all personnel who learn that they have been involved in a medication error without regard for how recently the error occurred;
6. Establish procedures to inform and follow up with patients and their families about a medication error;
7. Understand that reporting medication errors and adverse drug reactions is a responsibility that should be shared by all health care providers. However, health systems may designate a person or committee specifically responsible for reporting and investigating medication errors and adverse drug reactions. In investigational drug studies, a study's principal investigator must report serious adverse events to the trial's sponsors (the drug manufacturer and the investigational new drug application holder) and to the institutional review board that oversees study conduct. Investigational drug sponsors are required to report to the FDA serious adverse effects associated with investigational agents, even if they are caused by a medication-use error; and
8. Encourage practitioners to report medication errors to a national medication-error tracking program. This allows other providers to learn how medication errors occur and how they can be prevented. Reporting mechanisms for medication-use systems should be standard-

ized by policy. Mechanisms must be developed for ongoing, interdisciplinary analysis and use of information that is reported to medication-error databases.[25]

Categorizing Medication Errors. In practice settings where a variety of disciplines provide patient care, serious potential and actual errors should be reported to an oversight committee composed of representatives of all the disciplines that provide care. By standardizing the way medication errors are reported, comparisons between reports and databases are facilitated, error trends are more easily identified, and system-based solutions can be developed.[26] Continuous oversight by a multidisciplinary quality-assurance committee promotes continuity and permits all primary patient care providers to evaluate system flaws and develop and improve the quality of processes and systems that safeguard patient care.[18] Medication-use oversight committees are advised to review medication-error reports from systems other than their own and evaluate their local medication-use system for design characteristics that may permit similar errors.[9,15]

"ASHP Guidelines on Preventing Medication Errors in Hospitals"[1] recommend adopting a system for categorizing medication-error severity such as the one developed by Myers and Hartwig et al.[25,26] Although this system is generally applicable to errors of occurrence with antineoplastic drugs, it categorizes errors by severity and prioritizes them without consideration for the frequency at which repeated errors occur. Accordingly, errors with the highest severity ranking receive the greatest efforts toward remediation. In contrast, potential errors are assigned a "zero"; ranking, the lowest severity level, as they do not reach patients. By relegating potential errors to the lowest priority category, this outcome severity-based system risks trivializing system-design flaws. Errors discovered before they reach patients could cause devastating consequences, yet serious nascent errors are often transformed into potential errors only by serendipitous discovery. Therefore, potential errors should be distinguished from errors of occurrence and subcategorized based on their potential to cause harm.[25,26] However, potential errors should not be taken less seriously than errors of occurrence. When serious potential errors are discovered, the systems and processes that contributed to the errors should be evaluated and their proximal causes identified. The greatest efforts toward remediation of potential errors and errors of occurrence should be concentrated on eliminating the causes of errors that could have and had, respectively, the greatest adverse effects on patients' health.

NCCMERP's definition for medication errors includes any event that may cause or lead to inappropriate medication use.[2] The definition is complemented by the *NCCMERP Taxonomy of Medication Errors,* a comprehensive expandable tool intended for use in developing databases and analyzing medication-error reports. The *Taxonomy* provides standardized language and structure for recording and tracking medication-error-related data for errors of occurrence and potential errors. NCCMERP permits interested persons to adopt it as it is presented or adapt it for use in a particular practice setting.

References

1. American Society of Hospital Pharmacists. ASHP guidelines on preventing medication errors in hospitals. *Am J Hosp Pharm.* 1993; 50:305–14.

2. National Coordinating Council on Medication Error Reporting and Prevention. About medication errors. www.nccmerp.org (accessed 2001 Jun 4).

3. Cohen MR, Anderson RW, Attilio RM, et al. Preventing medication errors in cancer chemotherapy. *Am J Health-Syst Pharm.* 1996; 53:737–46.

4. Attilio RM. Caring enough to understand: the road to oncology medication error prevention. *Hosp Pharm.* 1996; 31:17–26.

5. Beckwith MC, Tyler LS. Preventing medication errors with antineoplastic agents, part 1. *Hosp Pharm.* 2000; 35:511–23.

6. Beckwith MC, Tyler LS. Preventing medication errors with antineoplastic agents, part 2. *Hosp Pharm.* 2000; 35:732–47.

7. Kohler DR, Montello MJ, Green L, et al. Standardizing the expression and nomenclature of cancer treatment regimens. *Am J Health-Syst Pharm.* 1998; 55:137–44.

8. Berard CM, Mahoney CD, Welch DW, et al. Computer software for pharmacy oncology services. *Am J Health-Syst Pharm.* 1996; 53:733,752–6.

9. Kloth DD. Assuring safe care for cancer patients through an organized multidisciplinary team effort. *Hosp Pharm.* 1997; 32(suppl 1):S21–5.

10. Fischer DS, Alfano S, Knobf MT, et al. Improving the cancer chemotherapy use process. *J Clin Oncol.* 1996; 14:3148–55.

11. Lajeunesse JD. Quality assurance methods in chemotherapy production. *Hosp Pharm.* 1997; 32(suppl 1):S8–13.

12. Attilio RM. Strategies for reducing chemotherapy-related medication errors: improving the chemotherapy prescribing, dispensing, and administration process, and the patient's role in ensuring safety. *Hosp Pharm.* 1997; 32(suppl 1):S14–20.

13. Hutcherson DA, Gammon DC. Preventing errors with antineoplastic agents: a pharmacist's approach. *Hosp Pharm.* 1997; 32:194–202,209.

14. United Kingdom Joint Council for Clinical Oncology. Quality control in cancer chemotherapy. Managerial and procedural aspects. Oxford, England: Royal College of Physicians of London, 1994.

15. Cohen MR. Enhancing chemotherapy safety through medication system improvements. *Hosp Pharm.* 1997; 32(suppl 1):S1–7.

16. Leape LL, Bates DW, Cullen DJ, et al. Systems analysis of adverse drug events. *JAMA.* 1995; 274:35–43.

17. USP Quality Review. National council focuses on coordinating error reduction efforts.Rockville, MD: United States Pharmacopeial Convention, 1997 Jan.

18. Top-priority actions for preventing adverse drug events in hospitals. Recommendations of an expert panel. *Am J Health-Syst Pharm.* 1996; 53:747–51.

19. Pepper GA. Errors in drug administration by nurses. *Am J Health-Syst Pharm.* 1995; 52:390–5.

20. OSHA Training and Education Directive 1.15—Controlling exposure to hazardous drugs. Section V. Chap. 3. Washington, D.C.: U.S. Department of Labor, 1995 Sep 22.

21. Waddell JA, Solimando DA Jr, Strickland WR, et al. Pharmacy staff interventions in a medical center hematology–oncology service. *J Am Pharm Assoc.* 1998; 38:451–6.

22. Thorn DB, Sexton MG, Lemay AP, et al. Effect of a cancer chemotherapy prescription form on prescription completeness. *Am J Hosp Pharm.* 1989; 46:1802–6.

23. Lesar TS, Lomaestro BM, Pohl H. Medication-prescribing errors in a teaching hospital. A 9-year experience. *Arch Intern Med.* 1997; 157:1569–76.

24. Cohen MR. Drug product characteristics that foster drug-use-system errors. *Am J Health-Syst Pharm.* 1995; 52:395–9.

25. Myers CE. Needed: an interdisciplinary approach to drug misadventures. *Am J Health-Syst Pharm.* 1995; 52:367. Editorial.

26. Hartwig SC, Denger SD, Schneider PJ. Severity-indexed, incident report-based medication error-reporting program. *Am J Hosp Pharm.* 1991; 48:2611–6.

Developed through the ASHP Council on Professional Affairs and approved by the ASHP Board of Directors on April 19, 2002.

The bibliographic citation for this document is as follows: American Society of Health-System Pharmacists. ASHP guidelines on preventing medication errors with antineoplastic agents. *Am J Health-Syst Pharm.* 2002; 59:1648–68.

Recommendations from the National Coordinating Council for Medication Error Reporting and Prevention

Recommendations to Correct Error-Prone Aspects of Prescription Writing

The National Coordinating Council for Medication Error Reporting and Prevention emphasizes that illegibility of prescriptions and medication orders has resulted in injuries to, or deaths of patients. The Council, therefore, has made the following recommendations to help minimize errors.

- *All prescription documents must be legible. Prescribers should move to a direct, computerized, order entry system.*
- *Prescription orders should include a brief notation of purpose (e.g., for cough), unless considered inappropriate by the prescriber.* Notation of purpose can help further assure that the proper medication is dispensed and creates an extra safety check in the process of prescribing and dispensing a medication. The Council does recognize, however, that certain medications and disease states may warrant maintaining confidentiality.
- *All prescription orders should be written in the metric system except for therapies that use standard units such as insulin, vitamins, etc.* Units should be spelled out rather than writing "U." The change to the use of the metric system from the archaic apothecary and avoirdupois systems will help avoid misinterpretations of these abbreviations and symbols, and miscalculations when converting to metric, which is used in product labeling and package inserts.
- *Prescribers should include age, and when appropriate, weight of the patient on the prescription or medication order.* The most common errors in dosage result in pediatric and geriatric populations in which low body weight is common. The age (and weight) of a patient can help dispensing health care professionals in their double check of the appropriate drug and dose.
- *The medication order should include drug name, exact metric weight or concentration, and dosage form.* Strength should be expressed in metric amounts and concentration should be specified. Each order for a medication should be complete. The pharmacist should check with the prescriber if any information is missing or questionable.
- *A leading zero should always precede a decimal expression of less than one.* A terminal or trailing zero should never be used after a decimal. Ten-fold errors in drug strength and dosage have occurred with decimals due to the use of a trailing zero or the absence of a leading zero.
- *Prescribers should avoid use of abbreviations including those for drug names (e.g., MOM, HCTZ) and Latin directions for use.* The abbreviations in the chart below are found to be particularly dangerous because they have been consistently misunderstood and therefore, should never be used. The Council reviewed the uses for many abbreviations and determined that any attempt at standardization of abbreviations would not adequately address the problems of illegibility and misuse.
- *Prescribers should not use vague instructions such as "Take as directed" or "Take/Use as needed" as the sole direction for use.* Specific directions to the patient are useful to help reinforce proper medication use, particularly if therapy is to be interrupted for a time. Clear directions are a necessity for the dispenser to: (1) check the proper dose for the patient; and, (2) enable effective patient counseling.

Dangerous Abbreviations

Abbreviation	Intended Meaning	Common Error
U	Units	Mistaken as a zero or a four (4) resulting in overdose. Also mistaken for "cc" (cubic centimeters) when poorly written.
µg	Micrograms	Mistaken for "mg" (milligrams) resulting in a ten-fold overdose.
Q.D.	Latin abbreviation for every day	The period after the "Q" has sometimes been mistaken for an " I," and the drug has been given "QID" (four times daily) rather than daily.
Q.O.D.	Latin abbreviation for every other day	Misinterpreted as "QD" (daily) or "QID" (four times daily). If the "O" is poorly written, it looks like a period or "I ."
SC or SQ	Subcutaneous	Mistaken as "SL" (sublingual) when poorly written.
T I W	Three times a week	Misinterpreted as "three times a day" or "twice a week."
D/C	Discharge; also discontinue	Patient's medications have been prematurely discontinued when D/C, (intended to mean "discharge") was misinterpreted as "discontinue," because it was followed by a list of drugs.
HS	Half strength	Misinterpreted as the Latin abbreviation "HS" (hour of sleep).
cc	Cubic centimeters	Mistaken as "U" (units) when poorly written.
AU, AS, AD	Latin abbreviation for both ears; left ear; right ear	Misinterpreted as the Latin abbreviation "OU" (both eyes); "OS" (left eye); "OD" (right eye)

In summary, the Council recommends:

Don't Wait ... Automate!
When In Doubt, Write It Out!
When In Doubt, Check It Out!
Lead, Don't Trail!

Recommendations on Labeling and Packaging to Industry (Manufacturers of Pharmaceuticals and Devices)

The Council recommends that industry not use any printing on the cap and ferrule of injectables except to convey warnings.

The Council encourages industry to employ failure mode and effects analysis in its design of devices, and the packaging and labeling of medications and related devices.

The Council encourages industry to employ machine-readable coding (e.g. bar coding) in its labeling of drug products. The Council recognizes the importance of standardization of these codes for this use.

The Council encourages printing the drug name (brand and generic) and the strength on both sides of injectables, and IV bags, containers, and overwraps. For large volume parenterals and IV piggybacks (minibags), the name of the drug should be readable in both the upright and inverted positions.

The Council encourages industry to support the development of continuing education programs focusing on proper preparation and administration of its products.

The Council encourages industry to use innovative labeling to aid practitioners in distinguishing between products with very similar names, for example, the use of tall letters such as VinBLAStine and VinCRIStine.

The Council encourages industry to avoid printing company logos and company names that are larger than the type size of the drug name.

The Council encourages collaboration among industry, regulators, standards-setters, health care professionals, and patients to facilitate design of packaging and labeling to help minimize errors.

Adopted May 12, 1997 by the National Coordinating Council for Medication Error Reporting and Prevention.

Recommendations on Labeling and Packaging to Regulators and Standards-Setters

The Council recommends that FDA restrict the use of any printing on the cap and ferrule of injectables except to convey warnings.

The Council recommends the use of innovative labeling to aid practitioners in distinguishing between products with very similar names, for example, the use of tall letters such as VinBLAStine and VinCRIStine.

The Council recommends that FDA discourage industry from printing company logos and company names that are larger than the type size of the drug name.

The Council supports the recommendations of the USP-FDA Advisory Panel on Simplification of Injection Labeling.

Furthermore, the Council encourages USP/FDA to consider expansion of the concepts of simplification to apply to:

- Package inserts
- Labeling of other pharmaceutical dosage forms

The Council encourages further development of FDA's error prevention analysis efforts to provide consistent regulatory review of product labeling and packaging relative to the error-prone aspects of their design.

The Council encourages collaboration among regulators, standards-setters, industry, health care professionals, and patients to facilitate design of packaging and labeling to help minimize errors.

The Council encourages USP/FDA to examine feasibility and advisability of use of tactile cues in container design and on critical drugs. Such cues may be in the design of the container or embedded in the label.

The Council encourages the printing of the drug name (brand and generic) and the strength on both sides of injectables and IV bags, containers, and overwraps. For large volume parenterals and IV piggybacks (minibags), the name of the drug should be readable in both the upright and inverted positions.

Adopted May 12, 1997 by the National Coordinating Council for Medication Error Reporting and Prevention.

Recommendations to Health Care Organizations to Reduce Errors Due to Labeling and Packaging of Drug Products and Related Devices

The Council recommends the establishment of a systems approach to reporting, understanding, and prevention of medication errors in health care organizations. The organization's leaders should foster a culture and systems that include the following key elements:

a. An environment that is conducive to medication error reporting through the FDA MedWatch Program and/or the USP Practitioners'; Reporting Network.

b. An environment which focuses on improvement of the medication use process.

c. Mechanisms for internal reporting of actual and potential errors including strategies that encourage reporting.

d. Systematic approaches within the health care organization to identify and evaluate actual and potential causes of errors including Failure Mode and Effects Analysis (FMEA)[1] and root cause analysis.

e. Processes for taking appropriate action to prevent future errors through improving both systems and individual performance.

In addition, the Council makes the following recommendations to health care organizations to reduce errors due to labeling and packaging of drug products and related devices:

1. The Council recommends that health care organizations employ machine readable coding (e.g., bar coding) in the management of the medication use process.

2. The Council recommends reevaluation of existing storage systems for pharmaceuticals by health care organizations and establishment of mechanisms to insure appropriate storage and location throughout the organization from bulk delivery to point of use. The following issues should be considered when applicable:

- Storage and location that will help distinguish similar products from one another
- Storage and location of certain drugs, (e.g., concentrates, paralyzing agents) that have a high risk potential
- Scope, access, and accountability for floor stock medications
- Safety and accountability of access to pharmaceuticals in the absence of a pharmacist (e.g., floor stock, eliminate access to pharmacy after hours)
- Labeling and packaging of patient-supplied medications.

3. The Council recommends the development of policies and procedures for repackaging of medications that will clarify labeling to help avoid errors.

4. The Council encourages collaboration among health care organizations, health care professionals, patients, industry, standard-setters, and regulators to facilitate design of packaging and labeling to help minimize errors.

5. The Council recommends that health care organizations develop and implement (or provide access to) education and training programs for health care professionals, technical support personnel, patients, and caregivers that address methods for reducing and preventing medication errors.

Adopted March 30, 1998 by the National Coordinating Council for Medication Error Reporting and Prevention.

Recommendations to Health Care Professionals to Reduce Errors Due to Labeling and Packaging of Drug Products and Related Devices

The Council encourages health care professionals to routinely educate patients and caregivers to enhance understanding and proper use of their medications and related devices. Furthermore, the Council encourages health care professionals to regularly participate in error prevention training programs and, when medication errors do occur, to actively participate in the investigation.

In addition, the Council makes the following recommendations to health care professionals to reduce errors due to labeling and packaging of drug products and related devices:

1. The Council encourages health care professionals to use only properly labeled and stored drug products and to read labels carefully (at least three times—before, during, and after use).

2. The Council encourages collaboration among health care professionals, health care organizations, patients, industry, standard-setters, and regulators to facilitate design of packaging and labeling to help minimize errors.

3. The Council encourages health care professionals to take an active role in reviewing and commenting on proposed regulations and standards that relate to labeling and packaging (i.e., *Federal Register* and *Pharmacopeial Forum*).

4. The Council encourages health care professionals to report actual and potential medication errors to national (e.g., FDA MedWatch Program and/or the USP Practitioners' Reporting Network), internal, and local reporting programs.

5. The Council encourages health care professionals to share error-related experiences, case studies, etc., with their colleagues through newsletters, journals, bulletin boards, and the Internet.

Adopted March 30, 1998 by the National Coordinating Council for Medication Error Reporting and Prevention.

Recommendations to Reduce Errors Related to Administration of Drugs
Adopted June 29, 1999

1. The Council recommends that any order that is incomplete, illegible, or of any other concern should be clarified prior to administration using an established process for resolving questions.

2. The Council recommends that as one aspect of the overall medication use system, the following checks be performed immediately prior to medication administration: the right medication, in the right dose, to the right person, by the right route, at the right time.

3. The Council recommends that users of medication administration devices be knowledgeable about the device function and limitations.

4. The Council recommends that when electronic infusion control devices are employed, only those that prevent free-flow upon removal of the administration set should be used.

5. The Council encourages the use of linked automated systems (e.g., direct order entry, computerized medication administration record, bar coding) to facilitate review of prescriptions, increase the accuracy of administration, and reduce transcription errors.

6. The Council recommends that all persons who administer medications have adequate access to patient information, as close to the point of use as possible, including medical history, known allergies, prognosis, and treatment plan, to assess the appropriateness of administering the medication.

7. The Council recommends that all persons who administer medications have easily accessible product information as close to the point of use as possible, and are:

- Knowledgeable about indications for use of the medication as well as precautions and contraindications;
- Knowledgeable of the expected outcome from its use;
- Knowledgeable about potential adverse reactions and interactions with food or other medication;

- Knowledgeable of actions to take when adverse reactions or interactions occur; and,
- Knowledgeable about storage requirements.

8. The Council recommends that health care professionals administer only medications that are properly labeled and that during the administration process, labels be read three times: when reaching for or preparing the medication, immediately prior to administering the medication, and when discarding the container or replacing it into its storage location.

9. The Council recommends that at the time of administration, the name, purpose and effects of the medication be discussed with the patient and/or caregiver.

10. The Council recommends ongoing patient monitoring for desired and/or unexpected medication effects.

11. The Council recommends that the role of the work environment be considered when assessing safety of the drug administration process. Factors such as lighting, temperature control, noise-level, occurrence of distractions (e.g., telephone and personal interruptions, performance of unrelated tasks, etc.) should be examined. Sufficient resources must be provided for the given workload. The science of ergonomics (use dictionary definition) should be employed in the design of safe systems.

12. The Council recommends that data be collected regarding the actual and potential errors of administration for the purpose of continuous quality improvement.

Recommendations for Avoiding Error-Prone Aspects of Dispensing Medications

1. The Council recommends that prescriptions/orders always be reviewed by a pharmacist prior to dispensing. Any orders that are incomplete, illegible, or of any other concern should be clarified using an established process for resolving questions.

2. The Council recommends that patient profiles be current and contain adequate information that allows the pharmacist to assess the appropriateness of a prescription/order.

3. The Council recommends design of the dispensing area to prevent errors. Design should address fatigue-reducing environmental conditions (e.g., lighting, air conditioning, noise level, ergonomic fixtures); minimize distractions (e.g., telephone and personnel interruptions, clutter, unrelated tasks); and provide sufficient resources for workload.

4. The Council recommends that product inventory be arranged to help differentiate medications from one another. This may include the use of visual discriminators such as signs or markers. This is particularly important when confusion exists between or among strengths, similar looking labels, and similar sounding names.

5. The Council recommends that a series of checks be established to assess the accuracy of the dispensing process prior to the medication being provided to the patient. Whenever possible, an independent check by a second individual should be used. Other methods of checking include the use of automation, computer systems, and patient profiles.

6. The Council recommends that labels be read at least three times, for example, when selecting the product, when packaging the product, and when returning the product to the shelf.

7. The Council recommends that pharmacists counsel patients. Counseling should be viewed as an opportunity to verify the accuracy of dispensing and the patient's understanding of proper medication use.

8. The Council recommends that pharmacies collect data regarding actual and potential errors for the purpose of continuous quality improvement.

[1]Lieberman, P. Design failure mode and effects analysis and the industry. Automotive Engineering (AUTE). 1990; 31.

Approved by the National Coordinating Council for Medication Error Reporting and Prevention, March 19, 1999.

This document was endorsed by the ASHP Board of Directors in November 1999. That endorsement was reviewed in 2005 by the Council on Professional Affairs and by the Board of Directors and was found to still be appropriate.

Medication Therapy and Patient Care

Organization and Delivery of Services

Qualifications and Competencies Required to Prescribe Medications (1202)

Source: Council on Education and Workforce Development

To affirm that prescribing is a collaborative process that includes patient assessment, understanding of the patient's diagnoses, evaluation and selection of available treatment options, monitoring to achieve therapeutic outcomes, patient education, and adherence to safe and cost-effective prescribing practices; further,

To affirm that safe prescribing of medications, performed independently or collaboratively, requires competent professionals who complement each others' strengths at each step; further,

To explore the creation of prescribing standards that would apply to all who initiate or modify medication orders or prescriptions and that would facilitate development of competencies and training of prescribers; further,

To encourage research on the effectiveness of current educational processes designed to train prescribers.

Transitions of Care (1208)

Source: Council on Pharmacy Management

To recognize that continuity of patient care is a vital requirement in the appropriate use of medications; further,

To strongly encourage pharmacists to assume professional responsibility for ensuring the continuity of care as patients move from one setting to another (e.g., ambulatory care to inpatient care to home care); further,

To encourage the development, optimization, and implementation of information systems that facilitate sharing of patient-care data across care settings and providers; further,

To advocate that payers and health systems provide sufficient resources to support effective transitions of care; further,

To encourage the development of strategies to address the gaps in continuity of pharmacist patient care services.

This policy supersedes ASHP policy 0301.

Pharmacist Prescribing in Interprofessional Patient Care (1213)

Source: Council on Pharmacy Practice

To define pharmacist prescribing as follows: patient assessment and the selection, initiation, monitoring, adjustment, and discontinuation of medication therapy pursuant to diagnosis of a medical disease or condition; further,

To advocate that health care delivery organizations establish credentialing and privileging processes that delineate the scope of pharmacist prescribing within the hospital or health system and to ensure that pharmacists who prescribe are competent and qualified to do so.

Pharmacist's Role in Team-Based Care (1215)

Source: Council on Pharmacy Practice

To recognize that pharmacist participation in interprofessional health care teams as the medication-use expert increases the capacity and efficiency of teams for delivering high-quality care; further,

To advocate to policymakers, payers, and other stakeholders for the inclusion of pharmacists as care providers within team-based care; further,

To assert that pharmacists are responsible for coordinating the care they provide with that provided by other members of the health care team and are accountable to the patient and to the health care team for the outcomes of that care; further,

To urge pharmacists on health care teams to collaborate with other team members in establishing quality measures for care provided by those teams.

Collaborative Drug Therapy Management (1217)

Source: Council on Public Policy

To pursue the development of federal and state legislative and regulatory provisions that authorize collaborative drug therapy management by pharmacists; further,

To advocate expansion of federal and state legislative and regulatory provisions that optimize pharmacists' ability to provide the full range of professional services within their scope of expertise; further,

To acknowledge that as part of these advanced collaborative practices, pharmacists, as active members in team-based care, must be responsible and accountable for medication-related outcomes; further,

To support affiliated state societies in the pursuit of state-level collaborative drug therapy management authority for pharmacists.

This policy supersedes ASHP policy 9812.

Medication Adherence (1222)

Source: Council on Therapeutics

To recognize that improving medication adherence should be a key component of strategies to improve the quality and safety of patient care only when adherence improvement efforts include the following as required elements: (1) assessing the appropriateness of therapy, (2) providing patient education, and (3) ensuring patient comprehension of information necessary to support safe and appropriate use of prescribed therapies; further,

To advocate that pharmacists, because of their distinct knowledge, skills, and abilities, should take a leadership role in multidisciplinary efforts to develop, implement, monitor, and maintain effective strategies for improving medication adherence; further,

To recognize that clinicians, patients, and caregivers share accountability for the outcomes of medication therapies, and that the central role patients and their caregivers have in disease management includes responsibility for following instructions for safe and effective medication use; further,

To encourage development, evaluation, and dissemination of models that improve adherence, including those that combine existing strategies that have demonstrated effectiveness; further,

To discourage practices that inhibit education of or lead patients to decline education and clinical information regarding their medication therapy; further,

To support the development of mechanisms to document medication adherence interventions, including information technology solutions; further,

To advocate for payment models that facilitate an expanded role for pharmacists in medication adherence efforts.

Patient-Reported Outcomes Tools (1107)
Source: Council on Therapeutics
To advocate for expanded use of validated patient-reported outcomes (PRO) tools in clinical research and direct patient care; further,

To support development of validated PRO tools that are sensitive to differences in cultural and health literacy; further,

To encourage additional research on PRO tools, including studies to assess their correlation to overall patient outcomes; further,

To educate clinicians and patients about the appropriate use of PRO tools.

Pharmacist Accountability for Patient Outcomes (1114)
Source: Council on Pharmacy Practice
To affirm that pharmacists are obligated by their covenantal relationship with patients to ensure that medication use is safe and effective; further,

To declare that pharmacists, pursuant to their authority over a specialized body of knowledge, are autonomous in exercising their professional judgment and accountable as professionals and health care team members for safe and effective medication therapy outcomes; further,

To encourage pharmacists to define practices and associated measures of effectiveness that support their accountability for patient outcomes; further,

To promote pharmacist accountability as a fundamental component of pharmacy practice to other health care professionals, standards-setting and regulatory organizations, and patients.

Pharmacists' Role in Medication Reconciliation (1117)
Source: Council on Pharmacy Practice
To affirm that an effective process for medication reconciliation reduces medication errors and supports safe medication use by patients; further,

To advocate that pharmacists, because of their distinct knowledge, skills, and abilities, should take a leadership role in interdisciplinary efforts to develop, implement, monitor, and maintain effective medication reconciliation processes; further,

To encourage community-based providers, hospitals, and health systems to collaborate in organized medication reconciliation programs to promote overall continuity of patient care; further,

To declare that pharmacists have a responsibility to educate patients and caregivers on their responsibility to maintain an up-to-date and readily accessible list of medications the patient is taking and that pharmacists should assist patients and caregivers by assuring the provision of a personal medication list as part of patient counseling, education, and maintenance of an individual medical record.
This policy supersedes ASHP policy 0620.

Medication Therapy Management (1005)
Source: Council on Public Policy
To support medication therapy management (MTM) services as defined in Section 3503 of the Patient Protection and Affordable Care Act (PL 111-148); further,

To affirm that MTM is a partnership between the patient (or a caregiver) and a pharmacist, in collaboration with other health care professionals, that promotes the safe and effective use of medications.

Impact of Insurance Coverage Design on Patient Care Decisions (1017)
Source: Council on Pharmacy Management
To advocate that all health insurance policies be designed and coverage decisions made in a way that preserves the patient–practitioner relationship; further,

To oppose provisions in health insurance policies that interfere with established drug distribution and clinical services designed to ensure patient safety, quality, and continuity of care; further,

To advocate for the exclusion of hospital and health-system outpatient settings from restrictive reimbursement requirements.

Patient Access to Pharmacy Services in Small and Rural Hospitals (1022)
Source: Council on Pharmacy Practice
To advocate that critical-access hospitals (CAHs) and small and rural hospitals meet national medication management and patient safety standards, regardless of size or location; further,

To provide resources and tools to assist pharmacists who provide services to CAHs and small and rural hospitals in meeting standards related to safe medication use.
This policy supersedes ASHP policy 0503.

Scope and Hours of Pharmacy Services (1023)
Source: Council on Pharmacy Practice
To support the principle that all patients should have 24-hour access to a pharmacist responsible for their care, regardless of hospital size or location; further,

To advocate alternative methods of pharmacist review of medication orders (such as remote review) before drug administration when onsite pharmacist review is not available; further,

To support the use of remote medication order review systems that communicate pharmacist approval of orders electronically to the hospital's automated medication distribution system; further,

To promote the importance of pharmacist access to pertinent patient information, regardless of proximity to patient.
This policy supersedes ASHP policy 0403.

Health-System Use of Medications and Administration Devices Supplied Directly to Patients (0806)
Source: Council on Pharmacy Management
To encourage hospitals and health systems not to permit administration of medications brought to the hospital or clinic by the patient or caregiver when storage conditions or the source cannot be verified unless it is determined that the risk of not using such a medication exceeds the risk of using it; further,

To support care models in which medications are prepared for patient administration by the pharmacy and are obtained from a licensed, verified source; further,

To encourage hospitals and health systems not to permit the use of medication administration devices with which the staff is unfamiliar (e.g., devices brought in by patients) unless it is determined that the risk of not using such a device exceeds the risk of using it; further,

To advocate adequate reimbursement for preparation, order review, and other costs associated with the safe provision and administration of medications and use of related devices.

This policy supersedes ASHP policy 0706.

Standardization of Intravenous Drug Concentrations (0807)

Source: Council on Pharmacy Practice

To develop nationally standardized drug concentrations and dosing units for commonly used high-risk drugs that are given as continuous infusions; further,

To encourage all hospitals and health systems to use infusion devices that interface with their information systems and include standardized drug libraries with dosing limits, clinical advisories, and other patient-safety-enhancing capabilities.

Pharmacist's Leadership Role in Anticoagulation Therapy Management (0816)

Source: Council on Therapeutics

To advocate that pharmacists provide leadership in the interdisciplinary development, implementation, maintenance, effectiveness monitoring, and assurance of continuity of care of anticoagulation management programs; further,

To advocate that pharmacists be responsible for coordinating the individualized care of patients within anticoagulation management programs; further,

To encourage pharmacists who participate in anticoagulation programs to educate patients, caregivers, prescribers, and staff about anticoagulant medication uses, drug interactions, adverse effects, the importance of adhering to therapy, and recommended laboratory testing and other monitoring.

Standard Drug Administration Schedules (0707)

Source: Council on Pharmacy Management

To support the principle that standard medication administration times should be based primarily on optimal pharmacotherapeutics, with secondary consideration of workload, caregiver preference, patient preference, and logistical issues; further,

To encourage the development of hospital-specific or health-system-specific standard administration times through an interdisciplinary process coordinated by the pharmacy; further,

To encourage information technology vendors to adopt these principles in system design while allowing flexibility to meet site-specific patient needs.

This policy was reviewed in 2011 by the Council on Pharmacy Management and by the Board of Directors and was found to still be appropriate.

Universal Influenza Vaccination (0601)

Source: Commission on Therapeutics

To advocate universal administration of influenza vaccinations to the United States population.

This policy was reviewed in 2010 by the Council on Therapeutics and by the Board of Directors and was found to still be appropriate.

Integrated Team-Based Approach for the Pharmacy Enterprise (0619)

Source: Council on Professional Affairs

To advocate a high level of coordination of all components of the pharmacy enterprise in hospitals and health systems for the purpose of optimizing (1) the value of drug therapy and (2) medication-use safety; further,

To encourage pharmacy department leaders to develop and maintain patient-centered practice models that integrate into a team all components of the pharmacy enterprise, including general and specialized clinical practice, drug-use policy, product acquisition and inventory control, product preparation and distribution, and medication-use safety and other quality initiatives.

This policy was reviewed in 2010 by the Council on Pharmacy Practice and by the Board of Directors and was found to still be appropriate.

Health Care Quality Standards and Pharmacy Services (0502)

Source: Council on Administrative Affairs

To advocate that health care quality improvement programs adopt standard quality measures that are developed with the involvement of pharmacists, are evidence-based, and promote the demonstrated role of pharmacists in improving patient outcomes.

This policy was reviewed in 2009 by the Council on Pharmacy Practice and by the Board of Directors and was found to still be appropriate.

Health-System Facility Design (0505)

Source: Council on Administrative Affairs

To advocate the development and the inclusion of contemporary pharmacy specifications in national and state health care design standards to ensure adequate space for safe provision of pharmacy products and patient care services; further,

To promote pharmacist involvement in the design-planning and space-allocation decisions of health care facilities.

This policy was reviewed in 2009 by the Council on Pharmacy Management and by the Board of Directors and was found to still be appropriate.

Mandatory Tablet Splitting for Cost Containment (0525)

Source: Council on Professional Affairs

To oppose mandatory tablet splitting for cost containment in ambulatory care; further,

To encourage pharmacists, when voluntary tablet splitting is considered, to collaborate with patients, caregivers, and other health care professionals to determine whether tablet splitting is appropriate on the basis of the patient's ability to split tablets and the suitability of the medication (e.g., whether it is scored or is an extended-release product); further,

To urge pharmacists to promote dosing accuracy and patient safety by ensuring that patients are educated on how to properly split tablets; further,

To encourage further research by the United States Pharmacopeia and the Food and Drug Administration on the impact of tablet splitting on product quality.

This policy was reviewed in 2009 by the Council on Pharmacy Practice and by the Board of Directors and was found to still be appropriate.

Documentation of Pharmacist Patient Care Services (0407)

Source: Council on Administrative Affairs

To encourage the documentation of pharmacist patient care services in order to validate their impact on patient outcomes and total cost of care.

This policy was reviewed in 2008 by the Council on Pharmacy Management and by the Board of Directors and was found to still be appropriate.

Performance Improvement (0202)

Source: Council on Administrative Affairs

To encourage pharmacists to establish performance improvement processes within their practice settings that measure both operational and patient outcomes; further,

To encourage pharmacists to use contemporary performance improvement techniques and methods for ongoing improvement in their services; further,

To support pharmacists in their development and implementation of performance-improvement processes.

This policy was reviewed in 2011 by the Council on Pharmacy Management and by the Board of Directors and was found to still be appropriate.

Pharmacy Benefits for the Uninsured (0101)

Source: Council on Administrative Affairs

To support the principle that all patients have the right to receive care from pharmacists; further,

To declare that health system pharmacists should play a leadership role in ensuring access to pharmacists' services for indigent or low-income patients who lack insurance coverage and for patients who are underinsured; further,

To advocate better collaboration among health systems, community health centers, state and county health departments, and the federal Health Resources and Services Administration (HRSA) in identifying and addressing the needs of indigent and low-income patients who lack insurance coverage and of patients who are underinsured.

This policy was reviewed in 2010 by the Council on Pharmacy Management and by the Board of Directors and was found to still be appropriate.

Patient Satisfaction (0104)

Source: Council on Administrative Affairs

To encourage pharmacists to establish mechanisms within their practice settings that measure the level of satisfaction patients have with pharmacy services and with the outcomes of their drug therapy; further,

To construct such mechanisms in a manner that will (1) provide a system for monitoring trends in the quality of pharmacy services to patients, (2) increase recognition of the value of pharmacy services, and (3) provide a basis for making improvements in the process and outcomes of pharmacy services; further,

To facilitate a dialogue with and education of national patient satisfaction database vendors on the role and value of clinical pharmacy services.

This policy was reviewed in 2010 by the Council on Pharmacy Management and by the Board of Directors and was found to still be appropriate.

Patient Adherence Programs as Part of Health Insurance Coverage (0116)

Source: Council on Legal and Public Affairs

To support the pharmacist's role in patient medication adherence programs that are part of health insurance plans; further,

To support those programs that (1) maintain the direct patient-pharmacist relationship; (2) are based on the pharmacist's knowledge of the patient's medical history, indication for the prescribed medication, and expected therapeutic outcome; (3) use a communication method desired by the patient; (4) are consistent with federal and state regulations for patient confidentiality; and (5) are consistent with ASHP policy on confidentiality of patient health care information.

This policy was reviewed in 2010 by the Council on Public Policy and by the Board of Directors and was found to still be appropriate.

Pharmacist Validation of Information Related to Medications (9921)

Source: Council on Professional Affairs

To support consultation with a pharmacist as a primary means for consumers to validate publicly available information related to medications.

This policy was reviewed in 2008 by the Council on Pharmacy Practice and by the Board of Directors and was found to still be appropriate.

Collaborative Drug Therapy Management Activities (9801)

Source: House of Delegates Resolution

To support the participation of pharmacists in collaborative drug therapy management, which is defined as a multidisciplinary process for selecting appropriate drug therapies, educating patients, monitoring patients, and continually assessing outcomes of therapy; further,

To recognize that pharmacists participate in collaborative drug therapy management for a patient who has a confirmed diagnosis by an authorized prescriber; further,

To recognize that the activities of a pharmacist in collaborative drug therapy management may include, but not be limited to, initiating, modifying, and monitoring a patient's drug therapy; ordering and performing laboratory and related tests; assessing patient response to therapy; counseling and educating a patient on medications; and administering medications.

This policy was reviewed in 2007 by the Council on Pharmacy Practice and by the Board of Directors and was found to still be appropriate.

Multidisciplinary Action Plans for Patient Care (9804)

Source: Council on Administrative Affairs

To support pharmacists as integral participants in the development of multidisciplinary action plans for patient care (care MAPs), disease-management plans, and health-management plans.

This policy was reviewed in 2007 by the Council on Pharmacy Management and by the Board of Directors and was found to still be appropriate.

Medication Administration by Pharmacists (9820)

Source: Council on Professional Affairs

To support the position that the administration of medicines is part of the routine scope of pharmacy practice; further,

To support the position that pharmacists who administer medicines should be skilled to do so; further,

To support the position that pharmacists should be participants in establishing procedures in their own work settings with respect to the administration of medicines (by anyone) and monitoring the outcomes of medication administration.

This policy was reviewed in 2007 by the Council on Pharmacy Practice and by the Board of Directors and was found to still be appropriate.

ASHP Statement on Confidentiality of Patient Health Care Information

The American Society of Health-System Pharmacists (ASHP) believes that all medical information is sensitive and should be given the utmost protection. ASHP supports the adoption into federal law of a minimum standard for protection of individually identifiable patient health information and believes that states should retain the ability to adopt standards that are more stringent than federal law.

ASHP believes that patients should have the right to access and review their medical records and the ability to correct factual errors in those records. Patients should also have the right to know who has access to their medical records and to authorize how their medical information will be used.

The Health Insurance Portability and Accountability Act of 1996 (HIPAA) requires health systems to have written policies and procedures in place to guard against the unauthorized collection, use, or disclosure of individually identifiable patient health information and provide notice of such policies to their patients. All health-system personnel should be trained to understand and comply with those privacy standards.

ASHP strongly believes that pharmacists must have access to patient health records in order to provide quality care and ensure the safe use of medications. Within health systems, all authorized practitioners should be encouraged to communicate freely with each other while maintaining patient confidentiality and privacy. This includes pharmacists practicing across the continuum of practice settings in order to maintain continuity of care. Pharmacists recognize that with access to the patient's health record comes the pharmacist's professional responsibility to safeguard the patient's rights to privacy and confidentiality. Uniquely identifiable patient information should not be exchanged without the patient's authorization for any reason not directly related to treatment, payment, health care operations, or research conducted under an appropriately constituted institutional review board (IRB). ASHP advocates strict governmental protections, with appropriate civil or criminal penalties for violations, to prevent disclosure of individually identifiable patient information outside the health system (i.e., to an unauthorized third party) for any purposes not directly related to treatment, payment, health care operations, or research conducted under an appropriately constituted IRB.

Pharmacists participate extensively in research on drugs. ASHP believes that all research data must be recorded and stored in such a way that the subjects' rights of privacy and confidentiality are protected. IRBs have a responsibility to determine when informed consent is necessary and to establish procedures for obtaining informed consent. Patients should receive a statement describing the parties who may have access to patient-identifiable information (e.g., institutional personnel, business associates, researchers, personnel from study sponsors, employees of government agencies that monitor compliance with regulations). Patient authorization requirements under the privacy regulations of HIPAA must be followed, and patients always have the right to withdraw their consent at any time.

ASHP believes that there is no potential for a breach of patient confidentiality when patient information is aggregated for use in legitimate research or statistical measurement and is not uniquely identifiable. Therefore, specific authorization by individual patients for access to this information is not needed.

ASHP believes that pharmacy residency programs and other training programs must implement policies and procedures to ensure the confidentiality of patient medical records while allowing pharmacy students and residents access to these records in the course of their training and presentation of their research.

Developed through the ASHP Council on Public Policy and approved by the ASHP Board of Directors on February 22, 2008, and by the ASHP House of Delegates on June 10, 2008.

This statement supersedes the ASHP Statement on the Confidentiality of Patient Health Care Information dated April 21, 1999.

The bibliographic citation for this document is as follows: American Society of Health-System Pharmacists. ASHP statement on confidentiality of patient health care information. *Am J Health-Syst Pharm.* 2009; 66:411–2.

ASHP Statement on the Health-System Pharmacist's Role in National Health Care Quality Initiatives

Position

The American Society of Health-System Pharmacists (ASHP) believes that pharmacists who practice in hospitals and health systems ("health-system pharmacists") have a critical leadership role in national health care quality-improvement initiatives. Health-system pharmacists possess the knowledge of drug therapy and medication-use systems required to successfully implement quality-assurance and improvement programs. These pharmacists should use their authority over and accountability for medication management systems to align medication use in hospitals and health systems with the national health care quality agenda.

Background

Major reports from the Institute of Medicine (IOM) have demonstrated that the quality and safety environment across the health care industry needs significant transformation. *The Urgent Need to Improve Health Care Quality*[1] suggested that the quality of the health care system in the United States could be accurately measured and that the quality of care was being compromised by the underuse, overuse, and misuse of health care entities. *Crossing the Quality Chasm*[2] built a compelling case that the American health care delivery system requires major restructuring and proposed goals for improving six key dimensions of health care quality: safety, timeliness, effectiveness, efficiency, equity, and patient centeredness (the "STEEP" framework). To achieve these aims, IOM called for fundamental reforms, including new payment methodologies, public reporting, and transparency of quality-improvement data.

Since the release of these reports, health care policymakers, providers, purchasers, payers, consumers, and others have responded in ways that are beginning to change the U.S. health care delivery system. These changes are influenced by a growing number of private and public organizations, including the Joint Commission, Centers for Medicare and Medicaid Services (CMS), National Quality Forum, National Priorities Partnership, Agency for Healthcare Research and Quality, Institute for Healthcare Improvement, and American Health Quality Association, among others. These organizations, alone or in collaboration, identify health care quality measures to set the national health care quality agenda. These quality measures are collected and reported through both mandatory and voluntary reporting systems, and the outcome measurements of a health system may be linked to reimbursement (e.g., through CMS pay-for-performance programs).

Responsibilities of Health-System Pharmacists

Many national health care quality measures are related to medication use.[3] Health-system pharmacists are strategically positioned to integrate practices and procedures that support these quality measures into the medication-use system. To help align medication use in hospitals and health systems with the national health care quality agenda, health-system pharmacists should

- Become familiar with the organizations that influence the national health care quality agenda and monitor those organizations for changes in medication-use-related quality measures.
- Participate in the development, implementation, and evaluation of national and state health care quality-improvement initiatives related to medication use.
- Collaborate with other health care professionals to evaluate medication-use practices in their organizations and develop and implement programs that optimize patient outcomes, improve medication use, and align with the national health care quality agenda, including expanding the scope and reach of pharmacists' services when appropriate.
- Collect, analyze, and report data that measure health care quality related to medication use, and support the public availability of those data.
- Integrate and align information systems in their organizations with the national health care quality agenda.
- Educate other health care practitioners, health care executives, and the public about medication-related health care quality-improvement initiatives and the critical role pharmacists have in those initiatives (e.g., by publishing articles about innovative pharmacy services that improve patient outcomes or medication use).
- Encourage national pharmacy organizations to support, guide, and provide education related to the national health care quality agenda.

Conclusion

The number of mandatory and voluntary health care quality measures related to the use of medications is large and growing. As medication-use experts, health-system pharmacists have a responsibility to become knowledgeable about national health care quality-improvement initiatives and to align their practices accordingly. Because health-system pharmacists possess knowledge of drug therapy and medication-use systems and have authority over and accountability for medication management systems, they have a fundamental leadership role in the development, implementation, and evaluation of health care quality-improvement initiatives.

References

1. Chassin MR, Galvin RW. The urgent need to improve health care quality. Institute of Medicine National Roundtable on Health Care Quality. *JAMA.* 1998; 280:1000-5.
2. Institute of Medicine Committee on Quality of Health Care in America. Crossing the quality chasm: a new health system for the 21st century. Washington, DC: National Academy Press; 2001:43-56.

3. Bohenek WS, Grossbart SR. Pharmacists' role in improving quality of care. *Am J Health-Syst Pharm.* 2008; 65:1566-70.

Approved by the ASHP Board of Directors on April 17, 2009, and by the ASHP House of Delegates on June 16, 2009. Developed through the ASHP Council on Pharmacy Practice.

The contributions of Wayne S. Bohenek, Pharm.D., M.S., FASHP, and Jamie S. Sinclair, M.S., to this statement are gratefully acknowledged. The following organizations and individuals are acknowledged for reviewing draft versions of this statement (review does not imply endorsement): Academy of Managed Care Pharmacy (AMCP); Accreditation Council for Pharmacy Education (ACPE); American Pharmacists Association (APhA); South Carolina Society of Health-Systems Pharmacists (SCSHSP); John A. Armitstead, M.S., FASHP; Cathy Baker, Pharm.D.; Frank Briggs, Pharm.D., M.P.H.; Kimberly K. Daugherty, Pharm.D., BCPS; Jeanne Ezell, M.S., FASHP; Linda Gore Martin, Pharm.D., M.B.A., BCPS; Jody Jacobson Wedret, FASHP, FCSHP; Patricia Kienle, M.P.A., FASHP; Julie Kuhle, B.S.Pharm.; Greg Polk, M.B.A.; James A. Ponto, M.S., BCNP, FASHP; Mike Rouse, B.Pharm.(Hons), M.P.S. (ACPE); Marissa Schlaifer, M.S. (AMCP); Sue Skledar, M.P.H., FASHP; Darren M. Triller, Pharm.D.; and Bradley White, Pharm.D., R.N. (SCSHSP).

The bibliographic citation for this document is as follows: American Society of Health-System Pharmacists. ASHP Statement on the Health-System Pharmacist's Role in National Health Care Quality Initiatives. *Am J Health-Syst Pharm.* 2010; 67:578-9.

ASHP–SHM Joint Statement
on Hospitalist–Pharmacist Collaboration

Position

The American Society of Health-System Pharmacists (ASHP) and the Society for Hospital Medicine (SHM) believe that the rapidly emerging hospitalist model of inpatient care offers new and significant opportunities to optimize patient care through collaboration among hospitalists, hospital pharmacists (hereinafter, "pharmacists"), and other health care providers. The emerging model of care allows for deeper professional relationships among health care providers and promotes a shared interest in and responsibility for direct patient care, indirect patient care, and service activities. ASHP and SHM encourage hospitalists, pharmacists, and health care executives to seek out ways to foster collaboration between hospitalists and pharmacists.

The purpose of this consensus statement is to promote an understanding of the ways hospitalists and pharmacists can jointly optimize the care provided to patients in hospitals, examine opportunities for improving hospitalist–pharmacist alliances that enhance patient care, suggest future directions for collaboration, and identify aspects of such collaboration that warrant further research.

Background

Increases in health care spending and the expanding influence of managed care in the late 1980s and early 1990s resulted in calls for more efficient health care. The movement toward greater efficiency resulted in more emphasis on ambulatory care, fewer hospital admissions, shortened hospital stays, and an overall increase in the acuity of illness of hospitalized patients. The emphasis on ambulatory care increased the number and complexity of physician office visits, and the changing characteristics of office- and hospital-based care placed significant demands on primary care physicians and contributed to the rise of hospital medicine.

In 1996, the term "hospitalist" was introduced to the health care lexicon.[1] A hospitalist was defined as an inpatient physician who manages the care of hospitalized patients and facilitates the transfer of their care back to the primary care physician. The Society of Hospital Medicine has since defined a hospitalist as a physician whose primary professional focus is the general medical care of hospitalized patients and whose activities may include patient care, teaching, research, and leadership related to hospital medicine.[2]

The past decade has seen rapid growth in the number of hospitalists and the use of hospitalists by U.S. hospitals.[3] In 2005, 70% of hospitals with more than 200 beds used hospitalist services, and there were over 16,000 hospitalists in practice.[4] An estimated 20,000 hospitalists were practicing at over 2,600 U.S. hospitals in 2007.[5]

Initially, many physicians expressed concern about the potential for hospitalists to interfere in the relationship between the patient and the primary care physician, as well as about the potential negative impact on continuity of care.[6] However, subsequent studies demonstrated increasing acceptance of hospitalists by primary care physicians, with as many as 89% considering the hospitalist model to be superior to the historical model of hospital care being provided by primary care physicians or by specialists working on rotations.[7,8] Numerous studies demonstrate the value of hospitalists in improving quality of care, decreasing hospital costs and length of stay, and reducing hospital readmissions.[9–21]

As early as 1921, hospital pharmacists in the American Pharmaceutical Association (now the American Pharmacists Association) had formed a committee to address their distinct concerns. During the 1930s, hospital pharmacists began to organize state organizations and to adhere to a set of minimum standards of practice. In 1942, the American Society of Hospital Pharmacists (now the American Society of Health-System Pharmacists [ASHP]) was formed to establish minimum standards of pharmaceutical services in hospitals, provide interchange among pharmacists, promote new pharmaceutical techniques, and aid the medical profession in extending the economic and rational use of medications.[22] As of 2005, there were approximately 50,000 pharmacists practicing in U.S. hospitals.[23]

The modern mission of hospital pharmacy departments is to ensure optimal outcomes from the use of medicines.[24] Although the focus of hospital pharmacy has traditionally been on the safe dispensing of medications, direct patient care by pharmacists (clinical pharmacy) has always been a component of hospital pharmacy practice. Following the rise of pharmaceutical care in the 1980s,[25] these pharmacist services have expanded greatly. It has been estimated that 35–40% of hospital pharmacists are devoted to providing clinical services.[23] A systematic review in 2006 documented improved outcomes when clinical pharmacists interacted with the health care team on patient rounds, interviewed patients, reconciled medications, and provided discharge counseling and follow-up.[26] These findings support those of other studies in which specific clinical pharmacy services were associated with improved therapeutic and economic outcomes.[27–31]

Opportunities for Collaboration Between Pharmacists and Hospitalists

Pharmacists and hospitalists have shared interests that provide strong incentives for collaboration. All health care professionals share, first, a commitment to and responsibility for providing safe and effective patient care. Physicians, pharmacists, and other health care providers have long collaborated in providing direct patient care. The emerging hospitalist model of care offers more opportunities for collaboration because pharmacists and hospitalists also share interest in and responsibility for indirect patient care and service activities—developing the institutional policies, processes, and infrastructure that support patient care.

Direct patient care activities typically performed by hospitalists include obtaining patient histories, conducting physical examinations, making diagnoses, developing treatment plans, monitoring patients' responses to therapy, performing follow-up hospital visits, participating in family

meetings, and providing discharge instructions.[32] Specific clinical pharmacy services that have been associated with improved health care outcomes include providing drug information, managing medication protocols and adverse drug reactions, participating in medical rounds, gathering admission medication histories, interviewing patients, reconciling patient medications, and providing discharge counseling and follow-up.[26–31]

Pharmacists should be involved in the care of hospitalized patients and can collaborate with hospitalists in numerous ways, including

- Providing consultative services that foster appropriate, evidence-based medication selection (e.g., during rounds),
- Providing drug information consultation to physicians, nurses, and other clinicians,
- Managing medication protocols under collaborative practice agreements,
- Assisting in the development of treatment protocols,
- Monitoring therapeutic responses (including laboratory test results),
- Continuously assessing for and managing adverse drug reactions,
- Gathering medication histories,
- Reconciling medications as patients move across the continuum of hospital care, and
- Providing patient and caretaker education, including discharge counseling and follow-up.

Both hospitalists and pharmacists have a responsibility for ensuring continuity as patients move across settings of care.

In addition to their direct patient care activities, hospitalists add value through their efforts in hospital service activities, student and resident education, and research. Typical service activities include participating in quality-improvement and safety initiatives, developing institutional guidelines and protocols for the treatment of specific diseases, serving on hospital committees (e.g., the pharmacy and therapeutics [P&T] committee), and working with others to introduce new technologies to the hospital setting.[33,34]

Pharmacists also participate in hospital service activities, student and resident education, and research. For example, pharmacists serve on the P&T committee and are directly involved in managing the formulary system that guides an institution's medication use. As medication experts, pharmacists contribute to the development and implementation of patient care guidelines and other medication-use policies. Pharmacist expertise is also integral to many quality-improvement efforts (e.g., surgical infection prophylaxis) and to technology initiatives (e.g., bedside medication scanning and computerized prescriber-order-entry systems). Pharmacist provision of inservice education on medications and medication use is invaluable for all health care providers.

These overlapping responsibilities provide hospitalists and pharmacists with opportunities to collaborate on activities that can have a profound effect on care in the hospital. Hospitalists and pharmacists can work together to ensure that care is evidence-based, cost-effective, and adherent to national guidelines; establish an institutional culture of safety; develop and implement quality-improvement initiatives; meet accreditation standards; and, in many cases, foster the institution's education and research initiatives. Health professional education and research offer the opportunities to improve patient care provided not just by a single hospital but by other facilities as well.

Opportunities to Improve Collaboration

ASHP and SHM believe that there are opportunities for improving collaboration between hospitalists and pharmacists. Barriers to collaboration include real and perceived professional boundaries, poor integration of technology systems, inadequate pharmacist and hospitalist staffing, time constraints, inadequate funding and resources, lack of third-party compensation for clinical pharmacy services, and the competing obligations weighing on both professions.

Real and perceived professional boundaries can be addressed by clear communication and by enhanced interdisciplinary educational opportunities for all members of the health care team.[35–38] ASHP and SHM believe that, while hospitalists should serve as the primary leaders of hospital care teams, all health care professionals should be willing to assume a leadership role in treating patients and, when appropriate, accept leadership by other team members. Like all members of the care team, pharmacists require timely access to hospitalists for consultation, as well as access to patient information. The vital flow of information and communication among health care providers should be conducive to collaborating and improving patient outcomes. ASHP and SHM believe that properly applied, well-integrated technologies (e.g., electronic medical records and personal digital assistants with clinical decision support systems, including drug information) can enhance communication among all members of the health care team.

Hospitalists and pharmacists can work together to overcome limitations created by inadequate funding and staffing by providing evidence to health care executives of the value of clinical pharmacist positions and pharmacist–hospitalist collaboration. This evidence should examine the impact of these positions and such collaboration on therapeutic, safety, humanistic, and economic outcomes. Collaboration among all members of the health care team would also be encouraged by reforming the current fee-for-service reimbursement practices to base payment for care delivery on overall treatment goals (e.g., a payment rate based on diagnosis).

Conclusion

An interdisciplinary approach to health care that includes physicians, pharmacists, nurses, and other health care professionals will improve the quality of patient care. Hospitalists and pharmacists need to collaborate with each other and with other health care professionals to optimize outcomes in hospitalized patients. ASHP and SHM believe that hospitalist–pharmacist alliances should be encouraged and that the systems and technologies that enable collaboration, and the incentives for such collaboration, should be enhanced.

References

1. Wachter RM, Goldman L. The emerging role of "hospitalists" in the American health care system. *N Engl J Med.* 1996; 335:514–7.

2. Society of Hospital Medicine. Definition of a hospitalist. www.hospitalmedicine.org/Content/NavigationMenu/AboutSHM/DefinitionofaHospitalist/Definition_of_a_Hosp.htm (accessed 2007 May 29).

3. Kralovec PD, Miller JA, Wellikson L et al. The status of hospital medicine groups in the United States. *J Hosp Med.* 2006; 1:75–80.

4. AHA hospital statistics. Chicago: American Hospital Association; 2005.

5. Hospital medicine specialty shows 20 percent growth. SHM analysis of 2005 American Hospital Association survey data. www.hospitalmedicine.org/AM/Template.cfm?Section=Press_Releases&Template=/CM/ContentDisplay.cfm&ContentID=12507 (accessed 2007 May 29).

6. Sox HC. The hospitalist model: perspectives of the patient, the internist, and internal medicine. *Ann Intern Med.* 1999; 130:368–72.

7. Auerbach AD, Nelson EA, Lindenauer PK et al. Physician attitudes toward and prevalence of the hospitalist model of care: results of a national survey. *Am J Med.* 2000; 109:648–53.

8. Fernandez A, Grumbach K, Goitein L et al. Friend or foe? How primary care physicians perceive hospitalists. *Arch Intern Med.* 2000; 160:2902–8.

9. Wachter RM, Katz P, Showstack J et al. Reorganizing an academic medical service: impact on cost, quality, patient satisfaction, and education. *JAMA.* 1998; 279:1560–5.

10. Diamond HS, Goldberg E, Janosky JE. The effect of full-time faculty hospitalists on the efficiency of care at a community teaching hospital. *Ann Intern Med.* 1998; 129:197–203.

11. Stein MD, Hanson S, Tammaro D et al. Economic effects of community versus hospital-based faculty pneumonia care. *J Gen Intern Med.* 1998; 13:774–7.

12. Craig DE, Hartka L, Likosky WH et al. Implementation of a hospitalist system in a large health maintenance organization: the Kaiser Permanente experience. *Ann Intern Med.* 1999; 130:355–9.

13. Freese RB. The Park Nicollet experience in establishing a hospitalist system. *Ann Intern Med.* 1999; 130:350–4.

14. Rifkin WD, Connor DS, Silver A et al. Comparison of hospitalists and primary care internists in the care of patients with pneumonia. *J Gen Intern Med.* 1999; 14(suppl):S118.

15. Rifkin WD, Connor DS, Silver A et al. Comparing hospitalists' and community-based primary care physicians' care of patients with pneumonia. *J Gen Intern Med.* 2001; 16(suppl):S215.

16. Davis KM, Koch KE, Harvey JK et al. Effects of hospitalists on cost, outcomes, and patient satisfaction in a rural health system. *Am J Med.* 2000; 108:621–6.

17. Halpert AP, Pearson SD, LeWine HE et al. The impact of an inpatient physician program on quality, utilization, and satisfaction. *Am J Manag Care.* 2000; 6:549–55.

18. Bellet PS, Whitaker RC. Evaluation of a pediatric hospitalist service: impact on length of stay and hospital charges. *Pediatrics.* 2000; 105:478–84.

19. Landrigan C, Srivastava R, Muret-Wagstaff S et al. Outcomes of hospitalization in pediatric patients in-

sured by HMOs: comparison of care by hospitalists and traditional academic providers. *Pediatr Res.* 2000; 47:204A. Abstract.

20. Srivastava R, Landrigan C, Muret-Wagstaff S et al. Impact of a managed care hospitalist system in academic pediatrics. *Pediatr Res.* 2000; 47:228A. Abstract.

21. Srivastava R, Landrigan C, Muret-Wagstaff S et al. Cost savings for patients with acute conditions cared for by pediatric hospitalists in a tertiary care center. *Pediatr Res.* 2001; 49:125A. Abstract.

22. Zellmer WA. Overview of the history of pharmacy in the United States. In: Brown TR, ed. Handbook of institutional pharmacy practice. Bethesda, MD: American Society of Health-System Pharmacists; 2006:19–32.

23. Pedersen CA, Schneider PJ, Scheckelhoff DJ. ASHP national survey of pharmacy practice in hospital settings: dispensing and administration—2005. *Am J Health-Syst Pharm.* 2006; 63:327–45.

24. Zellmer WA. Perspectives on Hilton Head. *Am J Hosp Pharm.* 1986; 43:1439–43.

25. American Society of Hospital Pharmacists. ASHP statement on pharmaceutical care. *Am J Hosp Pharm.* 1993; 50:1720–3.

26. Kaboli PJ, Hoth AB, McClimon BJ et al. Clinical pharmacists and inpatient medical care: a systematic review. *Arch Intern Med.* 2006; 166:955–64.

27. Bond CA, Raehl CL, Franke T. Interrelationships among mortality rates, drug costs, total cost of care, and length of stay in United States hospitals: summary and recommendations for clinical pharmacy services and staffing. *Pharmacotherapy.* 2001; 21:129–41.

28. Bond CA, Raehl CL, Franke T. Clinical pharmacy services, hospital pharmacy staffing, and medication errors in United States hospitals. *Pharmacotherapy.* 2002; 22:134–47.

29. Bond CA, Raehl CL. Clinical pharmacy services, pharmacy staffing, and adverse drug reactions in United States hospitals. *Pharmacotherapy.* 2006; 26:735–47.

30. Schumock GT, Butler MG, Meek PD et al. Evidence of the economic benefit of clinical pharmacy services: 1996–2000. *Pharmacotherapy.* 2003; 23:113–32.

31. Kucukarslan SN, Peters M, Mlynarek M et al. Pharmacists on rounding teams reduce preventable adverse drug events in hospital general medicine units. *Arch Intern Med.* 2003; 163:2014–8.

32. O'Leary KJ, Liebovitz DM, Baker DW. How hospitalists spend their time: insights on efficiency and safety. *J Hosp Med.* 2006; 1:88–93.

33. Hauer KE, Wachter RM. Implications of the hospitalist model for medical students' education. *Acad Med.* 2001; 76:324–30.

34. Plauth WH III, Pantilat SZ, Wachter RM et al. Hospitalists' perceptions of their residency training needs: results of a national survey. *Am J Med.* 2001; 111:247–54.

35. Committee on the Health Professions Education Summit. Health professions education: a bridge to quality. Washington, DC: National Academy Press; 2003.

36. Cooper H, Carlisle C, Gibbs T et al. Developing an evidence base for interdisciplinary learning: a systematic review. *J Adv Nurs.* 2001; 31:228–37.

37. Horsburgh M, Lamdin R, Williamson E. Multiprofessional learning: the attitudes of medical, nursing, and pharmacy students to shared learning. *Med Educ.* 2001; 35:876–83.

38. Crawford GB, Price SD. Team working: palliative care as a model of interdisciplinary practice. *Med J Aust.* 2003; 179:S32–4.

Approved by the ASHP Council on Pharmacy Practice on September 24, 2007, by the ASHP Board of Directors on September 27, 2007, by the SHM Board of Directors on September 26, 2007. Developed through the American Society of Health-System Pharmacists Research and Education Foundation through a sponsorship from sanofi-aventis, Inc.

Daniel J. Cobaugh, Pharm.D., FAACT, DABAT (Corresponding Author, ASHP); Alpesh Amin, M.D., MBA, FACP (Corresponding Author, SHM); Thomas Bookwalter, Pharm.D. (ASHP, SHM); Mark Williams, M.D., FACP (SHM), Patricia Grunwald, Pharm.D. (ASHP); Cynthia LaCivita, Pharm.D. (ASHP); and Bruce Hawkins, B.A., B.S. (ASHP) are gratefully acknowledged for drafting this statement.

The bibliographic citation for this document is as follows: American Society of Health-System Pharmacists. ASHP–SHM joint statement on hospitalist–pharmacist collaboration. *Am J Health-Syst Pharm.* 2008; 65:260–3.

ASHP Statement on Pharmaceutical Care

The purpose of this statement is to assist pharmacists in understanding pharmaceutical care. Such understanding must precede efforts to implement pharmaceutical care, which ASHP believes merit the highest priority in all practice settings.

Possibly the earliest published use of the term pharmaceutical care was by Brodie in the context of thoughts about drug use control and medication-related services.[1,2] It is a term that has been widely used and a concept about which much has been written and discussed in the pharmacy profession, especially since the publication of a paper by Hepler and Strand in 1990.[3–5] ASHP has formally endorsed the concept.[6] With varying terminology and nuances, the concept has also been acknowledged by other national pharmacy organizations.[7,8] Implementation of pharmaceutical care was the focus of a major ASHP conference in March 1993.

Many pharmacists have expressed enthusiasm for the concept of pharmaceutical care, but there has been substantial inconsistency in its description. Some have characterized it as merely a new name for clinical pharmacy; others have described it as anything that pharmacists do that may lead to beneficial results for patients.

ASHP believes that pharmaceutical care is an important new concept that represents growth in the profession beyond clinical pharmacy as often practiced and beyond other activities of pharmacists, including medication preparation and dispensing. All of these professional activities are important, however, and ASHP continues to be a strong proponent of the necessity for pharmacists' involvement in them. In practice, these activities should be integrated with and culminate in pharmaceutical care provided by individual pharmacists to individual patients.

In 1992, ASHP's members urged the development of an officially recognized ASHP definition of pharmaceutical care.[9] This statement provides a definition and elucidates some of the elements and implications of that definition. The definition that follows is an adaptation of a definition developed by Hepler and Strand.[3]

Definition

The mission of the pharmacist is to provide pharmaceutical care. Pharmaceutical care is the direct, responsible provision of medication-related care for the purpose of achieving definite outcomes that improve a patient's quality of life.

Principal Elements

The principal elements of pharmaceutical care are that it is *medication related*; it is *care* that is *directly provided* to the patient; it is provided to produce *definite outcomes*; these outcomes are intended to improve the patient's *quality of life*; and the provider accepts personal *responsibility* for the outcomes.

Medication Related. Pharmaceutical care involves not only medication therapy (the actual provision of medication) but also decisions about medication use for individual patients. As appropriate, this includes decisions *not* to use medication therapy as well as judgments about medication selection, dosages, routes and methods of administration, medication therapy monitoring, and the provision of medication-related information and counseling to individual patients.

Care. Central to the concept of care is caring, a personal concern for the well-being of another person. Overall patient care consists of integrated domains of care including (among others) medical care, nursing care, and pharmaceutical care. Health professionals in each of these disciplines possess unique expertise and must cooperate in the patient's overall care. At times, they share in the execution of the various types of care (including pharmaceutical care). To pharmaceutical care, however, the pharmacist contributes unique knowledge and skills to ensure optimal outcomes from the use of medications.

At the heart of any type of patient care, there exists a one-to-one relationship between a caregiver and a patient. In pharmaceutical care, the irreducible "unit" of care is one pharmacist in a direct professional relationship with one patient. In this relationship, the pharmacist provides care directly to the patient and for the benefit of the patient.

The health and well-being of the patient are paramount. The pharmacist makes a direct, personal, caring commitment to the individual patient and acts in the patient's best interest. The pharmacist cooperates directly with other professionals and the patient in designing, implementing, and monitoring a therapeutic plan intended to produce definite therapeutic outcomes that improve the patient's quality of life.

Outcomes. It is the goal of pharmaceutical care to improve an individual patient's quality of life through achievement of definite (predefined), medication-related therapeutic outcomes. The outcomes sought are

1. Cure of a patient's disease.
2. Elimination or reduction of a patient's symptomatology.
3. Arresting or slowing of a disease process.
4. Prevention of a disease or symptomatology.

This, in turn, involves three major functions: (1) identifying potential and actual medication-related problems, (2) resolving actual medication-related problems, and (3) preventing potential medication-related problems. A medication-related problem is an event or circumstance involving medication therapy that actually or potentially interferes with an optimum outcome for a specific patient. There are at least the following categories of medication-related problems[3]:

- *Untreated indications.* The patient has a medical problem that requires medication therapy (an indication for medication use) but is not receiving a medication for that indication.

- *Improper drug selection.* The patient has a medication indication but is taking the wrong medication.

- *Subtherapeutic dosage.* The patient has a medical problem that is being treated with too little of the correct medication.

- *Failure to receive medication.* The patient has a medical problem that is the result of not receiving a medication (e.g., for pharmaceutical, psychological, sociological, or economic reasons).

- *Overdosage.* The patient has a medical problem that is being treated with too much of the correct medication (toxicity).

- *Adverse drug reactions.* The patient has a medical problem that is the result of an adverse drug reaction or adverse effect.
- *Drug interactions.* The patient has a medical problem that is the result of a drug–drug, drug–food, or drug–laboratory test interaction.
- *Medication use without indication.* The patient is taking a medication for no medically valid indication.

Patients may possess characteristics that interfere with the achievement of desired therapeutic outcomes. Patients may be noncompliant with prescribed medication use regimens, or there may be unpredictable variations in patients' biological responses. Thus, in an imperfect world, intended outcomes from medication-related therapy are not always achievable.

Patients bear a responsibility to help achieve the desired outcomes by engaging in behaviors that will contribute to—and not interfere with—the achievement of desired outcomes. Pharmacists and other health professionals have an obligation to educate patients about behaviors that will contribute to achieving desired outcomes.

Quality of Life. Some tools exist now for assessing a patient's quality of life. These tools are still evolving, and pharmacists should maintain familiarity with the literature on this subject.[10,11] A complete assessment of a patient's quality of life should include both objective and subjective (e.g., the patient's own) assessments. Patients should be involved, in an informed way, in establishing quality-of-life goals for their therapies.

Responsibility. The fundamental relationship in any type of patient care is a mutually beneficial exchange in which the patient grants authority to the provider and the provider gives competence and commitment to the patient (accepts responsibility).[3] Responsibility involves both moral trustworthiness and accountability.

In pharmaceutical care, the direct relationship between an individual pharmacist and an individual patient is that of a professional covenant in which the patient's safety and well-being are entrusted to the pharmacist, who commits to honoring that trust through competent professional actions that are in the patient's best interest. As an accountable member of the health-care team, the pharmacist must document the care provided.[4,7,12,13] The pharmacist is personally accountable for patient outcomes (the quality of care) that ensue from the pharmacist's actions and decisions.[1]

Implications

The idea that pharmacists should commit themselves to the achievement of definite outcomes for individual patients is an especially important element in the concept of pharmaceutical care. The expectation that pharmacists personally accept responsibility for individual patients' outcomes that result from the pharmacists' actions represents a significant advance in pharmacy's continuing professionalization. The provision of pharmaceutical care represents a maturation of pharmacy as a clinical profession and is a natural evolution of more mature clinical pharmacy activities of pharmacists.[14]

ASHP believes that pharmaceutical care is fundamental to the profession's purpose of helping people make the best use of medications.[15] It is a unifying concept that transcends all types of patients and all categories of pharmacists and

pharmacy organizations. Pharmaceutical care is applicable and achievable by pharmacists in all practice settings. The provision of pharmaceutical care is not limited to pharmacists in inpatient, outpatient, or community settings, nor to pharmacists with certain degrees, specialty certifications, residencies, or other credentials. It is not limited to those in academic or teaching settings. Pharmaceutical care is not a matter of formal credentials or place of work. Rather, it is a matter of a direct personal, professional, responsible relationship with a patient to ensure that the patient's use of medication is optimal and leads to improvements in the patient's quality of life.

Pharmacists should commit themselves to continuous care on behalf of individual patients. They bear responsibility for ensuring that the patient's care is ongoing despite workshift changes, weekends, and holidays. An important implication is that a pharmacist providing pharmaceutical care may need to work as a member of a team of pharmacists who provide backup care when the primary responsible pharmacist is not available. Another is that the responsible pharmacist should work to ensure that continuity of care is maintained when a patient moves from one component of a health-care system to another (e.g., when a patient is hospitalized or discharged from a hospital to return to an ambulatory, community status). In the provision of pharmaceutical care, professional communication about the patient's needs between responsible pharmacists in each area of practice is, therefore, essential. ASHP believes that the development of recognized methods of practicing pharmaceutical care that will enhance such communication is an important priority for the profession.

Pharmaceutical care can be conceived as both a purpose for pharmacy practice and a purpose of medication use processes. That is, a fundamental professional reason that pharmacists engage in pharmacy practice should be to deliver pharmaceutical care. Furthermore, the medication use systems that pharmacists (and others) operate should be designed to support and enable the delivery of pharmaceutical care by individual pharmacists. ASHP believes that, in organized health-care settings, pharmaceutical care can be most successfully provided when it is part of the pharmacy department's central mission and when management activity is focused on facilitating the provision of pharmaceutical care by individual pharmacists. This approach, in which empowered frontline staff provide direct care to individual patients and are supported by managers, other pharmacists, and support systems, is new for many pharmacists and managers.

An important corollary to this approach is that pharmacists providing pharmaceutical care in organized health-care settings cannot provide such care alone. They must work in an interdependent fashion with colleagues in pharmacy and other disciplines, support systems and staff, and managers.[7] It is incumbent on pharmacists to design work systems and practices that appropriately focus the efforts of all activities and support systems on meeting the needs of patients. Some patients will require different levels of care, and it may be useful to structure work systems in light of those differences.[16,17] ASHP believes that the provision of pharmaceutical care and the development of effective work systems to document and support it are major priorities for the profession.

In the provision of pharmaceutical care, pharmacists use their unique perspective and knowledge of medication therapy to evaluate patients' actual and potential medication-related problems. To do this, they require direct access to clinical information about individual patients. They make

judgments regarding medication use and then advocate optimal medication use for individual patients in cooperation with other professionals and in consideration of their unique professional knowledge and evaluations. Pharmaceutical care includes the active participation of the patient (and designated caregivers such as family members) in matters pertinent to medication use.

The acknowledgment of pharmacists' responsibility for therapeutic outcomes resulting from their actions does not contend that pharmacists have exclusive authority for matters related to medication use. Other health-care professionals, including physicians and nurses, have valuable and well-established, well-recognized roles in the medication use process. The pharmaceutical care concept does not diminish the roles or responsibilities of other health professionals, nor does it imply any usurping of authority by pharmacists. Pharmacists' actions in pharmaceutical care should be conducted and viewed as collaborative. The knowledge, skills, and traditions of pharmacists, however, make them legitimate leaders of efforts by health-care teams to improve patients' medication use.

Pharmaceutical care requires a direct relationship between a pharmacist and an individual patient. Some pharmacists and other pharmacy personnel engage in clinical and product-related pharmacy activities that do not involve a direct relationship with the patient. Properly designed, these activities can be supportive of pharmaceutical care, but ASHP believes it would be confusing and counterproductive to characterize such activities as pharmaceutical care. ASHP believes that clinical and product-related pharmacy activities are essential, however, and are as important as the actions of pharmacists interacting directly with patients.

Pharmaceutical educators must teach pharmaceutical care to students.[18] Providers of continuing education should help practicing pharmacists and other pharmacy personnel to understand pharmaceutical care. Students and pharmacists should be taught to conceptualize and execute responsible medication-related problem-solving on behalf of individual patients. Curricula should be designed to produce graduates with sufficient knowledge and skills to provide pharmaceutical care competently.[8,18] Initiatives are under way to bring about these changes.[8] Practicing pharmacists must commit their time as preceptors and their workplaces as teaching laboratories for the undergraduate and postgraduate education and training necessary to produce pharmacists who can provide pharmaceutical care.[8]

Research is needed to evaluate various methods and systems for the delivery of pharmaceutical care.

Pharmaceutical care represents an exciting new vision for pharmacy. ASHP hopes that all pharmacists in all practice settings share in this vision and that the pharmaceutical care concept will serve as a stimulus for them to work toward transforming the profession to actualize that vision.

References

1. Brodie DC. Is pharmaceutical education prepared to lead its profession? The Ninth Annual Rho Chi Lecture. *Rep Rho Chi.* 1973; 39:6–12.
2. Brodie DC, Parish PA, Poston JW. Societal needs for drugs and drug-related services. *Am J Pharm Educ.* 1980; 44:276–8.
3. Hepler CD, Strand LM. Opportunities and responsibilities in pharmaceutical care. *Am J Hosp Pharm.* 1990; 47:533–43.
4. Penna RP. Pharmaceutical care: pharmacy's mission for the 1990s. *Am J Hosp Pharm.* 1990; 47:543–9.
5. Pierpaoli PG, Hethcox JM. Pharmaceutical care: new management and leadership imperatives. *Top Hosp Pharm Manage.* 1992; 12:1–18.
6. Oddis JA. Report of the House of Delegates: June 3 and 5, 1991. *Am J Hosp Pharm.* 1991; 48:1739–48.
7. American Pharmaceutical Association. An APhA white paper on the role of the pharmacist in comprehensive medication use management; the delivery of pharmaceutical care. Washington, DC: American Pharmaceutical Association; 1992 Mar.
8. Commission to Implement Change in Pharmaceutical Education. A position paper. Entry-level education in pharmacy: a commitment to change. *AACP News.* 1991; Nov (Suppl):14
9. Oddis JA. Report of the House of Delegates: June 1 and 3, 1992. *Am J Hosp Pharm.* 1992; 49:1962–73.
10. Gouveia WA. Measuring and managing patient outcomes. *Am J Hosp Pharm.* 1992; 49:2157–8.
11. MacKeigan LD, Pathak DS. Overview of health-related quality-of-life measures. *Am J Hosp Pharm.* 1992; 49:2236–45.
12. Galinsky RE, Nickman NA. Pharmacists and the mandate of pharmaceutical care. *DICP Ann Pharmacother.* 1991; 21:431–4.
13. Angaran DM. Quality assurance to quality improvement: measuring and monitoring pharmaceutical care. *Am J Hosp Pharm.* 1991; 48:1901–7.
14. Hepler CD. Pharmaceutical care and specialty practice. *Pharmacotherapy.* 1993; 13:64S–9S.
15. Zellmer WA. Expressing the mission of pharmacy practice. *Am J Hosp Pharm.* 1991; 48:1195. Editorial.
16. Smith WE, Benderev K. Levels of pharmaceutical care: a theoretical model. *Am J Hosp Pharm.* 1991; 48:540–6.
17. Strand LM, Cipole RJ, Morley PC, et al. Levels of pharmaceutical care: a needs-based approach. *Am J Hosp Pharm.* 1991; 48:547–50.
18. O'Neil EH. Health professions education for the future: schools in service to the nation. San Francisco, CA: Pew Health Profession Commission; 1993.

This statement was reviewed in 1998 by the Council on Professional Affairs and the ASHP Board of Directors and was found to still be appropriate.

Approved by the ASHP Board of Directors, April 21, 1993, and by the ASHP House of Delegates, June 9, 1993. Developed by the ASHP Council on Professional Affairs.

The bibliographic citation for this document is as follows: American Society of Hospital Pharmacists. ASHP statement on pharmaceutical care. *Am J Hosp Pharm.* 1993; 50:1720–3.

ASHP Guidelines on Documenting Pharmaceutical Care in Patient Medical Records

Purpose

The professional actions of pharmacists that are intended to ensure safe and effective use of drugs and that may affect patient outcomes should be documented in the patient medical record (PMR). These guidelines describe the kinds of information pharmacists should document in the PMR, how that information should be documented, methods for obtaining authorization for pharmacist documentation, and the important role of training and continuous quality improvement (CQI) in documentation.

Background

Pharmaceutical care is the direct, responsible provision of medication-related care for the purpose of achieving definite outcomes that improve a patient's quality of life.[1] A core principle of pharmaceutical care is that the pharmacist accepts professional responsibility for patient outcomes.[2] Integrating pharmaceutical care into a patient's overall health care plan requires effective and efficient communication among health care professionals. As an integral member of the health care team, the pharmacist must document the care provided. Such documentation is vital to a patient's continuity of care and demonstrates both the accountability of the pharmacist and the value of the pharmacist's services. Moreover, because clinical services (e.g., those incident to a physician's services) are generally considered reimbursable only when they are necessary for the medical management of a patient and when the service provided and the patient's response are carefully documented, thorough documentation may increase the likelihood of reimbursement. Early implementation of such documentation practices may help health-system pharmacies cope with documentation requirements in the event pharmacists' clinical services become reimbursable.

The PMR's primary purpose is to convey information for use in patient care; it serves as a tool for communication among health care professionals. Information in the PMR may also be used in legal proceedings (e.g., as evidence), education (e.g., for training students), research (e.g., for evaluating clinical drug use), and quality assurance evaluations (e.g., to ascertain adherence to practice standards).[3]

Clinical recommendations made by a pharmacist on behalf of the patient, as well as actions taken in accordance with these recommendations, should be documented in a permanent manner that makes the information available to all the health care professionals caring for the patient. ASHP believes that, to ensure proper coordination of patients' medication therapies, health care systems must be designed to enable, foster, and facilitate communication and collaboration among health care providers.[2] Health care systems must not erect barriers to that communication or to the exercise of the professional judgment of health care providers.

Although telephone calls and other oral communication may be necessary for immediate interventions, they do not allow for the dissemination of information to care providers who are not a part of the conversation. Such interventions should be documented in the PMR as soon as possible after the acute situation has settled. For less urgent and routine recommendations, timely documentation is also preferred, because delays in response to telephone calls or pager messages may lead to miscommunicated or undocumented recommendations. Unofficial, temporary, or removable notes placed in the PMR do not provide a standard of acceptable communication or documentation and therefore are discouraged. Documentation that is not a part of the PMR (e.g., documentation in pharmacy records) may provide a degree of risk reduction; however, such documentation does not provide important information to other care providers and can interrupt continuity of care when the patient is discharged or transferred.

Documenting Pharmaceutical Care

Pharmacists should be authorized and encouraged to make notations in the PMR for the purpose of documenting their findings, assessments, conclusions, and recommendations.[2] ASHP believes that all significant clinical recommendations and resulting actions should be documented in the appropriate section of the PMR. The pharmacy department should establish policies and procedures for documenting information in the PMR. Such policies and procedures will help pharmacists exercise good judgment in determining what information to document in the PMR and how to present it.

Examples of information a pharmacist may need to document in the PMR include, but are not limited to, the following:

1. A summary of the patient's medication history on admission, including medication allergies and their manifestations.
2. Oral and written consultations provided to other health care professionals regarding the patient's drug therapy selection and management.
3. Physicians' oral orders received directly by the pharmacist.
4. Clarification of drug orders.
5. Adjustments made to drug dosage, dosage frequency, dosage form, or route of administration.
6. Drugs, including investigational drugs, administered.
7. Actual and potential drug-related problems that warrant surveillance.
8. Drug therapy-monitoring findings, including
 a. The therapeutic appropriateness of the patient's drug regimen, including the route and method of administration.
 b. Therapeutic duplication in the patient's drug regimen.
 c. The degree of patient compliance with the prescribed drug regimen.
 d. Actual and potential drug–drug, drug–food, drug–laboratory test, and drug–disease interactions.
 e. Clinical and pharmacokinetic laboratory data pertinent to the drug regimen.
 f. Actual and potential drug toxicity and adverse effects.

g. Physical signs and clinical symptoms relevant to the patient's drug therapy.
9. Drug-related patient education and counseling provided.

Documentation by pharmacists should meet established criteria for legibility, clarity, lack of judgmental language, completeness, need for inclusion in the PMR (versus an alternative form of communication), appropriate use of a standard format (e.g., SOAP [subjective, objective, assessment, and plan] or TITRS [title, introduction, text, recommendation, and signature]), and how to contact the pharmacist (e.g., a telephone or pager number).[4]

The authority to document pharmaceutical care in the PMR comes with a responsibility to ensure that patient privacy and confidentiality are safeguarded and the communication is concise and accurate. Local, state, and federal guidelines and laws (including the Health Insurance Portability and Accountability Act of 1996 [HIPAA]) and risk management sensitivities should be considered. Nonjudgmental language should be used, with care taken to avoid words that imply blame (e.g., *error, mistake, misadventure,* and *inadvertent*) or substandard care (e.g., *bad, defective, inadequate, inappropriate, incorrect, insufficient, poor, problem,* and *unsatisfactory*).[3] Facts should be documented accurately, concisely, and objectively; such documentation should reflect the goals established by the medical team.

Documentation of a formal consultation solicited by a physician or other health care provider may include direct recommendations or suggestions as appropriate. However, unsolicited informal consultations, clinical impressions, findings, suggestions, and recommendations should generally be documented more subtly, with indirect recommendations presented in a way that allows the provider to decline the suggestion without incurring a liability. For example, the phrase "may want to consider" creates an opportunity for the suggestion to be acted upon or not, depending on presenting clinical factors.

Obtaining Authorization to Document Pharmaceutical Care

The authority to document pharmaceutical care in the PMR is granted by the health care organization in accordance with organizational and medical staff policies. Although documenting pharmaceutical care in the PMR is a pharmacist's professional responsibility, physicians and other health care professionals may not be accustomed to or open to this practice.

The following steps are recommended for obtaining authorization to document pharmaceutical care in the PMR:

1. Determine the existing organizational and medical staff policies regarding authority for documentation in the PMR. These policies may provide specific guidance on how to proceed.
2. Ascertain whether other nonphysician and nonnurse providers in the organization or affiliated organizations have been granted authority to document patient care activities in the PMR. If so, consult them regarding the process used to establish the authority.
3. Identify physicians in the organization who are willing to support documentation of pharmaceutical care in the PMR.

4. Identify the committees in the organization whose recommendations or decisions will be required to establish authority for pharmacists to document pharmaceutical care in the PMR. Determine the necessary sequence of these approvals. Committees typically involved include the pharmacy and therapeutics (P&T) committee, the executive committee of the medical staff, a quality-assurance committee (e.g., the CQI committee), and the medical records committee.
5. Determine the accepted method and format for submitting a proposal requesting authority to document pharmaceutical care in the PMR. In some organizations, a written proposal may be required. If so, determine the desired format (length, style, and necessary justification) and deadlines for proposal submission. An oral presentation to the deciding bodies may be required. If so, determine in advance the desired presentation format and supporting materials desired by these bodies.
6. Draft a written plan describing
 a. Examples of information to be documented in the PMR. It may be helpful to describe how this important information may be lost or miscommunicated if it is not documented in the PMR.
 b. The locations within the PMR where documentation will be made and any special format or forms proposed. New forms will have to comply with HIPAA regulations and will require review and approval by specific organizational or medical staff committees. To achieve the goal of effective communication among all the members of the health care team, compartmentalization of the PMR should be avoided.
 c. The persons who will be documenting pharmaceutical care in the PMR (i.e., pharmacists, residents, or students). If pharmacy residents or students will be making notations in the PMR, procedures regarding authority and cosignatures will also have to be described.
7. Review the draft plan with the chair of the P&T committee, the director of nursing, the director of medical records, and other appropriate administrative personnel, such as the organization's risk management officer and legal counsel.
8. Seek the endorsement and recommendation of the P&T committee.
9. In appropriate sequence, seek the endorsement or decision of any other committees necessary for ultimate approval. Monitor the proposal's course through the various committees and provide assistance, clarification, or additional data as necessary.
10. When the final approving body grants PMR documentation authority, participate in the required policy development and the communication of the new policy to the individuals or departments in the organization that will be affected by the change (e.g., nurses, the medical staff, the quality-assurance staff, and the medical records department).

Training and CQI

Pharmacist documentation in the PMR is a skill that requires ongoing training and evaluation.[4] A temporary committee may be formed to manage the initial training required to implement pharmacist documentation in the PMR. That

committee may consider offering presentations by physicians or other members of the health care team to provide their perspective on how to effectively communicate using the PMR. The information in those presentations may be reinforced by workshops on documentation skills. Presentation and workshop topics may include the choice of communication method (i.e., when documentation in the PMR is preferred to other means of communication), the documentation format (e.g., SOAP or TITRS), documentation etiquette, and legal requirements.[4] Documentation skills should be demonstrated before a pharmacist is allowed to make notations in the PMR.[4] The ASHP Clinical Skills Program is another tool for training pharmacists to use the PMR.[3]

Documentation of pharmaceutical care should also be one of the many functions addressed in CQI efforts. Pharmacy department CQI efforts should include the development of quality indicators that can be used to evaluate pharmacist documentation in the PMR.[4] Other CQI efforts might analyze and improve systemwide policies and procedures for documenting medication use.[5] Periodic review of organizational policies and procedures will allow for their revision in response to changes in health care and advances in technology, including the availability of an electronic PMR.[6,7]

References

1. Hepler CD, Strand LM. Opportunities and responsibilities in pharmaceutical care. *Am J Hosp Pharm.* 1990; 47:533–43.

2. American Society of Hospital Pharmacists. ASHP statement on pharmaceutical care. *Am J Hosp Pharm.* 1993; 50:1720–3.

3. Shepherd MF. Professional conduct and use of patient medical records. In: ASHP Clinical Skills Program, module 1: reviewing patient medical charts. Bethesda, MD: American Society of Hospital Pharmacists; 1992:38–41.

4. Lacy CF, Saya FG, Shane RR. Quality of pharmacists' documentations in patients' medical records. *Am J Health-Syst Pharm.* 1996; 53:2171–5.

5. Matuschka P. Improving documentation of preoperative antimicrobial prophylaxis. *Am J Health-Syst Pharm.* 1998; 55:993–4.

6. Lau A, Balen RM, Lam R, et al. Using a personal digital assistant to document clinical pharmacy services in an intensive care unit. *Am J Health-Syst Pharm.* 2001; 58:1229–32.

7. Gordon W, Malyuk D, Taki J. Use of health-record abstracting to document pharmaceutical care activities. *Can J Hosp Pharm.* 2000; 53:199–205.

These guidelines were reviewed in 2008 by the Council on Pharmacy Practice and by the Board of Directors and were found to still be appropriate.

Approved by the ASHP Board of Directors, February 20, 2003. Revised by the ASHP Council on Professional Affairs. Supercedes the ASHP Guidelines for Obtaining Authorization for Documenting Pharmaceutical Care in Patient Medical Records dated November 16, 1988.

The bibliographic citation for this document is as follows: American Society of Health-System Pharmacists. ASHP guidelines on documenting pharmaceutical care in patient medical records. *Am J Health-Syst Pharm.* 2003; 60:705–7.

ASHP Guidelines on Pharmacist-Conducted Patient Education and Counseling

Purpose

Providing pharmaceutical care entails accepting responsibility for patients' pharmacotherapeutic outcomes. Pharmacists can contribute to positive outcomes by educating and counseling patients to prepare and motivate them to follow their pharmacotherapeutic regimens and monitoring plans. The purpose of this document is to help pharmacists provide effective patient education and counseling.

In working with individual patients, patient groups, families, and caregivers, pharmacists should approach education and counseling as interrelated activities. ASHP believes pharmacists should educate and counsel all patients to the extent possible, going beyond the minimum requirements of laws and regulations; simply offering to counsel is inconsistent with pharmacists' responsibilities. In pharmaceutical care, pharmacists should encourage patients to seek education and counseling and should eliminate barriers to providing it.

Pharmacists should also seek opportunities to participate in health-system patient-education programs and to support the educational efforts of other health care team members. Pharmacists should collaborate with other health care team members, as appropriate, to determine what specific information and counseling are required in each patient care situation. A coordinated effort among health care team members will enhance patients' adherence to pharmacotherapeutic regimens, monitoring of drug effects, and feedback to the health system.

ASHP believes these patient education and counseling guidelines are applicable in all practice settings—including acute inpatient care, ambulatory care, home care, and long-term care—whether these settings are associated with integrated health systems or managed care organizations or are freestanding. The guidelines may need to be adapted; for example, for use in telephone counseling or for counseling family members or caregivers instead of patients. Patient education and counseling usually occur at the time prescriptions are dispensed but may also be provided as a separate service. The techniques and the content should be adjusted to meet the specific needs of the patient and to comply with the policies and procedures of the practice setting. In health systems, other health care team members share in the responsibility to educate and counsel patients as specified in the patients' care plans.

Background

The human and economic consequences of inappropriate medication use have been the subject of professional, public, and congressional discourse for more than two decades.[1–5] Lack of sufficient knowledge about their health problems and medications is one cause of patients' nonadherence to their pharmacotherapeutic regimens and monitoring plans; without adequate knowledge, patients cannot be effective partners in managing their own care. The pharmacy profession has accepted responsibility for providing patient education and counseling in the context of pharmaceutical care to improve patient adherence and reduce medication-related problems.[6–9]

Concerns about improper medication use contributed to the provision in the Omnibus Budget Reconciliation Act of 1990 (OBRA '90) that mandated an offer to counsel Medicaid outpatients about prescription medications. Subsequently, states enacted legislation that generally extends the offer-to-counsel requirement to outpatients not covered by Medicaid. Future court cases may establish that pharmacists, in part because of changing laws, have a public duty to warn patients of adverse effects and potential interactions of medications. The result could be increased liability for pharmacists who fail to educate and counsel their patients or who do so incorrectly or incompletely.[10]

Pharmacists' Knowledge and Skills

In addition to a current knowledge of pharmacotherapy, pharmacists need to have the knowledge and skills to provide effective and accurate patient education and counseling. They should know about their patients' cultures, especially health and illness beliefs, attitudes, and practices. They should be aware of patients' feelings toward the health system and views of their own roles and responsibilities for decision-making and for managing their care.[11]

Effective, open-ended questioning and active listening are essential skills for obtaining information from and sharing information with patients. Pharmacists have to adapt messages to fit patients' language skills and primary languages, through the use of teaching aids, interpreters, or cultural guides if necessary. Pharmacists also need to observe and interpret the nonverbal messages (e.g., eye contact, facial expressions, body movements, vocal characteristics) patients give during education and counseling sessions.[12]

Assessing a patient's cognitive abilities, learning style, and sensory and physical status enables the pharmacist to adapt information and educational methods to meet the patient's needs. A patient may learn best by hearing spoken instructions; by seeing a diagram, picture, or model; or by directly handling medications and administration devices. A patient may lack the visual acuity to read labels on prescription containers, markings on syringes, or written handout material. A patient may be unable to hear oral instructions or may lack sufficient motor skills to open a child-resistant container.

In addition to assessing whether patients know *how* to use their medications, pharmacists should attempt to understand patients' attitudes and potential behaviors concerning medication use. The pharmacist needs to determine whether a patient is willing to use a medication and whether he or she intends to do so.[13,14]

Environment

Education and counseling should take place in an environment conducive to patient involvement, learning, and acceptance—one that supports pharmacists' efforts to establish caring relationships with patients. Individual patients, groups, families, or caregivers should perceive the counseling environment as comfortable, confidential, and safe.

Education and counseling are most effective when conducted in a room or space that ensures privacy and opportunity to engage in confidential communication. If such an isolated space is not available, a common area can be restructured to maximize visual and auditory privacy from other patients or staff. Patients, including those who are disabled, should have easy access and seating. Space and seating should be adequate for family members or caregivers. The design and placement of desks and counters should minimize barriers to communication. Distractions and interruptions should be few, so that patients and pharmacists can have each other's undivided attention.

The environment should be equipped with appropriate learning aids, e.g., graphics, anatomical models, medication administration devices, memory aids, written material, and audiovisual resources.

Pharmacist and Patient Roles

Pharmacists and patients bring to education and counseling sessions their own perceptions of their roles and responsibilities. For the experience to be effective, the pharmacist and patient need to come to a common understanding about their respective roles and responsibilities. It may be necessary to clarify for patients that pharmacists have an appropriate and important role in providing education and counseling. Patients should be encouraged to be active participants.

The pharmacist's role is to verify that patients have sufficient understanding, knowledge, and skill to follow their pharmacotherapeutic regimens and monitoring plans. Pharmacists should also seek ways to motivate patients to learn about their treatment and to be active partners in their care. Patients' role is to adhere to their pharmacotherapeutic regimens, monitor for drug effects, and report their experiences to pharmacists or other members of their health care teams.[12,15] Optimally, the patient's role should include seeking information and presenting concerns that may make adherence difficult.

Depending on the health system's policies and procedures, its use of protocols or clinical care plans, and its credentialing of providers, pharmacists may also have disease management roles and responsibilities for specified categories of patients. This expands pharmacists' relationships with patients and the content of education and counseling sessions.

Process Steps

Steps in the patient education and counseling process will vary according to the health system's policies and procedures, environment, and practice setting. Generally, the following steps are appropriate for patients receiving new medications or returning for refills[12–21]:

1. Establish caring relationships with patients as appropriate to the practice setting and stage in the patient's health care management. Introduce yourself as a pharmacist, explain the purpose and expected length of the sessions, and obtain the patient's agreement to participate. Determine the patient's primary spoken language.
2. Assess the patient's knowledge about his or her health problems and medications, physical and mental capability to use the medications appropriately, and attitude toward the health problems and medications. Ask open-ended questions about each medication's purpose and

what the patient expects, and ask the patient to describe or show how he or she will use the medication.

Patients returning for refill medications should be asked to describe or show how they have been using their medications. They should also be asked to describe any problems, concerns, or uncertainties they are experiencing with their medications.

3. Provide information orally and use visual aids or demonstrations to fill patients' gaps in knowledge and understanding. Open the medication containers to show patients the colors, sizes, shapes, and markings on oral solids. For oral liquids and injectables, show patients the dosage marks on measuring devices. Demonstrate the assembly and use of administration devices such as nasal and oral inhalers. As a supplement to face-to-face oral communication, provide written handouts to help the patient recall the information.

 If a patient is experiencing problems with his or her medications, gather appropriate data and assess the problems. Then adjust the pharmacotherapeutic regimens according to protocols or notify the prescribers.
4. Verify patients' knowledge and understanding of medication use. Ask patients to describe or show how they will use their medications and identify their effects. Observe patients' medication-use capability and accuracy and attitudes toward following their pharmacotherapeutic regimens and monitoring plans.

Content

The content of an education and counseling session may include the information listed below, as appropriate for each patient's pharmacotherapeutic regimen and monitoring plan.[8,9,20] The decision to discuss specific pharmacotherapeutic information with an individual patient must be based on the pharmacist's professional judgment.

1. The medication's trade name, generic name, common synonym, or other descriptive name(s) and, when appropriate, its therapeutic class and efficacy.
2. The medication's use and expected benefits and action. This may include whether the medication is intended to cure a disease, eliminate or reduce symptoms, arrest or slow the disease process, or prevent the disease or a symptom.
3. The medication's expected onset of action and what to do if the action does not occur.
4. The medication's route, dosage form, dosage, and administration schedule (including duration of therapy).
5. Directions for preparing and using or administering the medication. This may include adaptation to fit patients' lifestyles or work environments.
6. Action to be taken in case of a missed dose.
7. Precautions to be observed during the medication's use or administration and the medication's potential risks in relation to benefits. For injectable medications and administration devices, concern about latex allergy may be discussed.
8. Potential common and severe adverse effects that may occur, actions to prevent or minimize their occurrence, and actions to take if they occur, including notifying the prescriber, pharmacist, or other health care provider.
9. Techniques for self-monitoring of the pharmacotherapy.

10. Potential drug–drug (including nonprescription), drug–food, and drug–disease interactions or contraindications.
11. The medication's relationships to radiologic and laboratory procedures (e.g., timing of doses and potential interferences with interpretation of results).
12. Prescription refill authorizations and the process for obtaining refills.
13. Instructions for 24-hour access to a pharmacist.
14. Proper storage of the medication.
15. Proper disposal of contaminated or discontinued medications and used administration devices.
16. Any other information unique to an individual patient or medication.

These points are applicable to both prescription and nonprescription medications. Pharmacists should counsel patients in the proper selection of nonprescription medications.

Additional content may be appropriate when pharmacists have authorized responsibilities in collaborative disease management for specified categories of patients. Depending on the patient's disease management or clinical care plan, the following may be covered:

1. The disease state: whether it is acute or chronic and its prevention, transmission, progression, and recurrence.
2. Expected effects of the disease on the patient's normal daily living.
3. Recognition and monitoring of disease complications.

Documentation

Pharmacists should document education and counseling in patients' permanent medical records as consistent with the patients' care plans, the health system's policies and procedures, and applicable state and federal laws. When pharmacists do not have access to patients' medical records, education and counseling may be documented in the pharmacy's patient profiles, on the medication order or prescription form, or on a specially designed counseling record.

The pharmacist should record (1) that counseling was offered and was accepted and provided or refused and (2) the pharmacist's perceived level of the patient's understanding.[9] As appropriate, the content should be documented (for example, counseling about food–drug interactions). All documentation should be safeguarded to respect patient confidentiality and privacy and to comply with applicable state and federal laws.[10]

References

1. Smith MC. Social barriers to rational drug therapy. *Am J Hosp Pharm.* 1972; 29:121–7.
2. Priorities and approaches for improving prescription medicine use by older Americans. Washington, DC: National Council on Patient Information and Education; 1987.
3. Manasse HR Jr. Medication use in an imperfect world: drug misadventuring as an issue of public policy, part 1. *Am J Hosp Pharm.* 1989; 46:929–44.
4. Manasse HR Jr. Medication use in an imperfect world: drug misadventuring as an issue of public policy, part 2. *Am J Hosp Pharm.* 1989; 46:1141–52.
5. Johnson JA, Bootman JL. Drug-related morbidity and mortality: a cost-of-illness model. *Arch Intern Med.* 1995; 155:1949–56.
6. Summary of the final report of the Scope of Pharmacy Practice Project. *Am J Hosp Pharm.* 1994; 51:2179–82.
7. Hepler CD, Strand LM. Opportunities and responsibilities in pharmaceutical care. *Am J Hosp Pharm.* 1990; 47:533–42.
8. Hatoum HT, Hutchinson RA, Lambert BL. OBRA 90: patient counseling—enhancing patient outcomes. *US Pharm.* 1993; 18(Jan):76–86.
9. OBRA '90: a practical guide to effecting pharmaceutical care. Washington, DC: American Pharmaceutical Association; 1994.
10. Lynn NJ, Kamm RE. Avoiding liability problems. *Am Pharm.* 1995; NS35(Dec):14–22.
11. Herrier RN, Boyce RW. Does counseling improve compliance? *Am Pharm.* 1995; NS35(Sep):11–2.
12. Foster SL, Smith EB, Seybold MR. Advanced counseling techniques: integrating assessment and intervention. *Am Pharm.* 1995; NS35(Oct):40–8.
13. Bond WS, Hussar DA. Detection methods and strategies for improving medication compliance. *Am J Hosp Pharm.* 1991; 48:1978–88.
14. Felkey BG. Adherence screening and monitoring. *Am Pharm.* 1995; NS35(Jul):42–51.
15. Herrier RN, Boyce RW. Establishing an active patient partnership. *Am Pharm.* 1995; NS35(Apr):48–57.
16. Boyce RW, Herrier RN, Gardner M. Pharmacist-patient consultation program, unit I: an interactive approach to verify patient understanding. New York: Pfizer Inc.; 1991.
17. Pharmacist-patient consultation program, unit II: counseling patients in challenging situations. New York: Pfizer Inc.; 1993.
18. Pharmacist-patient consultation program, unit III: counseling to enhance compliance. New York: Pfizer Inc.; 1995.
19. Boyce RW, Herrier RN. Obtaining and using patient data. *Am Pharm.* 1991; NS31(Jul):65–70.
20. Herrier RN, Boyce RW. Communicating risk to patients. *Am Pharm.* 1995; NS35(Jun):12–4.
21. APhA special report: medication administration problem solving in ambulatory care. Washington, DC: American Pharmaceutical Association; 1994.

This guideline was reviewed in 2011 by the Council on Pharmacy Practice and by the ASHP Board of Directors and was found to still be appropriate.

Approved by the ASHP Board of Directors, November 11, 1996. Revised by the ASHP Council on Professional Affairs. Supersedes the ASHP Statement on the Pharmacist's Role in Patient-Education Programs dated June 3, 1991, and ASHP Guidelines on Pharmacist-Conducted Patient Counseling dated November 18, 1992.

The bibliographic citation for this document is as follows: American Society of Health-System Pharmacists. ASHP guidelines on pharmacist-conducted patient education and counseling. *Am J Health-Syst Pharm.* 1997; 54:431–4.

ASHP Guidelines on the Pharmacist's Role in the Development, Implementation, and Assessment of Critical Pathways

Purpose

The purpose of these guidelines is (1) to describe the pharmacist's role in the development, implementation, and assessment of critical pathways (CPs) and (2) to help pharmacists prepare for that responsibility. Because pharmacotherapy is a central component of many CPs, pharmacists should take leadership roles in the development, implementation, and assessment of CPs. By assuming leadership roles, pharmacists can help improve patient outcomes, contribute to cost-effective patient care, and promote multidisciplinary approaches to patient care and performance improvement. Although pharmacist involvement in the early stages of CP development is crucial to success, CP development is generally cyclical, and pharmacists should seek opportunities to become involved at any stage in the cycle of CP development, implementation, and assessment.

Background

The development of CPs has been stimulated by the desire to improve patient outcomes by applying evidence-based clinical practice guidelines; increased interest in measuring and improving the quality of health care, including continuous-quality-improvement (CQI) initiatives; and managed care and other market-driven health care reforms. CPs can be defined as patient care management plans that delineate key steps along an optimal treatment timeline to achieve a set of predetermined intermediate and ultimate goals for patients who have clearly defined diagnoses or require certain procedures.[1] CPs have also been called care guides, clinical pathways, clinical care plans, and care maps.[2] CPs derive from the industrial engineering concept of critical paths[3] and were originally associated with inpatient acute care and used primarily by nurses. CPs have evolved to incorporate the spectrum of patient care providers and settings and to include CQI concepts.[4] CPs and similar tools are developed in many facilities for many purposes.[5–20] Although dismissed by some critics as "cookbook medicine," CPs have in some cases been shown to improve patient outcomes[21–26] and to reduce health care expenses.[27–36] ASHP believes that carefully developed and skillfully managed CPs can improve the care of patients across the spectrum of health-system settings, as well as improve the allocation of scarce health care resources.

Typical CP Process

Each health system will use a process of CP development, implementation, and assessment that meets its own needs within its own structure, culture, practice settings, and policies and procedures, but these processes do share common elements. Typically, once a disease or procedure is selected for CP development, a multidisciplinary team analyzes its current management (including process variances, costs, and outcomes), evaluates the scientific literature, and develops a plan of care. The planned actions for each discipline on the health care team are mapped on a timeline for the specific

Summary of guidelines. Because pharmacotherapy is a central component of many critical pathways, pharmacists should take leadership roles in their development, implementation, and assessment.

Pharmacists can improve the development of critical pathways by ensuring the evidence-based selection of medications, establishing measures for monitoring patients for drug efficacy and adverse effects, and evaluating the proposed critical pathway for patient safety.

Pharmacists can improve the implementation of critical pathways by documenting processes and outcomes, ensuring proper patient selection and medication use, monitoring patients for drug efficacy and adverse effects, and providing for continuity of care. Pharmacists can improve the assessment of critical pathways by measuring and analyzing processes and outcomes, disseminating the results of those analyses, and reviewing the critical pathways' pharmacotherapy to keep pace with changes in best practices.

disease or procedure.[37] Pharmacists perform the following functions in a typical CP: oversee the selection of medications by using an evidence-based approach, develop the criteria for medication selection or dosages, monitor patients for drug efficacy and adverse effects (or establish parameters for monitoring), and ensure continuity of care across the health system. The following describes common steps in the development, implementation, and assessment of CPs.[3]

1. *Select diagnoses and procedures.* Diagnoses and procedures selected for CP development usually include those with high process variability, high cost, high patient volume, and high risk. CPs can be developed for common or specialized diagnoses (e.g., myocardial infarction, diabetes mellitus) or procedures (e.g., transurethral prostatectomy, coronary artery bypass grafting), for diagnoses that are likely to cause changes in health status (e.g., uncontrolled asthma), and for diseases requiring complicated pharmacotherapeutic regimens (e.g., AIDS). The criteria for selection should be developed with input from administrative and clinical leaders to ensure institutionwide acceptance and should be based on scientific evidence.

2. *Appoint a development team.* The development team should include key health care providers from all organizational components involved in the CP. The importance of a multidisciplinary approach to CP development cannot be overemphasized. If possible, consideration should be given to including a patient representative on the CP development team. Although insurance carriers and managed care providers may not have representatives on the development team, their protocols or guidelines should be evaluated by the team for inclusion in the CP as appropriate.

3. *Conduct a search of the scientific literature.* A literature and database search conducted early in the process will help identify measures for assessing current processes and outcomes and will help ensure an evidence-based approach to the CP.

4. *Document current processes and outcomes.* The current processes, costs, variances, and outcomes need to be documented, usually through flow charting of the current process, retrospective chart review, and benchmarking. Benchmarking may be internal or external to the health system. Depending on the health system's resources, benchmarking may rely on chart review or may use computerized databases that compare physicians' use of resources, health-system costs, and outcomes for specific diagnosis-related groups. This step identifies the health system's practice and compares it with published clinical guidelines that are preferably consensus based (e.g., guidelines from the Agency for Healthcare Research and Quality or the American Heart Association). The team developing the CP should use an evidence-based approach to identify, discuss, and resolve the gaps between clinical guidelines and current local practice. Input from the practitioners who will be involved in the CP is crucial to the success of this process evaluation and CP development in general.

5. *Develop the CP.* Multidisciplinary, standardized development of the CP ensures integration of care and elimination of duplication and oversights. The CP should state its goals, define actions essential to achieving those goals, provide for patient education, outline assessment of patient safety, identify measures of conformance and outcomes, and describe required documentation. The actions and resources required for implementation should be discussed and agreed upon by all disciplines involved.

 a. Goals and outcomes
 * Define the specific goals or measurable outcomes of the CP (e.g., decreased length of stay, decreased ventilator time, reduced overall patient cost, decreased pain scores, early ambulation).
 * Select the areas of focus or categories of actions essential to achieving the goals and outcomes. To ensure consistency and continuity, these areas of focus should be standardized for all CPs developed within a health system; examples of focus areas are treatments, medications, and patient education and counseling.
 * Determine the appropriate time frame. This will vary according to the disease or procedure being addressed and the practice setting (e.g., emergency room, ambulatory care clinic, acute care hospital). The time frame may be specified in minutes, hours, days, or phases. A workload assessment may be required to develop appropriate time frames.
 * Define the activity for the focus area under the appropriate time frame (e.g., "pharmacist provides medication-use education and counseling on discharge day").

 b. Patient education
 * Modify the CP, using lay terms in the patient's primary language, to educate the patient about activities to be performed, time frames, and

expected outcomes. In some practice settings, the patient may be an active partner in CP decision-making and implementation.

 c. Patient safety
 * Identify potential risks to the patient that may arise from use of the CP. For example, the CP could be subjected to the institution's failure-mode and effects analysis, or the medication safety self-assessment tool of the Institute for Safe Medication Practices could be used to assess the safety of the practices outlined in the CP.[38]

 d. Monitoring
 * Identify measures of conformance and variance so that the CP and the resulting outcomes can be continuously improved. Variances are deviations from the CP that may be positive or negative, avoidable or unavoidable, consequential or inconsequential. Sources of variances include patient responses to medications, physician decisions, and system breakdowns.

 e. Documentation
 * Develop a single, multidisciplinary work sheet or other tool that describes the CP's actions and time frames and provides spaces for documenting that actions were performed.[12] Describe how this tool will be used and how data will be collected.

6. *Obtain approval for the CP and educate participants.* To ensure global acceptance among all health care provider groups, the CP should be approved by appropriate committees, especially those of the medical staff. The impact of CP implementation on practitioner workloads will require careful consideration, and departmental policies or procedures may need to be modified. The pharmacy and therapeutics (P&T) committee should review pharmacotherapeutic issues associated with the CP early enough during development that therapeutic concerns can be addressed as they arise rather than after the CP is implemented. After the CP is approved, all health care team members involved in the care of the patients affected by the CP should be educated about the anticipated outcomes, specific actions and time frames, and professional responsibilities associated with the CP.

7. *Implement the CP.* After the necessary education and training of providers, the CP is available for use. Starting the CP as a pilot project for a small number of patients may provide valuable initial assessments that will facilitate wider implementation. Staff members should be designated to identify patients suitable for the CP and to guide their enrollment and the CP's use. Patients enrolled in a CP are assigned to a health care team whose members have specific responsibilities for actions and time frames.

8. *Assess the CP.* Because not all consequences of a CP are foreseeable, CPs require periodic assessment. Assessments after a few days or weeks of use may gauge only the feasibility of the CP and not its success in achieving desired goals, but they should identify unexpected problems that may require modifications to the CP. Surveys of health care practitioners may be useful in such initial assessments. Assessments after a few months of use may provide an initial perspective

on the CP's success but may not be sufficient to fully evaluate outcomes. Assessments after longer periods should produce evidence supporting the CP's original goals. Regular analysis of the results and variances, as well as new information (e.g., new indications for medications) and technologies (e.g., new pharmacotherapy), provides data for a root-cause analysis and continuous improvement of the CP.

9. *Disseminate the results of the assessment.* The results of the assessment should be shared not just with health-system managers or members of the CP development or oversight committees but with all staff involved in the CP. Widespread dissemination allows for more suggestions for improvement from all members of the health care team and encourages acceptance of any alterations in the CP required by the assessment. Publishing the results in a journal, sharing the experience with a practice network, or presenting the results at a meeting expands the general pool of knowledge concerning CPs.

Pharmacist Involvement

These guidelines suggest actions to help prepare pharmacists and pharmacy departments for involvement in the development, implementation, and assessment of CPs at various levels of care and in different practice settings. The applicability of these guidelines depends on a pharmacist's or pharmacy department's current level of involvement in patient care and CPs. Pharmacists should focus on incorporating contemporary pharmaceutical care principles (e.g., assessing medication orders, developing pharmacotherapeutic regimens and monitoring plans, educating and counseling patients, calculating doses according to pharmacokinetic principles, conducting medication-use evaluations [MUEs], and managing anticoagulation therapy) in the development, implementation, and assessment of CPs.[39–42]

Preparing for Involvement in CP Development. Pharmacists should learn about their health system's approach to CP development and assess their readiness for involvement. They should

1. Review the health system's current strategic plan with respect to CPs. Because CPs are inherently collaborative, pharmacists should try to understand this strategic plan from the perspective of other health care providers, seeking advice from them when necessary. When reviewing the strategic plan, pharmacists should also consider the needs of specific patient populations served by their institutions.

2. Educate the pharmacy staff on the purposes and processes of CP development and the contents of CPs. The patient care decisions required in CPs demand clinical knowledge, and the pharmacotherapy involved should be based on evidence in the scientific literature. This clinical knowledge is fundamental to the CP. An effective contributor to the CP process needs to first acquire the clinical knowledge on which the CP is based and then use CQI, teamwork, negotiation, and administrative skills to develop, implement, and assess the CP.

3. Discuss CP experiences with pharmacy colleagues within and outside the health system. Pharmacists should create a forum within the health system for ongoing dialogue about CPs; for example, CPs could be made a regular agenda

item for the P&T committee meeting and for other multidisciplinary clinical and departmental meetings.

4. Monitor pharmacy, nursing, quality management, health-system, health care, and management literature for ideas on CP development, implementation, and assessment. CPs from other institutions may be used as examples of and frameworks for mapping care, but they should not be adopted directly, because acceptance and use are greater when CPs are developed or adapted by their users.

5. Identify opportunities for contributing, through the provision of pharmaceutical care, to the health system's patient care delivery and improvement efforts.

Initiating Involvement. Pharmacists should begin their involvement in the CP process in ways most appropriate to their health system's structure, culture, practice settings, and policies and procedures. Involvement may vary substantially from one health system to another, but in general pharmacists should

1. Develop relationships with nursing, medical, dietary, laboratory, quality management, risk management, respiratory care, and other personnel through routine meetings, nursing and medical forums, and other multidisciplinary opportunities. These relationships should be used to promote pharmacists' contributions to collaborative patient care. The pharmacy department should support the use of CPs as an effective way to integrate and align services, processes, and costs.

2. Support or initiate the implementation of a multidisciplinary team for CP development and oversight and ensure that the pharmacy department and the P&T committee are represented on the oversight committee.

3. Seek leadership roles on the health system's CP oversight committee and development teams but be willing to accept subordinate roles. For example, pharmacists should be willing to lead or assist with literature evaluation for the health system's CP development teams.

4. Identify qualities required for the pharmacist's role and develop a consistent process for selecting the most appropriate pharmacists to participate on the various CP development teams.

5. Ensure the ongoing involvement of the P&T committee in the CP process. The P&T committee can facilitate the process by
 - Reviewing and endorsing the pharmacotherapy proposed for inclusion in each CP.
 - Establishing a standing P&T subcommittee or liaison position to assist CP development teams. The subcommittee or liaison would have the opportunity to educate the CP team about the formulary process, the process for MUE, the appropriate use of restricted medications, and other critical medication-use issues.
 - Publishing CPs and information about the health system's experiences with CPs in the P&T committee newsletter.
 - Developing the drug therapy portion of the CP assessment into an MUE.

6. Emphasize to pharmacists, other health care providers, and health-system administrators pharmacists' responsibility for implementing CP steps that involve pharmacotherapeutic regimens and monitoring, medication distribution, and patient education and counseling.

7. Initiate, after appropriate approvals, the development of the pharmacotherapeutic components of CPs.
8. Offer to evaluate and adapt the pharmacotherapeutic components of existing protocols and guidelines for CPs under development. Maintain a pharmacotherapy database to facilitate CP updates when new medications and pharmacotherapeutic alternatives become available.
9. Develop patient education and counseling materials for the pharmacotherapeutic components of CPs and develop plans for pharmacists or other members of the health care team to provide education and counseling to patients.
10. Advocate the development and use of preprinted medication orders (hard copy or electronic) and consistent use of terminology (e.g., generic drug names, decimals and units of measurement, and standardized terms and abbreviations) within the CP.
11. Be proactive in anticipating alternative processes or drug regimens that may be required in unusual circumstances, such as drug shortages.

Maintaining Involvement. Pharmacists' continued involvement in CPs will depend on their ability to demonstrate their contributions to patient care delivery and improvement to the CP oversight committee and development teams and to the health system's administration. To accomplish this, pharmacists can

1. Monitor the literature of pharmacy, nursing, quality management, health systems, health care, and management for ideas on CP development, implementation, and assessment.
2. Identify new areas for CP development on the basis of medication-use data (e.g., medication error data and MUE findings).
3. Incorporate CPs into the pharmacy department's culture by building responsibilities and performance expectations for CP development, implementation, and assessment into pharmacists' job descriptions.
4. Identify and train pharmacy staff on their roles and responsibilities for implementing the pharmaceutical care components of CPs.
5. Provide objective clinical input that is based on scientific evidence.
6. Ensure consistent use of terminology (e.g., generic drug names, decimals and units of measurement, and standardized terms and abbreviations), rational medication use, and appropriate monitoring. This could be done by the P&T committee or by a pharmacist who coordinates and reviews the pharmacotherapeutic efforts of all CPs.
7. Maintain good working relationships with CP development teams. The pharmacist member should be confident, assertive, cooperative, and effective in communicating with other health care providers.
8. Develop and maintain clinical and management skills through ongoing self-education.

Contributing to the CQI Aspects of CPs. The pharmacist should ensure that the pharmaceutical care actions of the CP contribute to patient satisfaction, desired clinical outcomes, and financial goals by

1. Monitoring the literature for best-practice results relating to specific disease states (as defined by federal diagnosis-related-group classification) and comparing these results with the health system's experience.
2. Ensuring that an internal system of CP tracking and therapeutic review is in place for the rapid insertion of new, more effective therapies into the CP and that CPs are integrated into the institution's CQI processes.
3. Assisting the development of patient satisfaction surveys.
4. Monitoring the results of the CPs and using them to perform MUEs.[42] Since patients enrolled in CPs are receiving predetermined pharmacotherapeutic regimens and monitoring, this is an excellent opportunity to perform disease- and outcome-oriented MUEs. The pharmacist should review the variances and outcomes associated with the CP, determine the effects of pharmacotherapy, and use this analysis to modify the CP. The pharmacotherapeutic component must be specific enough (e.g., specifying the medication and dosage) that its influence on the outcomes can be determined with confidence.
5. Ensuring that CPs are updated when there are changes in institutional practices (e.g., formulary changes) or when external practices change (e.g., guidelines are revised, dosage or monitoring recommendations are revised).

Ensuring the Continuity of a CP. Many CPs require continuity of care across various levels of care and practice settings. Such CPs should specify referral patterns among the levels of care and practice settings. To help accomplish this, pharmacists can

1. Ensure that members of all organizational components are included in the development and assessment of the CP as appropriate for the particular disease or procedure. Included might be personnel in the emergency department, the operating room, the intensive care unit, the step-down unit, the general nursing unit, the rehabilitation unit, the long-term-care facility, the ambulatory care clinic, the laboratory, and the home care service.
2. Develop relationships with ambulatory care, home care, and long-term-care pharmacists and other health care providers to foster the seamless provision of pharmaceutical care by inviting pharmacist members of managed care organizations to participate in CP development, exchanging CPs with the managed care organizations, and creating work teams to ensure the continuity of care.
3. Organize interdisciplinary sharing of information (e.g., recent laboratory test results) and documentation that are useful to all health care providers.
4. Develop a plan to communicate and monitor both internal and external CPs so that pharmacists have a full understanding of the CP process and can evaluate and adjust the CP as necessary when new therapeutic modalities emerge. Optimize this by using electronic and Internet technology to rapidly insert new pharmacotherapies into CPs when appropriate and evaluate which pharmacotherapies are included in which CPs to ensure consistency in medication management.
5. Initiate dialogue among pharmacists to ensure the continuity of the individual patient's CP. For example, when a patient is admitted, the hospital pharmacist should, if necessary and with the patient's permission, contact the patient's community pharmacist or managed care company to obtain information as allowed

under local, state, and federal laws (e.g., the Health Insurance Portability and Accessibility Act). The pharmacist should document an accurate medication history (prescription and nonprescription products, dietary supplements, and home remedies), the patient's history of adverse drug reactions and allergies, the patient's medication-taking behaviors (adherence, health beliefs, and social and cultural issues), and any self-monitoring. This does not obviate the requirement for the pharmacist to establish a professional relationship with the patient and to obtain information directly. When the patient is discharged, the hospital pharmacist could (in accordance with the institution's policies and procedures and with the patient's permission) prepare an original discharge summary or append to the physician's discharge summary any necessary notes regarding medications. An appropriate member of the discharge team should forward the discharge summary to relevant health care providers (e.g., physicians, home care nurses, and community or home care pharmacists). The summary should include the patient's chief complaint, the patient's height and weight, a history of the present illness (including the hospital course), pregnancy and lactation status, prescription and nonprescription medications on admission and at discharge, patient education and counseling, the monitoring plan (including patient self-monitoring and a plan for long-term monitoring of the patient's pharmacotherapeutic regimen), and a person to contact if the patient has questions. The pharmacist should check any discharge prescriptions against the indications listed in the discharge summary.

The Pharmacist's Responsibility

Carefully developed and skillfully managed CPs can improve the quality of care and the allocation of health care resources. Because pharmacotherapy is a central component of many CPs, pharmacists can help improve patient outcomes, contribute to cost-effective patient care, and promote team approaches to patient care and performance improvement by incorporating contemporary pharmaceutical care principles, activities, and services into the development, implementation, and assessment of CPs. Health systems will develop CPs in ways that are most appropriate to their patient populations, organizational structure, culture, and environment, so it is the responsibility of health-system pharmacists to identify opportunities to become involved in and improve the CPs in their institutions.

References

1. Darer J, Pronovost P, Bass E. Use and evaluation of critical pathways in hospitals. *Eff Clin Pract.* 2002; 5:114–9.
2. Lumsdon K, Hagland M. Mapping care. *Hosp Health Netw.* 1993; 67:34–40.
3. Coffey RJ, Richards JS, Remmert CS, et al. An introduction to critical paths. *Qual Manag Health Care.* 1992; 1:45–54.
4. Jaggers LD. Differentiation of critical pathways from other health care management tools. *Am J Health-Syst Pharm.* 1996; 53:311–3.
5. Koch KE. Opportunities for pharmaceutical care with critical pathways. *Top Hosp Pharm Manag.* 1995; 14:1–7.
6. Stevenson LL. Critical pathway experience at Sarasota Memorial Hospital. *Am J Health-Syst Pharm.* 1995; 52:1071–3.
7. Gousse GC, Rousseau MR. Critical pathways at Hartford Hospital. *Am J Health-Syst Pharm.* 1995; 52:1060–3.
8. Shane R, Vinson B. Use of critical pathways and indicators in pharmacy practice. *Top Hosp Pharm Manag.* 1995; 14:55–67.
9. Gouveia WA, Massaro FJ. Critical pathway experience at New England Medical Center. *Am J Health-Syst Pharm.* 1995; 52:1068–70.
10. Saltiel E. Critical pathway experience at Cedars-Sinai Medical Center. *Am J Health-Syst Pharm.* 1995; 52:1063–8.
11. Nelson SP. Critical pathways at University of Iowa Hospitals and Clinics. *Am J Health-Syst Pharm.* 1995; 52:1058–60.
12. Marrie TJ, Lau CY, Wheeler SL, et al. A controlled trial of a critical pathway for treatment of community-acquired pneumonia. CAPITAL Study Investigators. Community-Acquired Pneumonia Intervention Trial Assessing Levofloxacin. *JAMA.* 2000; 283:749–55.
13. Cannon CP, Hand MH, Bahr R, et al. Critical pathways for management of patients with acute coronary syndromes: an assessment by the National Heart Attack Alert Program. *Am Heart J.* 2002; 143:777–89.
14. Jones S. A clinical pathway for pediatric gastroenteritis. *Gastroenterol Nurs.* 2003; 26:7–18.
15. Nierman DM. A structure of care for the chronically critically ill. *Crit Care Clin.* 2002; 18:477–91.
16. Kercsmar CM, Myers TR. Clinical pathways in treatment of asthma. *Curr Opin Allergy Clin Immunol.* 2002; 2:183–7.
17. Mavroukakis SA, Muehlbauer PM, White RL Jr, et al. Clinical pathways for managing patients receiving interleukin 2. *Clin J Oncol Nurs.* 2001; 5:207–17.
18. Zevola DR, Raffa M, Brown K. Using clinical pathways in patients undergoing cardiac valve surgery. *Crit Care Nurse.* 2002; 22:31–9, 44–50.
19. Rymer MM, Summers D, Soper P. Development of clinical pathways for stroke management: an example from Saint Luke's Hospital, Kansas City. *Clin Geriatr Med.* 1999; 15:741–64.
20. Bisanz A, DeJesus Y, Saddler DA. Development, implementation, and ongoing monitoring of pathways for the treatment of gastrointestinal cancer at a comprehensive cancer center. *Gastroenterol Nurs.* 1999; 22:107–14.
21. Sesperez J, Wilson S, Jalaludin B, et al. Trauma case management and clinical pathways: prospective evaluation of their effect on selected patient outcomes in five key trauma conditions. *J Trauma.* 2001; 50:643–9.
22. Mamolen NL, Brenner PS. The impact of a burn wound education program and implementation of a clinical pathway on patient outcomes. *J Burn Care Rehabil.* 2000; 21:440–5.

23. Crane M, Werber B. Critical pathway approach to diabetic pedal infections in a multidisciplinary setting. *J Foot Ankle Surg.* 1999; 38:30–3.

24. Baker CM, Miller I, Sitterding M, et al. Acute stroke patients comparing outcomes with and without case management. *Nurs Case Manag.* 1998; 3:196–203.

25. Holtzman J, Bjerke T, Kane R. The effects of clinical pathways for renal transplant on patient outcomes and length of stay. *Med Care.* 1998; 36:826–34.

26. Petitta A, Kaatz S, Estrada C, et al. The transition to medication system performance indicators. *Top Hosp Pharm Manag.*1995; 14:20–6.

27. Johnson KB, Blaisdell CJ, Walker A, et al. Effectiveness of a clinical pathway for inpatient asthma management. *Pediatrics.* 2000; 106:1006–12.

28. Philbin EF, Rocco TA, Lindenmuth NW, et al. The results of a randomized trial of a quality improvement intervention in the care of patients with heart failure. The MISCHF Study Investigators. *Am J Med.* 2000; 109:443–9.

29. Murphy M, Noetscher C, Lagoe R. A multihospital effort to reduce inpatient lengths of stay for pneumonia. *J Nurs Care Qual.* 1999; 13:11–23.

30. Dzwierzynski WW, Spitz K, Hartz A, et al. Improvement in resource utilization after development of a clinical pathway for patients with pressure ulcers. *Plast Reconstr Surg.* 1998; 102:2006–11.

31. Boykin JV Jr, Crossland MC, Cole LM. Wound healing management: enhancing patient outcomes and reducing costs. *J Healthc Resour Manag.* 1997; 15:22,24–6.

32. Leibman BD, Dillioglugil O, Abbas F, et al. Impact of a clinical pathway for radical retropubic prostatectomy. *Urology.* 1998; 52:94–9.

33. Bailey R, Weingarten S, Lewis M, et al. Impact of clinical pathways and practice guidelines on the management of acute exacerbations of bronchial asthma. *Chest.* 1998; 113:28–33.

34. Uchiyama K, Takifuji K, Tani M, et al. Effectiveness of the clinical pathway to decrease length of stay and cost for laparoscopic surgery. *Surg Endosc.* 2002; 16:1594–7.

35. Wilson SD, Dahl BB, Wells RD. An evidence-based clinical pathway for bronchiolitis safely reduces antibiotic overuse.*Am J Med Qual.* 2002; 17:195–9.

36. Smith DM, Gow P. Towards excellence in quality patient care: a clinical pathway for myocardial infarction. *J Qual Clin Pract,* 1999; 19:103–5.

37. Kirk JK, Michael KA, Markowsky SJ, et al. Critical pathways: the time is here for pharmacist involvement. *Pharmacotherapy.* 1996; 16:723–33.

38. Institute for Safe Medication Practices. Medication safety self-assessment. www.ismp.org/pages/mssacaprdf. html (accessed 2003 May 16).

39. American Society of Hospital Pharmacists. ASHP statement on pharmaceutical care. *Am J Hosp Pharm.* 1993; 50:1720–3.

40. American Society of Hospital Pharmacists. ASHP statement on principles for including medications and pharmaceutical care in health care systems. *Am J Hosp Pharm.* 1993; 50:756–7.

41. American Society of Health-System Pharmacists. ASHP guidelines on a standardized method for pharmaceutical care. *Am J Health-Syst Pharm.* 1996; 53:1713–6.

42. American Society of Health-System Pharmacists. ASHP guidelines on medication-use evaluation. *Am J Health-Syst Pharm.* 1996; 53:1953–5.

These guidelines were reviewed in 2009 by the Council on Pharmacy Practice and by the Board of Directors and were found to still be appropriate.

Approved by the ASHP Board of Directors on April 15, 2004. Developed by the ASHP Council on Professional Affairs. Supersedes the "ASHP guidelines on the pharmacists' role in the development of clinical care plans" dated November 16, 1996.

The bibliographic citation for this document is as follows: American Society of Health-System Pharmacists. ASHP guidelines on the pharmacist's role in the development, implementation, and assessment of critical pathways. *Am J Health-Syst Pharm.* 2004; 61:939–45.

ASHP Guidelines on a Standardized Method for Pharmaceutical Care

Need for a Standardized Method

The purpose of this document is to provide pharmacists with a standardized method for the provision of pharmaceutical care in component settings of organized health systems. Since the introduction of the pharmaceutical care concept[1] and the development of the ASHP Statement on Pharmaceutical Care,[2] considerable variation in pharmacists' provision of pharmaceutical care has been noted. ASHP believes pharmacists need a standardized method for providing pharmaceutical care.

This document describes a standardized method based on functions that all pharmacists should perform for individual patients in organized health systems. The use of this method would foster consistency in the provision of pharmaceutical care in all practice settings. It would support continuity of care both within a practice setting (e.g., among pharmacists on different work shifts caring for an acutely ill inpatient) and when a patient moves among practice settings (e.g., when an inpatient is discharged to home or ambulatory care). Further, a standardized method would establish consistent documentation so that patient-specific and medication-related information could be shared from pharmacist to pharmacist and among health professionals.

The need to identify the functions involved in pharmaceutical care and the critical skills necessary to provide it was discussed at the San Antonio consensus conference in 1993.[3] Functions for the provision of pharmaceutical care were identified by the practitioner task force of the Scope of Pharmacy Practice Project.[4] Those functions have been defined in more detail in the pharmacotherapy series of the ASHP Clinical Skills Program.[5-9]

These Guidelines are not specific to any practice setting. ASHP believes this standardized method can be used in acute care (hospitals), ambulatory care, home care, long-term care, and other practice settings. Functions can be tailored as appropriate for a given practice setting. It is recognized that the degree of standardization and tailoring appropriate for a given work site will depend on the practice environment, the organization of services (e.g., patient-focused or department-focused), working relationships with other health professionals, the health system's and patient's financial arrangements, and the health system's policies and procedures. ASHP believes the use of the systematic approaches encouraged by these guidelines will assist pharmacists in implementing and providing pharmaceutical care in their work sites.

Functions of Pharmaceutical Care

ASHP believes that a standardized method for the provision of pharmaceutical care should include the following:

- Collecting and organizing patient-specific information,
- Determining the presence of medication-therapy problems,
- Summarizing patients' health care needs,
- Specifying pharmacotherapeutic goals,
- Designing a pharmacotherapeutic regimen,
- Designing a monitoring plan,
- Developing a pharmacotherapeutic regimen and corresponding monitoring plan in collaboration with the patient and other health professionals,
- Initiating the pharmacotherapeutic regimen,
- Monitoring the effects of the pharmacotherapeutic regimen, *and*
- Redesigning the pharmacotherapeutic regimen and monitoring plan.

These major functions have been adapted, in part, from the pharmacotherapy series of the ASHP Clinical Skills Program and the final report of the ASHP Model for Pharmacy Practice Residency Learning Demonstration Project.

Collecting and Organizing Pertinent Patient-Specific Information. Information should be collected and used as a patient-specific database to prevent, detect, and resolve the patient's medication-related problems and to make appropriate medication-therapy recommendations. The database should include the following sections, each containing specific types of information to the extent that it is relevant to medication therapy:

Demographic
 Name
 Address
 Date of birth
 Sex
 Religion and religious affiliation
 Occupation

Administrative
 Physicians and prescribers
 Pharmacy
 Room/bed numbers
 Consent forms
 Patient identification number

Medical
 Weight and height
 Acute and chronic medical problems
 Current symptoms
 Vital signs and other monitoring information
 Allergies and intolerances
 Past medical history
 Laboratory information
 Diagnostic and surgical procedures

Medication therapy
 Prescribed medications
 Nonprescription medications
 Medications used prior to admission
 Home remedies and other types of health products used
 Medication regimen
 Compliance with therapy
 Medication allergies and intolerances
 Concerns or questions about therapy

Assessment of understanding of therapy
Pertinent health beliefs

Behavioral/lifestyle
 Diet
 Exercise/recreation
 Tobacco/alcohol/caffeine/other substance use or abuse
 Sexual history
 Personality type
 Daily activities

Social/economic
 Living arrangement
 Ethnic background
 Financial/insurance/health plan

Objective and subjective information should be obtained directly from patients (and family members, other caregivers, and other health professionals as needed). A physical assessment should be performed as needed. In addition, information can be obtained by reviewing the patient's health record and other information sources.

Information in the patient's health record should be understood, interpreted, and verified for accuracy before decisions are made about the patient's medication therapy. With access to the patient's health record comes the professional responsibility to safeguard the patient's rights to privacy and confidentiality. The Privacy Act of 1974,[10] professional practice policies,[11,12] and policies and procedures of organized health systems provide guidance for the pharmacist in judging the appropriate use of patient-specific information.

The patient (as well as family members, caregivers, and other members of the health care team as needed) should be interviewed. This is necessary for the pharmacist to establish a direct relationship with the patient, to understand the patient's needs and desired outcome, to obtain medication-related information, and to clarify and augment other available information. Pharmacists in many practice settings, including ambulatory care, may need to perform physical assessments to collect data for assessing and monitoring medication therapy.

Information, including clinical laboratory test results, gathered or developed by other members of the health care team may not be in the patient's health record. Therefore, to ensure that the patient information is current and complete, other sources should be checked. Other sources may include medication profiles from other pharmacies used by the patient.

Although it is ideal to have a comprehensive database for all patients, time and staffing limitations may necessitate choices regarding the quantity of information and the number of patients to follow. Choices could be determined by the health system's policies and procedures, by clinical care plans, or by disease management criteria in the patient's third-party health plan.

Systems for recording patient-specific data will vary, depending on pharmacists' preferences and practice settings. Electronic documentation is recommended. Some information may already be in the patient's health record. Therefore, when authorized, the additional information gathered by the pharmacist should be recorded in the patient's health record so that it can be shared with other health professionals. Abstracted summaries and work sheets may also be useful.

Determining the Presence of Medication-Therapy Problems. Conclusions should be drawn from the integration of medication-, disease-, laboratory test-, and patient-specific information. The patient's database should be assessed for any of the following medication-therapy problems:

- Medications with no medical indication,
- Medical conditions for which there is no medication prescribed,
- Medications prescribed inappropriately for a particular medical condition,
- Inappropriate medication dose, dosage form, schedule, route of administration, or method of administration,
- Therapeutic duplication,
- Prescribing of medications to which the patient is allergic,
- Actual and potential adverse drug events,
- Actual and potential clinically significant drug–drug, drug–disease, drug–nutrient, and drug–laboratory test interactions,
- Interference with medical therapy by social or recreational drug use,
- Failure to receive the full benefit of prescribed medication therapy,
- Problems arising from the financial impact of medication therapy on the patient,
- Lack of understanding of the medication therapy by the patient, and
- Failure of the patient to adhere to the medication regimen.

The relative importance of problems must be assessed on the basis of specific characteristics of the patient or the medication. Checklists, work sheets, and other methods may be used to determine and document the presence of medication-therapy problems. The method should be proactive and should be used consistently from patient to patient.

Summarizing Patients' Health Care Needs. The patient's overall needs and desired outcomes and other health professionals' assessments, goals, and therapy plans should be considered in determining and documenting the medication-related elements of care that are needed to improve or prevent deterioration of the patient's health or well-being.

Specifying Pharmacotherapeutic Goals. Pharmacotherapeutic goals should reflect the integration of medication-, disease-, laboratory test-, and patient-specific information, as well as ethical and quality-of-life considerations. The goals should be realistic and consistent with goals specified by the patient and other members of the patient's health care team. The therapy should be designed to achieve definite medication-related outcomes and improve the patient's quality of life.

Designing a Pharmacotherapeutic Regimen. The regimen should meet the pharmacotherapeutic goals established with the patient and reflect the integration of medication-, disease-, laboratory test-, and patient-specific information; ethical and quality-of-life considerations; and pharmacoeconomic principles. It should comply with the health system's medication-use policies, such as clinical care plans and disease management plans. The regimen should be designed for optimal medication use within both the health system's and the patient's capabilities and financial resources.

Designing a Monitoring Plan for the Pharmacotherapeutic Regimen. The monitoring plan should effectively evaluate achievement of the patient-specific pharmacotherapeu-tic goals and detect real and potential adverse effects. Measurable, observable parameters should be determined for each goal. Endpoints should be established for assessing whether the goal has been achieved. The needs of the patient, characteristics of the medication, needs of other health care team members, and policies and procedures of the health care setting will influence the monitoring plan.

Developing a Pharmacotherapeutic Regimen and Corresponding Monitoring Plan. The regimen and plan developed in collaboration with the patient and other health professionals should be systematic and logical and should represent a consensus among the patient, prescriber, and pharmacist. The approach selected should be based on consideration of the type of practice setting, its policies and procedures, practice standards, and good professional relations with the prescriber and patient. The regimen and monitoring plan should be documented in the patient's health record to ensure that all members of the health care team have this information.

Initiating the Pharmacotherapeutic Regimen. Depending on the regimen and plan, the pharmacist could, as appropriate, implement all or portions of the pharmacotherapeutic regimen. Actions should comply with the health system's policies and procedures (e.g., prescribing protocols) and correspond to the regimen and plan. Orders for medications, laboratory tests, and other interventions should be clear and concise. All actions should be documented in the patient's health record.

Monitoring the Effects of the Pharmacotherapeutic Regimen. Data collected according to the monitoring plan should be sufficient, reliable, and valid so that judgments can be made about the effects of the pharmacotherapeutic regimen. Changes in patient status, condition, medication therapy, or nonmedication therapy since the monitoring plan was developed should be considered. Missing or additional data should be identified. Achievement of the desired endpoints should be assessed for each parameter in the monitoring plan. A judgment should be made about whether the pharmacotherapeutic goals were met. Before the pharmacotherapeutic regimen is adjusted, the cause for failure to achieve any of the pharmacotherapeutic goals should be determined.

Redesigning the Pharmacotherapeutic Regimen and Monitoring Plan. Decisions to change the regimen and plan should be based on the patient's outcome. When clinical circumstances permit, one aspect of the regimen at a time should be changed and reassessed. Recommendations for pharmacotherapeutic changes should be documented in the same manner used to document the original recommendations.

Pharmacist's Responsibility

An essential element of pharmaceutical care is that the pharmacist accepts responsibility for the patient's pharmacotherapeutic outcomes. The same commitment that is applied to designing the pharmacotherapeutic regimen and monitoring plan for the patient should be applied to its implementation.

The provision of pharmaceutical care requires monitoring the regimen's effects, revising the regimen as the patient's condition changes, documenting the results, and assuming responsibility for the pharmacotherapeutic effects.

References

1. Hepler CD, Strand LM. Opportunities and responsibilities in pharmaceutical care. *Am J Hosp Pharm.* 1990; 47:533–43.
2. American Society of Hospital Pharmacists. ASHP statement on pharmaceutical care. *Am J Hosp Pharm.* 1993; 50:1720–3.
3. Implementing pharmaceutical care. Proceedings of an invitational conference conducted by the American Society of Hospital Pharmacists and the ASHP Research Foundation. *Am J Hosp Pharm.* 1993; 50: 1585–656.
4. Summary of the final report of the Scope of Pharmacy Practice Project. *Am J Hosp Pharm.* 1994; 51:2179–82.
5. Shepherd MF. Clinical skills program pharmacotherapy series module 1. Reviewing patient medical charts. Bethesda, MD: American Society of Hospital Pharmacists; 1992.
6. Mason N, Shimp LA. Clinical skills program pharmacotherapy series module 2. Building a pharmacist's patient data base. Bethesda, MD: American Society of Hospital Pharmacists; 1993.
7. Mason N, Shimp LA. Clinical skills program–module 3. Constructing a patient's drug therapy problem list. Bethesda, MD: American Society of Hospital Pharmacists; 1993.
8. Jones WN, Campbell S. Clinical skills program pharmacotherapy series module 4. Designing and recommending a pharmacist's care plan. Bethesda, MD: American Society of Hospital Pharmacists; 1994.
9. Frye CB. Clinical skills program pharmacotherapy series module 5. Monitoring the pharmacist's care plan. Bethesda, MD: American Society of Hospital Pharmacists; 1994.
10. PL 93-579. 5 U.S.C.A. 552a (88 Stat. 1896).
11. ASHP guidelines for obtaining authorization for documenting pharmaceutical care in patient medical records. *Am J Hosp Pharm.* 1989; 46:338–9.
12. Principles of practice for pharmaceutical care. Washington, DC: American Pharmaceutical Association; 1995.

Approved by the ASHP Board of Directors, April 24, 1996. Developed by the ASHP Council on Professional Affairs.

The bibliographic citation for this document is as follows: American Society of Health-System Pharmacists. ASHP guidelines on a standardized method for pharmaceutical care. *Am J Health-Syst Pharm.* 1996; 53:1713–6.

Specific Practice Areas

Pharmacist's Role in Accountable Care Organizations (1214)

Source: Council on Pharmacy Practice

To recognize that pharmacist participation in collaborative health care teams improves outcomes from medication use and lowers costs; further,

To advocate to health policymakers, payers, and other stakeholders for the inclusion of pharmacists as health care providers within accountable care organizations (ACOs) and other models of integrated health care delivery; further,

To advocate that pharmacist-provided care (including care coordination services) be appropriately recognized in reimbursement models for ACOs; further,

To advocate that pharmacists be included as health care providers in demonstration projects for ACOs; further,

To encourage comparative effectiveness research and measurement of key outcomes (e.g., clinical, economic, quality, access) for pharmacist services in ACOs; further,

To encourage pharmacy leaders to develop strategic plans for positioning pharmacists in key roles within ACOs.

Criteria for Medication Use in Geriatric Patients (1221)

Source: Council on Therapeutics

To support medication therapy management, including assessment of physiologic and pharmacokinetic factors, as a central component of providing safe and effective drug therapy to geriatric patients; further,

To oppose use of the Beers criteria or similar criteria by the Centers for Medicare & Medicaid Services and other accreditation and quality improvement entities as the sole indicator to assess the appropriateness of prescribing for geriatric patients based on known limitations in the evidence evaluating the association between use of medications listed in such criteria and subsequent adverse drug events; further,

To advocate for the development, refinement, and validation of new criteria that consider drug-, disease-, and patient-specific factors and demonstrate the ability to decrease the occurrence of adverse drug events in geriatric patients; further,

To support research to assess the clinical application of existing and proposed criteria, including assessment of their correlation to patient outcomes and strategies for implementation; further,

To encourage inclusion of validated criteria in clinical decision support systems and other information technologies to facilitate prescribing for geriatric patients; further,

To acknowledge that such criteria are intended as a guide and should not replace the clinical judgment of pharmacists and other clinicians.

Tobacco and Tobacco Products (1224)

Source: Council on Therapeutics

To discourage the use, distribution, and sale of tobacco and tobacco products in and by pharmacies; further,

To advocate for tobacco-free environments in hospitals and health systems; further,

To seek, within the bounds of public law and policy, to eliminate the use and distribution of tobacco and tobacco products in meeting rooms and corridors at ASHP-sponsored events; further,

To promote the role of pharmacists in tobacco-cessation counseling and medication therapy management; further,

To join with other interested organizations in statements and expressions of opposition to the use of tobacco and tobacco products.

This policy supersedes ASHP policy 0713.

Safe and Effective Use of IV Promethazine (1105)

Source: Council on Therapeutics

To recognize intravenous (IV) promethazine as a treatment alternative in limited clinical circumstances; further,

To support health-system efforts to restrict use of IV promethazine by encouraging alternate routes of administration or use of therapeutic alternatives when appropriate; further,

To encourage health systems to establish medication-use processes that reflect nationally recognized best practices to limit the potential for patient harm when IV promethazine use is medically necessary.

Pain Management (1106)

Source: Council on Therapeutics

To advocate fully informed patient and caregiver participation in pain management decisions as an integral aspect of patient care; further,

To advocate that pharmacists actively participate in the development and implementation of health-system pain management policies and protocols; further,

To support the participation of pharmacists in pain management, which is a multidisciplinary, collaborative process for selecting appropriate drug therapies, educating patients, monitoring patients, and continually assessing outcomes of therapy; further,

To advocate that pharmacists lead efforts to prevent inappropriate use of pain therapies, including engaging in strategies to detect and address patterns of abuse and misuse; further,

To encourage the education of pharmacists, pharmacy students, and other health care providers regarding the principles of pain management and methods to minimize drug diversion.

This policy supersedes ASHP policy 0306.

Safety and Effectiveness of Ethanol for Treatment of Alcohol Withdrawal Syndrome (1010)

Source: Council on Therapeutics

To oppose the use of oral or intravenous ethanol for the prevention or treatment of alcohol withdrawal syndrome (AWS) because of its poor effectiveness and safety profile; further,

To support hospital and health-system efforts that restrict or prohibit the use of oral or intravenous ethanol therapies to treat AWS; further,

To educate clinicians about the availability of alternative therapies for AWS.

Pharmacist's Role in Providing Care for an Aging Population (0902)

Source: Council on Pharmacy Practice

To encourage expansion of geriatric health care services; further,

To foster expanded roles for pharmacists in caring for geriatric patients; further,

To support successful innovative models of team-based, interdisciplinary geriatric care; further,

To increase training of pharmacists in caring for geriatric patients within college of pharmacy curricula, in ASHP-accredited postgraduate-year-one residencies, and through the expansion of the number of ASHP-accredited postgraduate-year-two geriatric pharmacy residency programs.

Pharmacist Role in the Health Care (Medical) Home (0908)

Source: Council on Public Policy

To advocate to health policymakers, payers, and other stakeholders for the inclusion of pharmacists as a care provider within the health care (medical) home model; further,

To ensure that there are appropriate reimbursement mechanisms for the care that pharmacists provide (including care coordination services) within the health care home model; further,

To advocate to the Centers for Medicare & Medicaid Services that pharmacists be included in demonstration projects for the health care home model; further,

To encourage comparative effectiveness research and measurement of key outcomes (e.g., clinical, economic, quality, access) for pharmacist services in the health care home model.

Safe and Effective Use of Heparin in Neonatal Patients (0912)

Source: Council on Therapeutics

To support the development and use of nationally standardized concentrations of heparin when used for maintenance and flush of peripheral and central venous lines in neonatal patients; further,

To advocate that hospitals and health systems use manufacturer-prepackaged heparin flush products to improve the safe use of heparin in neonatal patients.

Role of Pharmacists in Sports Pharmacy and Doping Control (0710)

Source: Council on Pharmacy Practice

To encourage pharmacists to engage in community outreach efforts to provide education to athletes on the risks associated with the use of performance-enhancing drugs; further,

To encourage pharmacists to advise athletic authorities and athletes on medications that are prohibited in competition; further,

To advocate for the role of the pharmacist in all aspects of sports pharmacy and doping control.

This policy was reviewed in 2012 by the House of Delegates and by the Board of Directors and was found to still be appropriate.

Pharmacist Support for Dying Patients (0307)

Source: Council on Professional Affairs

To support the position that care for dying patients is part of the continuum of care that pharmacists should provide to patients; further,

To support the position that pharmacists have a professional obligation to work in a collaborative and compassionate manner with patients, family members, caregivers, and other professionals to help fulfill the patient care needs, especially the quality-of-life needs, of dying patients of all ages; further,

To support research on the needs of dying patients; further,

To provide education to pharmacists on caring for dying patients, including education on clinical, managerial, professional, and legal issues; further,

To urge the inclusion of such topics in the curricula of colleges of pharmacy.

This policy was reviewed in 2007 by the Council on Pharmacy Practice and by the Board of Directors and was found to still be appropriate.

Pharmacists' Role in Immunization and Vaccines (0213)

Source: Council on Educational Affairs

To affirm that pharmacists have a role in promoting and administering proper immunizations to patients and employees in all settings; further,

To encourage pharmacists to seek opportunities for involvement in disease prevention through community immunization programs; further,

To advocate the inclusion of the pharmacist's role in immunization in college of pharmacy curricula; further,

To strongly encourage pharmacists to use available opportunities and materials to educate at-risk patients, their caregivers, parents, guardians, and health care providers about the importance of immunizations.

This policy was reviewed in 2011 by the Council on Education and Workforce Development and by the Board of Directors and was found to still be appropriate.

Interventions to Reduce High-Risk Behavior in Intravenous Drug Users (9711)

Source: House of Delegates Resolution

ASHP supports the use of needle and syringe exchange programs, drug abuse treatment, and community outreach programs for substance abusers to reduce the risk of transmission of the human immunodeficiency virus (HIV), hepatitis B virus, and hepatitis C virus in intravenous drug users.

This policy was reviewed in 2011 by the Council on Pharmacy Practice and by the Board of Directors and was found to still be appropriate.

Primary and Preventive Care (9407)

Source: Council on Professional Affairs

To support primary and preventive care roles for pharmacists in the provision of pharmaceutical care; further,

To collaborate with physician, nursing, and health-system administrator groups in pursuit of these goals.

This policy was reviewed in 2011 by the Council on Pharmacy Practice and by the Board of Directors and was found to still be appropriate.

ASHP Statement on the Pharmacist's Role in Antimicrobial Stewardship and Infection Prevention and Control

Position

The American Society of Health-System Pharmacists (ASHP) believes that pharmacists have a responsibility to take prominent roles in antimicrobial stewardship programs and participate in the infection prevention and control programs of health systems. This responsibility arises, in part, from pharmacists' understanding of and influence over antimicrobial use within the health system. Further, ASHP believes that the pharmacist's ability to effectively participate in antimicrobial stewardship and infection prevention and control efforts can be realized through clinical endeavors focused on proper antimicrobial utilization and membership on multidisciplinary work groups and committees within the health system. These efforts should contribute to the appropriate use of antimicrobials, ultimately resulting in successful therapeutic outcomes for patients with infectious diseases, and reduce the risk of infections for other patients and health care workers.

Background

Antimicrobial stewardship is utilized in practice settings of health systems to improve patient outcomes while minimizing the unintended consequences of antimicrobial use. The goals of antimicrobial stewardship programs include attenuating or reversing antimicrobial resistance, preventing antimicrobial-related toxicity, and reducing the costs of inappropriate antimicrobial use and health care-associated infections. Guidelines published by the Infectious Diseases Society of America and the Society for Healthcare Epidemiology of America and endorsed by ASHP and other organizations describe an evidence-based approach to antimicrobial stewardship in health systems and the important role pharmacists with infectious diseases training have in leading stewardship efforts.[1]

Identifying and reducing the risks of developing, acquiring, and transmitting infections among patients, health care workers, and others are an important part of improving patient outcomes. In order to maximize outcomes, antimicrobial stewardship should be used in combination with infection prevention and control practices.[1] Most health systems maintain an infection prevention and control program directed by a multidisciplinary committee. The specific program and responsibilities of the infection prevention and control committee (or its equivalent) may differ among health systems.

Typically, the infection prevention and control committee develops organizational policies and procedures addressing

1. The management and provision of patient care and employee health services regarding infection or infection prevention and control.
2. The education of staff, patients, family members, and other caregivers in the prevention and control of infections.

3. Surveillance systems to track the occurrence and transmission of infections.
4. Surveillance systems to track the use of antimicrobials and the development of antimicrobial resistance.
5. Promotion of evidence-based practices and interventions to prevent the development of infections.

Responsibilities of Pharmacists

Pharmacists' responsibilities for antimicrobial stewardship and infection prevention and control include promoting the optimal use of antimicrobial agents, reducing the transmission of infections, and educating health professionals, patients, and the public.

Promoting Optimal Use of Antimicrobial Agents. An important clinical responsibility of the pharmacist is to ensure the optimal use of antimicrobial agents throughout the health system. Functions related to this responsibility may include

1. Encouraging multidisciplinary collaboration within the health system to ensure that the prophylactic, empirical, and therapeutic uses of antimicrobial agents result in optimal patient outcomes. These activities may include antimicrobial-related patient care (e.g., aiding in appropriate selection, optimal dosing, rapid initiation, and proper monitoring and de-escalation of antimicrobial therapies) as well as the development of restricted antimicrobial-use procedures, therapeutic interchange, treatment guidelines, and clinical care plans.[2]
2. Working within the pharmacy and therapeutics committee (or equivalent) structure, which may include infectious disease-related subcommittees, to ensure that the number and types of antimicrobial agents available are appropriate for the patient population served. Such decisions should be based on the needs of special patient populations and microbiological trends within the health system. High priority should be given to developing antimicrobial-use policies that result in optimal therapeutic outcomes while minimizing the risk of the emergence of resistant strains of microorganisms.
3. Operating a multidisciplinary, concurrent antimicrobial stewardship program that uses patient outcomes to assess the effectiveness of antimicrobial-use policies throughout the health system.
4. Generating and analyzing quantitative data on antimicrobial drug use to perform clinical and economic outcome analyses.
5. Working with the microbiology laboratory personnel to ensure that appropriate microbial susceptibility tests are reported on individual patients in a timely manner, and collaborating with the laboratory, infectious diseases specialists, and infection preventionists in compiling susceptibility reports (at least annually) for

distribution to prescribers within the health system to guide empirical therapy.

6. Utilizing information technology to enhance antimicrobial stewardship through surveillance, utilization and outcome reporting, and the development of clinical decision-support tools.

7. Facilitating safe medication management practices for antimicrobial agents by utilizing efficient and effective systems to reduce potential errors and adverse drug events.

Reducing the Transmission of Infections. Pharmacists should participate in efforts to prevent or reduce the transmission of infections among patients, health care workers, and others within all of the health system's applicable practice settings. This may be accomplished through

1. Participating in the infection prevention and control committee (or its equivalent).

2. Establishing internal pharmacy policies, procedures, and quality-control programs to prevent contamination of drug products prepared in or dispensed by the pharmacy department. This is of paramount importance in the preparation and handling of sterile products.[3] Other considerations include (but are not limited to) provisions for cleaning pharmaceutical equipment (e.g., laminar-airflow hoods and bulk-compounding equipment) and establishment of appropriate personnel policies (e.g., limiting the activities of staff members who exhibit symptoms of a viral respiratory illness or other infectious condition).

3. Encouraging the use of single-dose packages of sterile drug products rather than multiple-dose containers, except in sterile environments.

4. Recommending proper labeling, dating, and storage of sterile products and multiple-dose sterile-product containers (if used).

5. Encouraging routine immunization (e.g., influenza vaccination) of hospital staff and others who impact the patient care environment, and promoting periodic screening for selected transmissible diseases (e.g., tuberculosis) in accordance with health-system policy and federal, state, or local regulations.

6. Promoting adherence to standard precautions by health care workers, patients, and others who impact the patient care environment.[4]

7. Collaborating in the development of guidelines for risk assessment, treatment, and monitoring of patients and health care workers who have been in contact with persons with a transmissible infectious disease.

8. Striving for zero tolerance of health care-associated infections, including surgical site infections, catheter-associated bloodstream infections, catheter-associated urinary tract infections, and ventilator-associated pneumonia.

Educational Activities. The pharmacist's role includes providing education and information about antimicrobial stewardship and infection prevention and control to health professionals, patients, and members of the public who come in contact with the health system's practice settings. Incorporating active intervention techniques, such as for-

mulary restriction and preauthorization, enhances the effectiveness of educational activities in the patient care setting.[1] Specific activities may include

1. Providing clinical conferences, newsletters, and other types of educational forums for health professionals on topics such as antimicrobial use and resistance, decontaminating agents (disinfectants, antiseptics, and sterilants), aseptic technique and procedures, and sterilization methods.

2. Educating and counseling inpatients, ambulatory care patients, home care patients, and their families and caregivers in the following areas: adherence to prescribed directions for antimicrobial use, storage and handling of medications and administration devices, and other infection prevention and control procedures (e.g., medical waste disposal).

3. Participating in public health education and awareness programs aimed at controlling the spread of infectious diseases by
 a. Promoting prudent use of antimicrobials,
 b. Providing immunization access for children and adults, an
 c. Promoting appropriate infection prevention and control measures (e.g., proper hand hygiene techniques).

4. Providing exposure to antimicrobial stewardship and infection prevention and control practices through experiential and didactic training for practicing health-system pharmacists, students, residents, and research fellows.

Education and Training of Pharmacists

ASHP recognizes that the current shortage of pharmacists with advanced training in infectious diseases and the limited number of training opportunities may require pharmacists without such training to assume some of the responsibilities described above. ASHP supports the expansion of pharmacy education and postgraduate residency training on infectious diseases in order to develop an adequate supply of pharmacists trained to deliver these essential services.

Conclusion

ASHP believes that pharmacists have a responsibility to take prominent roles in antimicrobial stewardship and infection prevention and control programs in health systems. Pharmacists should participate in antimicrobial stewardship and infection prevention and control efforts through clinical endeavors focused on proper antimicrobial utilization and membership on relevant multidisciplinary work groups and committees within the health system.

References

1. Dellit TH, Owens RC, McGowen JE et al. Infectious Diseases Society of America and the Society for Healthcare Epidemiology of America guidelines for developing an institutional program to enhance antimicrobial stewardship. *Clin Infect Dis.* 2007; 44:159-77.

2. American Society of Health-System Pharmacists. ASHP guidelines on the pharmacist's role in the development, implementation, and assessment of critical pathways. *Am J Health-Syst Pharm.* 2004; 61:939-45.

3. American Society of Health-System Pharmacists. ASHP guidelines on quality assurance for pharmacy-prepared sterile products. *Am J Health-Syst Pharm.* 2000; 57:1150-69.

4. Siegel JD, Rhinehart E, Jackson M et al. 2007 guideline for isolation precautions: preventing transmission of infectious agents in healthcare settings, June 2007. www.cdc.gov/ncidod/dhqp/pdf/guidelines/Isolation2007.pdf (accessed 2009 Feb 18).

Suggested Readings

Centers for Disease Control and Prevention. Guideline for disinfection and sterilization in healthcare facilities, 2008. Accessed 15 December 2008. www.cdc.gov/ncidod/dhqp/pdf/guidelines/Disinfection_Nov_2008.pdf.

Centers for Disease Control and Prevention [CDC]. Guidelines for environmental infection control in health-care facilities: recommendations of CDC and the Healthcare Infection Control Practices Advisory Committee (HICPAC). *MMWR.* 2003; 52(No. RR-10):1-48.

Diekema DJ, Doebbeling BN. Employee health and infection control. *Infect Control Hosp Epidemiol.* 1995; 16:292-301.

Gardner P, Schaffner W. Immunization of adults. *N Engl J Med.* 1993; 328:1252-8.

Goldmann DA, Weinstein RA, Wenzel RP et al. Strategies to prevent and control the emergence and spread of antimicrobial-resistant microorganisms in hospitals. A challenge to hospital leadership. *JAMA.* 1996; 275:234-40.

Kollef M, Shapiro S, Fraser V et al. A randomized trial of ventilator circuit changes. *Ann Intern Med.* 1995; 123:168-74.

MacDougall C, Polk RE. Antimicrobial stewardship programs in health care systems. *Clin Microbiol Rev.* 2005 Oct; 18(4):638-56.

Sepkowitz KA. Occupationally acquired infections in health care workers. *Ann Intern Med.* 1996; 125:826-34,917-28.

Shlaes DM, Gerding DN, John JF Jr. et al. SHEA and IDSA Joint Committee on the Prevention of Antimicrobial Resistance: guidelines for the prevention of antimicrobial resistance in hospitals. *Clin Infect Dis.* 1997; 25:584-99.

This statement supersedes the ASHP Statement on the Pharmacist's Role in Infection Control dated June 3, 1998.

Approved by the ASHP Board of Directors on April 17, 2009, and by the ASHP House of Delegates on June 16, 2009. Developed through the ASHP Council on Pharmacy Practice.

Curtis D. Collins, Pharm.D., M.S., is gratefully acknowledged for drafting this statement.

The bibliographic citation for this document is as follows: ASHP Statement on the Pharmacist's Role in Antimicrobial Stewardship and Infection Prevention and Control. *Am J Health-Syst Pharm.* 2010; 67:575-7.

ASHP Statement on the Pharmacist's Role in Clinical Pharmacokinetic Monitoring

The American Society of Health-System Pharmacists (ASHP) believes that clinical pharmacokinetic monitoring is a fundamental responsibility of all pharmacists providing pharmaceutical care. Clinical pharmacokinetic monitoring is an integral component of pharmaceutical care for selected patients based on their specific pharmacotherapy, disease states and related factors, and treatment goals. ASHP believes that clinical pharmacokinetic monitoring is essential to achieving positive outcomes for these patients across the continuum of care and in all practice settings of health systems. Examples of such outcomes include decreased mortality, decreased length of treatment, decreased length of hospital stay, decreased morbidity (either improved symptoms of disease or improved recuperation), and decreased adverse effects from drug therapy.

Background

Clinical pharmacokinetics is the process of applying pharmacokinetic principles to determine the dosage regimens of specific drug products for specific patients to maximize pharmacotherapeutic effects and minimize toxic effects. Application of these principles requires an understanding of the absorption, distribution, metabolism, and excretion characteristics of specific drug products in specific diseases and patient populations. The influence of factors such as age, sex, diet, pathophysiologic conditions, and concomitant use of other drug products must also be understood. The development of patients' individualized dosage regimens should be based on integrated findings from monitoring both the drug concentration-versus-time profiles in biological fluids and the pharmacologic responses to these drug products.

Within the pharmaceutical care process, pharmacists' clinical functions include appropriate and cost-conscious therapeutic drug monitoring and provision of clinical pharmacokinetic assessments. Clinical pharmacokinetic monitoring is necessary when the range between minimal effectiveness and toxicity is narrow and the results of the drug assay provide significant information for clinical decision-making. In the absence of drug concentration measurements, patient-specific characteristics and physiological markers should be used to provide clinical pharmacokinetic assessments and make dosage-regimen recommendations.

Responsibilities

The following responsibilities should be part of clinical pharmacokinetic services or monitoring conducted by pharmacists:

1. Designing patient-specific drug dosage regimens based on the pharmacokinetic and pharmacologic characteristics of the drug products used, the objectives of drug therapy, concurrent diseases and drug therapy, and other pertinent patient factors (e.g., demographics, laboratory data) that improve the safety and effectiveness of drug therapy and promote positive patient outcomes.
2. Recommending or scheduling measurements of drug concentrations in biological fluids (e.g., plasma, serum, blood, cerebrospinal fluid) or tissues in order to facilitate the evaluation of dosage regimens.
3. Monitoring and adjusting dosage regimens on the basis of pharmacologic responses and biological fluid and tissue drug concentrations in conjunction with clinical signs and symptoms or other biochemical variables.
4. Evaluating unusual patient responses to drug therapy for possible pharmacokinetic and pharmacologic explanations.
5. Communicating patient-specific drug therapy information to physicians, nurses, and other clinical practitioners and to patients orally and in writing, and including documentation of this in the patient's health record.
6. Educating pharmacists, physicians, nurses, and other clinical practitioners about pharmacokinetic principles and appropriate indications for clinical pharmacokinetic monitoring, including the cost-effective use of drug concentration measurements.
7. Developing quality assurance programs for documenting improved patient outcomes and economic benefits resulting from clinical pharmacokinetic monitoring.
8. Promoting collaborative relationships with other individuals and departments involved in drug therapy monitoring to encourage the development and appropriate use of pharmacokinetic principles in pharmaceutical care.

Pharmacists with specialized education, training, or experience may have the opportunity to assume the following additional responsibilities:

1. Designing and conducting research to expand clinical pharmacokinetic knowledge and its relationship to pharmacologic responses, exploring concentration–response relationships for specific drugs, and contributing to the evaluation and expansion of clinical pharmacokinetic monitoring as an integral part of pharmaceutical care.
2. Developing and applying computer programs and point-of-care information systems to enhance the accuracy and sophistication of pharmacokinetic modeling and applications to pharmaceutical care.
3. Serving as an expert consultant to pharmacists with a general background in clinical pharmacokinetic monitoring.

Readers are referred to ASHP's more thorough publications on the subject of clinical pharmacokinetic monitoring,

including *Clinical Pharmacokinetics Pocket Reference* and *Concepts in Clinical Pharmacokinetics: A Self-Instructional Course.*

This statement was reviewed in 2008 by the Council on Pharmacy Practice and by the Board of Directors and was found to still be appropriate.

Approved by the ASHP Board of Directors, November 15, 1997, and by the ASHP House of Delegates, June 3, 1998. Revised by the ASHP Council on Professional Affairs. Supersedes a previous version approved by the House of Delegates on June 5, 1989.

The bibliographic citation for this document is as follows: American Society of Health-System Pharmacists. ASHP statement on the pharmacist's role in clinical pharmacokinetic monitoring. *Am J Health-Syst Pharm.* 1998; 55:1726–7.

ASHP Statement on the Pharmacist's Role in Hospice and Palliative Care

Position

The American Society of Health-System Pharmacists (ASHP) believes that pharmacists have a pivotal role in the provision of hospice and palliative care and that pharmacists should be integral members of all hospice interdisciplinary teams. Pharmacists practicing in U.S. health systems have been active in defining and providing palliative care since the introduction of hospice through a demonstration project supported by the National Cancer Institute and conducted in New Haven, Connecticut, between 1974 and 1977.[1]

Palliative care has been defined by the World Health Organization (WHO) as "the active total care of patients whose disease is not responsive to curative treatment."[2] WHO notes that control of pain, other symptoms, and psychological, social, and spiritual problems is paramount. The goal of palliative care is achievement of the best quality of life for patients and their families.

Pharmaceutical care is defined as the direct, responsible provision of medication-related care for the purpose of achieving definite outcomes that improve a patient's quality of life.[3] Medication therapy is the cornerstone of most—but not all—symptom control in palliative care. The goals of palliative care and pharmaceutical care are consistent, with the latter being a necessary component of good palliative care.

Hospice is a philosophy and program that delivers palliative care. Hospice care is provided by an interdisciplinary team, which provides expert medical care, pain management, and emotional and spiritual support expressly tailored to the patient's wishes. Emotional and spiritual support are also extended to the family of the patient. In U.S. hospice programs, care is usually provided in the patient's home or in a homelike setting operated by a hospice program. Hospice and palliative care share the same core values and philosophies.

The purpose of this statement is to describe pharmacist's responsibilities and to promote understanding of the various ways in which pharmacists provide or contribute to the provision of care to patients who might be nearing the end of life.

Background

Currently, there are over 3100 operational or planned hospice programs in the 50 states, the District of Columbia, Puerto Rico, and Guam.[4] According to the National Hospice and Palliative Care Organization, 42% of hospices were freestanding in 2000 and 33% were affiliated with hospitals, 22% with home health agencies, and 9% with hospital systems. Over 700,000 patients were served in 2000, and that number is growing annually. In that same year, 73% of hospices were nonprofit, 20% were for-profit institutions, and 7% were run by government.

In 2000, 2.4 million Americans died from all causes. Hospices admitted approximately 700,000 patients. Of those, 600,000 died while under hospice care. Patients are discharged from hospices typically because of stabilization of disease, moving to an area or facility not served by a hospice, and patient and family preference. Over half of patients who die of

cancer in the United States are cared for by a hospice. Hospices across the country are caring for increasing numbers of patients with cardiac disease, AIDS, renal disease, end-stage pulmonary disease, dementia, amyotrophic lateral sclerosis, Parkinson's disease, and other degenerative neurologic diseases.

Hospice care is covered by Medicare Part A, private health insurance, and Medicaid in most states for patients who meet certain criteria. Any Medicare beneficiary who has a terminal illness with a prognosis of less than six months is, if the disease runs its normal course as certified by the attending physician and the hospice medical director, eligible for the hospice Medicare benefit.[5] Ninety-one percent of U.S. hospices have met Medicare certification requirements to provide this benefit to Medicare beneficiaries at no cost to the beneficiaries. Many hospices receive charitable contributions to cover the cost of care for terminally ill patients who cannot afford to pay for their care.

Palliative care should be provided in conjunction with curative care at the time of diagnosis of a potentially terminal illness. Palliative care alone may be indicated when attempts at a cure are judged to be futile. Admissions to hospice and palliative care programs often come too late for optimal services to be provided.[6] The mean length of stay is 50 days, and the median is 25 days.[4] Many hospice patients die within days to a week after admission to a program.

A nationwide Gallup survey conducted in 1996 indicated that 9 out of 10 adults, if terminally ill and with six months or less to live, would prefer to be cared for at home. A majority of adults would be interested in a comprehensive program of care, such as hospice. When asked to name their greatest fear associated with death, most respondents cited being a burden to family and friends. Pain was the second most common fear. Effective hospice programs address these concerns.

Pharmaceutical services provided by pharmacists in U.S. hospices were surveyed qualitatively and quantitatively in 1979 and 1991.[7,8]

While many pharmacists continue to serve hospice programs as volunteer consultants to the interdisciplinary team, a growing number of those who work with hospice programs are now considered integral staff and are paid for their services. Inhouse pharmacies have increased since the mid-1990s, and the number continues to grow. A hospice that can support its own pharmacy typically has an average daily census of 200 patients. Most pharmacists who provide pharmaceutical services to hospice programs are not employed directly by the hospices but by a provider of pharmaceutical services, such as a home health pharmacy or hospital. Many are employees of pharmacies that have contracts with hospices to provide drug products and services. In recent years, specialized hospice pharmacy services have been developed in several parts of the United States, and such programs are growing rapidly.

The Hospice Interdisciplinary Team. According to Medicare hospice regulations, a hospice interdisciplinary team should include a doctor of medicine or osteopathy, a registered nurse, a social worker, and a pastoral or other counselor.

Many other professionals and support persons often serve on such teams. In addition, Medicare regulations state that the hospice must "employ a licensed pharmacist; or have a formal agreement with a licensed pharmacist to advise the hospice on ordering, storage, administration, disposal, and recordkeeping of drugs and biologicals." According to the two published surveys of pharmacist activities in hospices, the hospice pharmacist typically is a full member of the interdisciplinary team.[7,8]

By regulation, a patient's plan of care must be reviewed and updated at specified intervals. If a hospice has more than one team, then it must designate the team by which a particular patient will be cared for. Hospice teams typically meet for one or two hours two to four times a month to review patients' care, status, and needs. Treatment plan modifications, determinations of need for additional services, and planning for consultations with specialists, changes in care settings, imminent death, and other important events are discussed. Education and training are often provided at these meetings as well.

The hospice medical director is a doctor of medicine or osteopathy who is responsible for the medical component of the patient's care. The director also serves as a consultant to the patient's primary care physicians and the hospice program staff. Pharmacists coordinate pharmacotherapy by making recommendations for appropriate therapy, educating patients and the hospice team about medications, monitoring therapeutic responses, and performing other medication-related functions. Adjusting drug therapy in accordance with treatment algorithms is a new role for pharmacists in some hospice and palliative care settings.

A registered nurse coordinates the implementation of each patient's plan of care. After certified nursing assistants, who may provide personal care on a daily basis, nurses make the largest number of home visits. Social workers are responsible for the psychosocial care of patients and their families, and they arrange bereavement care for families after patients die. The volunteer director recruits, trains, and coordinates volunteers—another essential component of hospice care. Volunteers provide needed relief for family caregivers and a broad range of services to patients and their families.

Chaplains address spiritual and existential issues. Hospice chaplaincy is typically nondenominational and is often provided in coordination with patients' own clergy. Other frequent participants in team meetings include nursing assistants, home health aides, dietitians, physical therapists, occupational therapists, speech therapists, and hospice administrative personnel. Students and postgraduate trainees from a variety of professions, including pharmacy, often attend as well.

Value of the Pharmacist's Care. Most hospice and palliative care is reimbursed through a capitation plan. Therefore, fees for service generally do not apply. Pharmacists can improve the cost-effectiveness of pharmacotherapy for symptom control in hospice care through patient-specific monitoring for drug therapy outcomes, recommending alternative drug products and dosage forms, minimizing duplicative and interacting medications, compounding medications extemporaneously, improving drug storage and transportation, and educating staff, patients, and families about the most efficient ways of handling and using medications. Systems for documenting these activities and determining cost-effectiveness and the cost–benefit and cost–utility ratios of medications used in the care of terminally ill patients are needed.

Avoidance of admissions to hospitals or long-term-care facilities through improved symptom control is a highly desirable and cost-effective outcome of pharmaceutical care for hospice and palliative care patients.

The Pharmacist's Responsibilities

High-quality hospice and palliative care requires both traditional and expanded pharmacist activities, including a variety of clinical, educational, administrative, and support responsibilities:

1. *Assessing the appropriateness of medication orders and ensuring the timely provision of effective medications for symptom control.* Pharmacists maintain patient medication profiles and monitor all prescription and nonprescription medication use for safety and effectiveness. Pharmacists provide patients with essential medications within a time frame that ensures continuous symptom control (especially pain relief) and avoids the need for emergency medical services.

2. *Counseling and educating the hospice team about medication therapy.* Pharmacists attend hospice team meetings to advise other team members about medication therapy, including dosage forms, routes of administration, costs, and availability of various drug products. This is done through regularly scheduled educational sessions. Pharmacists develop and maintain a library of contemporary references about medications, dietary supplements, and alternative and complementary therapies. Pharmacists advise members of the hospice team about the potential for toxicity from and interactions with dietary supplements and alternative and complementary therapies.

3. *Ensuring that patients and caregivers understand and follow the directions provided with medications.* Pharmacists ensure that all medication labeling is complete and understandable by patients and their caregivers. Hospice pharmacists communicate with patients, either through the team or in person, about the importance of adhering to the prescribed drug regimen. Pharmacists explain the differences among addiction, dependence, and tolerance and dispel patient and caregiver misconceptions about addiction to opiate agonists. Pharmacists ensure the availability of devices and equipment to permit accurate measurement of liquid dosage forms by patients and their caregivers. Pharmacists counsel patients about the role and potential toxicity of alternative and complementary therapies. When needed, hospice pharmacists visit patients' homes to communicate directly with patients and their caregivers and to make necessary assessments.

4. *Providing efficient mechanisms for extemporaneous compounding of nonstandard dosage forms.* Hospice pharmacists communicate with pharmaceutical manufacturers to determine the availability of nonstandard dosage forms. Medication-compounding needs in hospice care include the preparation of dosage forms to ease administration (e.g., concentrated sublingual solutions, topical medications), flavoring medications to promote compliance, eliminating or adjusting ingredients that patients cannot tolerate, and preparing or changing drug concentrations. Whenever possible, pharmacists compound formulations for which stability and bioavailability data are available.

5. *Addressing financial concerns.* Hospice benefits usually cover medications. However, patients may lack insurance coverage or benefits may not cover medications that are not considered strictly palliative. Pharmacists communicate with pharmaceutical manufacturers to obtain medications through patient assistance programs.

6. *Ensuring safe and legal disposal of all medications after death.* Medications dispensed to patients are "owned" by the patients and, in most states, cannot be used for other patients. Medications remaining in patients' homes fall under a variety of hazard categories. Pharmacists are able to assist families with the removal of the medications from the home in compliance with federal and state drug control and environmental protection laws and regulations.

7. *Establishing and maintaining effective communication with regulatory and licensing agencies.* Because hospice patients often require large quantities of controlled substances, open communication with both state and federal controlled-substance agencies is important. Pharmacists ensure compliance with laws and regulations pertaining to medications.

Pharmacists' Scope of Practice

The pharmacist may have a range of practice privileges that vary in their level of authority and responsibility. Pharmacists who participate in hospice and palliative care should meet the health care organization's competency requirements to ensure that they provide appropriate quality and continuity of patient care. They should demonstrate required knowledge and skills, which may be obtained through practice-intensive continuing education and pharmacy practice and specialty residencies.

The specific practice of pharmacists should be defined within a scope-of-practice document or a similar tool or protocol developed by the health care organization. The scope-of-practice document defines activities that pharmacists would provide within the context of collaborative practice as a member of the interdisciplinary team, as well as limitations where appropriate. The document should indicate referral and communication guidelines, including the documentation of patient encounters and methods for sharing patient information with collaborating medical providers.

Also included in the scope-of-practice document should be references to activities that will review the quality of care provided and the methods by which the pharmacist will maintain continuing professional competency for functions encompassed by the scope-of-practice document. A process should be in place, and responsible parties identified, to review and update the scope-of-practice document as appropriate.

Documentation of Services

As members of the interdisciplinary health care team, pharmacists should have access to patients' health records and authority to make entries necessary for the team's coordinated care of the patient. With access to the patient's health record comes the pharmacist's professional responsibility to safeguard the patient's rights to privacy and confidentiality. Patients should be informed that pharmacists, as well as other members of the team, have access to their records.

Pharmacists should routinely sign patient-review records at interdisciplinary team meetings. Pharmacist documentation in patient records should include drug therapy recommendations, monitoring of medication effects, patient and family education and counseling activities, and other activities as indicated. Medication profiles should be maintained and should include information about prescription and nonprescription drug products, dietary supplements, and alternative and complementary therapies. Pharmacists also should maintain detailed formulation files for all extemporaneously compounded dosage forms. Other records should be maintained in compliance with applicable federal and state laws and regulations.

References

1. Lipman AG. Drug therapy in terminally ill patients. *Am J Hosp Pharm.* 1975; 32:270–6.
2. World Health Organization Expert Committee. Cancer pain relief and palliative care. Technical report series 804. Geneva, Switzerland: World Health Organization; 1990.
3. American Society of Hospital Pharmacists. ASHP statement on pharmaceutical care. *Am J Hosp Pharm.* 1993; 50:1720–3.
4. National Hospice and Palliative Care Organization. NHPCO facts and figures on hospice care in America. www.nhpco.org (accessed 2002 Apr 11).
5. Gage B, Miller SC, Coppola K et al. Important questions for hospice in the next century. www.aspe.hhs.gov/daltcp/Reports/impques.htm#execsum (accessed 2001 Nov 27).
6. Lipman AG. Evidence-based palliative care. *J Pharm Care Pain Symptom Control.* 1999; 7(4):1–9.
7. Berry JI, Pulliam CC, Caiola SM et al. Pharmaceutical services in hospices. *Am J Hosp Pharm.* 1981; 38:1010–4.
8. Arter SG, Berry JI. The provision of pharmaceutical care to hospice patients: results of the National Hospice Pharmacist Survey. *J Pharm Care Pain Symptom Control.* 1993; 1(1):25–42.

Suggested Readings

1. Lipman AG, Berry JI. Pharmaceutical care of terminally ill patients. *J Pharm Care Pain Symptom Control.* 1995; 3(2):31–56.
2. Arter SG, Lipman AG. Hospice care: a new opportunity for pharmacists. *J Pharm Pract.* 1990; 3:28–33.
3. Lipman AG. Pain management in the home care and hospice patient. *J Pharm Pract.* 1990; 3:1–11.
4. Wilkins C. Pharmacy and hospice: a personal experience. *Consult Pharm.* 1988; 3:462–5.
5. Arter SG, DuBe J, Mahoney J. Hospice care and the pharmacist. *Am Pharm.* 1987; NS27:616–24.
6. Murphy DH. The delicate art of caring: treating the whole person. *Am Pharm.* 1984; NS24:388–90.
7. Quigley JL, Quigley MA, Gumbhir AK. Pharmacy and hospice: partners in patient care. *Am Pharm.* 1982; NS22:420–3.
8. Berry JI. Pharmacy services in hospice organizations. *Hosp Formul.* 1982; 17:1333–8.
9. Mullan PA. Pharmacy and hospice: opportunities for service. *Am Pharm.* 1982; NS22:424–6.
10. Oliver CH. Pharmacy and hospice: talk with the dying patient. *Am Pharm.* 1982; NS22:429–33.

11. DuBe JE. Hospice care and the pharmacist. *US Pharm.* 1981; Apr:25–38.
12. Gable FB. Death with dignity: the pharmacist's role in hospice care. *Apothecary.* 1980; Sep/Oct:62–7.
13. Hammel MI, Trinca CE. Patient needs come first at Hillhaven hospice: pharmacy services essential for pain control. *Am Pharm.* 1978; NS18:655–7.
14. Nee D. Pharmacy practice in a hospice setting. *Fla Pharm Today.* 1995; Apr:19–23.

Approved by the ASHP Board of Directors in April 2002 and ASHP House of Delegates in June 2002. Developed through the ASHP Council on Professional Affairs.

The bibliographic citation for this document is as follows: American Society of Health-System Pharmacists. ASHP statement on the pharmacist's role in hospice and palliative care. *Am J Health-Syst Pharm.* 2002; 59:1770–3.

ASHP Statement on the Pharmacist's Role in Medication Reconciliation

Position

The American Society of Health-System Pharmacists (ASHP) believes that an effective process for medication reconciliation reduces medication errors and supports safe medication use by patients. ASHP encourages hospitals and health systems, including community-based providers and managed care systems, to collaborate in organized, multidisciplinary medication reconciliation programs to promote continuity of patient care. ASHP further believes that pharmacists, because of their distinct knowledge, skills, and abilities, are uniquely qualified to lead interdisciplinary efforts to establish and maintain an effective medication reconciliation process in hospitals and across health systems. Pharmacists should lead or assume key roles in the following essential components of medication reconciliation: developing policies and procedures, implementing and continuously improving medication reconciliation processes, training and assuring the continuing competency of those involved in medication reconciliation, providing operational and therapeutic expertise in the development of information systems that support medication reconciliation, and advocating for medication reconciliation programs in the community. Pursuant to their leadership role, pharmacists share accountability with other hospital and health-system leaders for the ongoing success of medication reconciliation processes across the continuum of care.

Background

The term "medication reconciliation" is defined by The Joint Commission (TJC) as "the process of comparing the medications a patient is taking (and should be taking) with newly ordered medications" in order to resolve discrepancies or potential problems.[1] The goals of medication reconciliation are to obtain and maintain accurate and complete medication information for a patient and use the information within and across the continuum of care to ensure safe and effective medication use. Although it is sometimes associated with survey and accreditation activities, medication reconciliation is an important component of patient safety and has demonstrated effectiveness in preventing adverse drug events. When organizations do not consistently and reliably reconcile patient medications across the continuum of care, medication errors and adverse drug events occur: approximately half of all hospital-related medication errors and 20% of all adverse drug events have been attributed to poor communication at the transitions and interfaces of care.[2,3]

In 1999, the Institute of Medicine (IOM) report *To Err Is Human: Building a Safer Health System*[4] identified medication errors as the most common type of health-system error, contributing to several thousand deaths each year. The fiscal impact of these errors is also significant. With reported costs of $2595–4685 per adverse drug event, drug-related morbidity and mortality was estimated to be over $177 billion in 2000 alone.[5]

Reports and studies such as these had a profound impact on the medical community, and the call for action was immediate. Organizations such as the Institute for Healthcare Improvement (IHI), the Agency for Healthcare Research and Quality (AHRQ), and TJC launched initiatives for performance improvement and established higher expectations through new regulatory standards for improved communication between providers and patients and across health care systems.

In 2005, TJC made medication reconciliation a focus of one of its National Patient Safety Goals. The initial goal included a number of detailed and specific requirements, which made implementation challenging and resulted in numerous findings of noncompliance during survey. In response, TJC affirmed the importance of the goal but suspended it in 2009 and 2010 for extensive revision. After a comprehensive literature review and analysis of data collected by surveyor teams, a modified goal was released in 2011, and scoring of the goal began in July 2011.[6] The revised goal sets an expectation for maintaining accurate medication information at critical risk points in the medication-use process while allowing organizations latitude to define processes and encouraging performance improvement.

The purpose of this statement is to describe pharmacists' responsibilities and accountabilities in medication reconciliation practices.

Pharmacists' Responsibilities

When performed by pharmacists, medication reconciliation can reduce the frequency and severity of hospital medication errors that could potentially result in patient harm.[7] Pharmacists have demonstrated high rates of patient interventions; interventions per patient; and documentation of medications, medication interactions, drug-related admissions, and previous drug failures.[8]

ASHP and the American Pharmacists Association (APhA) began a collaborative effort in 2007 and 2008 to create a shared vision for the role of the pharmacist in medication reconciliation processes.[9] That vision recognizes that pharmacists should take a leadership role in improving medication reconciliation, acting as both advocates and medication experts, to provide information to and educate patients and health care providers. Specifically, pharmacists' responsibilities were described as including but not being limited to:

- providing leadership in designing and managing patient-centered medication reconciliation systems,
- educating patients and health care professionals about the benefits and limitations of the medication reconciliation process, and
- serving as patient advocates throughout transitions of care.

Using this vision as a guide, ASHP has developed the following recommendations for pharmacists' functions in medication reconciliation activities.

Pharmacists' Functions

Although medication reconciliation is required at key transitions of care, activities associated with medication reconciliation should be considered part of ongoing care provided to a patient. Beyond active participation in medication reconciliation activities, pharmacists have five fundamental functions in medication reconciliation: developing policies and procedures regarding medication reconciliation processes, implementing and continuously improving those processes, training and assuring the continuing competency of those involved in medication reconciliation, providing operational and therapeutic expertise in the development of information systems that support medication reconciliation, and advocating for medication reconciliation programs in the community. The extent of pharmacist involvement in these functions will depend on the resources available.

Policy and Procedure Development. Pharmacists should provide leadership and participate in establishing policies and procedures that encourage (a) provision of patient-care services that include medication reconciliation processes, (b) implementation and operation of an evidence-based medication reconciliation system that optimizes available resources, (c) education of organization staff on the importance of medication reconciliation as a patient safety initiative, and (d) promotion of medication reconciliation as a focus of performance improvement activities.

Implementation and Performance Improvement. Pharmacists should lead or participate in organizational implementation of and performance improvement efforts regarding medication reconciliation activities. These activities may include but are not limited to: (a) establishing a medication reconciliation implementation task force or redesign team; (b) creating a vision and expectations for medication reconciliation activities; (c) securing executive-level commitment to or sponsorship of medication reconciliation resource needs; (d) identifying barriers that are preventing, or potential barriers that may prevent, safe and effective medication reconciliation procedures within their practice model, as well as possible solutions; (e) guiding workflow development that integrates operational and clinical needs; (f) establishing roles and responsibilities of health care providers in medication reconciliation processes, including pharmacy technicians, pharmacy students, and other medical support personnel; (g) ensuring that competency-based training for all personnel involved in medication reconciliation procedures is established; (h) creating or assisting in the development of standardized documentation templates for medication lists and reconciliation; (i) ensuring that established procedures meet regulatory requirements and organizational policy; and (j) developing a method for ongoing medication reconciliation system evaluation.

Training and Competency Assurance. Pharmacists should lead or participate in (a) identifying all health care providers and support staff involved in medication reconciliation activities; (b) creating competency training and skills assessment that are specific to each staff member's roles and responsibilities in medication reconciliation (e.g., conducting a medication interview, taking a medication history, performing medication reconciliation); (c) providing education and performing assessments to ensure the competency of those who document and perform medication reconciliation activities; and (d) providing didactic or simulated training for medication history and reconciliation procedures.

Information Systems Development. As more organizations adopt computerized provider order entry, electronic medical records, and other information systems, pharmacists should ensure that the systems support medication reconciliation throughout the continuum of care. Consideration should be given to establishing methods for data extraction from the medical record that allow for internal and external reporting of measures related to medication reconciliation.

Advocacy. Pharmacists should provide information about medication reconciliation to health care providers, patients, and the community, and they should evaluate the effectiveness of these advocacy efforts on the medication reconciliation process. Activities may include clinical grand rounds, professional conferences, patient counseling, or mass communications such as newsletters or public service announcements. These efforts should (a) demonstrate the effectiveness of sound medication reconciliation processes in improving patient safety and reducing health care costs; (b) emphasize the importance of timely and accurate communication of medication information between patients and their health care providers; (c) clarify and describe the important role of technology and electronic medical records that support medication reconciliation documentation and reconciliation; (d) provide strategies for preventing medication adverse events related to overuse, misuse, omission, duplication, or other discrepancies found during medication reconciliation processes; (e) highlight the importance of completing a full and accurate medication history, including supplement use, prior to prescribing or administering a new medication; and (f) describe opportunities for pharmacist extenders, such as pharmacy technicians and students, to participate in medication reconciliation activities.

Resource Constraints. Although the literature demonstrates the important role of pharmacists in successful medication reconciliation processes across the continuum of care, significant resources are needed to perform medication reconciliation skillfully and efficiently, which suggests opportunities for expanding the roles of pharmacy residents, students, and technicians. When properly trained, these individuals can participate in the documentation of medication histories, which should then be reviewed by the pharmacist for accuracy prior to medication reconciliation, as described in the ASHP Pharmacy Practice Model Initiative Summit Recommendations.[10] In one study, potential errors due to incomplete or incorrect information, illegible orders, and serious drug interactions were reduced by 82% by having pharmacy technicians obtain medication histories.[11]

When confronted with limited resources, pharmacists should at a minimum participate in and guide interdisciplinary efforts to develop and define policies and procedures for their organizations, standardize workflows for electronic documentation, promote safe practices to the

community, and, most importantly, engage health care leadership in efforts to ensure medication reconciliation processes are successful.

Conclusion

An effective process for medication reconciliation reduces medication errors and supports safe medication use. Pharmacists are uniquely qualified to lead interdisciplinary efforts to establish and maintain an effective medication reconciliation process in hospitals and across health systems and should lead or assume key roles in the essential components of medication reconciliation. Because of their crucial role, pharmacists share accountability with other hospital and health-system leaders for the ongoing success of medication reconciliation processes across the continuum of care.

References

1. The Joint Commission. National Patient Safety Goals Effective January 1, 2012. NPSG.03.06.01. www.jointcommission.org/assets/1/6/NPSG_Chapter_Jan2012_HAP.pdf. (accessed 02 Feb 2012).

2. Barnsteiner JH. Medication reconciliation: transfer of medication information across settings: keeping it free from error. *J Infus Nurs.* 2005; 28(2 suppl):31–6.

3. Rozich J, Roger R. Medication safety: one organization's approach to the challenge. *J Clin Outcomes Manag.* 2001; 8:27–34.

4. Kohn LT, Corrigan JM, Donaldson MS (Eds.). To err is human: building a safer health system. Washington, DC: National Academy Press; 1999.

5. Bates DW, Spell N, Cullen DJ, et al. The cost of adverse drug events in hospitalized patients. *JAMA.* 1997; 277:307–11.

6. The Joint Commission. 2011 National Patient Safety Goals. www.jointcommission.org/standards_information/npsgs.aspx. (accessed 13 Dec 2011).

7. Gleason KM, Groszek JM, Sullivan C, et al. Reconciliation of discrepancies in medication histories and admission orders of newly hospitalized patients. *Am J Health-Syst Pharm.* 2004; 61:1689–95.

8. Gurwich EL. Comparison of medication histories acquired by pharmacists and physicians. *Am J Hosp Pharm.* 1983; 40:1541–2.

9. Chen D, Burns A. ASHP–APhA Medication Reconciliation Initiative Workgroup Meeting, February 12, 2007: Summary and Recommendations. www.ashp.org/s_ashp/docs/files/MedRec_ASHP_APhA_Wkgrp_MtgSummary.pdf (accessed 01 Feb 2012).

10. American Society of Health-System Pharmacists. Pharmacy Practice Model Initiative Summit Recommendations. Recommendation D3a. February 1, 2011. www.ashp.org/DocLibrary/PPMI/Summit-Recommendations.aspx (accessed 01 Feb 2012).

11. Michels R, Meisel S. Program using pharmacy technicians to obtain medication histories. *Am J Health-Syst Pharmacy.* 2003; 60:1982–6.

Approved by the ASHP Board of Directors on April 13, 2012, and by the ASHP House of Delegates on June 10, 2012. Developed through the ASHP Council on Pharmacy Practice.

Michelle M. Thoma, Pharm.D., is gratefully acknowledged for drafting this statement.

Note: This statement had not been published in the *American Journal of Health-System Pharmacy* (*AJHP*) when *Best Practices for Hospital & Health-System Pharmacy 2012–2013* went to press. Some minor editorial differences may exist between this document and the official one that will eventually appear in *AJHP* and subsequent editions of this publication.

ASHP Statement on the Pharmacist's Role in Primary Care

Position

The American Society of Health System Pharmacists (ASHP) believes that pharmacists have a role in meeting the primary care needs of patients by fulfilling their responsibilities to provide pharmaceutical care and, in states where it is authorized, through their expanded responsibilities in collaborative drug therapy management.

Pharmaceutical care is the direct, responsible provision of medication-related care for the purpose of achieving definite outcomes that improve a patient's quality of life.[1] Pharmacists establish relationships with patients to ensure the appropriateness of medication therapy and patients' understanding of their therapy, and to monitor the effects of that therapy. In collaborative drug therapy management, pharmacists enter agreements with physicians and other prescribers that may authorize pharmacists, for patients who have a confirmed diagnosis, to select appropriate medication therapies and regimens and adjust them on the basis of patients' responses.

National and international organizations, states, and health care organizations, among others, may have differing or overlapping definitions of primary care. Primary care is a concept intended to improve the quality of care received by everyone in the United States.[2] For the purposes of this document, primary care is defined as the provision of integrated, accessible health care services by clinicians who are accountable for addressing a majority of personal health care needs, developing a sustained partnership with patients, and practicing in the context of family and community. Primary care services should be comprehensive, coordinated, and continuously provided over time by individuals or a team of health care professionals according to the patient's needs. Services should be accessible to patients by telephone or at sites of care provision. Clinicians who provide these services are responsible for the quality of care, the satisfaction of patients, and the efficient use of resources, as well as for their own ethical behavior.[3]

Practice elements of pharmaceutical care and collaborative drug therapy management are consistent with the intents and evolving forms of primary care. ASHP supports the development of definitions and working models of primary care that recognize and incorporate the services of pharmacists for meeting primary care needs of patients. In general, pharmacists contribute to the provision of primary care through the delivery of pharmaceutical care and in collaboration with other health care providers.[4-9] Furthermore, pharmacists may directly provide a limited range of primary care functions in addition to those encompassed by pharmaceutical care, either independently or in collaboration with other members of a primary care team.[10,11] High-quality, coordinated, and continuous medication management for patients should be measurable as a result of the provision of pharmaceutical care within a primary care delivery model. The benefits to patients are valuable access to medication information, the prevention and resolution of medication-related problems, improved outcomes, and increased satisfaction.[12] Pharmacists are able to use medication-related encounters with patients to provide information and either resolve or make a referral for other health care needs.

The purposes of this statement are to promote understanding of the various ways in which pharmacists provide or contribute to the provision of primary care in integrated health systems and to clarify future directions for pharmacists in efforts to expand patient care services in primary care.

Background

Changes in the nation's health care system, especially the growth of managed care and integrated health systems, are stimulating adoption of primary care as a way of meeting basic health care needs and managing access to specialty services. Integrated health systems are organized to deliver acute, intermediate, long-term, home, and ambulatory care. They are intended to seamlessly provide care across practice settings through appropriate use of individual health professionals and teams.[13] Integrated systems offer opportunities for pharmacists and other health care providers to detect and respond to the medication-related needs of patients in transition between settings (e.g., from inpatient to ambulatory care). As integrated systems expand to offer more intensive ambulatory care services and cover broader geographic areas, primary care will become more prominent. Improving patients' access to and continuity of care, implementing disease management, and focusing on quality-related outcomes contribute to optimizing drug costs within the total costs of patient care.[14] Pharmacists involved in primary care contribute to all of these.

Pharmacists participate in primary care services in a variety of practice settings within integrated health systems, including the acute (inpatient), physician office, clinic, pharmacy, long-term, and home settings. A growing number of acute care hospitals have pharmacists participating in patient care activities in ambulatory care clinics and hospital-based home health care services.[15] Along with other providers, pharmacists are expanding and further defining practice models to meet the pharmaceutical and primary care needs of patients throughout the continuum of care.

Responsibilities

Pharmacists involved in primary care participate with other team members in the management of patients for whom medications are a focus of therapy. Pharmacists' responsibility is to optimize patients' medication therapy. Primary care pharmaceutical services should be designed to support the various components of the medication-use process (ordering, dispensing, administering, monitoring, and educating) as individual steps or as they relate to one another in the continuum of care. Pharmacists should evaluate all components of the medication-use process to optimize the potential for positive patient outcomes.

Functions. In general, pharmacists who participate in providing primary care to individual patients perform the following functions in collaboration with physicians and other members of the primary care team:

- Perform patient assessment for medication-related factors.

- Order laboratory tests necessary for monitoring outcomes of medication therapy.
- Interpret data related to medication safety and effectiveness.
- Initiate or modify medication therapy care plans on the basis of patient responses.
- Provide information, education, and counseling to patients about medication-related care.
- Document the care provided in patients' records.
- Identify any barriers to patient compliance.
- Participate in multidisciplinary reviews of patients' progress.
- Communicate with payers to resolve issues that may impede access to medication therapies.
- Communicate relevant issues to physicians and other team members.

Expanded Functions. Expanded primary care functions of pharmacists include all the functions previously described as well as:

- Provide individualized health promotion and disease prevention, including administration of immunizations where this is legally and organizationally authorized.
- Perform limited physical assessment and supervise medication therapy with appropriate collaborative drug therapy management authority.

Pharmacists' Scope of Practice. The pharmacist may have a range of practice privileges that vary in their extent of authority and responsibility. Pharmacists who participate in collaborative primary care practice should meet the health care organization's competency requirements to ensure that they provide appropriate quality and continuity of patient care. They should demonstrate required knowledge and skills that may be obtained through practice-intensive continuing education and pharmacy practice and specialty residencies. The specific practice of pharmacists who participate in collaborative primary care should be defined within a scope-of-practice document or a similar tool developed by the health care organization. The scope-of-practice document defines activities that pharmacists would provide within the context of collaborative primary care practice, as well as limitations where appropriate. The document should indicate referral and communication guidelines, including the documentation of patient encounters and methods for sharing patient information with collaborating medical providers. Also included should be references to activities that will review the quality of care provided and the methods by which the pharmacist will maintain continuing professional competency for functions within the scope-of-practice document. A process should be in place to review and update the scope-of-practice document as appropriate.

Description of Services Provided. The services offered by the pharmacist range from consulting with the health care team to providing direct support of the patient while working in collaboration with the health care team. The pharmacist provides medication therapy outcomes management as part of the patient's ongoing care. The level of intensity of services varies as the patient's needs change. For chronic illnesses, services may range from health maintenance care to active management of treatment; for acute illnesses, services may range from facilitating access to medical care to providing initial management. In this context, health maintenance may

include counseling (e.g., abuse of alcohol, tobacco, and other drugs; use of seat belts) and ordering screening procedures (e.g., blood lipids and glucose, fecal occult blood). The complexity of services provided varies according to patient need and support from within the integrated health system.

Areas of primary care pharmacy practice that have previously been demonstrated to be cost-effective and to improve outcomes include participation on primary care teams and primary care clinics for medication monitoring and refill in the management of general or specific pharmacotherapy (e.g., for asthma, hypertension, dyslipidemia, anticoagulation, dermatologic diseases, diabetes, and psychotherapeutics).[16–23]

Documentation of Pharmacists' Care. Pharmacists in each setting should routinely document the quantity and quality of services provided and the estimated effect on patient outcomes. Pharmacists must safeguard patients' rights to privacy and confidentiality. Patient information should be shared only with members of the health care team and others with authorized access as needed for the care of patients.

Methods for referral to other health care providers and documentation of care provided should be defined and must occur as a routine part of the daily functions of a pharmacist's practice. When more than one pharmacist is involved in delivering care, practice standards for the group should be adopted and should serve as a guide for all. Pharmacists must also establish methods of communication among themselves in order to provide and ensure continuity of pharmaceutical care on behalf of patients served.

Value of Pharmacist's Care. Methods for obtaining compensation or economic and professional credit for value-added services must continue to be addressed. Structures designed to measure the practitioner's effectiveness as part of an innovative team should be instituted. The pharmacy profession should embrace these activities in the form of well-structured research. Integrated health systems will need to receive adequate support to expand the availability of pharmacists to provide pharmaceutical care as an essential component of primary care.

References

1. American Society of Health System Pharmacists. ASHP statement on pharmaceutical care. *Am J Hosp Pharm.* 1993; 50:1720–3.
2. Rubin E. Beyond the rhetoric: ensuring the availability of primary care. Report of an AHC/FASHP retreat. *Am J Pharm Educ.* 1993; 57:191–3.
3. Donaldson MS, Yordy KD, Lohr KN, et al., eds. Primary care: America's health in a new era. Committee on the Future of Primary Care, Division of Health Services, Institute of Medicine. Washington, DC: National Academy Press; 1996.
4. Koecheler JA, Abramowitz PW, Swim SE, et al. Indicators for the selection of ambulatory patients who warrant pharmacist monitoring. *Am J Hosp Pharm.* 1989; 46:729–32.
5. Lobas LH, Lepinski PW, Abramowitz PW. Effects of pharmaceutical care on medication cost and quality of patient care in an ambulatory-care clinic. *Am J Hosp Pharm.* 1992; 49:1681–8.
6. Chrischelles EQ, Helling DK, Aschoff CR. Effect of clinical pharmacy services on the quality of family

practice physician prescribing and medication costs. *Drug Intell Clin Pharm.* 1989; 23:417–21.

7. Monson R, Bond CA, Schuna A. Role of the clinical pharmacist in improving drug therapy: clinical pharmacists in outpatient therapy. *Arch Intern Med.* 1981; 141:1441–4.

8. Bond CA, Monson R. Sustained improvement in drug documentation, compliance, and disease control: a four-year analysis of an ambulatory care model. *Arch Intern Med.* 1984; 114:1159–62.

9. Jameson J, VanNoord G, Vanderwoud K. The impact of a pharmacotherapy consultation on the cost and outcome of medical therapy. *J Fam Pract.* 1995; 41:469–72.

10. Dong BJ, Echaves SA, Brody RV, et al. Pharmacist provision of preventive health services in a hypertension clinic. *Am J Health-Syst Pharm.* 1997; 54:564–6.

11. Furmaga EM. Pharmacist management of a hyperlipidemia clinic. *Am J Hosp Pharm.* 1993; 50:91–5.

12. Galt KA, Skrabal MA, Abdouch I, et al. Using patient expectations and satisfaction data to design a new pharmacy service model in a primary care clinic. *J Manage Care Pharm.* 1997; 3:531–40.

13. American Society of Health-System Pharmacists. Vision statement. American Society of Health-System Pharmacists. *Am J Health-Syst Pharm.* 1996; 53:174.

14. Chamberlain MA. The vertically integrated pharmacy department. *Am J Health-Syst Pharm.* 1998; 55:669–75.

15. Raehl CL, Bond CA, Pitterle ME. Ambulatory pharmacy services affiliated with acute care hospitals. *Pharmacotherapy.* 1993; 13:618–25.

16. Chandler C, Barriuso P, Rozenberg-Ben- Dror K, et al. Pharmacists on a primary care team at a Veterans Affairs medical center. *Am J Health-Syst Pharm.* 1997; 54:1280–7.

17. Oke TO. Primary health care services with a functional ambulatory care clinical pharmacy in a low income housing project clinic. *J Natl Med Assoc.* 1994; 86:465–8.

18. Alsuwaidan S, Malone DC, Billups SJ, et al. Characteristics of ambulatory care clinics and pharmacists in Veterans Affairs medical centers. *Am J Health-Syst Pharm.* 1998; 55:68–72.

19. Libby EA, Laub JJ. Economic and clinical impact of a pharmacy-based antihypertensive replacement program in primary care. *Am J Health-Syst Pharm.* 1997; 54:2079–83.

20. Konzem SL, Morreale AP, Kaplan LA. Pharmacist-managed primary care dermatology clinic. *Hosp Pharm.* 1996; 31:823–5,834.

21. Wilson Norton JL, Gibson DL. Establishing an outpatient anticoagulation clinic in a community hospital. *Am J Health-Syst Pharm.* 1996; 53:1151–7.

22. Lacro JP, Kodsi A, Dishman B, et al. Primary care role of psychopharmacists in an ambulatory care setting. *Calif J Health-Syst Pharm.* 1995; 7:9–10.

23. Galt KA. Cost avoidance, acceptance, and outcomes associated with a pharmacotherapy consult clinic in a Veteran's Affairs medical center. *Pharmacotherapy.* 1998; 18:1103–11.

Approved by the ASHP Board of Directors, April 21, 1999, and by the ASHP House of Delegates, June 7, 1999. Developed by the Council on Professional Affairs.

Kimberly A. Galt, Pharm.D., FASHP, Richard F. Demers, and Richard N. Herrier, Pharm.D., are gratefully acknowledged for drafting this document.

The bibliographic citation for this document is as follows: American Society of Health-System Pharmacists. ASHP statement on the pharmacist's role in primary care. *Am J Health-Syst Pharm.* 1999; 56:1665–7.

ASHP Statement on the Pharmacist's Role in Substance Abuse Prevention, Education, and Assistance

Position

The American Society of Health-System Pharmacists (ASHP) believes that pharmacists have the unique knowledge, skills, and responsibilities for assuming an important role in substance abuse prevention, education, and assistance. Pharmacists, as health care providers, should be actively involved in reducing the negative effects that substance abuse has on society, health systems, and the pharmacy profession. Further, ASHP supports efforts to rehabilitate pharmacists and other health-system employees whose mental or physical impairments are caused by dependency on psychoactive drugs.

Background

The term "substance abuse," as used in this Statement, includes those diseases described by the American Psychiatric Association's Diagnostic and Statistical Manual of Mental Disorders, fourth edition, text revision (DSM-IV-TR) criteria as "psychoactive substance use disorders."[1] Psychoactive substances are abused primarily to depress, stimulate, or distort brain activity. Examples include alcohol, tobacco, "street" drugs (e.g., marijuana, lysergic acid diethylamide [LSD], cocaine, methamphetamine, inhalants, methylenedioxymethamphetamine [MDMA], gammahydroxybutyrate [GHB], heroin), and the nonmedical use or the overuse of psychoactive and other prescription and nonprescription drugs (e.g., oxycodone, ketamine, methadone, and dextromethorphan).

Substance abuse is a major societal problem. The 2000 National Household Survey on Drug Abuse, a primary source of statistical information on the use of illegal drugs by the U.S. population, estimated that (a) 4.3 million Americans (or 1.9% of the total population) ages 12 years or older were current illicit drug users, (b) 7.1 million Americans (or 3.2% of the total population) were dependent on illicit drugs or alcohol, and (c) 5.1 million Americans (or 2.3% of the total population) were dependent on alcohol.[2] A study of psychiatric disorders in America suggested a lifetime prevalence of substance abuse disorders of 16.4%, of alcohol abuse or dependency of 13.3%, and of other drug abuse or dependency of 5.9%.[3] Studies suggest that the prevalence of drug abuse among health professionals appears to be similar to that in the general population.[4-6] Given their access, however, health professionals abuse prescription drugs more often and "street" drugs less often than does the general population.

Substance abuse frequently coexists with and complicates other psychiatric disorders, and it is a common and often unrecognized cause of physical morbidity. Intravenous drug abuse is a major factor in the spread of HIV and hepatitis. Alcohol is a major factor in cirrhosis of the liver, and tobacco is a key contributor to emphysema and lung cancer. Collectively, substance abuse contributes significantly to morbidity and mortality in our population and to the cost of health care.

Substance abuse is also a serious workplace problem. The Substance Abuse and Mental Health Services Adminis-

tration reported that approximately 70% of those reporting illicit drug use within the past month were currently employed full-time and that 1 in 12 full-time employees reports current use of illicit drugs.[7] Substance abuse by employees of health care organizations leads to reduced productivity, increased absenteeism, drug diversion, and, almost certainly, increased accidents and medication misadventures. Consequently, it affects the quality of patient care, liability, and operational and health care costs.

Pharmacists have unique, comprehensive knowledge about the safe and effective use of medications and about the adverse effects of their inappropriate use. The provision of pharmaceutical care to individual patients involves pharmacists assessing the appropriateness of pharmacotherapy, counseling, and monitoring medication-use outcomes. Health-system pharmacists have organizational responsibilities for contributing to the (a) development of the health care organization's medication-use policies, including input into the decisions of the pharmacy and therapeutics committee, (b) development of clinical care plans and other types of protocols, and (c) investigation and prevention of adverse medication events. Furthermore, pharmacists have legal and organizational responsibilities for medication distribution and control across the continuum of practice settings within health care organizations. With this combination of knowledge and organizational responsibilities, pharmacists are prepared to serve in leadership and service roles in substance abuse prevention and education and assist in a variety of patient care, employee health, and community activities.

Responsibilities

The scope of substance abuse responsibilities of pharmacists varies with the health care organization's mission, policies and procedures, patient population, and community. The responsibilities listed below should be adapted to meet local needs and circumstances. Each responsibility is intended to be applicable to any substance of abuse; therefore, specific substances are generally not mentioned. Pharmacists should be involved in substance abuse prevention, education, and assistance by performing the following activities:

Prevention

1. Participating in or contributing to the development of substance abuse prevention and assistance programs within health care organizations. A comprehensive program should consist of (a) a written substance abuse policy, (b) an employee education and awareness program, (c) a supervisor training program, (d) an employee assistance program, (e) peer support systems, such as pharmacist recovery networks, and (f) drug testing.[8]
2. Participating in public substance abuse education and prevention programs (e.g., in primary and secondary schools, colleges, churches, and civic organizations)

and stressing the potential adverse health consequences of the misuse of legal and use of illegal drugs.

3. Discouraging pharmacist involvement in the sale of alcohol and tobacco products.

4. Establishing a multidisciplinary controlled-substance inventory system that discourages diversion and enhances accountability that complies with statutory and regulatory requirements. Where helpful, for example, procedures might require the purchase of controlled substances in tamper-evident containers and maintenance of a perpetual inventory and ongoing surveillance system.

5. Working with local, state, and federal authorities in controlling substance abuse (e.g., complying with controlled-substance reporting regulations and cooperating in investigations that involve the misuse of controlled substances, especially diversions from a health care organization).

6. Working with medical laboratories to (a) identify substances of abuse by using drug and poison control information systems, (b) establish proper specimen collection procedures based on knowledge of the pharmacokinetic properties of abused substances, and (c) select proper laboratory tests to detect the suspected substances of abuse and to detect tampering with samples.

Education

1. Providing information and referral to support groups appropriate to the needs of people whose lives are affected by their own or another person's substance abuse or dependency.

2. Providing recommendations about the appropriate use of mood-altering substances to health care providers and the public, including those persons recovering from substance dependency and their caregivers.[9]

3. Fostering the development of undergraduate and graduate college of pharmacy curricula and pharmacy technician education on the topic of substance abuse prevention, education, and assistance.[10]

4. Providing substance abuse education to fellow pharmacists, other health care professionals, and other employees of their health care organization.

5. Instructing drug abuse counselors in drug treatment programs about the pharmacology of abused substances and medications used for detoxification.

6. Promoting and providing alcohol risk-reduction education and activities.

7. Maintaining professional competency in substance abuse prevention, education, and assistance through formal and informal continuing education.

8. Conducting research on substance abuse and addiction.

Assistance

1. Assisting in the identification of patients, coworkers, and other individuals who may be having problems related to their substance abuse, and referring them to the appropriate people for evaluation and treatment.

2. Participating in multidisciplinary efforts to support and care for the health care organization's employees and patients who are recovering from substance dependency.

3. Supporting and encouraging the recovery of health professionals with alcoholism or other drug addictions. Major elements of an employer's support program might include (a) a willingness to hire or retain employees, (b) participating in monitoring and reporting requirements associated with recovery or disciplinary contracts, (c) maintaining an environment supportive of recovery, (d) establishing behavioral standards and norms among all employees that discourage the abuse of psychoactive substances, including alcohol, and (e) participating in peer assistance programs.

4. Collaborating with other health care providers in the development of the pharmacotherapeutic elements of drug detoxification protocols.

5. Providing pharmaceutical care to patients being treated for substance abuse and dependency.

6. Maintaining knowledge of professional support groups (e.g., state- and national-level pharmacist recovery networks) and other local, state, and national organizations, programs, and resources available for preventing and treating substance abuse (see "Other resources").

7. Refusing to allow any student or employee, including health professionals, to work, practice, or be on-site for rotations within the health care organization while his or her ability to safely perform his or her responsibilities is impaired by drugs, including alcohol. The refusal should follow the organization's policies and procedures, the principles of ethical and responsible pharmacy practice, and statutory requirements. Practice should not be precluded after appropriate treatment and monitoring, if approved by the treatment provider or contract monitor (or both, when applicable).

References

1. American Psychiatric Association. Diagnostic and statistical manual of mental disorders. 4th ed. Washington, DC: American Psychiatric Association; 2000:198–9.

2. Epstein JF. Substance dependence, abuse and treatment: findings from the 2000 National Household Survey on Drug Abuse. Rockville, MD: U.S. Department of Health and Human Services, 2002; DHHS publication no. SMA 02-3642 (Series A-16).

3. Robins L, Regier D. Psychiatric disorders in America: the epidemiologic catchment area study. New York: Free Press; 1991:81–154.

4. McAuliffe WE, Santangelo SL, Gingras J, et al. Use and abuse of controlled substances by pharmacists and pharmacy students. *Am J Hosp Pharm.* 1987; 44:311–7.

5. Sullivan E, Bissell L, Williams E. Chemical dependency in nursing: the deadly diversion. Menlo Park, CA: Addison-Wesley; 1988.

6. Bissell L, Haberman PW, Williams RL. Pharmacists recovering from alcohol and other drug addictions: an interview study. *Am Pharm.* 1989; NS29(6):19–30. [Erratum, *Am Pharm.* 1989; NS29(9):11.]

7. Office of Applied Studies, Substance Abuse and Mental Health Services Administration. An analysis of worker drug use and workplace policies and programs. Rockville, MD: U.S. Department of Health and Human Services; 1997.

8. Center for Substance Abuse Prevention, Substance Abuse and Mental Health Services Administration. Making your workplace drug free: a kit for employers. Rockville, MD: U.S. Department of Health and Human Services; 1994.

9. Davis NH. Dispensing and prescribing cautions for medical care during recovery from alcohol and drug addiction. *J Pharm Pract.* 1991; 6:362–8.

10. Baldwin JN, Light K, Stock C, et al. Curricular guidelines for pharmacy education: substance abuse and addictive disease. *Am J Pharm Educ.* 1991; 55:311–6.

Other Resources

1. Hogue MD, McCormick DD, eds. Points of light: a guide for assisting chemically dependent health professional students. Washington, DC: American Pharmaceutical Association; 1996.

2. AACP Special Interest Group on Pharmacy Student and Faculty Impairment. American Association of Colleges of Pharmacy guidelines for the development of psychoactive substance use disorder policies for colleges of pharmacy. *Am J Pharm Educ.* 1999; 63:28S–34S.

3. Tucker DR, Gurnee MC, Sylvestri MF, et al. Psychoactive drug use and impairment markers in pharmacy students. *Am J Pharm Educ.* 1988; 52:42–7.

4. Miederhoff PA, Voight FB, White CE. Chemically impaired pharmacists: an emerging management issue. *Top Hosp Pharm Manage.* 1987; 7(Nov):75–83.

5. Kriegler KA, Baldwin JN, Scott DM. A study of alcohol and other drug use behaviors and risk factors in health profession students. *J Am Coll Health.* 1994; 42:259–65.

6. Haberman P. Alcoholism in the professions. Troy, MI: Performance Resource; 1991.

7. Bissell L, Royce JE. Ethics for addiction professionals. Center City, MN: Hazelden Foundation; 1994.

8. Colvin R. Prescription drug addiction: the hidden epidemic. Omaha, NE: Addicus; 2002.

9. Crosby L, Bissell L. To care enough: intervention with chemically-dependent colleagues. Minneapolis: Johnson Institute; 1989.

10. Johnson VE. Intervention: how to help someone who doesn't want help. A step-by-step guide for families and friends of chemically-dependent persons. Minneapolis: Johnson Institute; 1989.

11. Rinaldi RC, Steindler EM, Wilford BB, et al. Clarification and standardization of substance abuse terminology. *JAMA.* 1988; 259:555–7.

12. Brown ME, Trinkoff AM, Christen AG, et al. Impairment issues for health care professionals: review and recommendations. *Subst Abus.* 2002; 23S:155–65.

13. Dole EJ, Tommasello AC. Recommendations for implementing effective substance abuse education in pharmacy practice. *Subst Abus.* 2002; 23S:263–71.

14. National Clearinghouse for Alcohol and Drug Information (NCADI). The clearinghouse is a federally funded service that assists in finding information on all aspects of substance abuse. Many publications and educational materials are available free of charge from NCADI. Telephone, 800-729-6686; Web site, http://store.health.org/.

15. Center for Substance Abuse Prevention (CSAP) Workplace Helpline (for employers). Telephone, 800-967-5752; e-mail, helpline@samhsa.gov.

16. National Association of State Alcohol and Drug Abuse Directors (NASADAD). The association coordinates and encourages cooperative efforts between the federal government and state agencies on substance abuse. NASADAD serves as a resource on state drug programs and can provide contacts in each state. Web site, www.nasadad.org.

17. Community organizations are available to help with drug or alcohol problems. Treatment counselors may be valuable in developing assistance policies and in providing professional education about treatment and referral systems. Community drug-abuse-prevention organizations may be helpful in prevention efforts, in-cluding community drug education. Check your local telephone directory under headings such as Alcoholism Information and Treatment, Drug Abuse Information and Treatment, and Counselors.

18. Twelve-step groups (usually available locally unless otherwise noted; listed telephone numbers and Web sites are for national headquarters):
 a. Adult Children of Alcoholics (ACOA); for adults who, as children, lived with alcoholic parents. Telephone, 310-534-1815; Website, www.adultchildren.org/.
 b. Al-Anon; provides information on alcoholism and alcohol abuse and refers callers to local Al-Anon support groups established to help people affected by others' alcohol misuse. Telephone, 888-425-2666; Web site, www.al-anonorg/.
 c. Alateen; for adolescents affected by alcoholics. Web site, www.al-anon.org/alateen.html.
 d. Alcoholics Anonymous (AA); provides information and support to recovering alcoholics. Telephone, 212-870-3400; Website, www.alcoholics anonymous.org.
 e. Cocaine Anonymous (CA); for individuals with cocaine dependencies. Telephone, 310-559-5833; Web site, www.ca.org/.
 f. International Pharmacists Anonymous (IPA); for pharmacists in recovery (a national group that often holds support-group meetings at national and regional conferences). Contact IPA List Keeper, 319 East 5th Street, Ogallala, NE 69153-2201; telephone, 308-284-8296; Website, http://mywebpages.comcast.net/ipa/ipapage.htm.
 g. Nar-Anon; for helping people affected by another's drug misuse. Telephone, 310-547-5800.
 h. Narcotics Anonymous (NA); provides information and support to recovering substance abusers. Telephone, 818-773-9999; Web site, www.na.org.

19. Advocacy and professional substance abuse education:
 a. American Pharmacists Association (APhA) Pharmacy Recovery Program; for information sharing, education, and advocacy. Telephone, 800-237-2742. The American Dental Association, American Medical Association, and American Nurses Association have similar programs.
 b. The Pharmacy Section (cosponsored by APhA and APhA Academy of Students of Pharmacy) of the University of Utah School on Alcoholism and

Other Drug Dependencies (a one-week seminar each summer); for learning to deal with substance abuse problems as they affect the profession. Telephone, 801-538-4343; Web site, www.med. utah. edu/ads/.

This statement was reviewed in 2008 by the Council on Pharmacy Practice and by the Board of irectors and was found to still be appropriate.

Approved by the ASHP Board of Directors on April 15, 2003, and by the ASHP House of Delegates on June 1, 2003. Developed through the ASHP Council on Professional Affairs. Supersedes the ASHP Statement on the Pharmacist's Role in Substance Abuse Prevention, Education, and Assistance approved by the ASHP Board of Directors, April 22, 1998, and revised and approved by the ASHP House of Delegates and the ASHP Board of Directors, June 3, 1998.

The bibliographic citation for this document is as follows: American Society of Health-System Pharmacists. ASHP statement on the pharmacist's role in substance abuse prevention, education, and assistance. *Am J Health-Syst Pharm.* 2003; 60:1995–8.

ASHP Statement on the Pharmacist's Role in the Care of Patients with HIV Infection

Position

The American Society of Health System Pharmacists (ASHP) believes that pharmacists have a role in the care of patients infected with human immunodeficiency virus (HIV). Pharmacists have a responsibility to provide pharmaceutical care to these patients and, in states where it is authorized, can expand on that responsibility through collaborative drug therapy management.

Pharmaceutical care is the direct, responsible provision of medication-related care for the purpose of achieving definite outcomes that improve a patient's quality of life.[1] Pharmacists establish relationships with patients to ensure the appropriateness of medication therapy and patients' understanding of their therapy and to monitor the effects of that therapy. In collaborative drug therapy management, pharmacists enter into agreements with physicians who may authorize pharmacists to select appropriate medication therapies for patients who have a confirmed diagnosis and adjust them on the basis of patients' responses.[2]

Clinicians who provide these services are responsible for the quality of care, the satisfaction of patients, and the efficient use of resources, as well as their own ethical behavior.[3] High-quality, coordinated, and continuous medication management for patients should be measurable as a result of the provision of these services. The potential benefits to patients include access to medication information, the prevention and resolution of medication-related problems, improved outcomes, and increased satisfaction.[4] Pharmacists are able to use medication-related encounters with patients to provide information and either resolve problems or make a referral for health care needs.

The purposes of this statement are to promote an understanding of the various ways in which pharmacists can provide or contribute to the provision of care for patients infected with HIV in integrated health systems and to suggest future directions for pharmacists to expand patient care services.

Background

HIV infection, like many other chronic illnesses, affects nearly every organ system of the body. HIV is pathogenic in some instances, and superinfection by bacteria, other viruses, or fungi is common in the advanced stages of HIV infection. Unlike some other illnesses, HIV infection can be prevented by curbing high-risk behaviors,[5] so the illness still carries a social stigma among some who believe that they are not at risk. Among those at high risk for HIV infection are intravenous drug users and the severely mentally ill,[6] whose conditions may discourage testing for HIV infection or disclosure of HIV status and can also hinder treatment. Discrimination against HIV-infected individuals in housing and employment persists and may impede the delivery of health care by disrupting the stability of home and work life.

Our understanding of the basic pathophysiology and immunology of HIV infection continues to evolve on an almost-daily basis, and drug development occurs at a rapid pace. Since 1990, the Food and Drug Administration (FDA) has averaged one new antiretroviral agent approval per year; several years have seen the approval of two or three new antiretrovirals.[7] With these rapidly changing and complex therapeutic options, it is a challenge for many primary care providers to keep abreast of state-of-the-art strategies for managing HIV infection and provide comprehensive treatment for a relatively small population of patients. General practitioners know intuitively what has been shown in the literature: patients who are cared for by physician experts in HIV infection have better outcomes.[8-10] The advent of effective antiretroviral therapies has increased the need for clinicians with a broad knowledge of and experience managing HIV infection's concomitant diseases. In addition, important drug–drug interactions exist between antiretroviral agents and drugs used to treat opportunistic infections, between antiretroviral agents and drugs used to treat non-HIV-related comorbidities, and among the antiretroviral agents themselves. Failure to recognize these drug–drug interactions may result in additional or exacerbated adverse effects, nonadherence, therapeutic failure, or irreversible drug resistance. HIV-infected patients require extraordinary counseling and education regarding their treatment, from the importance of adherence to ways to recognize and cope with long-term consequences of therapy. The complexity of pharmacotherapy for patients with HIV infection presents special challenges and opportunities for pharmacists interested in developing a specialized knowledge base about HIV treatment.

There are a range of places within integrated health systems where pharmacists are likely to interact directly with patients infected with HIV: outpatient pharmacies, ambulatory care clinics, inpatient settings, dialysis units, hospices, and home infusion and home health care companies. Pharmacists are often considered the most accessible health professional; they are frequently at the frontline in helping HIV-infected patients deal with barriers to medication access, managing adverse effects and drug interactions, and adhering to medication regimens. Because many HIV-infected patients feel disconnected from the community, compassion on the part of the pharmacist can forge a strong bond with the patient and perhaps enhance patient adherence to antiretroviral treatment.

Patients' ability to adhere to antiretroviral regimens is essential to achieving the goals of drug therapy. Although the exact degree of adherence needed to ensure successful outcomes from drug therapy is not known, one study found that patients must take 95% of their doses to maintain drug levels that will achieve viral suppression, prevent drug resistance, and avert treatment failure.[11] Lack of adherence is often cited as the most common cause of the development of drug resistance and reduced effectiveness or therapeutic failure.[12] Mutations that lead to resistance to one drug may confer resistance to other drugs in the same therapeutic class, severely limiting future treatment options.[13,14]

Causes of nonadherence are multifactorial and differ greatly from patient to patient. In general, adherence has not been related to patient age, race, sex, education level, socioeconomic status, or history of substance abuse.[15] The principal factors associated with nonadherence to antiretroviral

therapies appear to be patient-related, and include mental illness (particularly untreated depression), unstable housing, active substance abuse, and major life crises.[16,17] Some patients stop or reduce the dosage of antiretroviral medication because of adverse effects.[17–19] Other factors that have been shown to negatively affect adherence include inconvenient frequency of drug administration, dietary restrictions, and pill burden.[17] A health care professional's assessment of a patient's ability to adhere to a medication regimen is a notoriously poor predictor of actual adherence.[20,21] In one study, the most important predictor of a patient's lack of success with an antiretroviral regimen was the patient's inability to keep appointments with the health care practitioner.[22]

Responsibilities

Pharmacists involved in the care of HIV-infected patients participate with other members of the health care team (e.g., physicians, physician assistants, nurse practitioners, nurses, dietitians, social workers, case managers, and pastoral care providers) in the management of patients for whom medications are a focus of therapy. The pharmacist's responsibility is to optimize the patient's medication therapy. Because of the rapid changes in HIV treatment, pharmacists involved in the care of HIV-infected patients should commit themselves to weekly if not daily education from journals or other sources. Pharmacy services should be designed to support the various components of the medication-use process (ordering, dispensing, administering, monitoring, and educating) as individual steps or as they relate to one another in the continuum of care. Pharmacists should evaluate all components of the medication-use process to optimize the potential for positive patient outcomes.[2] Particular care is needed in the prescribing and dispensing phases because the names of many antiretroviral agents sound and look similar, especially when they are handwritten, and some physicians continue to refer to antiretroviral agents by their chemical or investigational names. Verification of the appropriateness of the antiretroviral cocktail and its dosages is important because dosing recommendations change frequently as more becomes known about individual drug pharmacokinetics and because drug–drug interactions may be used clinically to simplify or increase the efficacy of drug regimens. Pharmacists should screen the medication profile for potential drug–drug and drug–food interactions. A number of antiretroviral drugs cannot be taken with certain foods, and it is the responsibility of the pharmacist to ensure that the patient and caregivers (dietitians, nurses, family members, and friends) are aware of these dietary restrictions.

Pharmacists are responsible for assessing patients' readiness to adhere to drug therapy, assisting in the design of therapeutic plans to increase the likelihood of adherence, assisting the patient in successful implementation of drug therapy, intervening when the patient states or intimates that he or she cannot or will not adhere to treatment, and providing ongoing monitoring of adherence. The public health implications of inconsistent adherence are much greater with antiretroviral agents than with other chronic medications. The pharmacist can promote patient adherence by considering the patient's history of adverse effects when recommending a regimen; helping to develop a daily medication administration schedule that accommodates the patient's sleep, work, and meal schedules; providing memory aids for medication

taking; recruiting an adherence coach; and educating and motivating patients and caregivers.[23] To ensure a consistent supply of antiretroviral medications, patients need to be counseled to plan for medication refills so they are never without these medications. Pharmacists, along with other health care professionals, are responsible for postmarketing surveillance of adverse drug events. Suspected adverse drug events should be reported to the patient's primary care provider and to FDA's MedWatch program. Many antiretroviral medications were marketed with scant data about their long-term effects because FDA's accelerated drug approval process allows certain drugs to be approved with only six months of clinical (Phase III) data. Pharmacists should also be aware of the potential for adverse events or drug interactions caused by dietary supplements and should report those as well.

Pharmacists' ability to recognize potential opportunistic infections or other HIV-associated complications and appropriately refer the patient for evaluation and management by a physician is critical. In addition, pharmacists have an obligation and an opportunity to educate members of the community about prevention of HIV infection and may be in a position to recognize persons undertaking high-risk behaviors. The pharmacist should recommend testing of persons at high risk for HIV infection and help educate patients infected with HIV about how to modify their behavior to prevent disease transmission.

The advent of effective antiretroviral therapies has made the treatment of hospitalized patients with acute HIV-related conditions more complex. Pharmacists still need to be prepared to recognize, prevent, and treat the acute opportunistic infections associated with advanced AIDS. The extended survival of those undergoing antiretroviral therapies introduces new comorbidities, such as diseases of the liver, malignancies, hyperlipidemia, and diabetes mellitus, which pharmacists must take into account as they provide pharmaceutical care.

Care for dying patients is also part of the continuum of pharmaceutical care that pharmacists should provide to patients. Pharmacists have a professional obligation to work in a collaborative and compassionate manner with patients, family members, caregivers, and other health care professionals to help fulfill the pharmaceutical care needs—especially nutrition support; the management of diarrhea, electrolyte imbalances, pain, and depression; and other quality-of-life needs—of dying patients.[24,25]

When more than one pharmacist is involved in delivering care, practice standards for the group should be adopted and should serve as a guide for all. Pharmacists should also establish methods of communication among themselves in order to provide and ensure continuity of pharmaceutical care on behalf of the patients served.[2] Methods for referral to other health care providers should also be defined.

Functions. In general, pharmacists perform the following functions in collaboration with physicians and other members of the health care team[2]:

1. Perform patient assessment for medication-related factors.
2. Order or recommend laboratory tests necessary for monitoring outcomes of medication therapy and potential drug toxicities, and cancel unnecessary laboratory tests.

3. Provide drug information to physicians and other members of the health care team.

4. Identify potential and actual drug–drug interactions and make recommendations for dosage modification or alternative therapies, if appropriate.

5. Interpret data related to medication safety and effectiveness.

6. Initiate or modify medication therapy or patient care plans on the basis of patient responses.

7. Provide information, education, and counseling to patients about medication-related care.

8. Document the care provided in patients' records.

9. Identify any barriers to patient adherence to medication regimens.

10. Communicate with prescribers known instances of nonadherence to medication therapy and propose strategies to the prescriber and patient to improve the likelihood of success of subsequent regimens.

11. Communicate relevant issues to physicians and other members of the health care team.

12. Participate in multidisciplinary reviews of patients' progress. Hospice caregivers and volunteer community service organizations should be included in this review as appropriate.

13. Communicate with payers to resolve issues that may impede access to medication therapies.

Expanded Functions. In addition to the aforementioned functions, pharmacists practicing in some settings and with some interdisciplinary relationships may engage in the following activities:

1. Monitoring efficacy of the regimen by tracking $CD4^+$ T lymphocyte counts and viral load and providing input about patients' response to therapy to other members of the health care team.

2. Providing individualized health promotion recommendations and disease prevention advice and activities, including administration of immunizations where authorized by law and institutional policies.

3. Assessing patient knowledge about HIV infection and its treatment and educating patients about the pathophysiology and natural history of HIV infection and progression to AIDS; the goals, mechanism of action, and duration of antiretroviral drug therapy; potential adverse effects from and interactions with antiretroviral drug therapy and ways to manage adverse effects; the concept of drug resistance and the importance of adherence to the therapeutic regimen; laboratory monitoring of therapeutic response to antiretroviral drug therapy; and therapeutic strategies for overcoming therapeutic failure.

4. Recognizing (using accepted guidelines) when patients are at risk for opportunistic infections, recommending initiation or discontinuation of prophylaxis, and intervening to ensure evaluation and management by a physician or other practitioner (e.g., physician assistant, nurse practitioner, or clinical pharmacist).

5. Performing limited physical assessment and supervising medication therapy with appropriate collaborative drug therapy management authority.

6. Assessing the indications for HIV drug-resistance testing, the appropriateness of timing for sample collection, interpreting test results, and designing a new antiretroviral regimen in consultation with an expert in drug resistance.

7. Referring patients to other health care or social service providers, such as psychologists, psychiatrists, social workers, case managers, and chemical dependency providers or support groups (e.g., Alcoholics Anonymous or Narcotics Anonymous) in conjunction with the patient's primary care provider.

8. Educating the community about modes of HIV transmission and effective techniques for prevention of transmission.

9. Encouraging public policy decisions that reduce the risk of transmission of HIV, hepatitis B, hepatitis C, and other sexually transmitted diseases.[26]

10. Performing research related to antiretroviral therapy (e.g., adherence, quality of life, pharmacokinetics).

Pharmacists' Scope of Practice. The pharmacist may have a range of practice privileges that varies in its extent of authority and responsibility. Pharmacists who participate in the collaborative care of patients with HIV should meet the health care organization's competency requirements to ensure that they provide appropriate quality and continuity of patient care. They should demonstrate required knowledge and skills that may be obtained through practice-intensive continuing education, pharmacy practice, and specialty residencies. The specific practice of pharmacists who participate in collaborative practice should be defined within a scope-of-practice document or similar tool or protocol developed by the health care organization. The scope-of-practice document should define activities that pharmacists would provide within the context of collaborative practice, as well as limitations when appropriate. The document should indicate referral and communication guidelines, including the documentation of patient encounters and methods for sharing patient information with collaborating medical providers.[2] Pharmacists participating in collaborative practice should remember that, although diagnosing is not within the pharmacist's scope of practice, the pharmacist must be able to recognize the manifestations of opportunistic infections and complications of HIV infection and treatment in order to know when to refer a patient to the appropriate practitioner. Also included in the scope-of-practice document should be references to activities that will review the quality of care provided and the methods by which the pharmacist will maintain continuing professional competency for functions encompassed by the scope-of-practice document. A process should be in place, and responsible parties identified, to review and update the scope-of-practice document as appropriate.

Description of Services Provided. The services offered by the pharmacist range from consulting with the health care team to providing direct support to the patient while working in collaboration with the health care team. The pharmacist provides medication therapy outcomes management as part of the patient's ongoing care. The level of intensity of services varies as the patient's needs change and the disease progresses. For patients who suspect HIV infection, the pharmacist should refer the patient for confidential or anonymous testing (anonymous testing is not available in every state in the United States). Pharmacists also have an important responsibility to ensure the availability of emergency antiretroviral therapy in postexposure prophylaxis and

provide counseling and education to the exposed person. For persons who are newly diagnosed with HIV infection, the pharmacist may facilitate access to medical care or refer a patient to a provider who specializes in the care of patients with HIV infection. The pharmacist may be called on to assess the patient's readiness and ability to adhere to antiretroviral therapy, provide initial or follow-up education on HIV-related disease and complications, as well as antiretroviral medications, and evaluate adherence to a therapeutic regimen. The pharmacist should maintain a current knowledge of antiretroviral therapy and may be called on to recommend and monitor the patients' antiretroviral therapy in collaboration with primary care providers or other members of the health care team. When collaborating with HIV specialists, the pharmacist is often asked to conduct follow-up visits with patients whose disease is stable or make an early follow-up telephone call or visit with patients just starting antiretroviral therapy. For patients with known HIV infection of longer duration, the pharmacist may be expected to ensure that the patient is monitored for long-term complications of antiretroviral therapy, such as diabetes mellitus or metabolic, cardiovascular, or hepatic complications. In the absence of a dietitian, the pharmacist may also monitor for changes in the patient's weight and appetite. The complexity of services provided varies according to the patient's needs and support from within the integrated health system, as well as the availability of other health care professionals on the team. In many situations, the pharmacist may play (or supplement) the role of financial counselor or social worker to facilitate access to medications. To deliver uninterrupted antiretroviral drug therapy, the pharmacist will often need to be knowledgeable about financial resources available to patients with HIV infection.

Documentation of Pharmacists' Care. The professional actions of pharmacists that are intended to ensure safe and effective use of drugs and that may affect patient outcomes should be documented in the patients' medical records.[27] Pharmacists in every practice setting should routinely document the quantity and quality of services provided and the estimated effect on patient outcomes.

Confidentiality of medical data is protected by common law and by constitutional rights to privacy. Confidentiality for the HIV-infected person is a critical issue because of the stigma that is sometimes still associated with the illness. Pharmacists should always take extreme care in discussing drug therapy to ensure that confidential medical information is not overheard by other individuals. Information about medications should be disclosed only to appropriate individuals and only with authorized consent from the patient, preferably in writing. Before counseling anyone other then the patient about medications, the pharmacist needs to ascertain that the person with whom he or she is speaking has been authorized by the patient. Pharmacists are urged to explore their local and state laws that may apply to the confidentiality of medical records.

Value of Pharmacists' Care. Methods for obtaining compensation or economic and professional credit for value-added services must continue to be addressed. Structures designed to measure the practitioner's effectiveness as part of an innovative team should be instituted. The pharmacy profession should embrace these activities in the form of well-structured research.[2] Integrated health systems, as well as other treatment settings, will need to receive adequate

support to expand the availability of pharmacists to provide pharmaceutical care as an essential component of the care of HIV-infected patients. Therefore, aggressive research must be pursued to demonstrate the importance and effectiveness with respect to outcomes of the pharmacist's role in educating the patient about his or her disease and medications.[2] Because many patients with HIV infection are eventually disabled and disenfranchised, few patients are able to pay out-of-pocket for drug therapy management services, as some patients do for diabetes education or smoking-cessation programs. Third-party payers who cover patients with HIV infection (e.g., private health insurance, state AIDS drug assistance programs, and Medicaid) must begin to cover the cost of patient education and adherence monitoring.

References

1. American Society of Hospital Pharmacists. ASHP statement on pharmaceutical care. *Am J Hosp Pharm.* 1993; 50:1720–3.
2. American Society of Health-System Pharmacists. ASHP statement on the pharmacist's role in primary care. *Am J Health-Syst Pharm.* 1999; 56:1665–7.
3. Donaldson MS, Yordy KD, Lohr KN, et al., eds. Primary care: America's health in a new era. Washington, DC: National Academy Press; 1996:33.
4. Galt KA, Skrabal MA, Abdouch I, et al. Using patient expectations and satisfaction data to design a new pharmacy service model in a primary care clinic. *J Manage Care Pharm.* 1997; 3:531–40.
5. Centers for Disease Control and Prevention. HIV/AIDS surveillance report, 2001; 13(2):14–5.
6. Rosenberg SD, Goodman LA, Osher FC, et al. Prevalence of HIV, hepatitis B, and hepatitis C in people with severe mental illness. *Am J Public Health.* 2001; 91:31–7.
7. Food and Drug Administration. Antiretroviral drugs approved by FDA for HIV. www.fda.gov/oashi/aids/virals.html (accessed 2003 Feb 24).
8. Zuger A, Sharp VL. HIV specialists: the time has come. *JAMA.* 1997; 278:1131–2.
9. Valenti WM. The HIV specialist improves quality of care and outcomes. *AIDS Read.* 2002; 12:202–5.
10. Gardner LI, Holmberg SD, Moore J, et al. Use of highly active antiretroviral therapy in HIV-infected women: impact of HIV specialist care. *J Acquir Immune Defic. Syndr* 2002; 29:69–75.
11. Paterson D, Swindells S, Mohr J, et al. Adherence to protease inhibitor therapy and outcomes in patients with HIV infection. *Ann Intern Med.* 2000; 133:21–30.
12. Deeks SG, Hecht FM, Swanson M, et al. HIV RNA and CD4 cell count response to protease inhibitor therapy in an urban AIDS clinic: response to both initial and salvage therapy. *AIDS.* 1999; 13:F35–43.
13. Report of the NIH Panel to Define Principles of Therapy of HIV Infection. *Ann Intern Med.* 1998; 128(12, pt. 2):1057–78.
14. Dybul M, Fauci AS, Bartlett JG, et al. Guidelines for using antiretroviral agents among HIV-infected adults and adolescents: *Ann Intern Med.* 2002; 137(5, pt. 2):381–433.
15. Sacett DL, Snow JS. The magnitude of compliance and non-compliance. In: Haynes RB, Tayloe DW, Sackett DL, eds. Compliance in health care. Baltimore, MD: Johns Hopkins University Press; 1979:31.

16. Besch CL. Compliance in clinical trials. *AIDS*. 1995; 9:1–10.

17. Chesney MA. Factors affecting adherence to antiretroviral therapy. *Clin Infect Dis.* 2000; 30(suppl 2):S171–6.

18. Ammassari A, Murri R, Pezzotti P, et al. Self-reported symptoms and medication side effects influence adherence to highly active antiretroviral therapy in persons with HIV infection. *J Acquir Immune Defic Syndr.* 2001; 28:445–9.

19. Heath KV, Singer J, O'Shaughnessy MV, et al. Intentional nonadherence due to adverse symptoms associated with antiretroviral therapy. *J Acquir Immune Defic Syndr.* 2002; 31:211–7.

20. Crespo-Fierro M. Compliance/adherence and care management in HIV disease. *J Assoc Nurses AIDS Care.* 1997; 8:43–54.

21. Bangsberg DR, Hecht FM, Clague H, et al. Provider assessment of adherence to HIV antiretroviral therapy. *J Acquir Immune Defic Syndr.* 2001; 26:435–42.

22. Lucas GM, Chaisson RE, Moore RD. Highly active antiretroviral therapy in a large urban clinic: risk factors for virologic failure and adverse drug reactions. *Ann Intern Med.* 1999; 131:81–7.

23. Bartlett JA. Addressing the challenges of adherence. *J Acquir Immune Defic Syndr.* 2002; 29:S2–10.

24. American Society of Health-System Pharmacists. Medication therapy and patient care: specific practice areas: position 9816 (appropriate pharmacy support for dying patients). In: Deffenbaugh JH, ed. Best practices for health-system pharmacy: positions and guidance documents of ASHP. 2002–2003 ed. Bethesda, MD: 2002; 200.

25. Joint Commission on Accreditation of Healthcare Organizations. Pain assessment and management standards—hospitals. www.jcrinc.com (Accessed 2003 Jul 22).

26. American Society of Health-System Pharmacists. ASHP statement on the pharmacist's role in infection control. *Am J Health-Syst Pharm.* 1998; 55:1724–6.

27. American Society of Health-System Pharmacists. ASHP guidelines on documenting pharmaceutical care in patient medical records. *Am J Health-Syst Pharm.* 2003; 60:705–7.

Other Resources

Web Site Resources

General HIV Care and Treatment Information
- Healthcare Communication Group-Clinical Care Options for HIV (www.healthcg.com/hiv)
- U.S. Department of Health and Human Services AIDSinfo Web site (www.aidsinfo.nih.gov)
- Medscape-AIDS(www.hiv.medscape.com/home/topics/aids)
- HIV Insite Home (www.hivinsite.ucsf.edu)
- HIV Insite International AIDS Society (www.hivinsite.ucsf.edu/medical/iasusa)

Clinical Practice Guidelines and Recommendations
- *Morbidity and Mortality Weekly Report* (www.cdc.gov/epo/mmwr)
- U.S. Department of Health and Human Services AIDSinfo Web site (www.aidsinfo.nih.gov)

Drug Interactions
- Clinical Management of HIV–AIDS Drug Interactions (www.healthcg.com/hiv/treatment/interactions)
- Georgetown University Medical Center Division of Clinical Pharmacology (www.dml.georgetown.edu/depts/pharmacology)
- University of California at San Francisco (http://arvdb.ucsf.edu)

Clinical Trials
- U.S. Department of Health and Human Services AIDSinfo Web site (www.aidsinfo.nih.gov)

Hotlines

- University of California at San Francisco Warmline (800) 933-3413

HIV Certificate Programs

- SouthEast AIDS Training and Education Center, Atlanta GA
- Charlotte AHEC, Charlotte NC (800) 874-2417

This statement was reviewed in 2008 by the Council on Pharmacy Practice and by the Board of Directors and was found to still be appropriate.

Developed through the ASHP Council on Professional Affairs. Approved by the ASHP Board of Directors on April 15, 2003, and by the ASHP House of Delegates on June 1, 2003.

The bibliographic citation for this document is as follows: American Society of Health-System Pharmacists. ASHP statement on the pharmacist's role in the care of patients with HIV infection *Am J Health-Syst Pharm.* 2003; 60:1998–2003.

ASHP Statement on Pharmacy Services to the Emergency Department

Position

The American Society of Health-System Pharmacists (ASHP) believes every hospital pharmacy department should provide its emergency department (ED) with the pharmacy services that are necessary for safe and effective patient care. Although the nature of these services will vary with each institution's needs and resources, the pharmacist's role may include

- Working with emergency physicians, emergency nurses, and other health care professionals to develop and monitor medication-use systems that promote safe and effective medication use in the ED, especially for high-risk patients and procedures,
- Collaborating with emergency physicians, emergency nurses, and other health care professionals to promote medication use in the ED that is evidence based and aligned with national quality indicators,
- Participating in the selection, implementation, and monitoring of technology used in the medication-use process,
- Providing direct patient care as part of the interdisciplinary emergency care team,
- Participating in or leading emergency-preparedness efforts and quality-improvement initiatives,
- Educating patients, caregivers, and health care professionals about safe and effective medication use, and
- Conducting or participating in ED-based research.

ASHP supports the expansion of pharmacy education and postgraduate residency training to include an emphasis on emergency care.

The purposes of this statement are to promote understanding of the pharmacist's contributions to the care of patients in the ED and to suggest future roles for pharmacists in providing that care.

Background

EDs across the nation treat approximately 114 million patients annually.[1] EDs are overcrowded because of a high percentage of uninsured patients, increased patient volume, increased complexity of patients in the ED, and a hospital bed shortage that frequently results in the boarding of inpatients in the ED. The combination of interruptions, intense pressure, and a fast-paced environment can lead to medication errors and fewer error interceptions.[1] The Institute of Medicine (IOM) has estimated that as many as 98,000 people die each year as a result of medical errors and that adverse drug events (ADEs) occurred in 3.7% of hospitalizations.[2] Hafner et al.[3] reported a similar frequency of ADEs in the ED. Chin et al.[4] found that 3.6% of patients received an inappropriate medication in the ED and 5.6% were prescribed an inappropriate medication at discharge.

Pharmacy services in the ED have been documented since the 1970s.[5-8] These services initially focused on inventory control, cost containment, and participation on resuscitation teams but have since expanded to include clinical pharmacy services.[9] The effectiveness of clinical pharmacy services has been well documented in other settings. The participation of pharmacists in intensive care units and on internal medicine teams has improved patient outcomes by reducing preventable ADEs by 66% and 78%, respectively.[10-12] Similar effectiveness with pharmacist participation on emergency medicine teams has also been documented.[13] Despite this evidence, the 2005 ASHP national survey found that only 3.5% of the hospitals surveyed had a pharmacist assigned to the ED for any period of time, and only 5% had a formal policy requiring that pharmacists review and approve medication orders before administration in EDs.[14]

Pharmacy Services in the ED

All health care professionals share a commitment to and responsibility for providing safe and effective patient care. These shared objectives provide strong incentives for collaboration. Pharmacists and other health care professionals can collaborate in developing and monitoring medication-use systems that promote safe and effective medication use in the ED, including medication use in high-risk ED patients and procedures. By working together, pharmacists and other health care professionals can ensure that medication use in the ED is evidence based, cost-effective, and adherent to national guidelines; develop and implement emergency-preparedness plans and quality-improvement efforts; and, in many cases, foster the institution's education and research initiatives. The department of pharmacy should assume a leadership role in ensuring these collaborations.

When making decisions regarding pharmacy services to the ED, hospital leadership should consider the ED's need for medication therapy management services, medication-allergy assessment and clarification, medication-interaction assessment, reporting of and intervention on medication errors and ADEs, timely provision of drug information, and participation in formulary decision making. Institutions should also keep in mind the Joint Commission's pharmacist first-review requirement[15] and national patient safety goals,[16] the hospital's quality indicators related to medication selection, timing, and delivery; the potential effects of patient flow and technology on medication safety in the ED; and contributions pharmacists can make to continuity of care from ED admission through hospital discharge.

Patient Care. The IOM report, Hospital-Based Emergency Care: At the Breaking Point, recommends the inclusion of clinical pharmacists on the ED care team to ensure patients' medication needs are appropriately met, to lead system changes in order to reduce or eliminate medication errors, and to evaluate the cost effectiveness of medication therapy for the patient and hospital.[1] As part of the interdisciplinary ED care team, pharmacists can provide care to critically ill patients by

- Participating in resuscitation efforts,
- Providing consultative services that foster appropriate evidence-based medication selection,
- Providing consultation on patient-specific medication dosage and dosage adjustments,
- Providing drug information consultation to emergency physicians, emergency nurses, and other clinicians,
- Monitoring for patient allergies and drug interactions,
- Monitoring patient therapeutic responses (including laboratory values),
- Continuously assessing for and managing adverse drug reactions, and
- Gathering or reviewing medication histories and reconciling patients' medications.

In addition, pharmacists can provide care to ambulatory patients in the ED by

- Modifying medication regimens based on collaborative-practice agreements for the management of specific patient populations that return to the ED,
- Providing vaccination screening, referral, and administration,
- Offering patient and caregiver education, including discharge counseling and follow-up, and
- Providing information on obtaining medications through patient assistance programs, care funds, and samples.

The boarding of patients in the ED until an inpatient bed becomes available poses challenges for patients, caregivers, and health care professionals. The department of pharmacy should work with the health care professionals involved in the care of these patients to provide a seamless medication-use process.

Emergency-Preparedness Planning. ASHP believes that all hospital and health-system pharmacists must assertively exercise their responsibilities to prepare for and respond to disasters.[17] ASHP has insisted that emergency-response planners at the federal, regional, state, and local levels call on pharmacists to participate in the full range of planning issues related to pharmaceuticals. Hospital emergency-preparedness plans, including ED components, must be developed with the assistance of departments of pharmacy. Pharmacists should play a pivotal role in emergency-preparedness planning and as members of the health care team that provides care to victims. Ensuring the efficacy and safety of the medication-use process is a natural role for pharmacists because treatment of disaster victims almost always involves the use of pharmacologic agents.[18,19]

Quality-Improvement Initiatives. The department of pharmacy can collaborate with other health care professionals on a variety of quality-improvement initiatives in the ED, including

- Guiding the development of evidence-based treatment protocols, algorithms, and clinical pathways that are congruent with nationally accepted practice guidelines and quality indicators,

- Assisting in the development, implementation, and assessment of various technologies used throughout the ED's medication-use process,
- Conducting failure mode and effects analysis and root-cause analysis on error-prone aspects of the medication-use process,
- Participating in ED-based and hospitalwide committees (e.g., pharmacy and therapeutics, infection control, disaster) whose decisions affect medication use in the ED,
- Maintaining compliance with standards of national accrediting bodies, such as the Joint Commission, and
- Assisting in surveillance and reporting of adverse drug reactions.

Education. The pharmacy department should support the pharmacist's role in providing education and information to health care professionals, patients, and the public in ED service areas. Specific activities could include

- Conducting educational forums for health care professionals and students on topics such as emergency preparedness, disaster management, poisoning prevention and treatment, immunizations, and use of medications in the ED and emergency situations,
- Providing health literacy-sensitive education to patients and caregivers regarding medication use, disease-state management, and prevention strategies, and
- Offering ED-based educational opportunities to pharmacy students and residents.

The ED offers an enormous number of services, activities, and opportunities to train future pharmacists in all aspects of the medication-use process. Students and residents could participate in longitudinal experiences in ED-based services such as clinics, community services (e.g., health fairs), and satellite pharmacies and could study topics as varied as cultural follow-up, ADE monitoring and reporting, or toxicology services. Introductory experiences could focus on student training on specific skills or competencies, such as taking medication histories, medication reconciliation, or discharge counseling. Residency training of pharmacists in emergency care would provide more rewarding educational experiences, foster pharmacist involvement in emergency-medicine research, and ultimately improve the quality of patient care. Such residencies should meet ASHP-accredited residency quality standards.[20] Achievement of the goals, objectives, and expected outcomes of such training would be supported by around-the-clock or on-call clinical pharmacist services in the ED.

ED-Based Research. Research on and publications about ED pharmacy, though plentiful, usually focus on specific clinical settings, such as toxicology, drug interactions, and infectious disease epidemiology. The literature lacks a broad representation of the varied scope and range of ED pharmacy practices. ASHP believes that there should be more research and publications regarding medication use in the ED and ED-based pharmacy activities. Studies that generate data on therapeutic, safety, humanistic, and economic outcomes of pharmacist-mediated process changes are urgently needed.

Professional Development of Pharmacists in Emergency Care

ASHP believes there should be an increase in the number of ED-based training opportunities for pharmacists, pharmacy students, and residents. Schools and colleges of pharmacy are encouraged to provide ED-based educational opportunities for students. Hospitals and health systems are encouraged to support ED-based educational programs that produce experts in the field. Postgraduate training of pharmacists will provide a pipeline of clinicians, educators, leaders, and scientists who are experts in and committed to quality emergency care.

Conclusion

Every pharmacy department should provide the ED with the pharmacy services required to ensure safe and effective patient care. These services must be tailored to match each institution's needs and resources; therefore, pharmacy departments must decide the best way to safely provide medications to ED patients. ASHP supports the expansion of pharmacy education and postgraduate residency training to include emphasis on emergency care in order to develop an adequate supply of pharmacists who are trained to deliver these essential pharmacy services.

References

1. Institute of Medicine of the National Academies. Hospital-based emergency care: at the breaking point. www.iom.edu/CMS/3809/16107/35007.aspx (accessed 2006 Sep 5).
2. Kohn LT, Corrigan JM, Donaldson MS, eds. To err is human: building a safer health system. Washington, DC: National Academy Press; 1999:26.
3. Hafner JW Jr, Belknap SM, Squillante MD et al. Adverse drug events in emergency department patients. *Ann Emerg Med.* 2002; 39:258–67.
4. Chin MH, Wang LC, Jin L et al. Appropriateness of medication selection for older persons in an urban academic emergency department. *Acad Emerg Med.* 1999; 6:1232–42.
5. Elenbaas RM, Waeckerle JF, McNabney WK. The clinical pharmacist in emergency medicine. *Am J Hosp Pharm.* 1977; 34:843–6.
6. Schwerman E, Schwartau N, Thompson CO et al. The pharmacist as a member of the cardiopulmonary resuscitation team. *Drug Intell Clin Pharm.* 1973; 7:299–308.
7. Kasuya A, Bauman JL, Curtis RA et al. Clinical pharmacy on-call program in the emergency department. *Am J Emerg Med.* 1986; 4:464–7.
8. Powell MF, Solomon DK, McEachen RA. Twenty-four hour emergency pharmaceutical services. *Am J Hosp Pharm.* 1985; 42:831–5.
9. Fairbanks RJ, Hays DP, Webster DF et al. Clinical pharmacy services in an emergency department. *Am J Health-Syst Pharm.* 2004; 61:934–7.
10. Leape LL, Cullen DJ, Clapp MD et al. Pharmacist participation on physician rounds and adverse drug events in the intensive care unit. *JAMA.* 1999; 282:267–70. [Erratum, JAMA. 2000; 283:1293.]
11. Kane SL, Weber RJ, Dasta JF. The impact of critical care pharmacists on enhancing patient outcomes. *Intensive Care Med.* 2003; 29:691–8.
12. Kucukarslan SN, Peters M, Mlynarek M et al. Pharmacists on rounding teams reduce preventable adverse drug events in hospital general medicine units. *Arch Intern Med.* 2003; 163:2014–8.
13. Ling JM, Mike LA, Rubin J et al. Documentation of pharmacist interventions in the emergency department. *Am J Health-Syst Pharm.* 2005; 62:1793–7.
14. Pedersen CA, Schneider PJ, Scheckelhoff DJ. ASHP national survey of pharmacy practice in hospital settings: dispensing and administration—2005. *Am J Health-Syst Pharm.* 2006; 63:327–45.
15. Medication Management Standard MM.4.10—preparing and dispensing. In: Comprehensive accreditation manual for hospitals. Oakbrook Terrace, IL: Joint Commission on the Accreditation of Healthcare Organizations: 2006:MM-10.
16. Joint Commission. National patient safety goals. www.jointcommission.org/PatientSafety/National PatientSafetyGoals (accessed 2007 May 25).
17. American Society of Health-System Pharmacists. ASHP statement on the role of health-system pharmacists in emergency preparedness. *Am J Health-Syst Pharm.* 2003; 60:1993–5.
18. Burda AM, Sigg T. Pharmacy preparedness for incidents involving weapons of mass destruction. *Am J Health-Syst Pharm.* 2001; 58:2274–84.
19. Setlak P. Bioterrorism preparedness and response: emerging role for health-system pharmacists. *Am J Health-Syst Pharm.* 2004; 61:1167–75.
20. American Society of Health-System Pharmacists. ASHP residency accreditation regulations and standards. www.ashp.org/Import/ACCREDITATION/Residency Accreditation/RegulationsStandards.aspx (accessed 2008 Sep 24).

Developed through the ASHP Council on Pharmacy Practice and approved by the ASHP Board of Directors on September 28, 2007, and by the ASHP House of Delegates on June 10, 2008.

Roshanak Aazami, Pharm.D.; Elizabeth A. Clements, Pharm.D.; Daniel J. Cobaugh, Pharm.D., FACCT, DABAT; and Frank P. Paloucek, Pharm.D., are gratefully acknowledged for drafting this statement. The ASHP Section of Clinical Specialists and Scientists Section Advisory Group on Emergency Care is also gratefully acknowledged for reviewing drafts and providing advice on the development of this statement.

The drafters have declared no conflict of interest.

The bibliographic citation for this document is as follows: American Society of Health-System Pharmacists. ASHP statement on pharmacy services to the emergency department. *Am J Health-Syst Pharm.* 2008; 65:2380–3.

ASHP Statement on Racial and Ethnic Disparities in Health Care

Position

Health disparities continue to be a major public health problem confronting the U.S. health care system. These disparities arise from a complex set of factors, including social and economic inequality, cultural and linguistic barriers, and persistent racial and ethnic discrimination. Evidence continues to emerge, however, that some health disparities are attributable to differences in the quality of health care provided to different racial and ethnic groups. The American Society of Health-System Pharmacists (ASHP) believes that all patients, regardless of race, ethnicity, sex, age, sexual orientation, religion, physical or mental disability (or impairment), education, socioeconomic status, diagnosis, or limitations in access, have the right to high-quality health care that reflects knowledge of, sensitivity to, and respect for their differences.

Pharmacists who practice in hospitals and health systems ("health-system pharmacists"), working individually and in coordination with interested organizations and other health care professionals, can play a leading role in building culturally competent systems of care to reduce racial and ethnic disparities in health care by

- Increasing awareness of these disparities among health care providers, health-system administrators, legislators, regulators, third-party payers, and the public,
- Promoting a more diverse and culturally competent health care work force and environment,
- Ensuring effective communication with patients and among providers,
- Fostering consistent use of multidisciplinary teams and evidence-based guidelines for patient care,
- Collecting and reporting data on health care access, utilization, and outcomes by racial and ethnic minorities and measuring progress toward reducing health care disparities, and
- Researching, identifying, and disseminating best practices for providing culturally competent care and reducing disparities in health care.

Background

The Institute of Medicine (IOM) defines racial and ethnic disparities in health care as "racial or ethnic differences in the quality of healthcare that are not due to access-related factors or clinical needs, preferences, and appropriateness of intervention."[1] IOM states that "evidence of racial and ethnic disparities in healthcare is . . . remarkably consistent across a range of illnesses and healthcare services." More than 600 articles documenting racial or ethnic variations in health care have been published in the past three decades.[2] With the majority of U.S. population growth between now and 2050 expected to come from racial and ethnic minority Americans and immigrants, our health care system must soon learn how to address the effects that race and ethnicity can have on health care. Eliminating health disparities is so important that it is one of only two overarching goals for the Healthy People 2010 objectives.[3]

Culture has been defined by IOM as "the accumulated store of shared values, ideas (attitudes, beliefs, values, and norms), understandings, symbols, material products, and practices of a group of people."[1] Ethnicity refers to "a shared culture and way of life, especially as reflected in language, folkways, religious and other institutional forms, material culture such as clothing and food, and cultural products such as music, literature, and art."[1] An ethnic group is a collection of people "socially distinguished or set apart, by others or by itself, primarily on the basis of cultural or national-origin characteristics."[1] Like ethnicity, race has been described as a sociocultural concept used to distinguish groups of people (in this case, those who share certain physical characteristics) and treat them differently.

ASHP recognizes the need to address all forms of health disparities and believes that health-system pharmacists can take an important step in addressing these broader disparities by assuming a leadership role in the national campaign to eliminate racial and ethnic disparities in health care. Health-system pharmacists, like other health professionals, have espoused a tradition of nondiscriminatory health care practice.[4,5] Because medication therapy management is central to many of the health disparities cited by IOM (e.g., treatment for pain, HIV infection, diabetes, end-stage renal disease, kidney transplantation),[1] health-system pharmacists have opportunities to directly address these disparities. As health-system administrators and members of multidisciplinary health care teams, health-system pharmacists have an important role to play in implementing the institutional changes necessary to eliminate racial and ethnic disparities in health care. ASHP believes that health-system pharmacists have a professional and moral responsibility to address racial and ethnic disparities in health care.

General Principles

The following three principles should guide the actions of health-system pharmacists in efforts to eliminate racial and ethnic disparities in health care: (1) all patients have the right to high-quality care, (2) medication-use practices should reflect knowledge of, sensitivity to, and respect for the race and culture of the patient, and (3) health-system pharmacists have a vital role to play in eliminating racial and ethnic disparities in health care.

All Patients Have the Right to High-Quality Care. A long-standing policy position of ASHP holds that "all patients have the right to . . . high-quality pharmaceutical care."[4] ASHP believes that all patients have the right to receive care from pharmacists and that health-system pharmacists should play a leadership role in ensuring patient access to pharmacists' services.[6] The Code of Ethics for Pharmacists issued by the American Pharmacists Association states that the pharmacist "places concern for the well-being of the patient at the center of professional practice" and "seeks justice in

the distribution of health resources."[5] Racial and ethnic disparities in health care are antithetical to the core principles of pharmacy and must be eliminated.

Medication-Use Practices Should Reflect Knowledge of, Sensitivity to, and Respect for the Race and Culture of the Patient. Culture strongly influences how a person interacts with the world. Failing to account for the patient's race or cultural beliefs and values in health care decisions can lead to negative health consequences. Providers may miss screening opportunities because they are unfamiliar with the prevalence of conditions among racial or ethnic groups. They may fail to consider different responses to medications that exist in different populations. Potential harmful interactions between medications and traditional remedies used by the patient may be overlooked. Finally, miscommunication due to cultural, linguistic, or literacy differences between providers and patients regarding symptoms, medications, supplements, or the use of devices may lead to faulty diagnoses, unnecessary laboratory testing, medication-related errors, decreased adherence to therapy, or missed opportunities for early detection and preventive measures.[7]

The Code of Ethics for Pharmacists states that "in all cases" the pharmacist "respects personal and cultural differences among patients."[5] Clinicians who want to provide the best care for their patients must understand the role of culture and its potential impact on health outcomes and the provider–patient relationship.

Health-System Pharmacists Have a Vital Role to Play in Eliminating Racial and Ethnic Disparities in Health Care. In their roles as medication-use experts, patient care providers, and health-system administrators, health-system pharmacists have the knowledge, skills, and opportunities to contribute to efforts to eliminate racial and ethnic disparities in health care.

Pharmacists' Roles in Eliminating Disparities

IOM has made recommendations to eliminate racial and ethnic disparities in health care.[1] The IOM recommendations most relevant to health-system pharmacists are listed in the appendix. ASHP would add to that list that pharmacists can and should engage in research on disparities in health care. ASHP encourages all health care professionals and administrators to embrace these recommendations and urges health-system pharmacists to take the following actions to help eliminate health care disparities.

Increase Awareness of Disparities. One elemental barrier to eliminating racial and ethnic disparities in health care may be a lack of awareness of their existence and their impact on society. Polls show that a significant majority of Americans believe that African Americans receive the same quality of health care as whites,[1,8] despite ample evidence to the contrary.[1] Efforts to eliminate racial and ethnic disparities in health care must begin with the acknowledgment that there is a problem. Health-system pharmacists should lead efforts to increase awareness of health disparities among health care providers, health-system administrators, legislators, regulators, third-party payers, and the public. Pharmacists

can increase awareness of health disparities by encouraging their health care organizations to make the elimination of disparities in health care a key component of the organization's mission. They can help their institutions foster an environment that promotes input from and involvement by all members of the organization in addressing this component of the organizational mission. In addition, pharmacists can help develop inhouse and community programs to promote cultural understanding and appreciation of the importance of diversity. They can also partner with community groups, governmental agencies, health care provider organizations, payers, and others to increase awareness of specific diseases among certain populations and encourage innovation and creativity in evaluating and disseminating approaches to eliminating disparities in health care.

Create a More Diverse Health Care Work Force. Increased racial and ethnic diversity among health care professionals may be associated with improved access to care for racial and ethnic minority patients, greater patient choice of and satisfaction with health care professionals, more effective patient–clinician communication, and enhanced educational experiences for students in the health professions.[9] Racial and ethnic diversity in the health care work force has been well correlated with the delivery of quality care to diverse patient populations. For minority patients, racial concordance between patient and physician is associated with greater patient satisfaction and higher self-rated quality of care.[10] Spanish-speaking patients, for example, report more satisfaction with care from Spanish-speaking providers.[11]

In 2002, the American Hospital Association's Commission on Workforce for Hospitals and Health Systems reported that although the national labor force is becoming more diverse, hospital employees remain disproportionately female and Caucasian.[12] The Commission recommended working aggressively to develop a work force that more fully represents changing U.S. demographics. IOM has also cited a continuing shortage of minorities among health care professionals.[9]

ASHP is committed to developing a diverse work force of health-system pharmacists.[13] In June 2003, the ASHP Board of Directors established the Ad Hoc Committee on Ethnic Diversity and Cultural Competence, which has recommended six major goals and developed long-term strategic action plans for each goal.[14] ASHP members are encouraged to participate in these efforts and to monitor their progress at ASHP's Health Disparities Web Resource Center (www.ashp.org/s_ashp/cat1c.asp?CID=4266&DID=7523).

Promote Culturally Competent Care and Services. Many cultures take a different approach to health than is found in allopathic ("western") medicine. Perceptions of illness and disease vary by culture, and culture may influence a person's health-seeking behavior, approach to seeking out health care providers, and treatment preferences. As allopathic medicine increasingly emphasizes evidence-based approaches, health care practitioners will more frequently confront the cultural divide between the demands of their profession and the closely held beliefs of their patients. Cultural competency is rapidly becoming a quality and risk management issue for hospitals and health systems. ASHP is committed

to developing a culturally sensitive, competent, and respectful work force.[15]

The Department of Health and Human Services (HHS) states that a culturally competent health care practitioner is

- Knowledgeable about cultural differences and their impact on attitudes and behaviors,
- Sensitive, understanding, nonjudgmental, and respectful in dealings with peoples whose culture is different from one's own, and
- Flexible and skillful in responding and adapting to different cultural contexts and circumstances.[16]

HHS's Office of Minority Health has developed a set of standards for culturally and linguistically appropriate services in health care to provide a consistent and comprehensive approach to cultural and linguistic competence in health care.[17] These standards offer a framework for implementing services and organizational structures to help health care organizations and providers, including pharmacists, respond to the cultural and linguistic issues presented by diverse populations. ASHP believes these standards should be used to assess staff competence and to guide organizations' educational programming and strategic planning. Education on cultural competency issues is encouraged in preceptor training sessions, residency standards, and leadership orientation at ASHP and affiliate levels. The Accreditation Council for Pharmaceutical Education now requires that schools and colleges of pharmacy include cultural competency in their curricula.[18] Approaches to the subject could include standalone courses in health disparities and cultural competence, inclusion of traditional healers in the educational process, and infusion of the concept of cultural competence throughout the curriculum (e.g., through case studies that include diverse populations). ASHP believes that experiential learning should also include practice experiences with racial and ethnic minorities, medically underserved populations, and patient populations whose cultures incorporate the use of traditional healers and complementary or alternative medicine (e.g., folk medicine, home remedies).

The Code of Ethics for Pharmacists states that "A pharmacist maintains professional competence."[5] ASHP believes that cultural competence is among the competencies that pharmacists, residents, fellows, students, and technicians have an obligation to develop and maintain.

Ensure Effective Communication with Patients and Among Providers. The Code of Ethics for Pharmacists states that "a pharmacist communicates with patients in terms that are understandable."[5] ASHP guidelines recommend that pharmacists "know about their patients' cultures, especially health and illness beliefs, attitudes, and practices," and "adapt messages to fit patients' language skills and primary languages, through the use of teaching aids, interpreters, or cultural guides if necessary."[19] Persons with the most health problems and the greatest need for self-management skills often have the poorest health literacy. Health-system pharmacists providing direct patient care should be able to assess the health literacy of patients and provide appropriate education.[20]

Lack of interpretation services or culturally and linguistically appropriate health education materials is associated with patient dissatisfaction, poor comprehension and compliance, and ineffective or lower quality of patient care.[21–23] Health care providers rely heavily on the use of the written word to communicate, a circumstance that contributes to health care disparities.[1] When interpretation services are used, practitioners should ensure their quality. Fluency in language is not necessarily sufficient to provide adequate interpretation of the complex concepts involved in medical decision-making. Interpretation by family members also raises issues of patient confidentiality and autonomy.

Communication with patients needs to be culturally and linguistically appropriate. For example, although Spanish is the primary language of many cultures, simply translating educational material into Spanish may not provide the cultural context to make the education effective.

Health-system pharmacists should also utilize their medication-use expertise to help their institutions and communities develop culturally and linguistically appropriate public education campaigns. These campaigns could address health risks prevalent in racial and ethnic minority populations served by the hospital and explain preventive measures and health care services available to those populations.

Health care professionals also need to recognize that racial and cultural differences may affect communication among providers. Health-system pharmacists should take steps to ensure that provider-to-provider communication is effective and reflects the respect for colleagues expressed in the Code of Ethics for Pharmacists.[5]

Utilize Multidisciplinary Teams and Evidence-Based Guidelines. Multidisciplinary team approaches to health care improve health outcomes for majority and minority patients being treated for a range of diseases.[1] ASHP believes pharmacists should be integral participants in the development of multidisciplinary action plans for patient care, disease management plans, and health management plans.[24] Evidence-based guidelines "offer the advantages of consistency, predictability, and objectivity,"[1] but their use must be balanced with the need for clinical flexibility, especially when there is evidence of different outcomes or responses among racial or ethnic groups.

Collect and Monitor Data on Health Disparities. Standardized collection of data regarding access to medications, drug utilization, and medical and cost-effectiveness outcomes from medication therapy management by racial and ethnic minorities would promote research on disparities in health care and help institutions monitor the progress of their efforts to eliminate those disparities.[25] Pharmacists should be active partners with health care administrators and other health professionals in developing measures of progress against health care disparities in institutional performance measures, which should be a key component of the organization's mission.[26]

Research Disparities in Health Care. Health-system pharmacists can research, identify, and disseminate best practices for providing culturally competent care and reducing disparities in health care. Priority areas for research include racial and ethnic groups' access to medications, drug utilization, and medical and cost-effectiveness outcomes from medication therapy management. Pharmacists must keep pace with research regarding disparities in health care, programs to provide culturally competent care to patients, and new educational approaches to improving patient care. It is also important that pharmacy develop researchers to investi-

gate health care disparities and cutting-edge practitioners to translate those research findings into practice.

Conclusion

ASHP believes racial and ethnic disparities in health care are antithetical to the core principles of pharmacy. All patients have the right to high-quality health care that reflects knowledge of, sensitivity to, and respect for their differences. Health-system pharmacists, working individually and in coordination with interested organizations and other health care professionals, can and must play a vital role in efforts to eliminate racial and ethnic disparities in health care.

References

1. Smedley BD, Stith AY, Nelson AR, eds. Unequal treatment: confronting racial and ethnic disparities in health care. Washington, DC: National Academy Press; 2003.
2. Rubenstein LS. Racial disparities and health: Physicians for Human Rights testimony to Congressional Black Caucus. March 18, 2003. www.phrusa.org/research/methics/caucus_0303.html (accessed 2006 Dec 1).
3. U.S. Department of Health and Human Services. Healthy People 2010. www.healthypeople.gov/default.htm (accessed 2005 Nov 4).
4. ASHP policy position 9006: nondiscriminatory pharmaceutical care. In: Hawkins B, ed. Best practices for hospital and health-system pharmacy: positions and guidance documents of ASHP. Bethesda, MD: American Society of Health-System Pharmacists; 2006:82.
5. American Pharmacists Association. Code of Ethics for Pharmacists. www.pharmacist.com/AM/PrinterTemplate.cfm?Section=Search1&template=/CM/HTMLDisplay.cfm&ContentID=2903 (accessed 2008 Jan 7).
6. ASHP policy position 0101: pharmacy benefits for the uninsured. In: Hawkins B, ed. Best practices for hospital and health-system pharmacy: positions and guidance documents of ASHP. Bethesda, MD: American Society of Health-System Pharmacists; 2006:161.
7. Brach C, Fraser I. Can cultural competency reduce racial and ethnic health care disparities? A review and conceptual model. Med Care Res Rev. 2000; 57(suppl 1):181–217.
8. Harvard Forums on Health. Americans speak out on disparities in health care. www.phsi.harvard.edu/health_reform/poll_media_report_disparities.pdf (accessed 2004 Dec 10).
9. Committee on Institutional and Policy-Level Strategies for Increasing the Diversity of the U.S. Healthcare Workforce. In the nation's compelling interest: ensuring diversity in the health care workforce. Washington, DC: National Academy Press; 2004.
10. Saha S, Komaromy M, Koepsell TD et al. Patient-physician racial concordance and the perceived quality and use of health care. Arch Intern Med. 1999; 159:997–1004.
11. Morales LS, Cunningham WE, Brown JA et al. Are Latinos less satisfied with communication by health care providers? J Gen Intern Med. 1999; 14:409–17.
12. American Hospital Association Commission on Workforce for Hospitals and Health Systems. In our hands: how hospital leaders can build a thriving workforce. www.aha.org/aha/key_issues/workforce/commission/InOurHands.html (accessed 2004 Dec 10).
13. ASHP policy position 0409: cultural diversity among health care providers. In: Hawkins B, ed. Best practices for hospital and health-system pharmacy: positions and guidance documents of ASHP. Bethesda, MD: American Society of Health-System Pharmacists; 2006:253.
14. Report of the ASHP Ad Hoc Committee on Ethnic Diversity and Cultural Competence. Am J Health-Syst Pharm. 2005; 62:1924–30.
15. ASHP policy position 0314: cultural competence. In: Hawkins B, ed. Best practices for hospital and health-system pharmacy: positions and guidance documents of ASHP. Bethesda, MD: American Society of Health-System Pharmacists; 2006:75.
16. Department of Health and Human Services Administration on Aging. Achieving cultural competence: a guidebook for providers of services to older Americans and their families. www.aoa.gov/prof/adddiv/cultural/CC-guidebook.pdf (accessed 2004 Dec 10).
17. U.S. Department of Health and Human Services. Final report: national standards for culturally and linguistically appropriate services in health care (2001). www.omhrc.gov/omh/programs/2pgprograms/finalreport.pdf (accessed 2004 Dec 10).
18. Accreditation standards and guidelines for the professional program in pharmacy leading to the doctor of pharmacy degree. Chicago: Accreditation Council for Pharmaceutical Education; 2006.
19. American Society of Health-System Pharmacists. ASHP guidelines on pharmacist-conducted patient education and counseling. Am J Health-Syst Pharm. 1997; 54:431–4.
20. ASHP policy position 0510: communication among health-system pharmacy practitioners, patients, and other health care providers. In: Hawkins B, ed. Best practices for hospital and health-system pharmacy: positions and guidance documents of ASHP. Bethesda, MD: American Society of Health-System Pharmacists; 2006:74.
21. Erizinger S. Communication between Spanish-speaking patients and their doctors in medical encounters. Cult Med Psychiatry. 1991; 15:91–101.
22. Carrasquillo O, Orav EJ, Brennan TA et al. Impact of language barriers on patient satisfaction in an emergency department. J Gen Intern Med. 1999; 14:82–7.
23. Perez-Stable EJ, Napoles-Springer A, Miramontes JM. The effects of ethnicity and language on medical outcomes of patients with hypertension or diabetes. Med Care. 1997; 35:1212–9.
24. ASHP policy position 9804: multidisciplinary action plans for patient care. In: Hawkins B, ed. Best practices for hospital and health-system pharmacy: positions and guidance documents of ASHP. Bethesda, MD: American Society of Health-System Pharmacists; 2006:161.
25. Ver Ploeg M, Perrin E, eds. Eliminating health disparities: measurement and data needs. Washington, DC: National Academy Press; 2004.

26. The Commonwealth Fund. Enhancing public hospitals' reporting of data on racial and ethnic disparities in care. www.cmwf.org/publications/publications_show.htm?doc_id=452681&#doc452681 (accessed 2007 Jan 31).

Appendix—Institute of Medicine Recommendations Most Pertinent to Hospital and Health-System Pharmacy Practice[1]

General Recommendations

Recommendation 2-1. Increase awareness of racial and ethnic disparities in healthcare among the general public and key stakeholders.

Recommendation 2-2. Increase healthcare providers' awareness of disparities.

Legal, Regulatory, and Policy Interventions

Recommendation 5-3. Increase the proportion of underrepresented U.S. racial and ethnic minorities among healthcare professionals.

Health-System Interventions

Recommendation 5-6. Promote the consistency and equity of care through use of evidence-based guidelines.

Recommendation 5-9. Support the use of interpretation services where community need exists.

Recommendation 5-11. Implement multidisciplinary treatment and preventive care teams.

Patient Education and Empowerment

Recommendation 5-12. Implement patient education programs to increase patients' knowledge of how to best access care and participate in treatment decisions.

Cross-Cultural Education in the Health Professions

Recommendation 6-1. Integrate cross-cultural education into the training of all current and future health professionals.

Data Collection and Monitoring

Recommendation 7-1. Collect and report data on healthcare access and utilization by patients' race, ethnicity, socioeconomic status, and, where possible, primary language.

Recommendation 7-2. Include measures of racial and ethnic disparities in performance measurement.

Recommendation 7-3. Monitor progress toward the elimination of healthcare disparities.

Recommendation 7-4. Report racial and ethnic data by OMB categories, but use subpopulation groups where possible.

Developed through the ASHP Council on Pharmacy Practice and approved by the ASHP Board of Directors on April 16, 2007, and by the ASHP House of Delegates on June 24, 2007.

The bibliographic citation for this document is as follows: American Society of Health-System Pharmacists. ASHP statement on racial and ethnic disparities in health care. *Am J Health-Syst Pharm.* 2008; 65:728–33.

This statement was reviewed in 2011 by the Council on Pharmacy Practice and by the Board of Directors and was found to still be appropriate.

ASHP Statement on the Role of Health-System Pharmacists in Emergency Preparedness

The United States has experienced and remains vulnerable to many events that cause large numbers of casualties. The tragic events of September 11, 2001, and the subsequent anthrax exposures and deaths also awakened the nation to the threat of homeland terrorist attacks.

As the United States began to enhance counterterrorism measures in response to the homeland terrorist attacks of September 11, 2001, it became clear that hospital and health-system pharmacists have an essential role in emergency preparedness.

Position

The American Society of Health-System Pharmacists (ASHP) believes that hospital and health-system pharmacists must assertively exercise their responsibilities in preparing for and responding to disasters, and the leaders of emergency planning at the federal, regional, state, and local levels must call on pharmacists to participate in the full range of issues related to pharmaceuticals. For the purposes of this Statement, disasters include natural disasters (e.g., floods, hurricanes, tornadoes, earthquakes, and forest fires); industrial accidents (e.g., explosions, fires, chemical releases, radiation escape from nuclear power plants, and airplane or train crashes); and terrorist attacks with weapons of mass destruction (WMD), including biological and chemical agents and radiological, nuclear, and explosive devices.

General Principles

1. On the basis of their education, training, experience, and legal responsibilities, pharmacists should have a key role in the planning and execution of (a) pharmaceutical distribution and control and (b) drug therapy management of patients during disasters.
2. The expertise of the pharmacist should be sought in (a) developing guidelines for the diagnosis and treatment of casualties and exposed individuals, (b) selecting pharmaceuticals and related supplies for national and regional stockpiles and local emergency inventories in emergency-preparedness programs, (c) ensuring proper packaging, storage, handling, labeling, and dispensing of emergency supplies of pharmaceuticals, (d) ensuring appropriate deployment of emergency supplies of pharmaceuticals, and (e) ensuring appropriate education and counseling of individuals who receive pharmaceuticals from an emergency supply in response to a disaster.
3. Pharmacists should be in a position to advise public health officials on appropriate messages to convey to the public about the use of essential pharmaceuticals in response to disasters, giving consideration to issues such as adverse effects, contraindications, the effectiveness of alternative pharmaceuticals, and the potential development of drug-resistant infectious agents.
4. In the event of a disaster, pharmacists should be called on to collaborate with physicians and other prescribers in managing the drug therapy of individual victims.

Advice to Hospital and Health-System Pharmacy Directors

Every hospital and health-system pharmacy director (or designee) should

1. Become well informed about the local history of and potential for natural disasters and industrial accidents, as well as the threat of terrorist attacks with WMD, including potential agents that could be used and the related diagnostic and treatment issues;
2. Become thoroughly informed of federal, regional, state, local, and institutional plans for emergency-preparedness, especially those related to the distribution, control, and use of pharmaceuticals;
3. Ensure that the pharmaceutical components of the institution's emergency plans are coordinated with the overall local preparedness plans involving other institutions, community pharmacies, and wholesalers, as well as coordinated with federal, regional, and state plans;
4. Ensure that the appropriate pharmaceuticals and related equipment and supplies are in stock at the institution, consistent with the overall local emergency-preparedness plan, which should account for the interim between the occurrence of a disaster and the receipt of federal or state assistance;
5. Ensure that information about the appropriate use of pharmaceuticals in response to a disaster is available to the health professionals in the institution;
6. Ensure that the institution does not engage in stockpiling of pharmaceuticals without regard to local emergency-preparedness plans that are designed to meet the needs of the whole community; and
7. Ensure that pharmacy personnel are trained to implement the institution's emergency plans.

Advice to Hospital and Health-System Pharmacists

Every hospital and health-system pharmacist should

1. Become well informed about the local history of and potential for natural disasters and industrial accidents, as well as the threat of terrorist attacks with WMD, including potential agents that could be used and the related diagnostic and treatment issues;
2. Become thoroughly informed of local and institutional plans for emergency preparedness, especially those related to the distribution, control, and use of pharmaceuticals;
3. Share with professional colleagues and patients evidence-based information on pharmaceuticals used to respond to disasters;
4. Act assertively to prevent and allay panic and irrational responses to disasters;

5. Strongly discourage individuals from developing personal stockpiles of pharmaceuticals for use in the event of chemical, biological, or nuclear terrorism;

6. Consider volunteering in advance of a disaster to assist in (a) distributing emergency supplies of pharmaceuticals, (b) dispensing and administering medications and immunizations, and (c) managing the drug therapy of individual victims; and

7. Develop and maintain first-aid skills and complete and maintain basic cardiac life support (BCLS) certification. BCLS certification may be required for administering injectable medications, such as vaccines.

Advice to Hospital and Health-System Administrators

Hospital and health-system administrators should

1. Ask the pharmacy director to participate in preparing the institution's emergency-preparedness plan and to consider participating in the development of local, state, regional, and federal emergency-preparedness plans;

2. Consult with the pharmacy director to coordinate the institution's participation in the building of emergency pharmaceutical supplies for use in the community;

3. Refrain from building institutional stockpiles of pharmaceuticals that are not coordinated with the local plan;

4. Encourage local preparedness-planning officials to involve pharmacists in the full range of issues related to pharmaceuticals; and

5. Encourage and enable pharmacy personnel employed by the institution to participate in local, state, regional, and federal emergency-preparedness planning and to volunteer for community service in the event of a disaster.

Advice to Emergency-Preparedness Planners

Emergency-preparedness planners at the federal, regional, state, and local levels should

1. Consult with qualified pharmacists in all areas in which the pharmacist's expertise would contribute to the creation and execution of workable plans;

2. Inform pharmacists, through national and state pharmacy organizations, of plans for deployment of emergency pharmaceutical supplies so that appropriate plans can be made at the local level; and

3. Consult with qualified pharmacists on messages that should be conveyed to the public about the appropriate use of pharmaceuticals in the event of a disaster.

Advice to State Societies of Health-System Pharmacists

State societies of health-system pharmacists should

1. Offer their assistance to state and local emergency-preparedness planning officials, especially in identifying

qualified pharmacists to participate in emergency-preparedness planning;

2. Advise their members of information unique to the state regarding pharmacists' participation in emergency-preparedness planning and deployment efforts; and

3. Establish a volunteer network of health-system pharmacists for deployment in the event of a terrorist attack.

Commitments Made by ASHP

In support of the efforts of health-system pharmacists in emergency preparedness and counterterrorism, ASHP will

1. Maintain an electronic communications network of hospital pharmacy department directors that can be used to transmit urgent information related to emergency preparedness and counterterrorism;

2. Disseminate promptly to ASHP members important new information related to pharmacist involvement in emergency preparedness and counterterrorism;

3. Disseminate to ASHP members and others in the health care community timely evidence-based information about pharmaceuticals used when responding to disasters; and

4. Meet with government officials and others when necessary to clarify promptly important issues that affect the involvement of health-system pharmacists in emergency preparedness and counterterrorism.

This statement was reviewed in 2008 by the Council on Pharmacy Practice and by the Board of Directors and was found to still be appropriate.

Approved by the ASHP Board of Directors on February 21, 2003, and by the ASHP House of Delegates on June 1, 2003. Developed through the ASHP Council on Professional Affairs. Supersedes the ASHP Statement on the Role of Health-System Pharmacists in Counterterrorism approved by the ASHP Board of Directors, November 27, 2001, and revised and approved (as the ASHP Statement on the Role of Health-System Pharmacists in Emergency Preparedness) by the ASHP House of Delegates and the ASHP Board of Directors, June 2, 2002.

The bibliographic citation for this document is as follows: American Society of Health-System Pharmacists. ASHP statement on the role of health-system pharmacists in emergency preparedness. *Am J Health-Syst Pharm.* 2003; 60:1993–5.

ASHP Statement on the Role of Health-System Pharmacists in Public Health

Position

Pharmacists who practice in hospitals and health systems (health-system pharmacists) play a vital role in maintaining and promoting public health. The American Society of Health-System Pharmacists (ASHP) believes that all health-system pharmacists have a responsibility to participate in global, national, state, regional, and institutional efforts to promote public health and to integrate the goals of those initiatives into their practices. Furthermore, health-system pharmacists have a responsibility to work with public health planners to ensure their involvement in public health policy decision-making and in the planning, development, and implementation of public health efforts.

The primary objectives of this statement are to (1) increase awareness of health-system pharmacists' contributions to public health, (2) describe the role of health-system pharmacists in public health planning and promotion, and (3) identify new opportunities for health-system pharmacists' involvement in future public health initiatives. This statement does not provide an exhaustive review of health-system pharmacists' public health activities. Its intent is to stimulate dialogue about the role that health-system pharmacists can play in providing care that improves public health in the United States.

Background

Public health has been defined simply as "what we as a society do to assure the conditions in which people can be healthy."[1] In contrast to medicine, public health initiatives "emphasize the prevention of disease and the health needs of the population as a whole."[2]

Public health services have been characterized as occurring on two levels: the planning ("macro") level and the implementation ("micro" or "provider") level.[3] Macro-level public health services focus on the well-being of the population as a whole and emphasize the assessment and prioritization of a community's health-related needs as well as planning to address those needs. Such services include working with community representatives in identifying health-related community problems; setting community health priorities; formulating community health programs and policies; managing, administering, and evaluating community health-promotion programs; educating the community in ways that promote public health; and researching, presenting, and publishing information about public health activities.[3] These macro-level activities are carried out by public health professionals with varying backgrounds, degrees, and interests.

Micro-level public health services include all the activities required to implement public health initiatives. Many of these services are performed on a provider-to-patient or a program-to-population basis, usually with a specific health-related outcome in mind.[4] Examples of such services include disease screening, immunization, counseling for at-risk populations, and tobacco-cessation programs.

One concept underlying many public health activities is prevention, which is commonly categorized into three types: primary prevention (reducing the actual incidence and occurrence of diseases, injuries, and disability), secondary prevention (decreasing the severity or progression of the disease, injury, and disability), and tertiary prevention (treatment or rehabilitation to return the disease, injury, or disability to the initial or baseline state).[5] Public health efforts on the macro and micro levels can fall anywhere along the prevention spectrum and can reinforce each other. For example, Healthy People 2010 (a macro-level public health policy) aims to reduce the number of hospital admissions attributable to drug therapy management problems (primary prevention).[6] Policies implemented by individual hospitals (on the micro level) will allow clinicians to quickly identify such adverse drug events (ADEs) and prevent them from worsening (secondary prevention), as well as treat the affected patients (tertiary prevention). Pooling and evaluating these clinical experiences can lead to the development of dispensing guidelines or utilization studies that could be used as a primary prevention tool on the macro level.

The health-system pharmacist's role in public health, and the distinction between individualized patient care and public health efforts, can be illustrated by several examples. Providing optimal pharmacotherapy to a single patient has great value. Nonetheless, lessons learned from the management of individual patients can have an even greater impact when they result in practice guidelines or health policies that affect the larger population. Such policy development requires careful evaluation and synthesis of health information using epidemiologic principles. Similarly, identification of a specific ADE is an important patient care service routinely performed by health-system pharmacists. The pharmacoepidemiologic study of ADEs across a population, coupled with action to prevent or mitigate such events, can have a significant impact on public health. Counseling a patient on the proper use of a medication helps that patient. When that knowledge is systematically evaluated and used to develop better behavioral outcomes, general public health can be improved. Finally, a health-system pharmacist who dispenses medications as a member of an emergency-response team has a limited impact on public health. However, the same health-system pharmacist working with emergency-preparedness planners to develop policies and programs that ensure proper utilization of the full range of pharmacy services during a disaster can have an enormous effect on the health of the affected population.

Public Health Activities of Health-System Pharmacists

In 1981, the American Public Health Association (APHA) outlined the public health role of the pharmacist in a pioneering statement.[7] This succinct policy position, building on a previous APHA publication,[8] declared that pharmacists were an underutilized resource in promoting public health

and described an array of functions that could be performed by pharmacists, from providing direct personal health care services to planning for health care for communities or wider geographic areas. In 2004, the American Association of Colleges of Pharmacy recognized the important role pharmacists can play in public health by including population-based care and public health in its Center for Advancement in Pharmaceutical Education (CAPE) Educational Outcomes.[9] These outcomes also emphasized the pharmacist's role in the public health components of "health improvement, wellness, and disease prevention" and the need for pharmacist involvement to ensure the "availability of effective, quality health and disease prevention services," as well as the urgency to "develop public health policy."[9]

The public health duties that an individual health-system pharmacist performs will vary, based on the individual's experience, abilities, training, and work setting. ASHP believes that all health-system pharmacists, working alone or in collaboration with health care colleagues and administrators, can contribute to the promotion of public health. ASHP believes that health-system pharmacists have specific public-health-related responsibilities in infection control[10]; substance abuse prevention, education, and treatment[11]; immunization[12]; tobacco cessation[13]; and emergency preparedness and response.[14] The following are examples of other activities that health-system pharmacists can engage in to promote public health:

- Providing population-based care,
- Developing disease prevention and control programs (including medication safety programs) in their institutions and communities,
- Developing health-education policies and programs within their institutions that address the needs of patients, other health care professionals, community leaders, and the public,
- Collaborating with state and local authorities, including local and state health departments and boards of health, to address local and regional health care needs (including environmental hazard and emergency-preparedness programs),
- Advocating for sound legislation, regulations, and public policy regarding disease prevention and management, and
- Engaging in population-based research and initiating campaigns to disseminate new knowledge.

Population-Based Care. The Institute of Medicine, in *Crossing the Quality Chasm: A New Health System for the 21st Century,* presented the problems of health care quality in the United States and provided recommendations for change.[15] Subsequent follow-up reports, including *Priority Areas for National Action: Transforming Health Care Quality,* have provided additional direction related to population-based care.[16] The CAPE Educational Outcomes recommended that pharmacists engage in both patient-centered and population-based care, suggesting that a core competency of pharmacists is the ability to develop "population-specific, evidence-based disease management programs and protocols based upon analysis of epidemiologic and pharmacoeconomic data, medication use criteria, medication use review and risk reduction strategies."[9]

Over the past two decades, the expanding role of health-system pharmacists in patient care has allowed them to support public health efforts by designing and providing disease management programs. ASHP urges health-system pharmacists to build on this foundation by leading their institutions' efforts to provide population-based care. By working with their health care colleagues through such institutional mechanisms as the pharmacy and therapeutics committee and using tools such as medication-use evaluation, health-system pharmacists can contribute to population-specific, evidence-based disease management programs tailored to fit the needs of the institutions and communities they serve. Health-system pharmacists can participate in quality reviews and ensure that evidence-based treatments are used for all patients to help alleviate health care disparities.

Disease Prevention and Medication Safety. Health-system pharmacists can be involved in disease prevention and control in many ways. For example, they can help develop institutional screening programs to check immunization status and identify undiagnosed medical conditions (e.g., hypertension, diabetes, hyperlipidemia, depression). The health-system pharmacist's role in medication safety and error prevention is in keeping with the national public health goals outlined in the federal government's Healthy People 2010 initiative, which include reducing the number of hospital admissions resulting from drug therapy mismanagement and fostering programs to intercept counterfeit medications.[6] Medication reconciliation programs are one example of the tools pharmacists can encourage their facilities to use to achieve these goals.

Health Education. Health-system pharmacists can promote public health by developing patient education programs on safe and effective medication use[17] and other public health-related topics, such as tobacco cessation, exercise, and healthy nutrition. Pharmacists should support the education and training of the population at an early age, such as through school health programs, to help children develop good health behaviors that can continue into adulthood. Furthermore, health-system pharmacists can improve society's use of medications by educating their health care colleagues about safe and effective medication use. Health-system pharmacists can also use their knowledge and expertise to educate community leaders (e.g., legislators, regulators, public officeholders, school officials, religious leaders) about and involve them in public health initiatives.

Public Health Policy. Health-system pharmacists should be encouraged to participate in public health policy development, from local boards of health to national programs. By linking disease prevalence, drug utilization, and the determinants of disease, health-system pharmacists can place prevention within a larger context. Drugs play a central role in health, and health policy, especially policy directed at chronic disease, must be formulated with a better understanding of the relationship of drug therapy to the many other factors that affect disease outcomes. Since medication use increases as patients age, health-system pharmacists will face increasing responsibilities to ensure appropriate and cost-effective medication use as the average age of the U.S. population rises.

Health-system pharmacist participation in emergency planning and service delivery is critical. Requirements for new and enlarged inventories of specialized pharmaceuticals to provide prophylaxis and treatment to communities during emergencies are growing. The Centers for Disease Control and Prevention's Strategic National Stockpile (SNS) program, for example, includes 12-hour push packages, vendor-managed inventory, "chempacks," vaccines, and medical supplies.[18] Hospital and health-system pharmacies are essential in planning for accommodation of supplies, such as antibiotics and antidotes needed in the initial 24 hours following a crisis, before state and federal assets become available. Community-based planning efforts for mass immunization, prophylaxis, and treatment, including pandemic response to biological, chemical, radiological, or explosive agents, are an ongoing process, as is planning for utilization of the SNS. Medication management is a critical component of all these contingencies, yet many of the plans do not address pharmacy participation. Involvement of health-system pharmacists is critically important to reliably address medication issues.

ASHP encourages pharmacists to serve on National Disaster Medical System assistance teams (http://ndms.dhhs. gov), the National Pharmacy Response Team (www.ndms. dhhs.gov/nprt.html), or local units of the Medical Reserve Corps (www.medicalreservecorps.gov) to assist in distributing emergency supplies of pharmaceuticals, dispensing and administering medications and immunizations, and managing the drug therapy of individual victims.[14] The development, implementation, and revision of local emergency operations plans, which include public health management of emergencies, require pharmacist input. Health-system pharmacists need to be actively involved in planning for procurement, distribution, and dispensing of medications, as well as ongoing management of patient medication issues.

Pharmacists should also work with health-system administrators to develop policies and initiatives that heighten awareness of the applicable laws and best management practices in the proper handling and disposal of hazardous drugs.

As medication-use experts and experienced health-system administrators, health-system pharmacists can and should contribute to the development of public-health-related legislation and regulation and should be involved in public program oversight and administration. Legislators, regulators, and program managers at all levels of government should be educated to utilize this expertise. Health-system pharmacists, as individuals and through their professional associations, state and local boards of health, and state boards of pharmacy, are encouraged to participate in legislative, regulatory, and oversight processes.

Research and Training. To assume a greater responsibility in public health, health-system pharmacists must receive adequate education and training. Pharmacy curricula should include advanced coursework in public health and research design. Health-system pharmacists need to be proficient in research methodology, pharmacoepidemiology, and biostatistics and their applications to public health decision-making. Knowledge and experience in the design, conduct, and interpretation of clinical studies (both observational and experimental) are essential. Health-system pharmacists have the opportunity to participate in collaborative research and serve on institutional review boards, data monitoring and safety committees, and expert medication advisory committees. Experiential and didactic training for practicing health-system pharmacists, students, residents, and research fellows should include exposure to research in public health policy, pharmacoepidemiology, pharmacoeconomics, health-related quality of life, and evidence-based medicine. Health-system pharmacists should also work directly with public health policymakers and other key stakeholders, such as professional organizations, medical centers, academic institutions, governmental agencies, and third-party payers, to promote optimal pharmacotherapy.

Future Roles

Revolutionary progress in basic biomedical sciences, including human genomics, stem-cell biology, immunology, biomedical engineering, and bioinformatics, has provided an unprecedented supply of information for improving human health. The rapidly emerging fields of population genetics and pharmacogenomics highlight the significance of molecular techniques in the clinical diagnostic laboratory and the potential for application in patient-directed pharmacotherapy. Medication-prescribing decisions will increasingly rely on the results of genotyping of drug-metabolizing enzymes. New technology and practices will allow health-system pharmacists to reduce treatment failures and prevent adverse drug reactions through the proper application of pharmacogenetic principles.[19] Advances in informatics will permit aggregation and application of population- and patient-specific clinical data in ways that will encourage development of population-specific, evidence-based disease management programs. As medication-use experts, health-system pharmacists will need to apply these new tools not simply to improve patient-specific pharmacotherapy but to advance public health. Similarly, innovations in medication delivery technology will allow more complex therapies to be administered outside institutional settings. Patients, caregivers, and health professionals will require education about the safe use of such technologies, as will the legislators and other officials responsible for regulating their use.

Conclusion

Health-system pharmacists play a vital role in maintaining and promoting public health. ASHP believes that all health-system pharmacists have a responsibility to participate in global, national, state, regional, and institutional efforts to promote public health and to integrate them into their practices and that health-system pharmacists should be involved in public health policy decision-making and in the planning, development, and implementation of public health efforts. Health-system pharmacists can improve public health by providing population-based care; developing disease prevention and control programs; providing health education; collaborating with state and local authorities to address local and regional health care needs, including emergency preparedness and response; advocating for sound legislation, regulations, and public policy regarding disease prevention and management; and engaging in public health research.

References

1. Committee for the Study of the Future of Public Health. The future of public health. Washington, DC: National Academies Press; 1988:1.
2. Higher education for public health. New York: Milbank Memorial Fund; 1976.
3. Bush PJ, Johnson KW. Where is the public health pharmacist? *Am J Pharm Educ.* 1979; 43:249–53.
4. Bush PJ, ed. The pharmacist role in disease prevention and health promotion. Bethesda, MD: ASHP Research and Education Foundation; 1983:3.
5. Ives TJ, DerMarderosian AH. Pharmacists and public health. In: Hendrickson R, Beringer P, DerMarderosian AH et al., eds. Remington: the science and practice of pharmacy. 21st ed. Philadelphia: Lippincott Williams & Wilkins; 2006:51.
6. Office of Disease Prevention and Health Promotion. Healthy People 2010. www.healthypeople.gov/document/HTML/Volume2/17Medical.htm (accessed 2007 Dec 27).
7. American Public Health Association. APHA policy 8024: the role of the pharmacist in public health. *Am J Public Health.* 1981; 71:213–6.
8. Cain RM, Kahn JS. The pharmacist as a member of the health team. *Am J Public Health.* 1971; 61:2223–8.
9. Center for Advancement in Pharmaceutical Education (CAPE) Educational Outcomes 2004. www.aacp.org/Docs/MainNavigation/Resources/6075_CAPE2004.pdf (accessed 2007 Nov 27).
10. American Society of Health-System Pharmacists. ASHP statement on the pharmacist's role in infection control. *Am J Health-Syst Pharm.* 1998; 55:1724–6.
11. American Society of Health-System Pharmacists. ASHP statement on the pharmacist's role in substance abuse prevention, education, and assistance. *Am J Health-Syst Pharm.* 2003; 60:1995–8.
12. American Society of Health-System Pharmacists. ASHP guidelines on the pharmacist's role in immunization. *Am J Health-Syst Pharm.* 2003; 60:1371–7.
13. American Society of Health-System Pharmacists. ASHP therapeutic position statement on smoking cessation. *Am J Health-Syst Pharm.* 1999; 56:460–4.
14. American Society of Health-System Pharmacists. ASHP statement on the role of health-system pharmacists in emergency preparedness. *Am J Health-Syst Pharm.* 2003; 60:1993–5.
15. Committee on Quality of Health Care in America. Crossing the quality chasm: a new health system for the 21st century. Washington, DC: National Academy Press; 2001.
16. Adams K, Corrigan JM, eds. Priority areas for national action: transforming health care quality. Washington, DC: National Academies Press; 2003.
17. American Society of Health-System Pharmacists. ASHP guidelines on pharmacist-conducted patient education and counseling. *Am J Health-Syst Pharm.* 1997; 54:431–4.
18. Centers for Disease Control and Prevention. Strategic National Stockpile. www.bt.cdc.gov/stockpile/ (accessed 2007 Nov 20).
19. Spear BB, Health-Chiozzi M, Huff J. Clinical applications of pharmacogenetics. *Trends Mol Med.* 2001; 7:201–4.

Other Resources

Pharmacists looking for further involvement in public health have many options. First, training and competence in public health disciplines are invaluable in understanding the field of public health and its applications to pharmacy practice. Accredited schools of public health offer traditional didactic classes, and some have courses or continuing education available on-line that will give the beginner a clearer understanding of the four traditional areas of public health practice: health administration and policy, health education, biostatistics, and epidemiology. Pharmacists who wish to pursue a degree in public health can also do so on-line at a growing number of schools of public health (www.asph.org/document.cfm?page=718).

Pharmacists with an interest in federal public health initiatives can start with one of three main points of access. The first is the Centers for Disease Control and Prevention (www.cdc.gov), the largest repository of documents, program descriptions, and contacts in the realm of prevention. Major efforts aimed at disease surveillance, infectious disease control, immunization, health education, chronic disease maintenance, and disease-related data management provide an ample and readily available source of information. The second major source of information is the Office of Disease Prevention and Health Promotion (http://odphp.osophs.dhhs.gov), which provides access to Healthy People 2010, a health information clearinghouse, national dietary guidelines, and information about health observances. Finally, the Agency for Healthcare Research and Quality (www.ahrq.gov) provides information on evidence-based clinical practice, the Guide to Clinical Preventive Services (www.ahrq.gov/clinic/pocketgd.htm), and quality measurement of health care. Virtually the entire realm of public health within the U.S. Public Health Service can be accessed or linked via these three websites.

State government websites provide public health information for their respective states. State entities serve as the main policymaking entity for public health priorities and strategies, provide a conduit for federal public health dollars, and are the main repository of health information and data for the state. States often organize a range of advisory groups, task forces, and planning committees whose output shapes their public health agenda. These entities also provide input and direction for state legislative bodies to address, legislate, and fund.

On the local level, boards of health serve as the main government entities involved in public health. Aside from their usual routine of immunizations and restaurant inspections, these boards serve as the policymakers for disaster response and provision of primary care to underserved populations. They receive federal and state dollars that are used to fund public health efforts. They are closest to the general population both in their makeup and in their efforts at improving the public's health. Pharmacists interested in learning more about public health and the types of activities that community public health agencies are involved in can register for a free interactive tutorial at www.nynj-phtc.org/orientation.

Below is a list of websites that provide information related to public health.

Public Health Organizations

- World Health Organization (www.who.int)
- Pan American Health Organization (www.paho.org)
- American Public Health Association (www.apha.org)
- Association of State and Territorial Health Officials (www.astho.org)
- National Association of County and City Health Officials (www.naccho.org)
- Public Health Foundation (www.phf.org)
- Association of Schools of Public Health (www.asph.org)

Federal Health Agencies

- U.S. Department of Health and Human Services (www.dhhs.gov)
- Office of the Surgeon General, Public Health Priorities (www.surgeongeneral.gov/publichealthpriorities.html)
- Centers for Disease Control and Prevention (www.cdc.gov)
- Food and Drug Administration (www.fda.gov)
- Health Resources and Services Administration (www.hrsa.gov)
- National Institutes of Health (www.nih.gov)
- Agency for Healthcare Research and Quality (www.ahrq.gov)
- Environmental Protection Agency (www.epa.gov)

Developed through the ASHP Council on Pharmacy Practice and approved by the ASHP Board of Directors on January 12, 2007, and by the ASHP House of Delegates on June 24, 2007.

The bibliographic citation for this document is as follows: American Society of Health-System Pharmacists. ASHP statement on the role of health-system pharmacists in public health. *Am J Health-Syst Pharm.* 2008; 65:462–7.

This statement was reviewed in 2011 by the Council on Pharmacy Practice and by the Board of Directors and was found to still be appropriate.

ASHP Statement on the Use of Dietary Supplements

Position

The American Society of Health-System Pharmacists (ASHP) believes that the widespread, indiscriminate use of dietary supplements presents substantial risks to public health and that pharmacists have an opportunity and a professional responsibility to reduce those risks. ASHP recognizes that patients may choose to use legally available dietary supplements, but believes that the decision to use substances that may be pharmacologically active should always be based on reliable information about their safety and efficacy. The current regulatory framework governing dietary supplements does not provide consumers or health care providers with sufficient information on safety and efficacy to make informed decisions. Furthermore, standards for product quality are currently inadequate. ASHP recognizes the concerns raised by the dietary supplement industry regarding regulating dietary supplements as nonprescription drugs because of the industry's inability to patent product ingredients. Still, ASHP urges Congress to amend the Dietary Supplement Health and Education Act of 1994 (DSHEA) to require that the Food and Drug Administration (FDA) develop a regulatory scheme to ensure that dietary supplements are safe and effective. ASHP believes that dietary supplements, at a minimum, should (1) receive FDA approval for evidence of safety and efficacy, (2) meet manufacturing standards for identity, strength, quality, purity, packaging, and labeling, and (3) undergo mandatory postmarketing reporting of adverse events, including drug interactions.

ASHP strongly encourages in vitro and clinical studies of interactions between dietary supplements and medications. Because of the demonstrated risk of these interactions, ASHP discourages the concurrent use of dietary supplements and drug therapy, especially those therapies for which failure may have irreversible consequences (e.g., immunosuppressive therapy, cancer chemotherapy, treatment for human immunodeficiency virus infection, anticoagulation therapy, and hormonal contraceptive therapy).

ASHP believes that the criteria used to evaluate dietary supplements for inclusion in health-system formularies should be as rigorous as those established for nonprescription drugs and that the self-administered use of dietary supplements during a health-system stay may increase risks to patients and liabilities to health care professionals and institutions.

ASHP urges pharmacists and other health care practitioners to integrate awareness of dietary supplement use into everyday practice and encourages pharmacists to increase efforts to prevent interactions between dietary supplements and drugs. ASHP also supports the education of pharmacists and other health care practitioners in the taxonomy, formulation, pharmacology, and pharmacokinetics of dietary supplements and believes that such education should be required in college of pharmacy curricula.

Background

Dietary supplements are defined in DSHEA as products "intended to supplement the diet" that contain vitamins, minerals, herbs or other botanicals, amino acids; "a dietary substance for use by man to supplement the diet by increasing the total daily intake"; or "a concentrate, metabolite, constituent, extract, or combinations of these ingredients."[1]

Evidence of variability in dietary supplement content[2-8] has spurred efforts to standardize products. Current federal regulations regarding the manufacture of dietary supplements are not adequate.[9] Some manufacturers voluntarily follow good manufacturing practices (GMPs) devised by their own trade groups (e.g., the National Nutritional Foods Association GMP Certification Program[10]), and the U.S. Pharmacopeia (USP) has created voluntary standards for a handful of dietary supplements.[11] Manufacturers that wish to carry the "USP approved" seal on their product labels have to subject their products to testing by USP. The creation of these voluntary programs reflects a widespread concern, even on the part of dietary supplement manufacturers, that production processes must be regulated. Although FDA has had the authority to establish dietary supplement GMPs for almost a decade, it issued its first proposed rule on the topic in 2003. [12]

DSHEA does not require FDA to review evidence of the efficacy or safety of dietary supplements, so manufacturers have no burden to prove that their products are effective or safe. Although dietary supplement labeling cannot claim activity in the treatment of a specific disease or condition, claims that suggest an effect on the "structure or function of the body" are allowed.[1] For example, dietary supplements containing echinacea can be labeled as supporting immune health (as a "function") but cannot be labeled as preventing or ameliorating colds (treating a disease). Regardless of this distinction between function and treatment, consumers are bombarded by the lay press (and even some scientific literature) with what can only be described as specific-disease indications for dietary supplements (e.g., glucosamine for osteoarthritis, black cohosh for menopausal symptoms, and St. John's wort for depression).

The health claims allowed in dietary supplement labeling by current interpretation of DSHEA create further confusion for consumers. FDA's attempt to hold these health claims to the same scientific standard required for conventional foods was struck down in *Pearson* v. *Shalala,* so FDA must permit dietary supplement labels to carry "qualified" health claims based on equivocal scientific evidence.[13]

Although DSHEA does require that dietary supplements be safe, it does not require prospective testing to ensure safety. To remove a product from the market, FDA must prove that the product is unsafe. Under DSHEA, some dietary supplements that were banned from the U.S. market because of concerns about their safety have been allowed to return (e.g., sassafras tea, dehydroepiandrosterone). Demonstrably unsafe products have made their way onto the market, and fatal adverse reactions have been reported.[14,15]

Establishing the safety record of dietary supplements has been complicated by the lack of systematically collected data about their adverse reactions. The MedWatch system has been used to a limited extent to report adverse events related to dietary supplement use, but, nine years after the passage of DSHEA, FDA is still developing an adverse-reaction-reporting system for dietary supplements. Despite the limited data, however, the number of case reports of interactions between dietary supplements and medications is growing.[16-21] The safety of dietary supplements for special populations (e.g., children, pregnant women, people with impaired organ or immunologic function) has also not been demonstrated.

Dangers to Public Health

It has been estimated that 40% of the U.S. population uses dietary supplements often and that almost twice as many have used at least 1 of the estimated 29,000 dietary supplements on the market.[22] Out-of-pocket expenditures on dietary supplements total approximately $18 billion annually.[23] Such widespread and indiscriminate use of dietary supplements presents five dangers to the public health:

1. Some dietary supplements are inherently unsafe when ingested orally (e.g., chaparral, ephedra, comfrey, tiractricol, aristolochic acid, pennyroyal).[24–28]
2. Lax regulation of dietary supplement manufacturing presents the risk of contamination or adulteration with harmful substances, including carcinogens,[29–32] and of dangerous variability in active ingredient content among products.[2–8]
3. The use of dietary supplements may compromise, delay, or supplant treatment with therapies of proven efficacy.[16–21,25]
4. Dietary supplements may present dangers to special populations (e.g., children, pregnant women, patients undergoing surgery, patients with impaired organ or immunologic function).
5. Spending on dietary supplements represents an enormous health-related expenditure of unsubstantiated value.[33]

Since the mid-19th century, the federal government has exercised its responsibility to protect Americans from hazardous or adulterated foods and medicines. ASHP believes that, with the passage and implementation of DSHEA, the federal government has abandoned its duty to create a regulatory scheme for dietary supplements that adequately protects the health of consumers. Under DSHEA, consumers and health care practitioners are not provided with the information they need to use dietary supplements safely. To reduce the dangers posed by the current regulatory framework, Congress should amend DSHEA to

1. Require that dietary supplements undergo FDA approval for evidence of safety and efficacy,
2. Mandate FDA-approved dietary supplement labeling that describes safe use in a clear, standardized format, including the potential for interaction with medications and cautions for special populations,
3. Require FDA to promulgate and enforce GMPs for dietary supplements,
4. Require that dietary supplements meet FDA-established standards for identity, strength, purity, and quality, and
5. Empower FDA to establish and maintain an adverse-event-reporting system specifically for dietary supplements, and require dietary supplement manufacturers to report suspected adverse reactions to FDA.

Implications for Practice

Although examples of persons rejecting potentially life-saving medical interventions in favor of alternative therapies can be found in the medical and lay press,[34] the presumption that most users of dietary supplements reject traditional treatments is unfounded. One survey found that most individuals who use alternative therapies for a specific symptom or disease are also receiving care and prescription medications from a physician or surgeon.[35] In a more recent nationwide survey, almost 20% of adults taking prescription drugs reported that they were taking at least one dietary supplement, not including vitamin or mineral supplements.[36]

Pharmacists and other health care practitioners therefore have an opportunity to reduce the risks associated with dietary supplement use. Health care providers face unfamiliar challenges in this effort, however, because much of the information they typically use to establish pharmaceutical treatment regimens is lacking for dietary supplements. Product content is not standardized, therapeutic goals are vague, and evidence of efficacy and safety is absent or ambiguous. ASHP believes that pharmacists, as medication-use experts and accessible members of the health care team, are uniquely qualified and positioned to counsel patients using or considering the use of dietary supplements. Despite their professional responsibility to provide patients with sound advice, pharmacists (like other health care providers) are frustrated by the lack of reliable information about the safety and efficacy of dietary supplements. Pharmacists have shown that they can improve medication safety by identifying and preventing adverse drug events,[37] and they could play a similar role in preventing adverse events due to dietary supplement use if they had sound, evidence-based professional resources.

Incorporate Awareness of Dietary Supplement Use into Practice. ASHP urges pharmacists and other health care practitioners to integrate awareness of dietary supplement use into everyday practice. ASHP believes that all health systems should have an institutional policy regarding the use of dietary supplements. Such policies should allow pharmacists and other health care practitioners to exercise their professional judgment and try to balance patient autonomy and institutional concerns.

Patient Counseling. Although most consumers of alternative therapies also take prescription medications,[35] one survey found that 72% of respondents who used alternative therapies did not report that use to their health care providers.[38] Pharmacists and other health care practitioners must therefore routinely inquire about a patient's current or planned use of dietary supplements, providing examples so that patients understand what is meant (e.g, asking "Do you use dietary supplements, such as St. John's wort or gingko?").[39] This information will allow pharmacists and other health care practitioners to counsel the patient about dietary supplement use and monitor for adverse reactions and drug interactions.

When counseling patients about dietary supplements, the concept of *caveat emptor* (buyer beware) must be emphasized because the content and safety of dietary supplements are not well regulated. ASHP believes that all pharmacists, at a minimum, should be familiar with the pharmacology and pharmacokinetics of common dietary supplements that might contraindicate concurrent use with a therapeutic regimen (i.e., proven and potential pharmacokinetic and pharmacodynamic interactions with prescription and nonprescription medications) to the extent that sound evidence exists. To provide informed counsel to patients using or considering the use of dietary supplements, pharmacists further need to be familiar with the following:

- The typical uses of common dietary supplements and the scientific literature regarding their efficacy and safety,
- The proven and potential interactions between common dietary supplements and prescription and nonprescription medications,
- The methods of therapeutic monitoring for common dietary supplements, including signs and symptoms of potential adverse effects and toxicities,
- The proven and potential effects of certain disease states on supplement absorption, distribution, and elimination, and
- The safety of using dietary supplements before or after surgery.

Despite the shortcomings of the data on dietary supplements, the limited references on the topic that are available should be consulted.[40–45]

Patients stabilized on a combination of a supplement and medication should be cautioned not to suddenly discontinue the use of either without first consulting with the prescriber. The potential for adverse effects from an interaction exists both when a dietary supplement is discontinued and when it is initiated.

Dietary supplement sales have a very high potential for profit. Despite the expectation that pharmacies should receive a profit from the sale of products, professional ethics mandate that any recommendations or purchasing suggestions be made with the well-being of the customer or patient as the primary concern. Pharmacists should also review promotional and reference materials promulgated in or by their workplaces to ensure that these materials are evidence based and not misleading or deceptive. The scientific literature about the safety and efficacy of dietary supplements is updated continually. Pharmacists have a responsibility to continually monitor that literature and incorporate the evolving knowledge into their care for and advice to patients.

Inclusion in Formularies. ASHP believes that the criteria used to evaluate dietary supplements for inclusion in health-system formularies should be as rigorous as those established for prescription and nonprescription drugs. The Joint Commission on Accreditation of Healthcare Organizations (JCAHO) has recommended that medical staff weigh the patient care implications of dietary supplements with the same rigor applied to prescription and nonprescription medications,[46] and all JCAHO medication management standards apply to dietary supplements, as well as prescription and nonprescription drugs.[47] ASHP believes that the decision to include any product in a health-system formulary should be based on comparative data regarding efficacy, adverse effects, cost, and potential therapeutic advantages and deficiencies.[48] The lack of definitive evidence of efficacy and safety and the demonstrated variability in product content make most dietary supplements unsuitable for inclusion in health-system formularies.[49] More research is needed to determine the relative effectiveness of dietary supplements and their safety for all patient populations, especially drug–supplement interactions.

The shortcomings that make most dietary supplements unsuitable for inclusion in formularies also argue strongly against their self-administered use by patients during a health-system stay. ASHP believes that the use of self-administered medications should be avoided to the extent possible[50] and that pharmacists should identify all drug products before their use.[15] There is currently no way to definitively determine the content of dietary supplements brought into health systems. In addition, discontinuing supplement use may be advisable as part of the diagnostic workup, and the possibility that supplement use may have contributed to hospitalization should be considered.

If an institution decides, as a matter of patient autonomy, to allow the use of dietary supplements, such use should require a prescribed order for the specific dietary supplement in the patient medical record and pharmacist review and verification of the order. Health systems should be aware that the use of dietary supplements may expose patients to risks, and the health system and staff should take steps to reduce potential liability (e.g., require patients to sign a liability waiver for dietary supplement use) and decrease those risks.

Conclusion

Current regulation of the manufacture and labeling of dietary supplements fails to address substantial risks to the public health. As the activity of some dietary supplements has become apparent, so have their dangers and the shortcomings of the current regulatory framework. These laws and regulations should be revised, with the primary goal of providing consumers and health care practitioners with the information they need to use dietary supplements safely and effectively. In short, dietary supplements should be regulated in a manner that ensures that they are safe and effective. Regardless of the shortcomings of the current regulatory framework, pharmacists have an opportunity and a professional responsibility to reduce the risks presented by dietary supplement use.

References

1. Dietary Supplement Health and Education Act of 1994 (SB 784). http://thomas.loc.gov/ (accessed 2003 Apr 1).
2. Gurley BJ, Wang P, Gardner SF. Ephedrine-type alkaloid content of nutritional supplements containing *Ephedra sinica* (Ma-huang) as determined by high performance liquid chromatography. *J Pharm Sci.* 1998; 87:1547–53.
3. Harkey MR, Henderson GL, Gershwin ME, et al. Variability in commercial ginseng products: an analysis of 25 preparations. *Am J Clin Nutr.* 2001; 73:1101–6.
4. Parasrampuria J, Schwartz K, Petesch R. Quality control of dehydroepiandrosterone dietary supplement products. *JAMA.* 1998; 280:1565. Letter.
5. Feifer AH, Fleshner NE, Klotz L. Analytical accuracy and reliability of commonly used nutritional supplements in prostate disease. *J Urol.* 2002; 168:150–4.
6. De los Reyes GC, Koda RT. Determining hyperforin and hypericin content in eight brands of St. John's wort. *Am J Health-Syst Pharm.* 2002; 59:545–7.
7. Glisson JK, Rogers HE, Abourashed EA, et al. Clinic at the health food store? Employee recommendations and product analysis. *Pharmacotherapy.* 2003; 23:64–72.
8. Gurley BJ, Gardner SF, Hubbard MA. Content versus label claims in ephedra-containing dietary supplements. *Am J Health-Syst Pharm.* 2000; 57:963–9.
9. Fontanarosa PB, Rennie D, DeAngelis CD. The need for regulation of dietary supplements—lessons from ephedra. *JAMA.* 2003; 289:1568–70. Editorial.

10. National Nutritional Foods Association. NNFA GMP certification program overview. www.nnfa.org/services/science/gmp.htm (accessed 2003 Dec 12).

11. U.S. Pharmacopeia. U.S. Pharmacopeia dietary supplement verification program. www.usp-verified.org (accessed 2004 May 13).

12. Food and Drug Administration. Current good manufacturing practice in manufacturing, packing, or holding dietary ingredients and dietary supplements. Proposed rule. *Fed Regist.* 2003; 68:12157–263.

13. *Pearson* v. *Shalala,* 164 F.3d 650 (D.C. Cir. 1999).

14. Food and Drug Administration. Illnesses and injuries associated with the use of selected dietary supplements. www. cfsan.fda.gov/~dms/ds-ill.html (accessed 2003 Feb 14).

15. Palmer ME, Haller C, McKinney PE, et al. Adverse events associated with dietary supplements: an observational study. *Lancet.* 2003; 361:101–6.

16. Williamson EM. Drug interactions between herbal and prescription medicines. *Drug Saf.* 2003; 26:1075–92.

17. Fugh-Berman A. Herb–drug interactions. *Lancet.* 2000; 355: 134–8.

18. Yue QY, Bergquist C, Gердén B. Safety of St. John's wort *(Hypericum perforatum). Lancet.* 2000; 355:576–7. Letter.

19. Brazier NC, Levine MA. Drug–herb interaction among commonly used conventional medicines: a compendium for health care professionals. *Am J Ther.* 2003; 10:163–9.

20. Izzo AA, Ernst E. Interactions between herbal medicines and prescribed drugs: a systematic review. *Drugs.* 2001; 61:2163–75.

21. Piscitelli SC, Burstein AH, Chaitt D, et al. Indinavir concentrations and St. John's wort. *Lancet.* 2000; 355:547–8. Letter. [Erratum, *Lancet.* 2001;357:1210.]

22. Office of the Inspector General. Dietary supplement labels: key elements. Report OEI-01-01-00120. http://oig.hhs.gov/oei/reports/oei-01-01-00120.pdf (accessed 2004 May 13).

23. Annual overview of the nutrition industry VII. *Nutr Bus J.* 2002; 7(May/Jun):1–11.

24. Food and Drug Administration. Dietary supplements: warnings and safety information. www.cfsan.fda.gov/~dms/ds~warn.html (accessed 2004 May 21).

25. De Smet PA. Herbal remedies. *N Engl J Med.* 2002; 347:2046–56.

26. Blumenthal M, ed. The complete German Commission E monographs—therapeutic guide to herbal medicines. Austin, TX: American Botanical Council; 1998:116,125–6.

27. Nortier JL, Martinez MC, Schmeiser HH, et al. Urothelial carcinoma associated with the use of a Chinese herb (*Aristolochia fangchi*). *N Engl J Med.* 2000; 342:1686–92.

28. Shekelle PG, Hardy ML, Morton SC, et al. Efficacy and safety of ephedra and ephedrine for weight loss and athletic performance: a meta-analysis. *JAMA.* 2003; 289:1537–45.

29. Slifman NR, Obermeyer WR, Musser SM, et al. Contamination of botanical dietary supplements by *Digitalis lanata. N Engl J Med.* 1998; 339:806–11.

30. Food and Drug Administration. Letter to health care professionals: FDA concerned about botanical products, including dietary supplements, containing aristolochic acid. http://vm.cfsan.fda.gov/~dms/ds-botl2.html (accessed 2003 Apr 1).

31. De Smet PA. Toxicological outlook on the quality assurance of herbal remedies. In: De Smet PA, Keller K, Hansel R, et al., eds. Adverse effects of herbal drugs. Vol. 1. Berlin: Springer-Verlag; 1992:1–72.

32. De Smet PA. The safety of herbal products. In: Jonas WB, Levin JS, eds. Essentials of complementary and alternative medicine. Philadelphia: Lippincott Williams & Wilkins; 1999:108–47.

33. De Smet PA. Health risks of herbal remedies. *Drug Saf.* 1995; 13:81–93.

34. Eisenberg DM, Davis RB, Ettner SL, et al. Trends in alternative medicine use in the United States, 1990–1997: results of a follow-up national study. *JAMA.* 1998; 280:1569–75.

35. Astin JA. Why patients use alternative medicine: results of a national study. *JAMA.* 1998; 279:1548–53.

36. Kaufman DW, Kelly JP, Rosenberg L, et al. Recent patterns of medication use in the ambulatory adult population of the United States: the Slone survey. *JAMA.* 2002; 287:337–44.

37. Leape LL, Cullen DJ, Clapp M, et al. Pharmacist participation on physician rounds and adverse drug events in the intensive care unit. *JAMA.* 1999; 282:267–70.

38. Eisenberg DM, Kessler RC, Van Rompay MI, et al. Perceptions about complementary therapies relative to conventional therapies among adults who use both: results from a national survey. *Ann Intern Med.* 2001; 135:344–51.

39. Ang-Lee MK, Moss J, Yuan CS. Herbal medicines and perioperative care. *JAMA.* 2001; 286:208–16.

40. Chambliss WG, Hufford CD, Flagg ML, et al. Assessment of the quality of reference books on botanical dietary supplements. *J Am Pharm Assoc.* 2002; 42:723–34.

41. Haller CA, Anderson IB, Kim SY, et al. An evaluation of selected herbal reference texts and comparison to published reports of adverse herbal events. *Adverse Drug React Toxicol Rev.* 2002; 21:143–50.

42. Kemper KJ, Amata-Kynvi A, Sanghavi D, et al. Randomized trial of an internet curriculum on herbs and other dietary supplements for health care professionals. *Acad Med.* 2002; 77:882–9.

43. Sweet BV, Gay WE, Leady MA, et al. Usefulness of herbal and dietary supplement References. *Ann Pharmacother.* 2003; 37:494–9.

44. Office of Dietary Supplements. International Bibliographic Information on Dietary Supplements (IBIDS) database. http://ods.od.nih.gov/showpage.aspx? pageid=48 (accessed 2003 Dec 11).

45. Memorial Sloan-Kettering Cancer Center. AboutHerbs Web site. www.mskcc.org/mskcc/html/11570.cfm (accessed 2003 Dec 11).

46. Rich DS. Ask the Joint Commission: understanding JCAHO requirements for hospital pharmacies. St. Louis: Facts and Comparisons; 2002:132–3.

47. Medication management standards. In: Comprehensive accreditation manual for hospitals, 2004 update. Oakbrook Terrace, IL: Joint Commission on Accreditation of Healthcare Organizations; 2004:MM1–20.

48. American Society of Hospital Pharmacists. ASHP technical assistance bulletin on the evaluation of drugs for formularies. *Am J Hosp Pharm.* 1988; 45:386–7.

49. Ansani NT, Ciliberto NC, Freedy T. Hospital policies regarding herbal medicines. *Am J Health-Syst Pharm.* 2003; 60:367–70.

50. American Society of Hospital Pharmacists. ASHP technical assistance bulletin on hospital drug distribution and control. *Am J Hosp Pharm.* 1980; 37:1097–1103.

51. American Society of Health-System Pharmacists. ASHP guidelines: minimum standard for pharmacies in hospitals. *Am J Health-Syst Pharm.* 1995; 52:2711–7.

This statement was reviewed in 2009 by the Council on Pharmacy Practice and by the Board of Directors and was found to still be appropriate.

Approved by the ASHP Board of Directors on April 14, 2004, and by the ASHP House of Delegates on June 20, 2004. Developed through the ASHP Council on Professional Affairs. Supersedes ASHP policies 0223, 0304, and 0324.

The bibliographic citation for this document is as follows: American Society of Health-System Pharmacists. ASHP statement on the use of dietary supplements. *Am J Health-Syst Pharm.* 2004; 61:1707–11.

ASHP Guidelines on Emergency Medicine Pharmacist Services

Emergency medicine (EM) is an ever-changing, rapidly evolving practice specialty. The formal emergency department (ED) has its roots in the 1950s, when full-time emergency services were established in the United States.[1] Since then, the rate of mortality from accidental and traumatic injuries has significantly declined as a result of the development of regional trauma centers and improved training in the care of trauma patients.[2,3] The first descriptions of pharmacy services provided in the ED appeared in the 1970s.[4-6] These early reports detail services primarily related to medication distribution. Since that time, the literature has detailed the development of EM pharmacy services as they evolved to address changing needs in the ED.[7-23] In recent years, the number of EM pharmacists (EMPs) has dramatically increased,[24] likely as a result of several factors, including an increased focus on preventing medication errors in the ED and the EMP's role in error prevention, changing medication management standards from regulatory and accrediting agencies, and emerging literature on a variety of critical illnesses that emphasizes the need for early, goal-directed therapy. Furthermore, initial research indicates that ED health care providers highly value the services provided by EMPs.[25]

Purpose

In 2008, ASHP published a statement on services that the pharmacy department should provide to the ED.[26] These guidelines extend beyond the scope of that document and are intended to define the role of the EMP, to suggest goals for providing services to meet institution-specific needs, and to establish a definition of best practices for the ED. These guidelines are based on the primary literature, therapeutic and practice guidelines, national standards, and the consensus of experts in the field of EM pharmacy practice.

Two levels of EMP services are described: essential services, which should be the basis of the practice specialty, and desirable services, which would optimize pharmacotherapy outcomes through the highest level of practice, teaching, and research and should be considered in addition to essential services. The services are further delineated by either a direct patient care or an administrative focus.

The services provided by EMPs will depend on the level of services provided by the ED. Optimal EMP coverage would provide consistent pharmacy services through a physical presence in the ED 24 hours per day, seven days per week. However, such coverage is not possible in every institution, nor may it be ideal based on institutional needs. Coverage and services provided by EMPs will therefore vary from institution to institution and should be designed to best meet the needs of the institution's emergency and pharmacy departments. In concert with ED and pharmacy administrators and providers, each EMP should use his or her professional judgment to individually weigh the factors that determine which services should be provided. These factors include the patient populations served, the number of pharmacists and time dedicated to services provided to the ED, whether corresponding duties are required of EMPs in other areas of the hospital, and the extent of time provided for administrative duties and obligations outside the ED. Finally, it should be noted that the many services described in these guidelines could not be provided by a single EMP. When used in these guidelines, the phrase "the EMP" should not be interpreted to imply that a single EMP could or should be expected to provide every service detailed herein.

The target audience for these guidelines includes EMPs, health-system administrators, physicians, emergency nurses and other emergency clinical staff, accreditors, and regulators. In addition, pharmacists and health-system administrators may find these guidelines helpful in establishing new pharmacy services in the ED. Because some of these readers may not require as much detail as others, the services are briefly summarized in Appendix A. Those seeking more information should consult the appended list of recommended readings, references, and resources (Appendix B).

Essential Direct Patient Care Roles of EMPs

The essential direct patient care roles of EMPs include optimizing medication use through participation in direct patient care rounds, medication order review, medication therapy monitoring, participation in procedures that utilize high-risk medications, resuscitation, medication procurement and preparation, provision of medication information, and documentation of associated interventions.

Direct Patient Care Rounds. Because the large majority of medication errors occur in the prescribing and administration phases of the medication-use process, it is critical for EMPs to be involved in direct patient care activities, including medication selection and the prescribing process.[22,27-29] For the purposes of these guidelines, rounding is broadly defined as conducting bedside patient care evaluations; working as a visible, well-integrated member of the multidisciplinary ED team; and participating in traditional rounding services when applicable (e.g., in EDs with EM residency programs for physicians). When conducting patient care rounds, EMPs should focus on providing direct patient care; they will be most effective in doing this when physically present in the ED. EMPs, in collaboration with other ED providers, should be accountable for ensuring optimized medication therapy regimens and therapeutic outcomes based on emerging literature, treatment guidelines, and quality measures established by accrediting bodies. Depending on the number of patients seen in the ED and the number of pharmacists dedicated to the ED, EMPs should create a triage system to focus their patient care efforts on patients with critical illnesses or urgent needs, on high-risk patient populations, or on specific classes of medications most associated with medication errors.

Medication Order Review. Medication order review in the ED must comply with federal, state, and local regulations and accreditation requirements. The Joint Commission's stan-

dards state that all medication orders should undergo prospective order review by a pharmacist prior to administration of the medication to the patient, with three exceptions: (1) in an emergency situation, (2) if a delay in administration would harm the patient, and (3) if a licensed independent practitioner is present to oversee the ordering, preparation, and administration of the medication.[30] Although many medication orders in the ED fall under the above exceptions, the level of assessment during medication order review should be consistent with that provided for patients elsewhere in the hospital. The process through which ED medication orders are reviewed should be determined by each institution based on its needs, staffing structure, and systems, as well as the interpretation of requirements by regulatory and accrediting organizations.

The role of an EMP in medication order review will vary, depending on the number of patient visits per day, particularly during peak patient utilization; the hours of EMP coverage; and the method of medication order entry. The role of an EMP should not focus on the medication order review process alone but rather should parallel the role of other pharmacy specialists providing direct patient care services within the institution.[24,31–33] A process should be developed to ensure that other pharmacists are accountable to review those orders that are not reviewed by an EMP.[3] Medication order review by EMPs may be performed in a manner other than traditional medication order review. When at the bedside, an EMP is able to quickly complete a review of medication orders and make medication selection and dosing recommendations based on patient-specific factors. Having a physical presence in the ED provides EMPs with the information needed to prioritize patient orders based on need and time demands. To allow EMPs to review medication orders while maintaining a physical presence in the ED, institutions should consider employing portable hand-held technology for use by the ED patient care team, including EMPs.

The majority of medication orders in the ED are one-time orders, so an EMP's intervention is most valuable if performed prior to medication administration. Ideally, all orders for high-risk medications would receive prospective review, but optimal medication use in the ED requires a balance between ensuring patient safety and preventing delays in patient care. EMPs should develop a triage system to focus the medication order review process on high-risk medications, high-risk patient populations, and emergent situations. When evaluating medication orders, EMPs should focus on key factors such as appropriateness of the medication and dose, potential medication interactions, and patient-specific factors (e.g., age, weight, medication allergies, disease states, current clinical condition).[30] If time and other patient care activities allow, EMPs may be involved in the review process of routine medication orders, including cost-saving initiatives, formulary compliance, and therapeutic substitutions.

In an institution with computerized provider order entry (CPOE), centrally located or designated pharmacists could work collaboratively with the EMP to assist in the medication order review process for routine ED medication orders, as well as admitting orders for boarded patients. If time permits, EMP participation in CPOE medication database maintenance should also be considered. In an institution that relies on written medication orders, a process should be developed to address the medication order review process through collaboration between the pharmacy and emergency

departments. An alert system should be developed to notify the EMP to any medication orders requiring immediate pharmacist intervention, while all other routine medication orders would be sent to the central pharmacy for review, processing, and preparation.

Medication Therapy Monitoring. The development and assessment of monitoring parameters related to medication therapy are essential steps in the medication-use process; they will determine whether the therapy selected was safe and effective, was suboptimal, or failed and whether changes to the regimen are needed. Research on pharmacist participation in monitoring medication therapy has demonstrated improved clinical outcomes in a variety of settings, including the treatment, management, and monitoring of chronic disease states such as diabetes mellitus, hypertension, and hyperlipidemia, and from therapeutic medication monitoring of antimicrobial and anticoagulant therapy in the hospital setting.[34–37]

Several medication classes administered in the ED exert an immediate therapeutic effect and therefore can be monitored shortly after administration. EMPs should be familiar with the pharmacokinetic parameters of medications commonly administered in the ED, as well as the recommended monitoring parameters associated with each therapeutic agent. Monitoring should also be provided for medications the patient has taken prior to arrival in the ED, whether administered by emergency medical services or by the patient as part of a home medication regimen. Medication therapy monitoring should include both subjective (e.g., patient-reported pain score) and objective (e.g., blood pressure, heart rate) elements.

EMPs should provide recommendations for monitoring parameters for both the effectiveness and safety of medications administered in the ED. Much of this assessment can be completed by EMPs and used in combination with information gathered from the patient's medical record. EMPs should subsequently suggest revisions to medication regimens based on the results of monitoring parameters and the established goals for therapy. In addition, EMPs should incorporate medication therapy monitoring parameters in the development of treatment protocols used in the ED, and they may provide education to other health care providers regarding appropriate monitoring of medication therapies.

Patient Care Involving High-Risk Medications and Procedures. A number of high-risk medications and procedures are utilized in the ED. A procedure may be considered high risk for a variety of reasons. Procedures performed on patients considered at high risk due to critical illness or instability may qualify, or the procedure may involve medications with a narrow therapeutic index or with serious potential for adverse effects (i.e., high-alert medications).[38] EMPs should be present at the bedside to assist in the delivery of patient care involving high-risk medications or procedures. Participation should include assisting in the appropriate selection of medications and corresponding doses, preparation of medications, and patient monitoring.

EMPs should also participate in efforts to improve the safety of procedures that utilize high-risk medications. EMPs should evaluate current processes associated with the use of high-risk medications and should assist in the development of processes and systems to improve current practices and prevent potential harm and errors. The EMP's role may

include assisting in the development of policies and protocols, with a focus on appropriate medication selection, use, monitoring, and management. Several recommendations for reducing errors associated with high-risk medications and procedures have been suggested.[29,39–41] For example, use of medication infusion systems with smart infusion technology software and double checks on high-alert medications may be considered.[39,40] In addition, EMPs should provide education and training related to high-risk medications to ED health care providers.

Resuscitation. EMPs should be present during all resuscitations in the ED. Initial evaluations of the role of EMPs in the resuscitation of trauma patients have revealed improved patient safety by decreasing preventable adverse medication events and expedited time to medication administration.[7,42–44] The role of EMPs in resuscitation may vary, depending on such factors as the clinical scenario or the practice setting, but may involve preparing medications for immediate administration; ensuring appropriate medication selection and dose; ensuring appropriate administration of medications; obtaining medications that are not readily available in the ED; making recommendations for alternative routes of administration when appropriate; answering medication information questions; assisting physicians with differential diagnosis, particularly when related to a potential medication-related cause; and completing resuscitation documentation.[45,46] In addition, EMPs should ensure that processes are in place to maintain an appropriate and readily available supply of emergency medications in the ED.

Toxicologic emergencies present resuscitation scenarios in which the knowledge of EMPs is highly valuable. Pharmacist involvement in toxicologic emergencies has been described for more than 30 years.[47,48] EMPs should be familiar with the recognition and treatment of patients experiencing a toxicologic emergency, including recognition of characteristic physical signs and symptoms noted in the physical examination, laboratory parameters, and other diagnostic evaluations (e.g., toxidromes), that can result from a wide range of substances, including prescription and over-the-counter medications, illicit drugs, natural occurring poisons (e.g., those from plants, mushrooms, or envenomations), and various chemicals.[49] When a patient with a suspected toxicologic emergency presents to the ED, EMPs should assist in obtaining a thorough and accurate medication history and a history of present illness, as well as in identifying potential causative agents; should assist in the selection and administration of specific antidotes and other supportive therapies; may assist in the preparation of antidotes; and should provide recommendations for monitoring antidote effectiveness and safety. These services should be provided in collaboration with clinical and medical toxicologists, when available, or local and regional poison control centers. Finally, EMPs should serve as a resource to the pharmacy department in ensuring that an adequate inventory of toxicologic antidotes is available in the institution.[50]

In preparing to become a member of the resuscitation team, EMPs should seek out training and certification in the conditions applicable to their practice settings. Several training opportunities and certification programs are available, including but not limited to the American Stroke Association National Institutes of Health Stroke Scale, American Heart Association (AHA) Basic Life Support (BLS), AHA Advanced Cardiac Life Support (ACLS), AHA Pediatric Advanced Life Support (PALS), American College of Surgeons Advanced Trauma Life Support, American Academy of Clinical Toxicology Advanced HAZMAT Life Support (AHLS), and board certification as a Diplomate of the American Board of Applied Toxicology (DABAT). At a minimum, all EMPs should achieve and maintain up-to-date certification in BLS, ACLS, and PALS.

Medication Procurement and Preparation. Medication procurement in the ED presents challenges that differ significantly from those in other areas of the hospital. Because of the urgent treatment needs of patients in the ED, several critical medications must be readily available. EMPs should be an integral part of the medication procurement and preparation process for medications used in the ED, as dispensing medications is one of the five stages of the medication-use process that EMPs can impact to prevent medication errors.[29] EMPs may serve as consultants to the pharmacy department and ED regarding the development or revision of processes associated with medication procurement, or they may play a more active role in medication procurement and preparation.

The options available for medication procurement vary widely among EDs and depend on such factors as patient volume and acuity, the physical limitations of the ED, and processes established by the pharmacy department. Medications may be available in automated dispensing cabinets, in emergency kits, from the inpatient central pharmacy department, or from a satellite pharmacy within the ED. A satellite pharmacy with compounding ability may best serve the needs of an ED by providing prompt preparation of medications, though this is not considered a requirement. While a sterile room for preparation of intravenous medications may not be a possibility for most EDs, a laminar flow hood would aid in the preparation of most intravenous medication requests. In an ED with no satellite pharmacy, the central pharmacy should have processes in place to assist with rapid preparation and delivery of medications.[26] In this model, EMPs should work with the central pharmacy to ensure understanding of urgent medication needs. Finally, EMPs should be competent and responsible for preparation of medications needed for emergency use at the bedside as an exception to the *United States Pharmacopeia* 797 standards.[51] Competency should include methods of compounding, knowledge of potential medication interactions, intravenous medication compatibility, rates of administration, and skill in using references on these topics.

A full review of medications used in the ED, including commonly used medications, high-risk medications, and antidotes, should be performed regularly (e.g., annually or as required by institution policy). EMPs should be involved in the decision-making process regarding which medications will be made available immediately within the ED.[52] Medications identified as appropriate and necessary for frequent use in the ED should be stored in automated dispensing cabinets or another location as designated safe by the institution, with appropriate alerts to prevent medication errors.[52] EMPs may assist in the evaluation and management of these medications, including monitoring for appropriate usage, inventory levels, and medication storage according to both hospital and regulatory body requirements. Optimization of available medications should be based on changes in prescribing practices, guideline or protocol recommendations,

medication availability, and formulary changes. Inventory and storage replacement should be maintained by technician support and should not be the responsibility of EMPs.

Finally, EMPs should be involved with the institution's formulary review and process-improvement committees to assist with medication reviews of new formulary agents and for revisions to the current formulary regarding medications used in the ED. Further, data from medication-use evaluations, safety monitoring, and monitoring for adherence to national quality indicators should be used to assist in evaluating medication procurement and preparation processes.

Medication Information. The most common cause of medication errors is a lack of information related to medication therapy.[53] Provision of medication information is therefore a vital role in the practice of all pharmacists, including EMPs. Numerous studies in the ED demonstrate that medication information is an important service provided by EMPs.[9,10,25,54] A survey of pharmacy departments revealed that only 50.4% of respondents provide medication information services to the ED.[54] In addition, ED health care providers report that they are more likely to utilize the resources of a pharmacist when that pharmacist is located in the ED rather than the central pharmacy department.[25] These statistics suggest a strong role in medication information for the EMP.

The medication information needs of the ED cover a broad spectrum of clinical scenarios and may include questions related to medication selection, dose, and administration; adverse medication reactions; intravenous compatibility; medication interactions; and identification of unknown medications.[55] EMPs should ensure that access to appropriate primary, secondary, and tertiary references is available as needed to respond to medication information requests. EMPs must be able to quickly and accurately retrieve the answers to medication information questions using readily available resources, programs for personal digital assistants, textbooks, or electronic resources to provide urgently needed medication information.

Documentation. Research on pharmacist interventions in the inpatient setting has demonstrated improvement in patient outcomes through optimized pharmacotherapy regimens, improved monitoring of medication therapy, and avoidance of adverse medication events.[36] In addition, pharmacist participation in patient care has been shown to significantly reduce the costs associated with medication therapy.[56,57] Research has detailed EMP interventions in the ED, describing improvements to the medication-use process and patient care by EMPs recommending improvements in medication therapy, serving as a medication information resource, and improving patient safety.[4,5,9,11,13,18,20,22,58] Several of these publications have shown dramatic cost avoidance.[8,17,19,21,23] More detailed studies on the role of EMPs in managing specific disease states and a definitive evaluation of improvement in patient outcomes are needed.

EMPs should be diligent in documenting interventions provided during patient care and other activities (e.g., education). They should regularly review intervention documentation to identify trends, which may indicate a need to educate ED health care providers or change medication-use procedures. Finally, cost-avoidance documentation may provide the justification needed for further expansion of EMP services.

Health care institutions should support EMPs by providing the means to document interventions. Different media have been used to document interventions, including personal digital assistants, software programs on institutional intranets, and manual paper systems.[59-64] Electronic systems offer more complete, readily retrievable documentation and shorter entry times than manual systems, without the risk of loss associated with paper records.[65,66] In addition, electronic documentation systems offer the benefit of associating cost avoidance with the documented intervention.[19] Although determining true cost avoidance can be difficult, there is research available to provide some guidance for quantifying the cost avoidance of pharmacist interventions.[6,10,56,57,67-69] In addition to these benefits, electronic documentation of EMP interventions may improve communication with other health care providers caring for the patient after admission (e.g., "hand-off") if the documentation system allows the documentation to follow the patient.

Desirable Direct Patient Care Roles of EMPs

Desirable direct patient care roles of EMPs include the care of boarded patients, obtaining medication histories, and medication reconciliation.

Care of Boarded Patients. ED overcrowding is a common occurrence.[70,71] Not only are more patients seeking primary care services in the ED, but a significant number of EDs have closed over the past decade, increasing ED patient volumes.[72,73] Because there are many obstacles and processes that hinder the timely transfer of admitted patients from the ED to an inpatient bed,[74] overcrowding in the ED often results in bottlenecks that force EDs to provide care to patients for long periods of time while they await admission or physical transfer to an inpatient bed or to another institution for a different level of care ("boarding").[75] The needs of a boarded patient can vary from simple requests for as-needed medications to such complex needs as critical care management.

Processes should be developed, based on institutional resources, to designate the pharmacist who will be accountable for providing care to boarded patients (i.e., an EMP or the pharmacist assigned to the area to which the patient will be admitted). The EMP's primary role in ensuring the safety and effectiveness of the medication-use process of the ED should not be compromised to provide care for boarded patients if alternatives exist. When staffing levels are insufficient (e.g., when only a single EMP is present in the ED) or when the boarding area is physically separated from the ED, the responsibility of caring for boarded patients should be assigned to the inpatient pharmacist. (Ideally, to ensure continuity of care, the inpatient pharmacist would be the same pharmacist responsible for providing care to the patient after admission.) The services provided to boarded patients by EMPs will depend on the level of services offered by the institution. At a minimum, EMPs should review the medication profile of critical patients, with a focus on high-risk medications, medication dosing and procurement, and monitoring, as necessary. When it is necessary to initiate an admitting order for a boarded patient, the responsible pharmacist should review medications administered in the ED and those taken prior to arrival at the ED to prevent duplications in therapy.

Medication Histories and Medication Reconciliation.
Research on medication reconciliation has identified several barriers to obtaining an accurate medication history in the ED.[76-82] In many cases, ED staff are required to contact multiple sources, including primary care physician offices, pharmacies, and family members, to obtain a medication history, and even these burdensome efforts may not result in an accurate home medication list. There have been significant changes in medication reconciliation practices, with the most recent recommendations from The Joint Commission that complete medication reconciliation needs only be performed by the receiving unit for patients admitted to the hospital and that "screening" reconciliations be performed in the ED, unless otherwise requested by the treating physician.[30]

Although research has shown that pharmacists are the providers who obtain the most accurate home medication list,[83-85] dedicating a pharmacist solely to medication reconciliation is not the best allocation of pharmacist resources in the ED. EMPs should assist in the development and implementation of a risk-stratification protocol for identifying and determining which ED patients need a medication history. In general, medication histories may be obtained for patients with known or suspected toxicologic emergencies, with known or suspected adverse events from home medications, or with complicated medication histories that will influence ED clinical decision-making.

Auxiliary pharmacy staff (pharmacy students hired through work/study programs and pharmacy technicians) can also be effective in obtaining accurate home medication histories; when possible, they should be incorporated into medication reconciliation procedures.[86-89] Quality reviews of medication histories completed by pharmacy technicians should be conducted to assess accuracy and to provide guidance for further training opportunities.

Essential Administrative Roles of EMPs

The administrative duties of EMPs will vary, depending on such factors as the availability of other EMPs to provide direct patient care activities in the ED or to distribute committee involvement among other EMPs. The essential administrative roles of EMPs include involvement in medication and patient safety initiatives, quality-improvement activities, professional leadership, and emergency preparedness.

For EMPs to succeed in fulfilling their administrative responsibilities without compromising patient care in the ED, pharmacy management must provide support that will allow EMPs to participate in committee meetings, pursue related projects, and develop proposals with action plans. Ideally, another pharmacist would be made available to provide coverage for direct patient care activities in the ED.

Medication and Patient Safety. EMPs play an important role in monitoring and ensuring patient and medication safety in the ED. The environment of the ED is naturally at high risk for patient and medication safety lapses. EMPs should encourage and assist in maintaining a safe environment for medication and patient safety, which should be continuously reviewed for potential process improvements. This review can include proactive and continuous monitoring of medication practices; identification of errors and high-risk medications for monitoring; addressing hazardous conditions with poten-

tial for harm; and documentation and review of medication errors, adverse medication events, and near misses.[22,27,28,90]

Medication errors that occur in the ED should be reviewed by EMPs in collaboration with other health care providers and hospital executives to identify potential sources of error, contributing factors related to the error, and potential solutions for preventing similar errors. Performance of a root cause analysis could identify potential error trends or system failures and contribute to the development of safe medication practices and processes for prevention of future events. In addition, a review of medication errors should result in education and future policy or guideline development. Finally, EMPs should be responsible for the development and provision of education to ED health care providers on the source of the error, the risks associated with the error, and ways to prevent similar errors in the future.

Quality-Improvement Initiatives. As a practitioner in the ED setting, an EMP is able to recognize those aspects of patient care, medication safety, compliance with hospital and regulatory policies, and adherence to national practice recommendations and guidelines that could be improved. EMPs or other pharmacy representatives should be extensively involved with quality-improvement initiatives in the ED. Involvement with a multidisciplinary committee of ED health care providers and hospital administrators will provide EMPs with an avenue for improving the quality of care in the ED.

EMPs should participate in ongoing efforts to optimize pharmacotherapy regimens through medication-use evaluations and through the development and implementation of medication-use guidelines and pathways. A medication-use evaluation may be beneficial in reviewing medications commonly used in the ED, as well as those medications associated with errors.[91,92] The results of a medication-use evaluation can be used to further guide education for other ED health care providers.

Leadership Duties and Professional Service. The leadership role of EMPs should include responsibilities to both the pharmacy department and ED. Involvement in administrative processes of both departments allows EMPs to serve as a liaison between the groups to support joint endeavors. This role would ideally include participation in departmental meetings, medication-use committees, quality-improvement and process-improvement committees, medication safety committees, and research meetings for both departments. Involvement in such meetings ensures that the needs of both departments are met and provides EMPs with an avenue for improving both patient care and medication use. In addition, involvement in ED-specific research projects increases pharmacy involvement, pharmacy publication and recognition, and grant funding potential.

Membership and active participation in local, state, and national professional pharmacy organizations are essential for the continued growth of the practice of EM pharmacy. As a relatively young area of practice, EM pharmacy is continually developing and growing. One way to support this development and strengthen the presence of EM pharmacy is through participation in professional organizations. At the local level, EMPs may collaborate to develop a local support network for training and research and can provide new practitioners with avenues for learning. At the state

level, legislative and professional advocacy may help educate government officials and other health care professionals about EM pharmacy practice. At the national level, collaboration among EMPs increases the strength as a group, serves to challenge existing programs to improve, assists new programs in their development, and allows collaboration as a group to affect the stature, practice, and further development of EM pharmacy practice. A final source of support for the development of the profession is involvement with national EM organizations. Traditionally designed for physicians, nurses, and emergency medical technicians, EM organizations provide an avenue for education, networking, and publication for EMPs.

Emergency Preparedness. As experts in pharmacology and toxicology, EMPs have the skills and knowledge to serve as active participants in emergency situations, such as natural disasters; disease outbreaks; biological, radiological, or chemical exposures; and acts of terrorism. It is essential that EMPs, in conjunction with the department of pharmacy, participate in emergency preparedness planning.[93,94] Planning and involvement should occur at a minimum at the institutional level, with participation potentially expanding to include local, state, and national emergency preparedness efforts. Knowledge of local, state, and national emergency preparedness plans, programs, and support systems is paramount in the development of institution-specific emergency preparedness plans. These plans and programs should be used to develop recommendations and policies regarding decontamination, medication acquisition, stockpiles, storage, distribution, and use.[93]

Actively participating in emergency preparedness events will strengthen the knowledge and skills EMPs need to effectively lead in emergency situations. EMPs and executives in the pharmacy department should work together in the development of pharmacy-specific plans to coincide with institution-specific plans. Education of ED and pharmacy staff related to emergency preparedness should be among the responsibilities of EMPs.

To further develop strengths in emergency preparedness, EMPs should seek out training and certification in emergency preparedness, such as certification for AHLS, Basic Disaster Life Support, Advanced Disaster Life Support, and the National Incident Management System.

Desirable Administrative Roles of EMPs

Education of pharmacists and other health care providers, pharmacy students and residents, and ED patients and their caregivers and participation in research are desirable administrative roles for EMPs.

Education. The role of EMPs in education can be variable and broad, and it has been mentioned in conjunction with other responsibilities throughout these guidelines. It is desirable for EMPs to participate in the education of other health care providers, including pharmacists and pharmacy staff, pharmacy students, pharmacy residents, physicians, medical residents, midlevel practitioners, nurses, and emergency medical support personnel. The types and levels of education will vary with patient care and administrative workload.

Provision of education to ED health care staff should, at a minimum, include information on the appropriate use of medications, improvement in quality and effective medication use, and patient and medication safety. Education may include formal sessions (e.g., in-service or didactic presentation at a conference) or participation in courses such as BLS, ACLS, or PALS. Participation in formal education sessions may strengthen the relationship with other ED health care providers and serves as a method of continuous learning for EMPs. Informal education may also be provided through interaction in the ED, particularly at the bedside, which is a time-efficient, effective tool for education of staff.

Participation in the didactic and experiential education of doctor of pharmacy students is also a desirable activity that supports the development of the profession. Precepting pharmacy residents in EM learning experiences supports the overall development of direct patient care practitioners and provides exposure to the practice of EM pharmacy. To support the continued development of EM pharmacy services, the development of EM residency training programs is highly desirable. With the expansion of EM pharmacy service locations and hours and the increasing role of EMPs in administrative activities, the need for additional qualified pharmacists increases. New EMPs should focus on developing current services with plans to develop advanced (e.g., postgraduate year two) residency training programs after the program is established and the practice experience is significant. Additionally, education and development of currently practicing pharmacists are desirable, as education and development of existing pharmacists will provide additional EMP coverage.

Having medication therapy expertise, EMPs are uniquely qualified to provide medication education and information to patients and their caregivers in the ED and should play a key role in the delivery of medication information. In some cases, the education of ED patients and their families and caregivers may be independently considered among the essential roles of the EMP. EMPs may develop a system of triage for patient education so that counseling is focused on patients who will be discharged from the ED with a new or high-risk medication or on patients whose visit to the ED was the result of a medication adverse event or error. In addition to developing a triage system for identifying the patients with the greatest need for education, EMPs may also rely on other ED health care providers to identify patients in need of medication education. The medication education provided to patients and caregivers in the ED is diverse and may include information related to the use of a new device, the importance of medication adherence, or a potential adverse medication event. Education can include oral or written materials and should be documented in the patient's medical record. EMPs should confirm patient and caregiver understanding of the medication education provided.

Research and Scholarly Activity. The Institute of Medicine has described three aspects of emergency care research.[95] These aspects include EM research, defined as research conducted in either the prehospital or ED setting by EM specialists; trauma and injury control research, defined as the research of the acute management of traumatic injury; and research contributions that affect the ED but are attributed to other practice specialties. EM research can be further subdivided into basic science, clinical, and health services research. A number of research priorities in the prehospital and ED settings have been described.[96–100]

There is also an urgent need for research in EM pharmacy, both for pharmacotherapy and pharmacy practice. Such research would be facilitated by the development of a practice-based research network, which is a group of practitioners located locally, regionally, or nationally that collaborates on pursuits of scholarly activity.[101] Practice research networks can be effective, as a larger group of researchers represents a larger patient population that is more diverse than a single medical center. Practice-based research networks have been successful in other areas of practice and among a wide variety of health care practitioners, including interdisciplinary health care teams.

The role of the pharmacist in research has been described and can be applied to the ED setting.[102,103] EMPs may participate in ongoing clinical and practice-based research being conducted in the institution, including identifying a research question, providing assistance with patient recruitment and randomization, assisting with research medications, and completing data collection and analysis. EMPs could also assist in securing funding for conducting research in the ED, and, after the completion of research projects, EMPs could participate in the scholarly activities related to research efforts.

Conclusion

EMPs provide many vital services within the ED. The central role of the EMP is to improve patient outcomes by improving patient safety, preventing medication errors, and providing optimized pharmacotherapy regimens and therapeutic outcomes through participation in direct patient care activities and quality-improvement initiatives in the ED. In addition, EMPs can provide education to members of the pharmacy department and other health care providers, as well as patients and their caregivers, and EMPs may participate in research and scholarly activities in the ED.

References

1. Institute of Medicine of the National Academies Committee on the Future of Emergency Care in the United States Health System. Historical development of hospital-based emergency and trauma care. In: Hospital-based emergency care: at the breaking point. Washington, DC: National Academy Press; 2006:353–64.
2. Cales RH, Trunkey DD. Preventable trauma deaths. A review of trauma care systems development. *JAMA.* 1985; 254:1059–63.
3. Gruen RL, Jurkovich GJ, McIntyre LK, et al. Patterns of errors contributing to trauma mortality: lessons learned from 2,594 deaths. *Ann Surg.* 2006; 244:371–80.
4. Elenbaas RM, Waeckerle JF, McNabney WK. The clinical pharmacist in emergency medicine. *Am J Hosp Pharm.* 1977; 34:843–6.
5. Elenbaas RM. Role of the pharmacist in providing clinical pharmacy services in the emergency department. *Can J Hosp Pharm.* 1978; 31:123–5.
6. Spigiel RW, Anderson RJ. Comprehensive pharmaceutical services for the emergency room. *Am J Hosp Pharm.* 1979; 36:52–6.
7. Patanwala AE, Hays D. Pharmacist's activities on a trauma response team in the emergency department. *Am J Health-Syst Pharm.* 2010; 67:1536–8.
8. Fairbanks RJ, Hays DP, Webster DF, et al. Clinical pharmacy services in an emergency department. *Am J Health-Syst Pharm.* 2004; 61:934–7.
9. Wymore ES, Casanova TJ, Broekemeier RL, et al. Clinical pharmacist's daily role in the emergency department of a community hospital. *Am J Health-Syst Pharm.* 2008; 65:395–6, 398–9.
10. Whalen FJ. Cost justification of decentralized pharmaceutical services for the emergency room. *Am J Hosp Pharm.* 1981; 38:684–7.
11. Culbertson V, Anderson RJ. Pharmacist involvement in emergency room services. *Contemp Pharm Pract.* 1981; 4:167–76.
12. Powell MF, Solomon DK, McEachen RA. Twenty-four hour emergency pharmaceutical services. *Am J Hosp Pharm.* 1985; 42:831–5.
13. Kasuya A, Bauman JL, Curtis RA, et al. Clinical pharmacy on-call program in the emergency department. *Am J Emerg Med.* 1986; 4:464–7.
14. Schauben JL. Comprehensive emergency pharmacy services. *Top Hosp Pharm Manage.* 1988; 8:20–8.
15. Laivenieks N, McCaul K, O'Brodovich M. Clinical pharmacy services provided to an emergency department. *Can J Hosp Pharm.* 1992; 45:113–5.
16. Berry NS, Folstad JE, Bauman JL, et al. Clinical pharmacy services provided to an emergency department. *Ann Pharmacother.* 1992; 26:476–80.
17. Levy DB. Documentation of clinical and cost-saving pharmacy interventions in the emergency room. *Hosp Pharm.* 1993; 28:630–4, 653.
18. Mialon PJ, Williams P, Wiebe RA. Clinical pharmacy services in a pediatric emergency department. *Hosp Pharm.* 2004; 39:121–4.
19. Ling JM, Mike LA, Rubin J, et al. Documentation of pharmacist interventions in the emergency department. *Am J Health-Syst Pharm.* 2005; 62:1793–7.
20. Weant KA, Sterling E, Winstead PS, et al. Establishing a pharmacy presence in the ED. *Am J Emerg Med.* 2006; 24:514–5.
21. Lada P, Delgado G Jr. Documentation of pharmacists' interventions in an emergency department and associated cost avoidance. *Am J Health-Syst Pharm.* 2007; 64:63–8.
22. Brown JN, Barnes CL, Beasley B, et al. Effect of pharmacists on medication errors in an emergency department. *Am J Health-Syst Pharm.* 2008; 65:330–3.
23. Aldridge VE, Park HK, Bounthavong M, et al. Implementing a comprehensive, 24-hour emergency department pharmacy program. *Am J Health-Syst Pharm.* 2009; 66:1943–7.
24. Pederson CA, Schneider PJ, Scheckelhoff DJ. ASHP national survey of pharmacy practice in hospital settings: dispensing and administration—2008. *Am J Health-Syst Pharm.* 2009; 66:926–46.
25. Fairbanks RJ, Hildebrand JM, Kolstee KE, et al. Medical and nursing staff highly value clinical pharmacists in the emergency department. *Emerg Med J.* 2007; 24:716–8.
26. American Society of Health-System Pharmacists. ASHP statement on pharmacy services to the emer-

gency department. *Am J Health-Syst Pharm.* 2008; 65:2380–3.

27. Patanwala AE, Warholak TL, Sanders AB, et al. A prospective observational study of medication errors in a tertiary care emergency department. *Ann Emerg Med.* 2010; 55:522–6.

28. Flynn EA, Barker K, Barker B. Medication-administration errors in an emergency department. *Am J Health-Syst Pharm.* 2010; 67:347–8.

29. Peth HA. Medication errors in the emergency department: a systems approach to minimizing risk. *Emerg Med Clin N Am.* 2003; 21:141–58.

30. The Joint Commission. 2011 comprehensive accreditation manual for hospitals: the official handbook. Oakbrook Terrace, IL: Joint Commission Resources; 2011.

31. Bond CA, Raehl CL, Franke T. Clinical pharmacy services and hospital mortality rates. *Pharmacotherapy.* 1999; 19:556–64.

32. Bond CA, Raehl CL. Clinical pharmacy services, pharmacy staffing, and hospital mortality rates. *Pharmacotherapy.* 2007; 27:481–93.

33. Bond CA, Raehl CL. Clinical pharmacy services, pharmacy staffing, and adverse drug reactions in United States hospitals. *Pharmacotherapy.* 2006; 26:735–47.

34. Tully MP, Seston EM. Impact of pharmacists providing a prescription review and monitoring service in ambulatory care or community practice. *Ann Pharmacother.* 2000; 34:1320–31.

35. Coast-Senior EA, Kroner BA, Kelley CL, et al. Management of patients with type 2 diabetes by pharmacists in primary care clinics. *Ann Pharmacother.* 1998; 32:636–41.

36. Kaboli PJ, Hoth AB, McClimon BJ, et al. Clinical pharmacist and inpatient medical care: a systematic review. *Arch Intern Med.* 2006; 166:955–64.

37. Chisholm-Burns MA, Graff Zivin JS, Lee JK, et al. Economic effects of pharmacists on health outcomes in the United States: a systematic review. *Am J Health-Syst Pharm.* 2010; 67:1624–34.

38. Institute for Safe Medication Practices. ISMP's list of high-alert medications (2008). www.ismp.org/Tools/highalertmedications.pdf (accessed 2010 Oct 20).

39. The Joint Commission. High-alert medications and patient safety. *Sentinel Event Alert.* 1999; 11:1–3.

40. Wilson K, Sullivan M. Preventing medication errors with smart infusion technology. *Am J Health-Syst Pharm.* 2004; 61:177–83.

41. Federico F. Preventing harm from high-alert medications. *Jt Comm J Qual Patient Saf.* 2007; 33:537–42.

42. Kalina M, Tinkoff G, Gleason W, et al. A multidisciplinary approach to adverse drug events in pediatric trauma patients in an adult trauma center. *Pediatr Emerg Care.* 2009; 25:444–6.

43. Kelly-Pisciotti SJ, Hays DP, O'Brien TE, et al. Pharmacists enhancing patient safety during trauma resuscitations. Presented at the American Society of Health-System Pharmacists Midyear Clinical Meeting. Las Vegas, NV: Dec 2009.

44. Acquisto NM, Hays DP, Fairbanks RJ, et al. The outcomes of emergency pharmacist participation during acute myocardial infarction. *J Emerg Med.*

Epub ahead of print. 2010 Aug 31 (DOI 10.1016/j.jemermed.2010.6.011).

45. Draper HM, Eppert JA. Association of pharmacist presence on compliance with advanced cardiac life support guidelines during in-hospital cardiac arrest. *Ann Pharmacother.* 2008; 42:469–74.

46. Shimp LA, Mason NA, Toedter NM, et al. Pharmacist participation in cardiopulmonary resuscitation. *Am J Health-Syst Pharm.* 1995; 52:980–4.

47. Czajka PA, Skoutakis VA, Wood GC, et al. Clinical toxicology consultation by pharmacists. *Am J Hosp Pharm.* 1979; 36:1087–9.

48. Roberts RW, Russell WL. A pharmacist-based toxicology service. 1978. *Ann Pharmacother.* 2007; 41:1719–24.

49. Bronstein AC, Spyker DA, Cantilena LR, et al. 2008 annual report of the American Association of Poison Control Centers' National Poison Data System (NPDA): 26th annual report. *Clin Tox.* 2009; 47:911–1084.

50. Dart RC, Borron SW, Caravati EM, et al. Expert consensus guidelines for stocking antidotes in hospitals that provide emergency care. *Ann Emerg Med.* 2009; 54:386–94.

51. U.S. Pharmacopeial Convention. USP <797> guidebook to pharmaceutical compounding—sterile preparations. 2nd ed. Rockville, MD: U.S. Pharmacopeial Convention; 2008.

52. American Society of Health-System Pharmacists. ASHP guidelines on the safe use of automated dispensing devices. *Am J Health-Syst Pharm.* 2010; 67:483–90.

53. Leape LL, Bates DW, Cullen DJ, et al. Systems analysis of adverse drug events. *JAMA.* 1995; 274:35–43.

54. Thomasset KB, Faris R. Survey of pharmacy services provision in the emergency department. *Am J Health-Syst Pharm.* 2003; 60:1561–4.

55. Rosenberg JM, Koumis T, Nathan JP, et al. Current status of pharmacist-operated drug information centers in the United States. *Am J Health-Syst Pharm.* 2004; 61:2023–32.

56. McMullin ST, Hennenfent JA, Ritchie DJ, et al. A prospective, randomized trial to assess the cost impact of pharmacist-initiated interventions. *Arch Intern Med.* 1999; 159:2306–9.

57. Kinky DE, Erush SC, Laskin MS, et al. Economic impact of a drug information service. *Ann Pharmacother.* 1999; 33:11–6.

58. Rothschild JM, Churchill W, Erickson A, et al. Medication errors discovered by emergency department pharmacists. *Ann Emerg Med.* 2010; 55:513–21.

59. Reilly JC, Wallace M, Campbell MM. Tracking pharmacist interventions with a hand-held computer. *Am J Health-Syst Pharm.* 2001; 58:158–61.

60. Silva MA, Tataronis GR, Maas B. Using personal digital assistants to document pharmacist cognitive services and estimate potential reimbursement. *Am J Health-Syst Pharm.* 2003; 60:911–5.

61. Simonian AI. Documenting pharmacist interventions on an intranet. *Am J Health-Syst Pharm.* 2003; 60:151–5.

62. Lau A, Balen RM, Lam R, et al. Using a personal digital assistant to document clinical pharmacy services in

an intensive care unit. *Am J Health-Syst Pharm.* 2001; 58:1229–32.

63. Bosinski TJ, Campbell L, Schwartz S. Using a personal digital assistant to document pharmacotherapeutic interventions. *Am J Health-Syst Pharm.* 2004; 61:931–4.

64. Mason RN, Pugh CB, Boyer SB, et al. Computerized documentation of pharmacists' interventions. *Am J Hosp Pharm.* 1994; 51:2131–8.

65. Schumock GT, Hutchinson RA, Bilek BA. Comparison of two systems for documenting pharmacist interventions in patient care. *Am J Hosp Pharm.* 1992; 49:2211–4.

66. Zimmerman CR, Smolarek RT, Stevenson JG. A computerized system to improve documentation and reporting of pharmacists' clinical interventions, cost savings, and workload activities. *Pharmacotherapy.* 1995; 15:220–7.

67. Mutnick AH, Sterba KJ, Peroutka JA, et al. Cost savings and avoidance from clinical interventions. *Am J Health-Syst Pharm.* 1997; 54:392–6.

68. Schneider PJ, Gift MG, Lee YP, et al. Cost of medication-related problems at a university hospital. *Am J Health-Syst Pharm.* 1995; 52:2415–8.

69. Kopp BJ, Mrsan M, Erstad BL, et al. Cost implications of and potential adverse events prevented by interventions of a critical care pharmacist. *Am J Health-Syst Pharm.* 2007; 64:2483–7.

70. Olshaker JS, Rathlev NK. Emergency department over-crowding and ambulance diversion: the impact and potential solutions of extended boarding of admitted patients in the emergency department. *J Emerg Med.* 2006; 30:351–6.

71. Andrulis DP, Kellermann A, Kintz EA, et al. Emergency departments and crowding in United States teaching hospitals. *Ann Emerg Med.* 1991; 20:980–6.

72. Brennan TA, Leape LL, Laird NM, et al. Incidence of adverse events and negligence in hospitalized patients: results of the Harvard medical practice study I. *New Engl J Med.* 1991; 324:370–6.

73. Weiss SJ, Ernst AA, Nick TG. Comparison of the national emergency department overcrowding scale and the emergency department work index for quantifying emergency department crowding. *Acad Emerg Med.* 2006; 13:513–8.

74. Kulstad EB, Sikka R, Sweis RT, et al. ED overcrowding is associated with an increased frequency of medication errors. *Am J Emerg Med.* 2010; 28:304–9.

75. American College of Emergency Physicians. Emergency department crowding: high impact solutions. www.acep.org/practres.aspx?id=32050 (accessed 2010 Oct 20).

76. Santel JP. Reconciliation failures lead to medication errors. *Jt Comm J Qual Patient Saf.* 2006; 32:225–9.

77. Tam VC, Knowles SR, Cornish PL, et al. Frequency, type, and clinical importance of medication history errors at admission to hospital: a systematic review. *Can Med Assoc J.* 2005; 173:510–5.

78. Cornish PL, Knowles SR, Marchesano R, et al. Unintended medication discrepancies at the time of hospital admission. *Arch Intern Med.* 2005; 165:424–9.

79. Gleason KM, Groszek JM, Sullivan C, et al. Reconciliation of discrepancies in medication histo-

ries and admission orders of newly hospitalized patients. *Am J Health-Syst Pharm.* 2004; 61:1689-95.

80. Miller SL, Miller S, Balon J, et al. Medication reconciliation in a rural trauma population. *Ann Emerg Med.* 2008; 52:483–91.

81. Schenkel S. The unexpected challenges of accurate medication reconciliation. *Ann Emerg Med.* 2008; 52:493–5.

82. Eppert HD, Eppert JA. In response to "the unexpected challenges of accurate medication reconciliation." *Ann Emerg Med.* 2009; 53:548–9.

83. Carter MK, Allin DM, Scott LA, et al. Pharmacist-acquired medication histories in a university hospital emergency department. *Am J Health-Syst Pharm.* 2006; 63:2500–3.

84. Reeder TA, Mutnick A. Pharmacist- versus physician-obtained medication histories. *Am J Health-Syst Pharm.* 2008; 65:857–60.

85. Nester TM, Hale LS. Effectiveness of a pharmacist-acquired medication history in promoting patient safety. *Am J Health-Syst Pharm.* 2002; 59:2221–5.

86. Lubowski TJ, Cronin LM, Pavelka RW, et al. Effectiveness of a medication reconciliation project conducted by PharmD students. *Am J Pharm Educ.* 2007; 71:94.

87. Mersfelder TL, Bickel RJ. Inpatient medication history verification by pharmacy students. *Am J Health-Syst Pharm.* 2008; 65:2273–5.

88. Michels RD, Meisel SB. Program using pharmacy technicians to obtain medication histories. *Am J Health-Syst Pharm.* 2003; 60:1982–6.

89. Hayes BD, Donovan JL, Smith BS, et al. Pharmacist-conducted medication reconciliation in an emergency department. *Am J Health-Syst Pharm.* 2007; 64:1720–3.

90. Ratz Y, Shafir I, Berkovitch S, et al. The importance of the pharmacist in reporting adverse drug reactions in the emergency department. *J Clin Pharm.* 2010; 50:1217–21.

91. American Society of Health-System Pharmacists. ASHP guidelines on medication-use evaluation. *Am J Health-Syst Pharm.* 1996; 53:1953–5.

92. American Society of Health-System Pharmacists. ASHP guidelines on the pharmacist's role in the development, implementation, and assessment of critical pathways. *Am J Health-Syst Pharm.* 2004; 61:939–45.

93. American Society of Health-System Pharmacists. ASHP statement on the role of health-system pharmacists in emergency preparedness. *Am J Health-Syst Pharm.* 2003; 60:1993–5.

94. Setlak P. Bioterrorism preparedness and response: emerging role for health-system pharmacists. *Am J Health-Syst Pharm.* 2004; 61:1167–75.

95. Institute of Medicine of the National Academies Committee on the Future of Emergency Care in the United States Health System. Enhancing the emergency care research base. In: Hospital-based emergency care: at the breaking point. Washington, DC: National Academy Press; 2006:291–320.

96. Aghababian RV, Barsan WG, Bickell WH, et al. Research directions in emergency medicine. *Am J Emerg Med.* 1996; 14:681–3.

97. Maio RF, Garrison HG, Spaite DW, et al. Emergency medical services outcomes project I (EMSOP I): prioritizing conditions for outcomes research. *Ann Emerg Med.* 1999; 33:423–32.

98. Seidel JS, Henderson D, Tittle S, et al. Priorities for research in emergency medical services for children: results of a consensus conference. *Ann Emerg Med.* 1999; 33:206–10.

99. Becker LB, Weisfeldt ML, Weil MH, et al. The PULSE initiative: scientific priorities and strategic planning for resuscitation research and life saving therapies. *Circulation.* 2002; 105:2562–70.

100. Hoyt DB, Holcomb J, Abraham E, et al. Working group on trauma research program summary report: National Heart Lung Blood Institute (NHLBI), National Institute of General Medical Sciences (NIGMS), and National Institute of Neurological Disorders and Stroke (NINDS) of the National Institutes of Health (NIH), and the Department of Defense (DOD). *J Trauma.* 2004; 57:410–5.

101. Lipowsi EE. Pharmacy practice-based networks: Why, what, who, and how. *J Am Pharm Assoc.* 2008; 48:142–52.

102. American Society of Hospital Pharmacists. ASHP statement on pharmaceutical research in organized health-care settings. *Am J Hosp Pharm.* 1991; 48:1781.

103. Fagan SC, Touchette D, Smith JA, et al. The state of science and research in clinical pharmacy. *Pharmacotherapy.* 2006; 26:1027–40.

Appendix A—Summary of Recommendations

Essential Direct Patient Care Roles of EMPs

Direct patient care rounds: It is critical for EMPs to be accountable for and involved in direct patient care activities, including medication selection and the prescribing process. EMPs should focus on providing direct patient care and will be most effective in doing this when physically present in the ED, working as visible and well-integrated members of the multidisciplinary ED team.

Medication order review: Review of medication orders in the ED should provide the same level of assessment provided to patients elsewhere in the hospital. The role of an EMP in medication order review will vary, depending on site-specific factors. The EMP should develop a triage system to focus the medication order review process on high-risk medications, high-risk patient populations, and emergent situations. The EMP must not be the sole party responsible for ensuring that medication order review occurs in the ED; the pharmacy department should ensure that adequate processes are in place to ensure that all medication orders are reviewed in compliance with federal, state, and local regulations and accreditation requirements. Each institution should strive to identify the optimal balance between accountability for prospective medication order review and direct patient care activities in the ED.

Medication therapy monitoring: EMPs should ensure that medication therapy administered in the ED is safe and ef-

fective by designing monitoring plans for medications administered both in the ED and prior to arrival. EMPs should subsequently provide recommendations for modifications to medication regimens based on the results of monitoring parameters and established goals for therapy.

Patient care involving high-risk medications and procedures: Whenever possible, EMPs should be present at the patient's bedside to assist in the delivery of patient care that utilizes high-risk medications or procedures. EMPs should review the use of high-risk medications in the ED and should assist in the development of processes and procedures to improve patient safety and avoid errors. In addition, EMPs should provide education to ED health care providers related to the use of high-risk medications.

Resuscitation: EMPs should be present during all resuscitations in the ED, including trauma, cardiopulmonary arrest, and toxicologic emergencies. In the resuscitation setting, EMPs should prepare medications for immediate administration, ensure the appropriate administration and dose of medications, obtain medications that are not readily available in the ED, make recommendations for alternative routes of medication administration, answer medication information questions, assist with differential diagnosis, and complete resuscitation documentation. EMPs should be familiar with the recognition and treatment of toxicologic emergencies and should assist in identifying causative agents, with the selection and administration of antidotes and other supportive therapies, and with recommendations for monitoring antidote therapy in conjunction with toxicologists and poison control centers. EMPs should seek training programs relevant to the conditions treated in their EDs.

Medication procurement and preparation: Although the role of EMPs will vary, depending on the needs and resources of the institution, EMPs should be an integral part of the medication procurement and preparation process in the ED. EMPs should be involved in selecting medications stocked in the ED, should ensure safe storage and usage of these medications, should ensure timely turnaround for medications obtained from the central pharmacy, and may assist in the preparation of urgently needed medications. EMPs should be involved with the institution's formulary review and process-improvement committees to assist with formulation of policies regarding medications used in the ED.

Medication information: Medication information is a vital role of EMPs. The medication information needs of the ED cover a broad spectrum of clinical scenarios and patient cases. EMPs should ensure access to appropriate primary, secondary, and tertiary references as needed to respond to medication information requests and must be able to quickly and accurately retrieve the answers to medication information questions using those resources.

Documentation: EMPs should document interventions provided in the ED to allow measurement of improvement in patient outcomes and potential cost avoidance. EMPs should regularly review intervention documentation to identify trends, which may indicate a need to educate ED health care providers or change medication-use procedures. Health care

institutions should support EMPs by providing means to document those interventions.

Desirable Direct Patient Care Roles of EMPs

Care of boarded patients: Based on institutional resources, processes should be developed to identify the pharmacist accountable for providing care to boarded patients. These processes should not compromise the EMP's primary role in ensuring safe and effective use of medications for new patients presenting to the ED. When possible, responsibility for the care of boarded patients should be assigned to the pharmacist who will be responsible for providing care to the patient after admission to ensure continuity of care. At a minimum, the responsible pharmacist should review the medication profile of critical patients, review any high-risk medications, assist with medication dosing, assist with medication procurement, and provide monitoring as necessary.

Medication histories and medication reconciliation: EMPs may assist in the development of a risk-stratification protocol for determining which medication histories will be obtained in the ED. In general, a focus on patients with known or suspected toxicologic emergencies, with known or suspected adverse events from home medication regimens, or with complicated medication histories that will influence ED clinical decision-making should be considered.

Essential Administrative Roles of EMPs

Medication and patient safety: In collaboration with physicians, nurses, and hospital executives, EMPs should assist in reporting medication errors, reviewing reported medication errors, and identifying error trends. EMPs should further assist in developing safe medication practices and processes for prevention of errors, assist in implementing system improvements, and provide staff education when needed.

Quality-improvement initiatives: EMPs or other pharmacy representatives should be extensively involved with quality-improvement initiatives in the ED. EMPs should participate in ongoing efforts to optimize pharmacotherapy regimens through medication-use evaluation and development of medication-use guidelines and pathways.

Leadership duties and professional service: The leadership duties and professional service of EMPs may include involvement at the hospital level, which provides EMPs with an avenue for improving both patient care and medication use. Involvement with local, state, and national professional pharmacy organizations, as well as with other professional health care organizations, will allow for collaboration, leading to further development of EM pharmacy practice and the role of the EMP as an integral member of the ED health care team.

Emergency preparedness: The role of EMPs in emergency preparedness should include education, training, and certification; knowledge of federal, state, and local emergency preparedness and response policies; involvement with institutional emergency preparedness policy development; planning of and participation in planned disaster drills; and education of pharmacy and ED staff.

Desirable Administrative Roles of EMPs

Education: It is desirable that EMPs provide education to fellow pharmacists; other health care providers; pharmacy students and residents; and ED patients, their families, and caregivers.

Research and scholarly activity: There is an urgent need for research in EM pharmacy, both for pharmacotherapy and pharmacy practice. EMPs can be valuable researchers in the ED and should be encouraged to participate in the completion of research projects and scholarly activities. The establishment of pharmacy practice research networks to facilitate the completion of pharmacy-based research projects in the ED setting should also be encouraged.

Appendix B—Recommended Readings, References, and Resources

The following list represents suggested readings that would be useful to readers and should be considered in addition to those references and resources provided in the guidelines. The suggested readings are categorized into applicable categories and are then listed in alphabetical order by the primary author. For additional resources related to specific areas of emergency medicine pharmacist (EMP) service development, implementation, and best practices, please refer to the ASHP Section of Clinical Specialists and Scientists Section Advisory Group on Emergency Care Internet Resource Center (www.ashp.org/EmergencyCare.aspx). In addition to these resources and references, interested parties should seek out relevant resources and references related to local, regional, state, and national regulatory and accrediting agencies.

Internet Resources

1. American Society of Health-System Emergency Medicine Pharmacist Practice Internet Resource Center. www.ashp.org/EmergencyCare.aspx
2. American Society of Health-System Pharmacy Medication Reconciliation Toolkit. www.ashp.org/Import/PRACTICEANDPOLICY/PracticeResourceCenters/PatientSafety/ASHPMedicationReconciliationToolkit_1.asp
3. Institute for Healthcare Improvement: Prevent Adverse Drug Events (Medication Reconciliation). www.ihi.org/IHI/Programs/Campaign/ADEsMedReconciliation.htm

Primary Literature

Initial descriptions of EMP services

1. Berry NS, Folstad JE, Bauman JL, et al. Follow-up observations on 24-hour pharmacotherapy services in the emergency department. *Ann Pharmacother.* 1992; 26:476–80.
2. Culbertson V, Anderson RJ. Pharmacist involvement in emergency room services. *Contemp Pharm Pract.* 1981; 4:164–76.
3. Elenbaas RM. Role of the pharmacist in providing clinical pharmacy services in the emergency department. *Can J Hosp Pharm.* 1978; 31:123–5.
4. Elenbaas RM, Waeckerle JF, McNabney WK. The clinical pharmacist in emergency medicine. *Am J Hosp Pharm.* 1977; 34:843–6.

5. High JL, Gill AW, Silvernale DJ. Clinical pharmacy in an emergency medicine setting. *Contemp Pharm Pract.* 1981; 4:227–30.

6. Kasuya A, Bauman JL, Curtis RA, et al. Clinical pharmacy on-call program in the emergency department. *Am J Emerg Med.* 1986; 4:464–7.

7. Laivenieks N, McCaul K, O'Brodovich M. Clinical pharmacy services provided to an emergency department. *Can J Hosp Pharm.* 1992; 45:113–5.

8. Powell MF, Solomon DK, McEachen RA. Twenty-four hour emergency pharmaceutical services. *Am J Hosp Pharm.* 1985; 42:831–5.

9. Schauben JL. Comprehensive emergency pharmacy services. *Top Hosp Pharm Manage.* 1988; 8:20–8.

10. Spigiel RW, Anderson RJ. Comprehensive pharmaceutical services in the emergency department. *Am J Hosp Pharm.* 1979; 36:52–6.

11. Whalen FJ. Cost justification of decentralized pharmaceutical services for the emergency room. *Am J Hosp Pharm.* 1981; 38:684–7.

12. Whalen FJ. Cost containment of emergency room prescriptions. *Am J Hosp Pharm.* 1982; 39:312–3.

Recent descriptions of EMP services

13. Aldridge VE, Park HK, Bounthavong M, et al. Implementing a comprehensive, 24-hour emergency department pharmacy program. *Am J Health-Syst Pharm.* 2009; 66:1943–7.

14. American Society of Health-System Pharmacists. ASHP statement on pharmacy services to the emergency department. *Am J Health-Syst Pharm.* 2008; 65:2380–3.

15. Bednall R, McRobbie D, Duncan J, et al. Identification of patients attending accident and emergency who may be suitable for treatment by a pharmacist. *Fam Pract.* 2003; 20:4–7.

16. Cohen V, Jellinek SP, Hatch A, et al. Effect of clinical pharmacists on care in the emergency department: a systematic review. *Am J Health-Syst Pharm.* 2009; 66:1353–61.

17. Fairbanks RJ, Hays DP, Webster DF, et al. Clinical pharmacy services in an emergency department. *Am J Health-Syst Pharm.* 2004; 61:934–7.

18. Fairbanks RJ, Hildebrand JM, Kolstee KE, et al. Medical and nursing staff highly value clinical pharmacists in the emergency department. *Emerg Med J.* 2007; 24:716–9.

19. Mialon PJ, Williams P, Wiebe RA. Clinical pharmacy services in a pediatric emergency department. *Hosp Pharm.* 2004; 39:121–4.

20. Patanwala AE, Hays D. Pharmacist's activities on a trauma response team in the emergency department. *Am J Health-Syst Pharm.* 2010; 67:1536–8.

21. Szczesiul JM, Fairbanks RJ, Hildebrand JM, et al. Survey of physicians regarding clinical pharmacy services in academic emergency departments. *Am J Health-Syst Pharm.* 2009; 66:576–9.

22. Thomasset KB, Faris R. Survey of pharmacy services provision in the emergency department. *Am J Health-Syst Pharm.* 2003; 60:1561–4.

23. Weant KA, Sterling E, Winstead PS, et al. Establishing a pharmacy presence in the ED. *Am J Emerg Med.* 2006; 24:514–5.

24. Witsil JC, Aazami R, Murtaza UI, et al. Strategies for implementing emergency department pharmacy services: results from the 2007 ASHP Patient Care Impact Program. *Am J Health-Syst Pharm.* 2010; 67:375–9.

25. Wymore ES, Casanova TJ, Broekemeirer RL, et al. Clinical pharmacist's daily role in the emergency department of a community hospital. *Am J Health-Syst Pharm.* 2008; 65:395–6, 398–9.

Resuscitation

26. Acquisto NM, Hays DP, Fairbanks RJ, et al. The outcomes of emergency pharmacist participation during acute myocardial infarction. *J Emerg Med.* 2010 [epub ahead of print 2010 Aug 31].

27. Draper HM, Eppert JA. Association of pharmacist presence on compliance with advanced cardiac life support guidelines during in-hospital cardiac arrest. *Ann Pharmacother.* 2008; 42:469–74.

28. Schwerman E, Schwartau N, Thompson CO, et al. The pharmacist as a member of the cardiopulmonary resuscitation team. *DICP.* 1973; 7:299–308.

29. Shimp LA, Mason NA, Toedter NM, et al. Pharmacist participation in cardiopulmonary resuscitation. *Am J Health-Syst Pharm.* 1995; 52:980–4.

Toxicology

30. Czajka PA, Skoutakis VA, Wood GC, et al. Clinical toxicology consultation by pharmacists. *Am J Hosp Pharm.* 1979; 36:1087–9.

31. Dart RC, Borron SW, Caravati EM, et al. Expert consensus guidelines for stocking antidotes in hospitals that provide emergency care. *Ann Emerg Med.* 2009; 54:386–94.

32. Roberts RW, Russell WL. A pharmacist-based toxicology service. 1978. *Ann Pharmacother.* 2007; 41:1719–24.

Automated medication dispensing systems

33. American Society of Health-System Pharmacists. ASHP guidelines on the safe use of automated dispensing devices. *Am J Health-Syst Pharm.* 2010; 67:483–90.

34. Conners GP, Hays D. Emergency department drug orders: does drug storage location make a difference? *Ann Emerg Med.* 2007; 50:414–8.

35. Gordon JO, Hadsall RS, Schommer JC. Automated medication-dispensing system in two hospital emergency departments. *Am J Health-Syst Pharm.* 2005; 62:1917–23.

Documentation and cost avoidance

36. Bosinski TJ, Campbell L, Schwartz S. Using a personal digital assistant to document pharmacotherapeutic interventions. *Am J Health-Syst Pharm.* 2004; 61:931–4.

37. Kopp BJ, Mrsan M, Erstad BL, et al. Cost implications of and potential adverse events prevented by interventions of a critical care pharmacist. *Am J Health-Syst Pharm.* 2007; 64:2483–7.

38. Lada P, Delgado G Jr. Documentation of pharmacists' interventions in an emergency department and associated cost avoidance. *Am J Health-Syst Pharm.* 2007; 64:63–8.

39. Lau A, Balen RM, Lam R, et al. Using a personal digital assistant to document clinical pharmacy services in an intensive care unit. *Am J Health-Syst Pharm.* 2001; 58:1229–32.

40. Levy DB. Documentation of clinical and cost-saving pharmacy interventions in the emergency room. *Hosp Pharm.* 1993; 28:624–7, 630–4, 653.

41. Ling JM, Mike LA, Rubin J, et al. Documentation of pharmacist interventions in the emergency department. *Am J Health-Syst Pharm.* 2005; 62:1793–7.

42. Mason RN, Pugh CB, Boyer SB, et al. Computerized documentation of pharmacists' interventions. *Am J Hosp Pharm.* 1994; 51:2131–8.

43. McMullin ST, Hennenfent JA, Ritchie DJ, et al. A prospective, randomized trial to assess the cost impact of pharmacist-initiated interventions. *Arch Intern Med.* 1999; 159:2306–9.

44. Mutnick AH, Sterba KJ, Peroutka JA, et al. Cost savings and avoidance from clinical interventions. *Am J Health-Syst Pharm.* 1997; 54:392–6.

45. Reilly JC, Wallace M, Campbell MM. Tracking pharmacist interventions with a hand-held computer. *Am J Health-Syst Pharm.* 2001; 58:158–61.

46. Schumock GT, Hutchinson RA, Bilek BA. Comparison of two systems for documenting pharmacist interventions in patient care. *Am J Hosp Pharm.* 1992; 49:2211–4.

47. Schneider PJ, Gift MG, Lee YP, et al. Cost of medication-related problems at a university hospital. *Am J Health-Syst Pharm.* 1995; 52:2415–8.

48. Simonian AI. Documenting pharmacist interventions on an intranet. *Am J Health-Syst Pharm.* 2003; 60:151–5.

49. Silva MA, Tataronis GR, Maas B. Using personal digital assistants to document pharmacist cognitive services and estimate potential reimbursement. *Am J Health-Syst Pharm.* 2003; 60:911–5.

50. Zimmerman CR, Smolarek RT, Stevenson JG. A computerized system to improve documentation and reporting of pharmacists' clinical interventions, cost savings, and workload activities. *Pharmacotherapy.* 1995; 15:220–7.

Medication histories and medication reconciliation

51. Ajdukovic M, Crook M, Angley C, et al. Pharmacist elicited medication histories in the emergency department: identifying patient groups at risk of medication misadventure. *Pharm Pract.* 2007; 5:162–8.

52. Akwagyriam I, Goodyer LI, Harding L, et al. Drug history taking and the identification of drug related problems in an accident and emergency department. *J Accid Emerg Med.* 1996; 13:166–8.

53. Carter MK, Allin DM, Scott LA, et al. Pharmacist-acquired medication histories in a university hospital emergency department. *Am J Health-Syst Pharm.* 2006; 63:2500–3.

54. Cornish PL, Knowles SR, Marchesano R, et al. Unintended medication discrepancies at the time of hospital admission. *Arch Intern Med.* 2005; 165:424–9.

55. Gleason KM, Groszek JM, Sullivan C, et al. Reconciliation of discrepancies in medication histories and admission orders of newly hospitalized patients. *Am J Health-Syst Pharm.* 2004; 61:1689–95.

56. Hayes BD, Donovan JL, Smith BS, et al. Pharmacist-conducted medication reconciliation in an emergency department. *Am J Health-Syst Pharm.* 2007; 64:1720–3.

57. Lubowski TJ, Cronin LM, Pavelka RW, et al. Effectiveness of a medication reconciliation project conducted by PharmD students. *Am J Pharm Educ.* 2007; 71:94.

58. Mersfelder TL, Bickel RJ. Inpatient medication history verification by pharmacy students. *Am J Health-Syst Pharm.* 2008; 65:2273–5.

59. Michels RD, Meisel SB. Program using pharmacy technicians to obtain medication histories. *Am J Health-Syst Pharm.* 2003; 60:1982–6.

60. Miller SL, Miller S, Balon J, et al. Medication reconciliation in a rural trauma population. *Ann Emerg Med.* 2008; 52:483–91.

61. Nester TM, Hale LS. Effectiveness of a pharmacist-acquired medication history in promoting patient safety. *Am J Health-Syst Pharm.* 2002; 59:2221–5.

62. Reeder TA, Mutnick A. Pharmacist- versus physician-obtained medication histories. *Am J Health-Syst Pharm.* 2008; 65:857–60.

63. Santel JP. Reconciliation failures lead to medication errors. *Jt Comm J Qual Patient Saf.* 2006; 32:225–9.

64. Schenkel S. The unexpected challenges of accurate medication reconciliation. *Ann Emerg Med.* 2008; 52:493–5.

65. Tam VC, Knowles SR, Cornish PL, et al. Frequency, type, and clinical importance of medication history errors at admission to hospital: a systematic review. *Can Med Assoc J.* 2005; 173:510–5.

Medication and patient safety

66. Bizovi KE, Beckley BE, McDade MC, et al. The effect of computer-assisted prescription writing on emergency department prescription errors. *Acad Emerg Med.* 2002; 9:1168–75.

67. Brown JN, Barnes CL, Beasley B, et al. Effect of pharmacists on medication errors in an emergency department. *Am J Health-Syst Pharm.* 2008; 68:330–3.

68. Case LL, Paparella S. Safety benefits of a clinical pharmacist in the emergency department. *J Emerg Nurs.* 2007; 33:564–6.

69. Federico F. Preventing harm from high-alert medications. *Jt Comm J Qual Patient Saf.* 2007; 33:537–42.

70. Flynn E, Barker K, Barker B. Medication-administration errors in an emergency department. *Am J Health-Syst Pharm.* 2010; 67:347–8.

71. Gruen RL, Jurkovich GJ, McIntyre LK, et al. Patterns of errors contributing to trauma mortality: lessons learned from 2,594 deaths. *Ann Surg.* 2006; 244:371–80.

72. The Joint Commission. High-alert medications and patient safety. *Sentinel Event Alert.* 1999; 11:1–3.

73. Juarez A, Gacki-Smith J, Bauer MR, et al. Barriers to emergency departments' adherence to four medication safety-related Joint Commission National Patient Safety Goals. *Jt Comm J Qual Patient Saf.* 2009; 35:49–59.

74. Kraus DM, Stifter J, Hatoum HT. Program to improve nurses' knowledge of pediatric emergency medications. *Am J Hosp Pharm.* 1991; 48:97–101.

75. Kulstad EB, Sikka R, Sweis RT, et al. ED overcrowding is associated with an increased frequency of medication errors. *Am J Emerg Med.* 2010; 28:304–9.

76. Peth HA. Medication errors in the emergency department: a systems approach to minimizing risk. *Emerg Med Clin N Am.* 2003; 21:141–58.

77. Risser DT, Rice MM, Salisbury ML, et al. The potential for improved teamwork to reduce medical errors in the emergency department. *Ann Emerg Med.* 1999; 34:373–83.

78. Rothschild JM, Churchill W, Erickson A, et al. Medication errors discovered by emergency department pharmacists. *Ann Emerg Med.* 2010; 55:513–21.

79. Schenkel S. Promoting patient safety and preventing medical error in emergency departments. *Acad Emerg Med.* 2000; 7:1204–22.

80. Taylor D, Walsham N, Taylor SE, et al. Potential for interaction between prescription drugs and complementary and alternative medicines amongst patients in the emergency department. *Pharmacotherapy.* 2006; 26:634–40.

81. Patanwala AE, Warholak TL, Sanders AB, et al. A prospective observational study of medication errors in a tertiary care emergency department. *Ann Emerg Med.* 2010; 55:522–6.

82. Wilson K, Sullivan M. Preventing medication errors with smart infusion technology. *Am J Health-Syst Pharm.* 2004; 61:177–83.

Adverse medication events

83. Aparasu RR. Drug-related injury visits to hospital emergency departments. *Am J Health-Syst Pharm.* 1998; 55:1158–61.

84. Croskerry P, Shapiro M, Campbell S, et al. Profiles in patient safety: medication errors in the emergency department. *Acad Emerg Med.* 2004; 11:289–99.

85. Dennehy CE, Kishi DT, Louie C. Drug-related illness in emergency department patients. *Am J Health-Syst Pharm.* 1996; 53:1422–6.

86. Hafner JW, Belknap SM, Squillante MD, et al. Adverse drug events in the emergency department. *Ann Emerg Med.* 2002; 39:258–67.

87. Kalina M, Tinkoff G, Gleason W, et al. A multidisciplinary approach to adverse drug events in pediatric trauma patients in an adult trauma center. *Pediatr Emerg Care.* 2009; 25:444–6.

88. Ratz Y, Shafir I, Berkovitch S, et al. The importance of the pharmacist in reporting adverse drug reactions in the emergency department. *J Clin Pharmacol.* 2010; 50:1217–21.

89. Schneitman-McIntire O, Farnen TA, Gordon N, et al. Medication misadventures resulting in emergency department visits at an HMO medical center. *Am J Health-Syst Pharm.* 1996; 53:1416–22.

90. Smith KM, McAdams JW, Frenia ML, et al. Drug-related problems in emergency department patients. *Am J Health-Syst Pharm.* 1997; 54:295–8.

Quality-improvement initiatives

91. American Society of Health-System Pharmacists. ASHP guidelines on medication-use evaluation. *Am J Health-Syst Pharm.* 1996; 53:1953–5.

92. American Society of Health-System Pharmacists. ASHP guidelines on the pharmacist's role in the development, implementation, and assessment of critical pathways. *Am J Health-Syst Pharm.* 2004; 61:939–45.

Emergency preparedness

93. American Society of Health-System Pharmacists. ASHP statement on the role of health-system pharmacists in emergency preparedness. *Am J Health-Syst Pharm.* 2003; 60:1993–5.

94. Burda AM, Sigg T. Pharmacy preparedness for incidents involving weapons of mass destruction. *Am J Health-Syst Pharm.* 2001; 58:2274–84.

95. Cohen V. Organization of a health-system pharmacy team to respond to episodes of terrorism. *Am J Health-Syst Pharm.* 2003; 60:1257–63.

96. Setlak P. Bioterrorism preparedness and response: emerging role for health-system pharmacists. *Am J Health-Syst Pharm.* 2004; 61:1167–75.

Research

97. Aghababian RV, Barsan WG, Bickell WH, et al. Research directions in emergency medicine. *Am J Emerg Med.* 1996; 14:681–3.

98. American Society of Hospital Pharmacists. ASHP statement on pharmaceutical research in organized health-care settings. *Am J Hosp Pharm.* 1991; 48:1781.

99. Becker LB, Weisfeldt ML, Weil MH, et al. The PULSE initiative: scientific priorities and strategic planning for resuscitation research and life saving therapies. *Circulation.* 2002; 105:2562-70.

100. Fagan SC, Touchette D, Smith JA, et al. The state of science and research in clinical pharmacy. *Pharmacotherapy.* 2006; 26:1027–40.

101. Lipowsi EE. Pharmacy practice-based networks: why, what, who, and how. *J Am Pharm Assoc.* 2008; 48:142–52.

102. Maio RF, Garrison HG, Spaite DW, et al. Emergency medical services outcomes project I (EMSOP I): prioritizing conditions for outcomes research. *Ann Emerg Med.* 1999; 33:423–32.

103. Seidel JS, Henderson D, Tittle S, et al. Priorities for research in emergency medical services for children: results of a consensus conference. *Ann Emerg Med.* 1999; 33:206–10.

Textbooks

1. Cohen V. Safe and effective medication use in the emergency department. Bethesda, MD: American Society of Health-System Pharmacists; 2009.

2. Institute of Medicine of the National Academies Committee on the Future of Emergency Care in the United States Health System. Hospital-based emergency care: at the breaking point. Washington, DC: National Academy Press; 2006.

3. Institute of Medicine of the National Academies Committee on the Future of Emergency Care in the United States. Hospital-based emergency care: at the breaking point. Washington, DC: National Academy Press; 2006.

Developed through the ASHP Section of Clinical Specialists and Scientists Advisory Group on Emergency Care and approved by the ASHP Board of Directors on July 8, 2011.

Heather Draper Eppert, Pharm.D., BCPS, and Alison Jennett Reznek, Pharm.D., BCPS, are gratefully acknowledged for authoring these guidelines. The authors and ASHP gratefully acknowledge Roshanak (Roshy) Aazami, Pharm.D., BCPS, Emergency Medicine Pharmacist, Cedars-Sinai Medical Center, for her substantial contribution and dedication to the completion of these guidelines.

The bibliographic citation for this document is as follows: American Society of Health-System Pharmacists. ASHP guidelines on emergency medicine pharmacist services. *Am J Health-Syst Pharm.* 2011; 68:e81–95.

ASHP Guidelines on the Pharmacist's Role in Immunization

Purpose

Pharmacists can play an important role in disease prevention by advocating and administering immunizations. Such activities are consistent with the preventive aspects of pharmaceutical care and have been part of pharmacy practice for over a century.[1,2] These guidelines address the pharmacist's role in promoting and conducting proper immunization of patients in all organized health care settings. The pharmacist's role in promoting disease prevention through participation in community efforts is also discussed.

Background

Each year, an average of 90,000 Americans die of vaccine-preventable infections such as influenza, pneumococcal disease, and hepatitis B.[3,5] Most of these people visited health care providers in the year preceding their deaths but were not vaccinated.[6–11] Influenza and pneumonia, considered together, are the fifth leading cause of death for Americans 65 years of age or older.[12] Although vaccination rates for U.S. children at the time they enter school exceed 95%, nearly 25% do not complete their primary series by the age of two years.[13] Most American adults are inadequately vaccinated, particularly against pneumococcal disease, influenza, hepatitis B, tetanus, and diphtheria.[6] Tens of millions of Americans remain susceptible to potentially deadly infections despite the availability of effective vaccines.

This long-standing failure to adequately immunize the U.S population helped prompt the inclusion of immunization as a leading health indicator for Healthy People 2010.[14] The renewed focus on immunization and the potential for increased vaccination needs in response to threats of bioterrorism should stimulate pharmacists, as well as other health care providers, to reassess what they and their institutions can do to improve immunization rates in their communities. Pharmacists can contribute to this effort by administering immunizations where scope of practice allows and by promoting immunization in other ways.

Immunization Administration

As health care providers, pharmacists can administer vaccines or host other health care professionals who can administer vaccines. Pharmacists must understand the legal and professional mechanisms by which authorization to administer vaccines is granted, as well as the additional responsibilities and considerations that accompany this expanded role. The feasibility of vaccine administration by pharmacists within a particular practice site or health care system can be determined by analyzing the issues of legal authority, training, and program structure.

Legal Authority. The pharmacist's authority to administer vaccines is determined by each state's laws and regulations governing pharmacy practice. At least 36 states permit vaccine administration by pharmacists as part of the scope of pharmacy practice.[15] The American College of Physicians–American Society of Internal Medicine supports pharmacists as sources of immunization information, hosts of immunization sites, and immunizers.[16] Vaccine administration may occur pursuant to individual prescription orders or through standing orders or protocols. The Centers for Disease Control and Prevention (CDC) Advisory Committee on Immunization Practices recommends the use of standing orders to improve adult immunization rates.[17] Its recommendations encourage pharmacists, among other providers, to establish standing-order programs in long-term-care facilities, home health care agencies, hospitals, clinics, workplaces, and managed care organizations. The Centers for Medicare and Medicaid Services (CMS) no longer requires a physician order for influenza or pneumoccocal immunizations administered in participating hospitals, long-term-care facilities, or home health care agencies.[18] Development of state-specific protocols or standing-order programs can be facilitated through partnerships with state pharmacy associations, boards of pharmacy, and health departments.

Training. Although legal authority to administer vaccines may be granted through pharmacy practice acts, pharmacists must achieve competency in all aspects of vaccine administration. A comprehensive training program should address the following:

1. The epidemiology of and patient populations at risk for vaccine-preventable diseases,
2. Public health goals for immunization (e.g., local, regional, state, and federal goals),
3. Vaccine safety (e.g., risk–benefit analysis),
4. Screening for contraindications and precautions of vaccination in each patient,
5. Vaccine stability and transportation and storage requirements,
6. Immunologic drug interactions,
7. Vaccine dosing (including interpreting recommended immunization schedules and patient immunization records and determining proper dosing intervals and the feasibility of simultaneous administration of multiple vaccines),
8. Proper dose preparation and injection technique,
9. Signs and symptoms of adverse reactions to vaccines, adverse reaction reporting, and emergency procedures, such as basic and advanced cardiac life support (BCLS and ACLS),
10. Documentation,
11. Reporting to the primary care provider or local health department, and
12. Billing.

Live and videotaped programming is available through some state and national pharmacy associations and offered in many college of pharmacy curricula. Information regarding immunizations can change rapidly. To maintain competency, pharmacists must have access to current immunization references (e.g., CDC's National Immunization Program publications, including the "Pink Book"[19]) and continuing-education programs to stay abreast of evolving guidelines and recommendations.

Program Structure. A vaccine administration program requires a solid infrastructure of appropriately trained staff, physical space, and written policies and procedures to ensure appropriate vaccine storage and handling, patient screening and education, and documentation. The structure of a vaccine administration program must also provide for storage and disposal of injection supplies, disposal of and prevention of exposure to biological hazards as dictated by the Occupational Safety and Health Administration (OSHA), and emergency procedures (e.g., BCLS and ACLS). Pharmacists should be fully immunized to protect their health and the health of their patients.[20]

Reimbursement. Immunization has repeatedly been shown to be cost-effective[21–24]; it may be the most cost-effective practice in medicine. However, third-party reimbursement policies often do not provide coverage for recommended vaccines despite this evidence. A major exception is Medicare Part B, which not only covers immunization services for its participants but also recognizes and compensates pharmacists as mass immunization providers. Enrollment as a Medicare provider is required to bill for covered services. Provider status can be obtained through local Medicare offices, which also process CMS claims for reimbursement (CMS-1500 claims). The CMS Web site (www.cms.hhs.gov) is a useful source for billing information. Pharmacists should continue to closely monitor other immunization reimbursement policies and advocate third-party coverage for immunizations as a cost-effective preventive measure. For patients without insurance coverage, requesting out-of-pocket payments from the patient remains a viable option for pharmacists to obtain compensation for their immunization services.

Immunization Promotion

Pharmacists who do not administer vaccines can promote immunization through six types of activities: (1) history and screening, (2) patient counseling, (3) documentation, (4) formulary management, (5) administrative measures, and (6) public education.[25,26] These promotional activities can also be integrated into or accompany a pharmacy-based immunization program.

History and Screening. Pharmacists can promote proper immunization by identifying patients in need of immunization. Tasks that support this objective include gathering immunization histories, encouraging use of vaccine profiles, issuing vaccination records to patients,[27–34] preventing immunologic drug interactions,[35,36] and screening patients for immunization needs.[28–33,37–39]

Immunization screening should be a component of all clinical routines, regardless of the practice setting. All health care institutions should implement consistent, systematic monitoring systems and quality indicators to ensure that all patients are assessed for immunization adequacy before they leave the facility. The health care provider designated to identify patient immunization needs should have the authority, knowledge, and responsibility to provide or arrange for the immunization service.[40] Clinics that provide treatment for a large number of patients at high risk for contracting vaccine-preventable diseases (e.g., diabetic, asthmatic, heart disease, and geriatric clinics) have a particular obligation to employ immunization screening and ensure appropriate vaccine use.

Screening for immunization needs may be organized in several ways; prototype screening forms are available.[39,41]

Pharmacists should seek out leadership roles in some or all of the following forms of immunization screening.

Occurrence screening. With this type of screening, vaccine needs are identified at the time of particular events, such as hospital or nursing home admission or discharge, ambulatory care or emergency room visits, mid-decade birthdays (e.g., years 25, 35, and 45),[42,43] and any contact with a health care delivery system for patients under 8 years or over 50 years of age.

Diagnosis screening. This screening reviews the vaccine needs of patients with conditions that increase their risk of preventable infections. Diagnoses such as diabetes, asthma, heart disease, acute myocardial infarction, congestive heart failure, chronic obstructive pulmonary disease, hemophilia, thalassemia, most types of cancer, sickle cell anemia, chronic alcoholism, cirrhosis, human immunodeficiency virus infection, and certain other disorders should prompt specific attention to the patient's vaccine needs.[12,33,42] The immunization rate for patients diagnosed with community-acquired pneumonia is considered a marker for quality by some accrediting bodies. Incorporating assessment of vaccination status into an institution's critical pathways has been shown to improve vaccination rates.[44]

Procedure screening. Immunization needs are assessed on the basis of medical or surgical procedures using this type of screening. These procedures include splenectomy, heart or lung surgery, organ transplantation, antineoplastic therapy, radiation therapy, immunosuppression of other types, dialysis, and prescription of certain medications used to treat conditions that increase patients' risk of preventable infections.[45,46] When designing and implementing automated prescription databases, pharmacy managers should consider specifications that allow retrieval of lists of patients receiving drugs that suggest the need for immunization.[33,37]

Periodic mass screening. This type of screening is a comprehensive assessment of immunization adequacy in selected populations at a given time. Such screening may be conducted, for example, during autumn influenza programs or outbreaks of certain vaccine-preventable illnesses (e.g., measles and meningococcal disease).[29,32,33] Schools and other institutions can perform mass screening when registering new students or residents. Mass screening may also be appropriate in areas where no comprehensive immunization program has been conducted recently. This type of screening helps improve vaccine coverage rates at a given time, but long-term benefits are much greater when such intermittent programs are combined with ongoing comprehensive screening efforts. Several states, including South Dakota, New Jersey, and Oklahoma, have enacted laws requiring that influenza and pneumococcal vaccines be offered annually to residents of nursing homes.

Occupational screening. This screening method focuses on the immunization needs of health care personnel whose responsibilities place them at risk of exposure to certain vaccine-preventable diseases or bring them into contact with high-risk patients (i.e., patients with those conditions listed in the *Diagnosis screening* section above). Health care providers who have contact with these patients should receive an annual influenza vaccination. Health care employers frequently provide immunization screening and vaccination of employees as part of employee health programs. OSHA requires that health care employers provide hepatitis B vaccination at no cost, on a voluntary basis, to all employees at risk for occupational exposure to blood borne pathogens.[47] Depending on their risk of exposure, it may be advisable for

members of the pharmacy staff to receive hepatitis B vaccination.

Screening for contraindications and precautions. After candidates for immunization have been identified, they should be screened for contraindications and precautions. A CDC-reviewed contraindication screening questionnaire is available.[48]

Patient Counseling. Patients in need of immunization should be advised of their infection risk and encouraged to accept the immunizations they need. Patient concerns about vaccine safety and efficacy should be discussed and addressed.[49,50] Health care providers can influence patients' attitudes regarding immunization.[51,52] Physicians should be informed of their patients' need for vaccination if standing orders or collaborative practice agreements are not in place. Patients who need immunizations should be vaccinated during the current health care contact unless valid contraindications exist. Delaying vaccination until a future appointment increases the risk that the patient will not be vaccinated.

Advising patients of their need for immunization can take several forms. In the ambulatory care setting, individualized or form letters can be mailed to patients, patients can be called by telephone, or an insert can be included with prescriptions informing patients of their infection risk and the availability and efficacy of vaccines.[30,33,53–55] Adhesive reminder labels can also be affixed to prescription containers for drugs used to treat conditions that may indicate the need for vaccination against influenza and pneumococcal disease (e.g., digoxin, warfarin, theophylline, and insulin[33]); these labels would be analogous to labels currently in widespread use (e.g., "Shake well" and "Take with food or milk"). Such labels might read, "You may need flu or pneumonia vaccine: Ask your doctor or pharmacist." Chart notes, consultations, messages to patients, one-on-one conversations, and similar means can be used to communicate with inpatients and institutional patients.[28,31,56]

Federal law requires that health care providers who administer diphtheria, tetanus, pertussis, measles, mumps, rubella, varicella, polio, *Haemophilus influenzae* type B, hepatitis B, and pneumococcal conjugate vaccines give the most recent version of the CDC-developed Vaccine Information Statement (VIS) to the adult or the parent or legal guardian of the child to be vaccinated.[57] VISs are available in many languages from state or local health departments or the CDC.[58] VISs are also available for other commonly used vaccines, such as influenza, pneumococcal polysaccharide, hepatitis A, meningococcal, and anthrax vaccines. Pharmacists should also ensure that informed consent is obtained in a manner that complies with state laws.[20]

Documentation. The National Childhood Vaccine Injury Act of 1986 (NCVIA) requires all health care providers who administer vaccines to maintain permanent vaccination records and to report occurrences of certain adverse events specified in the act.[57,59] The recipient's permanent medical record (or the equivalent) must state the date the vaccine was administered, the vaccine's manufacturer and lot number, and the name, address, and title of the person administering the vaccine. Pharmacists in organized health care settings may encourage compliance with this requirement by providing reminder notices each time doses of vaccines are dispensed.[60] Automated databases that allow for long-term storage of patient immunization information may provide an efficient method for maintaining and retrieving immunization records.[39] Efforts to develop electronic vaccination registries, especially for children, are under way by states collaborating with CDC.[61]

NCVIA also mandates that selected adverse effects noted after any inoculation be reported to the Vaccine Adverse Event Reporting System (www.vaers.org).[57,59,62] Because pharmacists have experience with adverse-drug-reaction reporting, they can take the lead in developing and implementing a program to meet this requirement, even if they are not responsible for administering the vaccine.

Patients should maintain personal immunization records that document all immunization experiences and function as a backup if the clinicians' immunization records are lost. Several personal immunization record forms are available. Public Health Service Form 731 (International Certificate of Vaccination), colloquially called the "yellow shot record," is used to document vaccines indicated for international travel but can also serve as a patient's personal record of vaccinations. The Immunization Action Coalition distributes a standard adult immunization record card developed in collaboration with CDC.[63] In addition, each state and the District of Columbia prints its own uniform immunization record form for pediatric immunizations, which may also be a suitable personal patient record. It has been recommended that adults carry personal immunization records in their wallets.[46]

Formulary Management. Formulary systems in organized health care settings should include vaccines, toxoids, and immune globulins available for use in preventing diseases in patients and staff. Decisions by the pharmacy and therapeutics committee (or its equivalent) on immunologic drug choices require consideration of relevant immunologic pharmaceutics, immunopharmacology, and disease epidemiology. Because of their expertise and training, pharmacists are well equipped to provide information and recommendations on which these decisions may be based.

It is the pharmacist's responsibility to develop and maintain product specifications to aid in the purchase of drugs under the formulary system.[64,65] The pharmacist should establish and maintain standards to ensure the quality, proper storage, and proper use of all pharmaceuticals dispensed. Pharmacists must choose between single dose or multidose containers of vaccines on the basis of efficiency, safety, economic, and regulatory considerations. Pharmacists in institutions should develop guidelines on the routine stocking of immunologic drugs in certain high-use patient care areas.

Proper transportation and storage are an important consideration for immunologic drugs, including vaccines, because many require storage at refrigerated or frozen temperatures. Pharmacists have an important responsibility to maintain the "cold chain" in the handling of these drugs. Detailed references on this topic have been published.[66–73] Storage considerations include the conditions in all areas in which immunologic drugs are kept, as well as a method for ensuring that immunologic drugs received by the pharmacy have been transported under suitable conditions.

It is important that methods be established for detecting and properly disposing of outdated and partially administered immunologic agents. Live viral (e.g., varicella, yellow fever, and smallpox) and live bacterial (e.g., bacille Calmette-Guérin) vaccines should be disposed of in the same manner as other infectious biohazardous waste.

Administrative Measures. Pharmacists on key committees (e.g., infection control and risk management) in organized health care settings can promote adequate immunization delivery among staff and patients by encouraging the development of sound organizational policies on immunization. Health care organizations should develop policies and protocols that address the following:

1. Hepatitis B preexposure prophylaxis for health care workers at risk for exposure to blood products and other contaminated items,[45,74-76]
2. Hepatitis B postexposure (e.g., needle stick) prophylaxis for previously unvaccinated patients, health care personnel, and personnel who have been vaccinated but do not have a previously documented serologic response,[45,74-76]
3. Rabies preexposure and postexposure prophylaxis,[77]
4. Wound management guidelines designed to prevent tetanus and diphtheria,[78,79]
5. Valid contraindications to vaccination to ensure patient safety and minimize inappropriate exclusions from vaccination,[78,80,81]
6. Requirements for employee immunization against measles, rubella, influenza, and other diseases,[42,82]
7. Tuberculosis screening of patients and staff,[83,84]
8. Immunization of persons at high risk (e.g., patients with diabetes, asthma, heart disease, and pregnant or immunocompromised patients). Current authoritative guidelines on this subject should be consulted,[42,46,58,85,86] and
9. Emergency measures in the event of vaccine-related adverse reactions. Such measures should address the availability of epinephrine and other emergency drugs, as well as BCLS and ACLS.

Public Education. Pharmacists have ample opportunities to advance the public health through immunization advocacy. Pharmacists can facilitate disease prevention strategies, because many potential victims of influenza and pneumococcal disease visit pharmacies and are seen by pharmacists daily. Pharmacists can lead local activities in observance of National Adult Immunization Week each October.[37] Working with local public health departments, state or national immunization coalitions, and other groups (e.g., state or local parent—teacher, diabetes, heart, lung, or retired persons' associations), pharmacists can promote vaccination among high-risk populations. Newsletters, posters, brochures, and seminars may be used to explain the risk of preventable infections to pharmacy staff, other health care personnel, and patients. Excellent resources are available from the Immunization Action Coalition and the National Coalition for Adult Immunization.

References

1. Hepler CD, Strand LM. Opportunities and responsibilities in pharmaceutical care. *Am J Hosp Pharm.* 1990; 47:533–43.
2. Grabenstein JD. Pharmacists and immunization: increasing involvement over a century. *Pharm Hist.* 1999; 41:137–52.
3. Prevention and control of influenza: recommendations of the Advisory Committee on Immunization Practices. *MMWR Recomm Rep.* 2002; 51(RR-3):1–31.
4. Prevention of pneumococcal disease: recommendations of the Advisory Committee on Immunization Practices (ACIP). *MMWR Recomm Rep.* 1997; 46(RR-8):1–24.
5. Thompson WW, Shay DK, Weintraub E, et al. Mortality associated with influenza and respiratory syncytial virus in the United States. *JAMA.* 2003; 289:179–86.
6. Williams WW, Hickson MA, Kane MA, et al. Immunization policies and vaccine coverage among adults. The risk for missed opportunities. *Ann Intern Med.* 1988; 108:616–25.
7. Fedson DS, Harward MP, Reid RA, et al. Hospital-based pneumococcal immunization. Epidemiologic rationale from the Shenandoah study. *JAMA.* 1990; 264:1117–22.
8. Fedson DS. Influenza and pneumococcal immunization strategies for physicians. *Chest.* 1987; 91:436–43.
9. Fedson DS. Improving the use of pneumococcal vaccine through a strategy of hospital-based immunization: a review of its rationale and implications. *J Am Geriatr Soc.* 1985; 33:142–50.
10. Magnussen CR, Valenti WM, Mushlin AI. Pneumococcal vaccine strategy. Feasibility of a vaccination program directed at hospitalized and ambulatory patients. *Arch Intern Med.* 1984; 144:1755–7.
11. Vondracek TG, Pham TP, Huycke MM. A hospital-based pharmacy intervention program for pneumococcal vaccination. *Arch Intern Med.* 1998; 158:1543–7.
12. Bratzler DW, Houck PM, Jiang H, et al. Failure to vaccinate Medicare inpatients: a missed opportunity. *Arch Intern Med.* 2002; 162:2349–56.
13. Barker L, Luman E, Zhao Z, et al. National, state, and urban area vaccination coverage levels among children aged 19–35 months—United States, 2001. *MMWR. Morb Mortal Wkly Rep.* 2002; 51(30):664–6.
14. Office of Disease Prevention and Health Promotion. Healthy people 2010. www.healthypeople.gov (accessed 2003 Mar 12).
15. American Pharmaceutical Association. States where pharmacists can immunize. www.aphanet.org/pharmcare/immunofact.html (accessed 2003 Mar 6).
16. Keely JL. Pharmacist scope of practice. *Ann Intern Med.* 2002; 136:79–85.
17. Use of standing orders programs to increase adult vaccination rates: recommendations of the Advisory Committee on Immunization Practices (ACIP). *MMWR Recomm Rep.* 2000; 49(RR01):15–26.
18. 42 C.F.R. §482–4.
19. Centers for Disease Control and Prevention. Epidemiology and prevention of vaccine-preventable diseases. 7th ed. Atlanta: U.S. Department of Health and Human Services; 2003.
20. Grabenstein JD. High expectations: standards and guidelines for immunization delivery. *Hosp Pharm.* 2000; 35:841–51.
21. Sisk JE, Moskowitz AJ, Whang W, et al. Cost-effectiveness of vaccination against pneumococcal bacteremia among elderly people. *JAMA.* 1997; 278:1333–9.
22. Van den Oever R, de Graeve D, Hepp B, et al. Pharmacoeconomics of immunisation: a review. *Pharmacoeconomics.* 1993; 3:286–308.
23. Nichol KL, Lind A, Margolis KL, et al. The effectiveness of vaccination against influenza in healthy, working adults. *N Engl J Med.* 1995; 333:889–93.
24. Nichol KL, Margolis KL, Wuorenma J, et al. The efficacy and cost-effectiveness of vaccination against influ-

enza among elderly persons living in the community. *N Engl J Med.* 1994; 331:778–84.

25. Grabenstein JD. Immunizations: what's a health-system pharmacy to do? Part 1. *Hosp Pharm.* 1998; 33:742,745–50,753.

26. Grabenstein JD. Immunizations: what's a health-system pharmacy to do? Part 2. *Hosp Pharm.* 1998; 33:870–2,876–80.

27. Huff PS, Hak SH, Caiola SM. Immunizations for international travel as a pharmaceutical service. *Am J Hosp Pharm.* 1982; 39:90–3.

28. Spruill WJ, Cooper JW, Taylor WJR. Pharmacist-coordinated pneumonia and influenza vaccination program. *Am J Hosp Pharm.* 1982; 39:1904–6.

29. Grabenstein JD, Smith LJ, Carter DW, et al. Comprehensive immunization delivery in conjunction with influenza vaccination. *Arch Intern Med.* 1986; 146:1189–92.

30. Williams DM, Daugherty LJ, Aycock DG, et al. Effectiveness of improved targeting efforts for influenza immunization in an ambulatory-care setting. *Hosp Pharm.* 1987; 22:462–4.

31. Morton MR, Spruill WJ, Cooper JW. Pharmacist impact on pneumococcal vaccination rates in long-term-care facilities. *Am J Hosp Pharm.* 1988; 45:73. Letter.

32. Grabenstein JD, Smith LJ, Watson RR, et al. Immunization outreach using individual need assessments of adults at an Army hospital. *Public Health Rep.* 1990; 105:311–6.

33. Grabenstein JD, Hayton BD. Pharmacoepidemiologic program for identifying patients in need of vaccination. *Am J Hosp Pharm.* 1990; 47:1774–81.

34. Grabenstein JD. Get it in writing: documenting immunizations. *Hosp Pharm.* 1991; 26:901–4.

35. Grabenstein JD. Drug interactions involving immunologic agents. Part I. Vaccine–vaccine, vaccine–immunoglobulin, and vaccine–drug interactions. *DICP.* 1990; 24:67–81.

36. Grabenstein JD. Drug interactions involving immunologic agents. Part II. Immunodiagnostic and other immunologic drug interactions. *DICP.* 1990; 24:186–93.

37. Grabenstein JD. Pneumococcal pneumonia: don't wait, vaccinate. *Hosp Pharm.* 1990; 25:866–9.

38. Grabenstein JD, Casto DT. Recommending vaccines to your patients' individual needs. *Am Pharm.* 1991; NS31:58–67.

39. Grabenstein JD. Immunization delivery: a complete guide. St. Louis: Facts and Comparisons; 1997.

40. Fedson DS, Houck P, Bratzler D. Hospital-based influenza and pneumococcal vaccination: Sutton's law applied to prevention. *Infect Control Hosp Epidemiol.* 2000; 21:692–9.

41. Immunization Action Coalition. Do I need any vaccinations today? www.immunize.org/catg.d/4036need.htm (accessed 2003 Mar 12).

42. Guide for adult immunization. 3rd ed. Philadelphia: American College of Physicians; 1994.

43. Slobodkin D, Zielske PG, Kitlas JL, et al. Demonstration of the feasibility of emergency department immunization against influenza and pneumococcus. *Ann Emerg Med.* 1998; 32:537–43.

44. Robke JT, Woods M, Heitz S. Pharmacist impact on pneumococcal vaccination rates through incorporation of immunization assessment into critical pathways in an acute care setting. *Hosp Pharm.* 2002; 37:1050–4.

45. Hepatitis B virus: a comprehensive strategy for eliminating transmission in the United States through universal childhood vaccination. Recommendations of the Immunization Practices Advisory Committee (ACIP). *MMWR Recomm Rep.* 1991; 40 (RR-13):1–25.

46. Canadian National Advisory Committee on Immunization. Canadian immunization guide. 5th ed. Ottawa, Ont.: Ministry of National Health and Welfare; 1998.

47. 29 C.F.R. §1910.1030.

48. Immunization Action Coalition. Screening questionnaire for adult immunization. www.immunize.org/catg.d/p4065scr.pdf (accessed 2003 Mar 12).

49. Grabenstein JD, Wilson JP. Are vaccines safe? Risk contamination applied to vaccination. *Hosp Pharm.* 1999; 34:713–4,717–8,721–3,727–9.

50. Kirk JK, Grabenstein JD. Interviewing and counseling patients about immunizations. *Hosp Pharm.* 1991; 26:1006–10.

51. Nichol KL, MacDonald R, Hauge M. Factors associated with influenza and pneumococcal vaccination behavior among high-risk adults. *J Gen Intern Med.* 1996; 11:673–7.

52. Gene J, Espinola A, Cabezas C, et al. Do knowledge and attitudes about influenza and its immunization affect the likelihood of obtaining immunization? *Fam Pract Res J.* 1992; 12:61–73.

53. Grabenstein JD, Hartzema AG, Guess HA, et al. Community pharmacists as immunization advocates: a clinical pharmacoepidemiologic experiment. *Int J Pharm Pract.* 1993; 2:5–10.

54. Grabenstein JD, Guess HA, Hartzema AG. People vaccinated by pharmacists: Descriptive epidemiology. *J Am Pharm Assoc.* 2001; 41:46–52.

55. Grabenstein JD, Guess HA, Hartzema AG, et al. Effect of vaccination by community pharmacists among adult prescription recipients. *Med Care.* 2001; 39:340–8.

56. Casto DT. Prevention, management, and control of influenza: roles for the pharmacist. *Am J Med.* 1987; 82(suppl 6A):64–7.

57. Health Services & Resources Administration. Vaccine injury table. *Fed Regist.* 1997; 62:7685–90.

58. Centers for Disease Control and Prevention. Vaccine Information Statements. www.cdc.gov/nip/publications/vis (accessed 2003 Mar 27).

59. Update on adult immunization. Recommendations of the Immunization Practices Advisory Committee (ACIP). *MMWR Recomm Rep.* 1991; 40(RR-12): 1–94.

60. Grabenstein JD. Compensation for vaccine injury: balancing society's need and personal risk. *Hosp Pharm.* 1995; 30:831–2,834–6.

61. Grabenstein JD. Vaccination records must be available to be used. *J Am Pharm Assoc.* 2000; 40:113.

62. Kapit RM, Grabenstein JD. Adverse events after immunization: reports and results. *Hosp Pharm.* 1995; 30:1031–2,1035–6,1038,1041.

63. Immunization Action Coalition. Adult immunization record card. www.immunize.org/adultizcards/index.htm (accessed 2003 Mar 12).

64. American Society of Hospital Pharmacists. ASHP technical assistance bulletin on hospital drug distribution and control. *Am J Hosp Pharm.* 1980; 37:1097–103.

65. ASHP statement on the pharmacist's responsibility for distribution and control of drug products. In:

Deffenbaugh JH, ed. Best practices for health-system pharmacy. Positions and guidance documents of ASHP. 2002–2003 ed. Bethesda, MD: American Society of Health-System Pharmacists; 2002:91.

66. Grabenstein JD. ImmunoFacts: vaccines and immunologic drugs. 28th ed. St Louis: Facts and Comparisons; 2002.

67. Centers for Disease Control and Prevention. Vaccine management: recommendations for handling and storage of selected biologicals. www.cdc.gov/nip/publications/vac_mgt_book.htm (accessed 2003 Mar 27).

68. Casto DT, Brunell PA. Safe handling of vaccines. *Pediatrics.* 1990; 87:108–12.

69. Ross MB. Additional stability guidelines for routinely refrigerated drug products. *Am J Hosp Pharm.* 1988; 45:1498–9. Letter.

70. Sterchele JA. Update on stability guidelines for routinely refrigerated drug products. *Am J Hosp Pharm.* 1987; 44:2698, 2701. Letter.

71. Miller LG, Loomis JH Jr. Advice of manufacturers about effects of temperature on biologicals. *Am J Hosp Pharm.* 1985; 42:843–8.

72. Vogenberg FR, Souney PF. Stability guidelines for routinely refrigerated drug products. *Am J Hosp Pharm.* 1983; 40:101–2.

73. Wolfert RR, Cox RM. Room temperature stability of drug products labeled for refrigerated storage. *Am J Hosp Pharm.* 1975; 32:585–7.

74. Update: recommendations to prevent hepatitis B virus transmission—United States. *MMWR Morb Mortal Wkly Rep.* 1995; 44:574–5.

75. Update: recommendations to prevent hepatitis B virus transmission—United States. *MMWR Morb Mortal Wkly Rep.* 1999; 48:33–4.

76. Prevention of hepatitis A through active or passive immunization: recommendations of the Advisory Committee on Immunization Practices (ACIP). *MMWR Recomm Rep.* 1999; 48(RR-12):1–37.

77. Human rabies prevention—United States, 1999. Recommendations of the Advisory Committee on Immunization Practices (ACIP). *MMWR Recomm Rep.* 1999; 48(RR-1):1–21.

78. Diphtheria, tetanus, and pertussis: recommendations for vaccine use and other preventive measures. Recommendations of the Immunization Practices Advisory Committee (ACIP). *MMWR Recomm Rep.* 1991; 40(RR-10):1–28.

79. Grabenstein JD. Stop buying tetanus toxoid (with one exception). *Hosp Pharm.* 1990; 25:361–2.

80. Pertussis vaccination: use of acellular pertussis vaccines among infants and young children. Recommendations of the Advisory Committee on Immunization Practices (ACIP). *MMWR Recomm Rep.* 1997; 46(RR-7):1–25.

81. American Academy of Pediatrics Committee on Infectious Diseases. The relationship between pertussis vaccine and brain damage: reassessment. *Pediatrics.* 1991; 88:397–400.

82. Immunization of health-care workers: recommendations of the Advisory Committee on Immunization Practices (ACIP) and the Hospital Infection Control Practices Advisory Committee (HICPAC). *MMWR Recomm Rep.* 1997; 46(RR-18):1–42.

83. Screening for tuberculosis and tuberculosis infection in high-risk populations: recommendations of the Advisory Council for the Elimination of Tuberculosis. *MMWR Recomm Rep.* 1995; 44(RR-11):19–34.

84. Anergy skin testing and tuberculosis [corrected] preventive therapy for HIV-infected persons: revised recommendations. *MMWR Recomm Rep.* 1997; 46(RR-15):1–10.

85. Health information for international travel, 2001–02. Washington, DC: Government Printing Office; 2001.

86. American College of Obstetricians and Gynecologists committee opinion. Immunization during pregnancy. *Obstet Gynecol.* 2003; 101:207–12.

These guidelines were reviewed in 2008 by the Council on Pharmacy Practice and by the Board of Directors and were found to still be appropriate.

Developed through the ASHP Council on Professional Affairs and approved by the ASHP Board of Directors on May 31, 2003.

The bibliographic citation for this document is as follows: American Society of Health-System Pharmacists. ASHP guidelines on the pharmacist's role in immunization. *Am J Health-Syst Pharm.* 2003; 60:1371–7.

ASHP Guidelines for Providing Pediatric Pharmaceutical Services in Organized Health Care Systems

Patient care consists of integrated domains of care, including medical care, nursing care, and pharmaceutical care. The provision of pharmaceutical care involves not only medication therapy but decisions about medication selection, dosages, routes and methods of administration, medication therapy monitoring, and the provision of medication-related information and counseling to individual patients.[1] The pediatric patient population poses some unique challenges to the pharmaceutical care provider in terms of these medication-related activities. These challenges include the lack of published information on the therapeutic uses and monitoring of drugs in pediatric patients; the lack of appropriate commercially available dosage forms and concentrations of many drugs for pediatric patients; and the resulting need to develop innovative ways of ensuring that the patient receives the drug in a manner that allows the intended therapeutic effect to be realized.[2] These guidelines are intended to assist pharmacists in meeting the special needs of the pediatric patient in any organized health care setting.

General Principles

The pharmacy service should be organized in accordance with the principles of good management. It should be under the direction of a pharmacist and be provided with sufficient physical facilities, personnel, and equipment to meet the pharmaceutical care needs of the pediatric population. Resources necessary for compounding and testing alternative doses and dosage forms of commercially available products are essential. The pharmacy should comply with all applicable federal, state, and local laws, codes, statutes, and regulations.[3] The setting should meet applicable accreditation criteria of the Joint Commission on Accreditation of Healthcare Organizations. Organizations such as the National Association of Children's Hospitals and Related Institutions, the American Academy of Pediatrics, and the Pediatric Pharmacy Administrative Group are useful sources of further information on pediatric health care services.

Orientation and Training Programs

Orientation, training, and staff development programs for pharmacists providing services to pediatric patients should emphasize dosage calculations, dosage-form selection appropriate to the patient's age and condition, and specialized drug preparation and administration techniques. Pharmacists should be familiar with the pharmacokinetic and pharmacodynamic changes that occur with age (e.g., in volume of distribution, protein binding, renal elimination, metabolism, muscle mass, and fluid requirements) and with disease-specific conditions that might affect drug choice or administration (e.g., short-gut syndrome, lactose intolerance). A sensitivity to the nature, frequency, and severity of medication-related errors in the pediatric population is important for all pharmacy personnel.[4]

Inpatient Services

A lack of availability of commercially prepared dosage forms, combined with the documented risk of calculation errors, requires the use of comprehensive unit dose drug distribution systems and intravenous (i.v.) admixture services for pediatric patients. Appropriate dosage standardization in both oral and parenteral drug distribution systems may facilitate the provision of these services.

Unit Dose System. The pediatric unit dose system must meet the original intent of these systems, which is to minimize errors and provide drugs to the patient care areas in ready-to-administer form. Multidose containers and stock medications should be avoided. An extemporaneous preparation service should facilitate the preparation and packaging of medications according to sound compounding principles.

I.V. Admixture Service. The drugs provided by the i.v. admixture service should include all i.v. push, i.v. minibag, intramuscular, and subcutaneous doses; large-volume injections; antineoplastic agents; parenteral nutrient fluids; ophthalmic products; peritoneal dialysis solutions; and irrigation fluids. Knowledge of pediatric fluid requirements and limitations, drug administration techniques and devices, and acceptable volumes for intramuscular injection is critical. Care should be taken when making dilutions to maximize concentrations of drug products (when safe to do so) for fluid-sensitive patients, as well as to minimize hyperosmolar solutions that might lead to destruction of vasculature or, in the neonate, intraventricular hemorrhage. Quality controls for both manually prepared and computer-driven preparation should exist to ensure that each product contains the ingredients ordered and that they are properly labeled. Knowledge of products that contain benzyl alcohol and the risks of this substance in neonates is essential in a pediatric i.v. admixture service.

The labels of all products should be evaluated for legibility, clarity of expression, and their potential for leading to a medication error.[5] Labels should include the drug name; the drug concentration; the route of administration; the expiration date or time; appropriate instructions for administration, additional preparation, and storage; and the lot number (if a batch-prepared product).[6]

Ambulatory Care Services

Ambulatory care pharmacy services should be attentive to the unique drug needs of the pediatric patient. These include the need for special dosage forms (e.g., liquids and chewable tablets), measuring devices, and detailed counseling on drug administration. When product stability is a problem, caregivers may have to be taught how to prepare an appropriate dosage form in the home. Consideration must be given to taste and the need for an extra prescription container to

be taken to school or daycare. Children should be included whenever possible in discussions concerning their medications. In the ambulatory care setting, the pharmacist is well positioned to play a role in preventive health care, including poison prevention and immunization.[7]

Drug Information

Drug information services should provide the pharmacist practicing in the pediatric setting with information unique to the pediatric population. References should include pediatric medical texts and current information on pediatric dosages, extemporaneous formulations, drug compatibilities and stability, poison control, and drug effects during pregnancy and lactation. Drug information should be available in areas where decisions are being made about drug therapy. Literature supporting the use of drugs for unlabeled uses in pediatric patients should also be available.[8] Pharmacists should provide other health care professionals with information on new and investigational drugs, adverse effects of and contraindications to drug therapy, compatibility and stability information, dosage computations, pharmacokinetics, and drug interactions. This may be accomplished through educational presentations, seeing patients in conjunction with other caregivers ("rounding"), and printed materials (e.g., newsletters).

Therapeutic Drug Monitoring

Therapeutic drug monitoring enables assessment of therapeutic outcomes and recognition at the earliest moment of an undesirable response to a drug. Both desired and undesired effects should be documented. The person performing therapeutic drug monitoring should take into consideration the age-related differences in dosage when recommending or reviewing drug therapy.

Pharmacokinetic Services

For both oral and injectable drugs, pharmacokinetic services should ensure that the drug has been administered appropriately before samples are taken for the measurement of serum drug concentrations. The frequency and timing of sampling should also be monitored to avoid excessive and traumatic sampling in children. Knowledge of age-related differences in absorption, distribution, metabolism, and elimination is essential for the pharmacist who is involved in pharmacokinetic services for pediatric patients. The collection and publication of accurate pharmacokinetic data on the pediatric population are encouraged.

Patient and Caregiver Education

Pharmacists should counsel and educate patients and caregivers about their medications, including the purpose of each medication, dosage instructions, potential drug interactions, potential adverse effects, and any specific age-related issues (e.g., compounding and diluting techniques, measuring and administration instructions). Caregivers should be informed of any drug products for which crushing, chewing, dividing, or diluting should be avoided. Suggestions about masking the taste of an unpleasant medication should also be provided. Administration of products, including ophthalmics, otics, inhalers, and injectables, should be demonstrated.

The prevention of accidental ingestion of medications should also be emphasized. The benefits of educational programs are best realized when a cooperative multidisciplinary approach is used. Sharing of pertinent information by all participants is fundamental to the success of patient education services.[9]

Medication Errors

Systems for the recognition, documentation, and prevention of medication errors are essential for the pediatric population. Pharmacist participation in quality-improvement committees and the participation of pharmacists, nurses, physicians, and risk managers are important in minimizing medication errors in pediatric patients. The development and enforcement of policies and procedures for minimizing medication errors are essential. Pediatric patients are especially vulnerable to errors caused by mistakes in calculations. Pharmacists should recognize that since some commercially available products are available in strengths that can be potentially toxic to a pediatric patient, special scrutiny of these products is necessary.[5]

Adverse Drug Reactions

Pediatric patients frequently have the same kinds of adverse drug reactions that adults have, but adverse reactions in the pediatric population may be harder to recognize or of greater or lesser intensity. The lack of literature on newly introduced therapeutic agents makes it imperative to monitor experience with new drugs initially used in the pediatric population. Comprehensive adverse drug reaction monitoring and reporting programs are important in reducing the occurrence of these reactions in pediatric patients.[10]

Drug-Use Evaluation

Drug-use evaluation should be directed at drugs with a low therapeutic index that require extensive monitoring, those that are responsible for serious medication errors in the institution, and those that are found to be associated with high frequency of preventable adverse drug reactions. Cost-related issues may also become important in the evaluations, since many expensive drugs are not available in package sizes appropriate for the pediatric patient.

Research

Pediatric patients have long been recognized as "therapeutic orphans" because of a relative absence of therapeutic trials in this patient population. The reasons for this are numerous and include ethical issues, potential adverse publicity, possible litigation, methodological hurdles, and an inability to justify such studies for economic reasons. Nonetheless, the need for timely and effective research on medication safety, efficacy, and practical application in the pediatric population is compelling. The paucity of pediatric drug information, the impact of new drug delivery systems, the expansion of adult diseases (such as AIDS) into the pediatric population, and expanded applications of new and established therapeutic agents are all areas warranting additional research. The pediatric pharmacist can be directly involved in collaboration with other health care providers in conducting pediatric

research. Examples of pediatric research topics include, but are not limited to, the following:

- Safety and efficacy of drug products in pediatric patients;
- Pharmacokinetics and pharmacodynamics of new medications;
- Stability, safety, and efficacy of extemporaneously compounded sterile and nonsterile drug products;
- Safety and efficacy of administration techniques;
- Comparative evaluations of medications addressing treatment regimens, outcomes of therapy, and their relative costs;
- Behavioral and socioeconomic compliance issues in pediatric pharmaceutical care; and
- New and existing pharmacy drug distribution systems and services for pediatric patients.

Examples of direct involvement include

- Serving as a member of an institutional review board;
- Maintenance, oversight, and dissemination of all information on investigational drug studies and comparative trials involving medications in the pediatric population; and
- Maintenance, coordination, and oversight of policies and procedures involving investigational drug studies and comparative trials involving medications in the pediatric population.

References

1. American Society of Hospital Pharmacists. ASHP statement on pharmaceutical care. *Am J Hosp Pharm.* 1993; 50:1720–3.
2. Pediatric Pharmacy Administration Group Committee on Pediatric Pharmacy Practice. Pediatric pharmacy practice guidelines. *Am J Hosp Pharm.* 1991; 48:2475–7.
3. American Society of Hospital Pharmacists. ASHP guidelines: minimum standard for pharmacies in institutions. *Am J Hosp Pharm.* 1985; 42:372–5.
4. Folli HL, Poole RL, Benitz WE, et al. Medication error prevention by clinical pharmacists in two children's hospitals. *Pediatrics.* 1987; 79:718–22.
5. American Society of Hospital Pharmacists. ASHP guidelines on preventing medication errors in hospitals. *Am J Hosp Pharm.* 1993; 50:305–14.
6. American Society of Hospital Pharmacists. ASHP technical assistance bulletin on single unit and unit dose packages of drugs. *Am J Hosp Pharm.* 1985; 42:378–9.
7. American Society of Hospital Pharmacists. ASHP technical assistance bulletin on the pharmacist's role in immunization. *Am J Hosp Pharm.* 1993; 50:501–5.
8. American Society of Hospital Pharmacists. ASHP statement on the use of medications for unlabeled uses. *Am J Hosp Pharm.* 1992; 49:2006–8.
9. American Society of Hospital Pharmacists. ASHP guidelines on pharmacist-conducted patient counseling. *Am J Hosp Pharm.* 1993; 50:505–6.
10. American Society of Hospital Pharmacists. ASHP guidelines on adverse drug reaction monitoring and reporting. *Am J Hosp Pharm.* 1989; 46:336–7.

Approved by the ASHP Board of Directors, April 27, 1994. Developed by the ASHP Council on Professional Affairs.

The bibliographic citation for this document is as follows: American Society of Hospital Pharmacists. ASHP guidelines for providing pediatric pharmaceutical services in organized health care systems. *Am J Hosp Pharm.* 1994; 51:1690–2.

ASHP Guidelines on the Provision of Medication Information by Pharmacists

Definition of Terms and Basic Concepts

The provision of medication information is among the fundamental professional responsibilities of pharmacists in health systems. The primary focus of this Guidelines document is to help pharmacists in various practice settings develop a systematic approach to providing medication information. Medication information may be patient specific, as an integral part of pharmaceutical care, or population based, to aid in making decisions and valuating medication use for groups of patients (e.g., medication evaluation for formulary changes, medication-use evaluations). The goal of providing carefully evaluated, literature-supported evidence to justify specific medication-use practices should be to enhance the quality of patient care and improve patient outcomes. To be an effective provider of medication information, the pharmacist must be able to[1]

1. Perceive and evaluate the medication information needs of patients and families, health care professionals, and other personnel, and
2. Use a systematic approach to address medication information needs by effectively searching, retrieving, and evaluating the literature and appropriately communicating and applying the information to the patient care situation.

Medication Information Activities

A variety of medication information activities may be provided, depending on the particular practice setting and need. The following activities, which are often performed in an organized health care setting, are enhanced by using a systematic approach to meeting medication information needs[2–5]:

1. Providing medication information to patients and families, health care professionals, and other personnel.
2. Establishing and maintaining a formulary based on scientific evidence of efficacy and safety, cost, and patient factors.
3. Developing and participating in efforts to prevent medication misadventuring, including adverse drug event and medication error reporting and analysis programs.
4. Developing methods of changing patient and provider behaviors to support optimal medication use.
5. Publishing newsletters to educate patients, families, and health care professionals on medication use.
6. Educating providers about medication-related policies and procedures.
7. Coordinating programs to support population-based medication practices (e.g., development of medication-use evaluation criteria and pharmacotherapeutic guidelines).
8. Coordinating investigational drug services.
9. Providing continuing-education services to the health care professional staff.
10. Educating pharmacy students and residents.
11. Applying health economic and outcome analysis.
12. Developing and maintaining an active research program.

An individual pharmacist may have full or partial responsibility for all or some of these activities. For example, preparing drug monographs for pharmacy and therapeutics committees was once considered almost exclusively the responsibility of the drug information center or drug information specialist. As pharmacy practice has evolved, the expertise and knowledge base of individual pharmacy practitioners have been integrated into this process. The pharmacist may prepare the monograph or, if a medication is adopted for use, may assist in designing the medication-use evaluation (MUE) criteria, collecting data, or educating health care professionals on appropriate use. Any of these activities may contribute to a larger medication policy management program coordinated by a medication information center or specialist. As pharmacists in various organized health care settings have become more involved in providing pharmaceutical care, their activities have become less distributive and more information based, requiring a higher level of competence by all pharmacists in meeting medication information needs.

Systematic Method for Responding to Medication Information Needs

The provision of medication information can be initiated by the pharmacist or requested by other health care professionals, patients and their family members, or the general public. The process is similar, regardless of how a medication information question is generated (e.g., by the pharmacist or by another health professional) or the context in which the information will be used (e.g., in a newsletter or for solving a patient-specific problem). The pharmacist must not only accumulate and organize the literature but also objectively evaluate and apply the information from the literature to a particular patient or situation.[6–8] Consideration should be given to the ethical and legal aspects of responding to medication information requests.[9,10] A systematic method can be outlined as follows:

1. To probe for information and develop a response with the appropriate perspective, consider the education and professional or experiential background of the requester.
2. Identify needs by asking probing questions of the patient, family members, or health care professional or by examining the medical record to identify the true question. This helps in optimizing the search process and assessing the urgency for a response.
3. Classify requests as patient-specific or not and by type of question (e.g., product availability, adverse drug event, compatibility, compounding/formulation, dosage/ administration, drug interaction, identification, pharmacokinetics, therapeutic use/efficacy, safety in pregnancy and nursing, toxicity and poisoning) to aid in assessing the situation and selecting resources.

4. Obtain more complete background information, including patient data, if applicable, to individualize the response to meet the patient's, family's, or health care professional's needs.

5. Perform a systematic search of the literature by making appropriate selections from the primary, secondary, and tertiary literature and other types of resources as necessary.

6. Evaluate, interpret, and combine information from the several sources. Other information needs should be anticipated as a result of the information provided.

7. Provide a response by written or oral consultation, or both, as needed by the requester and appropriate to the situation. The information, its urgency, and its purpose may influence the method of response.

8. Perform a follow-up assessment to determine the utility of the information provided and outcomes for the patient (patient-specific request) or changes in medication-use practices and behaviors.

9. Document the request, information sources, response, and follow-up as appropriate for the request and the practice setting.

Resources

It is the responsibility of the pharmacist to ensure that up-to-date resources, including representative primary, secondary, and tertiary literature, are available to assist in answering a variety of types of medication information requests. Pharmacists should be familiar with not only the components of the literature (e.g., primary) but also the features of individual resources in each component; this makes searching more efficient so that time can be used optimally in analyzing, applying, and communicating the information. The drug information modules of the ASHP Clinical Skills Program[6-8] describe the strengths and weaknesses of the different literature components and list frequently used resources and the types of information included in each publication. The following should be considered in purchasing literature resources:

1. Attributes of the literature (e.g., frequency of update, qualifications and affiliations of authors, year of publication, type of information, organization of material, type of medium, and cost).

2. Practice setting of the pharmacist (e.g., type of facility and needs of individuals within the environment).

3. Literature currently available and readily accessible.

4. Funds allocated for literature purchases.

The volume and sophistication of medication information, as well as the demand for it, are increasing, and human memory has limitations. Consideration should be given to using computers as a tool in the decision-making process. There are several areas in which computers can be valuable in the provision of medication information.[11] Databases are available for information management, retrieval, and communication. Information management databases include software for MUE, documentation of questions and responses, and preparation of reports of adverse drug events. Information retrieval sources include bibliographic databases (e.g., International Pharmaceutical Abstracts, Iowa Drug Information Service, MEDLINE) and full-text databases (e.g., Drug Information Fulltext).[12,13] Textbooks (e.g., *AHFS Drug Information*) and

journals can also be accessed through computer technology. Some information is available through electronic bulletin boards (e.g., PharmNet) and the Internet.[14-16] Computerized medical records can also be a valuable tool in assessing either individual patient needs or population-based needs.

Documentation and Quality Assessment

Individual practicing pharmacists should base their documentation of medication information requests and responses on the type and purpose of the request and the subsequent use of the documentation. For patient-specific medication information, requests and responses could be documented in the patient's medical record. Documentation may also be considered necessary for quality assessment and other performance improvement and management activities.

Documentation of medication information requests and responses should include, as appropriate for the purposes of the documentation, the following:

1. Date and time received.
2. Requester's name, address, method of contact (e.g., telephone or beeper number), and category (e.g., health care discipline, patient, public).
3. Person assessing medication information needs.
4. Method of delivery (e.g., telephone, personal visit, mail).
5. Classification of request.
6. Question asked.
7. Patient-specific information obtained.
8. Response provided.
9. References used.
10. Date and time answered.
11. Person responding to request.
12. Estimated time in preparation and for communication.
13. Materials sent to requesters.
14. Outcome measures suggested (e.g., impact on patient care, improvements in medication use, and requester satisfaction).

Responses to requests for medication information should be accurate, complete, and timely for maximal clinical usefulness and to establish credibility for pharmacist-provided information. Quality assessment of responses should be included in the medication information process; this could be selective for certain types of patient-specific requests, random by numbers of requests or for certain time periods, or on some other basis appropriate to meet the needs of the health system.

Keeping Current

It is the responsibility of the pharmacist to keep abreast of advancements both in the tools that can be used to systematically address information requests and in the information itself regarding pharmacotherapeutic or other issues affecting the practice of pharmacy.

References

1. Troutman WG. Consensus-derived objectives for drug information education. *Drug Inf J.* 1994; 28:791–6.

2. Rosenberg JM, Ruentes RJ, Starr CH, et al. Pharmacist-operated drug information centers in the United States. *Am J Health Syst-Pharm.* 1995; 52:991–6.

3. ASHP supplemental standard and learning objectives for residency training in drug information practice. In: Practice standards of ASHP 1994–95. Hicks WE, ed. Bethesda, MD: American Society of Hospital Pharmacists; 1994.

4. American Society of Hospital Pharmacists. ASHP accreditation standard for residency in pharmacy practice (with an emphasis on pharmaceutical care). *Am J Hosp Pharm.* 1992; 49:146–53.

5. American Society of Hospital Pharmacists. ASHP statement on the pharmacist's clinical role in organized health care settings. *Am J Hosp Pharm.* 1989; 46:2345–6.

6. Galt KA. Clinical skills program drug information series, module 1. Analyzing and recording a drug information request. Bethesda, MD: American Society of Hospital Pharmacists; 1994.

7. Smith GH, Norton LL, Ferrill MJ. Clinical skills program drug information series, module 2. Evaluating drug literature. Bethesda, MD: American Society of Health-System Pharmacists; 1995.

8. Galt KA, Calis KA, Turcasso NM. Clinical skills program drug information series, module 3. Responding to a drug information request. Bethesda, MD: American Society of Health-System Pharmacists; 1995.

9. Kelly WN, Krause EC, Krowinski WJ, et al. National survey of ethical issues presented to drug information centers. *Am J Hosp Pharm.* 1990; 47:2245–50.

10. Arnold RM, Nissen JC, Campbell NA. Ethical issues in a drug information center. *Drug Intell Clin Pharm.* 1987; 21:1008–11.

11. Dasta JF, Greer ML, Speedie SM. Computers in health care: overview and bibliography. *Ann Pharmacother.* 1992; 26:109–17.

12. Hoffman T. The ninth annual medical hardware and software buyers' guide. *MD Comput.* 1992; 9: 359–500.

13. Baker DE, Smith G, Abate MA. Selected topics in drug information access and practice: an update. *Ann Pharmacother.* 1994; 28:1389–94.

14. Gora-Harper ML. Value of pharmacy-related bulletin board services as a drug information resource. *J Pharm Technol.* 1995; 11:95–8.

15. Glowniak JV, Bushway MK. Computer networks as a medical resource. *JAMA.* 1994; 271:1934–9.

16. McKinney WP, Barnas GP, Golub RM. The medical applications of the Internet: information resources for research, education and patient care. *J Gen Intern Med.* 1994; 9:627–34.

Approved by the ASHP Board of Directors, April 24, 1996. Developed by the ASHP Council on Professional Affairs.

The bibliographic citation for this document is as follows: American Society of Health-System Pharmacists. ASHP guidelines on the provision of medication information by pharmacists. *Am J Health-Syst Pharm.* 1996; 53:1843–5.

ASHP Guidelines on Surgery and Anesthesiology Pharmaceutical Services

Purpose

In hospitals, surgery and anesthesiology generally have been without direct pharmacist involvement. Drugs have been available through a stock-distribution system maintained by operating-room (OR) personnel, and documentation of controlled-substance use has often been handled by personnel other than those administering the drugs. More important, without direct pharmacist involvement, patient-related issues that are best addressed by a pharmacist usually have been handled by other health care personnel out of necessity. ASHP believes that pharmaceutical services (including drug-use control) to these areas should be provided by pharmacists, ideally with their direct presence. In many hospitals this is accomplished through an onsite satellite pharmacy.[1-5]

The purpose of these guidelines is to help pharmacists identify services they could provide in the areas of surgery and anesthesiology, decide on the scope of these services, and develop performance improvement plans. In addition, the appendix provides guidance for justifying and implementing a satellite pharmacy. Some topics outlined in these guidelines are the subject of other ASHP practice standards, which should be referred to for additional information and guidance. Pharmacists should use professional judgment in assessing their organization's needs for pharmaceutical services in surgery and anesthesiology. The guidance should be adapted, as applicable, to meet those needs.

The term "surgery and anesthesiology pharmaceutical services" should not be interpreted too literally. Many satellite pharmacies serving surgery and anesthesiology areas also serve other areas. These may include cystoscopy and endoscopy suites, cardiac catheterization laboratories or suites, preoperative holding areas, postanesthesia care units (PACUs), labor and delivery rooms, freestanding surgical centers, and critical care areas. In general, these satellite pharmacies are termed "OR satellite pharmacies" and the pharmacist an "OR pharmacist." The guidelines do not distinguish among terms, because terms may be applied differently in various settings. The terms "satellite pharmacy" and "the pharmacist" are used in their broadest senses.

Pharmaceutical Services

The successful establishment of pharmaceutical services in surgery and anesthesiology will depend to a large extent on the OR pharmacist's ability to positively affect drug-use management, take a leadership role in all aspects of cost containment, and contribute to improving patient care and outcomes.

The performance of many activities and services may be improved in surgery and anesthesiology through the establishment of pharmaceutical services. Often these include the following:

1. Drug preparation and distribution;
2. Drug inventory control;
3. Waste reduction;
4. Drug cost reduction;
5. Improved revenue generation through accurate patient billing;
6. Improved documentation of drugs administered to patients;[6]
7. Clinical activities;
8. Formulary management;
9. Drug accountability and control, including adherence to organizational drug-use guidelines;
10. Quality assurance and continuous quality improvement;
11. Compliance with standards of the Joint Commission on Accreditation of Healthcare Organizations (JCAHO);
12. Informational, educational, and research activities;
13. Involvement with the use of drug administration devices; and
14. Enhanced interdisciplinary decision-making.

Drug Preparation and Distribution

In most ORs, the drug preparation and distribution functions can be improved by pharmacy personnel practicing in this setting. These activities should not be so labor-intensive as to exclude cognitive services being provided by the pharmacist. Technicians should be assigned most of the drug preparation and distribution activities, under the supervision of a pharmacist. Drug preparation and distribution can be accomplished in various ways. For non-anesthesiology drugs and drugs that are not case specific, a secure general supply of predetermined medications in limited quantities (e.g., in cart or cassette) can be provided, with the understanding that these drugs may be used for any patient. Anesthesiology medications could be supplied by case or by daily stock replenishment (e.g., an "anesthesia cart"). Increasingly, automated medication storage and distribution devices (e.g., Pyxis Medstation [Cardinal Health]) are being used to supply medications to the anesthesiology, nursing, and surgery staffs. With these devices, automatic and more accurate patient charging is often realized and pharmacy staff spend less time in distribution activities. The methods chosen may depend on the preferences and needs of the anesthesiologists and surgery staff, available resources, and whether there is a satellite pharmacy. The choice should be based on the method that will provide accurate and timely delivery of medications to meet the needs of patients. The common objectives for all methods, however, are reducing the time spent by nursing and anesthesiology staff in gathering and preparing medications and maximizing patient safety by limiting the selection of drugs, quantities, and dosage forms.

Drug Accountability and Control

The pharmacist should be responsible for all drugs and controlled substances dispensed and distributed in the setting. Pharmacy technicians could be assigned most of the responsibility for these daily activities. If there is a satellite pharmacy, all drug inventories, to the extent possible, should be centralized there. Minimal drug stock should be kept in each

surgical suite. Ideally, the satellite pharmacy should be staffed whenever the surgery and anesthesiology areas are normally staffed. If the satellite pharmacy is not open 24 hours a day, it may be necessary to establish an after-hours drug supply (e.g., a cart). The pharmacist should decide the drugs and quantities required for this supply and the accountability system to be used. The supply levels should be checked and replenished daily. With an OR pharmacy, trends in drug use or disappearance are more easily identified, noted, and reconciled. Systems to track drugs used, to adjust par levels as needed, and to monitor drug expiration dates should be devised.

Clinical Services

Provision of clinical services should be a major focus of pharmacists practicing in the surgery and anesthesiology areas. These services may be similar to those provided to all other patient care areas. Clinical services can be provided by a pharmacist even without a satellite pharmacy.

To make effective clinical contributions, the pharmacist should be familiar with all drugs used in the setting, including drugs for general and regional anesthesia, neuromuscular blockade, analgesia, preoperative management, hemodynamic control, diagnosis and manipulation during surgery, prevention of infection, treatment of intraoperative emergencies, control of bleeding, and postoperative nausea and vomiting (PONV). Knowledge may be gained by observation of surgery and anesthesia procedures, attendance at anesthesia and surgery conferences, assigned topics to be presented by each pharmacy team member, review of pertinent literature, and direct clinical involvement in patient care. Clinical services may include the following[7]:

Medication-Use Management. The pharmacist is especially suited to taking a leadership role in medication-use management in the OR. This could be accomplished through the development of pharmaceutical practice guidelines and critical pathways for select surgical procedures, including intraoperative drug use. Guidelines are routinely developed for the neuromuscular blocking agents, synthetic opioids, propofol, antiemetic agents, volatile inhalation agents, and anti-infectives for surgical prophylaxis. Additional guidelines could be developed on the basis of organizational needs. It has been demonstrated that pharmaceutical practice guidelines for anesthesia-related medications reduce costs without adversely affecting patient outcomes.[8–10] With or without established guidelines, the presence of an OR satellite pharmacy allows the pharmacist to reinforce the appropriate use of agents dispensed from the pharmacy and to monitor patient outcomes.

Medication-Regimen Review. Whenever possible, medication requests from surgery or anesthesiology staff should be evaluated before the drug is dispensed for appropriateness (e.g., allergies, disease states, adherence to pharmaceutical practice guidelines), dose, route of administration, timing of administration, and cost compared with other therapeutic alternatives. The pharmacist should review the surgery schedule and routinely screen patient profiles or charts before surgery for allergies (e.g., antimicrobials, narcotics, latex) and notify appropriate personnel of pertinent findings. In addition, doses, timing, and choices of prophylactic antimicrobials should be monitored. Profiles or charts should also be reviewed whenever possible for potential perioperative

drug—drug or drug—disease interactions and for proper continuation of maintenance medications and discontinuation of unnecessary medications postoperatively.

Medication-Use Evaluation. The pharmacist should take a leadership role in the performance of medication-use evaluations by establishing criteria, collecting data, analyzing the data, making recommendations, and performing follow-up. Data collection is often more easily accomplished prospectively or concurrently by coordination with surgery and anesthesiology staff. High-cost or high-use medications are good starting places for medication-use evaluations in the OR. Medication-use evaluations are especially useful for assessing compliance with established guidelines. In organizations with automated anesthesia record keepers, collection and manipulation of medication-use information is greatly facilitated.[11]

Drug Information. The pharmacist should provide timely and accurate drug information in response to known needs and random inquiries. Inquiries may originate from any type of staff, including surgery and recovery-room staff, anesthesia staff, residents, nurses, perfusionists, and students. Drug information may be provided in oral or written form, as appropriate. The preparation of responses could require detailed literature searches with accompanying interpretations. The satellite pharmacy should maintain a body of pharmaceutical literature containing current primary, secondary, and tertiary literature sources. Scientific and professional practice journals in pharmacy, anesthesiology, and surgery should be directly available or readily accessible to support clinical decision-making for patients in the OR. Online drug information and access to the Internet should also be readily available to OR pharmacists. Reference texts should be current and should provide detailed information in at least the following areas: drug action, adverse effects, dosages, drugs of choice, efficacy, formulations, incompatibilities, indications for use, drug interactions, laws and regulations, pharmacology, pediatric medication administration (if applicable), nonprescription drugs, drug use during pregnancy and lactation, pathophysiology, pharmacokinetics, toxicology, surgery, and anesthesia. The pharmacist may also develop and distribute a newsletter and make available specific articles of interest to others in the setting. The pharmacist should have access to a formal drug information center.

Formulary System. The pharmacist should continually evaluate the organization's formulary and advise the medical staff and pharmacy and therapeutics (P&T) committee about drug efficacy, adverse-effect experiences, cost, and ongoing need for formulary agents. OR pharmacists can enforce P&T committee-approved restrictions on anesthesiology and surgery drugs and educate OR personnel on these restrictions.

Drug Research. The pharmacist should strive to initiate and participate in research related to drug use in surgery and anesthesia. Pharmacists could be principal investigators or could support the studies of others (e.g., perform randomization, prepare drugs, assist in study design and data collection). Because the OR is one of the most medication-intensive areas of a hospital, it is an excellent setting for pharmacoeconomic analyses and outcome studies.[12–14] These studies are best accomplished when they are collaborative. Given that newer anesthetic agents are often more expensive than

older ones, studies are useful for learning whether a higher drug cost will result in a lower total cost for the patient.

Adverse-Drug-Reaction Monitoring and Reporting. The pharmacist should monitor, detect, document, report, and recommend appropriate management of adverse drug reactions that occur in the OR. OR health care providers should be asked to report suspected adverse drug reactions to the OR pharmacist for follow-up.

Education. Educational presentations on drug-related topics should be made regularly by the pharmacist to surgery and anesthesiology residents and staff, nursing staff, pharmacy staff, and other personnel. This could include information on drugs added to the organization's formulary, drug precautions, periodic reviews of drugs used during cardiac and respiratory arrest, pain management, and the management of malignant hyperthermia and latex allergy. The pharmacist should also educate OR personnel about drugs used in the setting, giving special attention to the synthetic opioids neuromuscular blocking agents, anesthetic gases, intravenous anesthetic agents, local anesthetics, antiemetics, and antimicrobials (surgical prophylaxis).

Formal educational rotations in the satellite pharmacy may be conducted for undergraduate and graduate pharmacy students, pharmacy residents, or pharmacy fellows. Specific learning and experiential goals and objectives should be developed. The student should learn about satellite pharmacy services and preoperative, intraoperative, and postoperative medication therapy through didactic instruction, observation, project participation, and selected readings. Rotations should be coordinated with the anesthesiology and nursing departments.

Rounds. When possible, the pharmacist should be an active participant with anesthesia, surgery, and PACU staff in patient care rounds. The pharmacist may limit rounds to specific types of patients (e.g., cardiothoracic surgery, transplant) for whom the pharmacist's preoperative or postoperative involvement may be most beneficial. The pharmacist should participate in anesthesia grand rounds, morbidity and mortality reviews, and other scheduled educational sessions as appropriate. Pharmacy grand rounds could be conducted by pharmacy staff to provide detailed drug information or to supplement anesthesia grand round topics.

Pain Management. The pharmacist should participate actively in epidural anesthesia, patient-controlled analgesia, and other pain-management programs. Participation could include the development of such a program, identification of appropriate patients, patient education, drug preparation, educational presentations to other staff, and participation in rounds with acute-pain-management teams as time permits.

Participation in Emergency Life Support. The pharmacist should be authorized to participate in the medication therapy for cardiac or respiratory arrests that occur in the OR. At a minimum, the pharmacist should have current certification in basic cardiac life support (BCLS) procedures and, preferably, training in advanced cardiac life support (ACLS). The pharmacist should also participate in the treatment of malignant hyperthermia by preparing and maintaining malignant hyperthermia emergency kits and preparing and administering medications used to treat malignant hyperthermia.

Pharmacokinetic Management and Consultation. The pharmacist should participate in the pharmacokinetic management of patients and should serve as a consultant to surgery and anesthesiology staff on pharmacokinetic of medications dosing.

Compliance with JCAHO Standards. The presence of pharmacy personnel in the surgery and anesthesiology areas, especially with an established satellite pharmacy, could help to ensure adherence to Joint Commission standards. Specifically, pharmacy plays a key role in compliance with the standards related to the medication-use process. These include reviewing medication orders; considering patient information when preparing and dispensing medication(s); ensuring pharmaceutical services are available when the pharmacy department is closed or pharmacy personnel are not available; controlling the preparation and dispensing of medication(s) (drugs should be secure from tampering, safe from patient-to-patient contamination, and properly labeled); ensuring that emergency medications are consistently available, controlled, and secure in the pharmacy and patient care areas; and monitoring the effects of medications on patients.

Documentation of Clinical Activities. The pharmacist should document clinical activities and identify activities leading to improved patient outcomes and cost reductions. This type of information is critical in order for the pharmacist to prove his or her value and the ongoing need for the services provided. The pharmacist is responsible for safeguarding the patient's rights to privacy and the confidentiality of the patient's clinical information.

Controlled Substances

All controlled-substance procedures should comply with applicable federal and state laws and regulations as well as the organization's policies and procedures. Procedures for the satellite pharmacy and the surgery and anesthesiology areas served should address the following:

1. Controlled substances (and other drugs) to be monitored;
2. Methods of distribution;
3. Records;
4. Ordering;
5. Storage, access, and inventory control;
6. Reconciliation and disposal;
7. Discrepancy reporting and disciplinary action; and
8. Performance of quality control checks.

The goal of the controlled-substance system is to prevent diversion yet be practical enough that patient care is not adversely affected. The system should limit exposure to controlled substances, be accountable and consistent, and contain an educational component for health care personnel.[15]

Controlled Substances (and Other Drugs) to Be Monitored. The pharmacist should be responsible for monitoring the use of all controlled substances. As required (e.g., because of abuse or diversion potential), drugs other than controlled substances (e.g., ketamine) could also be handled according to procedures similar or identical to those used for controlled substances.

Methods of Distribution

One of two primary methods could be used for distribution of controlled substances in the OR: a per-case method or a daily-supply method.

A per-case system is advantageous in that it minimizes the quantity of controlled substances available to the anesthesiologist and the anesthetist at any one time and allows for a good audit trail. Its major disadvantage is that it is very time intensive for an organization that performs many surgeries per day. This time may be better spent by the pharmacist in clinical activities.

Daily distribution of controlled substances is less time intensive and can be accomplished from a central pharmacy or an OR satellite pharmacy. Its disadvantages are that greater amounts of controlled substances are dispensed at one time and that these substances need to be kept secure throughout the day.

The various advantages and disadvantages of each method must be considered and the appropriate system selected on an organization-specific basis.

To the extent possible, controlled substances should be distributed only in response to signed orders or oral requests from prescribers. Given the urgency often present during surgical procedures, the necessity for prescribers to devote undivided attention to anesthesia procedures, and the use of sterility-safeguard procedures during surgery, it may not always be possible to comply with such a requirement. When it is possible, the organization's standard physician-order sheet or a special controlled-substance request form developed specifically for use in the surgical suite could be used. A par level of controlled substances needed per type of case or for the day could be devised; requests for controlled substances beyond this would be treated as special orders. Whatever the methods used, clear documentation that all controlled substances used were administered to the patient should be signed by the responsible prescribers at the end of each surgical procedure. Ideally, unused controlled substances drawn up by the anesthesiologist should be returned to the satellite pharmacy and wasted by the pharmacist. Alternatively, controlled substances could be disposed of by the anesthesiologist in the presence of a witness, with both parties documenting the disposal. No matter the system, disposal of contaminated controlled substances (e.g., with blood or other body fluid) should occur in the OR and be properly documented.

Records

Records should be kept of the following:

1. Controlled substances dispensed;
2. Controlled-substance inventories;
3. Controlled substances returned (including controlled substances drawn up but not used), and records reconciliation;
4. Controlled substances disposed; and
5. Controlled-substance use, categorized by prescriber.

If the satellite pharmacy does not provide 24-hour services, the documentation procedures for after-hours use should be as similar as possible to those used when the satellite pharmacy is staffed. This will help ensure staff efficiency and familiarity with the record-keeping requirements after hours. Forms specific to the setting and to the after-hours circumstance may have to be developed.

Ordering

The pharmacist should be responsible for ordering all controlled substances for the satellite pharmacy. Once received, the controlled substances should be added to the satellite pharmacy's stock and recorded in inventory records. If the satellite pharmacy does not provide 24-hour services, the pharmacist is responsible for ensuring that adequate supplies are available in a secure, specially designated after-hours location. The pharmacist should maintain controlled-substance inventory amounts sufficient only to meet the needs of the OR for a reasonable time. This time should depend on the frequency and timeliness with which controlled substances are available from the central pharmacy. Less inventory is required, for example, if controlled substances are ordered on a daily basis rather than less often. The inventory system should be perpetual in order to provide the most current record of controlled substances on hand.

Shortly after the initial opening of a satellite pharmacy and after drug use has stabilized, stock levels should be reassessed and adjusted as needed. During ordering, the pharmacist should note developing trends in use. Nonformulary controlled substances should be dispensed only by special request.

Storage, Access, and Inventory Control

Controlled substances should be stored in a locked space (e.g., cabinet, drawer, cart) within the satellite pharmacy. These storage spaces should remain locked when controlled substances are not being dispensed. Access to the space should be limited to satellite pharmacy personnel. If 24-hour satellite pharmacy services are not provided, a separate locked after-hours storage space will be required. Kits of after-hours controlled substances may be useful. No matter how they are configured or located, all after-hours supplies should be checked and all records reconciled by satellite pharmacy staff on the first working day after the after-hours supplies are entered.

If possible, one person per shift should be identified as being responsible for controlled substances (and related procedures) when the satellite pharmacy is not open. That person should have access (key or code) to locked after-hours supplies. This approach enables more consistent record keeping, limits the number of people with access to after-hours supplies, and enables more reliable monitoring of controlled-substance use. Individuals often assigned this responsibility include an "in-charge" nurse or the "first-call" anesthesiology resident.

Controlled-substance inventories should be verified by physical count at least once daily. If the satellite pharmacy is open for two shifts, an end-of-shift count by the morning pharmacist is recommended. The use of automated medication storage and distribution devices for controlled substances may be a timesaving benefit for maintaining a perpetual inventory. Unscheduled audits of controlled substances in the satellite pharmacy should be done by staff not normally assigned to this setting. The results should be documented.

Reconciliation and Disposal

A thorough system for reconciling controlled-substance use should be developed and include the following components[16–18]:

1. *Comparison of quantities dispensed with quantities documented as administered.* The quantity of controlled substances returned to the satellite pharmacy should be compared with the quantity dispensed. The amount dispensed should equal the amount returned (unopened and partially filled containers and partially used syringes) plus the amount documented as administered.
2. *Verification of use through review of the anesthesia record.* The anesthesia record should be reviewed to ensure that the amount documented as administered (in records returned to the satellite pharmacy) is identical to the amount documented in the patient's anesthesia record. This verification is ideally done for all cases but may be done by periodic audits of randomly selected cases if anesthesia records are not readily available for every case.
3. *Qualitative testing of returned controlled substances.* To verify that unadulterated drug is contained in partially used containers returned to the satellite pharmacy, a refractometer or other device can be used. It is important to randomly audit controlled-substance returns in order to detect trends in diversion. The organization's legal department should be consulted to make sure such testing is permitted.

The pharmacist should account for all controlled substances dispensed and should report all discrepancies to internal and external authorities as required.

Disposal of controlled substances (e.g., partially used syringes) should be done in the satellite pharmacy by a member of the pharmacy staff in the presence of a witness. This action should be documented in the satellite pharmacy's controlled-substance records.

Communication and Education

It is important that there are open lines of communication among the pharmacist, the chair of anesthesiology (or designee), and the head surgical nurse to allow sharing of information indicative of diversion (e.g., behavioral change). In addition, periodic continuing education for all members of the OR team on the potential for substance abuse may sensitize staff to this problem.[15]

Performance Improvement

The pursuit of continuous improvement in the quality of services provided should be a philosophy of practice of the pharmacist and the satellite pharmacy staff.[19] In that light, many activities may be seen as pertinent to performance improvement efforts. Some of these are the following:

1. Adverse-drug-reaction monitoring and reporting,
2. Medication-error monitoring and reporting,
3. Medication histories,
4. Periodic inspections of all drug storage sites,
5. Drug therapy monitoring related to improved patient outcome (e.g., decreased time in the PACU, decreased frequency of PONV),
6. Medication-use evaluations,
7. Drug-interaction monitoring,
8. Controlled-substance monitoring,
9. Quality control of compounded parenterals (e.g., cardioplegic solutions) and batch-prepared syringes,
10. Medication-waste monitoring, and
11. Allergy and patient demographic monitoring.

Some of these activities should not be difficult to implement in a satellite pharmacy, because ongoing procedures should already be developed for the organization overall. Sometimes, it may be necessary to develop new programs or variations of existing ones tailored to the surgery and anesthesiology areas.

Other Activities

Policies and Procedures. If there is a satellite pharmacy, the pharmacist should develop and maintain policies and procedures for the satellite pharmacy and its services. There should be policies and procedures for the preparation of drug kits (if applicable), medication distribution systems, controlled-substance handling, hours of operation, preparation of parenteral products, expiration-date checking and monthly inspections, recycling of products, monitoring of drug inventory levels, staff training, quality assurance activities, and after-hours drug distribution.

Interdisciplinary Interfaces. The pharmacist should function as a liaison between the pharmacy department and all staff in the setting served, including anesthesiology, nursing, and surgery staff; perfusionists; and management staff. The pharmacist should represent the pharmacy department on appropriate interdisciplinary committees charged with evaluating or making recommendations about services and medication selection and use in the surgery and anesthesiology areas. A committee specifically designed to focus on pharmacy matters may be appropriate.

Financial Analysis. The pharmacist should document drug costs, service costs, revenues, and savings attributable to the satellite pharmacy and the activities (clinical and distributive) of its staff. If there is no OR satellite pharmacy, some of the aforementioned items will not need to be included in the analysis. Financial reports should be prepared periodically (e.g., quarterly, annually) and provided to the hospital administration and the departments of anesthesiology, surgery, and pharmacy.

The Pharmacy Technician's Role

Pharmacy technicians assigned to the satellite pharmacy should be trained to perform their assigned functions. It is critical and appropriate for the technician to do most of the drug distribution-related activities in the satellite pharmacy. Within the total work force of pharmacy technicians in the organization, it is desirable to have some technicians trained as available back-up staff for the satellite pharmacy. Technicians should be trained and certified by the Pharmacy Technician Certification Board or equivalent. In general, technician training and experience should include parenteral drug preparation, drug distribution procedures, physician-order interpretation, anesthesia and OR record interpretation, computer order entry, and controlled-substance record keeping. Specific training should include a review of the following:

1. Procedures unique to surgical suites, including special apparel (e.g., caps, masks, foot covers) and restricted movements and areas within surgical suites;
2. Surgical-suite terms, including abbreviations and acronyms used to name surgical procedures;

3. Drug classes, indications for use, and proper handling of drugs routinely used in surgical suites (e.g., special packaging, preservative requirements for spinal and epidural drugs, infusion concentrations);
4. Controlled-substance procedures;
5. Emergency drugs typically used in surgical suites; and
6. A review of the role of the pharmacy technician in the OR pharmacy area.

Typical activities performed by pharmacy technicians in the satellite pharmacy under the supervision of the pharmacist are drug distribution, controlled-substance handling, sterile drug preparation, drug ordering and restocking, orientation and training of new staff, and quality assurance activities. Each of these will be discussed in greater detail.

Drug Distribution. The technician could distribute medications to storage sites in the setting and prepare per-case or per-prescriber kits of medications and distribute these after they have been checked by the pharmacist. If automated medication storage and distribution devices are used, the technician is responsible for all activities associated with restocking these. Given the nature of surgical procedures and the urgency of the need for the requested medications, distribution would be required in response to oral requests. The pharmacist should screen such requests to ensure proper choices of drugs for specific patients. The technician should be trained to ask about patient allergies and relay this information to the pharmacist before preparing a medication. The technician also should be taught which situations must be handled by the pharmacist (e.g., drug information, dose calculations).

The technician could return unused drugs to stock and charge patients or departments for medications used.

Another technician function could be to check and replenish after-hours drug supplies and charge medications used to appropriate patients or departments.

The technician could be responsible for monthly inspections of drug storage areas and drug supply areas in the satellite pharmacy. Technicians should be assigned their own inspection zone when drugs are stored in many places.

Controlled Substances. Other responsibilities of the technician could be the distribution of controlled substances and the creation of appropriate records according to the distribution procedures of the satellite pharmacy and according to federal and state laws and regulations. Typical activities could include helping with inventory counts, maintaining perpetual inventory records, disposing of controlled substances with the pharmacist, and participating in audits, assays, and preparation of reports.

Sterile Drug Preparation. The technician could aseptically compound, package, and label sterile drugs—for injection and for irrigation—and document all products made. Appropriate records of drug name, diluent, lot numbers, and expiration dates of batch-prepared products should be maintained by the technician.

Drug Ordering and Restocking of the Pharmacy Satellite. In addition, technicians could routinely order replenishment supplies of drugs for the satellite pharmacy, check supplies delivered in response to the orders, and place the stock in appropriate places. Requests for odd medications or unusual trends in medication demand should be reported to the pharmacist for further review.

Orientation and Training of New Staff. Helping with the orientation and training of new staff (including other technicians and pharmacy students) could also be a responsibility of the technician. An orientation checklist, workflow sheets, and task lists are helpful training tools. An OR pharmacy student module would be a helpful teaching tool for students on rotation in the satellite pharmacy.

Quality Assurance. The technician could be involved in quality assurance activities of the satellite pharmacy. Such activities may include regular controlled-substance audits or assays, microbiological monitoring of parenteral drugs prepared, and inspections of drug supplies (e.g., expiration dates).

Summary

Pharmaceutical services in surgery and anesthesiology should be the standard of practice in health care organizations across the United States. Although not essential, an onsite satellite pharmacy would help in the provision of these services. A majority of distribution-related activities should be done by technicians. The availability of automated devices and other technology may lessen, to some extent, the time devoted to drug distribution. It is important for the OR pharmacist to concentrate on the provision of clinical services, such as medication-use management, drug information services, medication-use evaluations, formulary management, and pharmacoeconomic analyses of anesthesia- related medications. These activities provide the best opportunity for the pharmacist to contribute to improving patient care and outcomes and containing costs. Finally, pharmaceutical services in surgery and anesthesiology should be periodically assessed for patient care and financial effectiveness.

References

1. Powell PJ, Maland L, Bair JN et al. Implementing an operating room pharmacy satellite. *Am J Hosp Pharm.* 1983; 40:1192–8.
2. Opoien D. Establishment of surgery satellite pharmacy services in a large community hospital. *Hosp Pharm.* 1984; 19:485–90.
3. Keicher PA, McAllister JC III. Comprehensive pharmaceutical services in the surgical suite and recovery room. *Am J Hosp Pharm.* 1985; 42:2454–62.
4. Buchanan EC, Gaither MW. Development of an operating room pharmacy substation on a restricted budget. *Am J Hosp Pharm.* 1986; 43:1719–22.
5. Vogel DP, Barone J, Penn F et al. Ideas for action: the operating room pharmacy satellite. *Top Hosp Pharm Manag.* 1986; 6:63–80.
6. Donnelly AJ. Multidisciplinary approach to improving documentation of medications used during surgical procedures. *Am J Hosp Pharm.* 1989; 46:724–8.
7. Shafer AS. Clinical pharmacy practice in the operating room. *J Pharm Pract.* 1993; 6:165–70.
8. Gora-Harper ML, Hessel E II, Shadick D. Effect of prescribing guidelines on the use of neuromuscular blocking agents. *Am J Health-Syst Pharm.* 1995; 52:1900–4.
9. Freund PR, Borolle TA, Posner KL, et al. Cost-effective reduction of neuromuscular-block drug expenditures. *Anesthesiology.* 1997; 87:1044–9.

10. Lubarsky DA, Glass PSA, Ginsberg B, et al. The successful implementation of pharmaceutical practice guidelines. *Anesthesiology*. 1997; 86:1145–60.

11. Lubarsky DA, Sanderson IC, Gilbert WC, et al. Using an anesthesia information management system as a cost containment tool. *Anesthesiology*. 1997; 86:1161–9.

12. Lorighlin KA, Weingarten CM, Nagelhout J, et al. A pharmacoeconomic analysis of neuromuscular blocking agents in the operating room. *Pharmacotherapy*. 1996; 16:942–50.

13. DeMonaco HJ, Shah AS. Economic considerations in the use of neuromuscular blocking drugs. *J Clin Anesth*. 1994; 6:383–7.

14. Tang J, Watcha MF, White PF. A comparison of costs and efficacy of ondansetron and droperidol as prophylactic antiemetic therapy for elective outpatient gynecologic procedures. *Anesth Analg*. 1996; 83:304–13.

15. Castellano FC. Developing methods for preventing and detecting substance abuse in the operating room: a disease approach. *J Pharm Pract*. 1993; 6:159–64.

16. Satterlee GB. System for verifying use of controlled substances in anesthesia. *Am J Hosp Pharm*. 1989; 46:2506–8.

17. Shovick VA, Mattei TJ, Karnack CM. Audit to verify use of controlled substances in anesthesia. *Am J Hosp Pharm*. 1988; 45:1111–3.

18. Gill DL, Goodwin SR, Knudsen AK, et al. Refractometer screening of controlled substances in an operating room satellite pharmacy. *Am J Hosp Pharm*. 1990; 47:817–8.

19. Hawkins PR. Quality improvement: pharmacy involvement in the operating room. *J Pharm Pract*. 1993; 6:171–6.

Appendix— Justifying and Implementing an Operating-Room Satellite Pharmacy

Justification of the need for a satellite pharmacy is a critical step in establishing pharmaceutical services in surgery and anesthesiology.[1,2]

The pharmacist's ability to positively affect medication-use management, to take a leadership role in all aspects of cost containment, and to contribute to improved patient care and outcomes must be highlighted.

Familiarization with Surgery and Anesthesiology Pharmaceutical Services. As an initial step, the person in charge of the project should become familiar with typical surgery and anesthesiology satellite pharmacy services. Review of pertinent literature, discussions with pharmacists in other organizations, and site visits to established satellite pharmacies are methods of accomplishing this step. The site visit is especially useful, because it can reinforce and further define information gained by other means. At the conclusion of this step, the pharmacist should have a realistic view of the types and scope of services typically provided.

Obtaining Support. If justification is to be successful, the support of key individuals from the major departments affected by the service should be obtained.[1] In most organizations, these are hospital administration, anesthesiology (anesthesiologists and certified registered nurse anesthetists), and surgery, operating-room (OR), and postanesthesia care unit nursing.

The support of the anesthesiology department is necessary because this department represents the major users of medications in the OR and has significant patient care responsibilities in this setting. Support for pharmaceutical services from anesthesiology department administration is important for the success of the project. If the request for satellite pharmacy services originates in the anesthesiology department, the justification process may be simpler and more collaborative. Data gathered during the preliminary review of the site and information obtained from the literature can be used when the project is discussed with anesthesiology administration. It may be valuable to solicit the support of any anesthesiologists who have been especially receptive to pharmacy involvement. Many anesthesiologists have had positive experiences with OR pharmaceutical services at other organizations. The proposal for a satellite pharmacy might then be presented jointly by pharmacy personnel and anesthesiologists. Once formalized, the proposal should be presented to hospital administration. The administration's opinion will provide some guidance on how to facilitate the approval process for the satellite pharmacy.

If conceptual support from these groups is obtained, development of a more formal proposal can begin. If there are still concerns about the benefits gained from OR satellite pharmacy services, it may be helpful to propose an interim step to expose more hospital staff to OR pharmaceutical services in order to keep the process moving forward. One possible approach is to suggest that a pilot project be conducted involving several ORs or one specific surgical specialty. The establishment of a permanent satellite pharmacy would depend on favorable results from the pilot project.

Initial Assessment of Setting. A general review of the surgery and anesthesiology areas to be served by the satellite pharmacy should be done after staff have become familiar with the project. At this time, it is not essential that detailed information be obtained. Useful information to collect includes the following:

1. All locations and quantities of drugs stored in the setting,
2. The location and storage of controlled substances,
3. Controlled-substance accountability systems used,
4. Drug preparation and distribution procedures used in the setting,
5. Billing systems used for all drugs,
6. Stock replenishment and rotation systems used, and
7. The role (or potential role) of automation in the involved areas.

The collection of this information could be speeded by a tour of the area and by inquiries through nurses, anesthesiologists, supply technicians, surgeons, and other OR personnel (e.g., perfusionists).

Formal Proposal. The development of a formal proposal is an important part of the justification process. It is essential that the proposal be well organized and factual. The writers of the proposal should expect the proposal to be examined in great detail by hospital administration and others during the decision-making process. The proposal should expand upon the information obtained in the initial review of the surgery and anesthesiology areas. Information that should be in the proposal includes the following:

1. The dollar value of current drug inventory,
2. The dollar value of drugs used per period (e.g., per year),

3. The dollar value of patient charges currently generated,
4. The estimated dollar value of increased revenue,
5. The average cost of drugs used per surgical case,
6. An estimated cost of drug waste per period,
7. The general quality and completeness of controlled-substance records,
8. The number of controlled-substance discrepancies reported per month,
9. The number of reports of drug-related incidents received per month,
10. The time personnel in the setting currently spend performing pharmacy-related activities,
11. The time pharmacy personnel currently spend performing activities for the setting, and
12. Opportunities for collaborative efforts by pharmacy–anesthesiology, pharmacy–nursing, pharmacy–perfusion, and pharmacy–surgery in drug-use management (e.g., development of pharmaceutical practice guidelines, performance of medication-use evaluations).

Collection of this information could be helped through the formation of a multidisciplinary team. Representatives of the departments of pharmacy, anesthesiology, nursing, and surgery should be included. This approach has several benefits. Data collection can be expedited, because the expertise of each individual can be used. The value of a satellite pharmacy will be continually reinforced to these individuals, and all groups will have input into the decision-making process.

A formal proposal should be prepared once the required information has been collected. Minimally, the proposal should contain the following sections[1]:

1. Introduction;
2. Statement of problems and anticipated benefits (and beneficiaries);
3. Summary of the proposed services;
4. Cost–benefit analysis, including staffing, estimated cost savings, revenue projections, and inventory savings; and
5. Implementation plan.

During preparation of these sections, it is important to be as specific as possible and to assign dollar values whenever these are available. The proposal should be endorsed by the members of the multidisciplinary team and should be submitted to the administration by the director of pharmacy. Careful planning, data collection, analysis, and presentation of the information gathered will make approval more likely.

Implementation. Implementation should begin as soon as possible after administrative approval.[1] Implementation steps should be planned and executed in a clear, concise manner. To guide planning, an implementation time line should be developed (e.g., Gantt chart), listing the steps to be taken, the task force member responsible for each step, and the expected amount of time required for each activity. The amount of time required for each activity may vary from organization to organization, but the order in which the steps should be performed will be reasonably standard.

The major implementation steps and an approximate order in which they should be completed are as follows[1]:

1. Obtain a formal commitment of space,
2. Assign a project leader (who should be responsible for the project's development and need not be the pharmacist who will be assigned to staff the satellite pharmacy; often, it is valuable for the project leader to be a supervisor or assistant director),
3. Identify construction and equipment needs,
4. Oversee construction work,
5. Obtain and install equipment,
6. Draft policies and procedures (e.g., controlled-substance accountability, medication distribution system, inventory control),
7. Develop job descriptions,
8. Select staff (pharmacists and support personnel),
9. Design and print forms,
10. Formalize policies and procedures,
11. Determine satellite pharmacy drug-stock levels,
12. Train staff,
13. Identify back-up and relief staff and orient them to the setting,
14. Educate nursing staff,
15. Educate anesthesiology department staff,
16. Educate surgeons,
17. Open the satellite pharmacy for operation,
18. Determine future goals for service, and
19. Determine systems for periodic analyses of the impact of the program.

Many of these steps can be expedited by a close working relationship with members of the anesthesiology and nursing departments.

The satellite pharmacy's services should be monitored and evaluated on an ongoing basis through workload statistics, data on controlled-substance discrepancies, financial data, and patient outcomes data. In addition, the satisfaction levels of the nursing and anesthesiology staffs should be assessed before the program is implemented, six months after implementation, and yearly after that.

References

1. Vogel DP, Barone J, Penn F, et al. Ideas for action: the operating room pharmacy satellite. *Top Hosp Pharm Manage.* 1986; 6:63–80.
2. Ziter CA, Dennis BW, Shoup LK. Justification of an operating-room satellite pharmacy. *Am J Hosp Pharm.* 1989; 46:1353–61.

These guidelines were reviewed in 2003 by the Council on Professional Affairs and by the Board of Directors and were found to still be appropriate.

Approved by the ASHP Board of Directors November 14, 1998. Developed through the ASHP Council on Professional Affairs. Supersedes the ASHP Technical Assistance Bulletin on Surgery and Anesthesiology Pharmaceutical Services dated November 14, 1990.

The bibliographic citation for this document is as follows: American Society of Health-System Pharmacists. ASHP guidelines on surgery and anesthesiology pharmaceutical services. *Am J Health-Syst Pharm.* 1999; 56:887–95.

Pharmaceutical Industry

Drug Products, Labeling, and Packaging

Standardized Clinical Drug Nomenclature (0920)
Source: Council on Pharmacy Management
To encourage federal agencies, the pharmaceutical industry, pharmacy and medical software providers, and purveyors of clinical data repositories and drug databases to explore the potential benefits of supplementing or modifying the National Drug Code with a coding system that can be used effectively to support patient care, research, and financial management; further,

To encourage that such a coding system encompass prescription drug products, nonprescription medications, and dietary supplements and include both active and inactive ingredients.

This policy supersedes ASHP policy 0801.

Disclosure of Excipients in Drug Products (0808)
Source: Council on Pharmacy Practice
To advocate that manufacturers declare the name and derivative source of all excipients in drug products on the official label.

(*Note: Derivative source* means the botanical, animal, or other source from which the excipient is originally derived.)

Patient Access to Orphan Drug Products (0715)
Source: Council on Public Policy
To encourage continued research, development, and marketing of orphan drug products; further,

To urge health policymakers, payers, and pharmaceutical manufacturers to develop innovative ways to ensure patient access to orphan drug products; further,

To support public policies that ensure that the cost of orphan drug products does not preclude reasonable patient access to these agents.

This policy was reviewed in 2011 by the Council on Public Policy and by the Board of Directors and was found to still be appropriate.

Standardizing Prefixes and Suffixes in Drug Product Names (0720)
Source: Council on Public Policy
To collaborate with others, including the United States Pharmacopeia and the Food and Drug Administration, in standardizing and defining the meaning of prefixes and suffixes for prescription and nonprescription drugs to prevent medication errors and ensure patient safety.

This policy was reviewed in 2011 by the Council on Public Policy and by the Board of Directors and was found to still be appropriate.

Elimination of Surface Contamination on Vials of Hazardous Drugs (0618)
Source: Council on Professional Affairs
To advocate that pharmaceutical manufacturers eliminate surface contamination on vials of hazardous drugs; further,

To inform pharmacists and other personnel of the potential presence of surface contamination on the vials of hazardous drugs; further,

To encourage health care organizations to adhere to published standards and regulations to protect workers from undue exposure to hazardous drugs.

This policy was reviewed in 2010 by the Council on Pharmacy Practice and by the Board of Directors and was found to still be appropriate.

Mandatory Labeling of the Presence of Latex (0501)
Source: Section of Inpatient Care Practitioners
To urge the Food and Drug Administration to mandate that manufacturers of medications and medication-device combination products include labeling information on whether any component of the product, including its packaging, contains natural rubber latex.

This policy was reviewed in 2009 by the Council on Pharmacy Practice and by the Board of Directors and was found to still be appropriate.

Ready-to-Use Packaging for All Settings (0402)
Source: Council on Professional Affairs
To advocate that pharmaceutical manufacturers provide all medications used in ambulatory care settings in unit-of-use packages; further,

To urge the Food and Drug Administration to support this goal; further,

To encourage pharmacists to adopt unit-of-use packaging for dispensing prescription medications to ambulatory patients; further,

To support continued research on the safety benefits and patient adherence associated with unit-of-use packaging and other dispensing technologies.

(*Note:* A *unit-of-use* package is a container–closure system designed to hold a specific quantity of a drug product for a specific use and intended to be dispensed to a patient without any modification except for the addition of appropriate labeling.)

This policy was reviewed in 2008 by the Council on Pharmacy Practice and by the Board of Directors and was found to still be appropriate.

Standardization, Automation, and Expansion of Manufacturer-Sponsored Patient-Assistance Programs (0404)
Source: Council on Administrative Affairs
To advocate standardization of application criteria, processes, and forms for manufacturer-sponsored patient assistance programs (PAP); further,

To advocate the automation of PAP application processes through computerized programs, including Web-based models; further,

To advocate expansion of PAPs to include high-cost drugs used in inpatient settings.

This policy was reviewed in 2008 by the Council on Pharmacy Management and by the Board of Directors and was found to still be appropriate.

Unit Dose Packaging Availability (0309)
Source: Council on Administrative Affairs
To advocate that pharmaceutical manufacturers provide all medications used in health systems in unit dose packages; further,

To urge the Food and Drug Administration to support this goal in the interest of public health and patient safety.

This policy was reviewed in 2007 by the Council on Pharmacy Management and by the Board of Directors and was found to still be appropriate.

Drug Shortages (0002)
Source: Council on Administrative Affairs
To declare that pharmaceutical manufacturers, distributors, group purchasing organizations, and regulatory bodies, when making decisions that may create drug product shortages, should strive to prevent those decisions from compromising the quality and safety of patient care.

This policy was reviewed in 2009 by the Council on Pharmacy Practice and by the Board of Directors and was found to still be appropriate.

Pediatric Dosage Forms (9707)
Source: Council on Professional Affairs
To support efforts that stimulate development of pediatric dosage forms of drug products.

This policy was reviewed in 2006 by the Council on Pharmacy Practice and by the Board of Directors and was found to still be appropriate.

Use of Color to Identify Drug Products (9608)
Source: Council on Professional Affairs
To support the reading of drug product labels as the most important means of identifying drug products; further,

To oppose reliance on color by health professionals and others to identify drug products; and further,

To oppose actions by manufacturers of drug products and others to promulgate reliance on color to identify drug products.

This policy was reviewed in 2008 by the Council on Pharmacy Practice and by the Board of Directors and was found to still be appropriate.

Expiration Dating of Pharmaceutical Products (9309)
Source: House of Delegates Resolution
To support and actively promote the maximal extension of expiration dates of pharmaceutical products as a means of reducing health care costs and to recommend that pharmaceutical manufacturers review their procedures to accomplish this end.

This policy was reviewed in 2011 by the Council on Pharmacy Practice and by the Board of Directors and was found to still be appropriate.

Tamper-Evident Packaging on Topical Products (9211)
Source: House of Delegates Resolution
ASHP should support the standardization and requirement of tamper-evident packaging on all topical products, including all dermatologicals and nonprescription products.

This policy was reviewed in 2011 by the Council on Pharmacy Practice and by the Board of Directors and was found to still be appropriate.

Drug Nomenclature (9011)
Source: House of Delegates Resolution
To work with the FDA, USP, and pharmaceutical industry to assure that drug products are named in a manner that clearly and without confusion permits identification of ingredients' strengths and changes.

This policy was reviewed in 2008 by the Council on Public Policy and by the Board of Directors and was found to still be appropriate.

Codes on Solid Dosage Forms of Prescription Drug Products (8709)
Source: Council on Legal and Public Affairs
To support efforts requiring manufacturers of solid dosage form prescription drug products to imprint a readily identifiable code indicating the manufacturer of the drug product and the product's ingredients; further,

To make information on transition of the codes readily available.

This policy was reviewed in 2011 by the Council on Public Policy and by the Board of Directors and was found to still be appropriate.

International System of Units (8612)
Source: Council on Professional Affairs
To not advocate, at this time, adoption of the International System of Units (SI units) as the exclusive labeling for drug dosages and concentrations; further,

To urge labelers to include: (1) units of mass, volume, or percentage concentrations and (2) moles or millimoles in labeling until the health professions and the public can be educated and be comfortable with use of SI units in prescribing and labeling drug products.

This policy was reviewed in 2008 by the Council on Pharmacy Practice and by the Board of Directors and was found to still be appropriate.

Elimination of Apothecary System (8613)
Source: Council on Professional Affairs
To recommend to all health professions and to the Pharmaceutical Manufacturers Association (PMA) [now the Pharmaceutical Research and Manufacturers of America (PhRMA)] that the apothecary system be eliminated in referring to dosage quantities and strengths.

This policy was reviewed in 2011 by the Council on Pharmacy Practice and by the Board of Directors and was found to still be appropriate.

Size, Color, and Shape of Drug Products (8310)
Source: Council on Legal and Public Affairs
To approve the authority of manufacturers to copy the size, shape, and color of generically equivalent drug products as a means of promoting better patient compliance (rational drug therapy), but only when the source and identity of the product are readily ascertainable from a uniform mark or symbol on the product.

This policy was reviewed in 2011 by the Council on Public Policy and by the Board of Directors and was found to still be appropriate.

Marketing

Direct-to-Consumer Advertising of Prescription and Nonprescription Medications (1119)
Source: Council on Public Policy
To oppose direct-to-consumer advertising unless it is educational in nature about prescription drug therapies for certain medical conditions and appropriately includes pharmacists as a source of information; further,

To oppose direct-to-consumer advertising of specific prescription drug products unless the following requirements are met: (1) that such advertising is delayed until postmarketing surveillance data are collected and assessed, (2) that the benefits and risks of therapy are presented in an understandable format at an acceptable literacy level for the intended population, (3) that such advertising promotes medication safety and allows informed decisions, (4) that a clear relationship between the medication and the disease state is presented, (5) that no such advertising or marketing information for prescription or nonprescription medication is directed toward minors, and (6) that such advertising include mechanisms that direct consumers to a medication adverse event reporting system (AERS); further,

To advocate that the Food and Drug Administration require an AERS reporting link in direct-to-consumer advertising material available on the Internet; further,

To support the development of legislation or regulation that would require nonprescription drug advertising to state prominently the benefits and risks associated with product use that should be discussed with the consumer's pharmacist or physician.

This policy supersedes ASHP policy 0609.

Regulation of Off-label Promotion and Marketing (1120)
Source: Council on Public Policy
To advocate for authority for the Food and Drug Administration to regulate the promotion and dissemination of information about off-label uses of medications by manufacturers; further,

To advocate that such promotion and dissemination be permitted only if manufacturers submit a supplemental new drug application for new use within a reasonable time after initial dissemination of information about off-label uses.

Pharmaceutical Distribution Systems (1016)
Source: Council on Pharmacy Management
To support wholesaler/distribution business models that meet the requirements of hospitals and health systems with respect to timely delivery of products, minimizing short-term outages and long-term product shortages, managing and responding to product recalls, fostering product-handling and transaction efficiency, preserving the integrity of products as they move through the supply chain, and maintaining affordable service costs.

This policy supersedes ASHP policy 0605.

Restricted Drug Distribution (0714)
Source: Council on Public Policy
To affirm support for the current system of drug distribution in which prescribers and pharmacists exercise their professional responsibilities on behalf of patients; further,

To acknowledge that there may be limited circumstances in which constraints on the traditional drug distribution system may be appropriate if the following principles are met: (1) the requirements do not interfere with the continuity of care for the patient; (2) the requirements preserve the pharmacist–patient relationship; (3) the requirements are based on scientific evidence fully disclosed and evaluated by prescribers, pharmacists, and others; (4) there is scientific consensus that the requirements are necessary and represent the least restrictive means to achieve safe and effective patient care; (5) the costs of the product and any associated product or services are identified for purposes of reimbursement, mechanisms are provided to compensate providers for special services, and duplicative costs are avoided; (6) all requirements are stated in functional, objective terms so that any provider who meets the criteria may participate in the care of patients; and (7) the requirements do not interfere with the professional practice of pharmacists, prescribers, and others; further,

To advocate that the Food and Drug Administration (FDA) be granted the authority to consult with practicing pharmacists and others when the establishment of a restricted distribution system is contemplated for a drug product; further,

To advocate that FDA be granted the authority to require that manufacturers disclose all of the considerations that led to the establishment of a restricted distribution system for a specific product; further,

To advocate that FDA be granted the authority to require that manufacturers include in each restricted distribution system a mechanism that will ensure medication reconciliation and continuity of care as patients transition from one level or site of care to another; further,

To advocate that FDA be granted the authority to require manufacturers to conduct a follow-up assessment of the impact of a restricted drug distribution system.

This policy was reviewed in 2011 by the Council on Public Policy and by the Board of Directors and was found to still be appropriate.

Medication Management for Patient Assistance Programs (0603)
Source: Council on Administrative Affairs
To support the principle that medications provided through manufacturer patient assistance programs should be stored, packaged, labeled, dispensed, and recorded using systems that ensure the same level of safety as prescription-based programs that incorporate a pharmacist-patient relationship.

This policy was reviewed in 2010 by the Council on Pharmacy Management and by the Board of Directors and was found to still be appropriate.

Drug Samples (9702)

Source: Council on Legal and Public Affairs

To oppose drug sampling or similar drug marketing programs that (1) do not provide the elements of pharmaceutical care, (2) result in poor drug control, allowing patients to receive improperly labeled and packaged, deteriorated, outdated, and unrecorded drugs, (3) provide access to prescription drugs by unauthorized, untrained personnel, (4) may encourage inappropriate prescribing habits, or (5) may increase the cost of treatment for all patients.

This policy was reviewed in 2011 by the Council on Public Policy and by the Board of Directors and was found to still be appropriate.

Manufacturer-Sponsored Patient-Assistance Programs (9703)

Source: Council on Legal and Public Affairs

To encourage pharmaceutical manufacturers to (1) extend their patient assistance programs to serve the needs of both uninsured and underinsured patients, (2) enhance access to and availability of such programs, and (3) incorporate the elements of pharmaceutical care into these programs.

This policy was reviewed in 2011 by the Council on Public Policy and by the Board of Directors and was found to still be appropriate.

ASHP Guidelines for Pharmacists on the Activities of Vendors' Representatives in Organized Health Care Systems

For purposes of this document, vendors' representatives are defined as agents who promote products and provide information and services to health care providers on behalf of manufacturers and suppliers. The narrow focus of this document is on those vendors who serve and interact with settings with respect to drug products, drug-related devices, and other equipment, supplies, and services purchased by pharmacies.

Each individual setting should develop its own specific policies and procedures relating to the activities of vendors' representatives. Such policies and procedures should supplement and complement applicable federal, state, and local laws and regulations (for example, statutes that address prescription drug-product sampling). The ASHP Guidelines on Pharmacists' Relationships with Industry, the ASHP Guidelines for Selecting Pharmaceutical Manufacturers and Suppliers, and setting-specific conflict-of-interest policies may be helpful in the development of policies and procedures.[1,2] The policies and procedures should be developed by the setting's pharmacy and therapeutics committee (or equivalent body) and approved by higher authorities in the setting as required. Depending on the individual setting, policies and procedures may be useful in the following areas.

1. *A defined scope of applicability.* The vendors' representatives to which any policies and procedures apply should be defined by the individual setting. For example, if the policies and procedures are applicable only to drug-product vendors' representatives and not to those promoting medical–surgical supplies, packaging equipment, or drug administration devices, this should be clearly stated.

2. *Orientation of representatives.* In some individual settings, vendors' representatives receive an orientation packet upon their initial visit to the setting. Such a packet might contain a copy of the setting's policies and procedures, a medical staff directory, and the formulary. Some settings provide a formal orientation program that includes meeting key individuals and touring the setting.

3. *Directory.* In some individual settings, a file of current vendor-contact information is maintained in the pharmacy. A form for recording such information might include the following:
 - The vendor's name and address;
 - The name, address, telephone number, and answering service number (if any), and drug-product assignment (purview) of each representative;
 - The name, address, and telephone number of the representative's manager;
 - The names, telephone numbers, and emergency telephone numbers of the vendor's directors of distribution, sales, and product information (titles may vary); and
 - The names and telephone numbers of the vendor's medical director and research director (titles may vary).

4. *Availability of vendor-contact information to professionals in the setting.* In some individual settings, the pharmacy department provides the setting's professional staff with the information in item 3, upon request.

5. *Registration while on premises.* In some individual settings, vendors' representatives register with the pharmacy department or other designated department upon each visit to the setting. At such time, the vendors' representatives document the time, purpose, and location of their appointments. In many settings, during the registration process, the representative is provided with a dated name badge to be prominently worn along with the representative's current vendor-supplied name tag (if any).

6. *Locations permitted.* In some individual settings, restriction (if any) from patient care and pharmacy storage and work areas in the setting are specified in the policies and procedures. Meetings with professional staff are conducted in areas convenient to staff and generally in non-patient-care areas.

7. *Appointments and purposes.* In some individual settings, representatives are encouraged to schedule appointments with appropriate pharmacy department staff to
 - Provide information useful for product evaluation. Representatives might be asked to include balanced scientific literature (journal reprints, for example) on drug-product safety and efficacy, as well as documentation of likely cost benefits.
 - Provide timely information on the vendor's products and services.
 - Facilitate procurement and crediting transactions.
 - Obtain and provide information necessary to support the setting's formulary system.
 - Facilitate informational activities for the pharmacy staff and other health care professionals with respect to the vendor's products.

8. *Exhibits.* In some individual settings, the pharmacy department provides opportunities for vendors' representatives to distribute informational material by arranging for organized, scheduled exhibits. Policies and procedures about the times, places, content, and conduct of such events are established.

9. *Dissemination of promotional materials.* In some individual settings, there are policies and procedures about the dissemination (by vendors' representatives) of information on formulary and nonformulary products, including the designation of appropriate categories of recipients of the information (e.g., attending physicians, department chairmen, house staff physicians). Representatives may be asked to promptly provide the pharmacy department with copies of all informational and promotional materials disseminated in the setting. The Food and Drug Administration (FDA) prohibits

the advertising and promotion of drug products for uses not reflected in FDA-approved product labeling ("unlabeled uses").[3] Pharmacists and other health care professionals should be aware of these laws and regulations when evaluating the content of promotional materials.

10. *Samples.* In some individual settings, there are policies and procedures with respect to product samples. ASHP urges that the use of drug samples within the institution be eliminated to the extent possible.[4,5]

11. *Noncompliance.* In some individual settings, policies and procedures exist to address noncompliance with the policies and procedures by either vendors' representatives or professional staff.

Each setting should have policies and procedures concerning research to be conducted on its premises. Pharmacists and vendors' representatives should clearly differentiate research from sales and promotional activities, applying appropriate policies and procedures accordingly.[6] Generally, scientific research involving drug products is coordinated through research departments of product manufacturers rather than through sales and promotional representatives.

References

1. American Society of Hospital Pharmacists. ASHP guidelines on pharmacists' relationships with industry. *Am J Hosp Pharm.* 1992; 49:154.

2. American Society of Hospital Pharmacists. ASHP guidelines for selecting pharmaceutical manufacturers and suppliers. *Am J Hosp Pharm.* 1991; 48:523–4.

3. American Society of Hospital Pharmacists. ASHP statement on the use of medications for unlabeled uses. *Am J Hosp Pharm.* 1992; 49:927–8.

4. American Society of Hospital Pharmacists. ASHP guidelines: minimum standard for pharmacies in institutions. *Am J Hosp Pharm.* 1985; 42:372–5.

5. Greenberg RB. The Prescription Drug Marketing Act of 1987. *Am J Hosp Pharm.* 1988; 45:2118–26.

6. American Society of Hospital Pharmacists. ASHP guidelines for pharmaceutical research in organized health-care settings. *Am J Hosp Pharm.* 1989; 46:129–30.

This guideline was reviewed in 1998 by the Council on Professional Affairs and by the ASHP Board of Directors and was found to still be appropriate.

Approved by the ASHP Board of Directors, November 17, 1993. Developed by the Council on Professional Affairs.

The bibliographic citation for this document is as follows: American Society of Hospital Pharmacists. ASHP guidelines for pharmacists on the activities of vendors' representatives in organized health care systems. *Am J Hosp Pharm.* 1994; 51:520–1.

Pharmacy Management

Pharmacy Management

Role of Corporate Pharmacist Leadership in Multifacility Organizations (1210)
Source: Council on Pharmacy Management
To advocate that a pharmacist must be responsible for leadership and have responsibility for standardization and integration of pharmacy services in multiple business units across the entire pharmacy enterprise of multifacility health systems and integrated delivery networks; further,

To educate health-system administrators about the importance of pharmacy leadership in setting system-wide policy regarding the safe and effective use of medications

Workload Monitoring and Reporting (0901)
Source: House of Delegates Resolution
To strongly discourage the use of pharmacy workload and productivity measurement systems ("pharmacy benchmarking systems") that are based solely upon dispensing functions (e.g., doses dispensed or billed) or a variant of patient days, because such measures do not accurately assess pharmacy workload, staffing effectiveness, clinical practice contributions to patient care, or impacts on costs of care, and therefore these measurement systems are not valid and should not be used; further,

To advocate the development and implementation of pharmacy benchmarking systems that accurately assess the impact of pharmacy services on patient outcomes and total costs of care; further,

To define pharmacy workload as all activities related to providing pharmacy patient care services; further,

To continue communications with health-system administrators, consulting firms, and professional associations regarding the value of pharmacists' services and the importance of using valid, comprehensive, and evidence-based measures of pharmacy workload and productivity; further,

To encourage practitioners and vendors to develop and use a standard protocol for collecting and reporting pharmacy workload data and patient outcomes; further,

To advocate to health-system administrators, consulting firms, and vendors of performance-measurement services firms the development and implementation of pharmacy benchmarking systems that accurately assess the impact of pharmacy services on patient outcomes and total costs of care.
This policy supersedes ASHP policy 0406.

Pharmacist Leadership of the Pharmacy Department (0918)
Source: Council on Pharmacy Management
To affirm the importance of an organizational structure in hospitals and health systems that places administrative, clinical, and operational responsibility for the pharmacy department under a pharmacist leader; further,

To affirm the role of the pharmacist leader in oversight and supervision of all pharmacy personnel; further,

To recognize the supporting role of nonpharmacists in leadership and management roles within pharmacy departments.
This policy supersedes ASHP policy 0606.

Pharmacy Staff Fatigue and Medication Errors (0504)
Source: Council on Administrative Affairs
To encourage pharmacy managers to consider workload fatigue, length of shifts, and similar performance-altering factors when scheduling pharmacy staff, in order to ensure safe pharmacy practices; further,

To oppose state or federal laws or regulations that mandate or restrict work hours for pharmacy staff; further,

To support research on the effects of shift length, fatigue, and other factors on the safe practice of pharmacy.

This policy was reviewed in 2009 by the Council on Pharmacy Management and by the Board of Directors and was found to still be appropriate.

ASHP Statement on the Roles and Responsibilities of the Pharmacy Executive

Position

The American Society of Health-System Pharmacists (ASHP) believes that complex hospitals and health systems benefit from having a pharmacy executive responsible for the design, operation, and improvement of their organization's medication-use process. This individual (sometimes referred to as the "chief pharmacy officer" but hereafter "the pharmacy executive") must be properly positioned within the organization to ensure the best utilization of his or her expertise in all decisions regarding medication use. To promote effective communication, collaboration, and teamwork with peers, the pharmacy executive should

- Be involved in the organization's strategic planning regarding all components of the medication-use process,
- Report directly to the organization's principal executive (e.g., chief executive officer [CEO], chief operating officer [COO]),
- Have a title internally consistent with others reporting at that organizational level,
- Participate in regularly scheduled CEO- or COO-level meetings, and
- Be a member of the medical executive committee (or its equivalent).

Background

Hospitals and health systems are complex organizations. Executive-level decisions that affect the medication-use system are made at a rapid pace, often with profound implications for patient care, patient safety, and the health system's fiscal well-being. The pharmacy executive must be properly positioned within an organization to ensure the best utilization of his or her expertise in decision-making that affects the policies, procedures, and systems that support safe, effective, and efficient medication use. When pharmacy leadership reports directly to the principal executive rather than through multiple layers of management, the quality and timeliness of information exchange improve significantly. Pharmacy leaders can more actively engage in critical decision-making and will be more effective in helping the health system anticipate and address rapid change.

Significant changes in pharmacy practice, health care, and health-system management over the past 20 years have dramatically transformed the traditional role of the pharmacy director.[1] More widespread use of the title "chief pharmacy officer" was first proposed in 2000 in an attempt to enhance the contribution pharmacy makes to patient care by creating organizational parity between the pharmacy executive and other chief officers (e.g., chief nursing, medical, and information officers).[2] When the pharmacy executive works collaboratively with others at this executive level, the pharmacy department is better positioned to effectively contribute to the organization's strategic initiatives and address system-wide issues regarding medications and medication use.

Qualifications and Responsibilities of the Pharmacy Executive

The pharmacy executive is a professionally competent, legally qualified pharmacist. He or she must be thoroughly knowledgeable about and have experience in hospital pharmacy practice and management. Additional qualifications might include completion of a pharmacy residency program accredited by ASHP, an advanced management degree (e.g., M.B.A., M.H.A.), or an administrative specialty residency.

What distinguishes the pharmacy executive from the established director of pharmacy position is a deeper knowledge of the organization's operations as well as a greater degree of involvement in the organization's strategic planning and decision-making processes. The pharmacy executive provides the organization with pharmacy's unique clinical and business perspectives in discussions and decisions related to changes in medical and surgical practice and operational changes.[3] He or she has experience leading evidence-based decision-making about drug use, controlling pharmaceutical expenses while maximizing patient benefit through the formulary system. The pharmacy executive has in-depth knowledge of the pharmaceutical supply chain, clinical therapeutics, physician prescribing habits, the medication-use process, medication-use policy, and the technology used to deliver and support patient care and about how those issues affect the overall success of the organization. The pharmacy executive understands the relationships between third-party requirements, coding, documentation, billing equations, pricing updates, and organizational resources and can provide quality assurance for all these functions, improving financial performance.[4]

The pharmacy executive's responsibilities include but are not limited to the following: strategic planning; designing, managing, and improving the medication-use system; ensuring quality outcomes through performance-improvement activities; leading drug-utilization efforts; optimizing use of information systems and technology; managing the pharmaceutical supply chain, pharmacy department financial operations, and human resources; ensuring compliance with regulatory and accreditation requirements; fulfilling the organization's research and educational missions; and providing institutional representation and leadership.[5] The pharmacy executive fulfills these responsibilities through his or her own actions, proper delegation to competent individuals on his or her staff, and collaborative efforts with other health care professionals.

Strategic Planning. The pharmacy executive assesses the health care environment, identifying opportunities to improve medication use and medication-use systems. In the organization's strategic planning, he or she provides pharmacy's perspective on how changes in the use of pharmaceuticals and related technology may affect systems in the future.

Medication-Use System Management. The pharmacy executive is responsible for overseeing the design, implementation, and management of a safe and effective medication-use system. He or she ensures that systems are developed and improved based on evidence and best practices, operate effectively and efficiently across the continuum of care, and are continuously evaluated and improved using contemporary quality-improvement methods. The pharmacy executive is responsible for developing plans for the continued operation of medication-use systems and for the provision of pharmaceutical services during emergencies and disasters.

Quality Outcomes and Performance Improvement. The pharmacy executive ensures that the medication-use system is continuously evaluated and improved using contemporary quality-improvement methods. The pharmacy executive provides leadership at the organizational level to ensure that pharmacists are positioned to improve the quality and safety of medication use throughout the health system. The pharmacy executive (or his or her designee) should be a member of all of the institution's key committees responsible for performance-improvement activities related to medication use and patient safety. The pharmacy executive and his or her staff must be intimately involved in all improvement initiatives involving medication use. The pharmacy executive should give particular attention to patients in high-risk areas (as identified by organizations such as the Centers for Medicare and Medicaid Services and the Joint Commission) to ensure that pharmacy services meet patient care needs and that drug therapy is as safe, effective, and economical as possible. The pharmacy executive (or a designee) is a member and active participant of the infection control committee and ensures that infection control principles are applied to the prescribing, dispensing, and administration of antimicrobials.

Drug-Utilization Management. The pharmacy executive collaborates with peers to develop drug-utilization and formulary initiatives that optimize therapeutic outcomes, reduce the risk of drug-related problems, and ensure the use of cost-effective pharmacotherapy throughout the health system. He or she identifies inappropriate utilization and leads efforts to modify practices to improve medication use.

Informatics and Technology. The pharmacy executive leverages technology and automated systems to optimize the medication-use system. He or she has responsibility for ensuring that information systems and technology used in the pharmacy and patient care environments maximize the safety, effectiveness, and efficiency of medication prescribing, dispensing, and administration. The pharmacy executive provides leadership at the organizational level regarding planning, purchasing, implementing, and maintaining information systems that support patient care (e.g., electronic health records, computerized prescriber-order-entry systems, smart pumps).

Supply Chain Management. The pharmacy executive is responsible for all pharmaceutical contracting, procurement, receiving, security, inventory control, diversion prevention, and distribution policies, including reverse distribution and other methods of pharmaceutical waste disposal. He or she ensures that the methods used to contract and obtain products are safe, cost-effective, and timely. The pharmacy executive is also responsible for emergency preparedness of the supply chain.

Financial Management. The pharmacy executive manages the health-system pharmacy's financial performance within the context of the broader health system. He or she develops budgets aligned with organizational and departmental objectives and monitors financial performance appropriately, performing financial audits and analysis as needed to ensure accurate, appropriate, and timely recording and classification of actual revenue capture and expenses.

Human Resources Management. The pharmacy executive manages the health-system pharmacy's human resource efforts. These efforts include determining the appropriate numbers and types of staff required to meet patient care needs, satisfy regulatory and accrediting requirements, and achieve the institution's mission. The pharmacy executive ensures effective and timely staff recruitment, orientation, training, education, mentoring, career development, performance review, and retention efforts.

Regulatory and Accreditation Compliance. The pharmacy executive ensures continued compliance with all national, state, and local regulations related to medications and their use. He or she is responsible for the implementation of Joint Commission medication management standards and National Patient Safety Goals related to medications; for maintaining ASHP accreditation, where applicable (e.g., residency and technician training); and for the implementation of best practices.

Research and Educational Missions. The pharmacy executive has an integral role in supporting the organization's research and educational missions by overseeing investigational drug services, fostering staff and resident research, and managing student and residency educational programs.

Institutional Representation and Leadership. The pharmacy executive demonstrates the personal leadership qualities and business acumen essential to operate effectively within the health system and to advance the profession and practice of pharmacy. He or she serves as the primary pharmacy representative on relevant committees of the organization's leaders to ensure that medication-use systems and pharmaceutical services meet the needs of patients and health care providers across the continuum of care. The pharmacy executive assumes a leadership role within the profession through active participation in local, state, and national professional associations.

Conclusion

Complex hospital and health systems should have a pharmacy executive responsible for the design, operation, and improvement of the organization's medication-use process. This individual must be properly positioned within the organization to ensure the best utilization of his or her expertise in all decisions regarding medication use.

References

1. Nold EG, Sander WT. Role of the director of pharmacy: the first six months. *Am J Health-Syst Pharm.* 2004; 61:2297–310.
2. Godwin HN. Achieving best practices in health-system pharmacy: eliminating the 'practice gap.' *Am J Health-Syst Pharm.* 2000; 57:2212–3.
3. Anderson RW. Health-system pharmacy: new practice framework and leadership model. *Am J Health-Syst Pharm.* 2002; 59:1163–72.
4. Mitchell CL, Anderson ER, Braun L. Billing for inpatient hospital care. *Am J Health-Syst Pharm.* 2003; 60(suppl 6):8–11.
5. Ivey MF. Rationale for having a chief pharmacy officer in a health care organization. *Am J Health-Syst Pharm.* 2005; 62:975–8.

Developed through the ASHP Council on Pharmacy Management and approved by the ASHP Board of Directors on March 7, 2008, and by the ASHP House of Delegates on June 10, 2008.

John E. Clark, Pharm.D., Rosario (Russ) J. Lazzaro, M.S., and Douglas A. Miller, Pharm.D., are gratefully acknowledged for drafting this statement.

The bibliographic citation for this document is as follows: American Society of Health-System Pharmacists. ASHP statement on the roles and responsibilities of the pharmacy executive. *Am J Health-Syst Pharm.* 2009; 66:499–502.

ASHP Statement on Standards-Based Pharmacy Practice in Hospitals and Health Systems

Position

Pharmacy practice leaders in hospitals and health systems have a distinguished history of advancing health-system pharmacy practice beyond the minimum required by law, regulation, and accreditation. The American Society of Health-System Pharmacists (ASHP) supports those efforts by developing and disseminating a comprehensive body of evidence-based, peer-reviewed descriptions of best practices in health-system pharmacy. ASHP believes that pharmacists who practice in hospitals and health systems ("health-system pharmacists") and pharmacy leaders in health systems can continuously improve the delivery of patient care by regularly assessing compliance with ASHP best practices, identifying gaps in practice, establishing practice improvement priorities appropriate for their unique circumstances, and working to close the targeted gaps.

Purpose

The purpose of this statement is to promote understanding of how health-system pharmacists use ASHP best practices to develop and promote in health systems a standard of practice that exceeds what is required by law, regulation, or accreditation.

Standards-Based Pharmacy Practice

A standard is "a statement that defines the performance expectations, structures, or processes that must be in place for an organization to provide safe and high quality care, treatment, and service."[1] In health care, practice standards serve as guideposts for a profession and as a way of communicating to peers, patients, policymakers, other professionals, and the public the roles and responsibilities of members of the profession. Practice standards also provide a benchmark for evaluating the quality of services and patient care.

Health-system pharmacists, like other health care professionals, practice under a number of mandated standards. These standards include state board of pharmacy regulations, public health requirements, Drug Enforcement Administration regulations, Joint Commission accreditation standards, Centers for Medicare and Medicaid Services conditions of participation, and the standards of other accrediting bodies and professional associations. Individual health care organizations also develop their own interdisciplinary practice policies and standards of care related to medication use, with health-system pharmacists serving as key participants in their development.

ASHP members have invested decades of effort in developing and maintaining an extensive body of policy positions, statements, and guidelines (hereinafter "ASHP best practices") that serve as a guide for effective, high-quality pharmacy practice in hospitals and health systems.[2] This comprehensive set of policies is unique in pharmacy.

ASHP best practices reinforce health-system pharmacists' established roles in health care and encourage development of responsibilities that answer the growing need and public demand for expanded involvement of pharmacists in patient care. ASHP best practices are based on professional and scientific literature and are developed with input from ASHP members, the public, regulatory bodies, other professional associations, and representatives of other health care disciplines. Peer groups of ASHP expert members systematically review ASHP best practices and compare them with the existing literature, the changing expectations of society, and changes in the professional and ethical challenges faced by health-system pharmacists. A compilation of these documents is published annually as *Best Practices for Hospital and Health-System Pharmacy* and made available to the public (www.ashp.org/bestpractices).

Most ASHP best practices represent the professional beliefs and aspirations of pharmacists practicing in health systems, based on evidence and expert opinion. Only three ASHP guidelines describe a minimum level of practice that all hospital pharmacy departments should consistently provide; these guidelines are designated as ASHP minimum standards.[3-5] Institutions that offer ASHP-accredited residencies are required to meet ASHP best practices to ensure the quality of the educational experience.

ASHP best practices represent a commitment by ASHP members to advancing the standard of pharmacy practice. ASHP believes that all health-system pharmacists have a role to play in raising health-system pharmacy practice to a level consistent with the best practices that have been developed and have gained acceptance by a peer-reviewed, consensus-based process. Practicing pharmacists and pharmacy leaders in health systems should use their professional judgment to regularly assess compliance with ASHP best practices, identify gaps in practice in their settings, establish practice improvement priorities appropriate for their unique circumstances, and work to close those practice gaps to ensure continuous improvement in the delivery of patient care.

Conclusion

Health-system pharmacy practice leaders have a long tradition of striving to advance practice beyond the minimum required by law, regulation, and accreditation. ASHP best practices embody those aspirations and provide health-system pharmacists with a means to continuously improve the delivery of patient care.

References

1. Comprehensive accreditation manual for hospitals. Oakbrook Terrace, IL: Joint Commission; 2007:GL-22.
2. Zellmer WA. Overview of the history of hospital pharmacy in the United States. In: Brown TR, ed. Handbook of institutional pharmacy practice. 4th ed.

Bethesda, MD: American Society of Health-System Pharmacists; 2006:19–32.

3. American Society of Health-System Pharmacists. ASHP guidelines: minimum standard for pharmacies in hospitals. *Am J Health-Syst Pharm.* 1995; 52:2711–7.

4. American Society of Health-System Pharmacists. ASHP guidelines: minimum standards for home care pharmacies. *Am J Health-Syst Pharm.* 1999; 56:629–38.

5. American Society of Health-System Pharmacists. ASHP guidelines: minimum standard for pharmaceutical services in ambulatory care. *Am J Health-Syst Pharm.* 1999; 56:1744–53.

Developed through the ASHP Council on Pharmacy Management and approved by the ASHP Board of Directors on March 7, 2008, and by the ASHP House of Delegates on June 10, 2008.

Scott Mark, Pharm.D., M.S., M.Ed., CHE, FASHP, FABC, is gratefully acknowledged for drafting this statement.

The bibliographic citation for this document is as follows: American Society of Health-System Pharmacists. ASHP statement on standards-based pharmacy practice in hospitals and health systems. *Am J Health-Syst Pharm.* 2009; 66:409–10.

ASHP Guidelines on Medication Cost Management Strategies for Hospitals and Health Systems

Because medication costs comprise the majority of health-system pharmacy budgets and continue to increase faster than other health care expenditures,[1] drug costs are a constant target for cost containment initiatives. The purpose of these guidelines is to provide guidance on medication-cost-management strategies.

These guidelines recommend techniques to manage drug costs in hospitals and health systems. The guidelines focus on drug use in inpatient settings and hospital clinics, where health-system pharmacies typically have responsibility for purchasing and distributing drugs. Strategies for other settings, such as managed care and ambulatory care settings, and strategies for revenue optimization are beyond the scope of this document. Although revenue optimization and medication cost management are complementary approaches to improving the financial performance of pharmacy departments, revenue optimization is best addressed through literature specific to that topic[2,3] and is not extensively reviewed in this document.

These guidelines examine methods for nonlabor pharmaceutical cost containment, focusing primarily on variable costs (costs dependent on patient volume) and direct drug costs. Fixed and indirect costs, such as labor to prepare or administer medication, nonpharmaceutical materials, and overhead, are also beyond the scope of these guidelines. There is also not an attempt to consider the impact of drug costs and drug-cost-management strategies on other hospital departments (e.g., laboratory, respiratory care) or on the total health care costs once the patient leaves the acute care setting. Although not discussed here, these shifts in drug costs are important to consider as drug therapies influence other health care costs, and pharmacists should lead efforts to promote the value medications provide across the hospital and health care system.

A broad range of drug-cost-management strategies exist throughout hospitals and health systems. Some approaches are relatively straightforward and can be implemented within the pharmacy. Other approaches are more complex and require high-level strategic planning and extensive collaboration throughout the hospital. Successful drug cost management requires systematic attention to and integration of both approaches. Because of the different nature of various drug-cost-management activities, these guidelines present information at different levels of complexity appropriate to the approach being described.

When selecting and implementing drug-cost-management strategies, it is essential that pharmacists remain mindful of patient safety and the quality of patient care.

Drug-cost-containment initiatives must never compromise the department's ability to provide the best possible care to patients. In many cases, it is prudent and necessary to monitor and evaluate the safety and outcomes of drug-cost-management projects. Fortunately, many drug-cost-containment strategies have little or no potential for detrimental effects on patient care, and efforts to improve the quality of drug use often coincide with cost-containment initiatives.

Trends in Medication Expenditures

Senior hospital administrators have recognized the importance of drug costs to the fiscal status of health systems. For example, a health care consultancy reported that in 1996, "managing hospital drug utilization and expenditures" was not ranked in the top 20 concerns for hospital CEOs.[4] When the survey was repeated in 2000; however, hospital CEOs ranked drug costs as their seventh most important concern. The 2000 survey also reported that among hospitals' greatest financial challenges, drug and technology costs were second only to decreased reimbursement, and hospital CEOs said that drugs offered the single greatest opportunity for cost savings.[4] Although somewhat dated, these data illustrate that drug-expenditure management presents health systems with an important challenge that is recognized by senior hospital administration.

Four primary factors drive growth in overall drug expenditures: price, utilization, mix, and innovation.[1]

Price inflation is an increase in the unit price of existing medications. Utilization is an increase in use of a drug, such as an increase in number of users, days of therapy, or dose per day of therapy. Mix changes when newer, more expensive therapies are used in place of older, less expensive but equally effective drugs. Finally, a blend of the utilization and mix factors increases drug expenditures when expensive, new medications become available to treat conditions previously untreatable with drug therapy (i.e., innovative therapy).

The United States spent over $250 billion dollars on prescription drugs in 2005, but total drug costs represent a relatively small portion of total U.S. health care spending (approximately 11%).[5] However, double-digit increases in prescription drug expenditures have been common (e.g., 15% in 2000, 18% in 2001, 12% in 2002, 11% in 2003, and 9% in 2004).[1,4,6] The rate of drug-expenditure growth has frequently been higher than inflation, increases in wages, and other health care spending, including spending for hospitals, physician services, and total health care expenditures. However, with the exception of 26% growth in 2001, the recent rate of growth in hospital drug expenditures has been less than the growth of total drug expenditures. Hospital drug expenditures grew 4.9% in 2000, 26% in 2001, 9.7% in 2002, 6.3% in 2003, 7.9% in 2004, and 5.7% in 2005.[1,5–7] However, the rate of growth in clinic drug expenditures has consistently exceeded the growth of total drug expenditures. Clinic drug expenditures grew 24.6% in 2000, 23% in 2001, 21.3% in 2002, 22.2% in 2003, 13.5% in 2004, and 12.4% in 2005.[1,5,7]

While the rate of increase in prescription drug expenditures moderated somewhat between 2004 and 2006, drug-expenditure growth remains substantial. Long-range forecasts suggest that the rate of increase in total prescription drug expenditures will continue to exceed the rate of increase for total health care expenditures through 2014. Because drug expenditures are the largest component of every health-system pharmacy's operating budget and often a meaningful portion of the entire hospital operating budget, drug expenses

attract significant attention from hospital leaders. For these reasons, it is apparent that drug-expenditure-management will remain an area of focus and responsibility for health-system pharmacists for the foreseeable future.[8]

Systematic Approach to Medication-Cost-Management Measures

A systematic approach to planning and prioritizing specific drug cost management strategies is essential when implementing initiatives that will influence drug expenditures in a health system. Annual financial planning (i.e., budgeting) is the most common planning approach, and specific drug-cost-management strategies should be considered a part of the budgeting process. However, longer-term strategic and programmatic planning activities also have an important role in managing drug expenditures.

A systematic approach to drug-cost containment requires specific and detailed data on both health-system drug purchases and actual drug-use patterns. Data must underlie all types of planning to manage medication expenditures. Systems should be established to have ready access to the data and continually review and monitor these data.

It is essential to interact and collaborate consistently with physician leaders from various specialties to successfully plan, prioritize, and implement medication-cost management efforts. Physician involvement must be sought during the annual financial planning process and when doing strategic or programmatic planning related to drug expenditures. Appropriate physician representatives must also be engaged in specific drug-cost-management initiatives. During the annual financial planning process, physicians can provide important information related to drug costs, such as anticipated use of key drugs in the pipeline, programmatic or new service implementation, anticipated recruitment of specialists who may require high-cost agents, projections for use of high-priority drugs, and insights for drug cost containment. Pharmacy leaders can also use this opportunity to update physicians on the pharmacy department's recent accomplishments and goals for the future.

Drug Budgeting. Although a complete discussion of the drug-budgeting process is beyond the scope of this document, several important suggestions are provided below. A general approach to systematically developing the annual drug budget is outlined in Table 1.[7] At the beginning of each calendar year, the *American Journal of Health-System Pharmacy* publishes a projection of drug expenditures for that year.[1,5–7]

Annual drug budgeting is a challenging exercise. Unanticipated situations that result in extreme increases in drug expenditures will likely occur and the pharmacy director should be prepared to explain those situations. Better data and more experience will improve a department's ability to forecast institutional drug expenditures. Regardless of the drug budget's accuracy in forecasting the institution's drug expenditures, a well-planned drug budget should help the department understand drug use patterns and identify opportunities for drug cost management. Specific reports that can be helpful in understanding drug use will be described below.

During the annual financial planning process, it is important to identify and focus on key drug expenditures. The

Table 1.
Steps for Developing Annual Drug Budget[7]

Collect and review data (e.g., drug purchase data, drug utilization data, workload and productivity data, other financial statements).
Develop budget for high-priority agents (top 50–60 drugs).
Identify relevant new drugs and build new agent budget.
Budget for nonformulary drugs and lower-priority drugs.
Establish a drug cost containment plan (identify drugs going off patent, opportunities for therapeutic interchange or protocol development).
Finalize and present the total drug budget.
Continue the budgeting process throughout the year through constant vigilance and monitoring of drug use.

Pareto Principle, or 80/20 rule, applies to drug budgeting and states that in nearly all cases, a few vital factors are important and many are trivial. A relatively small number of drugs (50–60) typically account for 80% of most hospital drug budgets. Therefore, budgeting and cost-containment efforts should focus on those drugs, and the cost-management plan should especially concentrate on those top drugs for which it is feasible to influence prescribing patterns. Much of this document focuses on the need to develop a cost-containment plan after initial estimates of drug costs are completed (Table 1).

Medication-cost-management projects should be carefully selected and prioritized as part of an ongoing financial planning process. Because drug-cost containment strategies must be customized to each health system's unique characteristics, a global assessment of the pharmacy department and the hospital must be conducted to identify opportunities for drug-cost-management. This assessment must go beyond a qualitative assessment of opportunities and must include retrieval and analysis of both drug purchase and drug-utilization data. Pharmacy departments may need to obtain and develop resources, such as personnel and software, to analyze these data.

Despite the need to customize the strategy and tactics to fit the needs of different hospitals and health systems, a systematic approach to identifying, prioritizing, and implementing medication-cost containment initiatives is necessary and can be applied in any setting. A clearly defined list of cost-containment targets should be established during each financial planning cycle. To be successful, the number of initiatives should be manageable and should focus on the institution's top expenditures. In many situations, multiple approaches for cost containment will be necessary.

The foundation for effective cost-management strategies, and the first stage of the systematic approach, begins with determining current costs of medications, both as ongoing expenses and those held as assets in inventory. Understanding and tracking key medication-cost indicators on an ongoing basis is necessary to determine the opportunities for medication-cost reduction. Examples of these indicators may include:

- Medication inventory per adjusted patient day
- Medication inventory turnover rate
- Contract coverage percentage
- Contract compliance percentage
- Intravenous-to-oral dosage ratio
- Volume-adjusted total medication costs (e.g., cost per adjusted patient day, discharge, etc.)

- Volume-adjusted drug category costs (e.g., antibiotics, anesthesia-related drugs, etc.)
- Descending-order total purchase histories, tracked over time

In addition, the use of external benchmarks may provide assistance in identifying medication-cost-reduction opportunities. External benchmarks may be available as a component of services provided by consulting organizations, the pharmacy's drug wholesaler or group-purchasing organization (GPO), or from professional published data. Benchmark data should be used with care; however, because there may be important limitations to the applicability of the data to a specific site. For example, difficulties may exist in adjusting the data for the specific pharmacy practice, such as models and intensity of services, and in finding an appropriate peer group.[9]

After cost-management opportunities are identified, they need to be quantified. Dollar values should be assigned to each opportunity, including inventory reduction, improvement in inventory turns, improving contract compliance, therapeutic interchange of various agents, and others. A specific goal and action plan should be set for each drug-cost-management target. For example, one goal might be to reduce expenditures for a drug class by 8% by establishing a contract for a new, preferred agent and implementing a therapeutic interchange program to shift use to the new agent. Alternatively, the goal might be to slow the rate of increase in use of a particular drug or drug class (e.g., based on current patterns, use of this drug class is expected to grow 15% in the next fiscal year, but the goal of interventions is to limit the rate of increase to 10%). Monitoring is essential, so drug cost containment targets should be consistently measured and evaluated. Identifying and quantifying the opportunities must be completed before prioritization and in-depth evaluation begins.

Assessment and Prioritization. Once opportunities for cost management have been identified and quantified, assessment and prioritization can occur. There are many methods of prioritization, but most of them contain two key elements: determining the potential benefit and estimating the relative ease or difficulty of attaining the benefit. Even though potential benefit may be clear-cut, the degree of difficulty is often hard to establish. Important points to consider when determining the relative degree of difficulty and likelihood of achieving benefits from a given drug-cost-management opportunity include (1) the amount of time pressure (the time available until the cost reductions occur), (2) key stakeholder (e.g., nurse, physician) sensitivity and willingness to collaborate, (3) extent of leadership support for the initiative, (4) resources required, and (5) existing level of expertise within the organization for the specific cost-management opportunity.

Drug-cost management strategies that are under the direct and exclusive purview of the pharmacy department (e.g., purchasing, inventory management, and waste reduction approaches) are generally easier to implement and provide more immediate benefits. These activities, however, often provide smaller or one-time financial benefits. Utilization management tactics (e.g., clinical practice guidelines and therapeutic interchange) generally provide greater financial benefits, but these efforts have correspondingly higher degrees of difficulty and complexity.

Because of the relative ease of implementation, cost-containment opportunities in areas that are primarily under the department's control will usually be pursued first. After these initiatives are underway, more complex techniques that require collaboration with the medical staff and others should be pursued.

These guidelines are structured so that the cost-management techniques are presented in the order in which health systems often implement them. Components of a cost-management program are listed in Table 2. An appendix that lists specific cost management opportunities is also provided. It is important to note that although these guidelines are separated into sections on purchasing and inventory management and medication-use management, both activities are integral and indivisible to drug-cost management planning and the practice of pharmacy in hospitals and health systems.

Purchasing and Inventory Management

When selecting drug-cost-containment initiatives, purchasing and inventory management procedures should be considered first.

Drug Product Costs and Procurement. At the most fundamental level, drug costs are a function of unit costs and

Table 2.
Components of a Cost-Management Program[a]

Pharmacy-Directed Activities
Purchasing
GPO contracts
Facility contracts
Wholesaler contracts
Inventory management
Wholesaler ordering
programs
Storage
Waste reduction
I.V. product waste
Returns

Interdisciplinary Activities
Medication utilization program
Clinical pharmacy services
Assessment of drug costs
Medical staff support
Formulary management
Therapeutic interchange
Guideline (protocol)
development
Pharmacist interventions
Plan implementation and
analysis

Reimbursement & Charging
Reimbursement
340B programs
CMS (DRG class)
Commercial insurance (payer
mix)
Outpatient infusion center
Charging
Coding and processing
Indigent care programs

[a]GPO = group purchasing organization, CMS = Centers for Medicare and Medicaid Services, DRG = diagnosis-related group.

utilization. Drug-unit costs are a function of acquisition costs (contracted or non-contracted), the external (in-bound) distribution fee, inventory management costs, and internal distribution costs.

Contracting. There are three main avenues for purchasing pharmaceuticals at discounted rates: GPO contracts, facility contracts, and wholesaler own-use contracts. All facilities should seek to maximize savings available from use of generic products, and some may have other considerations, such as use of 340B or indigent care programs.

GPO contracts. GPOs utilize the aggregate purchasing power of many facilities in negotiating pricing agreements with manufacturers. Most hospitals are members of a GPO. While there are GPOs that focus exclusively on drugs, the majority of GPOs offer contracts for medical and surgical supplies, food, and other support products and services in addition to pharmaceuticals. Most GPOs make their contract portfolio available to members via hard copy, and some GPOs have contract portfolios available on secure internet sites. Considerations in contracting with a GPO are listed in Table 3. It is also important to have routine surveillance, preferably an automated service, that ensures that contract prices are applied to all purchases.

GPOs are funded by one of two means. First, most, if not all, GPOs collect a contract administrative fee (CAF) from the manufacturers or distributors with which they contract. The CAF is rarely greater than 3% of the dollar volume of product purchased through the contract. Some GPOs return a portion or all of the CAF to its members. If any or all of the CAF for a particular drug product is returned to the facility by the GPO, it should be taken into account when calculating the net cost of the drug. The second method by which GPOs are funded is direct payment of fees by members to the GPO. In this arrangement, all of the CAF is returned to the facility.

Contracts through GPOs consider not only the unit cost of the pharmaceutical but also include the allowable distribution methods for the pharmaceutical, payment terms, returns policies, and supplier performance requirements. Many GPO contracts, especially those for multi-source generics, include simple line-item pricing, which only requires the purchaser to buy and pay for the product. Other contracts are more complicated, with incentive rebates for all purchases or rebates for achieving volume or market share targets.

Typically, market share agreements are utilized when two or more products can be used to treat the same disease and no generic equivalent exists. The incentive, such as a rebate, a lock-in of a current discount, or achievement of a higher discount, is contingent upon attaining a given market share for a particular product in the institution's market basket. To achieve the greatest financial advantage from the contract (lowest net drug cost), the pharmacy must work with the medical staff. This process requires a careful evaluation of comparative efficacy and safety of the product and its alternatives.

Some GPOs have multiple products on contract within categories of pharmaceuticals, allowing the facility to receive discounted pricing on similar agents when prescribing practices are not standardized to one agent. More aggressive GPOs will sometimes contract for a single agent within a particular class (e.g., for one fluoroquinolone or one liposomal amphotericin B product to the exclusion of others) in order to gain the maximum value for its members.

Successful use of GPO contracts requires a constructive and collaborative relationship between the member, the GPO, the manufacturer, and the distributor (i.e., wholesaler). Potential advantages of GPO contracts are listed in Table 4.

In addition to the contracting portfolio, GPOs offer services such as lost savings and compliance reports, rebate and contract administrative fee reports, clinical utilization management programs, and letters of commitment.

Lost savings and compliance reports. These reports provide data and analysis of missed savings opportunities in the user's purchase history (e.g., items purchased off-contract when a generically equivalent alternative item was on-contract). These reports may also indicate the compliance level, or the amount of purchases on-contract versus the amount of purchases that could have been made on-contract (drugs purchased on-contract plus the value of drugs purchased off-contract when alternatives were on-contract). These reports should be reviewed monthly to determine if purchasing practices are effective.

Rebate and contract administration fee report. These reports tally the amount of rebates and contract administration fees generated by the facility's purchases of specific products under contact. When evaluating the costs of two or more equivalent products, it is important to include any applicable rebates to arrive at net cost.

Clinical utilization management programs. These programs assist facilities in managing the utilization of various drug products and classes, often through evaluation and

Table 3.
Considerations in Group Purchasing Organization (GPO) Contracting

Fees (e.g., contract administrative fee)
Allowable distribution methods
Payment terms
Return policies
Supplier performance requirements
Rebates
Market-share agreements
Single-agent contracts
GPO services (e.g., lost savings and compliance reports, rebate and contract administration fee reports, clinical utilization management programs)
Letters of commitment

Table 4.
Potential Advantages of Group Purchasing Organization Contracts[10,11]

Standardization of products
Reduction of contract labor costs for institutions
Enhancement of member institution's purchasing program
Enhancement of information sharing
Enhancement of purchasing expertise
Protracted periods of price protection
Coordination of contracting and budgeting process
Reduction of duplication of purchasing efforts among institutions
Assistance identifying alternative or secondary products during drug shortage

comparison of product efficacy, safety, and cost, as well as therapeutic interchange programs.

Letters of commitment. Letters of commitment (LOC) available through GPOs should be evaluated and taken advantage of when appropriate. The LOCs usually contain requirements for the pharmacy to do one or more of the following in order to gain lower pricing or rebates:

- Declare that a particular drug is on formulary.
- Declare that a particular drug will be on formulary and will not be restricted.
- Achieve a target periodic volume.
- Achieve a target market share relative to competitive drugs for a given period of time.

The LOC may not require significantly more purchasing of the drug. If LOC requirements do not conflict with formulary and utilization management strategies, the LOC should be signed if there is a reasonable chance of meeting the requirements.

Facility contracts. The alternative to GPO contracting is individual contracting. This type of contracting may be done at the facility or the health-system level. In some cases, equal or better pricing than GPOs can be obtained by individual facilities when contracting, especially large facilities or integrated delivery networks (IDNs). Opportunities for better pricing through individual contracting may exist for specialized health systems (e.g., those focused on oncology or transplantation), that purchase a large volume of a selected drug and are able to commit to maintaining a market share for the drug.

It is important to carefully evaluate the benefits of individual contracting and its influence on the collective bargaining power of the GPO. Continual use of individual contracts that are in contravention to GPO contracts, in theory, will eventually erode the GPO's ability to consistently contract aggressively for its members. Because of larger GPO volume, manufacturers often will not offer the same pricing or other terms to individual facilities or IDNs that they offer to GPOs. Another factor to consider with individual contracting is that a facility may require contracts to be reviewed by attorneys, whereas the GPO acts as the contracting agent of the facility, obviating the need for legal review of each contract by the facility's counsel. Finally, the amount of time required to negotiate, write, and maintain an individual contract should be weighed against the incremental value gained over what a GPO contract would offer. In many situations, it may be more efficient and productive to voice contract concerns to GPO representatives and become involved in GPO committees rather than write multiple, individual contracts outside the GPO.

Some drug contracts, especially for sole-source awards to generic manufacturers, call for the manufacturer to reimburse the pharmacy for the difference in cost when the pharmacy must purchase a product off-contract because the manufacturer was not able to supply the contracted product. The manufacturer-unable-to-supply reimbursement process is time-consuming and the requirements can be rigid, but submitting reimbursement to manufacturers under these provisions can return additional funds to the pharmacy.

Wholesaler own-use contracts. Wholesalers are also able to take advantage of special pricing on certain branded and generic drugs and offer those products to their customers in the wholesaler's proprietary contract portfolio. This creates margin for the wholesalers that can be used to fund distribution discounts. Wholesalers also take advantage of cash discounts and quick-payment terms from manufacturers to increase their margin and to offer discounts to customers.

Generic Drug Savings Maximization. The expiration of patents on widely used branded drugs can result in large reductions in drug expenditures. It is important to be mindful of the opportunities presented by the first-time introduction of generics on high-spend branded drugs, both in budgeting and implementing rapid and effective uptake of generics when they are introduced.

Budgeting. There are several sources for monitoring patent expiration dates (off-patent dates) for branded drugs, includ-ing www.drugpatentwatch.com and the GPO. The GPO may also be able to estimate the potential initial savings from contracting for generic drugs that are first-time introductions. It is also important to determine when the first-time generic product will be available from multiple manufacturers. The initial savings differential between the branded and generic versions may be small because a single generic manufacturer often has a period of exclusivity before the generic drug becomes available from multiple sources. In some cases the savings may be so insignificant that health systems will choose to remain with the branded drug for safety reasons and consistency in product supply. Changing products several times within a short period of time could confuse caregivers, so pharmacy managers should weigh the benefits and risks of making such changes.

Operational considerations. Swift uptake of the generic product is necessary to maximize the savings after a branded drug comes off-patent and multiple generic versions are available. The following steps should be taken during any product conversion, but they are particularly important when converting from a brand name product to a first-time generic equivalent product.

- Contracting. Be sure that the health system has access to contract pricing on a generic product on the first date that the drug is available as a multisource item. The contract pricing will usually be through the health system's GPO, but in some cases, the health system may write its own contract for the generic product.
- Contract Price Loading. The contract pricing for the product must be loaded at the wholesaler with enough notice to become effective. Up to 30 days notice may be required before the contract pricing becomes effective through the wholesaler. Although the manufacturer or GPO typically send the contract information to the wholesalers, when the hospital or health system directly contracts for the generic drug, the contract information should be sent directly to the wholesaler by the hospital or health system.
- Demand Matching. Work with the wholesaler to ensure that there will be a sufficient supply of the generic product at the local wholesaler distribution center to match current purchases of the branded product, a process called demand matching. Wholesalers will need at least 30 days notice on demand matching to ensure sufficient stock of the generic product on the off-patent date. Working with the wholesaler on demand matching also improves overall supply chain management

by allowing the wholesaler to draw down inventory of products that will be in less demand.

- Autosubstitution. Some wholesalers allow pharmacies to institute autosubstitution rules in the wholesaler ordering system to substitute a preferred generic product for a branded product or non-preferred generic products. This process maximizes savings and contract compliance. Care must be exercised in creating autosubstitution rules to ensure correct product-to-product substitution in chemical entity, dosage form, package size, package form (unit dose, bulk oral, liquid), and so forth, especially in cases in which a brand-name drug goes off-patent. Autosubstitution rules may also be implemented in the wholesaler ordering system for medication safety reasons (e.g., reduction of sound-alike and look-alike drugs) in addition to savings optimization or contract compliance.

Other Considerations. Pharmacy managers should explore whether the hospital can obtain pharmaceuticals at advantageous pricing using 340B (disproportionate share) programs. Because hospitals and health systems must meet specific criteria to be designated as a 340B facility, pharmacy managers should collaborate with the chief financial officer and financial services department to determine if they can access 340B pricing for pharmaceuticals. Detailed descriptions of the qualifications and benefits of 340B programs are also available through the Health Resources and Services Administration Office of Pharmacy Affairs www.hrsa.gov/opa/; the Pharmacy Services Support Center, pssc.aphanet.org/; the Safety Net Hospitals for Pharmaceutical Access, safetynetrx.org; and ASHP 340B Information Site www.ashp.org/s_ashp/cat1c.asp? CID=3813&DID=6225.

Pharmaceutical manufacturers also continue to offer indigent patient care programs for select drugs for qualified patients on an individual basis. Although substantial savings can be realized through replacement drugs at no charge, the process can be arduous and complex. There are independent consulting services that specialize in assisting with coordination of the program for hospitals and typically require payment as a percentage of the savings. Patients eligible for Medicaid and other regional or local low-income health insurance do not usually qualify for the indigent care programs sponsored by the pharmaceutical industry.

Wholesalers and Distribution Fees. Most hospital pharmacies purchase 80% or more (by dollar volume) of their pharmaceutical needs from a drug distributor (wholesaler). Hospital pharmacies can lower their costs by ensuring that the distribution fee mark-up is as low as possible. To understand the cost that wholesalers charge for drugs, and the distribution fee charged to hospital pharmacies, it is necessary to understand wholesalers' revenue streams and expense drivers.

The adoption of the prime-vendor system, in which a pharmacy procures a very large portion of its pharmaceutical needs from one supplier, has led to great efficiencies in the pharmaceutical supply chain. Through these efficiencies, wholesalers are able to offer low incremental fees to their customers for distribution of pharmaceuticals. In many cases, they are able to offer discounts to the contracted price of the drug or "cost-minus" discounts to the wholesale acquisition cost of the drug if it is not contracted.

Through automated inventory, stock replacement, and order fulfillment, wholesalers have streamlined the delivery process and lowered pharmaceutical costs in the supply chain. In the past, wholesalers increased their margins through speculative buying, which is buying pharmaceuticals in large quantities and holding them past the date of future manufacturer price increases. The products would then be sold to customers at the higher price. These practices have reportedly decreased since 2004.[12] However, at the same time that speculative buying decreased, the wholesale drug industry instituted inventory management agreements with manufacturers, who in return for agreements regarding product supply and demand, pay the wholesalers a negotiated fee based on the percentage of the volume that the wholesalers purchase from them. These methods of creating margin through increasing revenue and decreasing expenses can be translated into a cost-minus fee structure for the hospital that is purchasing from the wholesalers.

Individual hospital factors that influence wholesaler fee structure. Several characteristics of individual hospital-pharmacy purchasing can affect a wholesaler's revenue and expenses and result in higher or lower distribution fees. To some degree, a higher purchasing volume results in a lower distribution fee. However, other factors, including deliveries per week, dollars per drop, dollars per line extension, numbers of delivery sites per location, payment terms, and special services, must also be considered. These factors should be considered collectively and not in isolation. In addition, most major wholesalers have supply, automation, and other service and equipment divisions, and an institutional contract with multiple divisions can provide additional savings.

Deliveries per week. The fewer deliveries from the wholesaler per week, the lower the expenses for the wholesaler, which can reduce the wholesaler distribution fee to the pharmacy. Some large hospitals have up to 11 deliveries per week, but other large hospitals are able to manage inventory so that patient care can be well-maintained with only 5. Inventory and patient care can be well maintained at less than five deliveries per week at small hospitals. Fewer deliveries may require additional purchasing discipline, but some wholesalers have programs to help pharmacies improve their purchasing practices.

Dollars per drop. This factor is important to wholesalers because the higher the number of delivery locations (drops), the higher the wholesalers' cost, and vice versa. For a given dollar value of pharmaceuticals purchased, a wholesaler's expenses are lower, and margin is higher, for a lower number of delivery points. This margin can be translated into lower distribution fees for the pharmacies, particularly for IDNs of multiple pharmacies.

Dollars per line extension. For each line of products on an invoice that a wholesaler fills and delivers to a pharmacy, there is an associated cost. The dollars per line extension is the total dollars purchased by a pharmacy over a given period of time divided by the number of lines of products ordered over the same period of time. Pharmacies with higher dollars per line extension purchased can sometimes have lower distribution costs than pharmacies with lower dollars per line extension because it costs relatively less for the wholesaler to service the pharmacy with the higher dollars per line extension.

Secondary wholesalers. Secondary wholesaler relationships should be avoided if inventory levels meet patient

care needs. Purchases from secondary wholesalers usually carry a much higher distribution fee. Such purchases also result in a higher primary wholesaler distribution fee because there are decreases for the pharmacy in its dollars per drop, dollars per line extension, and total volume. Wholesalers are increasingly requiring pharmacies to meet a minimum monthly volume to maintain an account, and the costs of maintaining the minimum volume at a significantly higher distribution fee can be prohibitive.

Expanding the use of the wholesaler within the health system may offer additional opportunities for cost savings. Hospital departments such as radiology, the clinical laboratory, interventional cardiology, and anesthesiology may procure pharmaceuticals directly from the manufacturer through the purchasing or materials management departments. Utilizing the pharmaceutical wholesaler for these products through a separate purchasing account does not change the process of procurement or distribution but reduces the unit cost through application of the wholesaler discount. Because some of these products may be relatively costly (e.g., contrast agents, blood factors, or anesthetic gases), there is a potential for additional savings if these purchases push the hospital into a higher tier of the wholesaler cost structure. Pharmacy directors should communicate with other department managers to determine how pharmaceuticals are purchased, and it is usually best if all drug purchases are managed by the pharmacy.

Payment method and frequency. Payment method and frequency can also affect the distribution fee. Many wholesalers offer a lower distribution fee to hospitals that pay by electronic fund transfer (EFT). Pharmacy managers should work with their accounts-payable departments to establish EFT, which is usually a more efficient method of payment for both the hospital and the wholesaler. In addition, the more frequent the payment, the lower the wholesaler distribution fee will generally be. Since 2004, the amount of speculative buying has waned and large discounts for more frequent payments have decreased. However, many wholesalers offer terms based on prepayment, or placing funds on deposit with the wholesaler, and then paying invoices on a go-forward basis. The advantage in lower distribution fee is clear, but this gain must be balanced against the time value of money for having the funds on deposit with the wholesaler rather than drawing a return for the health system.

Most GPOs have wholesaler-distribution agreements for use by their members. However, because of higher-than-average dollars per drop, dollars per line extension, and discipline in number of deliveries per week, large hospitals and health systems can often get better pricing and terms by dealing directly with wholesalers rather than through GPO wholesaler agreements.

Other wholesaler tools. Most wholesalers provide pharmacies with access to computer software or Web-based solutions for product ordering, reporting, and inventory management. The programs will allow the buyer to check for lower-priced alternatives and contract compliance prior to placing orders. Pharmacy managers should work with their wholesaler representatives to be sure that these features are available and utilized.

Some wholesalers produce contract compliance reports. These reports can be used to gauge the effectiveness of purchasing practices. Pharmacy managers should check with their wholesalers to determine if these reports are available.

If they are, they should be reviewed monthly for opportunities to improve contract purchasing.

Some wholesalers have automatic substitution programs to assist pharmacy buyers in selecting the correct product when multiple generic alternatives exist. These programs allow the pharmacy manager to direct purchases of less-preferred products (as determined by the pharmacy management) to more-preferred items. For example, if one brand of unit dose acetaminophen 325-mg tablet is on contract as a sole-source award, the autosubstitution program can allow for inadvertent orders for noncontract unit dose acetaminophen 325-mg tablets to be substituted with the preferred version. Such programs may not be available from all wholesalers, and they should receive careful consideration before being implemented.

Inventory Management. Inventory management is a balancing act. It involves meeting patient and internal customer needs while committing the least amount of dollars possible to drugs on the shelves or in automated cabinets. The rate of inventory turnover (defined as total annual drug expenses divided by the dollar value of the inventory assessed on an annual basis) is dependent on many factors. Typically, the pharmacies of smaller hospitals will have a lower drug inventory turnover (8–10 turns per year) than the pharmacies of larger hospitals (12–18 turns per year or higher) and some specialty hospitals.

Many wholesalers' ordering programs provide systematic methods for asset management (i.e., inventory value optimization and increasing turnover). Wholesaler representatives can assist in the initial setup of these programs. Inventory items should be divided into high-, medium-, and low-value products, and the minimum and maximum inventory levels for at least the high- and medium-value products should be established. At the same time, reorder points and reorder quantities should be established for at least the high- and medium-value products. Systematic use of these programs can decrease the time required for the ordering process and increase inventory turns. The minimum and maximum levels, as well as the reorder points and reorder quantities, should be reviewed on a routine schedule and revised when necessary.

When seeking to increase inventory turns, storage in the central pharmacy and automated dispensing cabinets should also be considered. Configuring pharmacy storage locations so that each drug product has only one storage location in the central pharmacy sometimes helps to free capital by reducing inventory. Automated cabinet inventories should be regularly reviewed for appropriate turnover. Most cabinet systems have report capabilities to optimize both the products and the quantities that should be in a particular cabinet based on the dispensing philosophy devised by pharmacy and nursing departments. Cabinet manufacturers have product specialists that consult with pharmacy management to optimize use of the cabinets.

I.V. product waste. Many pharmacies waste a significant quantity of drugs, particularly unused IV solutions, and many do not have an accurate valuation of the amount of waste because it is only sporadically monitored. Table 5 lists strategies for reduction of IV product waste.

Returns. Most pharmacies use a third party (reverse distributors or returns companies) to process wasted and expired drugs. However, not all pharmacies completely track

Table 5.
Strategies for Reducing I.V. Product Waste

Establish policies that are based on the most recent
 literature for maximum i.v. bag hang-times and i.v. set
 change frequency.
Institute an i.v.-to-oral switch program for both cost
 reduction and patient care benefits.
Periodically audit the amount of i.v. admixtures being wasted
 and log the date and time of waste, date and time of
 preparation, the i.v. fluid type and drug admixed, quantity
 of products, and the cost of the products. Review the log
 and determine the most common occurrences.
Reduce i.v. batch sizes (creating more, smaller batches)
 and reduce the amount of time between preparation of
 the i.v. dose and the actual administration time.
Routinely monitor the status of i.v. drips that are adjusted.
Routinely return all unused i.v. admixtures to the i.v.
 preparation area as soon as possible.
Consider the use of manufacturer premixed products where
 advantageous, both economically and for patient care.
Compare the quality, economic, and regulatory (e.g., *USP*
 chapter 797) differences within your practice site between
 different administration methods such as i.v. syringe
 infusion, i.v. intermittent infusion (i.v. piggyback), and
 volumetric drip chambers.
Establish standard concentrations, dosages, and base
 solutions for i.v. admixtures.
Ensure that there is an efficient process for communicating
 changes in i.v. admixtures (e.g., rate, fluid, dosage) or
 discontinuation.
Reduce total parenteral nutrition use by employing enteral
 nutrition when possible, and establish standardized
 total parenteral nutrient base solutions, hang times, and
 related policies and procedures.

and trend the drugs that are most commonly wasted, the dollar value of the expired and wasted drugs, or whether credits were received. The pharmacy manager and pharmacy buyer should work together to utilize reports from the reverse distributor to determine the opportunities for reducing the amount of expired and wasted drugs and insuring that all credits due to the pharmacy from the manufacturers are received.

Medication Utilization Management

Planning and Developing a Medication Utilization Management Program. An effective plan for medication utilization management must provide the health system with a road map for continuous improvement in pharmaceutical expense management, with specific goals and outcome measures of success. It is important to acknowledge that although one purpose of medication-utilization-management is to add economic value, the quality and safety of patient care are foremost in the mission of pharmacy services and should never be compromised for cost. Medication-utilization-management must integrate evidence-based science with the standards of medical practice within the health system.

Before embarking on a comprehensive medication-utilization-management plan, goals must be established, a reporting structure delineated, roles identified, measurement tools developed, and implementation procedures established. The successful plan is dependent on many levels of commitment, including commitment to administrative and clinical pharmacy management, the medical staff, and senior health-system management. The director of pharmacy provides leadership by facilitating the efforts of the medical staff, setting priorities for the clinical pharmacy staff, and cultivating the support of senior leadership. Clinical pharmacists with advanced training and education must have dedicated time to develop and implement the cost management initiatives. They must also be empowered to monitor the program and educate other staff to participate in therapeutic interchange, medication utilization review, and other interventions while encouraging the infusion of fresh ideas for pharmaceutical cost management.

Role of Clinical Pharmacy Services in Drug Cost Management. Clinical pharmacy services, activities in which pharmacists provide direct patient care, are an important foundation for a successful medication-utilization-management program that is focused on managing drug costs. Clinical pharmacy services have demonstrated an overall positive financial impact. In a systematic review of original assessments of clinical pharmacy services from 1988 to 1995, Schumock et al.[13] reported that 89% of 104 studies reviewed reported positive financial results. In the seven studies of clinical pharmacy services where sufficient information was available to calculate a benefit-to-cost ratio, the median benefit-to-cost ratio was 4.09:1. Therefore, in these studies, every dollar invested in clinical pharmacy services returned four dollars. The systematic review was updated in 2003 to review published assessments of clinical pharmacy services from 1995 to 2000, and once again, the value of clinical pharmacy services was demonstrated.[14] For this five-year period, benefit-to-cost ratios could be determined from 16 studies, and when these studies were combined, the median benefit:cost ratio was 4.68:1.

Some specific types of clinical pharmacy services have also been associated with decreased drug costs. Bond et al.[15] have used an extensive database of the outcomes of clinical pharmacy services to show that drug information services, medication admission histories, and drug protocol management are associated with lower drug costs.

In addition, clinical pharmacists' active involvement is crucial to the success of many drug-cost-management ini-tiatives. Many of the drug-cost-containment techniques can only be successful with diligent and often daily support from clinical pharmacists. For example, successful implementation of a clinical practice guideline as a drug-cost-management technique will require the expertise of the department's clinical pharmacists to develop the guideline, and will also require the pharmacy staff's consistent enforcement of the guideline in their interactions with prescribers. Similarly, it will often be the clinical pharmacist's responsibility to routinely carry out the hospital's therapeutic interchange policies.

Assessment of Drug Costs

A successful pharmaceutical-cost-management program must be data driven. GPOs, wholesalers, distributors, pharmaceutical manufacturers, and supply-chain divisions of multi-hospital systems need to track costs in a variety of ways. Advances in information technology have made drug usage data more accessible and sophisticated, and effort should be spent to manage and analyze these data. Pharmacy management must also take advantage of the data available in its own facility

through the materials management department, purchasing department, and finance department. Internal and external data sources are the foundation for the decision-making process for medication-utilization-management and must be examined closely prior to setting goals for cost-management initiatives.

Because each health system has a unique mix of patients, services, and centers of excellence, the drug-cost-assessment process must be customized to create a priority list of initiatives that will provide the greatest value. Key reports that should be considered are listed in Table 6. Once the formulas for denominator data are established as consistent across many facilities, a multihospital health system can effectively benchmark drug costs.

Medical Staff Support. Any program that involves altering prescribing patterns to improve the cost-effectiveness of drug therapy requires the support and engagement of the medical staff. Although health systems have the ability to negotiate discounted unit prices for pharmaceuticals, the efforts of the GPOs and the increased availability of generics have leveled the expense of many high-cost drug products used in hospitals. Cost-management programs have therefore become increasingly dependent on the hospital's ability to manage utilization and prescribing, which will ultimately influence market share and drug pricing. Several effective strategies that can harness physician knowledge, cultivate a collaborative relationship, and facilitate ownership of the process by the medical staff are described in Table 7.

Once the medical staff is engaged and there is a commitment from senior management for the medication-utilization-management program, a detailed procedure for initiative generation can be established. Key steps include the following:

- Designating clinical sub-groups based on categories of the initiatives,
- Identifying the lead physicians, clinical pharmacists, and other key practitioners for each group,
- Using evidence-based studies and the drug assessment data to make decisions,
- Defining the types and categories of the initiatives,
- Creating a dashboard and a clear and concise reporting format for communicating progress,
- Facilitating the infusion of ideas through brainstorming and other effective meeting and group techniques, and
- Defining measurable outcomes and benchmarks for evaluation.

Formulary Management. The guiding principles of a sound formulary management system are well described in two documents,[17,18] and are concisely summarized in the following statement: a well-managed formulary system ensures a close relationship between the organization's medication-use policies, the therapies offered by the organization, and the medication routinely stocked by the pharmacy.[18] Although the primary goal of a formulary system is to promote safe and effective drug therapy, it can be a valuable cost management tool and has inherent medical staff support through the actions of the pharmacy and therapeutics (P&T) committee. The medication-utilization-management program is highly dependent on an effective formulary system. Key aspects of formulary management in cost-management efforts are described in Table 8. Once again, the efforts of clinical pharmacists are crucial to successful implementation of the formulary system.

Methods of Pharmaceutical Cost Management. Pharmaceutical cost-management initiatives are typically categorized by therapeutic class or group or by method of implementation. The latter is usually subdivided into three or four different types: therapeutic interchange (therapeutic substitution), guideline (protocol)

Table 6.
Key Reports to Consider in Assessing Drug Costs

Report	Considerations
Wholesaler purchasing reports	For 80/20 analysis, by therapeutic class, and of top 200 drugs; drugs with multiple strengths and sizes need to be aggregated; wholesalers can also provide monthly trending reports and benchmarks from their customers.
Direct (nonwholesaler) purchase reports	Available from the purchasing or finance departments.
Interdepartmental purchasing reports	Available from materials management or other departments that have internal transfers.
Cost (total drug costs or specific drugs) per medical service or hospital area	Drug-utilization data will be needed to produce this report.
Cost per drug-related group reports	Available from internal sources (ideally) or fee-based external vendors; distinction must be made between using cost or charge data.
Cost per occupied bed, adjusted patient day, admission, discharge, or case mix index adjusted patient day	Adjusted patient days are calculated with a standard financial formula that modifies patient days with a ratio of outpatient to inpatient revenue to correct for volume changes and severity of illness.[16] External and internal benchmarking is dependent on these kinds of reports.
Pharmacy-adjusted patient days	Calculated using the same ratio of outpatient to inpatient revenue but for drugs only, and may also add specificity and value to comparative data.
Cost per case, procedure, or admission (e.g., surgical case, cardiac procedure, dialysis admission)	These are important based on the patient mix and the drugs that comprise the greatest costs within the health system. Physician participation in the dissemination of the data is essential.

Table 7.
Strategies to Involve Medical Staff in Cost-Management Efforts

Enlist the pharmacy and therapeutic (P&T) committee to review medication-utilization management issues as a standing agenda item.

Identify the centers of excellence and work with individual chiefs of service to gain support.

Meet with key medical staff departments and divisions, including infectious diseases, anesthesiology, cardiology, and oncology, as well as intensivists, hospitalists, and interventionalists as appropriate.

Develop prescriber reports on the targeted high-cost drugs and discuss methods for cost reduction.

Provide continuous feedback to the P&T committee and individual departments and divisions on cost management successes.

Provide hospitalwide expenditure data on the top 50 items to the P&T committee.

Utilize evidence-based research to propose changes in medication utilization.

Identify physician champions for specific initiatives.

Create a consistent procedure for developing prescribing guidelines, protocols, care paths, and preprinted orders.

Table 8.
Key Aspects of Formulary Management in Cost-Management Efforts

Policy for formulary drug addition and deletion through evidence-based product selection, including efficacy, safety, and pharmacoeconomic assessments

Policy for the use and monitoring of non-formulary medications

Policy for medication-use evaluation

Limitation on combination, sustained-release, and long-acting products

Policy for therapeutic interchange and prescribing guidelines

Reduction of drugs in the same therapeutic group or class

Periodic house cleaning to reduce under-used and discontinued line items

Policy for drug restriction

Procedure for consistently monitoring the use of new agents particularly if there are specific guidelines for use

System to provide the formulary electronically with timely updated information

Off-label or ad hoc use of medications

Restricted use (by indication, prescriber, patient care area, patient)

Dose adjustment or discontinuation based on clinical triggers or end points

Injectable to oral conversion

Therapeutic equivalence

development, and pharmacist interventions (clinical and operational), such as parenteral-to-oral conversions, renal-dose adjustments, drug restrictions, repackaging, dosage-form changes, waste reduction, and others. Although the terms are sometimes used interchangeably, therapeutic group refers to a broad classification (e.g., anesthetic agents, anti-infectives, or chemotherapeutic agents), whereas therapeutic class is a narrower designation (e.g., beta-lactam antibiotics, volatile anesthetic gases, serotonin antagonists). If the decision is made to use therapeutic class, then each of the methods of implementation are used as appropriate within the medication categories. An example would be selecting third-generation cephalosporins utilizing a therapeutic interchange for cefotaxime and ceftriaxone (therapeutic interchange method). Third-generation cephalosporins may also be the preferred class of antibiotics within a pneumonia protocol (guidelines method). Examples of using the implementation method rather than the therapeutic class would be to select several drug classes for therapeutic interchange, some for guideline development, and some for other intervention types.

Therapeutic interchange. ASHP defines therapeutic interchange (TI) as "an authorized exchange of therapeutic alternatives in accordance with previously established and approved written guidelines or protocols within a formulary system."[17] This definition stipulates that the interchange is between two or more drugs that are not generic equivalents. Although FDA defines the term *therapeutic equivalent* to include generically equivalent products, therapeutic interchange or substitution in the hospital setting generally refers to drugs that are not generically identical.

The American College of Clinical Pharmacy (ACCP) Guidelines for Therapeutic Interchange[19] contain a more recent definition of TI:

Therapeutic interchange is defined as the dispensing of a drug that is therapeutically equivalent to but chemically different from the drug originally prescribed. Although usually of the same pharmacological class,

drugs appropriate for therapeutic interchange may differ in chemistry or pharmacokinetic properties, and may possess different mechanism of action, adverse-reaction, toxicity, and drug interaction profiles. In most cases, the interchanged drugs have close similarity in efficacy and safety profiles.

The ACCP guidelines also describe a comprehensive five-part process for health-system TI implementation, with an emphasis on patient safety; an extensive review of drug classes appropriate for therapeutic interchange, including specific evidence-based examples; discussion of legal and regulatory issues; viewpoints of other professional organizations, including the American Medical Association, the American College of Physicians, and the Pharmaceutical Research and Manufacturers of America; and medical and pharmaceutical literature references.

The health system, through the action of the P&T committee, must decide on the general policy for a TI program, particularly regarding the authority and autonomy of the pharmacy staff. The committee may define TI as an automatic conversion by the pharmacist, may require contact with the prescriber before the change can occur, or may employ a combination of both. The prescriber may be informed orally before the drug is dispensed or through written communication in the medical record. Most commonly, TI implies pharmacist autonomy once the P&T committee has sanctioned the policy, but there may be exceptions based on the level of clinical judgment required. A survey of the prevalence of TI conducted in 2002 revealed that the vast majority (88%) of hospitals use TI programs, and most of those did not require the pharmacist to contact the prescriber before making the conversion.[20]

Categories of drugs that offer modest savings with minimal challenge include various non-prescription groups, such

as antacids, vitamins, nonsteroidal antiinflammatory drugs, topical products, and cold and cough remedies. To make significant gains in pharmaceutical cost savings, the health system must consider the drug classes that comprise the greatest proportion of drug expenditures, such as colony-stimulating factors, antiinfectives, cardiac agents, and drugs used in critical care settings. An abundance of literature supports the success of TI programs, both in terms of quality patient outcomes and economic benefit. Based on the literature, therapeutic classes offering the most opportunity for success with the medical staff, as well as significant cost savings, include histamine-2 antagonists, fluoroquinolones, hydroxymethylglutaryl–coenzyme A reductase inhibitors, serotonin antagonists, colony-stimulating factors, low molecular weight heparins, and proton pump inhibitors.[20-27] Although it is not the intent of these guidelines to delineate an exhaustive list of all potential TI opportunities, the appendix contains examples of the TIs that have proven successful.

Most of the evaluative studies on TI initiatives focus on the economic value and quality improvement related to standardization and formulary management. As the popularity of TI programs increases in the acute care, managed care, and ambulatory settings, an associated risk may also increase due to substitutions along the continuum of care and patient confusion regarding drug classes and duplicative therapy.[28,29] The Joint Commission standard requiring medication reconciliation can be partially traced to anecdotal reports of the potential for medication errors as a result of TI programs in various health care settings.[29] Pharmacists can play a vital role in supporting medication-reconciliation activities through medication history assessments and discharge counseling.[30,31]

Guidelines. A variety of terms are used to describe these tools, including prescribing guidelines, therapeutic position statements, therapeutic guidelines, clinical practice guidelines, protocols, or pathways. There may be subtle differences beween these tools, but they all seek to enhance patient safety, reduce variation in medical practice, and increase standardization.

Guidelines can focus on a disease state, a therapeutic class, or a specific drug.[32] Published guidelines are available for many drugs and drug classes.[33,34] The Agency for Health Care Research and Quality maintains an extensive online collection of published guidelines at www.guideline.gov. A 2004 ASHP survey found that 83% of U.S. hospitals use guidelines that include medications.[35] Successful implementation of such general guidelines often requires customization to meet the needs of individual health systems, however. For example, local guidelines should be developed that reflect the best available evidence, incorporate the opinions of local prescriber experts when necessary, and are applicable within the context of the individual health system.

Guidelines are also an important step leading to rules-based computerized prescriber order entry (CPOE), which is recommended by NQF in its 2006 Safe Practices.[36] CPOE facilitates guideline adherence during the ordering process.

Steps to implementing an effective pharmaceutical cost-containment program using drug-specific or drug class guidelines mirror those for TI and include:

- Utilization of evidence-based criteria,
- Adoption of published, evidence-based, and peer-reviewed guidelines from national organizations,

- Solicitation of thought leaders and clinical experts (e.g., physician specialists, chiefs of service, chief medical officers),
- Review and approval of the P&T committee,
- Education of clinical staff,
- Ongoing support from front line clinical pharmacist staff,
- Use of quantifiable measures, and
- Utilization of medication-use evaluation (MUE) to determine compliance.

The last step is an important distinction between TI and guidelines because what is approved by the medical staff and what is done in practice may differ. Conducting periodic MUEs with the approved criteria can determine the thoroughness and consistency of the guidelines and ultimately the success of this component of cost management. It should also be emphasized that although guidelines can be used to reduce drug costs, improving quality of care may require more spending rather than less.

When guidelines reduce inappropriate prescribing, drug costs will also be reduced. Due to the complex uses of some drugs and drug classes, such as low-molecular-weight heparins, guidelines may be more practical and effective in managing drug costs than TI and other approaches.[37] Drotrecogin alfa was one costly agent for which guidelines became the standard of care in most acute care settings.[38-40] Other successful guideline efforts have been demonstrated with a number of drugs and drug classes, such as third-generation cephalosporins,[41] statins,[42] antifungals,[43,44] albumin,[45] and serotonin-receptor antagonists.[46] Drug shortages can also be an impetus for the development and implementation of guidelines, as was the case with the use of parenteral pantoprazole, which may be used inappropriately and at a much higher cost in place of histamine-2 antagonists for stress ulcer prophylaxis.[47] Although volatile anesthetic agents are often a top-20 item in the pharmaceutical budget and offer a unique challenge for guidelines or TI implementation, accurate evaluation of cost savings can be accomplished by using the hourly cost to maintain a minimum alveolar concentration.[48]

Implementation of Medication Utilization Management Initiatives. Careful thought and attention to the implementation is required to successfully influence drug expenditures through medication utilization initiatives, and multifaceted interventions are often necessary. The active involvement and support of clinical pharmacists and the medical staff are crucial to effective implementation of these initiatives. It is necessary to seek out ways to integrate or hard-wire initiatives such as guidelines and TI into the care provided at the bedside. For example, passive guideline dissemination (e.g., simply posting to the hospital's intranet site) is rarely successful. Protocols, order sets, and pathways that reflect the evidence in the guideline should be used to integrate the guideline into daily patient care. The growing use of CPOE systems and other technologies can also be leveraged to implement medication-utilization-management endeavors. CPOE can be used to guide prescribing in such straightforward ways as leading prescribers to select formulary products or recommended dosing frequencies.[49] CPOE can also promote efficient medication use through more complex scenarios such as prompting therapeutic interchanges or requiring prescribers to follow interactive prescribing guide-

lines. For example, one institution established guidelines for activated protein C use and utilized an interactive computer order entry algorithm to implement the guideline.[50]

Data Analysis. To ensure the validity of the medication-utilization-management program, regardless of the method of implementation, the estimated and actual cost savings calculations must be grounded in accurate and consistent data analysis. Unfortunately, there is no standard regarding a method to determine the pharmaceutical cost savings with programs such as TI. Hospitals have struggled for years to balance practical considerations while striving for accuracy and completeness.[20] Hospitals have to decide early in the process whether to consider indirect costs such as devices and other non-pharmaceuticals, price changes during the review period, general drug price inflation, volume changes, and labor costs.

Equivalent doses for all drug alternatives for each TI must be established based on scientific evidence and current practice standards, which may not be the same as FDA-approved manufacturers' recommendations. Most of the references cited for TI above list the therapeutic equivalence for the drugs in a specific class. *Days of therapy* is the common method to compare equivalent costs of drug therapy within a therapeutic class, particularly for antibiotics and other classes that include scheduled drugs that are dosed multiple times per day. For classes that include drugs with extended half-lives and durations of action, weeks of therapy or cost per course of therapy may be more appropriate. Examples include colony-stimulating factors (e.g., epoetin versus darbopoetin and filgrastim versus pegfilgrastim). Correcting for equivalent strengths, sizes, and units of packaging is another important step in cost-savings calculations, particularly for liquid and parenteral products. The number of standard doses available from a container of liquid medication or a large volume parenteral medication varies based on the size of the container. Medical staff input is important in determining equivalent doses, particularly if there is a divergence between manufacturer's recommendations and published literature on dosing.

Once the methodology of data analysis is established, a drug savings matrix should be developed. This becomes the primary monitoring document that tracks the progress of each initiative based on the changes in utilization. Purchase data is the typical source for maintaining the cost savings matrix, but it is essential to adjust and scrub the data before matrix input. It is important to maintain a consistent common denominator. Utilization increases in certain targeted drugs may be due to patient volume and may be appropriate. Correcting for volume with denominator data and using effective MUE programs will assist with determining actual cost increases. The elements of a standard drug-savings matrix spreadsheet include the initiatives (TI and guidelines), savings targets, baseline purchase dollars corrected for volume, current purchase dollars (after implementation) corrected for volume, and actual savings monthly and year-to-date. It is important to be accurate and include both wholesaler and direct purchases, rebates, and wholesaler discounts.

To maintain commitment to and focus on the process, it is paramount to provide consistent feedback regarding the changes in the cost savings matrix to the P & T committee. Some health systems also establish a reporting structure to another oversight committee, such as a value analysis group or similar body that has overall responsibility for non-labor cost management.

Conclusion

Medication costs continue to rise and will continue to be a target for cost management. Drug costs make up a majority of health-system pharmacy budgets, and budgeting for these expenses is an important function, but longer-term programmatic and policy planning is also essential for successful cost management. An effective plan for medication utilization management must provide the health system with a road map for continuous improvement in pharmaceutical expense containment with specific goals and outcome measures of success. Gathering the data to understand drug expenditures and drug-use patterns is a prerequisite for cost-savings efforts, and constant vigilance and monitoring of these data are required.

A relatively small number of drugs usually makes up the majority of the drug budget. Cost-management efforts focused on these drugs will generally offer the best return. Cost-management strategies that fall completely under the pharmacy department's control (e.g., purchasing and inventory strategies) will be easiest to implement and should be pursued first. Strategies that require an interdisciplinary effort (e.g., use of protocols or guidelines, therapeutic interchange, IV-to-PO switches) can be led by pharmacists with the proper clinical background. Clinical pharmacy services, such as participation in rounds, pharmacokinetic monitoring, and renal dose adjustment, can also reduce drug expenses.

Cost management efforts should be coordinated. The programs should contain a clearly defined and manageable list of cost containment targets with a goal and specific targets for each initiative. Results should be measured and evaluated, and this information should be shared with the interdisciplinary team involved in the effort as well as with health-system administration.

When selecting and implementing drug-cost-management strategies, pharmacists must keep patient safety and the quality of patient care in mind. Cost-management initiatives must never compromise the pharmacy department's ability to provide the best possible care. Fortunately, there are many drug-cost-management opportunities that have little or no potential for detrimental effects on patient care, and efforts to improve appropriate use of a drug or drug class often also offer opportunities for cost containment.

References

1. Hoffman JM, Shah ND, Vermeulen LC et al. Projecting future drug expenditures—2006. *Am J Health-Syst Pharm.* 2006; 63:123–38.
2. Vogenberg FR, ed. Understanding pharmacy reimbursement. Bethesda, MD: American Society of Health-System Pharmacists; 2005:17–42.
3. ASHP Practice Resource Center for Pharmaceutical Reimbursement. www.ashp.org/s_ashp/cat1c.asp?CID=490&DID=532 (accessed 2007 Sep 10).
4. Clinical Initiative Center interviews. The Advisory Board Company. Washington, DC 2000:20–1.
5. Hoffman JM, Shah ND, Vermeulen LC et al. Projecting future drug expenditures—2007. *Am J Health-Syst Pharm.* 2007; 64:298–314.

6. Hoffman JM, Shah ND, Vermeulen LC et al. Projecting future drug expenditures 2004. *Am J Health-Syst Pharm.* 2004; 61:145–58.

7. Hoffman JM, Shah ND, Vermeulen LC et al. Projecting future drug expenditures 2005. *Am J Health-Syst Pharm.* 2005; 62:149–67.

8. Heffler S, Smith S, Keehan S et al. U.S. health spending projections for 2004–2014. *Health Aff (Millwood).* 2005; W5:74-WS-85.

9. Rough S, Saenz R. Benchmarking and productivity monitoring: practical strategies for pharmacy managers. www.ashp.org/s_ashp/docs/files/2004Leadership Summary.pdf (accessed 2007 Sep 10).

10. May BE, Herrick JD. Evaluation of drug-procurement alternatives. *Am J Hosp Pharm.* 1984; 41:1373–8.

11. Wetrich JG. Group purchasing: an overview. *Am J Hosp Pharm.* 1987; 44:1581–92.

12. Yost RD. New economics of the pharmaceutical supply chain. *Am J Health-Syst Pharm.* 2005; 62:525–6.

13. Schumock GT, Meek PD, Ploetz PA et al. Economic evaluations of clinical pharmacy services—1988–1995. *Pharmacotherapy.* 1996; 16:1188–208.

14. Schumock GT, Butler MG, Meek PD et al. Evidence of the economic benefit of clinical pharmacy services: 1996–2000. *Pharmacotherapy.* 2003; 23:113–32.

15. Bond CA, Raehl CL, Patry RL. Evidence-based core clinical pharmacy services in United States hospitals in 2020: services and staffing. *Pharmacotherapy.* 2004; 24:427–40.

16. Bond CA, Raehl CL. Clinical and economic outcomes of pharmacist-managed aminoglycoside or vancomycin therapy. *Am J Health-Syst Pharm.* 2005; 62:1596–605.

17. Coalition Working Group. Principles of a sound drug formulary system. In: Hawkins BH, ed. Best practices for hospital & health-system pharmacy. Bethesda, MD: American Society of Health-System Pharmacists; 2005:125–8.

18. American Society of Hospital Pharmacists. ASHP guidelines on formulary system management. *Am J Hosp Pharm.* 1992; 49:648–52.

19. Gray T, Bertch K, Galt K et al. Guidelines for therapeutic interchange - 2004. *Pharmacotherapy.* 2005; 25:1666–80.

20. Schachtner JM, Guharoy R, Medicis JJ et al. Prevalence and cost savings of therapeutic interchange among U.S. hospitals. *Am J Health-Syst Pharm.* 2002; 59:529–33.

21. Goldwater SH, Milkovich G, Morrison AJ Jr et al. Comparison of therapeutic interchange with standard educational tools for influencing fluoroquinolone prescribing. *Am J Health-Syst Pharm.* 2001; 58:1740–5.

22. Grace KA, Swiecki J, Hyatt R et al. Implementation of a therapeutic-interchange clinic for HMG-CoA reductase inhibitors. *Am J Health-Syst Pharm.* 2002; 59:1077–82.

23. Steiner MA, Yorgason RZ, Vermeulen LC et al. Patient outcomes after therapeutic interchange of dolasetron for granisetron. *Am J Health-Syst Pharm.* 2003; 60:1023–8.

24. Stull DM, Bilmes R, Kim H et al. Comparison of sargramostim and filgrastim in the treatment of chemotherapy-induced neutropenia. *Am J Health-Syst Pharm.* 2005; 62:83–7.

25. Bollinger KA, Vermeulen LC, Davis SN et al. Comparative effectiveness of low-molecular-weight heparins after therapeutic interchange. *Am J Health-Syst Pharm.* 2000; 57:368–72.

26. Nelson WW, Vermeulen LC, Geurkink EA et al. Clinical and humanistic outcomes in patients with gastroesophageal reflux disease converted from ome-prazole to lansoprazole. *Arch Intern Med.* 2000; 160:2491–6.

27. Sodorff MM, Galt KA, Galt MA et al. Patient perceptions of a proton pump inhibitor therapeutic interchange program across the continuum of care. *Pharmacotherapy.* 2002; 22:500–12.

28. Carroll NV. Formularies and therapeutic interchange: the health care setting makes a difference. *Am J Health-Syst Pharm.* 1999; 56:467–72.

29. Rodehaver C, Fearing D. Medication reconciliation in acute care: ensuring an accurate drug regimen on admission and discharge. *Jt Comm J Qual Patient Saf.* 2005; 31:406–13.

30. Gleason KM, Groszek JM, Sullivan C et al. Reconciliation of discrepancies in medication histories and admission orders of newly hospitalized patients. *Am J Health-Syst Pharm.* 2004; 61:1689–95.

31. Saunders SM, Tierney JA, Forde JM et al. Implementing a pharmacist-provided discharge counseling service. *Am J Health-Syst Pharm.* 2003; 60:1101,6,9.

32. American Society of Health-System Pharmacists. ASHP guidelines on the pharmacist's role in the development, implementation, and assessment of critical pathways. *Am J Health-Syst Pharm.* 2004; 61:939–45.

33. American Society of Health-System Pharmacists therapeutic position statements. www.ashp.org/s_ashp/cat1c.asp?CID=516&DID=558 (accessed 2007 Sep 10).

34. American Society of Health-System Pharmacists therapeutic guidelines. www.ashp.org/s_ashp/cat1c.asp?CID=516&DID=559 (accessed 2007 Sep 10).

35. Pedersen CA, Schneider PJ, Scheckelhoff DJ. ASHP national survey of pharmacy practice in hospital settings: prescribing and transcribing—2004. *Am J Health-Syst Pharm.* 2005; 62:378–90.

36. Safe practices for better healthcare: 2006 Update: A Consensus Report. Washington, DC: National Quality Forum (NQF). 2006:22.

37. Schumock GT, Nutescu EA, Walton SM et al. Survey of hospital policies regarding low-molecular-weight heparins. *Am J Health-Syst Pharm.* 2002; 59:534–8.

38. Bernard GR, Vincent JL, Laterre PF et al. Efficacy and safety of recombinant human activated protein C for severe sepsis. *N Engl J Med.* 2001; 344:699–709.

39. Matthay MA. Severe sepsis—a new treatment with both anticoagulant and antiinflammatory properties. *N Engl J Med.* 2001; 344:759–62.

40. Thompson CA. High-cost sepsis drug forces pharmacists to weigh patients' future. *Am J Health-Syst Pharm.* 2002; 59:692,697. News.

41. Dranitsaris G, Spizzirri D, Pitre M et al. A randomized trial to measure the optimal role of the pharmacist in promoting evidence-based antibiotic use in acute care hospitals. *Int J Technol Assess Health Care.* 2001; 17:171–80.

42. Fugit RV, Resch ND. Conversion of patients from simvastatin to lovastatin in an outpatient pharmacy clinic. *Am J Health-Syst Pharm.* 2000; 57:1703–8.

43. Mazzola JL, Belliveau PP, Cheeseman SH. Guidelines for liposomal amphotericin B. *Am J Health-Syst Pharm.* 2003; 60:1480–1.

44. Bower AN, Tang HM, Guglielmo BJ. Compliance in two medical centers with criteria for use of caspofungin and lipid-based amphotericin B. *Am J Health-Syst Pharm.* 2004; 61:915–20.

45. Vermeulen LC Jr, Ratko TA, Erstad BL et al. A paradigm for consensus. The University Hospital Consortium guidelines for the use of albumin, nonprotein colloid, and crystalloid solutions. *Arch Intern Med.* 1995; 155:373–9.

46. Lucarelli CD. Formulary management strategies for type 3 serotonin receptor antagonists. *Am J Health-Syst. Pharm.* 2003; 60:(10, suppl)S4–S11.

47. Devlin JW. Proton pump inhibitors for acid suppression in the intensive care unit: formulary considerations. *Am J Health-Syst Pharm.* 2005; 62:(10, suppl 2):24–30.

48. Chernin EL. Pharmacoeconomics of inhaled anesthetic agents: considerations for the pharmacist. *Am J Health-Syst Pharm.* 2004; 61:(suppl 4)S18–S22.

49. Teich JM, Merchia PR, Schmiz JL et al. Effects of computerized physician order entry on prescribing practices. *Arch Intern Med.* 2000; 160:2741–7.

50. Fischer MA, Lilly CM, Churchill WW et al. An algorithmic computerised order entry approach to assist in the prescribing of new therapeutic agents: case study of activated protein C at an academic medical centre. *Drug Saf.* 2004; 27:1253–61.

Appendix—Therapeutic Interchanges, Prescribing Guidelines, and Other Interventions

Therapeutic Interchanges

The following are some examples of drugs and drug classes for which health systems have successfully implemented therapeutic interchange protocols:

Angiotensin-converting-enzyme inhibitors
Adenosine–dipyridamole for cardiac stress test
Amphotericin, lipid-based
Angiotensin-receptor blockers
Benzodiazepine hypnotics
Beta-lactamase inhibitor antibiotics
Cephalosporins: first- (oral), second-, and third-generation
Cholesterol-lowering agents
Colony-stimulating factors (filgrastim and sargramostim, darbopoetin and epoetin alfa)
Fluroquinolones
Glycoprotein IIb/IIIa inhibitors
Hepatitis B vaccine, pediatric strength
Histamine H_2-receptor antagonists
Inhaled and intranasal corticosteroids
I.V. immune globulin
Insulins – various, including insulin aspart and insulin lispro

Iron products, injectable
Low-molecular-weight heparins
Narcotic analgesics (fentanyl group) in anesthesia
Neuromuscular blocking agents
Nonbenzodiazepine hypnotics
Proton-pump inhibitors
Respiratory agents (tiotropium interchanged with albuterol–ipratropium [Combivent, Boehringer Ingelheim], albuterol–ipratropium [Duoneb, Day] interchanged with individual drugs)
Respiratory spacers
Selective serotonin-reuptake inhibitors
Serotonin-receptor antagonists
Surfactants for newborns
Thrombolytics
Viscoelastic agents

Generic Substitutions

Generic products should be used routinely with few exceptions. The following are particularly important for cost savings:

Amiodarone
Fluconazole injection
Megestrol
Milrinone
Pamidronate
Propofol

Prescribing Guidelines

The following are some examples of drugs, drug classes, and diseases for which health-systems have developed prescribing guidelines, protocols, or pathways in collaboration with the medical staff and nursing staff.

Albumin
Anesthesia gas, low flow and guidelines for selection
Antibiotic surgical prophylaxis
Antibiogram and antibiotic guidelines
Antifungal (injectable) agents (voriconazole, itraconazole, caspofungin)
Aprotinin dosing
Carbapenems
Chemotherapy-induced nausea and vomiting
Colony-stimulating factor guidelines/monitoring
Drotrecogin alfa
Fosphenytoin
Heparin-induced thrombocytopenia
Intensive care unit sedation protocol
I.V. immune globulin
Levalbuterol
Nesiritide
Octreotide
Pneumonia protocol
Postoperative nausea and vomiting
Proton-pump inhibitors (i.v.)
Venous thromboembolism, use of anticoagulants in acute coronary syndrome
Ziprasidone injection

Interventions—Other

Other initiatives or activities that pharmacists can collaborate with the medical staff to reduce drug costs.

Cost per case in anesthesia
Antibiotic monitoring, laboratory reporting of sensitivities
Antibiotic restrictions
Eptifibatide waste reduction
Epoetin alfa waste reduction, prepare syringes
Pegfilgrastim is used in outpatients only

Approved by the ASHP Board of Directors on January 17, 2008. These guidelines supersede the ASHP Technical Assistance Bulletin on Assessing Cost-Containment Strategies dated September 27, 1991. Developed through the ASHP Council on Pharmacy Management.

ASHP gratefully acknowledges the expert panel that developed these guidelines: Michael Rubino, M.S., FASHP; James M. Hoffman, Pharm.D., M.S., BCPS; Larry J. Koesterer, M.B.A.; and Robert G. Swendrzynski, M.S.

The bibliographic citation for this article is as follows: American Society of Health-System Pharmacists. ASHP guidelines on medication cost management strategies for hospitals and health systems. *Am J Health-Syst Pharm.* 2008; 65:1368–84.

ASHP Guidelines on Outsourcing Pharmaceutical Services

Purpose

Health-system pharmacy, as an essential component in health care organizations, is challenged by changes in the structure and financing of health care to reduce costs and improve performance. One option being used to achieve these goals is outsourcing. Outsourcing is a formal arrangement by which a health care organization contracts with an outside company to obtain selected pharmaceutical services or comprehensive management of the organization's pharmacy. Through this arrangement, the organization negotiates a contract with a company to access its expertise, technologies, and resources.

ASHP believes that the organization's pharmacist-in-charge (e.g., a pharmacy director) must take complete responsibility for patient outcomes from all medication-related activities performed at or for the organization's work sites, whether they are carried out by the organization's or contractor's onsite staff or by the contractor off site. This responsibility should be explicitly stated in all outsourcing contracts.

Health care organizations considering outsourcing pharmaceutical services should have a clear understanding of what they want to accomplish. Consideration should include, at the least, an internal needs assessment, a cost analysis, and a careful review of possible contractors. The organization should examine the potential long-term consequences of outsourcing as well as the short-term outcomes expected during a contract's performance period.

The purpose of these guidelines is to provide an overview of factors and processes for health care organizations to consider when exploring outsourcing. The ideas presented in this document could be used for strategic planning with the organization's decision-makers, for drafting contract provisions, for comparing prospective contractors, for preparing for contract negotiations, or for evaluating a contractor's performance. These guidelines may be applied, for example, to independent and networked acute care hospitals, ambulatory care clinics, and home care providers.

This document includes ideas about reasons for outsourcing and reasons for not outsourcing, services available from contractors, the outsourcing process and outsourcing arrangements, and evaluation of contractor performance. The appendix provides a topical list of contract provisions, some of which relate to specific pharmaceutical services, pharmacy practices, or administrative functions that may be the subject of other ASHP practice standards. Organizations should refer to pertinent ASHP practice standards for additional information on which to base their contract provisions, agreements, and decisions. This document addresses representative outsourcing options and contract agreements and is not intended to cover all situations. Managers of pharmacy and health care organizations should use their professional judgment about applicability to their own needs and circumstances.

Environment

Various environmental influences and market forces that may contribute to outsourcing being considered as an option include the following.

Organizational and Operational

- Re-engineering and downsizing initiatives
- Consolidation and integration of health systems and departments within health systems
- Elimination of or reduction in the size of traditional departments
- Reorganization around patient-focused care
- Implementation of automated pharmacy systems and the attendant need to reorganize medication distribution functions

Staffing

- Shortage of nurses and other health care professionals
- Shortage of pharmacists with specific experience and capabilities

Financial and Cost-Control

- Restricted budgets
- Increased operating costs
- Increased drug costs
- Increased emphasis on measuring performance in terms of staffing and costs instead of clinical outcomes

Quality

- Increased expectations of and pressures from accreditation organizations and consumer groups to improve the quality of patient care

Governmental and Regulatory

- Increased numbers of individuals dependent on federal, state, and local governments for health care
- Reduced ability of federal, state, and local governments to finance health care
- Increased government controls on reimbursement for health care

Competitive

- Increased competition among health care organizations
- Increased competition among suppliers of pharmaceutical products and related services

Purposes of Outsourcing

Health care organizations that conduct in-depth assessments may decide that outsourcing either is or is not a good option for meeting their needs. Reasons for their decision will vary according to a variety of factors.

Reasons Health Care Organizations Outsource Pharmaceutical Services. Organizations tend to outsource pharmaceutical services when guided by a careful assessment of their capabilities of providing services themselves, when unsuccessful in

using their own resources to provide services, or, in some cases, when influenced by a consultant. Contracting with an outsourcing firm may produce one or more of the following results.

Organizational and operational
- Ease the consolidation of pharmaceutical services in integrated health systems
- Resolve operational inefficiencies (e.g., by improving medication distribution systems, designing new pharmacy workspaces, reducing medication dispensing and administration errors, and improving computer and information systems)
 - Enable the organization to acquire additional resources and expertise to carry out other changes (e.g., reallocation of existing staff to pharmaceutical care roles in patient care areas)
 - Provide educational programs for patients and their families and for health care staff

Staffing
- Help the organization to staff hard-to-fill pharmacy positions
- Allow the organization to reach optimal staffing levels for achieving productivity targets

Financial and cost-control
- Control or reduce the cost of the organization's services
- Control or reduce labor costs (e.g., by shifting the cost of employees, benefits, and liabilities to a contractor)
- Enable the organization to acquire a contractor who will share the risks associated with operating the pharmaceutical services
- Avoid the cost of purchasing and maintaining pharmacy equipment
- Avoid the cost of physical remodeling (e.g., by using an offsite contractor to provide specific services for which remodeling would be required)
- Increase the organization's financial operating margin (e.g., by allowing the organization to purchase drugs in bulk quantities, use group purchasing contracts, decrease lost charges, improve billing accuracy, decrease drug diversion and pilferage, improve drug formularies, and transfer drug inventory, equipment, and supply activities to a contractor)

Quality
- Enable the organization to maintain or improve the quality of patient care (e.g., by expanding clinical services and pharmaceutical care, establishing new services, and obtaining specialized expertise in pharmaceutical care)
- Provide support for the medical and nursing staffs and improve physician–nursing–pharmacy collaboration

Governmental and regulatory
- Correct regulatory and accreditation problems relating to pharmaceutical services
- Ensure continuing compliance with accreditation and certification standards

Competitive
- Enhance the organization's image
- Allow the organization to gain an edge on competitors through improvements in service, quality, or price

Reasons Health Care Organizations Do Not Outsource Pharmaceutical Services. An organization's choice to continue providing its own pharmaceutical services may be based on one or more of the following reasons.

Organizational and operational
- A belief that pharmaceutical services are well managed and are provided as effectively as or better than they could be by a contractor
- Negative experiences with outsourcing contractors (pharmacy or nonpharmacy) or awareness of other organizations' negative experiences with such contractors
- Concern that the decision to outsource pharmaceutical services can be reversed only with great difficulty
- A belief that the organization's needs are currently met cost-effectively and that changes are therefore unnecessary
- Concern about losing short-term and long-term control over decisions about pharmaceutical services
- Concern about reduced involvement of pharmacy leadership in organizationwide initiatives (e.g., development and implementation of information systems, clinical care plans or pathways, and disease management)

Staffing
- Concern that staff will be reduced to unacceptable levels
- Concern about potentially alienating relationships between pharmacists and other health care staff

Financial and cost-control
- An assessment that outsourcing would increase rather than decrease costs
- Concern that high-cost drugs might be excluded from contract agreements
- Concern that the organization may not be able to recapitalize pharmaceutical services if outsourcing is unsuccessful

Quality
- Concern that conflicting values and priorities of the outsourcing contractor and the organization will reduce quality
- Concern that clinical quality could be reduced as a result of a loss of continuity of pharmacy staffing and relationships with medical and nursing staffs

Professional responsibility
- Concern that outsourcing will confuse or dilute the onsite pharmacists' ultimate professional authority and responsibility for all medication-related activities and outcomes at the site

Pharmaceutical Services Provided by Contractors

Some contractors manage and provide comprehensive pharmaceutical services. Other contracors focus more on providing specialty services or carrying out specific tasks (e.g., drug information services, offsite preparation of sterile products). The needs of the health care organization should guide the identification of potential contractors

with the appropriate expertise and capabilities. Examples of services that may be available from contractors follow. (This list is likely to grow over time.)

Organizational and Operational

- Development of pharmacy policies, procedures, and processes
- Pharmacy record-keeping systems
- Productivity reviews
- Feasibility studies on expanding services (e.g., outpatient dispensing and home infusion)
- Unit dose medication distribution
- Pharmacy-based or offsite preparation of sterile products
- Pharmacokinetic monitoring and dosage determinations
- Medication therapy monitoring (e.g., for appropriate and effective use)
- Investigational drug programs
- Patient profile reviews
- Medication therapy-related consultation with physicians, nurses, and other health care professionals
- Assessment of patients' nutritional needs
- Guidance in purchasing and implementing automated pharmacy equipment
- Educational programs for patients, families, and caregivers
- Drug information services
- Packaging and repackaging of pharmaceuticals

Staffing

- Competency assessment and performance review
- Management, operational, and clinical training
- Recruitment and retention assistance

Financial and Cost-Control

- Billing
- Inventory control
- Formulary management

Quality

- Performance improvement (including improvement of medication use and reduction of medication errors)
- Quality assurance

Outsourcing Process

After the health care organization has completed an internal assessment of its needs and capabilities and decided to explore outsourcing, it should identify and contact reputable and experienced contractors. Some organizations simply identify prospective contractors and ask them to submit a proposal. A more thorough approach is to require prospective contractors to respond to a request for proposals (RFP). Although a formal RFP (and the contractor's formal proposal based on the RFP) may not be necessary, the information found in typical RFPs and proposals may be helpful for making a decision about outsourcing.

Contents of RFPs. RFPs often include the following information.

- A description of the organization (including statistical information)

- The organization's financial status (e.g., a current balance sheet and audited financial statement, the pharmacy's financial status)
- A description of the process the organization will use to select the contractor
- The organization's standard terms and conditions for contracting for services
- The names and telephone numbers of individuals in the organization who are involved in the outsourcing decision (the director of pharmacy should be included)
- A description of the specific outsourced services required of the contractor (e.g., pharmacy workspace design, intravenous admixture preparation, and implementation of an automated pharmacy system) and performance-measurement criteria or targets
- The date(s) on which the contractor can inspect the facility and the pharmacy
- The number of copies of the proposal to submit
- The name and address of the individual to whom the proposal is to be delivered
- Acceptable method(s) for delivery of the proposal (e.g., mail, delivery service, courier)
- A statement that the organization reserves the right to cancel its solicitation for services and reject any and all proposals
- A deadline date and time for receipt of the proposal
- The date on which the contractor would be expected to initiate services
- The date by which the selected contractor must provide a written contract
- Other requirements related to the proposal (e.g., that it be typewritten, that it include reference to an RFP number [if any], that it be signed by an officer of the firm who is authorized to contract)

Contents of Proposals. RFPs often require contractors to submit the following information with their proposals.

- A brief history of the contractor, including its mission, vision, and values
- The location of the contractor's offices and other facilities that would provide services to the organization
- The names, addresses, telephone numbers, and résumés or background information on the individual(s) who will provide the services
- Evidence that the contractor can provide qualified staff who are licensed or eligible for licensure by federal, state, and local agencies and a history of turnover in management, pharmacist, and support staff
- A history of the results of Joint Commission on Accreditation of Healthcare Organizations (JCAHO), Health Care Financing Administration, National Committee for Quality Assurance, state, or other accreditation or regulatory surveys conducted in the contractor's sites
- Proof of professional liability, general liability, and workers'-compensation insurance coverage (including the name, address, and telephone number of the insurance company) and a history of claims filed against the contractor
- Minimum-experience requirements (e.g., years of experience in providing outsourced pharmacy-management services, total number of clients served, current number of clients)

- A list of the requested services that the contractor can provide
- A list of the requested services that the contractor cannot provide and the reasons for the contractor's inability to provide them
- Evidence of organizational and staff experience and competence (including nature and extent) in the services the contractor can provide (e.g., pharmaceutical care, specialty clinical practice, antineoplastic medication preparation, enteral and parenteral nutrition solution preparation), as pertinent
- A copy of a standard or proposed contract
- A list of all fees and charges that would be billed under the contract and the detailed methods for their calculation, as well as a billing schedule
- A description of reports that the contractor will be expected to submit to the organization
- Information relating to the contractor's financial status and stability (e.g., balance sheets and audited financial statements for the past three years, bank references, lists of principal equity owners)
- The names, addresses, and telephone numbers of current clients receiving similar services
- The names, addresses, and telephone numbers of other clients served within the past two years and the reasons for all, if any, terminations of services
- Written references and copies of annual performance-improvement reports from clients of a similar size with similar types of patients

Visits to Contractors and Their Clients. Contractors should allow the organization's representatives to visit their corporate offices and production facilities and to tour pharmacies in the facilities of other clients. The contractor should provide ample opportunity for the organization's representatives to confer with the contractor's corporate and pharmacy staff.

Evaluating Proposals. A decision to outsource pharmaceutical services should be collaborative and should involve, as appropriate, the governing board, the chief executive officer (CEO), the chief financial officer (CFO), the chief operating officer (COO), the chief of the medical staff, the chair of the pharmacy and therapeutics committee, the director of nursing (DON), the director of pharmacy, and department heads, for example. The organization should scrutinize the following factors when evaluating proposals.

- Services offered versus services requested (including the contractor's ability to enhance current services)
- Professional experience (e.g., years of service; number, size, and types of clients; knowledge of the client's business)
- Financial stability (e.g., ability to absorb start-up expenses and to commit the resources needed to effect change)
- References and reputation (e.g., client-satisfaction reports, reputation in the health care industry, commitment to improving patient care)
- Technology or automated pharmacy systems (e.g., up-to-date hardware, proprietary software, the capability to interface with the organization's information systems)
- Education and training (e.g., internal and external continuing-education programs, educational allowances for professional and technical staff)

- Additional qualities (e.g., high employee morale, confidentiality, creativity, sensitivity to minorities and the community, willingness to share risks and rewards)
- Cost aspects of services (e.g., cost-effectiveness, ability to affect economies of scale)

The organization should assign an evaluation rating to each proposal. Ratings should be weighted appropriately with respect to professional services, experience, references, and cost of services. The organization should base its decision to outsource pharmaceutical services on its assessment of the contractor's ability to meet the organization's needs and fulfill the terms of the contract.

Negotiating the Contract. The organization should carefully review the proposal and clarify the provisions of the contract. Assistance from the organization's risk-management and legal counsel may be necessary. Negotiations can ensure a contract that best meets the needs of the organization and the contractor.

Signing the Contract. In some organizations the director of pharmacy may be authorized to sign contracts for outsourced services. If this is not the case, the director of pharmacy should be fully involved in negotiating the contract and advising the authorized signer(s).

Outsourcing Arrangement

The health care organization and the contractor should agree on the outsourcing arrangement that best meets their needs. Several outsourcing options are available to health care organizations. Variations and combinations of these options are common. The contract should clearly describe the outsourcing arrangement. Examples of outsourcing arrangements include the following.

Consulting. The contractor acts as a pharmacy consultant to the organization. Some consulting arrangements are limited to an assessment of all pharmaceutical services or to specific aspects of pharmaceutical services (e.g., clinical pharmacy services, productivity, compliance with JCAHO standards). Other consulting arrangements may include advising the pharmacy and helping it to improve its services.

Onsite Advisor. The contractor provides a full-time onsite advisor to the organization's director of pharmacy. The advisor works with the director of pharmacy and others, as needed, to carry out programs that will fulfill the contract provisions.

Management of Specific Pharmaceutical Services. The contractor provides one or more specific services (e.g., i.v. admixture preparation, drug information, stock replenishment, medication distribution). Services may be provided onsite or at an offsite location.

Comprehensive Management. The contractor assumes complete responsibility for operating the pharmacy and may provide some or all of the pharmacy staff.

Contract Provisions

A contract that meets the needs of the health care organization and of the contractor is the foundation for a successful

relationship. Contracts should include provisions of the outsourcing arrangement that describe agreements between the organization and the contractor concerning their respective responsibilities. These provisions will vary depending on the kind and scope of services outsourced. For example, contractors who prepare sterile products at an offsite location will not require onsite pharmacy space and utilities. Also, the assignment of responsibilities may vary. A contract may specify that the organization will purchase all drugs. Conversely, another contract may assign this responsibility to the contractor. See the appendix for examples of contract provisions.

Evaluation of Contractor's Performance

Health care organizations should evaluate and document their contractor's performance and assess their contractor's compliance with the terms of the contract. Objective and subjective evaluations should be regular (e.g., quarterly or annually). Evaluations should address all measurable standards of performance that are specified in the contract. Evaluations should be multidisciplinary and should involve, for example, the CEO, CFO, COO, DON, and medical staff representatives, as appropriate. An evaluation may include an assessment of how well the contractor performed the following functions.

- Improved the quality of patient care
- Responded to the organization's needs
- Helped the organization to achieve its financial and patient-outcome goals
- Evaluated the productivity and performance of pharmacy staff
- Provided continuing education for pharmacy staff
- Implemented and improved pharmacy clinical programs
- Improved pharmacy processes (e.g., medication dispensing and delivery)
- Reduced and controlled pharmacy costs without compromising patient care
- Worked and communicated effectively with the organization's staff and resolved interdepartmental problems
- Participated effectively in the organization's performance-improvement program

Suggested Reading

1. Curtis FR, Stai HC. Contract pharmacy services. In: Brown TR, ed. Handbook of institutional pharmacy practice, 3rd ed. Bethesda, MD: American Society of Hospital Pharmacists; 1992: 299–306.
2. Talley CR. Outsourcing drug distribution. *Am J Health-Syst Pharm.* 1997; 54:37. Editorial.
3. Schneider PJ. Outsourcing: a key to professional survival. *Am J Health-Syst Pharm.* 1997; 54:41–3.
4. Lazarus HL. Outsourcing: a success story. *Am J Health-Syst Pharm.* 1997; 54:43–4.
5. Puckett WH. Outsourcing: taking the first step. *Am J Health-Syst Pharm.* 1997; 54:45–8.
6. Kolar GR. Outsourcing: route to a new pharmacy practice model. *Am J Health-Syst Pharm.* 1997; 54:48–52.
7. Eckel FM. Outsourcing: at odds with pharmacy's professional foundation. *Am J Health-Syst Pharm.* 1997; 54:52–5.
8. Gates DM, Smolarek RT, Stevenson JG. Outsourcing the preparation of parenteral nutrient solutions. *Am J Health-Syst Pharm.* 1996; 53:2176–8.
9. Burruss RA, Carroll NV, Schraa C, et al. Outsourcing inpatient IV compounding: expense and medication error implications. *Pharm Pract Manage Q.* 1996; 16(3):52–9.
10. McAllister JC III. Collaborating with re-engineering consultants: maintaining resources for the future. *Am J Health-Syst Pharm.* 1995; 52:2676–80.
11. Anderson RJ. Clinical service contracts between hospital pharmacy departments and colleges of pharmacy. *Am J Hosp Pharm.* 1991; 48:1994–7.
12. Murphy JE, Ward ES, Job ML. Implementing and maintaining a private pharmacokinetics practice. *Am J Hosp Pharm.* 1990; 47:591–7.
13. Souhrada L. Contract management. *Hospitals.* 1990; 64(8):66–8.
14. Wagner M. Basic pitfalls can undermine hospital–service firm relationship. *Mod Healthc.* 1993; 23(8):32.
15. Wagner M. Contract-managed pharmacy departments are just the prescription at some hospitals. *Mod Healthc.* 1988; 18(8):36–40.

Appendix—Contract Provisions

The following are examples of contract provisions that, among others, the organization and contractor might adapt as needed and include in a contract, depending on the scope of services being considered. In addition, a contract would include provisions about the specific pharmaceutical services to be provided by the contractor. The language in contract provisions should be adapted to meet the needs of the health care organization and to comply with the organization's contracting policies and applicable laws and regulations.

Accreditation and Certification: A contract may include a requirement that services meet or exceed applicable accreditation and certification standards. These include, but are not limited to, the standards (or requirements) of the following organizations.
- Joint Commission on Accreditation of Healthcare Organizations
- American Osteopathic Association
- Health Care Financing Administration
- National Committee for Quality Assurance

After-Hours Pharmaceutical Services when 24-Hour Services Are Not Provided: The contractor may agree, for example, to provide an after-hours stock of drug products for authorized staff to use in filling urgent medication orders. In addition, the contractor may agree to ensure that a pharmacist is on call or available to return to the facility to provide pharmaceutical services.

Automation: A contract may outline responsibilities for the purchase or lease and the use of automated medication storage and distribution equipment and software associated with the equipment.

Choice of Law: There may be a statement that the contract is governed by the laws of the state in which patient care is provided.

Compensation for Contractor's Services: There may be compensation arrangements, which vary greatly but are often based on one or more of the following principles.

- Management fee(s)
- Fee per item dispensed or service performed
- Fixed fee per patient per patient day, admission, discharge, adjusted patient day, adjusted admission, or adjusted discharge

Besides agreeing on a compensation arrangement, the organization and the contractor may agree on ways for the contractor to share the financial risk of contract performance with the organization; these might include guarantees or incentives for meeting targets and penalties for underperformance.

Computer Equipment and Information Systems: A contract may outline responsibilities for the purchase, ownership, and maintenance of computer equipment and related software. Agreements might extend to personal computers used by pharmacy staff. There should be clear agreement about access to and use of data generated by the information system.

Confidentiality: There may be a requirement that information not generally available to the public (e.g., financial statements, medical records, market information) be kept confidential. Both parties must agree to safeguard access to computer databases and patient records to ensure that the patient's rights to privacy and confidentiality is protected. Use of the information should be limited solely to purposes specified in the contract.

Contractor Reports: The content and regularity of performance reports that the contractor will submit to the organization may be specified.

Controlled Substances: Responsibilities may be assigned for the procurement and security of controlled substances in compliance with Drug Enforcement Administration (DEA) and state regulations. For example, the organization may be required to

- Register with the DEA and any state equivalent for each site involved
- Assume complete responsibility for record keeping and security of controlled substances throughout the facility
- Ask the contractor to maintain proper records and provide adequate security for controlled substances as required by federal, state, and local laws and regulations and
- Verify that the contractor maintains proper records and provides adequate security for controlled substances

It may be necessary for the organization to grant power of attorney to the contractor to order and purchase controlled substances.

Similarly, the contractor may be required to

- Ensure that all registrations are current
- Order and maintain an adequate stock of controlled substances
- Ensure compliance with record-keeping and security requirements
- Inform the organization of problems with compliance

Cost Control: A contract may include objectives, methods, and performance measures for controlling costs.

Cytotoxic and Hazardous Drug Products: Responsibilities for ensuring the safety of the organization's staff and patients during the preparation and distribution of cytotoxic and hazardous drug products may be assigned. Either the organization or the contractor should pro-

vide a hazardous-materials handling program, including staff training, that meets Occupational Safety and Health Administration (OSHA) requirements.

Drug Inventory Disposition upon Termination of the Contract: A provision for the disposition of the drug inventory is based on inventory ownership. In cases in which the drug inventory may be purchased by either party, a mutually acceptable, independent appraiser could decide the purchase price. Legal advice may be needed to ensure that purchases comply with the Prescription Drug Marketing Act and other applicable laws and regulations.

Drug Inventory Ownership: If the contractor purchases the organization's inventory, a mutually acceptable, independent appraiser could decide the purchase price. Expired and other unusable drugs should be excluded from the purchase. The contractor could agree to obtain credit for the organization for expired and other unusable drugs if credit is obtainable. Legal advice may be needed to ensure that purchases comply with the Prescription Drug Marketing Act and other applicable laws and regulations.

Drug Ordering: A contract may assign responsibilities for selecting vendors and purchasing drug supplies for the organization. The contract should specify that all drugs used must be subject to approval by the organization's pharmacy and therapeutics (P&T) committee or its equivalent. The organization should understand how purchasing discounts are accounted for, recorded, and distributed. The impact of removing pharmacy items from group purchasing programs should be clear also.

Early Termination: There may be conditions for early termination of the contract.

Extension of Period of Performance: Conditions for extending the period of performance may be included in the contract.

Forms: Responsibilities for the design, approval, purchase, and storage of forms may be assigned.

Formulary System: A contract may assign responsibilities for evaluation of medications, collaboration with the P&T committee, and provision of formulary-related information services.

Hours of Pharmacy Operation: A contract may specify hours of operation that meet or exceed legal requirements and that are sufficient to serve patients' needs.

Laws, Rules, and Regulations: Requirements for services to meet or exceed federal, state, and local laws, rules, and regulations may be specified. These include but are not limited to those of FDA, DEA, OSHA, and the state board of pharmacy. The pharmacy should maintain (e.g., display, file) the appropriate licenses, permits, and records of equipment maintenance and certification. Any contractor required to be licensed as a manufacturer must be so licensed. The organization may agree to allow the contractor to act on the organization's behalf in communicating with the state board of pharmacy and other regulatory agencies.

Liability Insurance: Responsibilities for maintaining liability insurance coverage for the acts of employees may be assigned. The contract might specify, for example, that the contractor must maintain adequate liability insurance coverage for the acts of its employees.

Nondiscrimination: There might be a requirement that the contractor abide by all laws and regulations relating to discrimination in appointments, promotions, and terminations.

Ownership of Equipment, Fixtures, and Supplies: A contract may specify ownership of equipment, fixtures, and supplies and responsibilities for ensuring that equipment is maintained and certified according to applicable practice standards, laws, and regulations.

Performance Improvement: Responsibilities for establishing any performance-improvement programs and integrating them with the organization's performance-improvement activities may be included. Performance-improvement programs might be appropriate, for example, for the ordering, dispensing, and administering of medications and for the monitoring of medication effects and misadventures, including adverse drug reactions and adverse drug events.

Period of Performance: The contract might specify the period for which the contractor will provide services to the organization.

Pharmacy Staff Education and Training: Responsibilities for required ongoing staff education and training may be specified. For example, there might be an agreement that the contractor's staff will participate in the organization's education and training programs. In addition, the contractor may agree to provide specific training to ensure that all pharmacy personnel can perform any duties imposed by contractor-implemented functions.

Pharmacy Staff Employment: There may be a provision for the employment of pharmacists and technical and support personnel; this may specify those who will be employed by the organization and those who will be employed by the contractor. Whether employed by the organization or by the contractor, all staff should be competent and legally qualified. The organization should retain the right to assess, accept, or reject the performance of any of the contractor's staff who are used at the organization's work sites.

Pharmacy Staff Expenses: Responsibilities for any personnel expenses may be assigned. A contract might specify, for example, that the organization will be responsible for the salary, wages, and benefits of its employees whereas the contractor will be responsible for such expenses for its own employees. The contract might also allocate expenses for parking, meal discounts, and similar privileges for employees.

Pharmacy Staff Levels: There may be a requirement that the staffing levels for the contracted services be sufficient to meet the organization's needs.

Pharmacy Staff Orientation: A contract may assign responsibilities for orientation of all new pharmacy staff members to the organization and to the pharmacy, according to the organization's requirements.

Pharmacy Staff Performance: Responsibilities for pharmacy staff competency assessments and performance evaluations and for ensuring that assessments and evaluations are based on criteria in the individual's job description may be assigned.

Policies and Procedures: Responsibilities may be assigned for developing policies and procedures covering the outsourced services, all of which should comply with applicable laws, regulations, and accreditation or certification standards. The contract should specify that the policies and procedures must not conflict with those of the organization.

Purchasing and Accounts Payable: Responsibilities for maintaining the pharmacy's purchasing and accounts-payable functions, including ordering drugs, monitoring costs, and authorizing payment to vendors, might be specified.

Record Maintenance: A contract may assign responsibilities for maintaining and storing records. The contract should specify that all pertinent records must be kept for the time required by law and by the organization.

Space: Responsibilities for space required by the contractor to provide onsite services might be outlined. The organization should agree to provide space for the provision of onsite contractor services that is acceptable to the contractor and within the guidelines of the agencies that regulate the practice of pharmacy. Organizations might agree to provide the following facilities, depending on the contract's scope of services.
- Adequate square footage
- Space for preparing, compounding, packaging, and storing drugs under proper conditions
- Space for receiving and storing intravenous fluids and supplies
- Refrigerators and freezers
- Adequate space for maintaining and storing pharmacy records
- Laminar-airflow hoods and biological safety cabinets (if needed)

Sterile Products: A contract might include requirements for the quality of sterile products provided by the contractor. The contractor should ensure that sterile products (e.g., large-volume intravenous admixtures, total parenteral nutrient solutions) are prepared and labeled in a suitable environment by trained and competent employees. The contractor should provide quality-control information periodically and on demand. For services that involve deliveries, the contract should specify order cutoff and delivery times, any penalties for late deliveries, and arrangements for after-hours or emergency services and deliveries.

Successors: The rights of each party in the event that the organization or contractor merges or transfers its business or assets to a successor may be included in a contract.

Utilities: A contract may assign responsibility for utilities required by the contractor to provide onsite services. These utilities may include the following, as appropriate.
- Electrical service
- Water
- Heating and air conditioning
- Plumbing
- Janitorial services
- Internal and external telephone services (allowance might be made for a private external telephone line for the contractor)
- Security
- Waste disposal

These guidelines were reviewed in 2007 by the Council on Pharmacy Management and by the Board of Directors and were found to still be appropriate.

Approved by the ASHP Board of Directors, April 22, 1998. Developed through the Council on Administrative Affairs.

The bibliographic citation for this document is as follows: American Society of Health-System Pharmacists. ASHP guidelines on outsourcing pharmaceutical services. *Am J Health-Syst Pharm.* 1998; 55:1611–7.

ASHP Guidelines on Outsourcing Sterile Compounding Services

Purpose

Health care organizations considering outsourcing sterile compounding services should have a clear understanding of what they want to accomplish. Consideration should include, at the least, an internal needs assessment, a cost analysis, and a careful review of prospective compounding pharmacies. The organization should examine the potential long-term consequences of outsourcing as well as the short-term outcomes expected during a contract's performance period.

The purpose of these guidelines is to provide an overview of factors and processes for health care organizations to consider when exploring outsourcing of pharmacy sterile compounding. The ideas presented in this document could be used for strategic planning with the organization's decision-makers, for drafting contract provisions, for comparing prospective compounding pharmacies, for preparing for contract negotiations, or for evaluating a compounding pharmacy's performance.

This document includes ideas about reasons for outsourcing and reasons for not outsourcing, services available from compounding pharmacies, the outsourcing process and outsourcing arrangements, and evaluation of a compounding pharmacy's performance. The appendix provides a topical list of contract provisions, some of which relate to practices that are the subject of other American Society of Health-System Pharmacy (ASHP) guidelines. Organizations should refer to pertinent ASHP guidelines for additional information on which to base their contract provisions, agreements, and decisions.[1-3] This document addresses representative outsourcing options and contract agreements and is not intended to cover all situations. Managers of pharmacy and health care organizations should use their professional judgment about applicability to their own needs and circumstances.

Environment

There are various environmental influences and market forces that may contribute to a facility's decision to consider outsourcing. A list of some of those considerations follows.

Organizational and Operational

- Limited available technological resources to provide the specific desired services.
- Re-engineering and downsizing initiatives.
- Consolidation and integration of health systems and departments within health systems.
- Elimination of or reduction in the size of traditional pharmacy departments.
- Reorganization around patient-focused care.
- Implementation of automated pharmacy systems and the attendant need to reorganize medication preparation and distribution functions.

Staffing
- Shortage of pharmacists, nurses, and other health care professionals.

- Shortage of pharmacy personnel with specific experience and capabilities.

Financial and Cost Control

- Restricted budgets.
- Increased operating costs.
- Increased drug costs.
- Increased emphasis on measuring performance in terms of staffing and costs.

Quality Assurance

- Increased expectations of and pressures from payers, accreditation organizations, and consumer groups to improve the quality of patient care, reduce the incidence of hospital infections, and demonstrate compliance with applicable standards and regulations.

Governmental and Regulatory

- Reductions of federal, state, and local government reimbursement for health care.
- Increased numbers of individuals dependent on federal, state, and local governments for health care.
- Increased federal and state interest in standards for sterile compounding (i.e., *United States Pharmacopeia* [*USP*] chapter 797[4]).

Competitive

- Increased competition among healthcare organizations.
- Increased competition among suppliers of pharmaceutical products and related services.

Purposes of Outsourcing

Health care organizations that conduct in-depth assessments may decide that outsourcing either is or is not a good option for meeting their needs. Reasons for their decision will vary according to a variety of factors.

Reasons Health Care Organizations Outsource Sterile Compounding Services. Organizations tend to outsource sterile compounding services when guided by a careful assessment of their capabilities of providing services themselves, when unsuccessful in using their own resources to provide those services, or, in some cases, upon advice from a consultant. Contracting with an outsourcing firm may produce one or more of the following results.

Organizational and Operational

- Ease the consolidation of pharmaceutical services in integrated health systems.

- Resolve operational inefficiencies (e.g., batch compounding, staff scheduling, high-demand periods).
- Provide compounded preparations outside the scope of preparations routinely provided (e.g., complex or rarely compounded preparations).
- Enable the organization to acquire additional resources and expertise to carry out other priorities (e.g., reallocation of existing staff to roles in patient care areas).

Staffing

- Help the organization to staff hard-to-fill pharmacy positions and address staffing vacancies.
- Allow the organization to reach optimal staffing levels for achieving productivity targets.

Financial and Cost Control

- Control or reduce the cost of the organization's services (e.g., by shifting costs associated with i.v. admixture production from fixed to variable).
- Control or reduce labor costs (e.g., by shifting responsibility for employees, benefits, and liabilities to a compounding pharmacy).
- Enable the organization to acquire a business partner to share the risks and other associated liability by defining the responsibilities associated with operating sterile compounding services.
- Minimize the cost of facility remodeling (e.g., to meet *USP* 797 requirements).

Quality Assurance

- Provide consistent pharmacy and sterile compounding services, including documented beyond-use dating.
- Enable the organization to maintain or improve the quality of patient care (e.g., by expanding clinical services or establishing new services).
- Provide support for the medical and nursing staffs and improve physician–nursing–pharmacy collaboration.
- Improve organizational procedures by learning from the compounding pharmacy's experience and knowledge, especially with new technologies (e.g., labeling, bar-coding, or tamper-evidence technologies).

Governmental and Regulatory

- Assist and ensure compliance with legal, regulatory, certification, and accreditation requirements.

Competitive

- Allow the organization to gain an edge on competitors through improvements in service, quality, or price.

Reasons Health Care Organizations Do Not Outsource Sterile Compounding Services. An organization's choice to continue providing its own sterile compounding services may be based on one or more of the following reasons.

Organizational and Operational

- The organization demonstrates that its sterile compounding services are cost-effective, well managed, and provided as efficiently as or better than they could be by a compounding pharmacy.
- Negative experiences with outsourcing pharmacy (or even nonpharmacy) services, or awareness of other organizations' negative experiences with such outsourcing.
- Concern about time delays in receiving compounded preparations, especially products that are needed urgently or have poor stability or short beyond-use times.
- Concern that the compounding pharmacy may experience interruptions in service, perhaps with little notice, due to quality-control issues not related to services provided to the organization.
- Concern that the decision to outsource sterile compounding services can be reversed only with great difficulty.
- Concern about losing short-term and long-term control over decisions regarding or expertise in sterile compounding services.

Staffing

- Concern that staff will be reduced to unacceptable levels.

Financial and Cost Control

- An assessment that outsourcing would increase rather than decrease costs.
- Concern that high-cost drugs might be excluded from contract agreements.
- Concern that the organization may not be able to recapitalize sterile compounding services if outsourcing is unsuccessful.

Quality Assurance

- Concern that conflicting values and priorities of the compounding pharmacy and the organization will reduce quality.
- Concern about the qualifications or competencies of compounding pharmacy staff.

Professional Responsibility

- Concern that outsourcing sterile compounding will confuse or dilute the onsite pharmacists' ultimate professional and legal authority and responsibility for other medication-related activities and outcomes at the site.

Services Provided by Compounding Pharmacies

The needs of the health care organization should guide the identification of potential compounding pharmacies with the appropriate expertise and capabilities. Among the services that may be available from compounding pharmacies are

the preparation of implantable and external pump cartridges; total parenteral nutrition, dialysis, irrigation, or cardioplegia solutions; antibiotics; ophthalmic injectables and solutions; chemotherapy preparations; and analgesic preparations (patient-controlled analgesia, epidural, or regional nerve-block devices).

Compounding pharmacies are regulated in a number of ways. They may be registered as pharmacies and/or wholesalers in the states in which they dispense, as drug establishments and/or device manufacturers by the Food and Drug Administration (FDA), and/or as manufacturers by the Drug Enforcement Administration (DEA). FDA requires a device manufacturer registration for a compounding pharmacy to dispense devices such as dialysate solutions or heparin or citrate syringes. A compounding pharmacy registered as a drug establishment may apply for a labeler code that allows it to create National Drug Code (NDC) numbers for its products. These NDC numbers do not indicate FDA approval or that a New Drug Application has been filed, nor do they indicate a higher degree of quality (e.g., that terminal sterilization rather than an aseptic fill process has been used in compounding the preparation). Ascertaining that a preparation is labeled with an NDC number is therefore not a substitute for the due diligence required to verify a compounding pharmacy's quality processes (e.g., *USP* 797, current good manufacturing processes). Finally, compounding pharmacies are not permitted to prepare copies of commercial products. Dispensing of such products by compounding pharmacies will result in regulatory action, as FDA enforcement discretion does not apply to copies of commercial products.

Outsourcing Process

After the health care organization has completed an internal assessment of its needs and capabilities and decided to explore outsourcing, it should identify and contact reputable compounding pharmacies. Organizations that are part of a larger network (e.g., an integrated delivery network) may explore options that are available to them through the network or from other organizations in the network.

Some organizations simply identify prospective compounding pharmacies and ask them to submit a proposal. A more thorough approach is to require prospective compounding pharmacies to respond to a request for proposal (RFP). Although a formal RFP (and the compounding pharmacy's formal proposal based on the RFP) may not be necessary, the information found in typical RFPs and proposals may be helpful for making a decision about outsourcing.

Contents of RFPs. RFPs often include the following information:

- A description of the demographics of the organization making the RFP (e.g., number of hospitals, bed sizes, typical census).
- A description of the process the organization will use to select the compounding pharmacy.
- The organization's standard terms and conditions for contracting for services or, if available, a sample contract from the organization.
- The names and telephone numbers of individuals in the organization who are involved in the outsourc-

ing decision (the organization's director of pharmacy should be included).
- A description of the specific services required of the compounding pharmacy (e.g., volume, intravenous admixture preparation, automated pharmacy systems, existing intravenous delivery systems and devices) and performance-measurement criteria or targets.
- The dates on which the organization's representatives can inspect the compounding pharmacy's facility, with reasonable notice.
- The number of copies of the proposal to submit.
- The name and address of the individual to whom the proposal is to be delivered.
- Acceptable methods for delivery of the proposal (e.g., e-mail, mail, delivery service, courier).
- A statement that the organization reserves the right to cancel its solicitation for services and reject any and all proposals.
- A deadline date and time for receipt of the proposal.
- The date on which the compounding pharmacy would be expected to initiate services.
- The date by which the selected compounding pharmacy must provide a written contract.
- Other requirements related to the proposal (e.g., that it be in a specific file format, include reference to an RFP number [if any], or be signed by an officer of the firm who is authorized to contract or his or her designee).

Contents of Proposals. RFPs should require prospective compounding pharmacies to submit the following information with their proposals:

- A brief history of the compounding pharmacy, including its mission, vision, and values.
- The location of the compounding pharmacy's offices and other facilities that would provide services to the organization.
- The compounding pharmacy's regular business hours or hours of operation and emergency and after-hours contact information.
- The names, addresses, telephone numbers, and résumés or background information on individuals who will provide the outsourced services.
- Assurance that all pharmacists employed at the compounding facility are licensed as required.
- Evidence of the following documentation regarding the compounding pharmacy:
 - Proof of current liability insurance.
 - Current accreditation or certification certificates, if applicable.
 - State pharmacy licensure and other appropriate licenses.
 - Licensure documents if the compounding pharmacy is registered with FDA as a drug establishment or device manufacturer.
 - Current DEA registration as a manufacturer or wholesaler.
 - Licensure of pharmacists employed and verification that they are in good standing on file and available for review.
 - Registration of pharmacy technicians employed and verification that they are in good standing on file and available for review, if applicable.

- Pharmacist and pharmacy technician notarized statements stating they have never been convicted of a drug-related misdemeanor or felony on file and available for review.
- Standard operating procedures manual on file and available for review.
- Pharmacist training manual on file and available for review.
- Pharmacy technician training manual on file and available for review.
- Policies and procedures for sterility testing on file and available for review.
- Policies and procedures for pyrogen testing on file and available for review, if applicable.
- Examples of batch reports for products being considered for outsourcing.
- Examples of the quality-control reports.
- Stability documents and clinical references, as well as any materials that are used to determine beyond-use dates.
- A history of the results of all accreditation or regulatory surveys conducted of the compounding pharmacy's sites, including copies of significant regulatory actions.
- Proof of professional liability, general liability, and workers' compensation insurance coverage (including the name, address, and telephone number of the insurance company).
- Experience (e.g., years of experience in providing sterile compounding services, total number of clients served, current number of clients).
- A list of the requested services that the compounding pharmacy can provide and the normal terms of service, including but not limited to normal delivery cycles, availability and cost of emergency preparation and delivery, remedies for failure to perform to the contract, specific goods and services to be provided, and the infrastructure available at the compounding pharmacy for electronic ordering.
- A list of the requested sterile compounding services that the compounding pharmacy cannot provide and the reasons for its inability to provide them.
- A copy of a standard or proposed contract.
- A list of all fees and charges, including shipping, handling, and delivery charges, and any fees associated with order changes that would be billed under the contract and the billing methodology for their calculation.
- A billing schedule and a copy of a sample bill for each of the preparations compounded by the compounding pharmacy.
- A description of a routine delivery schedule (e.g., daily by a specified time) and options for nonroutine delivery (e.g., later the same day, after hours, weekends, holidays, during emergencies).
- Examples of reports that the compounding pharmacy will be expected to submit to the organization.
- Information relating to the compounding pharmacy's financial status and stability (e.g., balance sheets and audited financial statements for the past three years, bank references, lists of principal equity owners).
- The process for requesting new preparations from the compounding pharmacy.

- The names, addresses, and telephone numbers of
 - Current clients of a similar size or receiving similar types of compounded preparations, with written references and copies of annual performance-improvement reports, if possible.
 - Reference accounts served within the past two years and the reasons for all, if any, terminations of services.

Additional information to obtain from the prospective compounding pharmacy but not necessarily contained in the proposal may include

- Whether the compounding pharmacy has had product liability lawsuits filed against it for preparations it compounded. If so, the compounding pharmacy should be asked to provide a description of the lawsuits filed, the file date of the lawsuits, and the outcome.
- A description of the compounding pharmacy's formal procedures for conducting recalls and whether there have ever been recalls of any of its compounded preparations. If the compounding pharmacy has ever recalled any of its compounded preparations, it should be asked to provide the dates of recall, a description of the preparations recalled, and the reasons for the recall.
- Information related to the delivery process (especially in the case of severe weather).

Visits to Compounding Pharmacies and Their Clients. Compounding pharmacies should allow the organization's representatives to visit their corporate offices and compounding facilities. The compounding pharmacy should provide ample opportunity for the organization's representatives to confer with the compounding pharmacy's corporate, pharmacy, and compounding staff.

Evaluating Proposals. A decision to outsource sterile compounding services should be collaborative and may involve, as appropriate, the governing board, the chief executive officer (CEO), the chief financial officer (CFO), the chief operating officer (COO), the chief of the medical staff, the chair of the pharmacy and therapeutics (P&T) committee, the director of nursing (DON), the director of pharmacy, legal counsel, and department heads, for example. The organization should scrutinize the following factors when evaluating proposals:

- Services offered versus services requested (including the compounding pharmacy's potential to enhance currently offered sterile compounding services).
- Professional experience (e.g., years of service; number, size, and types of clients; knowledge of the organization's operations).
- Quality management program, specifically as it relates to facility cleaning and validation, staff training, and competency assessment.
- Financial stability (e.g., ability to absorb start-up expenses and to commit the resources needed to initiate service),
- References and reputation.
- Information systems and other technological infrastructure (e.g., the capability to interface with the organization's information and drug delivery systems, such

as infusion pumps or bar-coded medication administration systems).

- Demonstrated commitment to continually integrating technology and knowledge to improve patient safety.
- Education and training of compounding pharmacy's staff (e.g., internal and external continuing-education programs, educational allowances for professional and technical staff).
- The organization's and the compounding pharmacy's policies on specific compounding practices (e.g., references with real-time stability data supporting beyond-use dating, compliance with standards and regulations, use of USP–NF-grade ingredients or FDA-approved products in accordance with the organization's intended use).
- Risk assessment program to ensure that medication errors are not introduced by new or increased outsourced compounding activities and that the medications dispensed are compatible with the client's medication administration devices (e.g., bar-code labeling, smart pumps).
- Knowledge of the regulatory requirements and accreditation standards that the customer must meet and willingness to assist customers in meeting these standards.
- Inventory and supply chain issues (e.g., the organization's and compounding pharmacy's back-order policies).
- Emergency-preparedness implications (e.g., the ability of the organization and the compounding pharmacy to deliver services in the event of a disaster).
- Additional qualities (e.g., high employee morale, confidentiality, creativity, dedication to the community, collaborative spirit).
- Cost aspects of services (e.g., cost-effectiveness, ability to achieve economies of scale).

The compounding pharmacy should, at a minimum, be able to

- Provide assurance that each compounded sterile preparation meets applicable state and federal labeling requirements and is sterile and free of pyrogens and unintended particulate matter, according to professionally established and accepted quality monitoring data.
- If the compounding pharmacy is compounding high-risk preparations, provide documentation of the end-product testing processes used to determine that compounded sterile preparations are sterile and free of pyrogens and unintended particulate matter.
- Deliver appropriate compounded preparations in tamper-resistant packaging and in containers that will maintain proper storage temperature and (when required) protection from light during delivery and storage.
- Provide, upon request, batch records for any compounded sterile preparation.

The organization should assign an evaluation rating to each proposal. Ratings should be weighted appropriately with respect to services, experience, references, and cost. The organization should base its decision to outsource sterile compounding services on its assessment of the compounding facility's ability to meet the organization's needs and fulfill the terms of the contract.

Outsourcing Arrangement. The health care organization and the compounding facility should agree on the outsourcing arrangement that best meets their needs. The contract should clearly describe all aspects of the outsourcing arrangement. The health care organization's pharmacy should

- Ensure that the proper body of the health care organization (e.g., the organization's P&T committee) has developed a formal process to identify which preparations will (and which preparations will not) be prepared by the compounding pharmacy, based on the therapeutic needs of patients and logistical considerations associated with using a compounding pharmacy.
- Establish the components of the medication order or prescription.
- Determine whether patient consent must be obtained for use of preparations compounded outside the health care organization's pharmacy, consistent with state board of pharmacy regulations and prevailing law.
- Ensure that the agreement and the compounding pharmacy facility have been reviewed by all the necessary bodies in the pharmacy's health care organization (e.g., the organization's risk management team, legal counsel, P&T and infection control committees, epidemiology department staff).
- Determine how to handle situations in which a patient presents with a compounded medication that neither the health care organization's pharmacy nor the compounding pharmacy prepares under the existing agreement (e.g., medication in an implantable device, i.v. push medication, i.v. infusion) and that has not been previously considered by the P&T committee. Considerations include what the process will be for
 - Having the P&T committee consider outsourcing the compounding of such medications to a compounding pharmacy.
 - Acquiring such medications from a compounding pharmacy that the health care organization does not have an agreement with and how the associated liability risks will be addressed until the P&T committee decision is obtained regarding such medications.
 - Continuing to acquire such medications if the compounding pharmacy already under contract cannot or will not prepare them and how the associated liability risks will be addressed (e.g., whether the health care organization's pharmacy will negotiate an agreement with another compounding pharmacy that does compound the preparation) until the P&T committee decision is obtained regarding such medications.

Negotiating the Contract. The health care organization should carefully review the proposal and clarify the provisions of the contract. Active participation by the health care organization's risk management and legal counsel is highly recommended. Negotiations can ensure a contract that best meets the needs of the health care organization and the compounding pharmacy. ASHP believes that the health care organization's pharmacist-in-charge (e.g., a pharmacy director) must take complete responsibility for patient outcomes from all medication-related activities performed at or for the

organization's work sites, whether they are carried out by the organization's staff or by off-site contractors. This responsibility should be explicitly stated in all outsourcing contracts.

The signed contract between the parties should at a minimum

- Describe the term length of the agreement and the processes for the compounding pharmacy's billing to the health care organization, including methods of determining the charge for the compounded items, payment terms, and processes for resolution of disputed invoices.
- Contain a confidentiality clause and a Health Insurance Portability and Accountability Act business associate agreement, if applicable.
- Establish the pharmacy's right to inspect the premises of the compounding facility at any time with reasonable notice, including the right to inspect quality-control reports.
- Describe the method of communicating the medication order or prescription from the health care organization's pharmacy to the compounding pharmacy (e.g., telephone, fax, computer transmission, hard copy, electronic DEA form 222).
- Protect the health care organization from liabilities created by errors made by the compounding pharmacy and delineate the obligations of both parties.
- Establish preparation recall procedures that comply with hospital policy mandates and prevailing law should a preparation need to be recalled by the compounding pharmacy.
- Address documentation, regulatory and accreditation compliance, sterile compounding process, and compounded preparation considerations.
- Describe the pertinent situations and processes for the return of compounded preparations to the compounding pharmacy.
- Describe any requirements regarding the submission of quality reports by the compounding pharmacy.
- Describe the procedures for resolving preparation or delivery issues encountered by the organization or the compounding pharmacy.
- Describe the contents of ancillary agreements or addenda to the contract (e.g., the "expectations agreement" between the organization and the compounding pharmacy).

Organizations often find it convenient to outline expectations that are subject to frequent change in an addendum to the contract, because that allows the addendum to be updated rather than the entire contract. If such terms are not included in the contract, the expectation agreement should

- Delineate routine sterile compounding turnaround times (e.g., from receipt of the medication order or prescription by the compounding pharmacy to delivery to the health care organization) and describe acceptable deviations from the agreed-upon schedules (e.g., raw product availability problems, unique end-product testing requirements, compounded preparation stability characteristics, nonroutine and emergency requests).
- Describe the specific drugs provided, documentation flow, delivery methods, security considerations,

and time frames for the provision of controlled substances by the compounding pharmacy.
- Describe any special processes, documentation flow, delivery methods, security considerations, and time frames for the provision of hazardous drugs by the compounding pharmacy.

Signing the Contract. In some organizations the director of pharmacy may be authorized to sign contracts for outsourced services. If this is not the case, the director of pharmacy must be fully involved in negotiating the contract and advising the authorized signers.

Contract Provisions

A contract that meets the needs of the health care organization and of the compounding pharmacy is the foundation for a successful relationship. Contracts should specifically describe the respective responsibilities of the organization and the compounding pharmacy. See the appendix for examples of contract provisions.

Evaluation of Compounding Pharmacy's Performance

The health care organization should evaluate and document the compounding pharmacy's performance and assess the compounding pharmacy's compliance with the terms of the contract. The compounding pharmacy should regularly submit quality reports, and the organization should regularly perform objective and subjective evaluations (e.g., quarterly, annually). Evaluations should address all measurable standards of performance specified in the contract. Evaluations should be multidisciplinary and should involve, for example, the CEO, CFO, COO, DON, and medical staff representatives, as appropriate. An evaluation may include an assessment of how well the compounding pharmacy has

- Improved the quality of patient care.
- Responded to the organization's needs (e.g., invoicing, process adjustment).
- Helped the organization achieve its financial and patient-outcome goals.
- Improved the productivity and performance of pharmacy staff.
- Improved pharmacy processes (e.g., medication dispensing and delivery).
- Reduced and controlled pharmacy costs without compromising patient care.
- Worked and communicated effectively with the organization's staff and resolved problems.

Handling Performance or Quality Issues

The compounding pharmacy should provide the health care organization with information at least quarterly on its compliance with contract requirements and other information needed for the organization's quality-assurance programs. A mechanism should be in place for resolving preparation or delivery issues (e.g., delivery to the wrong location, late deliveries).

Conclusion

These guidelines offer an overview of factors and processes for health care organizations to consider when exploring the outsourcing of pharmacy sterile compounding. Such considerations include an internal needs assessment, a cost analysis, a careful review of prospective compounding pharmacies, and an examination of the potential long-term consequences of outsourcing as well as the short-term outcomes expected during a contract's performance period. The ideas presented can be used for strategic planning, drafting of initial contract provisions, comparing prospective compounding pharmacies, preparing for contract negotiations, or evaluating a compounding pharmacy's performance. These guidelines are intended to address representative outsourcing options and contract agreements and may not be applicable to all situations. Managers of pharmacy and health care organizations should exercise professional judgment about applicability to their own needs and circumstances.

References

1. American Society of Health-System Pharmacists. ASHP guidelines on outsourcing pharmaceutical services. *Am J Health-Syst Pharm.* 1998; 55:1611-7.
2. American Society of Health-System Pharmacists. ASHP guidelines on quality assurance for pharmacy-prepared sterile products. *Am J Health-Syst Pharm.* 2000; 57:1150-69.
3. American Society of Hospital Pharmacists. ASHP guidelines for selecting pharmaceutical manufacturers and suppliers. *Am J Hosp Pharm.* 1991; 48:523-4.
4. General information chapter 797: pharmaceutical compounding—sterile preparations. In: The United States pharmacopeia, 31st rev., and The national formulary, 26th ed. Rockville, MD: United States Pharmacopeial Convention; 2008:319-36.

Suggested Readings

Burruss RA, Carroll NV, Schraa C et al. Outsourcing inpatient IV compounding: expense and medication error implications. *Pharm Pract Manage Q.*1996;16(3):52-9.

Churchill WW. Determining your needs for outsourced compounding and selecting a service provider. *Pharm Purchas Prod.* www.pppmag.com/pp-p-october-2007-issue/outsourced-compounding.html (accessed 2008 Apr 16).

Curtis FR, Stai HC. Contract pharmacy services. In: Brown TR, ed. Handbook of institutional pharmacy practice, 3rd ed. Bethesda, MD: American Society of Hospital Pharmacists; 1992:299-306.

Douglass K, Kastango ES. Consolidation of pharmacy compounding services: an alternative to outsourcing. *Int J Pharm Compound.* 2001; 5:140-4.

Gates DM, Smolarek RT, Stevenson JG. Outsourcing the preparation of parenteral nutrient solutions. *Am J Health-Syst Pharm.* 1996; 53:2176-8.

Kastango ES. Sterile-product preparations: mix or buy? *Int J Pharm Compound.* 2001; 5:59-63.

Kupiec TC, Skinner R, Lanier L. Stability vs. potency testing: the madness is in the method. *Int J Pharm Compound.* 2008; 12 (1):50-3. Letter.

Ponto JA. Outsourcing radiopharmaceutical services. *Am J Health-Syst Pharm.* 1998; 55:2537.

Souhrada L. Contract management. *Hospitals.* 1990; 64(8):66-8.

Wagner M. Basic pitfalls can undermine hospital–service firm relationship. *Mod Healthcare.* 1993; 23(8):32.

Appendix—Contract Provisions

The following are examples of contract provisions that, among others, the organization and a compounding pharmacy might adapt as needed and include in a contract, depending on the scope of services being considered. In addition, a contract would include provisions about the specific compounding services to be provided by the compounding pharmacy. The language in contract provisions should always be adapted to meet the specific needs of the health care organization and to comply with the organization's contracting policies and applicable laws and regulations.

In reviewing the following list of suggested contract provisions, attention should be paid to the fact that listed provisions are not intended and should not be considered all-inclusive and do not constitute legal advice but rather are provided solely to convey general information related to legal issues commonly addressed in contracts for the outsourcing of sterile compounding services. The purpose of enumerating the following possible contract provisions is to provide a general understanding of the types of provisions that may be included in a contract. Because laws vary from jurisdiction to jurisdiction and are subject to varying interpretations, health care organizations considering outsourcing sterile compounding services should consult with professional legal counsel in their relevant jurisdictions regarding the drafting of contracts.

Accreditation and Certification. A contract should include a requirement that services meet or exceed applicable accreditation and certification standards. These include, but are not limited to, the standards (or requirements) of the following organizations.

- The Joint Commission
- American Osteopathic Association
- Center for Medicare and Medicaid Services
- Pharmacy Compounding Accreditation Board

After-Hours Access. This section describes the process and extent of access to off-site compounding pharmacy resources after normal business hours.

Choice of Law. The contract should state that the contract is governed by the laws of the state in which patient care is provided.

Compounding Pharmacy Indemnification. This section describes in detail the indemnities the compounding pharmacy owes the health care organization, such as

Contractor shall indemnify and defend Customer and its Affiliates, and each of their respective officers, directors, trustees, employees, agents, and representatives (collectively, the "Customer Indemnities") and hold them harmless from and against any and all Losses on account of any Claims asserted by a third party in connection with, arising from, or related to (a) any of the

acts or omissions to this Agreement attached hereto, (b) breach of Contractor's representations, (c) injuries to persons, including death, or damage to property caused by Contractor's agents, servants, or employees, or in any way attributable to Contractor's performance and prosecution of this Agreement, and (d) any sexual harassment or other illegal sexual advances upon any of Customer's employees, contractors, agents, or other personnel by any of Contractor's employees, independent contractors, or other personnel.

Compounding Pharmacy Performance Responsibilities. The off-site compounding center's responsibilities and commitments associated with proper federal and state licensure and regulatory requirements for all the preparations it compounds are outlined in this section (e.g., labeling). It further describes the compounding center's responsibilities to operate in accordance with applicable Good Manufacturing Practices, Drug Enforcement Agency (DEA) requirements (as applicable), *United States Pharmacopeia* (*USP*) 797 requirements, and company standard operating procedures.

Compounding Pharmacy Reports. The content and regularity of performance reports that the compounding pharmacy will submit to the organization may be specified.

Confidential Information. This section describes what information is considered confidential and actions that are required to prevent unauthorized distribution of such information. Both parties must agree to safeguard access to computer databases and patient records to ensure that the patient's rights to privacy and confidentiality are protected. Use of the information should be limited solely to purposes specified in the contract.

Customer Responsibilities. This section describes the health-system pharmacy's responsibilities for affirming that it has all required state, local, and federal licenses associated with the receipt of services being provided by the off-site compounding pharmacy. It may also describe the health care organization's responsibilities for determining clinical appropriateness of any compounded preparation it purchases from an off-site compounding pharmacy as well as the procedures to be used to ensure the traceability of compounded preparations.

Extension of Period of Performance. Conditions for extending the period of performance should be included in the contract.

Force Majeure. This section describes when neither party shall be liable for nonperformance or delays related to causes that are beyond one's reasonable control.

Forms. Responsibilities for the design, approval, purchase, and storage of forms may be assigned.

General Provisions. This section outlines a myriad of other contractual items, such as contract assignment, process for adding or changing compounding services, reference to other agreements, and reference to other applicable terms outside of the services agreement.

Hazardous Drug Preparations. Responsibilities for ensuring the safety of the organization's staff and patients during delivery and distribution of hazardous drug preparations may be assigned. Either the organization or the compounding pharmacy should provide a hazardous materials handling program, including staff training, that meets ASHP guidelines and Occupational Safety and Health Administration (OSHA) requirements.

Indemnification. This section describes specific conditions under which both parties will hold each other harmless for, and potentially defend, the actions of the other.

Information Transfer. This section describes the mechanisms by which the organization transfers orders and other information to the compounding pharmacy.

Laws, Rules, and Regulations. Requirements for services to meet or exceed federal, state, and local laws, rules, and regulations may be specified. These include but are not limited to those of FDA, DEA, OSHA, *USP*, and the state board of pharmacy. The compounding pharmacy should maintain (e.g., display, file) the appropriate licenses, permits, and records of equipment maintenance and certification. Any compounding pharmacy required to be licensed as a manufacturer must be so licensed.

Liability Insurance. This section describes the responsibility for maintaining liability insurance coverage. The contract might specify, for example, the specific level of liability insurance coverage that the health care organization and the compounding pharmacy must maintain.

Payment Terms. This section describes the agreed-upon number of days from receipt of an invoice by the health care organization's pharmacy until payment is due to the compounding pharmacy.

Period of Performance. This section specifies the period for which the compounding pharmacy will provide services to the organization.

Pricing. The price of each service the hospital pharmacy is interested in purchasing from the off-site compounding pharmacy along with conditions and methodology for price increases is described in this section. Shipping, handling, and delivery charges for both routine and non-routine deliveries should also be detailed.

Policies and Procedures. This section describes the required written policies and procedures covering the outsourced services, all of which should comply with applicable laws, regulations, and accreditation or certification standards. The contract should specify that the policies and procedures must not conflict with those of the organization.

Record Maintenance. The contract should specify that all pertinent records must be kept for the time required by law and by the organization and describe how, where, and by whom the record will be maintained.

Requirements. This section establishes a mutual understanding of annual purchase volume commitments between the health care organization's pharmacy and the compounding pharmacy.

Staff Education and Training. Responsibilities for required ongoing staff or compounding pharmacy education and training may be specified. For example, there might be an agreement that the compounding pharmacy's staff will participate in some of the organization's education and training programs. In addition, the compounding pharmacy may agree to provide specific training to ensure that all compounding pharmacy and health care organization personnel can perform the duties created by the compounding pharmacy's services.

Successors. The rights of each party in the event that the health care organization or compounding pharmacy merges or transfers its business or assets to a successor should be addressed in a contract.

Term of Agreement. This section communicates the length of time the agreement is in effect between the health care organization and the compounding pharmacy, including renewals.

Termination. This section describes how and when the contract will end or be terminated, including early termination. It should also address any penalties which may be appropriate or when the contract may be ended without penalty.

Developed through the ASHP Council on Pharmacy Management and approved by the ASHP Board of Directors on January 14, 2010.

ASHP gratefully acknowledges the expert panel that authored these guidelines. At the time of writing, members of the expert panel held the following positions. James R. Rinehart, M.S., FASHP, was Director of Pharmacy, and Susan Heckman, Pharm.D., was Pharmacy Sterile Products Manager, BryanLGH Medical Center, Lincoln, NE. Darrell Chan, Pharm.D., was Director of Pharmacy, West Anaheim Medical Center/La Palma Intercommunity Hospital, Anaheim, CA. Michael Cunningham, Pharm.D., was Medication Safety Coordinator, The Health Alliance, Pharmacy Services, Cincinnati, OH. Richard E. Geller, B.S.Pharm., was Pharmacy Manager, Cedars-Sinai Health System, West Hollywood, CA. Gary Grandfield, Pharm.D., M.B.A., was Director of Pharmacy, Central Admixture Pharmacy Services, Santa Fe Springs, CA. Rich Kruzynski, B.S.Pharm., M.B.A., was President, PharMEDium Services, Lake Forest, IL. Terry T. Nishizaki, Pharm.D., M.B.A., FCSHP, was Assistant Manager, Inpatient Pharmacy, UC Davis Medical Center, Sacramento, CA.

The bibliographic citation for this document is as follows: American Society of Health-System Pharmacists. ASHP guidelines on outsourcing sterile compounding services. *Am J Health-Syst Pharm.* 2010; 67:757-65.

Compensation and Reimbursement

Revenue Cycle Compliance and Management (1205)
Source: Council on Pharmacy Management
To encourage pharmacists to serve as leaders in the development and implementation of strategies to optimize medication-related revenue cycle compliance, which includes billing, finance, and prior authorization, for the health care enterprise; further,

To advocate for the development of consistent billing and reimbursement policies and practices by both government and private payers; further,

To advocate that information technology (IT) vendors enhance the capacity and capability of IT systems to support and facilitate medication-related billing and audit functions; further,

To investigate and publish best practices in medication-related revenue cycle compliance and management.

This policy supersedes ASHP policy 9902.

Payment Authorization and Verification Processes (1206)
Source: Council on Pharmacy Management
To advocate that public and private payers work together and in collaboration with providers to create standardized and efficient strategies for payment authorization and verification processes, such as local and national coverage determinations, that facilitate communication between patients, providers, and payers prior to therapy; result in timely coverage decisions; and do not disrupt patient care.

Value-Based Purchasing (1209)
Source: Council on Pharmacy Management
To support value-based purchasing reimbursement models when they are appropriately structured to improve health care quality, patient satisfaction, and clinical outcomes, and encourage medication error reporting and quality improvement; further,

To encourage pharmacists to actively lead in the design and interdisciplinary implementation of medication-related value-based purchasing initiatives.

This policy supersedes ASHP policy 0708.

Reimbursement for Unlabeled Uses of FDA-Approved Drug Products (0206)
Source: Council on Administrative Affairs
To support third-party reimbursement for FDA-approved drug products appropriately prescribed for unlabeled uses.

This policy was reviewed in 2011 by the Council on Pharmacy Management and by the Board of Directors and was found to still be appropriate.

Product Reimbursement and Pharmacist Compensation (0207)
Source: Council on Administrative Affairs
To pursue, in collaboration with public and private payers, the development of improved methods of reimbursing pharmacies for the cost of drug products dispensed and associated overhead; further,

To educate pharmacists about those methods; further,

To pursue, with federal and state health-benefit programs and other third-party payers, the development of a standard mechanism for compensation of pharmacists for patient care services and compounding and dispensing services; further,

To pursue changes in federal, state, and third-party payment programs to (1) define pharmacists as providers of patient care and (2) issue provider numbers to pharmacists that allow them to bill for patient care services; further,

To educate and assist pharmacists in their efforts to attain provider status and receive compensation for patient care services.

This policy was reviewed in 2006 by the Council on Pharmacy Management and by the Board of Directors and was found to still be appropriate.

Human Resources

Financial Management Skills (1207)

Source: Council on Pharmacy Management

To foster the systematic and ongoing development of management skills for health-system pharmacists in the areas of (1) health-system economics, (2) business plan development, (3) financial analysis, (4) metrics for clinical and distributive services, (5) pharmacoeconomic analysis, (6) diversified pharmacy services, (7) compensation for pharmacists' patient-care services, and (8) revenue cycle compliance and management; further,

To encourage colleges of pharmacy to incorporate these management areas in course work and experiential education; further,

To encourage financial management skills development in pharmacy residency training programs and new practitioner orientation.

This policy supersedes ASHP policy 0508.

Board Certification for Pharmacists (1225)

Source: Section of Clinical Specialists and Scientists

To support the principle that pharmacists who practice where a pharmacy specialty has been formally recognized by the profession should become board certified in the appropriate specialty area; further,

To recognize the Board of Pharmacy Specialties (BPS) as an appropriate organization through which specialties are formally recognized and specialty pharmacy certification should occur; further,

To advocate prioritization for recognition of new specialties in those areas where sufficient numbers of postgraduate year two residency training programs are established and where adequate numbers of pharmacists are completing accredited training programs to prepare them to practice in the specialty area; further,

To advocate for standardization of credentialing eligibility and recertification requirements to include consistent requirements for advanced postgraduate residency training; further,

To promote a future vision encouraging accredited training as an eventual prerequisite for board certification; further,

To encourage BPS to be sensitive to the needs of current practitioners as prerequisites evolve; further,

To actively encourage and support the development of effective training and recertification programs that prepare specialists for certification examination and ensure the maintenance of core competencies in their area of specialization.

Professional Socialization (1113)

Source: Council on Education and Workforce Development

To encourage pharmacists to serve as mentors to students, residents, and colleagues in a manner that fosters the adoption of: (1) high professional standards of pharmacy practice, (2) high personal standards of integrity and competence, (3) a commitment to serve humanity, (4) analytical thinking and ethical reasoning, (5) a commitment to continuing professional development, and (6) personal leadership skills.

This policy supersedes ASHP policy 0110.

Minimum Hiring Standards for Pharmacy Technicians (1015)

Source: Council on Education and Workforce Development

To encourage employers to hire pharmacy technicians who have successfully completed an ASHP-accredited pharmacy technician training program and are certified by the Pharmacy Technician Certification Board (PTCB); further,

To support employment practices that would permit hiring of pharmacy technician trainees only if those individuals (1) are required to both successfully complete an ASHP-accredited pharmacy technician training program and successfully complete PTCB certification within 24 months of employment, and (2) are limited to positions with lesser responsibilities until they successfully complete such training and certification; further,

To encourage employers to require ongoing PTCB certification as a condition of continued employment; further,

To encourage expansion of ASHP-accredited pharmacy technician training programs.

Credentialing and Privileging by Regulators, Payers, and Providers for Collaborative Drug Therapy Management (0905)

Source: Council on Public Policy

To advocate expansion of collaborative drug therapy management (CDTM) practices in which the prescriber and the licensed pharmacist agree upon the conditions under which the pharmacist initiates, monitors, and adjusts a patient's drug therapy; further,

To acknowledge that as a step toward the goal of universal recognition of and payment for pharmacist CDTM services, public or private third-party payers may require licensed pharmacists to demonstrate their competence to provide CDTM, before the payers authorize them to engage in or be paid for such clinical services; further,

To support (1) the development (as a professional initiative by pharmacist associations rather than as a government activity) of national standards for determining a pharmacist's competence to provide CDTM and (2) the appropriate use of these standards by clinical privileging systems, government authorities, and public or third-party payers; further,

To support the use of clinical privileging by hospitals and health systems to assess a licensed pharmacist's competence to engage in CDTM within the hospital or health system; further,

To advocate that state boards of pharmacy apply the principles of continuous quality improvement in assessing the quality, safety, and outcomes of CDTM.

(*Note: Privileging* is the process by which an oversight body of a health care organization or other appropriate provider body, having reviewed an individual health care provider's credentials and performance and found them satisfactory, authorizes that individual to perform a specific scope of patient care services within that setting.)

This policy supersedes ASHP policy 0318.

Intimidating or Disruptive Behaviors (0919)

Source: Council on Pharmacy Management

To affirm the professional responsibility of the pharmacist to ensure patient safety by communicating with other health care personnel to clarify and improve medication management; further,

To advocate that hospitals and health systems adopt zero-tolerance policies for intimidating or disruptive behaviors; further,

To encourage hospitals and health systems to develop and implement education and training programs for all health care personnel to encourage effective communication and discourage intimidating or disruptive behaviors; further,

To encourage colleges of pharmacy and residency training programs to incorporate training in communications and managing intimidating or disruptive behaviors; further,

To collaborate with other organizations to advocate codes of conduct that minimize intimidating or disruptive behavior in hospitals and health systems.

Education, Prevention, and Enforcement Concerning Workplace Violence (0810)

Source: Council on Public Policy

To advocate that federal, state, and local governments recognize the risks and consequences of workplace violence in the pharmacy community and enact appropriate criminal penalties; further,

To collaborate with federal, state, and local law enforcement and other government authorities on methods for early detection and prevention of workplace violence; further,

To encourage all workplace environments to develop and implement a policy for pharmacy personnel that (1) educates about prevention and deterrence of workplace violence, (2) identifies escalating situations that can lead to violence and instructs employees on protection and self-defense, and (3) provides continued support and care to heal personnel who were directly or indirectly involved in an incident of workplace violence; further,

To encourage the health care community to develop and maintain a communication network to share information about incidents of potential and real workplace violence.

Appropriate Staffing Levels (0812)

Source: Council on Public Policy

To advocate that pharmacists at each practice site base the site's pharmacist and technician staffing levels on patient safety considerations, taking into account factors such as (1) acuity of care, (2) breadth of services, (3) historical safety data, and (4) results of research on the relationship between staffing patterns and patient safety; further,

To advocate that regulatory bodies not mandate specific, uniform pharmacy personnel ratios but rather ensure that site-specific staffing levels optimize patient safety; further,

To encourage additional research on the relationship between pharmacy staffing patterns and patient safety.

This policy supersedes ASHP policy 0717.

Image of and Career Opportunities for Hospital and Health-System Pharmacists (0703)

Source: Council on Education and Workforce Development

To sustain and enhance the public information program promoting the professional image of hospital and health-system pharmacists to the general public, public policymakers, pay-

ers, other health care professionals, and hospital and health-system decision-makers; further,

To provide ASHP informational and recruitment materials identifying opportunities for pharmacy careers in hospitals and health systems.

This policy supersedes ASHP policy 0214.

Influenza Vaccination Requirements to Advance Patient Safety and Public Health (0615)

Source: Council on Professional Affairs

To advocate that hospitals and health systems require health care workers to receive an annual influenza vaccination except when (1) it is contraindicated, or (2) the worker has religious objections, or (3) the worker signs an informed declination; further,

To encourage all hospital and health-system pharmacy personnel to be vaccinated against influenza; further,

To encourage hospital and health-system pharmacists to take a lead role in developing and implementing policies and procedures for vaccinating health care workers and in providing education on the patient safety benefits of annual influenza vaccination; further,

To work with the federal government and others to improve the vaccine development and supply system in order to ensure a consistent and adequate supply of influenza virus vaccine.

This policy was reviewed in 2010 by the Council on Pharmacy Practice and by the Board of Directors and was found to still be appropriate.

Cultural Diversity Among Health Care Providers (0409)

Source: Council on Educational Affairs

To foster awareness of the cultural diversity of health care providers; further,

To foster recognition of the impact that cultural diversity of health care providers may have on the medication-use process; further,

To develop the cultural competencies of pharmacy practitioners, technicians, students, and educators.

This policy was reviewed in 2008 by the Council on Education and Workforce Development and by the Board of Directors and was found to still be appropriate.

Staffing for Safe and Effective Patient Care (0201)

Source: Council on Administrative Affairs

To encourage pharmacy managers to work in collaboration with physicians, nurses, health-system administrators, and others to outline key pharmacist services that are essential to safe and effective patient care; further,

To encourage pharmacy managers to be innovative in their approach and to factor into their thinking legal requirements, accreditation standards, professional standards of practice, and the resources and technology available in individual settings; further,

To support the following principles:

- Sufficient qualified staff must exist to ensure safe and effective patient care;
- During periods of staff shortages, pharmacists must exert leadership in directing resources to services that are the most essential to safe and effective patient care;
- Within their own organizations, pharmacists should develop contingency plans to be implemented in the

event of insufficient staff—actions that will preserve services that are the most essential to safe and effective patient care and will, as necessary, curtail other services; and

- Among the essential services for safe and effective patient care is pharmacist review of new medication orders before the administration of first doses; in settings where patient acuity requires that reviews of new medication orders be conducted at any hour and similar medication-use decisions be made at any hour, there must be 24-hour access to a pharmacist.

This policy was reviewed in 2011 by the Council on Pharmacy Management and by the Board of Directors and was found to still be appropriate.

Image of and Career Opportunities for Pharmacy Technicians (0211)
Source: Council on Educational Affairs
To promote the image of pharmacy technicians as valuable contributors to health care delivery; further,

To develop and disseminate information about career opportunities that enhance the recruitment and retention of qualified pharmacy technicians.

This policy was reviewed in 2011 by the Council on Education and Workforce Development and by the Board of Directors and was found to still be appropriate.

Pharmacist Recruitment and Retention (0218)
Source: Council on Legal and Public Affairs
To support federal and state incentive programs for new pharmacy graduates to practice in underserved areas; further,

To provide information and educational programming on strategies used by employers for successful recruitment and retention of pharmacists and pharmacy technicians; further,

To conduct regular surveys on trends in the health-system pharmacy work force, including retention rates for pharmacists and pharmacy technicians.

This policy was reviewed in 2011 by the Council on Public Policy and by the Board of Directors and was found to still be appropriate.

Professional Development as a Retention Tool (0112)
Source: Council on Educational Affairs
To recognize that pharmacy department staff development is an essential component of staff recruitment and retention as well as quality of work life; further,

To recognize that staff development encompasses more than formal inservice or external programs and includes informal learning among colleagues, mentoring, and other types of learning; further,

To strongly encourage pharmacy directors and health-system administrators to support staff development programs as an important benefit that aids in recruiting and retaining qualified practitioners; further,

To assist pharmacy directors with staff development initiatives by providing a variety of educational programs, services, and resource materials.

This policy was reviewed in 2010 by the Council on Education and Workforce Development and by the Board of Directors and was found to still be appropriate.

Pharmacist Credentialing (0006)
Source: Council on Educational Affairs
To support the position that credentialing is a voluntary professional activity distinct and separate from the licensing process; further,

To endorse the goals and the standards-based approach to credentialing being pursued by the Council on Credentialing in Pharmacy (CCP); further,

To support the position that all widely accepted post-licensure pharmacy credentialing programs must meet quality standards that are being established by CCP.

This policy was reviewed in 2009 by the Council on Education and Workforce Development and by the Board of Directors and was found to still be appropriate.

Drug Testing (9103)
Source: Council on Legal and Public Affairs
To recognize the use of pre-employment drug testing or drug testing for cause during employment based on defined criteria and with appropriate validation procedures; further,

To support employer-sponsored drug programs that include a policy and process that promote the recovery of impaired individuals.

This policy was reviewed in 2011 by the Council on Public Policy and by the Board of Directors and was found to still be appropriate.

Employee Testing (9108)
Source: Council on Legal and Public Affairs
To oppose the use of truth-verification testing such as polygraphs as routine employment practices because of the possible interference with the rights of individuals; further,

To recognize the limited use of such testing during employment where such testing may protect the rights of individuals against false witness.

This policy was reviewed in 2011 by the Council on Public Policy and by the Board of Directors and was found to still be appropriate.

ASHP Guidelines on the Recruitment, Selection, and Retention of Pharmacy Personnel

Purpose

These guidelines are intended to assist pharmacy managers in the recruitment, selection, and retention of qualified employees. The pharmacy manager working in an organized health care system will usually have to work with the system's human resources department and within the framework of the specific recruitment, selection, and hiring policies of the organization.

Recruitment

Position Descriptions. Well-developed job descriptions are extremely important in addressing many personnel issues. They are often used to establish salary ranges, define performance expectations, and write performance evaluations, but they can also be crucial tools in a successful recruitment effort.[1] The position description should contain detailed information on the knowledge, skills, experience, and abilities that an acceptable candidate should possess. The following information may be included in a position description:

- Position title and position control number (if applicable),
- Duties, essential job functions, and responsibilities of the position,
- Education, training, experience, and licensure required,
- Knowledge, skills, and abilities required to perform assigned duties,
- Reporting relationships,
- Pay grade and salary range (optional),
- Education and training required to maintain competence, and
- Other specifications of the position that may be required to meet legal requirements (e.g., the Americans with Disabilities Act) or the objectives of the organization (e.g., residency or certification requirements).

[*Note:* A variety of sample job descriptions can be found in Section 7.3 of the *Pharmacy Management Toolkit: Tools of the Trade for Pharmacy Managers and Directors* (CD-ROM) and in module 1 of *Competence Assessment Tools for Health-System Pharmacies* (online and print versions), both available from ASHP.]

A revised position description should be reviewed with staff members currently in that position and with the supervisor of that position. In many workplaces, human resources departments maintain a file of position descriptions and may require approval of all position descriptions in the organization. Procedures specific to the workplace should be followed. Staff with legal expertise should review revised position descriptions to determine compliance with organizational and legal requirements.

Recruitment Sources. Recruitment processes will depend on the type of position being filled. Strategies for filling a support staff position may not be appropriate when searching for a management candidate and vice versa. A recruitment plan

should be developed for each position being filled. This plan should incorporate strategies that have worked in the past while allowing for innovative ideas. Organizations that recruit frequently or have very limited candidate pools should consider a continuous recruitment plan so that a list of prospective candidates is available even before an opening occurs.

Recruitment of individuals from within the department or the organization (e.g., from another department) creates internal growth opportunities and may result in greater employee retention and staff loyalty. Internal recruitment may also be less disruptive and expensive. To facilitate internal recruitment, notice of a vacant position can be posted within the organization before the information is made available to outsiders. Posting can be accomplished by various means, including memoranda, e-mail, voice mail, newsletters, announcements at staff meetings, and bulletin boards.

Recruitment of outside candidates expands the number of potential candidates and the experience available to the organization. It brings in new talent and discourages a reliance on seniority as the primary basis for promotion. Budgetary constraints and the urgency to fill a position may affect the recruitment method selected for external candidates. When recruitment of individuals outside the organization becomes necessary, the following methods should be considered:

- Advertisements in professional journals, newspapers, state professional society newsletters, and electronic bulletin boards,
- Personnel placement services provided by national or state professional societies,
- Oral and written recommendations from colleagues. Some organizations offer a "finder's fee" for hires that result from an employee referral,
- Personal discussion or correspondence with potential candidates,
- Recruitment visits to colleges of pharmacy or to facilities that conduct technician-training programs,
- Professional recruiting firms, which typically charge the organization a percentage of the position's annual salary. In addition, recruitment advertising companies offer access to a list of job seekers for a fee,
- Familiarizing students with the organization by offering summer jobs or participating in college of pharmacy experiential rotations,
- Tuition assistance programs for students in exchange for future work commitments,
- A "prospect list" of individuals applying for previous job openings, which can often be supplied by the human resources department,
- Internet-job-site postings,
- Community job fairs and local or state welfare-to-work programs, and
- Organization-sponsored events such as continuing-education sessions, award presentations, or community outreach programs.

The ability to recruit qualified candidates will depend on a multitude of factors, including the financial stability and

location of the organization, the area's cost of living, the organization's compensation program (including salary, fringe benefits, and raise structure), the position's schedule and reporting structure, opportunities for professional growth and advancement, and the reputation and scope of pharmaceutical services offered. Only some of these factors are within the pharmacy manager's control.

Preinterview Information. The applicant's correspondence, resumé or curriculum vitae, letters of recommendation, academic records, and completed application form (if any) should be carefully evaluated on the basis of the position description to determine the suitability of the candidate for an interview.

There are certain legal restrictions on the type of information that may be requested from candidates on an application form. In general, an application form may request only information that relates directly to the evaluation of the applicant's ability to perform the job for which he or she is applying. If an application form different from that of the organization is used, it is advisable to have the human resources and legal departments review it before distribution to potential candidates.

Selection

Initial Screening Interview. An initial screening interview may be necessary if several qualified candidates have been identified. The screening interview is generally a brief interview conducted by the human resources department or the direct supervisor for the position; it offers a quick assessment of the suitability of the candidate for the position. This interview is often conducted by telephone, especially if the candidate lives far away. The screening interview should be documented and included in the applicant's file.

The Interview Process. A successful interview process is one that matches the best available candidate with a specific position. The process should allow the interviewers to predict the future performance of candidates as accurately as possible. One style of interview is the individual interview—one interviewer and one interviewee. Individual interviews offer the advantages of simplicity, ease of scheduling, and consistency of perspective. Because they are less intimidating to the candidate than group interviews, individual interviews may allow the interviewer to more accurately evaluate the applicant and provide the applicant with more opportunities to ask questions. The disadvantage of an individual interview is that it does not allow for multiple viewpoints and therefore increases the chance that something will be overlooked.

Another style, team interviewing, involves a group of interviewers. Members of the team may interview the candidate individually and then pool their results or they may interview the candidate as a group. The well-prepared team approach offers multiple perspectives within a standardized evaluation scheme. Its disadvantages are extra time consumed to train the team and conduct interviews and the intimidating effect it may have on candidates. Its advantage is that it incorporates more individuals into the process of analyzing a candidate's qualifications.[2] Team interviews foster the ideal of teamwork, and the involved employees share responsibility for the success or failure of the person hired. They also provide an opportunity to observe the candidate's ability to interact with groups, which may be important if the position will require that type of activity.

The composition of the interview team will depend on the position being filled. The team should include people with a common interest in the outcome of the selection process and people who have been in the organization long enough to share with the applicant some history of the organization and the department.[2]

Characteristics of an effective interview process include the following:

- Prior to the interview, the manager should provide the following to the candidate: information about the health-system institution, department, city, and state (if the applicant is not from the area); an agenda for the interview; the position description; travel directions to the facility; and clarification of expenses that will be incurred or reimbursed.
- The interview should be carefully planned. Consider the availability of those who need to participate in the process and allow adequate time for each event, including a tour of the facility (if needed).
- Interviewers should be well prepared. Preinterview information submitted by the candidate should be distributed to and reviewed by participants in advance of an interview.
- Carefully planned, open-ended questions should be developed in advance. Literature can be consulted to obtain sample questions and questions that are inadvisable or prohibited by law.[2–5] Human resources departments can usually assist in developing questions. (Refer to the appendix for sample questions.)
- To the extent possible, a core group of questions should be asked of all candidates as a means of comparing them. This does not negate the need to investigate different areas for each candidate or to pursue specific questions that surface during the interview.
- Questions should focus on predetermined criteria for the position and the qualifications of the candidates. The goal is to match the best candidate with the vacant position. Questions should focus on past performance, which is often a good indicator of future performance. In addition to questions regarding professional competency, the interview should contain questions that will help determine whether the applicant's attitudes and behaviors will be suitable for the job. Behavior-based selection criteria should be used when possible.
- The interviewer should give the candidate a realistic view of the position, including both favorable and unfavorable information. If the candidate is "oversold" on the position, dissatisfaction may set in when the truth becomes apparent.
- Performance standards and methods used for evaluation should be fully explained, and opportunities for professional growth should be presented.
- A description of employee benefits (e.g., medical insurance, vacation, sick leave, retirement benefits, and holidays) should be provided, either by the manager or by the human resources department.
- The initial salary and salary range for the position should be discussed with the candidate.
- The employee work schedule should be reviewed with the candidate.
- Any additional services or covered expenses the department offers should be outlined. Examples of these services of covered expenses include serving as a

provider of continuing-education programs, travel expenses and time off for continuing-education programs, payment of professional membership fees, and any other benefits that would attract the candidate to the position.

- A tour of the department should be provided.
- If the candidate is not from the area, a tour of the region should be given. Employees of the department or a real estate agency may show a candidate the area and describe the housing market and local schools.
- A follow-up letter is sent to the candidate after the interview to express thanks for interest in the position and the organization and to advise the candidate of the next steps. Timely and well-organized communication between recruiters and candidates is essential to a successful recruitment effort.

Each interview should be documented to keep track of each candidate's responses and to avoid confusion later. Documentation could include interview questions and the candidate's responses or simply a rating of the candidate's responses to specific questions. One person may be designated to collect and collate comments from a group interview. Documentation should occur immediately after the interview.[2] When considering a potential employee, the interviewer should examine punctuality, completeness and accuracy of the resumé or curriculum vitae, communication skills, compensation expectations, skills and knowledge pertinent to the position, and optimal fit with coworkers. The recruitment team should agree in advance on a systematic method for selecting the successful candidate.

Background Verification. The accuracy of information provided by the candidate should be verified by the human resources department. Information may be obtained from the following sources:

- Personal reference letters provided by the applicant,
- Letters of reference provided by previous employers or preceptors (with the applicant's permission),
- State board of pharmacy records,
- Academic records, and
- Legal background searches (when permitted by law and/or by the applicant).

Job Offer. The job offer should be made as quickly as possible after the interview process is completed. Offers should be made to candidates with enthusiasm and should include a deadline for response. Information about candidate selection should be kept confidential until the offer has been accepted. The organization may have specific policies and procedures regarding job offers.[2]

The salary offered to a candidate will usually be competitive with salaries for similar jobs in other organizations in the same market and compatible with the organization's existing salary structure. The market may vary, depending on the position. For example, the market for a pharmacy technician may be local, whereas the market for a pharmacist or pharmacy manager may be regional or national. To preserve equity within the organization, the salary offered to a candidate generally should be consistent with salaries of staff currently in that position. When exceptions are considered, it may become necessary to reassess the compensation of existing staff.

In addition to salary, other commitments made to a candidate should be expressed in writing as part of the formal job offer. These may include the following:

- Date on which employment will begin,
- Supervisor's name and position,
- Position description,
- Performance standards and evaluation system,
- Next performance review date,
- Next compensation increase date,
- Expected work schedule and whether it is subject to change depending on future needs of the department,
- Employee benefits (e.g., insurance, vacation, tuition assistance, sick leave, holidays, and retirement and pension benefits),
- Miscellaneous commitments (e.g., employment bonus, relocation expenses, licensure reimbursement, payment for professional association memberships, and payment for attendance at professional education programs), and
- Potential drug screening (as applicable and in keeping with the law) or employee physical examination and the dates of these activities.

Retention

Staff turnover is costly. The time required to recruit and train new employees has been shown to cause a temporary loss of productivity in the workplace.[6] Staff turnover also has a negative impact on staff morale, which may further reduce productivity and increase turnover. Because individuals have varied needs and wants that may change over time, there is no consistent formula for managers to apply to ensure employee retention.[7-9] Each organization's experience will depend on such factors as the age of employees, the employees' stages in life and career, the organizational structure, the work environment, and the work itself.

Retention may compete with recruitment. For example, creating staff positions with exclusively morning shifts may help retention but hurt recruitment, because fewer candidates are interested in evening shifts. When competing issues arise, pharmacy managers must balance them with the short- and long-term departmental goals and the current demand for employment.

Each organization should identify and assess retention factors by examining the unique aspects of the respective department and organization. For example, a committee broadly representing the organization could be established to determine major retention factors. On the basis of this assessment, a retention plan should be developed. The plan should be reviewed periodically as the needs of employees change; employee surveys may help determine these. The following factors may be considered in analyzing staff retention:

- *Training period.* The department should devote sufficient time and attention to training. Prepare for the new employee's first day by providing him or her with key material in advance and by developing an organized training schedule. Introduce the new employee to key people on the first day and have everyone in the department introduce themselves during the orientation period. Communicate with the new employee regularly during the training period and throughout the first three months.[10] Sufficient training time ensures that the new employee is comfortable in the new work environment and decreases the likelihood that he or she will become frustrated in the new position. Some organizations have developed a structured mentoring program in which a new employee is paired with a senior employee during the training period.

- *Intent to stay.* In several studies, this factor was the best predictor of staff retention.[11] Employees can simply be asked whether they intend to stay. Replies will reflect employee perceptions and should be considered in light of behavior (i.e., the actual turnover rate). Replies also may be influenced by the employees' fear of reprisal.

- *Job satisfaction.* Job satisfaction is a measure of the degree to which individuals like their jobs, their work environment, and relationships with their coworkers. Job satisfaction is important to retention, although the relationship may be direct or indirect. Employees can be asked how satisfied they are with their jobs; there are many survey instruments to assist pharmacy managers and directors in performing this task.[12] Job dissatisfaction does not necessarily lead to staff turnover if other factors are more important to the individual.[13,14]

- *Pay and benefits.* These refer to the remuneration for work performed and the organization's overall benefit plan. Pay may be hourly (a wage) or salaried and may include overtime premiums or bonuses and incentive plans. A benefit plan may include life, medical, dental, disability, and liability insurance; tuition payments; retirement packages; paid organizational membership dues; sick leave; paid vacation; child care; and prescription benefits. The value of specific benefits to an employee will likely change over time. Many organizations offer a benefits plan that gives the employee the option of choosing benefits individually suited to stages in his or her life and career.

- *Performance management.* Performance appraisal is a periodic assessment of an employee's performance throughout the year. Performance appraisal is only one step in a performance management process that includes appraisal, ongoing feedback, goal setting, and development. This process is important to the success of the manager, the employee, and the organization. The goal of performance management is to share information that will help the employee grow, both personally and professionally, and improve the organization. Periodic discussions with the employee are necessary to provide and receive feedback and to avoid surprises at the time of the scheduled performance appraisal.[15] Direct observation and evaluation by supervisors and coworkers can contribute to a meaningful appraisal.

- *Recognition and awards.* Employees often feel that recognition is lacking in the workplace.[7–10] New supervisors or managers should receive training in employee recognition, which includes both formal and informal feedback mechanisms, from structured employee of the month (or year) programs to a simple thank-you given in private or at a department meeting. Managers should identify how employees want to be recognized, through employee surveys or informal discussions.[10] Methods of employee recognition include

 - Thank-you notes,
 - Commendations,
 - Acknowledgment at department meetings,
 - Organization-wide events during National Pharmacy Week,
 - Employee of the month, quarter, or year,
 - Support for attendance at a professional meeting, and
 - Small awards such as movie tickets or gift certificates for coffee.[16]

- *Promotion opportunities.* These may be in the form of formal promotions, career advancement programs, training opportunities, or special project or committee appointments. Flat organizational structures provide fewer formal opportunities for staff promotion. Employees who have made personal investments in the organization—through expanded responsibilities associated with promotion—may have stronger feelings of loyalty that translate into increased retention. Succession planning is a key organizational strategy that ensures the availability of future leaders.

- *Job design.* This refers to the general tasks that an employee performs—the content of the work. Job design includes autonomy, the complexity of tasks, and the support and tools provided to the employee. Studies have found that job content is more highly correlated with retention as the level of an employee's education increases.[11] Motivational theories suggest that the job itself can motivate intrinsically and that success in the job can lead to increased employee satisfaction.

- *Peer relations.* This refers to working relationships with peers, nurses, physicians, and technical support staff. Peer relations are often rated highly as a reason for staying with an organization. It is difficult to predict during the interview process how a candidate's peer relations will develop, but past behaviors and discussion of hypothetical scenarios can provide some insight.

- *Kinship responsibilities.* This refers to family considerations, such as child care needs, spouse-employment transfers, and care for elderly relatives. Child and elder care needs are important for working parents. These considerations are also difficult to screen for during the interview process, and they will change over time. Legal restrictions prevent recruiters from asking some questions; the organization's human resources department should be able to offer advice on this issue.

- *Opportunity.* This refers to other options in the job market. Obviously, tight job markets (a relative lack of alternative positions) increase retention, whereas open job markets (those with many other open positions) may increase turnover. Managers should always be attentive to retaining good employees, but in open job markets they need to be especially attentive.

- *Staff-development opportunities.* This refers to job training, educational opportunities, and tuition reimbursement or other educational and personal growth opportunities for staff. Training and educational opportunities can affect recognition and awards, promotion opportunities, job design, and peer relations, so they can have a big impact on employee retention.

- *Management style.* This refers to the organizational structure and prevalent management style in the organization (e.g., on the spectrum from autocratic to participatory). The accessibility of management staff may be a factor as well as the extent to which staff input is encouraged. Each employee will prefer a particular management style; no one style will work equally well for all employees. Managers must be sensitive to the management styles that are effective for their staff.

- *Employee coaching.* This refers to the manager's mentorship role. Managers should provide feedback to employees regarding performance, teach specific job-related skills, hold formal and informal career discussions with employees, help employees achieve greater

self-awareness, advise employees on how best to prepare for career options, and assist employees in preparing a yearly career-development plan.[10] In addition, it is important that managers recognize and acknowledge the employee's contributions to the health system.

- *Management survey.* This refers to the organization's commitment to identifying opportunities for improving management. Such opportunities can be identified by surveying employees about their manager's performance. The survey should be conducted by each manager's supervisor. Managers should also complete the survey to see how their rating compares with that of their staff. Action plans should be established on the basis of the survey results.[10] Such "360-degree" surveys should be managed with caution, however; they may create animosity and foster unhealthy relationships between management and staff.
- *Physical working conditions.* This refers to the physical characteristics and safety of the workplace, such as space, equipment, noise levels, parking accommodations, and cleanliness.
- *Scheduling.* This refers to opportunities for varied scheduling, vacation time, shift rotation, job sharing, flexible hours, and part-time work.
- *Motivation.* Extrinsic motivators for change (such as salary, promotion, and recognition) can affect behavior, but they cannot change values and attitudes.[17] In the workplace, change occurs most readily when people are motivated by the desire to bring their professional activities in line with their personal and professional values and beliefs. Living vision and value statements offer employees an opportunity to shape an inspiring organizational culture. Although each employee's motivations will be different, some theories of motivation can help managers understand what contributes to job satisfaction. Maslow's[14] hierarchy of needs, for example, states that employees will be happiest when they are working toward self-actualization, which requires that their more basic needs for security, esteem, belonging, and knowledge be satisfied first. Herzberg et al.'s[18] motivation/hygiene theory explains that employees cannot be motivated by the "hygiene" aspects of their work (organization policies, supervision, salary, peer relations, and working conditions), but that dissatisfaction with those aspects can interfere with motivating factors (the work itself, responsibility, achievement, recognition, and advancement).
- *Exit interview.* An interview should be scheduled with a director of the department, the human resources department, and the exiting employee. The director should ask in-depth questions to identify why the employee is leaving. The exit interview should explore the employee's opinion of the company, department, his or her direct manager as well as any other issues the employee may have for leaving. Pharmacy managers should validate and share this information with the appropriate management staff to decrease the likelihood that another employee may leave for a similar reason.[14]

References

1. Poremba AC. Determining the department's staffing: writing job descriptions. In: Pharmacy management toolkit: tools of the trade for pharmacy managers and directors [CD-ROM]. Bethesda, MD: American Society of Health-System Pharmacists; 2001.
2. Nimmo CM, ed. Human resources management. ACCRUE level II. Bethesda, MD: American Society of Hospital Pharmacists; 1991.
3. Yate M. Hiring the best. 3rd ed. Holbrook, MA: Adams; 1990.
4. Wilson R. Conducting better job interviews. Hauppauge, NY: Barrons; 1991.
5. Smart B. The smart interviewer. New York: Wiley; 1989.
6. Donovan L. The shortage. *RN.* 1980; 8:21–7.
7. Smith SN, Stewart JE, Grussing PG. Factors influencing the rate of job turnover among hospital pharmacists. *Am J Hosp Pharm.* 1986; 43:1936–41.
8. Porter LW, Stears RM. Organizational work and personal factors in employee turnover and absenteeism. *Psychol Bull.* 1973; 80:151–76.
9. Loveridge CE. Contingency theory: explaining staff nurse retention. *J Nurs Adm.* 1988; 18:22–5.
10. Branham FL. Keeping the people who keep you in business. 1st ed. New York: Amacon; 2001.
11. Cavanagh SJ. Predictions of nursing staff turnover. *J Adv Nurs.* 1990; 15:373–80.
12. Section 7.5: employee satisfaction. In: Pharmacy management toolkit: tools of the trade for pharmacy managers and directors [CD-ROM]. Bethesda, MD: American Society of Health-System Pharmacists; 2001.
13. Johns G. Organizational behavior: understanding life at work. Glenview, IL: Scott, Foresman; 1983.
14. Maslow AH. Motivation and personality. 2nd ed. New York: Harper & Rowe; 1970.
15. Chrymko MM. How to do a performance appraisal. *Am J Hosp Pharm.* 1991; 48:2600–1.
16. Nelson B. 1001 ways to reward employees. New York: Workman Publishing; 1994.
17. Nimmo CM, Holland RW. The practice change model: an innovative pharmacy-specific approach to motivating staff change. In: Pharmacy management toolkit: tools of the trade for pharmacy managers and directors [CD-ROM]. Bethesda, MD: American Society of Health-System Pharmacists; 2001.
18. Herzberg F, Mausner B, Snyderman BB. The motivation to work. 2nd ed. New York: Wiley; 1959.

Appendix—Sample Questions to Ask of Job Candidates[2]

Questions for Experienced Pharmacists and Technicians

- How did you become interested in pharmacy?
- What skills or traits do you think a pharmacist needs to be successful?
- What is the single greatest contribution you have made in your present (or most recent) position?
- What is something you have recommended or tried in your present (or most recent) position that did not work? Why didn't it?
- How are you evaluated in your present (most recent) job?
- What would your present (most recent) employer say are your strong points? Your weak points?
- Why did you (do you want to) leave your last (present) job?

- Do you prefer working on a team or alone? Why?
- What part of the job did you like the best and least?

Questions for Recent College of Pharmacy Graduates

- What was your most rewarding college experience?
- Why did you want to study pharmacy?
- What would you change about your college experience if you could?
- Do you think your grades accurately reflect your academic achievements?
- What subjects did you like most and least? Why?

General Questions

- What qualities are you looking for in your next supervisor?
- What supervisory style do you think you have?
- What are your long-term career goals?
- How does this position fit in with your long-term career goals?
- What are you looking for in your next position that has been lacking in previous positions?

Subjects About Which You May Not Ask

- Race,
- National origin,
- Religion,

- Age,
- Marital or family status,
- Child care arrangements or childbearing plans,
- Arrest records (although convictions related to drug use would be appropriate),
- Credit rating and other financial information (unless the position involves financial responsibilities),
- Military discharge status, unless resulting from a military conviction, and
- General information that would point out handicaps or health problems unrelated to job performance.

Approved by the ASHP Board of Directors, September 27, 2002. Revised by the ASHP Council on Administrative Affairs. Supersedes the ASHP Technical Assistance Bulletin on the Recruitment, Selection, and Retention of Pharmacy Personnel dated April 27, 1994.

The bibliographic citation for this document is as follows: American Society of Health-System Pharmacists. ASHP guidelines on the recruitment, selection, and retention of pharmacy personnel. *Am J Health-Syst Pharm.* 2003; 60:587–93.

ASHP Long-Range Vision for the Pharmacy Work Force in Hospitals and Health Systems

Ensuring the Best Use of Medicines in Hospitals and Health Systems

Executive Summary

The ASHP Vision for the Pharmacy Workforce in Hospitals and Health Systems expresses a vision for building the workforce capacity of pharmacy departments in hospitals and health systems to meet the growing challenges related to optimizing the use of medicines in those settings.

Challenges

The scientific knowledge about drugs and the professional knowledge about pharmacy service delivery expand continuously. Many patients in hospitals and health systems in the United States have serious, complex, and urgent health problems that require advanced diagnostic evaluations, intricate medical procedures, and aggressive care. Medication use in hospitals and health systems is a prominent therapy for virtually all patients, and it is inherently complex and dangerous.

Pharmacy Functions

The objective of the overall pharmacy function in hospitals and health systems is to support sound patient care through the safe, evidence-based, and cost-beneficial use of medicines. Hospitals and health systems—in part because of demands by the government and external quality bodies—will require that pharmacists and pharmacy technicians possess and maintain sound credentials attesting to their competence to handle the tasks assigned to them. The overall pharmacy function in hospitals and health systems includes:

- Reviewing individual patients' medication orders for safety and effectiveness and taking corrective action as indicated.
- Collaboratively managing medication therapy for individual patients.
- Educating patients and caregivers about medications and their use.
- Leading continuous improvements in the medication-use process.
- Leading the interdisciplinary and collaborative development of medication-use policies and procedures.
- Acquiring quality drug products from trusted supply sources.
- Preparing medications in the doses and dosage forms needed.
- Distribution of medications to inpatients and outpatients.
- Ensuring the availability of quality drug information.
- Influencing drug administration policies, procedures, and the use of related devices.

- Conducting quality reviews of medication utilization in the hospital's or health system's population of patients and seeking improvements where indicated.
- Leading and influencing decisions about medication-related informatics, other technology (including drug administration devices), and automated processes in medication use.

The most effective pharmacy departments coordinate and integrate these functions into a cohesive whole, bringing together a team of pharmacists, pharmacy technicians, and others that have differentiated roles in management, patient care, medication-use policy, quality improvement, informatics, and drug product preparation and distribution.

Vision for Teamwork. Overall medication-use processes (which include prescribing, order review, dispensing, administration, monitoring, and adjusting therapy based on patient response) will be carried out by interdisciplinary teams, and pharmacists will continue to be the only health professionals with the depth and breadth of knowledge about, and the interest to focus their full time leadership attention on, the use of medicines.

Vision for Technology. Hospitals and health systems will continue to be technology-intensive environments. Shortages of pharmacists and pharmacy technicians qualified for work in hospitals and health systems are expected to be chronic. Technology will not eliminate these shortages. The use of technology will remain incomplete and nonstandardized (an important safety issue in itself) for some time.

Vision for Pharmacists' Responsibilities. Increasingly, pharmacists will apply their time to direct, interdisciplinary patient care to ensure the best use of medicines by individual patients. A growing number of pharmacists will work in highly specialized therapeutic areas. The expanded use of uniformly educated and certified pharmacy technicians will permit a larger portion of a pharmacy department's pharmacist staff to focus on direct patient care activities.

Credentials

Licensure alone will be insufficient for pharmacy practice in hospitals and health systems.

Vision for Residencies. Hospital and health-system employers will expect all entry-level pharmacists to have completed an ASHP-accredited first-year postgraduate pharmacy residency. First-year residency programs in hospitals and health systems concentrate on developing pharmacists that understand the organizational environment, can work in that environment to provide clinical care to individual patients, are capable of interdisciplinary professional work at both

an organizational and clinical level, understand the internal and external standards of quality that apply, and are adept at measuring and documenting metrics of success to manage quality.

Vision for Specialty Certification. Second-year ASHP-accredited postgraduate residencies will be required for pharmacists caring for highly specialized and complex patients. These programs prepare pharmacists to effectively interface with specialized physicians and nurses and manage pharmacy services and informatics. Pharmacists who provide services in an area in which specialty certification exists will be expected to be certified in that specialty.

Vision for Leadership. All hospital and health-system pharmacists will be required to refresh their credentials continuously and to engage actively in personal continuing professional development. Strong leadership will be required to provide and sustain comprehensive professional vision for pharmacy departments. Pharmacy managers will possess credentials appropriate to the scope of services and the size and complexity of the setting, including, in many cases, advanced graduate degrees in pharmacy or nonpharmacy disciplines. Pharmacy departments will be headed by pharmacists; nonpharmacist managers will handle many tasks that do not require the expertise or judgment of a pharmacist.

Vision for Pharmacy Technicians. Pharmacy technicians eventually will be defined in laws and regulations as those individuals working under a pharmacist's responsibility that (a) have completed an ASHP-accredited pharmacy technician training program, (b) are certified by the Pharmacy Technician Certification Board, and (c) are registered with state boards of pharmacy.

Achieving the Vision

ASHP is assessing what it and others need to do to achieve this vision for the pharmacy workforce in hospitals and health systems. Future programs and advocacy of ASHP will be based on this assessment.

Introduction

Medication use in hospitals and health systems is complex and inherently risky. The American Society of Health-System Pharmacists (ASHP) believes it is inevitable that public policymakers, hospital and health-system administrators, and others will seek to modify the roles and required credentials for the pharmacy work force in those settings to ensure that medication use is safe, effective, and appropriate. ASHP believes the decisions will be best guided by a long-range vision about the pharmacy work force for those settings.

This vision is consistent with the ASHP Vision Statement for Pharmacy Practice in Hospitals and Health Systems,[1] the ASHP Health-System Pharmacy 2015 Initiative,[2] and the future vision of pharmacy practice[3] developed by the Joint Commission of Pharmacy Practitioners. This document serves as

- An expression of ASHP's continuing aim to support the development of competence building, sound credentials, and credentialing and privileging processes for pharmacists and pharmacy technicians in hospitals and health systems,
- A guide for ASHP in its long-term development of policies, education, publications, and activities to help pharmacists and pharmacy technicians develop and maintain the competence and credentials needed to work in hospitals and health systems, and
- An advocacy tool to stimulate public policymakers, external quality standards groups, hospital and health-system trustees and administrators, hospital and health-system pharmacy directors, and leaders in other collaborative health professions to ensure that the pharmacy work force in hospitals and health systems is appropriately competent, has the appropriate credentials, and is appropriately privileged on the basis of credentialing processes.

Hospitals and Health Systems

Hospitals and health systems include individual hospitals, multiple-hospital systems, health maintenance organization clinics, hospital-affiliated predischarge and postdischarge clinics, hospital-based ambulatory care pharmacies, home care services, rehabilitation facilities, skilled-nursing facilities, and assisted-living facilities. Common to all of these settings are the health-system characteristics of (1) an interdependent and interdisciplinary work force, (2) collaboratively developed and evidence-based medication-use processes, (3) a governance structure that is accountable for safe, effective, and appropriate patient care, (4) multiple levels of care with continuity of care among these levels, and (5) an ongoing assessment of performance using externally established quality standards and accreditation requirements.

The Overall Pharmacy Function in Hospitals and Health Systems. Pharmacists and pharmacy departments bear professional and legal responsibility for all medication-use activities in hospitals and health systems. That responsibility is abundantly clear in professional standards, statutes, regulations, court precedents, and external quality standards. The overall pharmacy function in hospitals and health systems will continue to include

- Leading the interdisciplinary and collaborative development of medication-use policies and procedures within the setting, including pharmacy and therapeutics committee policies and therapeutic protocols,
- Reviewing patients' medication orders for safety and effectiveness,
- Collaboratively managing medication therapy for individual patients,
- Educating patients and caregivers about medications and their use,
- Leading continuous improvements in the quality of medication-use processes,
- Acquiring quality drug products from trusted supply sources,

- Preparing medications in the doses and dosage forms needed,
- Distributing medications to inpatients and outpatients,
- Integrating the work of staff in clinical and other functions to ensure coordinated attention to safe, effective, and appropriate care,
- Functioning as a gatekeeper with respect to the quality of drug information available to caregivers throughout the setting as a means to support up-to-date, evidence-based care,
- Influencing drug administration policies and procedures and the use of related devices,
- Conducting quality reviews of medication utilization in the hospital or health system's population of patients, and
- Leading and influencing decisions about medication-related informatics, other technology (including drug administration devices), drug administration, and automated medication-use processes.

Differentiation and Teamwork. In hospitals and health systems, the overall pharmacy function will be accomplished via a differentiated pharmacy work force that includes managers, pharmacists practicing in direct inpatient and outpatient clinical roles, pharmacists and pharmacy technicians in inpatient and outpatient drug preparation and logistical distribution, pharmacists leading informatics and other technology activities, pharmacy technicians, business and operations managers, and other personnel, including informatics assistants, secretarial and administrative assistants, clerks, stock-handling personnel, and couriers. Differentiation in the pharmacy work force will increase with the size and scope of hospitals and health systems. Differentiation will be most pronounced in academic health centers where there are additional missions of education and research. Overall medication-use processes will be conducted by interdisciplinary teams. Pharmacists will continue to be the only health professionals with the depth and breadth of knowledge about—and the interest to focus their full-time leadership attention on—the safe, effective, and appropriate use of medicines.

Technology. Hospitals and health systems will continue to be technology-intensive environments. Many of the technologies, including those for automated medication delivery, pharmaceutical compounding, pharmaceutical packaging and labeling, automated distribution and vending, bedside verification, drug administration (e.g., infusion pumps), electronic drug information, electronic communications, and electronic patient records, will influence medication use. Automation and information technology will be increasingly integrated into medication-use processes. Pharmacists with technology and informatics expertise will influence the choice and use of technologies to ensure patient safety, effectiveness of care, and efficiency.[4] As new technologies evolve, pharmacists will ensure that these preserve and enhance medication-use safety, effectiveness, and appropriateness.

Leadership. Ongoing pharmacy leadership and management will be required to provide and sustain a comprehensive professional vision and evidence-based medication use via an integrated and interdisciplinary work force and to apply limited resources to activities that will be the most effective. Leadership and management will be required

at all levels, including clinical practice, to ensure that the overall pharmacy function successfully influences the care of patients. In successful pharmacy departments, middle management positions will exist, and qualified personnel at all levels will be mentored for leadership and advanced-level positions. Hospitals and health systems in which this does not occur will be vulnerable to lapses in quality when inevitable turnover occurs in top management positions. Therefore, ongoing investment in succession planning will be essential. In large hospitals and multiple-facility systems, some pharmacists will be corporate-level directors (e.g., vice presidents). Some will have responsibility for departments in addition to pharmacy.

Pharmacies and pharmacy departments in hospitals and health systems will continue to be headed by pharmacists. In most cases, major positions below the department head level are currently occupied by pharmacists. However, it is likely that nonpharmacists will increasingly be employed below the department head level to handle various tasks that do not require the expertise or judgment of a pharmacist. These tasks may include secondary management, finance, personnel administration, quality assurance, informatics and technology, and supply and distribution logistics. Nonpharmacist positions of these types may be more common in large, complex hospitals and health systems where a differentiated work force is more necessary and possible.

Experiential Learning. Hospital and health-system pharmacists and pharmacy technicians will attain their knowledge, skills, and abilities in various ways. All pharmacists and pharmacy technicians will receive on-the-job orientation, training, and experiences that hone their knowledge and skills necessary for specific workplaces. New pharmacy college graduates will continue to be prepared primarily to deliver individual patient care. They will have in-depth knowledge about medications, their pharmacology, and their therapeutic uses. The Accreditation Council for Pharmacy Education's (ACPE's) accreditation standards for doctor of pharmacy degree programs require colleges to include experiential education in community pharmacy, ambulatory care, a hospital or health-system pharmacy, and inpatient or acute care general medicine.[5] These learning experiences are expected primarily to involve direct patient care rather than learning to navigate and fully influence the interdisciplinary and multidepartmental aspects of medication use within hospitals and health systems. Concerns exist about the capacity of hospitals and health systems to accommodate the growing volume of pharmacy students needing this experiential education. Most new graduates entering hospital and health-system practice will continue to require substantial further education in order to fully function in those settings. As a means to achieve that education, they should—at minimum—complete an ASHP-accredited pharmacy residency. Some hospitals and health systems may create mechanisms for existing staff to enroll in such residencies.

Pharmacists' Responsibilities

In hospitals and health systems, all pharmacists will be responsible for error prevention, patient safety, and patient outcomes related to medication therapy. Many will work at various supervisory and management levels in the acquisition, preparation, and dispensing of drug products, operating

facilities and equipment for those activities, ensuring the supply and integrity of drug products, providing evidence-based drug information to other professionals and patients, managing the technology applied to medication use, monitoring the quality of pharmacy services, and conducting medication-use-safety activities. Some pharmacists will be engaged in sterile compounding. Some will influence the selection and management of technology and information systems for medication use. Depending on the role of the hospital and health system in education, some pharmacists will educate and train pharmacy students, residents, and pharmacy technicians. All pharmacists will appropriately balance their roles as employees of the setting and their autonomous public professional obligations on behalf of patients.

Increasingly, and dependent partly on the expanded use of uniformly trained and educated pharmacy technicians certified by the Pharmacy Technician Certification Board (PTCB), pharmacists will apply their time to direct, interdisciplinary, and collaborative drug therapy to ensure that the medication therapy of individual patients is effective, evidence based, safe, and cost-effective.[6] Some pharmacists will work in highly specialized clinical areas. Specialists will train and support generalist pharmacists. To ensure a high level of coordination by all components of the pharmacy function in hospitals and health systems and appropriate medication use and safety, the work of clinical pharmacists will be integrated with other aspects of the overall medication-use process. Depending on the volume of clinical work required, most pharmacists will have some ongoing work assignments and responsibilities in medication distribution. Hospitals and health systems will require that all clinical pharmacists and faculty of colleges of pharmacy working in their facilities be credentialed through the routine processes used for all other pharmacy staff and be managed by the department of pharmacy.

Throughout the work setting, the acquisition of patient medication histories and the provision of discharge medication information to patients and downstream caregivers will be managed by pharmacists. This will facilitate continuity of care, reconciliation of medication regimens, and avoidance of medication-related problems. Pharmacists will ensure that necessary clinical monitoring of laboratory test values occurs pertinent to medication use for individual patients. They will engage in disease prevention activities on behalf of patients. Pharmacists will influence the selection of authoritative, evidence-based drug information that is made available to all caregivers in the workplace. They will engage in interdisciplinary development of systemwide policies, procedures, and therapeutic protocols about medica-tion use. They will engage in medication-related public health activities on behalf of their communities.

Medication-Use Process. Pharmacists will continuously improve and collaboratively redesign medication-use processes to optimize patient safety and improve patients' health-related quality of life. They will ensure that medication-use processes incorporate system characteristics of interdependency, checks, and immediate safety feedback mechanisms. In addition to caring for individual patients, pharmacists will ensure that the outcomes of medication therapy are assessed and managed on both a systemwide and patient population basis.

Interpersonal Skills. Pharmacists in hospitals and health systems will possess exceptional interpersonal skills, work well in interdisciplinary teams, and lead the development of medication-use policies and procedures to meet patients' needs. They will possess competence in caring for and effectively interacting with patients from a variety of cultures. They will engage in behavior and activities that promote the pharmacy profession and will represent the profession in a positive light and promote its goals.

Proliferation of Potent and Complex Medications

The scientific knowledge about drugs and the professional and managerial knowledge about pharmacy service delivery expand continuously. Further, many patients in hospitals and health systems in the United States have serious, complex, and urgent health problems that require advanced diagnostic evaluations, intricate medical procedures, and aggressive care. Even for nonurgent care, medication use in hospitals and health systems is a prominent (or at least adjunct) therapy for virtually all patients, and it is inherently complex and dangerous. The medications used are among the most potent, and many require complex administration procedures. Many of these medications are injectable products that pose both inherent pharmacologic and infection-control challenges and must be handled by individuals in multiple disciplines, some of whom have little education and training about medications. Even more potent and riskier medications are anticipated in the future, and medication use in hospitals and health systems is expected to become even more intense and complex. Medications for patient groups with specific genomic characteristics will evolve.

Public Demand

Medication-use problems (particularly errors) are well documented,[7–25] but the public is not yet sufficiently aware that there is available a professional (the pharmacist) with the expertise and interest to help prevent those problems and better ensure optimum medication therapy in hospitals and health systems.[26–34] However, an increasing public awareness and debate is evolving about medication-use safety and costs, including the cost of preventable errors.[35–44] This will ultimately function as an important driver of public demand that pharmacists and pharmacy technicians in hospitals and health systems be competent to achieve (and manage the achievement of) desired patient outcomes with respect to medication use.

Sound Credentials Required for Pharmacy Personnel in Hospitals and Health Systems

ASHP believes that every pharmacist and pharmacy technician working in hospitals and health systems will be required to possess and maintain sound credentials attesting to their competence. Hospitals and health systems will engage in ongoing systematic assessments of the credentials and experience of all pharmacists and pharmacy technicians.[45,46] Some local policies may, with good reason, allow privileges

for some pharmacists and pharmacy technicians who lack specific formal credentials; some of these practitioners may have well-documented experience and competence. As an ongoing investment in the safety and evidence-based effectiveness of medication use, hospitals and health systems will develop incentives to stimulate pharmacy staff to obtain desired credentials. Mechanisms will exist for acquisition of necessary credentials by entry-level pharmacists and pharmacy technicians and those in practice that aspire to expand their roles.

Residencies. ASHP believes that a variety of sound credentials will exist for pharmacists who practice in hospitals and health systems. ASHP-accredited postgraduate residency training exists to equip entry-level practitioners with the knowledge and skills they need to function safely and effectively and to successfully influence medication-use policies and procedures in their workplaces. First-year ASHP-accredited postgraduate residency programs in hospitals and health systems concentrate on developing pharmacists who (1) understand that organizational environment, (2) can work in that environment to provide clinical care to individual patients, (3) understand the academic health center environment (if the residency is conducted there), (4) are capable of interdisciplinary professional work at both an organizational and clinical level, (5) understand both the internal and external standards of quality that apply, and (6) are adept at measuring and documenting the metrics of success that are necessary for the management of quality in hospitals and health systems.[47-49]

Second-year ASHP-accredited postgraduate residencies are of several types. Some develop pharmacists capable of the care of highly specialized and complex patients, capable of effectively interacting with specialized physicians and nurses and conducting collaborative research. Others focus on hospital and health-system pharmacy management or informatics.[50,51,a]

Individuals enrolled in ASHP-accredited residency programs are licensed pharmacists. Similar to residencies in medicine, pharmacy residencies are intense, structured, "learn-by-doing" experiences that involve close work with preceptors and mentors. Pharmacy residents are fully accountable for the outcomes of their clinical and operational actions. Residencies are not "learn-by-observing" experiences, and they differ from internships, which are intended only to bring learners to a minimal competency for academic graduation or licensure. Among the benefits of residency training is the development of clinical skills and competency for work and leadership in hospitals and health systems. It is conceivable that future medication-use residencies may evolve that enroll pharmacists, physicians, and nurses and are conducted in an interdisciplinary fashion.

Hospital and health-system employers will expect new entry-level pharmacists in hospitals and health systems to have completed an ASHP-accredited first-year postgraduate pharmacy residency. ASHP believes that licensure alone will be insufficient for practice in hospitals and health systems.

Specialty Credentials. For some roles, pharmacists will be required to have completed ASHP-accredited second-year postgraduate pharmacy residencies for specialized clinical activities, informatics, and top management positions. Pharmacists who spend the majority of their time practic-

ing clinical specialties for which there is available certification by the Board of Pharmaceutical Specialties (BPS) or the American Society of Consultant Pharmacists (ASCP) Commission for Certification in Geriatric Pharmacy will be expected to be certified or to be working with appropriate promptness to become certified.[52,b] They will be expected to maintain the certification. Other sound certification credentials may evolve.

Continuous Professional Development. Hospital and health-system administrators, public policymakers, and pharmacists will insist that up-to-date, evidence-based medication use occurs in hospitals and health systems. Effective, evidence-based interdisciplinary care of hospital and health-system patients requires currentness in professional knowledge and skills. Therefore, all pharmacists will be required to refresh their credentials continuously and to engage actively in personal continuing professional development. Professionally motivated pharmacists will seek out some of the updating of their knowledge and skills on their own. In order to sustain pharmacy work force competence, hospitals and health systems will financially support staff development and will allow paid work time for it. The extent to which pharmacists and pharmacy technicians engage in activities to sustain and expand their competence will be a factor in ongoing local assessments of their credentials and their continued employment.

Evolving Credentials. Additional competence-building mechanisms will evolve to educate and train pharmacists for specific tasks in hospitals and health systems, including those involving complex and high-risk services for which in-depth knowledge is necessary. Sound credentials will evolve for those tasks, and pharmacists will be expected to obtain those credentials to do that work. Examples of special certification roles include diabetes education, advanced cardiac life support, emergency department care, handling of biological products and products hazardous to workers, sterile compounding, distribution logistics, informatics, and clinical research.

Current sound credentials specific for pharmacists include the following:

- Doctor of pharmacy degrees awarded by colleges of pharmacy accredited by ACPE. The current entry-level degree awarded by all colleges of pharmacy is the Doctor of Pharmacy degree. Until recently, colleges of pharmacy awarded bachelor of science degrees as the entry-level degree, which also are sound credentials,
- Graduate degrees in pharmacy,
- National Association of Boards of Pharmacy License Examination for state board of pharmacy licensure,
- Certification by BPS,[b]
- Certification by the ASCP Commission for Certification in Geriatric Pharmacy,[b] and
- Graduation from an ASHP-accredited pharmacy residency program.

Parallel with these sound credentials there likely will be purported "credentials" that are based on unsound approaches lacking ensured validity and depth. ASHP supports only sound credentials. In their own quality and liability interests, hospitals and health systems will come to understand that there is a quality spectrum of pharmacy credentials and

will insist on sound credentials for their pharmacy staff. The multiorganizational Council on Credentialing in Pharmacy (CCP) has created guiding principles for sound certification programs in pharmacy.[53]

Additional sound credentials in pharmacy may be recognized in the future, particularly for clinical specialties. BPS now certifies pharmacists in five specialties: pharmacotherapy (plus two "added qualifications" in infectious diseases and cardiology), nuclear pharmacy, nutrition support pharmacy, psychiatric pharmacy practice, and oncology pharmacy practice.[c] More BPS added qualifications may evolve. Hospitals and health systems will require pharmacists working in those areas to attain them. The Department of Veterans Affairs has established a mechanism for credentialing and privileging pharmacists to perform some tasks, including medication prescribing.[54–57] Privileging is defined as

the process by which an oversight body of a health care organization or other appropriate provider body, having reviewed an individual health care provider's credentials and performance and found them satisfactory, authorizes that individual to perform a specific scope of patient care services within that setting.[45]

It is conceivable that legislatures and regulatory bodies may establish additional required pharmacist licenses for specific activities.

Leadership Credentials. All pharmacy managers (whether pharmacists or nonpharmacists) will possess credentials appropriate to the scope of services and the size and complexity of the setting. Some pharmacists, particularly in large and complex settings and multiple-facility organizations, will have corporate-level administrative appointments higher than the department head level. Individuals with that authority will have sufficient management experience to have developed the skills and talents for that role and will possess appropriate advanced credentials, which may include graduation from an ASHP-accredited second-year postgraduate residency in management or advanced graduate degrees in pharmacy or nonpharmacy disciplines. The ASHP Research and Education Foundation has created a Center on Health-System Pharmacy Leadership. It is possible that this may lead to an available certification for pharmacy leaders in hospitals and health systems.

Pharmacy Technicians

In the pharmacy profession and in laws and regulations, pharmacy technicians eventually will be defined as those individuals working under a pharmacist who (1) have completed an ASHP-accredited pharmacy technician training program,[58–60] (2) are certified by PTCB, and (3) are registered with state boards of pharmacy. Other support staff will be employed in pharmacies in hospitals and health systems, but they will not be defined in laws and regulations as pharmacy technicians. All pharmacy technicians will be required to participate in continuing education offered by accredited providers of such continuing education. ACPE conducts a process to accredit such providers.

Role of Technicians. Most pharmacy technicians will be engaged in drug-product acquisition, preparation, dispensing,

and distribution under the physical supervision of pharmacists. Some pharmacy technicians will manage aspects of product acquisition and supply logistics. Some will manage the use of technology and quality assurance activities. Some will supervise other pharmacy technicians. Some will assist pharmacists in collecting and screening routine patient-specific clinical laboratory data and routine screening of clinical monitoring data to identify out-of-range findings that warrant pharmacist attention. Some will manage aspects of informatics.

Technician Credentials. Additional competence-building mechanisms will evolve to educate and train pharmacy technicians for specific tasks in hospitals and health systems, including those involving complex and high-risk services for which in-depth knowledge is necessary. Hospitals and health systems will require pharmacy technicians to obtain those credentials to do that work. Pharmacy technicians will continue to work under the supervision of pharmacists and will not be sanctioned to work independently. Although legislatures and regulatory bodies may establish licenses for pharmacy technicians, these will not be licenses for independent, unsupervised practice. Telepharmacy arrangements may evolve in which a supervising pharmacist may be physically remote from a pharmacy technician.

Sound credentials for pharmacy technicians currently include graduation from an ASHP-accredited pharmacy technician training program and certification by PTCB.

For pharmacy technicians, there also exists a spectrum in the quality of education and training available (some of which is unsound). Hospitals and health systems will be diligent in insisting on sound credentials. All pharmacy technicians will be registered with state boards of pharmacy.

Entry-Level Staff

Some entry-level staff will lack all the competencies and credentials needed to work fully in hospitals and health systems. Employers will require them to build competence and acquire appropriate credentials promptly. The initial work assignments of entry-level staff may be somewhat restricted until completion of the necessary competence building and acquisition of credentials.

Assumptions and Expectations

This vision is based on the following assumptions and expectations:

1. As scientific pharmacologic advances increase, mortality from various diseases will decrease. People will live longer and will have chronic conditions and more temporary acute conditions for which they will increasingly use hospital and health-system services. They will use more medications, necessitating greater numbers of qualified pharmacists and pharmacy technicians.
2. For reasons of quality assurance and compliance with accreditation requirements (such as Joint Commission standards[61]), hospitals and health systems will insist that pharmacists and pharmacy technicians demon-

strate that they are competent to perform the tasks set forth in their job descriptions.

3. Hospitals and health systems will establish systematic and ongoing processes to assess the competence and credentials of pharmacists and pharmacy technicians. Many hospitals and health systems will develop their own tools for assessing employee competence and credentials. Some will use external validation methods, such as BPS certification and graduation from an ASHP-accredited residency.

4. The quality of patient care in hospitals and health systems will be enhanced by pharmacists and pharmacy technicians with appropriate credentials.

5. To ensure safe, effective, and coordinated patient care, clinical and other pharmacy activities in hospitals and health systems will be staffed, conducted, and managed in an integrated fashion.

6. The public will increasingly wish to be able to distinguish pharmacists who are qualified to provide medication therapy management services from those who are not.

7. Governments and quality-standards organizations, such as the Joint Commission, will eventually insist on appropriate credentials for pharmacists and pharmacy technicians in hospitals and health systems.

8. Medicare provider status will evolve for pharmacists with appropriate credentials, enabling payment to hospitals and health systems for their medication therapy management. Medicare payments to hospitals and health system will be contingent on active local credentialing and privileging processes for all major health care workers in hospitals and health systems, including pharmacists.

9. Specialization will increase, and hospitals and health systems will look to sound credentials as indications of pharmacists' specialized competencies.

10. BPS will be urged to develop additional clinical credentialing processes in cooperation with professional associations.

11. In the face of shortages of qualified pharmacists and pharmacy technicians for hospital and health-system work, and in the face of the increasing need for qualified workers, accreditation bodies for hospitals and health systems will become increasingly insistent that the pharmacists and pharmacy technicians in those settings have appropriate credentials.

12. Compared with the chronic shortage of pharmacists across the entire pharmacy profession, the shortage of pharmacists competent to work in hospitals and health systems will continue to be more severe.[62–68]

13. The demographics of the pharmacy work force in hospitals and health systems are changing, and hospital and health-system employers will need to respond resourcefully and creatively to adjust to those changes.[69]

14. State laws and regulations will continue to require that pharmacists be graduates of colleges accredited by ACPE. However, some hospital and health-system employers in the United States will consider hiring graduates of foreign pharmacy schools. A process exists for foreign graduates to achieve a foreign pharmacy graduate equivalency certification.[70] Given that licensure alone will not be sufficient for successful work in hospitals and health systems, and given the advanced credentials needed for hospital and health-

system work, this avenue for recruitment will not likely be very effective for those settings.

15. Graduation from an ASHP-accredited pharmacy residency will become a minimum requirement by employers for pharmacists to work in hospitals and health systems.[d]

16. Graduation from an ASHP-accredited pharmacy technician training program, certification by PTCB, and registration with a state board of pharmacy will become minimum requirements for pharmacy technicians to practice in hospitals and health systems.[d]

17. Greater quality and consistency in the education and training of pharmacy technicians will allow for expanded roles for pharmacy technicians, similar to those seen in U.S. military facilities and to the legal allowances for the work of pharmacy technicians in several European and Nordic countries.

18. The demand for qualified pharmacy technicians with appropriate credentials will increase in the United States. State requirements for the credentials of pharmacy technicians are advancing rapidly.

19. Hospital and health-system pharmacy departments will continue to employ supportive personnel who are not legally defined as pharmacy technicians and are not legally authorized to perform the same functions as pharmacy technicians.

20. Technology will not eliminate pharmacy work-force shortages in hospitals and health systems. Moreover, the use of technology will remain incomplete and non-standardized (an important safety issue in itself) for some time.

21. As health care becomes increasingly collaborative and multidisciplinary, pharmacists' knowledge about medications will continue to be different from and more complete than that of other health care professionals.

Some Implications

Embedded in the following implications are numerous priorities that will influence ASHP's ongoing and long-term actions with respect to the pharmacy work force in hospitals and health systems. Other actions will evolve as well.

- Hospital and health-system trustees, administrators, and human resource, risk-management, and legal departments must be helped to understand that only qualified pharmacists and pharmacy technicians with appropriate credentials must comprise the pharmacy work force in hospitals and health systems.

- Mechanisms must be developed to help hospital and health-system employers readily discern sound pharmacy credentials from unsound ones.[53,71]

- Model local credentialing and privileging processes must be developed and implemented to assist hospitals and health systems in assessing whether pharmacists and pharmacy technicians possess the necessary credentials for the functions assigned to them.

- Colleges of pharmacy and pharmacies in hospitals and health systems must better articulate and integrate their respective roles in preparing graduates for ASHP-accredited pharmacy practice residencies.

- Since patient care in hospitals and health systems is inherently interdisciplinary, the education of pharma-

cists must be conducted in a more interdisciplinary manner.

- Sound credentials are needed for various subdepartment-level activities within hospitals and health systems (e.g., sterile compounding). ASHP and CCP should lead a prompt identification of the primary activities and develop a time-certain call for the profession to develop corresponding training and credentials for those activities.
- Public policymakers must be helped to understand the need for qualified pharmacists and pharmacy technicians within hospitals and health systems and to support mechanisms to educate and train practitioners for those roles.
- In cooperation with professional associations, BPS should expand the credentials for pharmacy practice and the number of pharmacists certified.
- Pharmacy technicians must receive uniform education and training before becoming PTCB certified.
- Pharmacy technicians must be registered with state boards of pharmacy.
- The National Association of Boards of Pharmacy should establish model laws and regulations to support state requirements for uniform education and training for pharmacy technicians and for PTCB certification of all pharmacy technicians.

Definitions

In this document, the following definitions apply, as published in 2006 by CCP.[71]

- *Accreditation:* Process by which a private association, organization or government agency, after initial and periodic evaluations, grants recognition to an organization, site or program that has met certain established criteria.
- *Certification:* Voluntary process by which a nongovernmental agency or an association grants recognition to an individual who has met certain predetermined qualifications specified by that organization. This formal recognition is granted to designate to the public that the individual has attained the requisite level of knowledge, skill, and/or experience in a well-defined, often specialized, area of the total discipline. Certification usually requires initial assessment and periodic reassessments of the individual's knowledge, skills and/or experience.
- *Credential:* Documented evidence of qualifications. Pharmacist credentials include diplomas, licenses, certificates, and certifications. For pharmacy technicians . . . CPhT . . . indicates certification by the Pharmacy Technician Certification Board. Credentials are reflected in a variety of abbreviations that pharmacists place after their names (e.g., Pharm.D. for "doctor of pharmacy," an earned academic degree; R.Ph. for "registered pharmacist," which indicates state licensure; and acronyms such as BCNSP for "Board-Certified Nutrition Support Pharmacist," which indicates that an individual has demonstrated advanced knowledge or skill in a specialized area of pharmacy).
- *Credentialing:* Process by which an organization or institution obtains, verifies, and assesses a pharma-

cist's qualifications to provide patient care services. [Similarly, credentialing can be applied to pharmacy technicians.]

[a]Federal funding is available to help support ASHP-accredited first-year residencies in hospitals caring for Medicare patients. To address the growing need in hospitals and health systems for pharmacists with advanced credentials, ASHP is seeking similar funding (which previously existed) for ASHP-accredited second-year residencies. ASHP is the accrediting body for pharmacy residencies. In early 2007, there were 714 ASHP-accredited postgraduate residency programs (481 first-year programs and 233 second-year programs). These programs graduate approximately 1400 residents per year. More ASHP-accredited residencies and residency graduates are needed to fulfill the work-force needs in hospitals and health systems.

[b]The processes used by BPS and ASCP for designating specialties and assessing the knowledge of individuals applying for certification are different.

[c]As of early 2007, BPS is engaged in a practice analysis in ambulatory care, which could lead to a sixth designation or "added qualifications."

[d]While this evolves to become a requirement by employers, a natural transition period will exist when pharmacists and pharmacy technicians who have achieved competence and successful experience in hospitals and health systems will continue to be employed.

References

1. American Society of Health-System Pharmacists. ASHP vision statement for pharmacy practice in hospitals and health systems. www.ashp.org/s_ashp?cat1c.asp?CID=2911&DID=4029 (accessed 2007 Mar 13).
2. American Society of Health-System Pharmacists. ASHP Health-System Pharmacy 2015 Initiative. www.ashp.org/s_ashp/quart1.asp?CID=218&DID=255 (accessed 2006 Dec 14).
3. Joint Commission of Pharmacy Practitioners. JCPP future vision of pharmacy practice, final version. www.aacp.org/Docs/MainNavigation/Resources/6725_JCPPFutureVisionofPharmacyPracticeFINAL.pdf (accessed 2006 Nov 28).
4. American Society of Health-System Pharmacists. ASHP statement on the pharmacist's role in informatics. *Am J Health-Syst Pharm.* 2007; 64:200–3.
5. Accreditation Council for Pharmacy Education. Accreditation standards and guidelines. www.acpe-accredit.org/standards/default.asp (accessed 2006 Dec 14).
6. Pharmacy Technician Certification Board. Pharmacy technician certification board (PTCB) announces milestone: 250,000 certified pharmacy technicians (CPhT). www.ptcb.org/AM/Template.cfm?Section=Home1&CONTENTID=2196&TEMPLATE=/CM/ContentDisplay.cfm (accessed 2007 Mar 13).
7. Leape LL, Bates DW, Cullen DJ et al. Systems analysis of adverse drug events. *JAMA.* 1995; 274:35–43.
8. Bates DW, Boyle DL, Vander Vliet MB et al. Relationship between medication errors and adverse drug events. *J Gen Intern Med.* 1995; 10:199–205.

9. Johnson JA, Bootman JL. Drug-related morbidity and mortality and the economic impact of pharmaceutical care. *Am J Health-Syst Pharm.* 1997; 54:554–8.

10. Bootman JL, Harrison DL, Cox E. The health care cost of drug-related morbidity and mortality in nursing facilities. *Arch Intern Med.* 1997; 157:2089–96.

11. Johnson JA, Bootman JL. Drug-related morbidity and mortality. A cost-of-illness model. *Arch Intern Med.* 1995; 155:1949–56.

12. Classen DC, Pestotnik SL, Evans RS et al. Adverse drug events in hospitalized patients. *JAMA.* 1997; 277:301–6.

13. Bates DW, Spell N, Cullen DJ et al. The costs of adverse drug events in hospitalized patients. *JAMA.* 1997; 277:307–11.

14. Lesar TS, Briceland L, Stein DS. Factors related to errors in medication prescribing. *JAMA.* 1997; 277:312–7.

15. Allan EL, Barker KN. Fundamentals of medication error research. *Am J Hosp Pharm.* 1990; 47:555–71.

16. Lesar TS, Lomaestro BM, Pohl H. Medication-prescribing errors in a teaching hospital. A 9-year experience. *Arch Intern Med.* 1997; 157:1569–76.

17. Bates DW, Cullen DJ, Laird N et al. Incidence of adverse drug events and potential adverse drug events. Implications for prevention. *JAMA.* 1995; 274:29–34.

18. Lazarou J, Pomeranz BH, Corey PN. Incidence of adverse drug reactions in hospitalized patients: a meta-analysis of prospective studies. *JAMA.* 1998; 279:1200–5.

19. Cohen MR, Proulx SM, Crawford SY. Survey of hospital systems and common serious medication errors. *J Healthc Risk Manag.* 1998; 18(1):16–27.

20. Barker KN, Flynn EA, Pepper GA et al. Medication errors observed in 36 health care facilities. *Arch Intern Med.* 2002; 162:1897–903.

21. Ernst FR, Grizzle AJ. Drug-related morbidity and mortality: updating the cost-of-illness model. *J Am Pharm Assoc.* 2001; 41:192–9.

22. Budnitz DS, Pollock DA, Weidenbach KN et al. National surveillance of emergency department visits for outpatient adverse drug events. *JAMA.* 2006; 296:1858–66.

23. Manasse HR Jr. Medication use in an imperfect world: drug misadventuring as an issue of public policy, part 1. *Am J Hosp Pharm.* 1989; 46:929–44.

24. Manasse HR Jr. Medication use in an imperfect world: drug misadventuring as an issue of public policy, part 2. *Am J Hosp Pharm.* 1989; 46:1141–52.

25. Davis TC, Wolf MS, Bass PF III et al. Literacy and misunderstanding prescription drug labels. *Ann Intern Med.* 2006; 145:887–94.

26. American Society of Health-System Pharmacists. Understanding and preventing drug misadventures. A multidisciplinary invitational conference sponsored by the ASHP Research and Education Foundation in cooperation with the American Medical Association, the American Nurses Association, and the American Society of Hospital Pharmacists. *Am J Health-Syst Pharm.* 1995; 52:369–416.

27. American Society of Health-System Pharmacists. Top-priority actions for preventing adverse drug events in hospitals. Recommendations of an expert panel. *Am J Health-Syst Pharm.* 1996; 53:747–51.

28. American Society of Hospital Pharmacists. ASHP guidelines on preventing medication errors in hospitals. *Am J Hosp Pharm.* 1993; 50:305–14.

29. Leape LL, Cullen DJ, Clapp MD et al. Pharmacist participation on physician rounds and adverse drug events in the intensive care unit. *JAMA.* 1999; 282:267–70. [Erratum, *JAMA.* 2000; 283:1293.]

30. Kucukarslan SN, Peters M, Mlynarek M et al. Pharmacists on rounding teams reduce preventable adverse drug events in hospital general medicine units. *Arch Intern Med.* 2003; 163:2014–8.

31. Schnipper JL, Kirwin JL, Cotugno MC et al. Role of pharmacist counseling in preventing adverse drug events after hospitalization. *Arch Intern Med.* 2006; 166:565–71.

32. Pearlman MD. Patient safety in obstetrics and gynecology: an agenda for the future. *Obstet Gynecol.* 2006; 108:1266–71.

33. Kaboli PJ, Hoth AB, McClimon BJ et al. Clinical pharmacists and inpatient medical care: a systematic review. *Arch Intern Med.* 2006; 166:955–64.

34. Manasse HR Jr, Thompson KK. Medication safety: a guide for health care facilities. Bethesda, MD: American Society of Health-System Pharmacists; 2006.

35. Kohn LT, Corrigan JM, Donaldson MS, eds. To err is human: building a safer health system. Washington, DC: National Academy Press; 1999.

36. Committee on Quality of Health Care in America. Crossing the quality chasm: a new health system for the 21st century. Washington, DC: National Academy Press; 2001.

37. Greiner AC, Knebel E, eds. Health professions education: a bridge to quality. Washington, DC: National Academies Press; 2003.

38. Aspden P, Wolcott JA, Bootman JL et al., eds. Preventing medication errors: quality chasm series. Washington, DC: National Academies Press; 2006.

39. Food and Drug Administration. Strategies to reduce medication errors: working to improve medication safety. www.fda.gov/fdac/special/testtubetopatient/safety.html (accessed 2006 Dec 15).

40. Food and Drug Administration. FDA's new drug safety initiative. www.fda.gov/cder/drugSafety.htm (accessed 2006 Dec 15).

41. National Quality Forum. Safe practices for better healthcare. www.qualityforum.org/projects/completed/safe_practices (accessed 2006 Dec 15).

42. National Quality Forum. Improving use of prescription medications. www.qualityforum.org/projects/completed/medications.asp (accessed 2006 Dec 15).

43. Joint Commission on Accreditation of Healthcare Organizations. Patient safety practices. An online resource for improving patient safety. www.jointcommission.org/PatientSafety/PSP (accessed 2006 Dec 15).

44. Joint Commission on Accreditation of Healthcare Organizations. 2007 National Patient Safety Goals. www.jointcommission.org/PatientSafety/NationalPatientSafetyGoals (accessed 2006 Dec 15).

45. American Society of Health-System Pharmacists. Policy: role of licensing, credentialing, and privileging in collaborative drug therapy management (0318).

www.ashp.org/s_ashp/bin.asp?CID=6&DID=4086&DOC=FILE.PDF (accessed 2006 Dec 14).

46. Galt KA. Credentialing and privileging for pharmacists. *Am J Health-Syst Pharm.* 2004; 61:661–70.

47. American Society of Health-System Pharmacists. Accreditation standards: postgraduate year one (PGY1) pharmacy residency programs. www.ashp.org/rtp/starting/ practice-residencies.cfm (accessed 2006 Nov 28).

48. American Society of Health-System Pharmacists. PGY1 educational goals and objectives. www.ashp.org/rtp/starting/specialized-residencies.cfm (accessed 2006 Nov 28).

49. Teeters JL, Brueckl M, Burns A et al. Pharmacy residency training in the future: a stakeholder's roundtable discussion. *Am J Health-Syst Pharm.* 2005; 62:1817–20.

50. American Society of Health-System Pharmacists. ASHP accreditation standard for postgraduate year two (PGY2) pharmacy residency programs. www.ashp.org/s_ashp/docs/files/RTP_PGY2AccredStandard.pdf (accessed 2007 Mar 13).

51. American Society of Health-System Pharmacists. PGY2 educational goals and objectives. www.ashp.org/rtp/Starting/PGY2.cfm (accessed 2006 Nov 28).

52. Board of Pharmaceutical Specialties. Recognized specialties. www.bpsweb.org (accessed 2006 Dec 14).

53. Council on Credentialing in Pharmacy. Guiding principles for certification of individuals in pharmacy. www.pharmacycredentialing.org/ccp/Files/CCP%20Guiding%20Principles%20for%20Certification%20Adopted%20January%202006.pdf (accessed 2006 Nov 28).

54. Department of Veterans Affairs. Credentialing and privileging. VHA handbook 1100.19. www1.va.gov/VHAPUBLICATIONS/ViewPublication.asp?pub_ID=357 (accessed 2006 Dec 15).

55. Department of Veterans Affairs. VHA Directive 2001-022. Implementation of VEPRO, VHA's national credentials databank. www1.va.gov/vhapublications/ViewPublication.asp?pub_ID=87 (accessed 2006 Dec 15).

56. American Society of Health-System Pharmacists. Medication prescribing authority for VA pharmacists to continue for 2 years. www.ashp.org/s_ashp/sec_news_article.asp?CID=167&DID=2024&id=2864 (accessed 2006 Dec 15).

57. Clause S, Fudin J, Mergner A et al. Prescribing privileges among pharmacists in Veterans Affairs medical centers. *Am J Health-Syst Pharm.* 2001; 58:1143–5.

58. American Society of Health-System Pharmacists. ASHP accreditation standard for pharmacy technician training programs. www.ashp.org/emplibrary/Accreditation%20Standard%20for%20Pharmacy%20Technician%20Training%202005%20.pdf (accessed 2006 Nov 27).

59. American Society of Health-System Pharmacists. ASHP-accredited technician training program directory. www.ashp.org/directories/technicians/directory-intro.cfm (accessed 2006 Nov 27).

60. American Society of Health-System Pharmacists. Model curriculum for pharmacy technician training. 2nd ed. www.ashp.org/technician/model_curriculum/index.cfm (accessed 2006 Nov 28).

61. Joint Commission on Accreditation of Healthcare Organizations. Standards. www.jointcommission.org/Standards (accessed 2006 Dec 14).

62. American Hospital Association. The state of America's hospitals—taking the pulse. Findings from the 2006 AHA Survey of Hospital Leaders. www.aha.org/aha/content/2006/PowerPoint/StateHospitalsChartPack2006.PPT (accessed 2006 Dec 15).

63. Department of Health and Human Services. The pharmacist workforce: a study of the supply and demand for pharmacists. http://bhpr.hrsa.gov/healthworkforce/reports/pharmacist.htm (accessed 2007 Mar 13).

64. American Society of Health-System Pharmacists. 2004 ASHP Pharmacy Staffing Survey results. www.ashp.org/emplibrary/04ASHPRxStaffSurvey.pdf (accessed 2006 May 3).

65. Knapp DA. Professionally determined need for pharmacy services in 2020. *Am J Pharm Educ.* 2002; 66:421–9.

66. White SJ. Will there be a pharmacy leadership crisis? An ASHP Foundation Scholar-in-Residence report. *Am J Health-Syst Pharm.* 2005; 62:845–55.

67. Mott DA, Doucette WR, Gaither CA et al. A ten-year trend analysis of pharmacist participation in the workforce. *Am J Pharm Educ.* 2002; 66:223–33.

68. Speedie MK, Manasse HR Jr. Pharmacists, pharmaceuticals and policy issues related to the workforce in pharmacy. Submitted for publication.

69. Report of the ASHP Task Force on Pharmacy's Changing Demographics. *Am J Health-Syst Pharm.* 2007; 64:1311–9.

70. National Association of Boards of Pharmacy. Foreign Pharmacy Graduate Equivalency Examination. www.nabp.net/index.html?target=/competency/intro.asp& (accessed 2007 Jan 4).

71. Council on Credentialing in Pharmacy. Credentialing in pharmacy. www.pharmacycredentialing.org/ccp/Files/CCPWhitePaper2006.pdf (accessed 2006 Nov 28).

Developed through the ASHP Council on Education and Workforce Development and approved by the ASHP Board of Directors on January 11, 2007.

The bibliographic citation for this document is as follows: American Society of Health-System Pharmacists. ASHP long-range vision for the pharmacy work force in hospitals and health systems. *Am J Health-Syst Pharm.* 2007; 64:1320–30.

White Paper on Pharmacy Technicians 2002: Needed Changes Can No Longer Wait

Introduction

The counting and pouring now often alleged to be the pharmacist's Chief occupation will in time be done by technicians and eventually by automation. The pharmacist of tomorrow will function by reason of what he knows, increasing the efficiency and safety of drug therapy and working as a specialist in his own right. It is in this direction that pharmaceutical education must evolve without delay.

—Linwood F. Tice, D.Sc.,
Dean, Philadelphia College of
Pharmacy and Science (1966)[1]

Health care and the profession of pharmacy have changed enormously since Dr. Tice articulated this vision more than 35 years ago. The role of the pharmacy technician has like-wise undergone substantial change. Technicians have increased in number. They may access a wide array of training opportunities, some of which are formal academic programs that have earned national accreditation. Technicians may now seek voluntary national certification as a means to demonstrate their knowledge and skills. State boards of pharmacy are increasingly recognizing technicians in their pharmacy practice acts.

Nonetheless, Dr. Tice' vision remains unrealized. Although pharmacy technicians are employed in all pharmacy practice settings, their qualifications, knowledge, and responsibilities are markedly diverse. Their scope of practice has not been sufficiently examined. Basic competencies have not been articulated. Standards for technician training programs are not widely adopted. Board regulations governing technicians vary substantially from state to state.

Is there a way to bring greater uniformity in technician competencies, education, training, and regulation while ensuring that the technician work force remains sufficiently diverse to meet the needs and expectations of a broad range of practice settings? This is the question that continues to face the profession of pharmacy today as it seeks to fulfill its mission to help people make the best use of medications.

The purpose of this paper is to set forth the issues that must be resolved to promote the development of a strong and competent pharmacy technician work force. Helping pharmacists to fulfill their potential as providers of pharmaceutical care would be one of many positive outcomes of such a development. The paper begins with a description of the evolution of the role of pharmacy technicians and of their status in the work force today. The next section sets forth a rationale for building a strong pharmacy technician work force. The paper then turns to three issues that are key to realizing the pharmacy technician' potential: (1) education and training, (2) accreditation of training institutions and programs, and (3) certification. Issues relating to state regulation of pharmacy technicians are then discussed. The paper concludes with a call to action and a summary of major issues to be resolved.

Many of the issues discussed in this report were originally detailed in a white paper developed by the American Pharmaceutical Association (APhA) and the American Society of Health-System Pharmacists (ASHP), which was published in 1996.[2] For this reason, this paper focuses primarily on events that have occurred since that time. Other sources used in the preparation of this paper include Institute of Medicine (IOM) reports,[3,4] report to the U.S. Congress on the pharmacy work force,[5] and input from professional associations representing pharmacists and technicians as well as from educators, regulators, and consumers.

The Pharmacy Technician: Past to Present

A pharmacy technician is "an individual working in a pharmacy [setting] who, under the supervision of a licensed pharmacist, assists in pharmacy activities that do not require the professional judgment of a pharmacist."[6] The technician is part of a larger category of "supportive personnel," a term used to describe all non-pharmacist pharmacy personnel.[7]

There have been a number of positive developments affecting pharmacy technicians in the past decade, including national certification, the development of a model curriculum for pharmacy technician training, and greater recognition of pharmacy technicians in state pharmacy practice acts. The role of the pharmacy technician has become increasingly well defined in both hospital and community settings. Technicians have gained greater acceptance from pharmacists, and their numbers and responsibilities are expanding.[8-11] They are starting to play a role in the governance of state pharmacy associations and state boards of pharmacy. Yet more needs to be done. There is still marked diversity in the requirements for entry into the pharmacy technician work force, in the way in which technicians are educated and trained, in the knowledge and skills they bring to the workplace, and in the titles they hold and the functions they perform.[12,13] absence of uniform national training standards further complicates the picture. Because of factors such as these, pharmacists and other health professionals, as well as the public at large, have varying degrees of understanding and acceptance of pharmacy technicians and their role in health care delivery.

An awareness of developments relevant to pharmacy technical personnel over the last several decades is essential to any discussion of issues related to current and future pharmacy technicians.[14,15] Policy statements of a number of national pharmacy associations are listed in the appendix. A summary of key events of the past half century follows.

1950s–1990s. Beginning in the late 1950s, hospital pharmacy and ASHP took the lead in advocating the use of pharmacy technicians (although the term "pharmacy technician" had not yet come into use), in developing technician training programs, and in calling for changes needed to ensure that the role of technicians was appropriately articulated in state laws and regulations.[16] Among the initial objectives was to make a distinction between tasks to be performed by professional and nonprofessional staff in hospital and community settings. This was largely accomplished by 1969.[14,17]

In the community pharmacy sector, chain pharmacies supported the use of pharmacy technicians and favored

on-the-job training. By contrast, the National Association of Retail Druggists (NARD, now the National Community Pharmacist Association [NCPA]), in 1974, stated its opposition to the use of technicians and other "subprofessionals of limited training" out of concern for public safety.[14]

Largely because of its origins, technician practice was initially better defined and standardized in hospitals than in community pharmacies. As the need for technicians in both settings became increasingly apparent, however, many pharmacists and pharmacy educators began to call for collaborative discussions and greater standardization on a number of issues related to pharmacy technicians, and in recent years, progress has been made toward this goal.

The Pharmacy Technician Work Force Today. Based on Pharmacy Technician Certification Board (PTCB) and Bureau of Labor Statistics (BLS) estimates, there are as many as 250,000 pharmacy technicians in the United States.[8,18] This is a significant increase over the 1996 estimate of 150,000.[2] BLS predicts that pharmacy technician employment will grow by 36% or more between 2000 and 2010.[8] This percentage of growth is "much faster than the average for all occupations," but in line with a majority of other supportive personnel in the health care sector.

Pharmacy technicians work in a wide variety of settings, including community pharmacies (approximately 70% of the total work force), hospitals and health systems (approximately 20%), long-term-care facilities, home health care agencies, clinic pharmacies, mail-order pharmacies, pharmaceutical wholesalers, managed care organizations, health insurance companies, and medical computer software companies.[8] The 2001 Schering Report found that 9 out of 10 community pharmacies employ pharmacy technicians.[10] Recent studies conducted in acute care settings indicate that this figure is nearly 100% for the hospital sector.[19]

What functions do technicians perform? Their primary function today, as in decades past, is to assist with the dispensing of prescriptions. A 1999 National Association of Chain Drug Stores (NACDS)/Arthur Andersen study revealed that, in a chain-pharmacy setting, pharmacy technicians' time was spent on dispensing (76%), pharmacy administration (3%), inventory management (11%), disease management (<1%), and miscellaneous activities, including insurance-related inquiries (10%).[21] Surveys conducted by PTCB have yielded similar results.[18,21] The nature of dispensing activities may be different in a hospital than in a community pharmacy. In hospitals, technicians may perform additional specialized tasks, such as preparing total parenteral nutrition solutions, intravenous admixtures, and medications used in clinical investigations and participating in nursing-unit inspections.[22]

In the past, pharmacists have traditionally been reluctant to delegate even their more routine work to technicians.[14] The 2001 Schering Report concluded that, in the past five years, pharmacists have become more receptive to pharmacy technicians. Indeed, much has changed in the scope of potential practice activities for pharmacy technicians and pharmacy's perception of the significant role technicians might play.[10,22] New roles for pharmacy technicians continue to emerge as a result of practice innovation and new technologies.[9,11] Despite their expanded responsibilities, many technicians believe that they can do more. For example, one study reported that 85% of technicians employed in chain pharmacies, compared with 58% of those working in independent pharmacies, felt that their knowledge and skills were being used to the maximum extent.[10]

Pharmacy Technicians: The Rationale

Several developments in health care as a whole, and in pharmacy in particular, have combined to create an increasing demand for pharmacy technicians. Three of significant importance are the pharmacist work force shortage, the momentum for pharmaceutical care, and increased concern about safe medication use.

Pharmacist Work Force Shortage. In 1995, a report by the Pew Health Professions Commission predicted that automation and centralization of services would reduce the need for pharmacists and that the supply of these professionals would soon exceed demand.[23] The predicted oversupply has failed to materialize; in fact, there is now a national shortage of pharmacists. A 2000 report of the federal Health Resources and Services Administration (HRSA) stated, "While the overall supply of pharmacists has increased in the past decade, there has been an unprecedented demand for pharmacists and pharmaceutical care services, which has not been met by the currently available supply."[5] The work force shortage is affecting all pharmacy sectors. Ongoing studies (by the Pharmacy Manpower Project and others) indicate that the pharmacy personnel shortages will not be solved in the short term.[24]

For pharmacy practitioners, the results of the work force shortage are clear: more work must be done with fewer pharmacist staff. Between 1990 and 1999, the number of prescriptions dispensed in ambulatory care settings increased by 44%, while the number of active pharmacists per 100,000 people increased by only about 5%.[5] Chain pharmacists now fill an average of 86 prescriptions during a normal shift—a 54% increase since 1993.[25] NACDS and IMS HEALTH estimate that, between 1999 and 2004, the number of prescriptions will increase by 36% while the number of pharmacists will increase by only 4.5% (Figure 1).[26]

Faced with greater numbers of prescriptions to dispense, pharmacists have less time to counsel patients. Working conditions and schedules have deteriorated, and job-related stress has risen.[10] Professional satisfaction has diminished. Perhaps most ominous, fatigue and overwork increase the potential for medication errors.[5,27]

Increased use of technicians is one obvious way of reducing workload pressures and freeing pharmacists to spend more time with patients. A white paper issued in 1999 by APhA, NACDS, and NCPA emphasized the need for augmenting the pharmacist's resources through the appropriate use of pharmacy technicians and the enhanced use of technology.[28]

The situation in pharmacy is not unique. A report from the IOM concluded that the health care system, as currently structured, does not make the best use of its resources.[4] Broader use of pharmacy technicians, in itself, will not solve the pharmacist work force crisis. It would ensure, however, that the profession makes better use of existing resources.

Momentum for Pharmaceutical Care. More than a decade ago, Hepler and Strand[29] expressed the societal need for pharmaceutical care. Since that time, the concept has been refined, and its impact on the health care system and patient care has been documented. Studies have shown that pharmaceutical care can improve patient outcomes, reduce the

Figure 1. Community prescriptions and pharmacists, 1992–2005. Rx = prescriptions, RPh (FTE) = registered pharmacist (full-time equivalent). Reprinted, with permission, from reference 26.

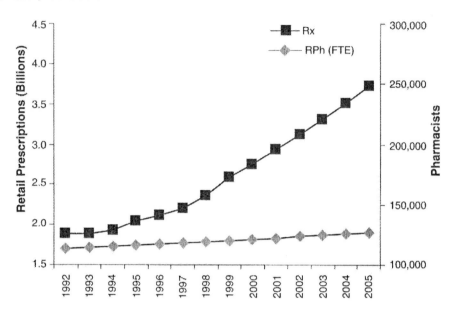

incidence of negative therapeutic outcomes, and avoid the economic costs resulting from such negative outcomes.[30-33] Nonetheless, other studies indicate that pharmacists continue to spend much of their time performing routine product-handling functions.[19,20] Widespread implementation of pharmaceutical care, a goal for the entire profession, has been difficult to achieve thus far.

Technicians are instrumental to the advancement of pharmaceutical care. As Strand[34,35] suggested, prerequisites to successful implementation of pharmaceutical care include enthusiastic pharmacists, pharmacy supportive personnel willing to work in a pharmacy where dispensing is done by technicians rather than pharmacists, and a different mindset i.e., the pharmacist will no longer be expected to "count and pour" but to care for patients.

In other words, implementation of pharmaceutical care requires a fundamental change in the way pharmacies operate. Pharmacists must relinquish routine product-handling functions to competent technicians and technology. This is a difficult shift for many pharmacists to make, and pharmacists may need guidance on how to do it. For example, they may need training in how to work effectively with technicians. Recognizing this need, some practice sites have developed successful practice models of pharmacy technicians working with pharmacists to improve patient care. Several of these sites have been recognized through PTCB's "Innovations in Pharmaceutical Care Award."[36]

Safe Medication Use. Used inappropriately, medications may cause unnecessary suffering, increased health care expenditures, patient harm, or even death.[33] Ernst and Grizzle[37] estimated that the total cost of drug-related morbidity and mortality in the ambulatory care setting in 2000 was more than $177 billion—more than the cost of the medications themselves. They stressed the urgent need for strategies to prevent drug-related morbidity and mortality.

The problems associated with inappropriate medication use have received broad publicity in recent years. For example, *To Err Is Human: Building a Safer Health System* drew attention to medical errors.[3] It criticized the silence that

too often surrounds the issue. Many members of the public were shocked to realize that the system in which they place so much trust was far from perfect.

Sometimes pharmacists have been implicated in medication errors. Technicians, too, have not escaped culpability.[38-43] Several studies, most of which were performed in hospitals, have, however, demonstrated that appropriately trained and supervised pharmacy technicians can have a positive effect on equalizing the distributive workload, reducing medication errors, allowing more time for clinical pharmacy practice, and checking the work of other technical personnel.[44,45] One study found that pharmacy technicians, when specially trained for the purpose, were as accurate as pharmacists in checking for dispensing errors.[46] The United States Pharmacopeia Medication Errors Reporting Program (USPMERP) has noted the contributions that pharmacy technicians can make to medication error prevention through their involvement in inventory management (e.g., identifying problems relating to "look-alike" labeling and packaging).[47] USPMERP also affirms that a "team approach" and "proactive attitudes" of pharmacists and technicians are important elements in reducing medication errors. The National Coordinating Council for Medication Error Reporting and Prevention advocates that a series of checks be established to assess the accuracy of the dispensing process and that, whenever possible, an independent check by a second individual (not necessarily a pharmacist) should be made.[48]

Reports such as these call for an expanded role for pharmacy technicians in a much-needed, systematic approach to medication error prevention.

Preparing Pharmacy Technicians for Practice

Historical Overview. Originally, all pharmacy technicians received informal, on-the-job training. The majority of pharmacy technicians are probably still trained this way.[8,18,49,50] Nevertheless, formal training programs, some of which are provided at the work site, are becoming more widespread. As state regulations, medications, record-keeping, and insurance

requirements have become more complex, there has been a move toward more formal programs.[51] Some employers have found that formal training improves staff retention and job satisfaction.[18,52] Another advantage of a formal training program is that it can confer a sense of vocational identity.[49]

Formal training programs for pharmacy technicians are not new; they were introduced in the armed forces in the early 1940s, and more structured programs were developed by the military in 1958. In the late 1960s, the Department of Health, Education, and Welfare recommended the development of "pharmacist aide" curricula in junior colleges and other educational institutions.[14] The first formal hospital-based technician training program was initiated around this time. Training programs proliferated in the 1970s as the profession sought to meet the need for a differentiated pharmacy work force.[53] Many of these programs were established in response to requests from hospital pharmacy administrators; at that time there was little interest in formally trained technicians in community pharmacies who continued to train technicians on the job.[54]

In the 1980s, ASHP issued training guidelines intended to help hospital pharmacists develop their own training programs.[7] ASHP recommended minimum entry requirements for trainees and a competency evaluation that included written, oral, and practical components. The guidelines were used not only by hospitals but by vocational schools and community colleges that wanted to develop certificate and associate degree programs.[49]

Acknowledging the importance of a common body of core knowledge and skills for all pharmacy technicians that would complement site-specific training, NACDS and NCPA developed a training manual, arranged into nine instructional sections and a reference section.[55] Each section has learning objectives, self-assessment questions, and competency assessment for the supervising pharmacist to complete. The manual focuses on the practical, legal, and procedural aspects of dispensing prescriptions, sterile-product compounding, patient interaction, and reimbursement systems. APhA and ASHP also produce technician training manuals and resource materials for pharmacy technicians.[56–60]

To date, most programs have referred to the "training" rather than the "education" of pharmacy technicians. Further discussion of the need for clarification of the education and training needs of pharmacy technicians is provided below.

Academic Training Programs. In 2002, approximately 247 schools and training institutions in 42 states offered a range of credentials, including associate degrees, diplomas, and certificates, to pharmacy technicians. The military also continues to provide formal training programs for pharmacy technicians.

Formal technician training programs differ in many respects, one of which is length. The *Accrediting Commission of Career Schools and Colleges of Technology School Directory* lists 36 "pharmacy" programs.[12] These programs vary in length from 540 to 2145 contact hours (24–87 weeks), with a median of 970 hours. ASHP, which accredits technician training programs, requires that programs have a minimum of 600 contact hours and a minimum duration of 15 weeks.[61] The Pharmacy Technicians Educators Council (PTEC), an association representing pharmacy technician educators, supports the ASHP minimum requirements.[62]

The minimum acceptable length of the program is a matter of debate. Some pharmacy technician educators deplore a move within the education system to get people into

the work force quickly. They believe that the pharmacy profession should make it clear that, while work force shortages and the needs of the marketplace are important considerations, rapid-training strategies do not seem appropriate for health care personnel whose activities directly affect the safe and effective use of medications.[51] There should be a clear relationship between the nature and intensity of education, training, and the scope of practice.

Entrance requirements for training programs also vary. Some have expressed concern that a substantial number of trainees may lack the necessary basic skills and aptitude to perform the functions expected of technicians.[51] The fact that about 30% of a certified pharmacy technician's time is spent performing tasks that require mathematical calculations reinforces the importance of suitably qualified training applicants.[21] ASHP acknowledged the need for minimum qualifications for training program applicants more than 20 years ago, but the issue continues to be a matter of debate.[7]

Progress Toward Standardization: The Model Curriculum. The absence of national training standards and the resultant variations in program content, length, and quality are barriers to the development of a strong technician work force. The problem is not unique to pharmacy technician training; other occupations in the health care sector also lack national standards. Nonetheless, it is ironic that persons in certain other occupations whose services have far less impact on public safety than do those of pharmacy technicians (e.g., barbers and cosmetologists) have training programs that, on average, are longer and less diverse than are pharmacy technician programs.[63] Reflecting a common sentiment on this issue, a 1999 PTEC survey concluded that "Expansion of the role of pharmacy technicians must be in tandem with standardizing training and establishment of competencies. Increased responsibilities should be commensurate with increased education."[64] Likewise, there was a consensus at the Third PTCB Stakeholders' Forum, held in June 2001, that national standards for pharmacy technician training are needed.[65]

Progress toward standardization has been facilitated by the *Model Curriculum for Pharmacy Technician Training.*[66] Having taken the initiative and the leadership role, ASHP collaborated with several other pharmacy associations (APhA, the American Association of Pharmacy Technicians, PTEC, the American Association of Colleges of Pharmacy [first edition only], and NACDS [second edition only]) to develop the *Model Curriculum.* The first edition, released in 1996, was based on the findings of the 1992–94 *Scope of Pharmacy Practice Project.*[67] Many of the revisions in the second edition, released in 2001, were based on a 1999 PTCB task analysis and accounted for changes in the scope of activities of today's pharmacy technicians as well as changes expected to occur over the next five years.[21,22] Significant changes were made, for example, in sections dealing with the technician's role in enhancing safe medication use, assisting with immunizations, and using "tech–check–tech" (a system in which pharmacy technicians are responsible for checking the work of other technicians with minimal pharmacist oversight).

The organizations that developed the model curriculum do not expect that every training program will cover every goal and objective of the curriculum; rather, the curriculum should be seen as a "menu" of possible learning outcomes. The model curriculum provides a starting point for identifying core competencies for pharmacy technicians.[22] It acknowledges the need

for a level of understanding of basic therapeutics, anatomy, physiology, and pharmacology. The curriculum does not include recommendations regarding the relative amount of time that should be allotted to each module, but such guidelines are under consideration.[68]

The Future Preparation of Pharmacy Technicians: Education Versus Training. Virtually all the consensus-development meetings and studies that have investigated training requirements for pharmacy technicians have called for the development of standardized training in some form.[51,69] APhA and ASHP concur with this position.[2,70,71]

Such a recommendation would best be accompanied by two important caveats. The first is that any national standards for education and training of pharmacy technicians will not eliminate the need for additional, site-specific training that focuses on local policies and procedures.[52,65] Second, standards-based education or training can conceivably be delivered successfully in a variety of different settings.

However, what exactly is meant when the terms education and training are applied to pharmacy technicians? They have tended in the past to be used somewhat interchangeably. However, a distinction needs to be made and a balance between the two needs to be reached to ensure that pharmacy technicians are adequately and appropriately prepared to perform, in a safe and efficient manner, the functions and responsibilities that are assigned to them—both now and in the future. As has already been noted in this paper, the roles and responsibilities of pharmacy technicians have evolved and expanded in recent years. While, in the main, pharmacy technicians perform routine tasks that do not require the professional judgment of a pharmacist, state pharmacy practice acts now recognize that pharmacy technicians are being assigned new and different functions in the practice setting, some of which may require a higher level of judgment or extensive product knowledge and understanding.

Training involves learning through specialized instruction, repetition and practice of a task or series of tasks until proficiency is achieved. Education, on the other hand, involves a deeper understanding of a subject, based on explanation and reasoning, through systematic instruction and teaching. People may be proficient in performing a task without knowing why they are doing it, why it is important, or the logic behind the steps being performed. While education (as described above) may involve a training component, both are vital to the learning (or preparation) of the technician. Barrow and Milburn[72] give a useful treatise on this subject. The education and training of pharmacy technicians and other supportive personnel must be commensurate with the roles they are performing. To ensure quality, both the education and training components should be standards based.

Accreditation of Pharmacy Technician Education and Training

The Council on Credentialing in Pharmacy (CCP) defines accreditation as "the process by which a private association, organization, or government agency, after initial and periodic evaluations, grants recognition to an organization that has met certain established criteria."[73] Accreditation is an integral aspect of ensuring a quality educational experience.

For pharmacy technician education and training, there are two types of accreditation: programmatic (also referred to as specialized) and institutional. Programmatic accreditation focuses specifically on an individual program, whereas insti-

tutional accreditation evaluates the educational institution as a whole, with less specific attention paid to the standards of individual programs offered by the institution. Institutional accreditors operate either on a regional or national basis; the latter usually has a more focused area of interest. A system of dual accreditation, in which institutional accreditation is conducted by regional accrediting bodies and programmatic accreditation is conducted by the American Council on Pharmaceutical Education (ACPE), has worked well for schools and colleges of pharmacy since the 1930s.

Based on information obtained from published directories, it is estimated that only 43% of the 247 schools and training institutions referred to earlier are accredited by bodies specializing in technical, allied health, and paraprofessional education; 36% have their programs accredited by ASHP; and 12% are accredited by both ASHP and one or more of the institutional accrediting bodies specializing in technical, allied health, and paraprofessional education.

Institutional Accreditation. For institutions offering pharmacy technician training, national institutional accreditation is carried out by at least four agencies: the Accrediting Commission of Career Schools and Colleges of Technology (ACCSCT), the Accrediting Bureau of Health Education Schools (ABHES), the Council on Occupational Education (COE), and the Accrediting Council for Independent Colleges and Schools (ACICS). All of these agencies are recognized by the U.S. Department of Education. None has a formal national affiliation with the profession of pharmacy.

Because there are no nationally adopted standards for pharmacy technician training, it is difficult for institutional accrediting bodies to set detailed program requirements. ACCSCT standards require programs to have an advisory committee, the majority of whose members represent employers in the field of training.[74] ABHES has a suggested curriculum outline for pharmacy technician programs. In an effort to improve the quality of their programs, COE and ABHES plan to switch from institutional to program accreditation.[75] Of some concern is the fact that such accreditation systems (for pharmacy technician training programs) would be outside the pharmacy profession and would not be based on national standards recognized by the profession.

Program Accreditation. Program accreditation for technician training is offered by ASHP. ASHP accreditation of technician training programs began in 1982 at the request of hospital pharmacists. Many hospital-based technician training programs were already using ASHP's guidelines and standards, but they expressed a need for a more formal method of oversight to ensure the quality of training. ASHP had already accredited pharmacy residency programs and moving into technician accreditation seemed a logical step.

Initially, nearly all ASHP-accredited programs were hospital based. This is no longer the case; of the 90 technician training programs currently accredited by ASHP, only 3 are hospital based. Over 90% of programs are located at vocational, technical, or community colleges.[76]

The objectives, standards, and regulations of the accreditation program, as well as a directory of accredited programs, are available on the ASHP Web site.[61,76–78] The accreditation standards are geared toward preparing technicians for all practice settings and require that pharmacy technicians be trained in a wide variety of practice environments and complete laboratory exercises before beginning their experiential training.

While accreditation is voluntary for both pharmacy degree programs and technician training programs, an important distinction exists. State boards of pharmacy and the National Association of Boards of Pharmacy (NABP) have recognized ACPE accreditation as an eligibility requirement for the North American Pharmacy Licensure Examination (NAPLEX).[79] Completion of an accredited program is not usually a prerequisite for employment, registration, or certification as a pharmacy technician. However, accreditation does bring a number of benefits. For the program, the benefits include enhanced recruitment potential for trainees, improved marketing, and the opportunity for peer review and quality improvement. For employers, completion of an accredited program may be an indication of the level of competence of a technician. Most importantly, accreditation provides all stakeholders with an objective, external, and independent evaluation of the quality of the education or training experience. Employers have a strong interest in the quality of training of their employees, not least of which is in terms of potential liability issues if the employer provides the training. Therefore, it would appear to be in the best interest of employers for the onus of quality assurance to rest with an independent party.

A New Role for ACPE? ASHP recognizes that the education, training, and utilization of pharmacy technicians now have broader professional implications than when it introduced its accreditation program began in 1982. For this reason, ASHP has asked ACPE to explore assuming responsibility for this function. Many people now believe that accreditation is best left to an independent agency that has no direct or indirect interest in the provision of training or in the activities of the graduates of the training program.[80]

Involving ACPE might have an additional advantage, should a decision be made to develop national training standards. ACPE, which has broad experience spearheading collaborative efforts to develop educational standards for pharmaceutical education, could be an appropriate organization to lead the process of developing uniform national standards for technician education and training. Responses to a 2000 ACPE survey indicate that more than 80% of respondents support further exploration of an ACPE role in this area.

Certification of Pharmacy Technicians

Certification is the process by which a nongovernmental agency or association grants recognition to an individual who has met certain predetermined qualifications specified by that agency or association.[2] For pharmacy, the PTCB, created in 1995, has been one of the most positive developments of the past decade.

"Certified pharmacy technician" (CPhT) is the only national credential available to pharmacy technicians. A credential is documented evidence of an individual's or program's qualifications or characteristics. Credentials may include diplomas, licenses, certificates, and certifications.[73] CCP was established in 1999. The development and application of credentialing standards for the pharmacy profession are integral components of CCP's vision and mission statements. PTCB was one of CCP's founding organizations. For a pharmacy technician, certification is an indication of the mastery of a specific core of knowledge.[2] Certification is mainly voluntary, although some state boards of pharmacy now require certification of technicians.

The PTCB examination is based on a task analysis that defined the work of pharmacy technicians nationwide: 64% of the exam is based on knowledge required to assist the pharmacist in serving patients, 25% on medication distribution and inventory control systems, and 11% on the administration and management of pharmacy practice.[21] By the end of 2001, more than 100,000 technicians had been certified with this program.[37] CPhTs must renew their certification every two years and complete at least 20 hours of pharmacy-related continuing education (including 1 hour of pharmacy law) during that period of time.

For many technicians, achieving PTCB certification is an important part of their professional development.[18] Many pharmacy chains have recognized the value of certification and provide assistance and incentives to staff to achieve certification, including reimbursement of costs, advancement to a higher grade, and a salary increase.[18] Studies have revealed that certified technicians remain in practice longer than do noncertified technicians.[81,82] Staff turnover, including both pharmacists and technicians, has decreased in pharmacies that employ certified technicians. Improved staff morale, higher productivity, reduced errors, and higher levels of customer satisfaction have also been noted. Additional benefits for employers include improved risk management, reduced technician training times, and lower training costs.[84] Some pharmacists feel more confident delegating dispensing activities to certified technicians than to technicians who are not certified.[10,21]

PTCB recognizes the need to reassess and modify its policies and procedures, as well as the examination, in response to the changing needs of pharmacy practice, the profession, and trends in the marketplace. To make such assessments, PTCB conducts research and seeks input from its stakeholders. PTCB also reviews its eligibility criteria for candidates who wish to sit for the certification examination. Under consideration are specialty certification assessments in areas such as preparation of intravenous admixtures and third-party-payment systems.

Regulation of Pharmacy Technicians

For many years, most state boards of pharmacy, often reflecting the attitudes of pharmacists, opposed recognizing technicians and expanding the scope of their activities.[52,14] As pharmacists' roles changed and use of supportive personnel expanded, these attitudes began to shift. Over the past five years, a majority of states have revised their pharmacy practice acts in areas related to technicians. Today, Ohio is the only state that does not formally address pharmacy technicians in state statutes or regulations.

NABP regularly surveys state pharmacy practice acts. The results of these surveys are bellwethers of change at the state level; collectively, they reveal trends. The most recent survey was conducted in 2001.[13] To highlight changes that have taken place since the publication of the 1996 "White Paper on Pharmacy Technicians,"[2] the results of NABP's 1996–1997[84] and 2001–2002[13] surveys were compared. NABP also appoints task forces to study and make recommendations on major issues. The deliberations of these task forces have resulted in, among other things, a call for formal recognition of pharmacy technicians, simplified state registration procedures, site-specific training, a national technician competency examination, and a disciplinary clearinghouse. Key developments in regulation, as

evidenced in the NABP surveys and in recent NABP task force recommendations and actions, are summarized below.

Changes in State Regulations: 1996–2001. *Terminology.* In the 1996–1997 NABP survey, at least 11 terms were used to describe pharmacy supportive personnel. At that time, 24 states used the term "pharmacy technician." By 2001, 38 states had adopted this designation.

Technician registration. In its "model act," designed to provide boards of pharmacy with model language that can be used when developing state laws or board rules, NABP advocates that pharmacists be licensed and that pharmacy technicians be registered.[85] "Registration" is defined as the process of making a list or being included on a list. It carries no indication or guarantee of the registrant's knowledge or skills. "Licensure" is the process by which an agency of government grants permission to an individual to engage in a given occupation upon finding that the applicant has attained the minimal degree of competency necessary to ensure that the public health, safety, and welfare will be reasonably well protected.[2] Like NABP, ASHP and APhA support registration and oppose licensure of pharmacy technicians. APhA and ASHP believe that licensed pharmacists must retain responsibility and accountability for the quality of service in a pharmacy.[72,73,86]

By 2001, 24 states required registration and 5 required licensure of pharmacy technicians, in accordance with NABP's recommendations. Although the term "license" is used in these regulations, in some cases the process would appear to more closely resemble "registration" in terms of the definitions used in this paper. The increase in the number of states (up from 14 in 1996) that now require either registration or licensure of pharmacy technicians is noteworthy.

Pharmacist-to-technician ratios. Since 1996, at least 25 states have liberalized their pharmacist-to-technician ratios (from a norm of 1:1 or 1:2 to 1:2 or 1:3). Some states further relaxed ratios in sites where certified pharmacy technicians are employed. In their 1996 white paper, APhA and ASHP called for a reassessment of mandated arbitrary pharmacist-to-technician ratios.[2] This stance reflects the organizations' conviction that pharmacists should be responsible and accountable for pharmacy technicians under their charge.[70,71] NACDS believes that each practice setting should be allowed to determine its own optimal ratio. Following the recommendation of a 1999 Task Force on Standardization of Technicians' Roles and Competencies,[88] NABP encouraged states to modify or eliminate ratios in pharmacy settings with quality assurance programs in place.

Standard training requirements. Between 1996 and 2001, the number of states that had incorporated training requirements into their regulations rose by 34% (from 19 to 26). Training requirements had been recommended in 1996 by an NABP task force.

The training requirements that state boards have put in place are, in some cases, minimal. Many states require nothing more than a training manual; there are no detailed minimum requirements. California, Kansas, Indiana, and Washington, on the other hand, have enacted competency-based regulations or well-defined standards for training program assessment. Some states require continuing education for renewal of registration or licensure; others are considering such a requirement.

Technician certification. Louisiana, New Mexico, Texas, Utah, Virginia, and Wyoming have made certification a requirement for registration or licensure. Texas was the first to introduce the requirement in 1996. The law was implemented in January 2001; a provision exists, however, for certain technicians to be exempted.[89] In Utah, the licensing authority has defined compliance with minimum training standards, as well as certification and the passing of a law examination, as requirements for licensure.[90] Alaska, Arizona, Kentucky, Massachusetts, Minnesota, North Carolina, Oregon, Tennessee, and Texas have altered pharmacist-to-technician ratios, responsibilities, supervision, or other requirements on the basis of a technician's certification status.

Levels of personnel and scope of practice. Based on findings of its 1999 task force, NABP has recognized two levels of supportive personnel: pharmacy technician and certified pharmacy technician, and specified the scope of practice that would be allowed for technicians working under the supervision of a pharmacist.[91] Activities that cannot be performed by a pharmacy technician include drug-utilization review, clinical conflict resolution, prescriber contact concerning prescription drug order clarification or therapy modification, patient counseling, dispensing-process validation, prescription transfer, and compounding. The following activities cannot be performed by a certified pharmacy technician: drug-utilization review, clinical conflict resolution, prescriber contact concerning prescription drug order clarification or therapy modification, patient counseling, dispensing-process validation, and receipt of new prescription drug order when communicating by telephone or electronically unless the original information is recorded so the pharmacist can review the order as transmitted. The task force had recommended a third, and higher, level of supportive personnel—the pharmacist assistant—but NABP did not adopt this recommendation. APhA and ASHP likewise oppose the creation of this category of supportive personnel.[70,71]

Many of the changes in state regulations are reflected in the functions that technicians perform. For example, the number of states allowing a pharmacy technician to call a physician for refill authorization increased by 41% (from 25 to 36) in hospital and institutional settings and by 47% (from 24 to 36) in a community setting between 1996 and 2001. Few states have traditionally allowed pharmacy technicians in any work setting to accept called-in (new) prescriptions from a physician's office, and there was little change in this area over the past five years. There was also little change in the dispensing-related activities that pharmacy technicians perform; however, the percentage of states allowing these activities was already high (>85% in 1996). The only dispensing-related activity to show a more than 15% increase (in the number of states that allow it) in the past five years is the reconstitution of oral liquids, which increased by 22% (from 41 to 51) in hospitals and by 23% (from 40 to 50) in community settings. In hospital and institutional settings, the number of states allowing technicians to compound medications for dispensing increased by 33% (from 34 to 46); the number increased by 24% (from 34 to 43) in the community setting.

Competency assessment. In May 2000, NABP resolved that it would (1) develop a national program to assess the competencies necessary for technicians to safely assist in the practice of pharmacy, (2) review existing technician certification programs to determine whether the development of its competence assessment program should be a cooperative effort with other groups, and (3) urge state boards to use this program as one criterion in determining the eligibility of technicians to assist in the

practice of pharmacy.[92] NABP has now joined PTCB on the national certification program for pharmacy technicians and will work with state boards of pharmacy to encourage acceptance of the PTCB certification program as a recognized assessment tool for pharmacy technicians.[93] The use of the PTCB certification program will also be incorporated into NABP's *Model State Pharmacy Act and Model Rules.*

The Need for Regulation. The difficulties stemming from lack of regulatory oversight over pharmacy technicians go further than one might initially foresee. For example, if state regulations do not recognize a class of personnel (through registration or licensure), it is difficult to discipline such personnel in the event of misconduct. Several state boards have reported that the absence of such regulation is creating problems (Rouse MJ, personal communication, 2001 Oct and Nov). For example, in the absence of adequate controls, pharmacy technicians who have committed an act of misconduct, such as drug diversion, can move from site to site, or state to state, without being traced or being held accountable. NABP and many state executives and pharmacists have called for better systems of control and measures to track disciplinary actions. By 2000, at least 25 states had incorporated disciplinary procedures for technicians in their regulations.[92]

Among the regulatory issues that remain in flux, none is more important than defining the roles and responsibilities of supportive personnel and the titles they are assigned. Pharmacy supportive personnel perform a wide array of services. Some state regulations recognize this and have differentiated levels of supportive personnel; some states have specific requirements for technicians-in-training. Multiple levels of pharmacy supportive personnel may continue to be required in the future, and the levels may vary among and within practice settings. The profession needs to determine what these levels should be and to define the role and function, competencies, education, training, and level of supervision appropriate for each.

Time for Action

Pharmacy faces a serious work force shortage at a time when the public and health care providers alike are looking to pharmacists to assume expanded responsibility for better medication use. Better use of human resources is essential. When pharmacists limit their direct involvement in the technical aspects of dispensing, delegate this responsibility to pharmacy technicians working under their supervision, and increase the use of automated dispensing technology, they can fully concentrate on the services for which they are uniquely educated and trained. Only then will Dr. Tice's vision of the future become reality.

The utilization, education, training, and regulation of pharmacy technicians have changed dramatically in the past five years. National certification has played a particularly important role in these changes. Nonetheless, many challenges remain. Because these challenges are interrelated, resolving them requires a coordinated approach. The profession needs a shared vision for pharmacy technicians and other supportive personnel. This vision will provide the framework within which further necessary change can take place. Beginning with that much-needed vision, the major issues to be discussed and resolved might be expressed as follows:

1. *Vision*
 a. Define a vision for pharmacy technicians as an integral part of the vision and mission of the profession of pharmacy.
 b. Develop goals, objectives, and strategies to realize this vision, including determining who will lead the process and the specific roles, present and future, of all parties.
 c. Communicate the vision and goals to all stakeholders, including policymakers and the public.
2. *Roles, responsibilities, and competencies*
 a. Define the different levels of pharmacy supportive personnel and the responsibilities or functions appropriate for individuals at each level.
 b. Determine the competencies required for high-level performance at each level.
3. *Education and training*
 a. Establish standards (including eligibility criteria) for the education and training of each level of pharmacy supportive personnel.
 b. Establish requirements for maintenance of competence, where applicable, and create the systems to achieve this.
 c. Consider the cost implications of any new training model, and devise appropriate strategies to address cost concerns.
4. *Credentialing and accreditation*
 a. Develop or enhance appropriate credentials, in collaboration with PTCB and CCP, to reflect what is happening and required in practice.
 b. Determine what the most appropriate systems of accreditation for education and training programs for pharmacy technicians are and who should lead this process on behalf of the profession.
5. *Regulation*
 a. Determine the appropriate regulatory framework under which pharmacy technicians can optimally contribute to the achievement of pharmacy's mission.
 b. Work to bring about further changes in state pharmacy practice acts and regulations in order to achieve the desired regulatory framework.
 c. Work to bring about the development and adoption of standardized definitions and terminology for pharmacy supportive personnel.

Conclusion

Change does not come easily, and it is seldom embraced by everyone. As Kenneth Shine put it, when discussing the need for change in the health system: "The issue . . . will be whether these needed changes occur only begrudgingly as a reaction to external forces, or whether they occur proactively as a result of professional leadership."[94] The profession of pharmacy is changing in response to internal as well as external influences. Both pharmacists and pharmacy technicians are, therefore, part of an evolving partnership. Pharmacy must respond to the changes that are already taking place and be sufficiently creative and flexible to anticipate and accommodate future developments. The need to address the issues surrounding pharmacy technicians in a timely manner cannot be overemphasized. Proper preparation of pharmacy technicians to work with pharmacists is

important in the promotion of public health and better use of medication. CCP, on behalf of its member organizations, offers this paper to provide a stimulus for professionwide action that can no longer wait.

References

1. Sonnedecker G, Kremers E. Kremers and Urdang's history of pharmacy. 4th ed. Madison, WI: American Institute of the History of Pharmacy; 1976:241.
2. American Society of Health-System Pharmacists. White paper on pharmacy technicians. *Am J Health-Syst Pharm.* 1996; 53:1793–6.
3. Kohn LT, Corrigan JM, Donaldson MS, eds. To err is human: building a safer health system. Washington, DC: National Academy Press; 1999.
4. Committee on Quality of Health Care in America. Crossing the quality chasm: a new health system for the 21st century. Washington, DC: National Academy Press; 2001.
5. Bureau of Health Professions. Report to Congress. The pharmacist workforce: a study of the supply and demand for pharmacists. Washington, DC: U.S. Department of Health and Human Services; 2000.
6. 1995 candidate handbook—national pharmacy technician certification examination. Washington, DC: Pharmacy Technician Certification Board; 1995:15.
7. American Society of Hospital Pharmacists. ASHP outcome competencies for institutional pharmacy technician training programs (with training guidelines). *Am J Hosp Pharm.* 1982; 39:317–20.
8. Bureau of Labor Statistics. Occupational outlook handbook. www.bls.gov/oco/ocos252.htm (accessed 2002 Apr 3).
9. Ervin KC, Skledar S, Hess MM, et al. Data analyst technician: an innovative role for the pharmacy technician. *Am J Health-Syst Pharm.* 2001; 58:1815–8.
10. Pharmacists, technicians, and technology: serving the patient. *Schering Report XXIII.* Kenilworth, NJ: Schering Laboratories; 2001.
11. Traynor K. Technician careers continue to evolve. *Newsl MD Society Health-Syst Pharm.* 2001; 24(4):1,4.
12. Accrediting Commission of Career Schools and Colleges of Technology directory. www.accsct.org/resource/resource_mainframe.html (accessed 2002 Apr 3).
13. 2001–2002 survey of pharmacy law. Park Ridge, IL: National Association of Boards of Pharmacy; 2001:34–44.
14. American Society of Hospital Pharmacists. Final report of the ASHP Task Force on Technical Personnel in Pharmacy. *Am J Hosp Pharm.* 1989; 46:1420–9.
15. American Society of Health-System Pharmacists. Chronology of ASHP activities for pharmacy technicians. www.ashp.org/technicians/chronology.html (accessed 2002 Mar 27).
16. Zellmer WA. Priorities for hospital pharmacy in the 1980s. *Am J Hosp Pharm.* 1980; 37:481. Editorial.
17. American Pharmaceutical Association. Report of the task force practitioner's and subprofessional's roles in pharmacy. *J Am Pharm Assoc.* 1969; 9:415–7.
18. Pharmacy Technician Certification Board: published and unpublished research, surveys, and employer consultations.
19. Ringold DJ, Santell JP, Schneider PJ. ASHP national survey of pharmacy practice in acute care settings:
dispensing and administration. *Am J Health-Syst Pharm.* 2000; 57:1759–75.
20. Arthur Andersen LLP. Pharmacy activity cost and productivity study. www.nacds.org/user-assets/PDF_files/arthur_andersen. PDF (accessed 2002 Mar 27).
21. Muenzen PM, Greenberg S, Murer MM. PTCB task analysis identifies role of certified pharmacy technicians in pharmaceutical care. *J Am Pharm Assoc.* 1999; 39:857–64.
22. Model curriculum for pharmacy technician training. 2nd ed. Bethesda, MD: American Society of Health-System Pharmacists; 2001:iv,1.
23. Pew Health Professions Commission. Critical challenges: revitalizing the health professions for the twenty-first century. San Francisco: Center for Health Professions; 1995.
24. Gershon SK, Cultice JM, Knapp KK. How many pharmacists are in our future? The Bureau of Health Professions projects supply to 2020. *J Am Pharm Assoc.* 2000; 40:757–64.
25. National Association of Chain Drug Stores. Pharmacy: playing a growing role in America's health care. www.nacds.org/wmspage.cfm?parm1=378 (accessed 2001 Nov 29).
26. IMS HEALTH and NACDS Economics Department. Used with permission.
27. Kelly WN. Pharmacy contributions to adverse medication events. Conference report: understanding and preventing drug misadventures. www.ashp.com/public/ proad/mederror/pkel.html (accessed 2002 Mar 27).
28. National Association of Chain Drug Stores, American Pharmaceutical Association, National Community Pharmacists Association. White paper. Implementing effective change in meeting the demands of community pharmacy practice in the United States; 1999.
29. Hepler CD, Strand LM. Opportunities and responsibilities in pharmaceutical care. *Am J Hosp Pharm.* 1990; 47:533–43.
30. American Pharmaceutical Association Foundation. Project ImPACT. www.aphafoundation.org/Project_Impact/Impact.htm (accessed 2002 Mar 28).
31. Johnson JA, Bootman JL. Drug-related morbidity and mortality: a cost-of-illness model. *Arch Intern Med.* 1995; 155:1949–56.
32. Johnson JA, Bootman JL. Drug-related morbidity and mortality and the economic impact of pharmaceutical care. *Am J Health-Syst Pharm.* 1997; 54:554–8.
33. Bootman JL, Harrison DL, Cox E. The health care cost of drug-related morbidity and mortality in nursing facilities. *Arch Intern Med.* 1997; 157:2089–96.
34. Strand LM. Building a practice in pharmaceutical care: Hoechst Marion Roussell lecture. *Pharm J.* 1998; 260:874–6.
35. Strand LM. Pharmaceutical care: Liverpool John Moores University seminar. *Pharm J.* 1998; 260:877–8.
36. Pharmacy Technician Certification Board Web site. www.ptcb.org/ (accessed 2002 Mar 28).
37. Ernst FR, Grizzle AJ. Drug-related morbidity and mortality: updating the cost-of-illness model. *J Am Pharm Assoc.* 2001; 41:192–9.
38. Lease D. Can you trust your pharmacist? http://speakout.com/activism/opinions/2850-1.html (accessed 2002 Mar 28).
39. Schuman D. When pharmacies make mistakes. www.news-sentinel.com (accessed 2002 Mar 28).

40. Levine J. Assistants' role in the spotlight: study finds mistakes by pharmacy technicians. http://my.webmd. com/content/article/1728.55198 (accessed 2002 Mar 28).

41. Stolberg SG. Death by prescription: the boom in medications brings rise in fatal risks. www.nytimes.com/library/national/science/060399sci-prescriptions.html (accessed 2002 Mar 28).

42. Hendren J. Pharmacy technicians dispense drugs: prescriptions often filled by lower paid technicians www.capecodonline.com/cctimes/archives/2000/mar/7/prescriptionsoften7.htm (accessed 2002 Mar 28).

43. Dooley K. 'Support personnel' handle pills: few standards regulate important job. *Lexington Herald-Leader.* 2001; Oct 22:11.

44. Kalman MK, Witkowski DE, Ogawa GS. Increasing pharmacy productivity by expanding the role of pharmacy technicians. *Am J Hosp Pharm.* 1992; 49:84–9.

45. Woller TW, Stuart J, Vrabel R, et al. Checking of unit dose cassettes by pharmacy technicians at three Minnesota hospitals: pilot study. *Am J Hosp Pharm.* 1991; 48:1952–6.

46. Ness JE, Sullivan SD, Stergachis A. Accuracy of technicians and pharmacists in identifying dispensing errors. *Am J Hosp Pharm.* 1994; 51:354–7.

47. Cowley E, Baker KR. Liability for errors in expanded pharmacy practice: issues for technicians and pharmacists. *J Am Pharm Assoc.* 2000; 40(suppl 1):S56–7.

48. National Coordinating Council for Medication Error Reporting and Prevention. Recommendations for avoiding error-prone aspects of dispensing medications. www.nccmerp.org/rec_990319.htm (accessed 2002 Apr 1).

49. Ray MD. Training hospital pharmacy technicians. *Am J Hosp Pharm.* 1984; 41:2595. Editorial.

50. Reeder CE, Dickson M, Kozma CM, et al. ASHP national survey of pharmacy practice in acute care settings—1996. *Am J Health-Syst Pharm.* 1997; 54:653–69.

51. Keresztes J, Palmer M, Lang SM, et al., eds. National pharmacy technician conference: looking toward the future. *J Pharm Technol.* 2001; 17 (suppl):S1–26.

52. Sanford ME, Faccinetti NJ, Broadhead RS. Observational study of job satisfaction in hospital pharmacy technicians. *Am J Hosp Pharm.* 1984; 41:2599–606.

53. American Society of Hospital Pharmacists. ASHP long-range position statement on pharmacy manpower needs and residency training. *Am J Hosp Pharm.* 1980; 37:1220.

54. Eichelberger BM. College-based technician training programs: producing without planning? *Am J Hosp Pharm.* 1979; 36:992–3.

55. Schafermeyer KW, Hobson EH, eds. The community retail pharmacy technician training manual. 3rd ed. Alexandria, VA: National Association of Chain Drug Stores and National Community Pharmacists Association; 1999.

56. Marks SM, Hopkins WA Jr. Pharmacy technician certification: quick-study guide. 2nd ed. Washington, DC: American Pharmaceutical Association; 2000.

57. Posey LM. Complete review for the pharmacy technician. Washington, DC: American Pharmaceutical Association; 2001.

58. Hopkins WA Jr. Complete MATH review for the pharmacy technician. Washington, DC: American Pharmaceutical Association; 2001.

59. Manual for pharmacy technicians. 2nd ed. Bethesda, MD: American Society of Health-System Pharmacists; 1998.

60. Pharmacy technician certification review and practice exam. Bethesda, MD: American Society of Health-System Pharmacists; 1998.

61. American Society of Health-System Pharmacists Commission on Credentialing. Accreditation standard for pharmacy technician training programs. www.ashp.org/technicians/techstnd.pdf (accessed 2002 Apr 1).

62. The Pharmacy Technician Educators Council. PTEC recommended pharmacy technology program content. www.rxptec.org/rptpc.html (accessed 2002 Apr 1).

63. Rouse MJ. Analysis of 36 pharmacy technician programs, 36 barbering and styling programs, and 34 cosmetology and styling programs listed in the ACCSCT Directory; 2001 Nov.

64. Moscou K. Pharmacy technician educators' attitudes toward education and training requirements for pharmacy technicians. *J Pharm Technol.* 2000; 16:133–7.

65. Pharmacy Technician Certification Board. Third Annual Stakeholder Forum; Leesburg, VA: 2001 Jun 13–14. (*Proceedings not yet published.*)

66. American Society of Health-System Pharmacists. Model curriculum for pharmacy technician training. www.ashp.org/technicians/model_curriculum/ (accessed 2002 Apr 1).

67. Summary of the final report of the Scope of Pharmacy Practice Project. *Am J Hosp Pharm.* 1994; 51:2179–82.

68. Rouse MJ. Personal communication with Nimmo CM, model curriculum committee leader. 2001 Oct.

69. Technical personnel in pharmacy: directions for the profession in society. Proceedings of an invitational conference conducted by the University of Maryland Center on Drugs and Public Policy and sponsored by the ASHP Research and Education Foundation. *Am J Hosp Pharm.* 1989; 46:491–557.

70. American Pharmaceutical Association Policy statements.

71. Professional policies adopted at the 54th annual session of the ASHP House of Delegates. *Am J Health-Syst Pharm.* 2002; 59:1563–7.

72. Barrow W, Milburn G, eds. A critical dictionary of educational concepts. 2nd ed. New York, NY: Teachers College Press; 1970.

73. Council on Credentialing in Pharmacy. Guiding principles or pharmacy credentialing activities. www.pharmacycredentialing.org/ (accessed 2002 Apr 1).

74. Accrediting Commission of Career Schools and Colleges of Technology. Getting accredited. www.accsct.org/getting/get_mainframe.html (accessed 2002 Apr 1).

75. Rouse MJ. (Letters to Eaton CJ, Associate Executive Director, Accrediting Bureau of Health Education Schools, and Puckett G, Associate Executive Director, Council on Occupational Education.) 2001 Nov.

76. American Society of Health-System Pharmacists. ASHP-accredited pharmacy technician training program directory. www.ashp.org/directories/technician/index.cfm (accessed 2002 Apr 1).

77. American Society of Health-System Pharmacists Commission on Credentialing. ASHP regulations on accreditation of pharmacy technician training programs. www.ashp.org/technicians/techregs.pdf (accessed 2002 Apr 1).

78. American Society of Health-System Pharmacists. Pharmacy technicians. www.ashp.org/technicians/index.html (accessed 2002 Apr 1).

79. Pharmacist.com. Getting your license. www.pharmacist.com/articles/l_t_0001.cfm (accessed 2002 Apr 1).
80. Association of Specialized and Professional Accreditors. Member code of good practice. www.aspa-usa.org/ (accessed 2002 Apr 1).
81. Burkhart A. Pharmacy's challenging environment: technicians as part of the solution. Paper presented at APhA Annual Meeting. San Francisco, CA; 2001 Mar 19.
82. Nouri L. The utilization of certified pharmacy technicians with automation and technology. Paper presented at APhA Annual Meeting. Washington, DC; 2000 Mar 12.
83. Murer MM. Innovations for enhancing patient safety and new roles for certified pharmacy technicians. Paper presented at ASHP Midyear Clinical Meeting. New Orleans, LA; 2001 Dec 4.
84. 1996–1997 Survey of pharmacy law. Park Ridge, IL: National Association of Boards of Pharmacy; 1997:32–40.
85. The Model state pharmacy act and model rules. Park Ridge, IL: National Association of Boards of Pharmacy; 2001.
86. Gans JA, Manasse HR. Memorandum to executive directors of state boards of pharmacy, state pharmacists associations, and state health-system pharmacists societies. Bethesda, MD: 1997 Oct 20.
87. National Association of Chain Drug Stores. Issue brief. 2002 Apr.
88. National Association of Boards of Pharmacy. Report of the Task Force on Standardization of Technicians' Roles and Competencies. 2000 May 8.
89. Texas State Board of Pharmacy. Rule §291.29: exemption from pharmacy technician certification requirements. www.tsbp.state.tx.us/Pharmacytechs.htm (accessed 2002 Apr 2).
90. Utah Division of Occupational and Professional Licensing. Pharmacy Practice Act. www.dopl.utah.gov/licensing/statutes_and_rules/58-17a.pdf (accessed 2002 Apr).
91. National Association of Boards of Pharmacy. Report of the NABP Committee on Law Enforcement/Legislation. 2000 Jan.
92. Madigan M. Regulatory evolution of pharmacy technicians. Paper presented at PTEC Annual Meeting. Toronto, Canada; 2001 Jul 10.
93. Pharmacy Technician Certification Board. News release 02-001. www.ptcb.org (accessed 2002 Apr 2).
94. Shine KI. President's report to the members. www.iom.edu/iom/iomhome.nsf/pages/2000+iom+president+report (accessed 2002 Apr 2).

Appendix—Policy Statements of National Associations

The following statements are published with the permission of the respective organizations and were accurate as of March 2002, with the exception of (d), which was accurate as of June 2002.

(a) The American Association of Colleges of Pharmacy
(b) The American Association of Pharmacy Technicians
(c) The American Pharmaceutical Association
(d) The American Society of Health-System Pharmacists
(e) The National Association of Chain Drug Stores
(f) The National Community Pharmacists Association
(g) The National Pharmacy Technician Association
(h) The Pharmacy Technicians Educators Council

The American Association of Colleges of Pharmacy

www.aacp.org/Docs/AACPFuntions/AboutAACP/4308_CumulativePolicies,1980-2001.pdf

Policies on Supportive Personnel

- AACP supports inclusion in the professional pharmacy curriculum of didactic and experiential material related to the supervision and management of supportive personnel in pharmacy practices. *(Source: Professional Affairs Committee, 1990)*
- Training for technicians in pharmacy must be based on competencies derived from tasks that are deemed appropriate by the profession and currently performed by technical personnel. *(Source: Professional Affairs Committee, 1989)*
- Pharmacy schools should offer their assistance to supportive personnel training programs to assure that programs meet appropriate educational objectives. *(Source: Professional Affairs Committee, 1987)*
- Training for supportive personnel in pharmacy must be based on sound educational principles with clearly established competency objectives. *(Source: Professional Affairs Committee, 1987)*

The American Association of Pharmacy Technicians

www.pharmacytechnician.com/

Code of Ethics for Pharmacy Technicians

Preamble
Pharmacy Technicians are healthcare professionals who assist pharmacists in providing the best possible care for patients. The principles of this code, which apply to pharmacy technicians working in any and all settings, are based on the application and support of the moral obligations that guide the pharmacy profession in relationships with patients, healthcare professionals and society.

Principles
- A pharmacy technician's first consideration is to ensure the health and safety of the patient, and to use knowledge and skills to the best of his/her ability in serving patients.
- A pharmacy technician supports and promotes honesty and integrity in the profession, which includes a duty to observe the law, maintain the highest moral and ethical conduct at all times and uphold the ethical principles of the profession.
- A pharmacy technician assists and supports the pharmacists in the safe and efficacious and cost effective distribution of health services and healthcare resources.
- A pharmacy technician respects and values the abilities of pharmacists, colleagues and other healthcare professionals.
- A pharmacy technician maintains competency in his/her practice and continually enhances his/her professional knowledge and expertise.
- A pharmacy technician respects and supports the patient's individuality, dignity, and confidentiality.

- A pharmacy technician respects the confidentiality of a patient's records and discloses pertinent information only with proper authorization.
- A pharmacy technician never assists in dispensing, promoting or distribution of medication or medical devices that are not of good quality or do not meet the standards required by law.
- A pharmacy technician does not engage in any activity that will discredit the profession, and will expose, without fear or favor, illegal or unethical conduct of the profession.
- A pharmacy technician associates with and engages in the support of organizations, which promote the profession of pharmacy through the utilization and enhancement of pharmacy technicians.

The American Pharmaceutical Association

www.aphanet.org

2001 Automation and Technical Assistance
APhA supports the use of automation for prescription preparation and supports technical and personnel assistance for performing administrative duties and facilitating pharmacist's provision of pharmaceutical care.

1996 Control of Distribution System (Revised 2001)
The American Pharmaceutical Association supports the pharmacists' authority to control the distribution process and personnel involved and the responsibility for all completed medication orders regardless of practice setting.
(*J Am Pharm Assoc.* NS36:396. June 1996)

1996 Technician Licensure and Registration
1. APhA recognizes, for the purpose of these policies, the following definitions:
 (a) Licensure: The process by which an agency of government grants permission to an individual to engage in a given occupation upon finding that the applicant has attained the minimal degree of competency necessary to ensure that the public health, safety, and welfare will be reasonably well protected. Within pharmacy, a pharmacist is licensed by a State Board of Pharmacy.
 (b) Registration: The process of making a list or being enrolled in an existing list.
2. APhA supports the role of the State Boards of Pharmacy in protecting the public in its interaction with the profession, including the Boards' oversight of pharmacy technicians, through their control of pharmacists and pharmacy licenses.
3. In States where the Board of Pharmacy chooses to exercise some direct oversight of technicians, APhA recommends a registration system.
4. APhA reaffirms its opposition to licensure of pharmacy technicians by statute or regulation.
 (*J Am Pharm Assoc.* NS36:396. June 1996)

1971 Sub-professionals: Functions, Standards and Supervision
The committee recommends that APhA endorse the use of properly supervised supportive personnel in pharmacy practice as a positive step toward improving the quality and quantity of pharmaceutical services provided by the profession.
(*J Am Pharm Assoc.* NS11:277. May 1971)

1966 Sub-professionals
The committee would be opposed to any assumption of the pharmacist's professional functions by sub-professionals or technicians. There is a need to determine exactly what these functions are and the relative position of the pharmacy intern. Under no circumstance should a sub-professional program in pharmacy create an individual such as the former "qualified assistant" still practicing in some states.
(*J Am Pharm Assoc.* NS6:332. June 1966)

The American Society of Health-System Pharmacists

www.ashp.org
See also www.ashp.org/public/hq/ (accessed 2002 Apr 4).
See also www.ashp.org/public/hq/policy/2001Policy Positions.pdf (accessed 2002 Apr 4).

[*Editor's note: ASHP policy positions 0224 and 0025 (below) have been superseded by ASHP policy positions 0322 and 0521, respectively, which are printed elsewhere in this book. ASHP policy positions are updated annually and can be accessed at ASHP's Web site at www.ashp.org/aboutashp/.*]

0224
Credentialing of Pharmacy Technicians
Source: Council on Legal and Public Affairs
To advocate and support registration of pharmacy technicians by state boards of pharmacy (registration is the process of making a list or being enrolled in an existing list; registration should be used to help safeguard the public by interstate and intrastate tracking of the technician work force and preventing individuals with documented problems from serving as pharmacy technicians); further,

To advocate and support mandatory certification of all current pharmacy technicians and new hires within one year of date of employment (certification is the process by which a nongovernmental agency or association grants recognition to an individual who has met certain predetermined qualifications specified by that agency or association); further,

To advocate the adoption of uniform standards for the education and training of all pharmacy technicians to ensure competency; further,

To oppose state licensure of pharmacy technicians (licensure is the process by which an agency of government grants permission to an individual to engage in a given occupation upon a finding that the applicant has attained the minimal degree of competency necessary to ensure that the public health, safety, and welfare will be reasonably well protected); further,

To advocate that licensed pharmacists should be held accountable for the quality of pharmacy services provided and the actions of pharmacy technicians under their charge.

0212
Pharmacy Technician Training
Source: Council on Educational Affairs
To support the goal that technicians entering the pharmacy work force have completed an accredited program of training; further,

To encourage expansion of accredited pharmacy technician training programs.

0211

Image of and Career Opportunities for Pharmacy Technicians

Source: Council on Educational Affairs

To promote the image of pharmacy technicians as valuable contributors to health care delivery; further,

To develop and disseminate information about career opportunities that enhance the recruitment and retention of qualified pharmacy technicians.

0209

Substance Abuse and Chemical Dependency

Source: Council on Educational Affairs

To collaborate with appropriate professional and academic organizations in fostering adequate education on substance abuse and chemical dependency at all levels of pharmacy education (i.e., colleges of pharmacy, residency programs, and continuing-education providers); further,

To support federal, state, and local initiatives that promote pharmacy education on substance abuse and chemical dependency; further,

To advocate the incorporation of education on substance abuse and chemical dependency into the accreditation standards for Doctor of Pharmacy degree programs and pharmacy technician training programs.

0025

Opposition to Creation of "Pharmacist Assistant" Category of Licensed Pharmacy Personnel

Source: House of Delegates

To reaffirm the following statement in the "White Paper on Pharmacy Technicians" (April 1996) endorsed by ASHP and the American Pharmacists Association:

"Although there is a compelling need for pharmacists to expand the purview of their professional practice, there is also a need for pharmacists to maintain control over all aspects of drug product handling in the patient care arena, including dispensing and compounding. No other discipline is as well qualified to ensure public safety in this important aspect of health care."

Further,

To note that some interest groups in pharmacy have advocated for the creation of a new category of licensed personnel called "Pharmacist Assistant" that would have (a) less education and training than pharmacists and (b) independent legal authority to perform many of the functions that are currently restricted to licensed pharmacists; further,

To support the optimal use of well trained, certified pharmacy technicians under the supervision of licensed pharmacists; further,

To oppose the creation of a category of licensed personnel in pharmacy such as "Pharmacist Assistant" that would have legal authority to perform independently those professional pharmacy functions that are currently restricted to licensed pharmacists.

8610

Pharmacy Technicians

Source: Council on Legal and Public Affairs

To work toward the removal of legislative and regulatory barriers preventing pharmacists from delegating certain technical activities to other trained personnel.

This policy was reviewed in 1997 by the Council on Legal and Public Affairs and by the Board of Directors and was found to still be appropriate.

The National Association of Chain Drug Stores

www.nacds.org

Issue Brief—Pharmacy Technicians (Issued October 2001; updated April 2002)

The Issue

Registration, training and certification of pharmacy support personnel (pharmacy technicians) and maximizing the duties that such pharmacy technicians can perform.

Background

Allowing pharmacy technicians to be utilized to the fullest extent possible without any ratio will:

- Enhance pharmacists availability to counsel patients and to confer with other health professionals;
- Improve overall service to patients;
- Ease workload and improve professional satisfaction for pharmacists; and,
- Enhance efficiency and improve resources available for meeting the increased prescription volume and addressing the pharmacist shortages.

Certification of Pharmacy Technicians

- Certification should be voluntary and not mandatory.
- "Certification" exams should be effective tools for evaluating pharmacy technicians at the various pharmacy practice sites, such as community retail pharmacies, hospital pharmacies, and other practice settings.
- If pharmacy technicians decide to be certified they should be permitted to perform expanded duties and responsibilities.
- Pharmacy technicians, even if not certified, should be permitted to do routine nonjudgmental dispensing functions including, but not limited to, handling nonjudgmental third party and other payment issues, offering the patient the availability of the pharmacist for counseling, placing telephone calls to prescribers for refill requests, taking phone calls from prescribers' offices authorizing refill prescriptions, and preparing prescriptions for pharmacist's final review.

Pharmacy Technician Training and Examinations

- Boards of Pharmacy should allow for employer-based pharmacy technician training programs and examination pursuant to a Pharmacy Technician Training Manual.
- Boards of Pharmacy should recognize that employer-based technician training programs prepare technicians to work in their own particular practice setting, and that

technician training programs should be designed to teach competencies relevant to the particular practice setting.

- Chain pharmacy technician training programs and examinations should receive Board approval.

NACDS Position

- Continue to permit an unlimited number of technicians and allow each practice setting to determine their optimal ratio.
- Allow technicians to perform non-judgmental tasks . . . those duties that do not require the expertise of a pharmacist.
- Allow technician training tailored to the pharmacy and to the company operations and standards.
- Allow certification to remain voluntary.
- Allow certified pharmacy technicians to perform additional duties and responsibilities commensurate with their competencies.
- Approve employer based training and examination pharmacy technician programs and recognize the importance of practice site specific training and examination programs such as community pharmacy based programs.
- Recognize the NACDS pharmacy technician training and examination program for certification of pharmacy technicians.

The National Community Pharmacists Association

www.ncpanet.org

NCPA supports the use of pharmacy technicians in community pharmacies to enhance the pharmacist's role in the provision of quality pharmacist care. NCPA believes the proper training and supervision of technicians by the pharmacist is critical to the health and safety of patients.

Technician Support and Technology:
Recognizing the current environment of regional shortages of pharmacists and the projected increase in prescription volume due to potential Medicare prescription drug benefit coverage and an aging population, NCPA recommends enhancing patient care and addressing manpower issues through the more efficient utilization of technician support and technology. NCPA strongly opposes the creation of any category of supportive personnel, which is not under the direct supervision of a licensed pharmacist.

The National Pharmacy Technician Association

www.pharmacytechnician.org/

Key Professional Issues
Medication Errors:
NPTA feels that the use of highly trained, educated and certified pharmacy technicians in the pharmacy profession will assist in efficiently and effectively reducing the occurrence of medication errors.

Technician Liability:
NPTA feels that with the emergence of national technician certification, producing increased roles and responsibilities, the issue of technician liability will become an evermore-

present factor. Currently, NPTA does not have a position statement on technician liability.

Technician Education and Training:
NPTA fully supports formalized education and training programs at institutions of higher education. NPTA feels strongly that at some point, pharmacy technicians should be required to obtain a degree/certificate to be allowed to practice as a pharmacy technician. At this point, NPTA does not have a position statement on whether this degree should be a one or two year degree, when this policy should be implemented, or an appropriate approach for those already practicing. The requirement of formal education for pharmacy technicians, which is not present in most states, will be an integral part of the advancement of pharmacy practice, patient safety and a more efficient/effective healthcare system.

Technician Certification, Regulation and Credentialing
National Certification:
NPTA fully supports legislated requirements of certification by pharmacy technicians across the United States. National Certification is an appropriate and effective first step towards the educational and training goals for pharmacy technicians of the future.

Continuing Education:
NPTA strongly believes that an independent organization should be setup to accredit and monitor providers of pharmacy technician level continuing education programs. NPTA feels that while certified pharmacy technicians should be allowed to utilize ACPE CE Programs, that no organization (local, state or national) should make ACPE programs a requirement, since currently all ACPE programs are designed at the pharmacist's level.

The Pharmacy Technicians Educators Council

www.rxptec.org/

PTEC Recommendations and Goals
PTEC strongly recommends that all pharmacy education and programs seek ASHP accreditation.

PTEC strongly recommends that all pharmacy technician-training programs have a minimum of 600 contact hours, in accordance with ASHP accreditation standards.

In the short term, PTEC will:

- Work with AACP to design and implement programs which would provide step-wise technician training curriculum credits which could be used towards pharmacist training and education.
- Advocate a PTEC representative attend AACP board meetings, and invite AACP officers to attend PTEC board meetings.

PTEC advocates that:

- Within 5 years, all technician-training programs have a *minimum* of 600 contact hours; and
- Within 10 years, all technician-training programs evolve into 2-year associate degree programs.

PTEC recognizes the need for, and supports the development and introduction of, appropriate credentials for pharmacy technicians, including at the specialty level.

PTEC will work with AACP to design and implement programs which would provide step-wise technician-training curriculum credits that could be used towards pharmacist training and education.

The PTEC recommended pharmacy technology program content is published on its website: www.rxptec.org/rptpc.html

———————

The following organizations have endorsed this document: Academy of Managed Care Pharmacy, American Association of Colleges of Pharmacy, American College of Apothecaries, American College of Clinical Pharmacy, Accreditation Council for Pharmacy Education, American Pharmacists Association, American Society of Consultant Pharmacists, American Society of Health-System Pharmacists, Board of Pharmaceutical Specialties, Commission for Certification in Geriatric Pharmacy, Pharmacy Technician Certification Board, and Pharmacy Technician Educators Council.

Development of this white paper was supported by an educational grant from PTCB.

The bibliographic citation for this document is as follows: American Society of Health-System Pharmacists. White paper on pharmacy technicians 2002: Needed changes can no longer wait. *Am J Health-Syst Pharm.* 2003; 60:37–51.

This document was also published in the *Journal of the American Pharmaceutical Association.*

Practice Settings

Practice Settings

Use of Two Patient Identifiers in the Outpatient Setting (1024)

Source: Council on Pharmacy Practice

To encourage the use of two identifiers to confirm patient identity when transferring filled prescriptions to the possession of the patient or patient's agent in outpatient settings.

Principles of Managed Care (0709)

Source: Council on Pharmacy Management

To recognize that the principles of managed care have many applications in hospital and health-system pharmacy practice; further,

To continue to include managed care topics in educational programming, publications, and professional-practice-development initiatives; further,

To continue to serve the professional needs of ASHP members who practice in managed care organizations.

This policy supersedes ASHP policy 0205.

Home Intravenous Therapy Benefit (0414)

Source: Council on Legal and Public Affairs

To support the continuation of a home intravenous therapy benefit under federal and private health insurance plans, and expand the home infusion benefit under Medicare Part B at an appropriate level of reimbursement for pharmacists' patient care services provided, medications, supplies, and equipment.

This policy was reviewed in 2008 by the Council on Public Policy and by the Board of Directors and was found to still be appropriate.

ASHP Guidelines: Minimum Standard for Home Care Pharmacies

Purpose

Home care pharmacies provide pharmaceutical products and clinical monitoring services to patients of all ages in their homes, including home infusion therapy, oral medications, home hospice pharmaceutical services, and parenteral and enteral nutrition. Pharmacists practicing in home care pharmacies provide a specialized form of pharmaceutical care to the patients they serve. Home care pharmacies, whether they are hospital-based, long-term-care pharmacies, community pharmacies, independent organizations, or multisite organizations, should be viewed as an integral component of the overall health care system.

Home care patients require systemwide continuity of care. Mechanisms should exist for appropriate and confidential sharing of patient information among responsible providers and caregivers across the continuum of care and in various components of health systems. Systemwide communication, through interfacing patient information systems, oral and written communication, and consistent product labeling, is important to optimize care and minimize the risk of health care misadventures.

The purpose of these guidelines is to outline the minimum requirements for the operation and management of pharmaceutical services to be provided by home care pharmacies. However, as noted, the provision of pharmaceutical care in the home care setting should be coordinated among other settings. Therefore, as applicable, these guidelines should be used in conjunction with minimum standards for other practice settings. Many of the topics outlined are the subject of other ASHP practice standards, which should be referred to for additional information and guidance. Because of differences in settings and in organizational arrangements and complexities, aspects of these guidelines may be more applicable to some settings than others. Managers of home care pharmacies should use their professional judgment in assessing and adapting these guidelines to meet their own needs and circumstances.

To ensure the safe, appropriate, and effective use of medications in the home, home care pharmacies should develop comprehensive services to address factors unique to home care. Caregivers such as family members, who often have no health care experience, should be trained to properly administer medications, operate medication administration devices, and monitor patients as necessary. Medications must be aseptically compounded, often in quantities sufficient for several days' use, and delivered under conditions that will ensure that product potency and purity are maintained. Vascular access should be maintained for the intended duration of therapy, which may range from days to years. Medication administration devices should be selected and maintained to accurately and safely administer a variety of therapeutic regimens. Potential complications should be anticipated, and a proactive plan of care should be established for monitoring, detecting, and managing complications. Economic considerations should be taken into account so that care is provided in the most cost-effective manner. Finally, home care pharmacies should have an effective organizational structure with the flexibility to meet the changing needs of patients, as well as to keep pace with the rapid growth of the industry and changes in health systems. As providers of pharmaceutical care in the home setting, pharmacists should be concerned with the outcomes of their services and not just the provision of these services. Effective management is necessary to ensure that quality outcomes of therapy are achieved.

The criteria for home care pharmacy that are covered in these guidelines are distributed among the following categories: (1) leadership and practice management, (2) drug information, education, and counseling, (3) care planning, monitoring, and continuity, (4) drug distribution and control, and (5) facilities, equipment, and information systems. Collectively, these criteria represent a minimum level of quality that all home care pharmacies should strive to provide consistently. While the scope of pharmaceutical services is likely to vary from site to site depending upon the needs of the patients served, these criteria are strongly linked to patient outcomes, and neglect of any one area may compromise quality.

Standard 1: Leadership and Practice Management

Effective leadership and practice management are necessary for the delivery of pharmaceutical services in a manner consistent with the needs of the home care patient, the needs of the home care organization and pharmacy, and the requirements for continuous improvement in patient care outcomes. The pharmacy manager should focus on the pharmacist's responsibility for providing pharmaceutical care and on the development of an infrastructure for supporting pharmaceutical care.

Managerial responsibilities include (1) setting the short-term and long-term goals of the pharmacy according to the needs of the patients served, (2) developing plans and schedules for achieving these goals, (3) directing implementation of the plans and the day-to-day activities associated with them, (4) determining whether the goals and schedules are being met, and (5) instituting corrective actions when necessary. The pharmacy manager, in carrying out these responsibilities, should supervise an adequate number of competent, qualified personnel. A part-time or contract manager has the same basic obligations and responsibilities as a full-time manager.

Managing the Pharmacy

Education and Training of the Home Care Pharmacy Manager. The home care pharmacy should be managed by a professionally competent, legally qualified pharmacist. The manager should be thoroughly knowledgeable about home care pharmacy practice and management. Completion of a pharmacy residency program and home care experience are desirable.

Pharmacy Mission. The pharmacy or its affiliated organization should have a written mission statement that, at a minimum, reflects both patient care and operational responsibilities.

The statement should be consistent with the mission of the home care organization and parent health system, if applicable. The mission should be understood by employees, contract staff, and other participants (e.g., students and residents) in the pharmacy's activities. The development and prioritization of goals, objectives, and work plans should be consistent with the mission statement.

Laws and Regulations. Compliance with local, state, and federal laws and regulations applicable to the home care pharmacy is required. The pharmacy should maintain written or computerized documentation of compliance concerning requirements for procurement and distribution of drug products, patient information, and related safety from the state board of pharmacy, Food and Drug Administration, Drug Enforcement Administration, Health Care Financing Administration, and Occupational Safety and Health Administration, among others. Home care pharmacies dispensing drugs across state boundaries shall comply with out-of-state licensure requirements, as well as other state and federal interstate laws and regulations.

Policy and Procedure Manual. A policy and procedure manual governing the scope of the home care pharmaceutical services (e.g., administrative, operational, and clinical) should be available and properly maintained. The manual should be reviewed and revised annually or whenever necessary to reflect changes in procedures specific to the sites where the pharmacy's products and services are provided. All personnel should be familiar with the contents of the manual. Appropriate mechanisms should be established to ensure compliance with the policies and procedures.

Practice Standards and Guidelines. The practice standards and guidelines of accrediting and professional organizations, such as the American Society of Health-System Pharmacists (ASHP) and the Joint Commission on Accreditation of Healthcare Organizations (JCAHO), should be assessed and adapted when applicable to the home care organization, the scope of pharmaceutical services, and the patient population served.

Managing Financial Resources

Financial Management. Oversight of workload and financial performance should be managed in accordance with the home care organization's requirements. Management should provide for (1) determination and analysis of pharmacy service costs, (2) analysis of budgetary variances, (3) capital equipment acquisition, (4) patient revenue projections, and (5) justification of personnel commensurate with workload productivity. The pharmacy manager should be an integral participant in the home care organization's financial management process.

Drug Expenditures. Specific policies and procedures for managing drug expenditures should address such methods as competitive bidding, group purchasing, utilization-review programs, inventory management, and cost-effective patient ser-vices.

Manufacturers and Suppliers. Criteria for selecting drug product manufacturers and suppliers should be established by the pharmacy to ensure the quality of drug products and the best prices.

Reimbursement. The manager of the pharmaceutical services or home care organization should be knowledgeable about reimbursements for home care pharmaceutical services, medications, supplies, durable medical equipment, and, if applicable, nursing services support. Processes should exist for routine verification of patient reimbursement benefits and for counseling patients about their anticipated financial responsibility for planned therapies. A process should also exist for responding to service requests from medically indigent patients.

Managing Pharmaceutical Care

Committee Involvement. A pharmacist should be a member of and actively participate on committees responsible for establishing policies and procedures for medication use, patient care, and performance improvement, among other things. Also, pharmacists should participate in the activities of similar committees of a parent home care organization or health system, as applicable.

Medication Therapy decisions. The pharmacist's prerogatives to initiate, monitor, and modify medication therapy for individual patients, consistent with laws, regulations, home care organization policy, and clinical protocols, should be clearly delineated and approved by the home care organization's authorized leadership.

Selection of Medications. Policies and procedures addressing the selection of medications should be available. These policies should be based on clinical appropriateness.

Home Care Medical Record Systems. Clinical actions and recommendations by pharmacists that are intended to ensure safe and effective use of medications and that have a potential effect on patient outcomes should be documented in patients' home care medical records. In addition, a patient medication profile should be maintained by all home care pharmacies regardless of where the dispensing of medications takes place. The home care medical record should include progress notes, laboratory test results, and other patient information related to determining the appropriateness of medications and monitoring their effects. The system should provide safeguards against the improper manipulation or alteration of records and provide an audit trail. An automated information system is preferred, but the system may be either manual or automated. If an automated information system is used, an auxiliary record-keeping procedure should be available for documenting medication information in case the automated system is inoperative.

Medication Histories. Pharmacists should prepare or have access to comprehensive medication histories for each patient's home care medical record and other databases (e.g., prescription and nonprescription medication profile), or both. A pharmacist-conducted medication history for each patient is desirable; however, a home care nurse may obtain and maintain current medication histories, provided this information is accessible to the pharmacist and other health care providers.

Patient Confidentiality. Patient confidentiality should be protected by safeguarding access to all sources of patient information, including financial (billing), medication profiles, and home care medical records. Patient information should

be shared only with health care providers within the home care pharmacy, home care organization, or health system authorized to care for the patient. Written policies and procedures for access to and dissemination of confidential patient information should be available. All employees should respect patient privacy and maintain confidentiality during home visits and deliveries.

Clinical Protocols. The pharmacist should be involved in the home care organization's initiatives to develop model clinical protocols, care plans, pathways, or disease management guidelines to ensure that pharmaceutical care elements are included. Clinical protocols should be used whenever appropriate to maximize the safety of medication use in the home.

Preventive and Postexposure Immunization Programs. The pharmacy should participate in the development of policies and procedures concerning preventive and postexposure programs for infectious diseases (including, but not limited to, HIV infection, tuberculosis, and hepatitis) for patients and employees.

Substance-Abuse Programs. The pharmacy should assist in the development of, and participate in, substance-abuse prevention, education, and employee and patient assistance programs.

Twenty-Four-Hour Pharmaceutical Services. Home care pharmaceutical services should be available 24 hours a day, seven days a week. A pharmacist should be available for consultation or dispensing after hours. Home care pharmacy staff may be supplemented by knowledgeable and experienced part-time or on-call personnel to extend pharmaceutical services coverage.

Pharmacy Security and Access After Hours. Only authorized pharmacy personnel should have access to the pharmacy area. Other home care organization personnel may be in the pharmacy area only when an authorized pharmacist is present, in accordance with the home care organization's policies or as required by laws and regulations. In an emergency situation in which a pharmacist is not present, such as a fire or security alarm, policies and procedures should guide safe access to the pharmacy area and provide for notification of the pharmacist in charge or a designee.

Disaster Situations. Policies and procedures should be available for providing pharmaceutical services in case of an areawide disaster affecting the home care pharmacy or patients' home care settings. Patients should be informed about what to do to safely continue needed home therapies in the event of a disaster.

Institutional Review Board. The manager of the pharmacy, or a designee, should be a member of the home care organization's or health system's institutional review board.

Managing Human Resources

Work Schedules and Assignments. The pharmacy manager should ensure that work schedules, procedures, and assignments make the best use of pharmacy personnel and other resources. Resources should be sufficient to ensure patient safety.

Position Descriptions. The responsibilities and related competencies for home care pharmacy employees should be clearly defined in written position descriptions for all job categories.

Performance Evaluation. Policies and procedures should define the ongoing performance evaluations of home care pharmacy personnel. All home care pharmacy personnel should receive regular and timely evaluations. Performance should be evaluated on the basis of position description requirements and expected competencies.

Support Personnel. Sufficient support personnel (pharmacy technicians and customer service, procurement, delivery, clerical, and administrative personnel) should be available to facilitate the delivery of pharmaceutical care and services. Pharmacy technician certification by the Pharmacy Technician Certification Board is desirable; alternatively, technicians should complete an equivalent state-approved pharmacy technician training program, if available. Appropriate supervisory controls should be maintained and documented consistent with federal and state laws and regulations.

Education and Training. All personnel should possess the education and training needed to fulfill their responsibilities, including specific knowledge related to home care. All personnel should participate in continuing-education programs and activities relevant to home care practice as necessary to maintain or enhance their competence.

Recruitment and Selection of Personnel. Personnel should be recruited and selected on the basis of the requirements in the established job descriptions and candidates' job-related qualifications and prior performance. The pharmacy manager should assist in identifying the relevant professional and technical qualifications and should participate in candidate interviews and selections.

Orientation of Personnel. There should be an established procedure for orienting new and current personnel to the pharmacy, the home care organization, the health systems that the home care pharmacy serves, respective positions, relevant home care services, community resources, and the parent organization.

Managing Performance Improvement

Performance Improvement. There should be an ongoing, systematic program for assessing the delivery of pharmaceutical care and services. Performance improvement activities based on assessments should be integrated with the home care organization's or health system's overall performance improvement activities. Operational and outcomes data should be benchmarked with those of other home care pharmacies of similar size and scope. Outcomes, including follow-up actions, of performance improvement efforts should be documented and provided to the home care organization's managers and others, as appropriate.

Medication-Use Evaluation. An ongoing medication-use-evaluation program should be in place to ensure that medications are used appropriately, safely, and effectively.

Adverse Drug Reactions. An ongoing program should be in place for monitoring, reporting, and preventing adverse drug

reactions. The pharmacist should submit reports of adverse drug reactions to FDA's MedWatch program and the drug's manufacturer, as appropriate.

Medication Errors. The home care organization should have an ongoing program to prevent medication errors. Pharmacists, physicians, nurses, and other appropriate home care personnel should monitor for and document medication errors. The home care organization should analyze the causes of medi-cation errors and implement corrective actions. Medication errors should be reported to voluntary national reporting systems and, as required, to accrediting organizations.

Drug Product Recalls. Procedures should be in place for responding to drug and device product recalls, for identifying patients who received or used a recalled product, and for removing the drug or device product from the pharmacy or home when the recall is at the user level.

Standard 2: Drug Information, Education, and Counseling

The home care pharmacist should provide accurate, comprehensive general and patient-specific drug information to patients, caregivers, other pharmacists, physicians, nurses, and other health care providers, as appropriate, in response to requests, in the delivery of pharmaceutical care, or through educational programs. Physicians and nurses should receive adequate information about a medication's therapeutic use, dosage, potential adverse effects, and safe administration in the home—in particular, stability requirements—before the medication is administered.

Information about the stability of drugs for home infusion should include administration via a variety of alternative delivery devices. These may include portable infusion pumps, syringe pumps, implantable infusion devices, and common peripheral and central-line administration.

Up-to-date drug information resources should be available in the home care pharmacy, including current periodicals, the latest editions of drug compendiums and textbooks in appropriate pharmaceutical and biomedical subject areas, and any references required by state boards of pharmacy. Availability of drug information on electronic media is desirable. Information may be accessed and provided in conjunction with medical libraries and other resources.

Drug Information Requests. Responses to general and patient-specific drug information requests should be accurate and prompt. Drug information requests and responses should be documented and monitored for accuracy and timeliness as part of performance improvement activities.

Patient Education and Counseling. Home care pharmacists should be available for and actively participate in patient education and counseling. The pharmacist is responsible for ensuring that the patient and, as appropriate, the caregiver receive information, are counseled, and understand the patient's medication therapy. Patient education and counseling should be coordinated with the patient's other health care providers. The content and form of the education and counseling should be specific to the patient's assessed needs, abilities, and readiness, consistent with care plans and services provided. Patient and caregiver compliance, understanding,

knowledge, and skills should be periodically reassessed. A home care pharmacist should be readily accessible to patients and caregivers if questions arise. Patient education and counseling should be performed in accordance with applicable federal and state laws and regulations and documented in the patient's home care record.

Medication Teaching Materials. Educational material tailored to the patient and the medication therapy should be provided to the patient and the caregiver for use at home. Specifically, medication teaching materials for drugs most often used in home care practice should be available for dissemination to patients, caregivers, and other health care providers. These materials should be based on information most appropriate for safe medication use in the home. Educational materials should contain, but not be limited to, the following: name and description of the medication; usual dose; dosage interval; duration of therapy; goals of drug therapy; importance of compliance; proper aseptic technique in preparation for use (if applicable); proper administration of medication; inspection of medication, containers, and related supplies before use; common severe adverse effects, drug–drug interactions, drug–nutrient interactions, and their management; proper use of medication-related equipment and supplies; emergency-response instructions; instructions for storing, handling, and disposing of the drug; and procedures to follow if a dose is missed.

Dissemination of Drug Information. Pharmacists should keep the home care organization's staff informed about the use of medications on an ongoing basis through appropriate consultations, publications, and presentations. Pharmacists should ensure the timely dissemination of drug product recall notices, safety alerts, market withdrawals, and labeling changes.

Pharmacist Consultations. Pharmacists should provide oral or written consultations to other health professionals regarding medication therapy selection and management. Consultations should be documented in the patient's home care medical record.

Investigational Drug Information. The home care pharmacist should have access to information on all investigational studies and similar research projects involving medications and medication-related devices used in the home care, hospital, or alternate-site setting. The pharmacist should provide pertinent written information (to the extent such information exists) about the safe and proper use of investigational drugs, including possible adverse effects and adverse drug reactions, to nurses, pharmacists, physicians, and other health care providers participating in clinical drug research.

Standard 3: Care Planning, Monitoring, and Continuity

An important aspect of pharmaceutical care is optimizing medication use for individual patients. This should include processes designed to ensure the safe and effective use of medications and to increase the probability of desired patient outcomes. The pharmacist, in collaboration with the patient, caregiver, physician, nurse, and other health care providers, should be responsible for developing an individualized care plan for each patient.

Care Plan. The care plan should be based on information obtained from the initial pharmacy assessment and other relevant information obtained from the patient, caregiver, physician, nurse, and other health care providers. At a minimum, the plan should include actual or potential medication therapy problems and proposed solutions, desired outcomes or goals of the medication therapy, and the objective and subjective parameters for monitoring outcomes or goals and medication therapy-related problems. The plan should be developed at the initiation of medication therapy, reviewed, and updated, if necessary, on a regular basis according to the home care organization's policies. The degree of detail of the plan should be based on the complexity of the patient's health problems and drug therapy. The pharmacist is responsible for ensuring that the medication therapy (pharmaceutical care) elements of the plan are communicated to appropriate parties involved in the patient's care. All the patient's health care providers should routinely share care plan information and actions. The plans and updates should be a part of the patient's home care medical record.

Initial Patient Assessment. The pharmacist should ensure that each patient referral for home care is assessed for appropriateness on the basis of formal, predetermined admission criteria, as outlined in the ASHP Guidelines on the Pharmacist's Role in Home Care.[1] Before the start of home care services, patients should be informed of their rights and responsibilities. These should be explained in detail and given in writing to the patient and a family member or other caregiver. Once a patient is accepted for home care services, but before the initiation of therapy, the organization should ensure that the patient's current clinical status, home environment, and support systems are assessed. A thorough pa-tient database should be prepared to identify pharmaceutical care needs and to provide the basis for ongoing medication therapy monitoring and for measuring patient outcomes. The patient database should be documented in the patient's home care medical record. Information that minimally should be included in the database is outlined in the ASHP Guidelines on the Pharmacist's Role in Home Care.[1] Information for the database can be gathered from the past and current medical record; laboratory test results; direct communication with the patient, caregiver, physician, nurse, and other health care providers; and the home care pharmacist's direct observations.

Medication Orders. Medication orders should be assessed by a pharmacist before the first dose is dispensed. A pharmacist should receive the physician's order. If not received by a pharmacist, the order should be verified by a pharmacist. The pharmacist should assess the order for the following:

1. Therapeutic appropriateness of the patient's medication regimen,
2. Therapeutic duplication in the patient's medication regimen,
3. Appropriateness of the route and method of administration of the medication,
4. Drug–drug, drug–nutrient, drug–laboratory test, and drug–disease interactions, and
5. Clinical and pharmacokinetic laboratory data for evaluating the efficacy of medication therapy and anticipating toxicity and adverse effects.

Any questions about the order should be resolved with the prescriber, and a written notation should be made in the patient's home care medical record or pharmacy copy of the prescriber's order. Information concerning changes should be communicated to the patient's other health care providers.

First-Dose Precautions. The pharmacist, in collaboration with other health care providers, should assess whether a first dose of a medication can be safely administered in the home or whether the patient should be referred to an alternative treatment site for the initiation of therapy. Policies and procedures should outline the situations and therapies for which medications for treating anaphylaxis should be dispensed so that the pharmacist can ensure that the appropriate medications are available when a first dose is to be administered.

Patient Education and Counseling. The home care pharmacist, or the nurse as the agent, should ensure that the patient, the caregiver, and other health care providers understand the proper use and administration of medications, including the intravenous access device and infusion device, as required. The home care pharmacist, or the nurse as the agent, should explain to the patient or the patient's agent the directions for use and any additional information. Also, prescriptions delivered outside the confines of the pharmacy should be discussed.

Medication Therapy Monitoring. After the initiation of medication therapy, the pharmacist collects and reviews data from physical and nutritional assessments, laboratory tests, and oral communication with the patient, caregiver, nurse, and physician (1) to evaluate the clinical status of the patient and the response to medication therapy, (2) to determine whether the patient's pharmaceutical care needs are being met, and (3) to ascertain whether the care plan designed for the patient is effective. The monitoring plan, which should be detailed in the care plan, guides medication therapy-monitoring activities and facilitates evaluation of the patient's progress by the pharmacist. Additionally, the pharmacist should, in collaboration with other professional staff members, monitor the following:

1. Functional status of the drug delivery system,
2. Patient utilization of medications, supplies, and equipment,
3. Patient compliance with the prescribed regimen,
4. Patient adaptation to delivery of care in the home, and
5. Patient satisfaction with the care and service delivered.

If the patient is responding and has no new identified pharmaceutical care needs or medication-related problems, but has not completed the course of therapy, pharmaceutical services should be continued as planned. If it is determined that the patient is not responding, or if new medication-related problems are identified, the plan should be revised and implemented.

Medical Emergencies. The home care pharmacist should participate in decisions about the emergency care of patients at home, including the development of protocols for using emergency drugs in the home.

Documentation of Pharmaceutical Care and Outcomes. The pharmacy should have an ongoing process for consistent documentation (and reporting to physicians, administrators, and others) of pharmaceutical care and patient outcomes resulting

from medication therapy and other pharmacy actions. Patient privacy and confidentiality must be protected at all times.

Continuity of Care. The pharmacist should routinely contribute to processes ensuring that each patient receives pharmaceutical care regardless of transitions that occur across different health care settings (for example, among different components of a health system and different types of home care services). When home care patients are admitted to a hospital, the home care pharmacy should inform the hospital about (1) the medications the patient is currently receiving from the home care pharmacy and (2) known allergies. The home care pharmacy should recognize hospital policy when considering whether properly stored medications and medical equipment from the home can be used during the home care patient's hospitalization.

Standard 4: Medication Distribution and Control

The home care pharmacy should be responsible for the procurement, storage, distribution, and control of all drug products it dispenses (including medication-related devices and pharmaceutical diagnostics). Policies and procedures governing these functions should be developed by the pharmacy manager in collaboration with other appropriate home care organization staff members.

Processing the Medication Order

Medication Orders. All patient medication orders should be documented in the patient's home care medical record. The home care pharmacist should obtain a signed original of the prescriber's order, a direct copy of the prescriber's order, an oral order from the prescriber or his authorized agent, or an electronically transmitted, prescriber-entered order consistent with applicable laws and regulations. Safeguards should be in place to ensure the security of electronically transmitted prescriber orders. All medication orders should be reviewed by a pharmacist and assessed in relation to the medication profile and, as appropriate, an established procedure for using an approved list of medications for specific treatment circumstances and emergencies. A system should exist to ensure that medication orders are not inappropriately continued.

Prescribing. Policies and procedures should be available to ensure that heath care providers meet applicable state licensure and home care organization authorization, if required, for prescribing medications. The pharmacy should advocate and foster conformance with standardized, approved terminology and abbreviations when medications are being prescribed.

Therapeutic Purpose. Prescribers should be encouraged to routinely communicate the condition being treated or the therapeutic purpose of medications with all prescription and medication orders.

Preparing, Packaging, and Labeling Medications

Sterile Products. Home care pharmacists are responsible for ensuring the quality of sterile products intended for use in the home. Guidance is available for developing an

adequately designed and equipped facility, training and validating employees, validating and documenting compounding procedures, practicing aseptic technique, monitoring the work environment, maintaining the facility and equipment, ensuring the quality of prepared products, and developing policies and procedures.[2,3]

Beyond-Use Dating. Home care pharmacies are often required to assign extended beyond-use dates to sterile products so that a multiple-day supply of medications can be dispensed and delivered. However, pharmacists should take into account circumstances that may affect the medication's potency and stability, including (1) delivery of sterile products to the home, either by the pharmacy's own vehicles or by a common carrier, (2) storage of sterile products in the home before use, (3) manipulation of sterile products in the home environment to add ingredients (such as vitamins) and to set up tubing and filters for administration, and (4) administration of products at temperatures that are warmer than controlled room temperature because of administration in outdoor or non-air-conditioned environments or the use of ambulatory infusion pumps worn close to the body.

Beyond-use dates should be based on the manufacturer's approved product labeling; however, information about the long-term stability of products for home use may not be included in the labeling. In addition, information may not accurately reflect the product's intended conditions of use in home care, including the concentration, diluent, container, and infusion conditions. The home care pharmacist should either consult the manufacturer for an appropriate beyond-use date or determine the date by reviewing the literature. Applying published stability data can introduce inaccuracies if the intended conditions of use differ greatly from the reported conditions. Pharmacists should maintain a record of the resources used for establishing beyond-use dates. A table or chart of accepted beyond-use dates, formulations, and conditions of use for commonly prepared products may be helpful in ensuring that assigned dates are consistent and appropriate. Patients should be trained to check products for current beyond-use dates prior to their use.

Packaging for Home Delivery. Products should be delivered in appropriate packaging to ensure that labeled storage requirements are met during transit under the expected environmental conditions. The pharmacy should develop and follow written procedures for packaging; these procedures should include privacy-protection considerations. Product confirmation after delivery should be used to ensure that the packaging procedures and materials used were effective in maintaining product integrity and temperature control during transit.

The stability of refrigerated products at room temperature should be taken into account when in the development of packaging procedures. A few refrigerated products have extended stability at room temperature and may be safely delivered without refrigerated packaging. Products that are stable for 24 hours or less at room temperature should always be delivered in temperature-controlled packaging (coolers, ice packs, etc.).

Labeling. Medications for home use should be labeled so that patients and caregivers can easily understand instructions for drug storage, preparation, and administration. Auxiliary labels should be used as necessary. When manipulation of medications is required before administration, labeling should clearly

state current contents and the steps for measuring, reconstituting, or adding other ingredients. Labels for compounded medications should state the total content of the medication or nutrient per container so that it can be clearly known in case the patient is transferred to another treatment setting.[4] If medications are to be administered with an infusion device, pump settings should be included on the label.

Delivery and Handling of Medications in the Patient's Home

Delivery. Policies and procedures should be available to ensure product integrity and temperature control during home delivery or patient pickup of supplies and drugs. Delivery to the patient should include inventory management to avoid excessive accumulation of supplies and drugs. Excesses may indicate poor compliance, inadequate patient training, failure to assess patient needs, or ineffective inventory management by the patient.

When common carriers are used, the pharmacy is responsible for ensuring that the carrier can provide timely delivery, proper handling, and external temperature control. Delivery personnel should know the shipping requirements for each package. If refrigerated products are packaged so that product labels containing storage instructions are concealed, an exterior "Refrigerate" label should be used. To protect patient confidentiality, prescription labels with medication names and directions should not be used to label boxes. Box labels should include only the patient's name and address, the storage requirements, and delivery instructions.

Additional precautions (such as double bagging [including at least one leakproof container] and cushioning) should be used to safeguard hazardous products from breaking and leaking. The delivery person, patient, and caregiver must be trained to recognize and manage accidental spills. Packages containing hazardous products should have appropriate precautionary labels.

Universal Precautions in Patients' Homes. Home care pharmacy personnel delivering medications or supplies to patients' homes should use universal precautions. Patients and caregivers should be instructed on the application of universal precautions in the home. The provision of instructions on universal precautions, as well as the provision of other information and counseling, should be documented. Personnel should always wash their hands before assisting patients with the handling of supplies in the home.

Storage in the Home. The pharmacy should take precautions to ensure that medications are properly stored with respect to temperature, light, and other labeled storage conditions. If sterile or other products require refrigeration, appropriate methods should be used to segregate them from food to avoid contaminating the outside of the container. Patients, caregivers, or delivery personnel should be trained to check the refrigerator on a regular basis to determine whether temperatures are within an acceptable range to ensure product integrity. If the patient does not have an appropriate environment for storage of medications, the pharmacy should make alternative arrangements so that medications are properly stored. Drugs and supplies that do not require refrigeration should be stored in a separate, restricted location not accessible to children and pets.

Waste Disposal. Patients receiving hazardous drugs in the home should be instructed in proper waste-disposal methods that comply with federal and state laws and regulations. Needles and other sharps should be placed in appropriate disposal containers, and a process should be established for the safe removal and disposal of the waste. Local codes may have specific disposal requirements.

Medication Administration. Policies and procedures on the administration of medications should be available. Only personnel who are authorized by the home care organization and are appropriately trained should be permitted to administer medications to a patient. Pharmacists, where legally permitted, may be authorized to administer medications after receiving appropriate training.

The Patient's Own Medications. Drug products and related devices not dispensed by the home care pharmacy that are to be used during the patient's course of therapy should be documented in the patient's home care medical record. When home care patients are admitted to a hospital, the home care pharmacy should inform the hospital about the medications the patient is currently receiving from the home care pharmacy and about any known allergies. The home care pharmacy should recognize hospital policy when considering whether properly stored medications and medical equipment from the home can be used during the home care patient's hospitalization.

Drug Samples. The use of drug samples should be eliminated to the fullest extent possible. However, if samples are permitted, the pharmacy should control these products to ensure proper storage, records, labeling, and product integrity.

Controlling Certain Categories of Medications

Cytotoxic and Hazardous Drug Products. Policies and procedures for storing, handling, and disposing of cytotoxic and other hazardous drug products should be available to ensure patient and employee safety in compliance with applicable local, state, and federal laws and regulations. Employees should be specially trained, and their handling and disposal of these products should be monitored. Spill kits should be available.[4]

Controlled Substances. Policies and procedures for the storage, distribution, use, and accountability of controlled substances should be available to ensure appropriate use and to prevent diversion in compliance with applicable local, state, and federal laws and regulations.

Investigational Drugs. Policies and procedures for the safe and proper use of investigational drugs should be established and followed. The pharmacy should be responsible for overseeing the distribution and control of all investigational drugs. Investigational drugs should be dispensed and administered to consenting patients in accordance with an approved protocol. Home care pharmacists should initiate, participate in, and support medical and pharmaceutical research appropriate to the goals, objectives, and resources of the home care organization.

Standard 5: Facilities, Equipment, and Information Resources

To ensure optimal operational performance and quality patient care, adequate space, equipment, and supplies should be available for all professional and administrative functions related to medication use. These resources should be located in areas that facilitate the provision of services to patients, nurses, prescribers, and other health care providers and should be integrated with the home care organization's communication and delivery or transportation systems. Facilities should be constructed, arranged, and equipped to promote safe and efficient work and to avoid damage to or deterioration of drug products.

Medication Storage and Preparation. Facilities should be available for storing and preparing medications in the home care pharmacy under proper conditions of sanitation, temperature, light, moisture, ventilation, segregation, and security to ensure medication integrity and personnel safety and to prevent drug diversion. Adequate refrigeration and freezer capacity should be provided within the secure pharmacy area.

Medication Storage Area Inspections. All stocks of medications stored in the home care pharmacy or in the organization's facilities should be inspected routinely to ensure the absence of recalled, outdated, unusable, or mislabeled products. Inspections should include storage conditions that would compromise medication integrity, storage arrangements that might contribute to medication errors, and storage locations that might be vulnerable to drug diversion efforts.

Compounding and Packaging. Designated space and equipment for compounding and packaging sterile and nonsterile drug products should be available.[2,5] The compounding environment should be monitored and maintained on an ongoing basis.

Cytotoxic and Hazardous Drug Products. Appropriate facility space, equipment, and supplies for compounding cytotoxic and hazardous drug products should be available (to include a biological safety cabinet, spill kits, eye-washing station, and protective garb).[6]

Drug Information. Adequate space, resources, and information handling and communication technology should be available to facilitate the provision of drug and related information to patients, caregivers, health care providers, multidisciplinary team members, and referring physicians.

Pharmacist–Patient Consultation. Home care pharmacists will primarily consult patients or caregivers over the telephone. Home visits should be considered for enhancing compliance or simplifying complex drug-related patient issues.

Office and Meeting Space. Office and meeting areas should be available for administrative, clinical, technical, and reimbursement staff. Ideally, interdisciplinary team members from pharmacy, nursing, and reimbursement are located within a proximate space. Sufficient educational and training activities should be established. Adequate facilities and equipment should be established for decontaminating, cleaning, and maintaining infusion devices, including durable medical equipment.

Drug Delivery Systems, Administration Devices, and Automated Dispensing Devices. Home care pharmacists should provide leadership and advice in organizational and clinical decisions about the selection of drug delivery systems, administration devices, and automated compounding and dispensing devices and should participate in the evaluation, use, and monitoring of these systems and devices. The potential for medication errors associated with such systems and devices must be thoroughly evaluated. Policies and procedures should be available for the certification (calibration) and maintenance of equipment and devices. Equipment should be adequately maintained and certified in compliance with applicable standards, laws, and regulations. Equipment maintenance and certification should be documented.

Record Maintenance. Adequate space should be available for maintaining and storing records, including medication profiles and other patient information, management information, equipment maintenance sheets, controlled-substances inventory sheets, and material safety data sheets, among others, to ensure compliance with laws, regulations, accreditation requirements, and sound management practices. Appropriate licenses, permits, and tax stamps should be available.

Information Technology. Computer resources should be used to maintain patient medication profiles, perform necessary patient billing procedures, manage drug product inventories, and interface with other available computerized systems to obtain patient-specific clinical information for drug therapy monitoring and other clinical functions and to facilitate the continuity of care after patients transfer to and from other care settings.

References

1. American Society of Hospital Pharmacists. ASHP guidelines on the pharmacist's role in home care. *Am J Hosp Pharm.* 1993; 50:1940–4.
2. American Society of Hospital Pharmacists. ASHP technical assistance bulletin on quality assurance for pharmacy-prepared sterile products. *Am J Hosp Pharm.* 1993; 50:2386–98.
3. The United States pharmacopeia, 23rd rev., and The national formulary, 18th ed. Rockville, MD: United States Pharmacopeial Convention; 1994:1963–75.
4. Mirtallo J, Driscoll D, Helms R, et al. Safe practices for parenteral nutrition feeding formulations. *JPEN J Parenter Enteral Nutr.* 1998; 22:49–66.
5. American Society of Hospital Pharmacists. ASHP technical assistance bulletin on compounding nonsterile products in pharmacies. *Am J Hosp Pharm.* 1994; 51:1441–8.
6. American Society of Hospital Pharmacists. ASHP guidelines on handling cytotoxic and hazardous drugs. *Am J Hosp Pharm.* 1990; 47:1033–49.

Suggested Reading

1. Monk-Tutor MR. The U.S. home infusion market. *Am J Health-Syst Pharm.* 1998; 55:2019–25.

2. Monk-Tutor MR. Home care practice as a model for providing pharmaceutical care. *Am J Health-Syst Pharm.* 1998; 55:486–90.

3. Andrusko-Furphy KT. Oryx and performance measurement in home care. *Am J Health-Syst Pharm.* 1998; 55:2299–301.

4. Scheckelhoff K. Understanding the dynamics of the integrated health system. *Infusion.* 1997; 3(Apr):18–22.

5. Haidar TA, Grillo JA. An interdisciplinary critical pathway for home intravenous antibiotic therapies. *Infusion.* 1997; 3(Apr): 38–50.

6. Bemus AM, Lindley CM, Sawyer WT, et al. Task analysis of home care pharmacy. *Am J Health-Syst Pharm.* 1996; 53:2831–9.

7. Andrusko-Furphy K. Why does home care require so much documentation? *Consult Pharm.* 1994; 9:581–2.

8. McPherson ML, Ferris R. Establishing a home health care consulting practice. *Am Pharm.* 1994; NS34 (Feb):42–9.

Approved by the ASHP Board of Directors, November 14, 1998. Developed by the ASHP Council on Professional Affairs.

Barbara McKinnon, Pharm.D., Karen E. Bertch, Pharm.D., Lawrence P. Carey, Pharm. D., Terry D. Leach, Larry D. Pelham, M.S., FASHP, Brian G. Swift, Pharm.D., and J. Scott Reid, Pharm.D., are gratefully acknowledged for drafting this document.

The bibliographic citation for this document is as follows: American Society of Health-System Pharmacists. ASHP guidelines on minimum standards for home care pharmacists. *Am J Health-Syst Pharm.* 1999; 56:629–38.

ASHP Guidelines: Minimum Standard for Pharmaceutical Services in Ambulatory Care

In recent years there has been an increasing emphasis in health care on the provision of ambulatory care services. This shift away from acute hospital care is due to several factors. Managed care has created incentives to decrease hospitalization rates and length of stay. The number of elderly patients with multiple chronic medical conditions that require longitudinal management is growing. There is more focus in medicine on preventive health and patient education. Appropriate medication therapy in the ambulatory care setting is often the most common and most cost effective form of treatment, yet the clinical, humanistic, and economic consequences of adverse drug events and the inappropriate use of medications in this setting could be catastrophic.[1] As providers of pharmaceutical care to patients in the ambulatory care setting, pharmacists should be concerned with and take responsibility for the outcomes of their services in addition to the provision of these services.

The provision of pharmaceutical services for ambulatory patients occurs in a variety of settings including free-standing pharmacies, ambulatory clinics, hospital outpatient departments, assisted living centers, and others. Pharmacists in ambulatory care settings could also provide some aspects of pharmaceutical services to patients through a mail-order prescription service, patients receiving home care, and patients residing in long-term care and other extended-care settings. Organizational arrangements may vary with the pharmaceutical services operating independently, or as components in local health care organizations that may be independent or affiliated with larger local and regional health systems.[2,3] Furthermore, in some settings the delivery of pharmaceutical care may be independent and separated from distributive services. For brevity, these guidelines will use the terms pharmaceutical services and organizations to imply any arrangement.

The primary purpose of these guidelines is to outline the minimum requirements for the operation and management of pharmaceutical services for patients in the ambulatory care setting. Pharmaceutical services, especially the provision of pharmaceutical care, in the ambulatory care setting should be coordinated among other settings, therefore, these guidelines should be used, as applicable, in conjunction with minimum standards for other practice settings. Rather than including detailed advice in this document, readers should refer to other ASHP documents that address many of the topics outlined for additional information and guidance. Because of differences in settings and organizational arrangements and complexity, aspects of these guidelines may not be applicable in some settings. Ambulatory care pharmacists should use their professional judgement in assessing and adapting these guidelines to meet the needs of their own practice settings.

In circumstances where a pharmacy or network of pharmacies are contracted to provide pharmaceutical services to the organization's patients, the following minimal standards should be incorporated into contract language.

The criteria for pharmaceutical services in the ambulatory care setting that are covered in these guidelines are distributed among the following categories: (1) leadership and practice management, (2) medication therapy and pharmaceutical care, (3) drug distribution and control, and (4) facilities, equipment, and other resources. Collectively, the criteria represent a minimum level of quality that pharmaceutical services for ambulatory patients should strive to provide on a consistent basis. While the scope of pharmaceutical services will likely vary from site to site, depending upon the needs of the patients served, the criteria are strongly linked to patient outcomes and neglect in any one may compromise quality.

Standard I: Leadership and Practice Management

Effective leadership and practice management skills are necessary for the delivery of pharmaceutical services in a manner consistent with the organization's and patients' needs and for the continuous improvement in patient care outcomes. Pharmaceutical service management should focus on the pharmacist's responsibility to provide pharmaceutical care and the development of the personnel, facilities, and other resources to support that responsibility. The guidelines use the term, director of ambulatory care pharmaceutical services or, director, to indicate the person responsible for managing services. Depending on the health care organization's structure and other factors, designations such as manager, pharmacist-in-charge, or responsible pharmacists are used.

The director of ambulatory care pharmaceutical services should be responsible for (1) setting the short- and long-term goals of the pharmacy based on the needs of the patients served, the specific needs of the pharmacy (and any organizational arrangement of which the pharmaceutical services may be a component), and developments and trends in health care and ambulatory care pharmacy practice, (2) developing plans and schedules for achieving these goals, (3) directing the implementation of the plans and the day-to-day activities associated with them, (4) determining whether the goals and schedule are being met, and (5) instituting corrective actions where necessary.[4,5] The director, in carrying out the aforementioned responsibilities, should employ an adequate number of competent, qualified personnel.

Managing Pharmaceutical Services

Education and Training, Director. Pharmaceutical services should be managed by a professionally competent, legally qualified pharmacist. The director of the ambulatory care pharmaceutical service should be thoroughly knowledgeable about and have experience in ambulatory care pharmacy practice and management. The director should have completed an applicable accredited pharmacy residency program or have equivalent training and experience. Completion of an advanced management degree (e.g., M.B.A., M.H.A., M.S.) and/or practice management residency is desirable.

Mission. The pharmaceutical service should have a written mission statement that, at a minimum, reflects patient care

and customer service responsibilities and, if applicable, is consistent with the mission of the organization of which the pharmacy may be a component. The mission should be understood by every employee and other participants (e.g., students and residents) involved with the pharmacy's activities. The development and prioritization of goals, objectives, and work tasks should be consistent with the mission statement.

Laws and Regulations. Compliance with local, state, and federal laws and regulations applicable to pharmaceutical services in the ambulatory care setting is required. The pharmacy shall maintain written or computerized documentation of compliance with requirements concerning procurement and distribution of drug products, patient information, and related safety from the board of pharmacy, Food and Drug Administration, Drug Enforcement Administration, Health Care Financing Administration, Occupational Health and Safety Administration, among others. Ambulatory care pharmacies dispensing medications across state boundaries shall comply with out-of-state licensure requirements, as well as other state and federal interstate laws and regulations.

Policies and Procedures Manual. A policies and procedures manual governing the scope of ambulatory care pharmaceutical services (e.g., administrative, operational, and clinical) should be available and properly maintained. The manual should be reviewed and revised annually or whenever necessary to reflect changes in policies and procedures, scope of services, organizational arrangements, and other factors. All personnel should be familiar with the contents of the manual. Appropriate mechanisms should be established to ensure compliance with the policies and procedures.

Practice Standards and Guidelines. The practice standards and guidelines of the American Society of Health-System Pharmacists, the National Committee on Quality Assurance (NCQA), the Health Plan Employer Data and Information Set (HEDIS), and the Joint Commission on Accreditation of Healthcare Organizations (JCAHO) or other appropriate accrediting body should be assessed and adapted, as applicable. The pharmacy should strive to meet these standards regardless of the particular financial and organizational arrangements by which pharmaceutical services are provided to the organization and its patients.

Managing the Medication-Use Process

Medication-Use Policy Development. Medication-use policy decisions should be based on clinical, quality-of-life, and pharmacoeconomic factors that result in optimal patient care. Committees within the organization (e.g., pharmacy and therapeutics, infection control) that make decisions concerning medication use should include the active and direct involvement of physicians, pharmacists, and other appropriate health care professionals. The pharmacy should prepare and present to these committees drug product evaluation reports that consider all aspects of safety, effectiveness, and cost.

Clinical Care Plans and Disease State Management. Pharmacists should be involved as part of an interdisciplinary team in the development and implementation of clinical care plans (clinical practice guidelines, critical pathways) and disease state management programs involving medication therapy, collaborative care agreements, and treatment protocols. Emphasis should be placed on clinical care plans, primary care, and medication treatment protocols that cover dosage calculations and limits, and use of medications frequently associated with adverse events, including medication errors.[6,7] Primary care protocols should consider whole patient needs for health promotion and disease prevention measures as well as appropriate patient assessments, management of medication-related care problems, and referrals for acute medical care. The targeting of diseases should consider the prevalence of the disease in the population served by the organization and the potential for impact on clinical and economic outcomes.[8]

Drug Information. Pharmacists should provide accurate, comprehensive, general and patient-specific drug information to patients, caregivers, other pharmacists, physicians, nurses, and other health care providers, as appropriate, in response to requests, in the delivery of pharmaceutical care, or through educational programs and publications.

Drug information sources should include current professional and scientific periodicals and the latest editions of textbooks in appropriate pharmaceutical and biomedical subject areas. Available information sources should support research on patient care issues and facilitate provision of pharmaceutical care and safety in the medication-use process. This information may be accessed in conjunction with medical libraries and other available resources. Appropriate drug information sources should be readily accessible to professional staff.

If applicable, pharmacists should have access to information on all investigational studies and similar research projects involving medications and medication-related devices used by the organization. Pharmacists should provide pertinent written information (to the extent known) about the safe and proper use of investigational drugs, including possible adverse effects, to nurses, pharmacists, physicians, and other health care providers involved in the care of patients admitted to the investigational drug protocols.

Development of Patient Care Services. Pharmacists should be involved in the development, implementation, and evaluation of new or changing patient care services within the organization, such as the development of new clinic or office sites. These efforts should promote the continuity of pharmaceutical care across the continuum of care, practice settings, and geographically dispersed facilities.

Preventive and Postexposure Immunization Programs. The pharmacy should participate in the development of policies and procedures concerning preventive and postexposure programs for infectious diseases (including, but not limited to, HIV, tuberculosis, and hepatitis) for patients and employees. As appropriate, pharmacists should promote the use of and may administer immunizations, when legally allowed.

Substance-Abuse Programs. The pharmacy should assist in the development of and participate in the organization's substance-abuse prevention, education, and employee and patient assistance programs.

Medical Emergencies. The pharmacy should participate in the development of policies and procedures to ensure the availabil-

ity, access, and security of emergency medications, including antidotes. Appropriately trained pharmacists should have an authorized role in responding to medical emergencies.

Institutional Review Board. Pharmacist's membership on the organization's institutional review board is preferred depending on the prevalence of clinical drug research.

Committee Involvement. A pharmacist should be a member of and actively participate in those committees responsible for establishing policies and procedures for medication-use, other aspects of patient care, and performance improvement and others, as appropriate. Also, pharmacists should participate in the activities of similar committees of a parent health system, as applicable.

Formulary Management and Integration. The pharmacy should maintain an up-to-date formulary of drug products approved by the medical staff. Drug products should be selected for the formulary through a medication-use policy development process (pharmacy and therapeutics committee or equivalent) that ensures the availability of the most appropriate drug products for the population served. The formulary should limit choices based on clinical evidence of efficacy and safety as well as cost to essential drug products with few duplicates. Drug products of marginal benefit should be eliminated or restricted, to the extent possible.

When applicable, the pharmacy should integrate the formularies (or approved drug lists) of third party payers into a patient care process that ensures optimal and cost-effective patient outcomes. Organizations with multiple practice settings such as acute inpatient and ambulatory care should coordinate formularies to promote continuity of care. A process should exist to obtain non-formulary drug products when medically necessary for the care of specific patients.

Disaster Services. Policies and procedures should exist for providing pharmaceutical services during facility, local, or area-wide disasters affecting the organization's patients. Appropriately trained pharmacists should be members of emergency preparedness teams and participate in drills. Patients should be informed about what to do in the event of a disaster to safely continue medication therapy.

Managing Performance Improvement

Performance Improvement. There should be an ongoing, systematic program for assessing the delivery of pharmaceutical care and services and of the utilization of medications in patient care.[9] Performance improvement activities based on assessments should be integrated with the organization's or health system's overall performance improvement activities, as applicable. Corrective actions should be planned and implemented for identified deficiencies and reassessed at appropriate time intervals. Operational and outcomes data should be bench-marked with those of other ambulatory care pharmaceutical services of similar size and scope. The results, including follow-up actions, of improvement efforts should be documented and provided to the organization's managers and others, as appropriate.

Medication-Use Evaluation. An ongoing program of monitoring drug utilization and costs should be in place to ensure that medications are used appropriately, safely, and effectively, and

to increase the probability of desired patient outcomes within defined populations of patients. The medication-use policy committee should define specific parameters for evaluation (disease state, pharmacological category, high-use/high cost drug products) as appropriate for the organization. Through the ongoing evaluation of medication-use, areas in need of improvement in medication prescribing and management can be identified and targeted for intervention.

Documentation and Measurement of Pharmaceutical Care, Interventions, and Outcomes. Pharmaceutical services should have an ongoing process for consistent documentation and measurement (and reporting to medical staff, administrators, and others) of pharmaceutical care, interventions, and patient outcomes from medication therapy (including patient satisfaction and quality of life) and pharmacists' contributions to patient care.[10]

Adverse Drug Reactions. An ongoing program should be in place for preventing, monitoring, and reporting adverse drug reactions. The program should include timely communications about the occurrences of adverse drug reactions to affected patients, their caregivers, and other providers. The pharmacy should submit adverse drug reaction reports to the FDA MedWatch program and drug products' manufacturers, as appropriate.

Medication Errors. The ambulatory care organization should have an ongoing program to prevent medication errors, including nonpunitive reporting and analysis. Pharmacists, physicians, nurses, and other health care personnel involved in the medication-use process should monitor for, document, and report medication errors. The organization, with the participation of pharmacists, should analyze the causes of medication errors and implement corrective actions. The occurrence of medication errors should be reported to voluntary national reporting systems (e.g., USP Medication Error Reporting Program and FDA MedWatch) and, as required, to accrediting organizations.

Integration of Population-Based and Patient-Specific Activities. A mechanism to ensure that the clinical and economic findings of population-based activities are appropriately incorporated into daily patient-specific practice should exist. Population-based activities provide insight and guidance in the treatment of the average patient, however, all variables identified in the patient-specific encounter should be considered in the therapeutic decision making for an individual patient.[11]

Managing Human Resources

Work Schedules and Assignments. The director should ensure that work schedules, procedures, and assignments optimize the use of personnel and other resources. Sufficient personnel should be available to ensure the safe and timely delivery of pharmaceutical services and patient care.

Position Descriptions. The responsibilities and related competencies of professional and supportive personnel should be clearly defined in written position descriptions. Pharmacists should be responsible for the provision of pharmaceutical care and for the supervision and management of support staff. Sufficient support staff (pharmacy technicians, clerical, secretarial) should be employed to facilitate the provision of pharmaceutical care. Technicians should be re-

sponsible for most aspects of drug distribution, including the processing of medication orders. This should be supervised and checked by a pharmacist. Roles of technicians and pharmacists should be clearly delineated to maximize the use of technicians in activities they can legally and safely perform.

Recruitment and Selection of Personnel. Personnel should be recruited and selected on the bases of requirements in established position descriptions. The personnel selection process should include an assessment of prior performance in job-related functions and the candidate's ability and willingness to contribute to achieving the pharmacy's mission. The director should assist in identifying the relevant professional and technical qualifications and should participate in candidate interviews and selections.

Performance Evaluation. Scheduled, periodic evaluations of performance should occur for all pharmacy personnel. Performance should be evaluated on the bases of position description requirements and expected competencies. Evaluations should include comments from professional and technical staff as well as other members of the health care team. Customer service should also be included in the evaluation process.

Education and Training. All personnel should possess the education and training needed to fulfill their responsibilities. All personnel should participate in relevant continuing education programs, staff development programs, and other activities as necessary to maintain or enhance their competence.

Pharmacist Licensure and Certification. All pharmacists shall possess a current state license to practice pharmacy. Board of Pharmaceutical Specialties' certification of pharmacists to provide specialty services to patients and selected patient care is encouraged, as applicable.

Technician Certification. Certification of pharmacy technicians by the Pharmacy Technician Certification Board should be strongly encouraged or required, as feasible. In addition, completion of an accredited training program is preferred.

Orientation of Personnel. All new personnel should be oriented to their positions' responsibilities and continued competencies, and applicable pharmacy and organization policies and procedures.

Managing Financial Resources

Budget Management. The pharmacy should have a budget consistent with the organization's financial management process that supports the scope of and demand for pharmaceutical services. Oversight of workload and financial performance should be managed in accordance with the organization's requirements. Management should provide for (1) determination and analysis of pharmaceutical service costs, (2) analysis of budgetary variances, (3) capital equipment acquisition, (4) patient revenue projections, and (5) justification of personnel commensurate with workload productivity.

Processes should enable the analysis of pharmaceutical services by unit-of-service and other parameters appropriate

to the organization (e.g., organization-wide costs by medication therapy, clinical service, specific disease management categories, and patient health plan enrollment). The director should have an integral part in the organization's financial management process.

Drug Expenditures. Specific policies and procedures for managing drug expenditures should address such methods as competitive bidding, group purchasing, utilization review programs, inventory management, and cost-effective patient services.

Revenue, Reimbursement, and Compensation. The director should be knowledgeable about revenues for pharmaceutical services including reimbursement for the provision of drug products and related supplies and compensation for pharmacists' cognitive services. Processes should exist for routine verification of patient benefits and for counseling patients about their anticipated financial responsibility for planned medication therapies. A process should also exist for responding to services requests from medically indigent patients. (For additional information, see: Coding and Reimbursement Guide for Pharmacists, St. Anthony Publishing; Directory of Prescription Drug Patient Assistance Programs, Pharmaceutical Research and Manufacturers Association.)

Standard II: Medication Therapy and Pharmaceutical Care

At a minimum, pharmacists are responsible for assessing the legal and clinical appropriateness of medication orders (or prescriptions), educating and counseling patients on the use of their medications, monitoring the effects of medication therapy, and maintaining patient profiles and other records. In the ambulatory care setting these responsibilities are best accomplished through the provision of pharmaceutical care whether in the context of collaborative agreements with physicians or independent of such agreements. The pharmaceutical care activities may vary, however, depending on whether agreements are in place, pharmacists have delegated authorities in patient care, and these are supported by provisions in the organization's policies and procedures. Individual state laws and regulations may establish specific requirements and limits.

Providing Pharmaceutical Care

Pharmaceutical care involves establishing a relationship with the patient; obtaining patient and medication history information; assessing the appropriateness of medication orders; preventing, identifying and resolving medication or other problems; educating and counseling patients; and monitoring the patient and medication effects.[12] When authorized for collaborative medication therapy or primary care, pharmacists may also participate in medication therapy decision-making and administering medications.

Pharmaceutical Care Plan. Pharmacists should maintain a comprehensive, on-going pharmaceutical care plan, either separately or as a component of a multidisciplinary care plan, for each patient based on level of responsibilities. The pharmaceutical care plan, if separate, should be accessible to prescribers, pharmacists, and other health care providers

involved in patient care. The pharmacist should be responsible for communicating the contents to the patient and other health care providers. The pharmaceutical care plan should, at a minimum, document the patient's medical and medication history, medication therapy assessment, and the medication therapy regimen, including drug name, strength, route of administration, indication of therapy, goal of therapy, monitoring parameters, and proposed length of therapy.

Depending on applicable laws and regulations and the organization's policies and procedures, the pharmaceutical care plan, or elements, may be a part of the patient's medical record or maintained in a separate pharmacy record or patient profile, preferably electronic.

Relationships with Patients. Patient-based medication therapy and pharmaceutical care begins with the relationship between the patient and the pharmacist. The ambulatory care pharmacist in the role of providing direct patient care should develop and maintain a level of rapport and trust with the patient and caregiver to effectively provide pharmaceutical care. The pharmacist should coordinate all aspects of the individual patient's pharmaceutical care and serve as a patient advocate. The pharmacist should be flexible and adapt to patient-specific variables such as the patient's perception of how their illness and/or symptoms impact his or her life and the patient's readiness for change.

Medication-Therapy Decisions. Pharmacists should actively participate in medication therapy decision-making and management through collaboration with the physician, patient, and other health care providers. By participating in collaborative drug therapy management, the pharmacist takes an active role in the initiation, management, and monitoring of medication therapy and takes responsibility for achieving desired therapeutic outcomes. The development of a collaborative care agreement between the pharmacist, prescriber, and the patient should occur in compliance with applicable laws and regulations and the organization's policies and procedures, as applicable.

Pharmacist Prescribing. When permitted by applicable state laws and regulations, pharmacist may be delegated prescriptive authority in accordance with established collaborative drug therapy management agreements.

Therapeutic Goals. The pharmacist and patient should work together and with other health care providers to set goals, timetables, and therapeutic milestones for all pharmacotherapy.

Patient and Medication History. Upon patient admission for ambulatory care services, a pharmacist should obtain, or conduct as necessary, a patient and medication history (or profile). The history should include, but not be limited to, known health problems and diseases, applicable measurements and laboratory values, known drug allergies and adverse drug experiences, and a comprehensive list of prescription and nonprescription medications and related medical devices currently being used. The history should be maintained and updated during subsequent patient encounters.

Medication Therapy Assessment. The pharmacist should assess medication orders, new and refill, prior to dispensing, to ensure safe and effective medication therapy. The assessment should include the appropriateness of the prescribed medication(s) for the patient's diagnosis and history, the identification of medication-related problems, and interventions for resolving the problems, if any. Problems should be resolved with the prescriber before further processing of the medication order. In addition, the assessment should produce a plan for monitoring patient adherence, therapeutic and adverse effects, and patient outcomes.

Patient Education and Counseling

Patient education and counseling are essential components of pharmaceutical care in the ambulatory care setting and pharmacists' provision should exceed the minimal legal requirements.[13] A simple offer to counsel is inconsistent with pharmacists' responsibilities. The pharmacist should ensure that the patient understands all information required for the safe and proper use of the medication and devices, as applicable. Directions for use should be clearly expressed. Supplementary written information should be provided as necessary to reinforce oral communications. Contingencies should be available to provide education, counseling, and written materials to non-English speaking patients, where applicable. Depending on need, this might require access to interpreters or bilingual pharmacists.

At a minimum, the pharmacist should verify that patients and caregivers, understand what medications (prescription, nonprescription, and alternative substances) they are using, why they are using them, how to use them, what therapeutic effects to expect, what potential adverse effects to watch for, and what actions to take if adverse effects occur. Counseling should also include the patients responsibility for adherence to and reporting on their experience with the medication therapy plan.

Medication Therapy Monitoring. The pharmacist should monitor patient understanding and adherence to their medication therapy plan and its effects and outcomes. During subsequent encounters with patients for medication order refills or follow up visits, pharmacists should obtain information, as appropriate, from patients, assess patient progress, identify any problems, and resolve problems either with the prescriber or in accord with a collaborative agreement.

Medication Administration. Only personnel who are permitted by law and regulation, authorized by the organization, and appropriately trained should administer medications to patients. Pharmacists should participate in establishing policies and procedures for medication administration in the ambulatory care setting. When legally permitted, medication administration by appropriately trained pharmacists may be within their scope of practice, depending on the ambulatory care setting's workload distribution among members of the health care team. As appropriate, pharmacists may witness now or one-time doses of medications self-administered by patients.

Supporting Pharmaceutical Care

Continuity of Care. Pharmacists should routinely contribute to processes that ensure each patient's pharmaceutical care is maintained regardless of transitions across the continuum of care and practice settings (e.g., between inpatient and community pharmacies or home care services).

Emergency Access to Pharmaceutical Care. Policies and procedures should exist within the organization to provide patients access to appropriate levels of pharmaceutical care during emergent situations 24 hours a day, including access to the pharmacist responsible for their care, if appropriate.

Medical Record Documentation. Clinical actions and recommendations by pharmacists that are designed to ensure safe and cost effective use of medications and that have a potential effect on patient outcomes should be documented in patients' medical records. Pharmacists' documentation in the patients' medical records may require organization-specific training and authorization.

Patient Confidentiality. Policies and procedures for access to and dissemination of confidential patient information should be available. Patient privacy and confidentiality should be protected by safeguarding access to all sources of patient information, including financial (billing), medication profiles, medical records, and organization reports, whether in computer databases or hard copy. Patient information should be shared only with authorized health care providers and others within the pharmacy or the organization as needed for the care of patients. Patient information should only be shared with family members and caregiver(s) upon the request of the patient. Privacy shall be maintained during all communication with a patient.

Standard III: Drug Distribution and Control

The pharmacy and/or contracted network pharmacies should be responsible for the procurement, distribution, and control of all drug products used in the treatment of the organization's patients. Policies and procedures governing medication distribution and control should be developed by the pharmacy in collaboration with other appropriate organization staff and committees.

Purchasing and Maintaining the Availability of Drug Products

Drug Product Availability. Drug products approved for routine use should be purchased, stored, and available in sufficient quantities to meet the needs of ambulatory care patients. Drug products not approved for routine use, but necessary to meet the needs of specific patients or categories of patients should be obtained in response to orders according to established policies and procedures.

Pharmaceutical Manufacturers and Suppliers. Criteria for selecting pharmaceutical manufacturers and suppliers or contracting with group purchasing organizations should be established by the pharmacy to ensure the quality and best price of drug products. Preference should be considered for manufacturers and suppliers that provide packaging and labeling designed to reduce vulnerability to medication errors (e.g., bar-coding).

Pharmaceutical Manufacturers' Representatives. Policies and procedures governing the activities of representatives (including related supplies and devices) within the pharmacy, ambulatory care setting, and organization should exist. Representatives should be provided written guidance on their activities. All promotional materials and activities should be reviewed and approved by the pharmacy. Representatives should not have access to patient care areas.

Samples. The use of drug product samples should be prohibited to the extent possible. However, if samples are permitted under certain circumstances, policies and procedures for their use should exist. The pharmacy should control samples to ensure proper storage, record keeping, and product integrity, if allowed by state law and regulation. Samples dispensed to patients should meet all applicable packaging and labeling laws and regulations and standards.

Drug Product Storage Area Inspections. All stocks of drug products whether located within or outside the pharmacy area should be inspected routinely and managed by pharmacy and location staff to ensure the absence of outdated, unusable, recalled, or mislabeled products. Storage conditions should be monitored to ensure compliance with environmental requirements and to assess, document, and correct any conditions that might foster medication deterioration and storage arrangements that might contribute to medication errors. Appropriate security must prevent the access of unauthorized staff and others (technical, health care provider, housekeeping, patients and caregivers) to stock medications and medication order forms (prescription blanks).

Patient Care Area Stock. Stocks of drug products held in nonpharmacy areas (e.g., nursing station, clinic, or physicians' offices) for direct administration to ambulatory patients should be minimal. To the extent possible, stocks should be limited to medications for emergency, diagnostic, and routine treatments, including certain injectables (e.g., local anesthetics and vaccines). The potential for medication errors and adverse effects should be considered for any drug product stocked outside of the pharmacy. Drug products shall be under control at all times to prevent unauthorized access and diversion.

Emergency Medications. The pharmacy should ensure the availability, access, and security of emergency medications, including antidotes. Pharmacists should have an authorized role in responding to medical emergencies.

Drug Recall and New Prescribing Information. An ongoing program should exist for timely intervention and dissemination of information regarding drug recalls and release of new prescribing or adverse drug reaction information on specific drug products. For situations in which the potential for an adverse event is possible, the pharmacy should have procedures in place to identify all patients of the organization using the product, to identify the prescribers of the product, and to intervene with specific alternatives to reduce the risk of adverse events.

Policies and procedures should exist for removing recalled drug products from all storage and patient care areas, and when the recall is to the user level, for notifying patients who have received recalled products and for replacing patients' supplies.

Processing the Medication Order

Prescribing. Policies and procedures should be available to ensure that health care providers meet applicable state licensure and, if required, organizational authorization for prescribing medications. Medications should be administered

and dispensed to ambulatory patients only upon the oral or written order of authorized prescribers. Oral new orders should be limited to non-routine and emergent situations and strongly discouraged for drug products and regimens prone to adverse events, including medication errors. A pharmacist should verify and reduce oral orders to writing as soon as possible.

The pharmacy should advocate and foster prescriber's conformance with the formulary, clinical care plans, and disease state management programs, and with standardized, approved terminology and abbreviations when prescribing medications. The pharmacy should advocate for the development and use of electronic prescribing systems (prescriber direct order entry).

Therapeutic Purpose. Prior to dispensing any medication, the pharmacist should substantiate the indication for which the medication was prescribed. Prescribers should be encouraged to routinely communicate the condition being treated or the therapeutic purpose of medications with all medication orders.

Medication Orders. Medication orders (or prescriptions) shall contain at a minimum the following information: patient name (and address), medication name, dose, frequency, route, quantity (duration), prescriber identification (and prescriber DEA number for controlled substances) and signature, and date. All medication orders shall be reviewed for legality and clinical appropriateness by a pharmacist before being dispensed. Any questions should be resolved with the prescriber, and a written notation made in the patient's pharmacy record or profile. Information concerning changes should be appropriately communicated to the patient, caregiver, and other involved health care providers.

Preparing, Packaging, and Labeling Medications

Preparation. The pharmacist should prepare or supervise the preparation, in a timely and accurate manner, those drug formulations, strengths, dosage forms, and packages prescribed, including those that are not commercially available but are needed in the care of patients.

Extemporaneous Compounding. Drug formulations, dosage forms, strengths, and packaging that are not available commercially but are deemed necessary for patient care should be prepared by appropriately trained personnel in accordance with applicable standards and regulations (e.g., FDA, U.S.P., state board of pharmacy). Adequate quality control and quality assurance procedures should exist for these operations. Commercially available products should be used to the maximum extent possible.

Sterile Products. All sterile medications for use in the ambulatory care facility or for use by patients in the home should be prepared in a suitable environment by appropriately trained personnel and labeled appropriately for the user. Quality control and quality assurance procedures for the preparation of sterile products should exist, including periodic assessment of personnel on aseptic technique.

Cytotoxic and Hazardous Drug Products. All cytotoxic and hazardous drug products for use in the ambulatory care facility or for use by patients in the home should be prepared in a suitable environment by appropriately trained personnel and labeled appropriately for the user. Special precautions, equipment, supplies (spill kits), and training for storage, handling, and disposal of cytotoxic and hazardous drug products should exist to ensure the safety of personnel, patients, and visitors. Quality control and quality assurance procedures for the preparation of cytotoxic and hazardous products should exist. Personnel handling cytotoxic and hazardous drug products should be monitored periodically for adverse effects.

Controlled Substances. Pharmacists are responsible for a lead role in the control of drug products that are subject to diversion and misuse. Pharmacists have primary responsibility for receipt, storage, security, distribution within the facility and to patients for home use, and disposal of controlled substances and for related records. Policies and procedures shall exist to ensure compliance with the Comprehensive Drug Abuse Prevention and Control Act of 1970 and with state laws and regulations that may be more stringent. Storage within the pharmacy and nonpharmacy (e.g., emergency room) areas are secure and have controlled access to only authorized personnel. Procedures are in place to detect and investigate inventory shrinkage.

Investigational Drugs. The pharmacy should be responsible for overseeing the distribution and control of all investigational drugs. Investigational drugs shall be approved for use by an institutional review board, and shall be dispensed and administered to consenting patients according to an approved protocol.

Non-FDA Approved Drugs. The pharmacy should seek and obtain documented authorization from appropriate organization committees for the pharmacologic use of any chemical substance that has not received FDA approval for any drug use. Documentation should exist to ensure that appropriate risk management measures (e.g., obtaining informed consent) have been taken.

Packaging. Medications dispensed to ambulatory care patients should be packaged and labeled in compliance with applicable federal and state laws and regulations and with USP and other standards. When feasible, dispensing in unopened manufacturers' and in tamper-evident packages is desirable. Packaging materials should be selected that preserve the integrity, cleanliness, and potency of compounded and commercially available drug products. Containers, including unit dose packages, for patient home use shall comply with the Poison Prevention Packaging Act.

Labeling. At a minimum, labels for patient home use of medications shall comply with applicable federal and state laws and regulations. Generally, labels contain: name, address, and telephone number of the pharmacy; date of dispensing; serial number of the prescription; patient's full name; name, strength, and dosage form of the medication; directions to the patient for use of the medication; name of the prescriber; precautionary information; authorized refills; and initials (or name) of the responsible pharmacist. Other information may be required by individual state law and regulation.

Drug Delivery Systems and Administration Devices.
Pharmacists should provide leadership and advice in organizational and clinical decisions regarding drug delivery systems and administration devices, and should participate in the evaluation, use, and monitoring of these systems and devices. The potential for medication errors associated with such systems and devices should be thoroughly evaluated.

Mail Distribution. The pharmacy may mail medications to patients, preferably when part of a comprehensive pharmaceutical care program, which provides patients access to a pharmacist. Mailed medications shall conform to all federal and state laws and regulations. Outer mailing packages and medication containers should protect the medication from heat, humidity, and other environmental conditions that would affect stability.[14] A toll-free telephone service should be provided that is answered during normal business hours to enable communication between a patient or a physician of a patient and a pharmacist with access to the patient's records. The pharmacy should have procedures for investigating, replacing, and reporting, as required, medications lost during delivery. Special requirements for mailing controlled substances vary by state law and regulation.

Standard IV: Facilities, Equipment, and Other Resources

To ensure optimal performance and quality patient care, adequate space, equipment, and other resources should be available for all professional and administrative functions relating to medication use. Pharmaceutical services operations should be located in areas that facilitate provision of services to patients, nurses, prescribers, and other health care providers. Facilities should be constructed, arranged, and equipped to promote safe and efficient work flow for staff and patients and to avoid damage to or deterioration of drug products.

Information Technology. Computer-based (electronic) information systems are preferred to maintain patient pharmaceutical care plans and medication profiles; perform necessary patient billing procedures; manage drug product inventories; and interface with other available computerized systems to obtain patient specific clinical information. Information is essential for medication therapy monitoring and other clinical functions, to facilitate the continuity of care to and from other care settings, and to produce drug utilization, cost, and related reports.

Medication Storage and Preparation Areas. Facilities should exist to store and prepare drug products and medications under proper conditions of sanitation, temperature, light, moisture, ventilation, segregation, and security throughout the pharmacy and other patient care areas. Monitored, adequate refrigeration and freezer capacity should be available within the secure pharmacy area and, as necessary, in nonpharmacy areas.

Compounding and Packaging. Designated space and equipment for compounding and packaging of sterile and nonsterile drug products, including hazardous drug products, should exist. The compounding and packaging areas should be clean and orderly and routinely monitored and maintained to minimize the risk of errors and contamination of drug products.

Patient Assessment and Counseling Area. A designated area for private patient assessment and counseling by pharmacists should be available to enhance patients' knowledge, understanding, and adherence to prescribed medication therapy regimens and monitoring plans. Space should accommodate the pharmacist and patient and, as appropriate, parents, caregivers, or chaperones.

Automation. There should be policies and procedures on the evaluation, selection, use, calibration and monitoring, and maintenance of all automated pharmacy systems.[15] Automated dispensing systems and software may be useful in promoting accurate and efficient medication ordering and preparation, dispensing, and distribution. The potential for medication errors associated with automated systems should be thoroughly evaluated and eliminated to the extent possible. Automated dispensing systems should support the pharmacist's assessment of medication orders (and opportunity to intervene) and checking of filled orders before dispensing.

Automated dispensing systems and automated storage and distribution devices should be controlled by the pharmacy's computer-based information system. An interface with the organization's information system is strongly encouraged. A pharmacist should supervise the stocking of medications in automated dispensing systems and in automated storage and distribution devices. The maintenance, calibration, and certification, as required by applicable standards, laws, and regulations, should be ongoing and documented.

Record and Equipment Maintenance. Adequate space should exist for maintaining and storing records (e.g., equipment maintenance, controlled substances inventory, material safety data sheets) to ensure compliance with laws, regulations, accreditation requirements, and sound management practices. Appropriate licenses, permits, and tax stamps and other documents should be on display or on file as required. All nonautomated equipment should be adequately maintained and certified in accordance with applicable standards, laws, and regulations. Equipment maintenance and certification should be documented.

Office and Meeting Area. Adequate office and meeting areas should be available for administrative, educational, and training activities.

References

1. Johnson JA, Bootman JL. Drug-related morbidity and mortality, a cost-of-illness model. *Arch Intern Med.* 1995; 155:1949–56.
2. Lewis RK, Carter BL, Glover DG, Hutchinson RA. Comprehensive services in an ambulatory care pharmacy. *Am J Health-Syst Pharm.* 1995; 52:1793–7.
3. Segarra-Newnham M, Soisson KT. Provision of pharmaceutical care through comprehensive pharmacotherapy clinics. *Hosp Pharm.* 1997; 32(Jun):845–50.
4. Crane VS, Hatwig CA, Hayman JN, Hoffman R. Developing a management planning and control system for ambulatory pharmacy resources. *Pharm Pract Manage Q.* 1998; 18(1):52–71.
5. Rosum RW. Planning for an ambulatory care service. *Am J Health-Syst Pharm.* 1997; 54:1584, 1587.
6. Kernodle SJ. Improving health care with clinical practice guidelines and critical pathways: implications for

pharmacists in ambulatory practice. *Pharm Pract Manage Q.* 1997; 17(3):76–89.

7. LaCalamita S. Role of the pharmacist in developing critical pathways with warfarin therapy. *J Pharm Pract.* 1997; 10:398–410.

8. Curtiss FR. Lessons learned from projects in disease management in ambulatory care. *Am J Health-Syst Pharm.* 1997; 54:2217–29.

9. MacKinnon N. Performance measures in ambulatory pharmacy. *Pharm Pract Manage Q.* 1997; 17(1): 52–62.

10. Borgsdorf LR, Mian JS, and Knapp KK. Pharmacist-managed medication review in a managed care system. *Am J Hosp Pharm.* 1994; 51:772–7.

11. Mutnick AH, Sterba KJ, Szymusiak-Mutnick BA. Integration of quality assessment and a patient-specific intervention/outcomes program. *Pharm Pract Manage Q.* 1998: 17(4):25–36.

12. Hepler CD, Strand LM. Opportunities and responsibilities in pharmaceutical care. *Am J Hosp Pharm.* 1990; 47:533–43.

13. Lewis RK, Lasack NL, Lambert BL, Connor SE. Patient counseling–a focus on maintenance therapy. *Am J Health-Syst Pharm.* 1997; 54:2084–98.

14. United States Pharmacopeia. General Notices and Requirements—Preservation, Packaging, Storage, and Labeling. *Pharmacopeial Forum.* Nov-Dec 1998; 24 (6):7205–12.

15. Glover DG. Automated medication dispensing devices. *J Am Pharm Assn.* 1997; NS37(May-Jun):353–60.

Approved by the ASHP Board of Directors, April 21, 1999. Revised by the Council on Professional Affairs. Supersedes an earlier version, ASHP Guidelines on Pharmaceutical Services for Ambulatory Patients, dated November 14, 1990.

Richard K. Lewis, Pharm.D., MBA, Bryan F. Yeager, Pharm.D., Darryl G. Glover, Pharm.D., Jennifer White, Pharm.D., Aimee Gelhot, Pharm.D., and Christopher A. Hatwig, M.S., are gratefully acknowledged for drafting this revision.

The bibliographic citation for this document is as follows: American Society of Health-System Pharmacists. ASHP guidelines: minimum standard for pharmaceutical services in ambulatory care. *Am J Health-Syst Pharm.* 1999; 56:1744–53.

ASHP Guidelines: Minimum Standard for Pharmacies in Hospitals

Purpose

The following minimum standard guidelines are intended to serve as a basic guide for the provision of pharmacy services in hospitals. These guidelines outline a minimum level of services that most hospital pharmacy departments should consistently provide. The reader is strongly encouraged to review the American Society of Health-System Pharmacy (ASHP) guidance documents referenced throughout these guidelines for more detailed descriptions. Certain elements of these guidelines may be applicable to other health care settings or may be useful in evaluating the scope and quality of pharmacy services.

Elements of Care

The mission of pharmacists is to help people make the best use of medications.[1] Therefore, pharmacists shall be concerned with not only the provision but the outcomes of pharmacy services. The elements of pharmacy services that are critical to safe, effective, and cost-conscious medication use in a hospital include (1) practice management; (2) medication-use policy development; (3) optimizing medication therapy; (4) drug product procurement and inventory management; (5) preparing, packaging, and labeling medications; (6) medication delivery; (7) monitoring medication use; (8) evaluating the effectiveness of the medication-use system; and (9) research. Although the scope of pharmacy services will vary from site to site, depending upon the needs of patients and the hospital as well as the resources available, these core elements are inextricably linked to successful outcomes. Failure to provide any of these services may compromise the quality of patient care.

Terminology

In these guidelines, the term "shall" is used to indicate a minimum standard of practice set forth in this document, in other ASHP policies, or in requirements established by laws, regulations, accrediting bodies, or other binding authorities. The term "should" is used to indicate a best practice that is strongly encouraged by ASHP but which may not be applicable to all institutions or in all circumstances.

Standard I. Practice Management

Effective leadership and practice management skills are necessary for the delivery of pharmacy services in a manner consistent with the hospital's and patients' needs. Such leadership should foster continuous improvement in patient care outcomes. The management of pharmacy services should focus on the pharmacist's responsibilities as a patient care provider and leader of the pharmacy enterprise through the development of organizational structures that support that mission. Development of such structures will require communication and collaboration with other departments and

services throughout the hospital, which every member of the pharmacy team should cultivate at every opportunity.

A. Pharmacy and Pharmacist Services
Pharmacy Mission, Goals, and Scope of Services. The pharmacy shall have a written mission statement that reflects both patient care and operational responsibilities. Other aspects of the pharmacy's mission may require definition as well (e.g., educational and research responsibilities). The mission statement shall be consistent with the mission of the hospital and, if applicable, aligned with the health system of which the hospital is a component. The development, prioritization, and implementation of the pharmacy's goals should be consistent with the mission statement. Determination of short- and long-term goals and the undertaking of implementation activities should be performed in collaboration with institutional leadership and other hospital staff (e.g., pharmacy, nursing, and medical staff), and these should be integrated with the goals of the hospital. The mission statement may also incorporate consensus-based national goals, such as those expressed in the recommendations from the ASHP Pharmacy Practice Model Initiative.[2]

The pharmacy shall also maintain a written document describing the scope of pharmacy services. These services should be consistent with the hospital's scope of services and should be applied throughout the hospital in all practice sites.

The mission, goals, and scope of services shall be clearly communicated to everyone involved in the provision of pharmacy services, including pharmacists, residents, students, technicians, and support staff.

24-Hour Pharmacy Services. Adequate hours of operation for the provision of needed pharmacy services shall be maintained; 24-hour pharmacy services should be provided when possible. Twenty-four hour pharmacy services should be employed in all hospitals with clinical programs that require intensive medication therapy (e.g., transplant programs, open-heart surgery programs, neonatal intensive care units, and trauma centers). When 24-hour pharmacy services are not feasible, a pharmacist shall be available on an on-call basis. Remote medication order processing may be employed (to the extent permitted by law and regulation) to help provide pharmacy services but is not a substitute for an on-call pharmacist.[3] Automated drug dispensing equipment and computer databases are also not a substitute for the skills and knowledge of a pharmacist and should not be considered alternatives to 24-hour pharmacy services.[4]

After-Hours Pharmacy Access. In the absence of 24-hour pharmacy services, access to a limited supply of medications shall only be available to authorized, licensed health care professionals for use in carrying out urgent medication orders. Access to such medications shall be carefully monitored and documented, and after-hours access shall be reviewed regularly to ensure appropriate use. The list of medications to be accessible and the policies and procedures to be used (including subsequent review of all activity by a

pharmacist) shall be developed a multidisciplinary committee of physicians, pharmacists, and nurses (e.g., by the pharmacy and therapeutics [P&T] committee or its equivalent).[5] Access to medications should be limited to cases in which the P&T committee (or its equivalent) determines that the urgent clinical need for the medication outweighs the potential risks of making the medication accessible. The potential safety risks of medications should be considered in the decision to make them accessible, and medications, quantities, dosage forms, and container sizes that might endanger patients should be limited whenever possible.

Routine after-hours access to the pharmacy by non-pharmacists for access to medications shall not be permitted. The use of well-designed night cabinets, after-hours medication carts, automated dispensing devices,[6] and other methods precludes the need for nonpharmacists to enter the pharmacy.[4]

Practice Standards and Guidelines. The standards and regulations of all relevant government bodies (e.g., state boards of pharmacy, departments of health) shall be met. The practice standards and guidelines of the American Society of Health-System Pharmacists, appropriate accrediting bodies (e.g., The Joint Commission [TJC], American Osteopathic Association Healthcare Facilities Accreditation Program [AOA HFAP], Det Norske Veritas [DNV], and the Centers for Medicare and Medicaid Services [CMS]) shall be viewed as applicable, and the hospital should strive to meet all applicable standards.

B. Laws and Regulations
Applicable local, state, and federal laws and regulations shall be met, and relevant documentation of compliance shall be maintained.

C. Policies and Procedures
Policy and Procedures Manual. There shall be a policy and procedures manual governing pharmacy functions (e.g., administrative, operational, and clinical), and all pharmacy personnel shall follow those policies and procedures. The manual may include a statement of the pharmacy's mission, philosophy, or values (e.g., the pharmacy's mission or vision statements), but it should concentrate on operational policies and procedures to guide and direct all pharmacy services. The pharmacy's policies and procedures should be consistent with the hospital's policies and procedures, and the manual should be reviewed by a designated medical staff committee for potential conflicts and other medical issues. The manual shall be reviewed by pharmacy staff on a regular basis and revised as necessary to reflect changes in procedures, organization, objectives, or practices. The manual shall be accessible to pharmacy department personnel as well as other hospital employees (e.g., through the hospital's intranet), and all pharmacy personnel should be familiar with its contents. Appropriate mechanisms to ensure compliance with the policies and procedures should be established.

Personnel Safety. Pharmacy employees should be involved in the development of the hospital's plans for emergency response, infection prevention and control, management of hazardous substances and waste, and incident reporting, and all pharmacy staff shall receive education about those plans.

Emergency Preparedness. Facility emergency preparedness plans shall describe the role of pharmacy staff in emergency response (including evacuation), and the facility's business continuity plan shall include procedures for providing safe and efficient pharmacy services in case of emergencies. Appropriately trained pharmacists should be members of emergency preparedness teams and participate in applicable preparations and drills.[7] The pharmacy shall establish, in conjunction with the hospital-wide emergency plan, policies and procedures for the safe and orderly evacuation of pharmacy personnel in the event of an emergency in the hospital.

Medical Emergencies. The pharmacy shall participate in hospital decisions about the contents of code carts, emergency medication kits and trays, and the role of pharmacists in medical emergencies. Pharmacists should serve on cardiopulmonary resuscitation (CPR) teams, and such pharmacists should receive appropriate training and maintain appropriate certifications (e.g., Basic Life Support [BLS], Advanced Cardiopulmonary Life Support [ACLS], Pediatric Acute Life Support [PALS]).

Immunization Programs. The pharmacy shall participate in the development of hospital policies and procedures concerning preventive and post-exposure immunization programs for patients and hospital employees.[8] When practical, pharmacists should participate as active immunizers for hospital and health-system based preventative immunization programs (e.g., influenza).

Substance Abuse Programs. The pharmacy shall assist in the development of and participate in hospital substance abuse education, prevention, identification, treatment, and employee assistance programs.[9]

D. Human Resources
Position Descriptions. Areas of responsibility within the scope of pharmacy services shall be clearly defined. The responsibilities and related competencies of professional and supportive personnel shall be clearly defined in written position descriptions. These position descriptions shall be reviewed and revised as required by the hospital's policies. Position descriptions should reflect more general aspects of performance (e.g., communication, motivation, teamwork) in addition to specific responsibilities and competencies.

Director of Pharmacy. The pharmacy shall be managed by a professionally competent, legally qualified pharmacist. The director of pharmacy should be thoroughly knowledgeable about and have experience in hospital pharmacy practice and management. An advanced management degree (e.g., M.B.A., M.H.A., or M.S.) or an administrative specialty residency[10] is desirable.

The director of pharmacy shall be responsible for

- establishing the mission, vision, goals and scope of services of the pharmacy based on the needs of the patients served, the needs of the hospital (and any health system of which the hospital may be a component) and developments and trends in health care and hospital pharmacy practice;
- developing, implementing, evaluating and updating plans and activities to fulfill the mission, vision, goals and scope of services of the pharmacy;

- actively working with or as a part of hospital or health-system leadership to develop and implement policies and procedures that provide safe and effective medication use for the patients served by the institution;
- mobilizing and managing the resources, both human and financial, necessary for the optimal provision of pharmacy services; and
- ensuring that patient care services provided by pharmacists and other pharmacy personnel are delivered in adherence to applicable state and federal laws and regulations, hospital privileging requirements, and national practice standards.

A part-time director of pharmacy shall have the same obligations and responsibilities as a full-time director.

Pharmacists. The pharmacy shall employ an adequate number of competent, legally qualified pharmacists to meet the specific medication-use needs of the hospital's patients. Pharmacists hired on a temporary or contract basis shall meet the same requirements as those employed by the hospital.

Support Personnel. Sufficient support personnel (e.g., pharmacy technicians and clerical or secretarial personnel) shall be employed to facilitate pharmacy services. Support positions shall have a written job description that includes a statement of the competencies required for that position. Support staff shall be properly trained and supervised, and professional development programs for them are desirable. Pharmacy technicians should have completed an ASHP-accredited pharmacy technician training program, should be certified by the Pharmacy Technician Certification Board, and shall meet the requirements of applicable laws and regulations. Pharmacy technicians working in advanced roles should have additional training and demonstrate competencies specific to the tasks to be performed.

Education and Training. All personnel shall possess the education and training required to fulfill their responsibilities, and shall participate in relevant continuing-education programs and activities as necessary to maintain or enhance their competence.[11]

Recruitment, Selection, and Retention of Personnel. Personnel should be recruited and selected by the pharmacy director on the basis of job-related qualifications and prior performance. An employee retention plan is desirable.[12]

Orientation of Personnel. There shall be an established, structured procedure for orienting new personnel to the pharmacy, the hospital, and their respective positions.[9] Evaluation of the effectiveness of orientation programs should be done in conjunction with the competency assessment required before a new hire can assume full responsibility for the new position.

Work Schedules and Assignments. The director of pharmacy shall ensure that work schedules, procedures, and assignments optimize the use of personnel and resources. There shall be a written departmental staffing plan that addresses how patients' needs will be met during periods of staff shortages and fluctuation in workload and/or patient acuity.

Remote medication order processing may be employed to help address staff shortages or workload fluctuations.[3]

Performance Evaluation. There shall be procedures for regularly scheduled evaluation of the performance of pharmacy personnel. The evaluation format should be consistent with that used by the hospital. The competencies of the position shall be well defined in the position description, short- and long-term goals should be established for each employee, and the employee's competency shall be assessed regularly. The pharmacy director shall ensure that an ongoing competency assessment program is in place for all staff, and each staff member should have a continuous professional development plan.

Effective Communication. There should be established methods for communicating important information to staff in a timely manner (e.g., electronic communications, staff meetings, newsletters, bulletin boards). The pharmacy should establish appropriate mechanisms to regularly assess the effectiveness of such communications.

Ethical Conduct. Standards of ethical conduct shall be established, and there shall be procedures for educating all pharmacy staff regarding these standards. The institution's conflict-of-interest and ethical conduct policies shall be clearly communicated to all staff, with appropriate staff acknowledgement of conformance with these policies.[13]

E. Facilities

Pharmacy. Adequate space, equipment, and supplies shall be available for all professional and administrative functions relating to pharmacy services. These resources shall meet all applicable laws and regulations, and shall be located in areas that facilitate the provision of services to patients, nurses, prescribers, and other health care providers and shall be integrated with the hospital's communication and delivery or transportation systems.

Medication Storage and Preparation Areas. There shall be suitable facilities to enable the receipt, storage, and preparation of medications under proper conditions of sanitation, temperature, light, moisture, ventilation, segregation, and security to ensure medication integrity and personnel safety throughout the hospital.[4]

Compounding Areas. There shall be suitable facilities to enable the compounding, preparation, and labeling of sterile and nonsterile products, including hazardous drug products, in accordance with established quality assurance procedures. The work environment should promote orderliness and efficiency and minimize the potential for medication errors and contamination of products.[14–20]

Patient Assessment and Consultation Area. In outpatient settings, a private area for pharmacist–patient consultations shall be available to confidentially enhance patients' knowledge of and adherence to prescribed medication regimens.[21]

Office and Meeting Space. Adequate office and meeting areas shall be available for administrative, educational, and training activities.

Automated Systems. There shall be policies and procedures for the evaluation, selection, use, calibration, monitoring, and maintenance of all automated pharmacy systems. Automated mechanical systems and software can promote safe, accurate, and efficient medication ordering and preparation, drug distribution, and clinical monitoring. Use of such systems and software shall be structured so as to not hinder the pharmacist's review of (and opportunity to intervene in) medication orders before the administration of first doses. The maintenance, calibration, and certification of all automated systems shall be performed and documented as required by all applicable laws, regulations, and standards.[6,22,23] All automated systems shall include adequate safeguards to maintain the confidentiality and security of patient records, and there shall be procedures to provide essential patient care services in case of equipment failure or downtime.

Information Technology. A comprehensive pharmacy computer system shall be employed and should be integrated to the fullest extent possible with other hospital information systems and software, including computerized provider order entry, medication administration, electronic health record, and patient billing systems. Computer resources should be used to support clerical functions, maintain patient medication profile records, provide clinical decision support, perform necessary patient billing procedures, manage drug product inventories, provide drug information, access the patient medical record, manage electronic prescribing, and interface with other computerized systems to obtain patient-specific clinical information for medication therapy monitoring and other clinical functions and to facilitate the continuity of care to and from other care settings. Pharmacists should be involved in the development and maintenance of order sets, templates, and dose ranges used in computerized provider order entry and clinical decision support systems. Pharmacy computer systems should be integrated with the hospital's clinical, financial, and administrative information systems. All computer systems shall include adequate safeguards to maintain the confidentiality and security of patient records, and a backup system should be available to continue essential computerized functions (e.g., those that support patient care) during equipment failure.

Drug Information. Adequate space, current resources, and information-handling and communication technology shall be available to facilitate the provision of drug information. The department of pharmacy shall select its drug information resources, and pharmacists shall play a leadership role in the selection of drug information resources used by other health care providers in the hospital. Up-to-date, objective drug information shall be available, including current print or electronic periodicals, newsletters, best practices guidelines, and recent editions of reference books in appropriate pharmaceutical and biomedical subject areas. Electronic drug information databases are preferred because they are frequently updated and can be made available to all health care professionals, but sufficient access to print information shall be available in case of equipment failure or downtime. Electronic and print drug information may be supplemented with medical libraries and other available resources. Appropriate drug information resources shall be readily accessible to pharmacists located in patient care areas.

Electronic databases and convenient methods of data dissemination (e.g., email and handheld devices) are desirable. If such tools are employed, they should be made available to all health care practitioners who require access to the data.

Record Maintenance. All records shall be maintained in accordance with applicable laws, regulations, and institutional policies. Adequate space shall exist for maintaining and storing records (e.g., equipment maintenance, controlled substances inventory, and material safety data sheets) to ensure compliance with laws, regulations, accreditation requirements, and sound management practices. Appropriate licenses and permits shall be on display or on file as required by law or regulation. Equipment shall be adequately maintained and certified in accordance with applicable practice standards, laws, and regulations. There shall be documentation of equipment maintenance and certification.

F. Committee Involvement
A pharmacist shall be a member of and actively participate in hospital and health-system committees responsible for establishing and implementing medication-related policies and procedures as well as those committees responsible for the provision of patient care, including the P&T, infection prevention and control, patient care, medication-use evaluation, medication safety, nutrition, and pain management committees (or their equivalents), as well as the institutional review board, quality improvement, and information technology committees (or their equivalents).[5,24–26]

Standard II. Medication-Use Policy Development

A. Medication-Use Policy Development
All committees that make decisions concerning medication management and use shall have at least one pharmacist as a member. This includes the pharmacy and therapeutics, infection control, patient care, medication-use evaluation, medication safety, nutrition, pain management, and information technology committees, as well as the institutional review board (or their equivalents).[5,24–26] Pharmacists shall be involved in the development, implementation, and assessment of care plans (protocols, critical pathways, disease statement management programs, or clinical practice guidelines), standing order, and order sets that involve medication therapy.[27]

B. Formulary
Formulary. A well-controlled formulary of approved medications shall be maintained and regularly updated by the P&T committee (or its equivalent). The impact of and compliance with the formulary should be periodically reviewed (e.g., through drug utilization reviews), and the P&T committee should regularly review the formulary for safety information. The P&T committee shall be responsible for developing and maintaining written criteria for drug product selection, which shall address formulary requests for medications intended for use in special populations (e.g., pediatric or geriatric populations). The P&T committee shall be responsible for developing and maintaining adequate product specifications to aid in the purchase of medications

and related supplies. The pharmacy shall disseminate the formulary by electronic (preferred) or other means to meet the needs of all health care professionals.

There shall be policies and procedures that address the use of dietary supplements and other alternative therapies.

There shall be policies and procedures for the procurement, control, and use of nonformulary medications required for patient care.[5]

Medication Therapy Monographs. Medication therapy monographs for medications under consideration for formulary addition or deletion shall be made available to the P&T committee for use in the decision-making process. These monographs should be based on evidence gathered through review and evaluation of the pertinent literature. Each monograph shall include a comparative therapeutic, economic, and risk assessment (inclusive of black-box warnings) of each medication. The risk assessment should address the likelihood of an error occurring and the risk of injury should that error occur.[5]

Nondrug Substances. There shall be policies and procedures that describe how the pharmacy shall seek and obtain documented authorization from appropriate medical staff and hospital committees prior to the medical use of any chemical substance that has not received FDA approval for use as a drug or medical nutrition therapy. All chemical or biological substances whose administration is intended for pharmacological or medical effect or as a substitute for or complement to approved drugs shall be under the control of the pharmacy. Documentation shall exist to ensure that appropriate risk management measures (e.g., obtaining informed consent) have been taken.

C. Drug Information
Drug Information Requests. The pharmacist shall provide patient-specific drug information and accurate and comprehensive information about drugs and drug therapy to health professionals, patients, and patients' caregivers as appropriate. Responses to general and patient-specific drug information requests shall be provided in an accurate and timely manner by a pharmacist, and there should be a process for assessing and ensuring the quality of responses.[28]

Dissemination of Drug Information. Pharmacists shall keep the hospital's staff and health care providers informed about the use of medications on an ongoing basis through appropriate publications, presentations, and programs. Pharmacists shall ensure timely dissemination of drug product information (e.g., recall notices, labeling changes, and changes in product availability). Electronic communications (e.g., websites, email newsletters, intranet postings) are preferred because of their timeliness and accessibility.[28]

Standard III. Optimizing Medication Therapy

An important responsibility of the pharmacist is optimizing medication use. Pharmacists, in collaboration with medical and nursing staff, shall develop policies and procedures based on demonstrated best practices for ensuring the quality of medication therapy. Clinical imperatives should be the primary determinant of medication-use decisions.

A. Creating a Relationship with the Patient
Pharmacist Role in Direct Patient Care. Hospital and pharmacy department policies should encourage pharmacists to provide direct patient care to the greatest extent possible in both inpatient and outpatient settings. Hospital and pharmacy department policies should encourage pharmacists to engage in medication therapy management,[29] collaborative drug therapy management, immunization, medication ordering and administration, and other patient care activities to the extent permitted by law, regulation, and hospital requirements.

Continuity of Care. Pharmacists should assume responsibility for continuity of care for patients' medication therapy. Pharmacists and pharmacy departments should take a leadership role in developing and implementing policies and procedures for admissions, discharges, and transfers so that patients' medication therapy is well managed regardless of patient transitions across care settings (e.g., among different components of a health system or between inpatient and community pharmacies or home care services).

Patient Confidentiality. Systems shall be in place to ensure that patient confidentiality is maintained in accordance with applicable laws and regulations. All pharmacy personnel shall respect and protect patient confidentiality by safeguarding access to all patient information. Patient information shall be shared only with authorized health professionals and others authorized within the hospital or health system as needed for the care of patients.[30] Pharmacy personnel should periodically receive training in how to comply with patient confidentiality laws and regulations.

B. Acquiring Essential Patient Data
Medication Histories. Pharmacists should obtain, prepare, or have immediate access to comprehensive medication histories for each patient, from the patient's medical record or other databases (e.g., a medication profile), or both. A pharmacist-conducted medication history for each patient is desirable. Electronic medical records should be constructed so that medication histories and other data required for medication management, including medication reconciliation, are available to all health professionals caring for a patient.

C. Consulting with Other Health Professionals about Medication Therapy
Pharmacist's Consultations. Pharmacists should provide oral and written consultations to other health professionals regarding medication therapy selection and management.[30]

Medical Record Documentation. There shall be policies and procedures for pharmacist review of and documentation in patients' medical records. Recommendations made by the pharmacist and actions taken in response to those recommendations should be documented in the patient's medical record so that other health care providers have access to that information.[30]

Medication Therapy Decisions. The pharmacist's prerogatives to initiate, monitor, and modify medication therapy for individual patients, and to order laboratory tests to exercise those responsibilities, consistent with laws, regulations, and hospital policy, shall be clearly delineated and approved by the appropriate committee (e.g., P&T, patient care, or medical executive committee).

Standard IV. Drug Product Procurement and Inventory Management

The pharmacy shall be responsible for the procurement, distribution, and control of all drug products used in the hospital for inpatient and ambulatory patients. Policies and procedures governing these functions shall be developed by the pharmacy with input from other appropriate hospital staff and committees.[4]

A. Selecting Sources of Pharmaceutical Products

Medication Acquisition. There shall be policies and procedures for managing medication acquisition. These policies and procedures should address such issues as formulary development (including initial evaluation for formulary consideration, medication utilization review programs, and therapeutic interchange), competitive bidding, group purchasing, best practices, medication shortages, outsourcing, and cost-effective patient services. Benchmarking of medication costs should be performed to determine whether medication expenses and the change in medication expenses over time are consistent with industry standards.[4,31,32]

Pharmaceutical Manufacturers and Suppliers. Criteria for selecting drug product manufacturers and suppliers shall be established by the pharmacy to ensure the highest quality of and the best price for drug products. Although these duties may be delegated in part to a group purchasing organization, the pharmacy maintains the sole responsibility for ensuring the quality of drug products used in the hospital.[31,32]

Pharmaceutical Manufacturers' Representatives. There shall be written policies governing the activities of manufacturers' representatives or vendors of drug products (including related supplies and devices) within the hospital. Representatives should not be permitted access to patient care areas, and should be provided with written guidance on permissible activities within the hospital. All promotional materials and activities shall be reviewed and approved by the pharmacy.[33]

B. Managing Inventory

Medication Storage. Medications shall be received, stored, and prepared under proper conditions of sanitation, temperature, light, moisture, ventilation, segregation, and security to ensure medication integrity and personnel safety.[4]

Drug Shortages. There shall be policies and procedures for managing drug product shortages. The pharmacy's inventory management system should be designed to detect subminimum inventory levels and alert the pharmacy to potential shortages, and pharmacy staff should monitor reliable sources of information regarding drug product shortages (e.g., the ASHP[34] and FDA[35] drug shortages web resource centers). The pharmacy should develop strategies for identifying alternative therapies, working with suppliers, collaborating with physicians and other health care providers, and conducting an awareness campaign in the event of a drug product shortage.[36]

Samples. The use of medication samples shall be eliminated to the extent possible. Medication samples shall never be used for inpatient treatment. If use of samples is otherwise permitted, there shall be policies and procedures to ensure their safe use. The pharmacy shall oversee the procurement, storage, and distribution of these products to ensure proper storage, maintenance of records, product integrity, and compliance with all applicable packaging and labeling laws, regulations, standards, and patient education requirements. Pharmacists should be involved in hospital efforts to secure safe and effective low-cost medications for low-income patients (e.g., through manufacturer patient assistance programs).[4,5,33]

Patient Care Area Stock. The proper use of automated dispensing devices reduces the need for medications to be stored in nonpharmacy areas.[6] Storage of medications in nonpharmacy areas (e.g., patient care and procedural areas) shall to the extent possible be limited to medications for emergency use and routinely used personal care items (e.g., mouthwash and antiseptic solutions). The list of medications to be accessible and the policies and procedures regarding their use shall be developed by a multidisciplinary committee of physicians, pharmacists, and nurses (e.g., the P&T committee).[5] Access to medications should be limited to cases in which the committee determines that the urgent clinical need for the medication outweighs the potential patient-safety risks of making the medication accessible. A separate assessment should occur for every location where a medication may be stocked.

Controlled Substances. There shall be policies and procedures to ensure control of the distribution and use of controlled substances and other medications with a potential for abuse. These policies and procedures shall be consistent with applicable laws and regulations, and shall include methods for preventing and detecting diversion.[4]

Patient's Own Medications. Drug products and related devices brought into the hospital by patients shall be identified by pharmacy and documented in the patient's medical record if the medications are to be used during hospitalization. They shall be administered only pursuant to a prescriber's order and according to hospital policies and procedures, which should ensure the pharmacist's identification and validation of the medication integrity as well as the secure and appropriate storage and management of such medications.

C. Inspecting Storage Areas and Inventory Items

Medication Storage Area Inspections. All stocks of medications shall be inspected routinely to ensure the absence of outdated, unusable, recalled, or mislabeled products. Storage conditions that would foster medication deterioration, storage arrangements that might contribute to medication errors, and other safety issues shall be assessed, documented, and corrected.[4]

D. Returning Recalled, Expired, Other Unusable Items

Drug Product Recalls. There shall be a written procedure for the timely handling and documentation of a drug product recall. These procedures should include an established process for removing from use any drugs or devices subjected to a recall, notifying appropriate health care professionals, identifying patients who may have been exposed to the recalled medication, and, if necessary, communicating available alternative therapies to prescribers. The pharmacy shall

be notified of any defective drug products or related supplies and equipment encountered by the nursing or medical staffs. All drug product defects should be reported to the FDA's MedWatch reporting program.[4]

Standard V. Preparing, Packaging, and Labeling Medications

A. Preparing Medications

Compounding. Drug formulations, dosage forms, strengths, and packaging that are not available commercially but are needed for patient care shall be prepared by appropriately trained personnel in accordance with applicable practice standards and regulations. The pharmacy shall provide adequate quality assurance procedures for these operations. Written master formulas and batch records (including product test results, as appropriate) shall be maintained, and a lot number or other method to identify each finished product with its production and control history shall be assigned to each batch.[14–20]

Sterile Preparations. When possible, manufactured sterile preparations should be preferred to compounding in the pharmacy. All sterile medications shall be prepared and labeled in a suitable environment by appropriately trained personnel in accordance with established quality assurance and expiration dating procedures.[14,19] The use of sterile medications compounded outside the pharmacy should be avoided to the extent possible; when they are used, there shall be procedures for aseptic preparation, quality assurance, expiration dating, and ongoing competency evaluations for compounding personnel.[14,19,37] Sterile compounding outside the pharmacy or satellite pharmacies (e.g., on nursing units) should be minimized and occur only in emergency situations.[14,19]

Hazardous Drug Products. There shall be policies and procedures that describe special precautions, equipment, and training for preparation, handling, storage, and disposal of hazardous drug products and products used in their preparation. These policies and procedures shall be consistent with applicable laws and regulations, and should be adequate to ensure the safety of staff, patients, visitors, the community, and the environment.[17]

B. Packaging Medications

Unit Dose Packaging. Whenever possible, medications shall be available for inpatient use in single-unit packages and in a ready-to-administer form. Manipulation of medications before administration (e.g., withdrawal of doses from containers, reconstitution of powdered drug products, labeling of containers, and splitting of tablets) by final users should be minimized.[15]

Bar-Coding of Unit Dose Packaging and Point of Care Administration. Unit-dose packages should contain a bar code, and that code should be used in inventory management, dose preparation and packaging, dispensing, and administration. It is the responsibility of the pharmacy department to ensure the quality of all aspects of bar-code medication administration, including scanability of bar codes and database management.[38,39]

Standard VI. Medication Delivery

A. Dispensing Medications

Prescribing. Medications shall be prescribed by individuals who have been granted appropriate clinical privileges in the hospital and are legally permitted to order medications. The pharmacy shall advocate and foster practitioners' conformance with standardized, approved, and safe terminology and abbreviations to be used throughout the hospital when prescribing medications and discourage use of nonstandard and unapproved terminology and abbreviations.[4]

Diagnostic or Therapeutic Purpose. Pharmacists should have immediate access to the patient's diagnosis or the intended therapeutic or medical purpose of medications.

Medication Orders. All patient medication orders shall be contained in the patient's medical record. A direct copy of the prescriber's order, either hard copy (including facsimile) or prescriber-entered electronic transmission (preferred method), shall be received by the pharmacist. Oral orders should be avoided to the extent possible. When oral orders are necessary, they shall follow the organization's established procedures for their use and documentation. Order transmittal safeguards should be used to ensure the security of the prescriber's order. Appropriate records of each medication order and its processing in the pharmacy shall be maintained in accordance with applicable laws and regulations.

A system shall exist to ensure that medication orders are not inappropriately continued.[4]

Review of Medication Orders. All medication orders shall be prospectively reviewed by a pharmacist and assessed in relation to pertinent patient and clinical information before the first dose is administered or made available in an automated dispensing device, except in emergent situations in which the treatment of the patient would be significantly compromised by the delay that would result from pharmacist review of the order. There shall be a procedure for retrospective review of these orders.

Any questions regarding an order shall be resolved with the prescriber prior to administration, and any action taken as a result of this intervention should be documented in the patient's medical record. Information concerning changes shall be communicated to the appropriate health professionals caring for the patient.[4]

Drug Delivery Systems, Administration Devices, and Automated Distribution Devices. The pharmacy shall have responsibility for developing policies, procedures, and quality assurance programs regarding drug delivery systems, administration devices, and automated distribution devices that ensure safety, accuracy, security, and patient confidentiality. The potential for medication errors associated with such systems and devices should be thoroughly evaluated.[4,6] Pharmacy personnel shall supervise the stocking and documentation of medications in automated dispensing devices.[6] Whenever possible, automated dispensing cabinets should employ profile-based technology integrated with remote medication order-entry capabilities.

Medication Administration. Only personnel who are authorized by the hospital in accordance with applicable laws

and regulations and appropriately trained shall be permitted to administer medications to a patient. All administered, refused, or omitted medication doses should be recorded in the patient's medical record according to an established procedure, and all medications that have not been administered should be returned to the pharmacy. No medication should be administered to a patient unless medical and nursing personnel have been provided with adequate information about, and are familiar with, its therapeutic use, method of administration, potential adverse effects, and dosage.

Standard VII. Monitoring Medication Use

A. Reviewing Patient Responses to Medication Therapy
Medication Therapy Monitoring. Medication therapy monitoring shall be conducted by pharmacists. Medication therapy monitoring includes a proactive assessment of patient problems and an assessment of

a. The therapeutic appropriateness of the patient's medication regimen.
b. Therapeutic duplication or omissions in the patient's medication regimen.
c. The appropriateness of the dose of the medication, as well as the route, method, and frequency of administration of the medication.
d. Patient adherence to the prescribed medication regimen.
e. Medication–medication, medication–food, medication–dietary supplement, medication–laboratory test, and medication–disease interactions.
f. Adverse drug reactions and other undesired effects.[40]
g. Patient medication allergies and sensitivities.
h. Clinical and pharmacokinetic laboratory data to evaluate the efficacy and safety of medication therapy and to anticipate toxicity and adverse effects.
i. Physical signs and clinical symptoms relevant to the patient's medication therapy.
j. Assessment of the effectiveness of the patient's medication therapy.

B. Educating and Counseling Patients and Family
Patient Education. Pharmacists shall be available to participate in patient education. Pharmacists should help to ensure that all patients are given adequate information about the medications they receive in order to help patients participate in their own health care decisions and encourage adherence to medication regimens. Patient education activities shall be coordinated with the nursing, medical, and other clinical staff as needed. Medication-related material developed by other services and departments as well as commercial sources should be reviewed by the pharmacy staff for accuracy, currency, literacy appropriateness, and completeness. If necessary, interpretative language services (written or oral) should be made available to patients.[21]

Standard VIII. Evaluating the Effectiveness of the Medication-Use System

There shall be an ongoing, systematic program for quality assessment and improvement of pharmacy services and the medication-use system. The program should include routinely evaluating the literature for new technologies or successful practices that have been demonstrated to enhance safety in other organizations to determine if such technologies or practices can improve the hospital's medication-use system. This program should be integrated with the hospital's or health system's quality assessment and quality improvement activities. Quality improvement activities related to the selection, prescription, procurement, storage, preparation, dispensing, distribution, administration, documentation, monitoring, and use of medications shall be routinely performed in cooperation with other health care providers. Feedback to appropriate individuals or entities about the quality achieved shall be provided.

A. Assessing Pharmacy Services and Practices
Documentation of Pharmacist-Provided Patient Care Services and Medication Therapy Outcomes. The pharmacy shall have an ongoing process for consistent documentation of the patient care services provided by pharmacists and patient outcomes from medication therapy.[30]

Workload and Financial Performance. A process shall exist to routinely monitor and document workload and financial performance. Metrics should encompass the full scope of patient care services provided by pharmacists and the pharmacy enterprise. This process should provide for the determination and analysis of hospital and system-wide costs of medication therapy. A pharmacist should be an integral part of the hospital's leadership teams (e.g., administrative, financial).

B. Improving the Medication-Use Process
Medication-Use Evaluation. There shall be an ongoing program for monitoring drug utilization and costs to ensure that medications are used appropriately, safely, and effectively, and to increase the probability of desired patient outcomes. The P&T committee (or its equivalent) should define specific parameters for evaluation (e.g., disease state, pharmacological category, or high-use/high-cost drug products) as appropriate for the organization. Through the ongoing evaluation of medication use, areas in need of improvement in medication prescribing and management can be identified and targeted for intervention.[32,41]

Medication Safety. Pharmacists should provide leadership to and participate in collaborative, multidisciplinary efforts to prevent, detect, and resolve drug-related problems that can result in patient harm. Pharmacists and other appropriate hospital personnel shall establish and regularly revise policies and procedures regarding medication error and adverse event prevention and reporting. Monitoring, detecting, review, and analysis of the hospital and health system's medication errors and near-misses should be an ongoing process in a *just culture* environment,[42] and corresponding corrective actions should be documented. An ongoing program for preventing, monitoring, resolving, and reporting adverse drug events shall be developed.[40] A pharmacist shall participate in appropriate organizational committees and work with physicians, nurses, administrators, and others to examine and improve systems to ensure that medication-use processes are safe.[41]

Antimicrobial Stewardship and Infection Prevention and Control. There shall be policies and procedures to promote

the optimal use of antimicrobial agents, reduce the transmission of infections, and educate health professionals, patients, and the public about these topics. Pharmacists should participate in antimicrobial stewardship and infection prevention and control efforts through clinical endeavors focused on proper antimicrobial utilization and membership on relevant multidisciplinary work groups and committees within the health system.

Pharmacists should monitor patients' laboratory reports of microbial sensitivities or applicable diagnostic markers and advise prescribers if microbial resistance is suspected, evaluate trends in microbial prescribing relative to changes in microbial resistance patterns, and assist in developing prescribing patterns to help minimize the development of drug resistance.[24]

Standard IX. Research

The pharmacist should initiate, participate in, and support clinical and practice-related research appropriate to the goals, objectives, and resources of the specific hospital.

Policies and Procedures. The pharmacist shall ensure that policies and procedures for the safe and proper use of investigational drugs and medication-related devices are established and followed, and that these policies and procedures meet all applicable laws and regulations. There shall be a procedure to assure that informed consent is obtained from the patient before the first dose of the study drug is administered.[5,44,45]

Procurement, Distribution, and Control of Investigational Drugs. The pharmacy shall be responsible for overseeing the procurement, distribution, and control of all investigational drugs. Investigational drugs shall be approved for use by an institutional review board and shall be dispensed and administered to consenting patients according to an approved protocol.[5,44,45]

Institutional Review Board. A pharmacist shall be a member of the hospital's institutional review board (or equivalent body), if one exists.[44]

Information Regarding Investigational Drugs. The pharmacy shall have access to information on all investigational studies and similar research projects involving medications and medication-related devices used in the hospital. The pharmacy shall provide pertinent written information (to the extent known) about the safe and proper use of investigational drugs, including possible adverse effects and adverse drug reactions, to nurses, pharmacists, physicians, and other health care professionals called upon to prescribe, dispense, and administer these medications.[44,45]

References

1. American Society of Health-System Pharmacists. Mission statement of the American Society of Health-System Pharmacists. *Am J Health-Syst Pharm.* 2001; 58:1524.
2. American Society of Health-System Pharmacists. The consensus of the Pharmacy Practice Model Summit. *Am J Health-Syst Pharm.* 2011; 68:1148–52.
3. American Society of Health-System Pharmacists. ASHP guidelines on remote medication order processing. *Am J Health-Syst Pharm.* 2010; 67:672–7.
4. American Society of Hospital Pharmacists. ASHP technical assistance bulletin on hospital drug distribution and control. *Am J Hosp Pharm.* 1980; 37:1097–103.
5. American Society of Health-System Pharmacists. ASHP guidelines on the pharmacy and therapeutics committee and the formulary system. *Am J Health-Syst Pharm.* 2008; 65:1272–83.
6. American Society of Health-System Pharmacists. ASHP guidelines on the safe use of automated dispensing devices. *Am J Health-Syst Pharm.* 2010; 67:483–90.
7. American Society of Health-System Pharmacists. ASHP statement on the role of health-system pharmacists in emergency preparedness. *Am J Health-Syst Pharm.* 2003; 60:1993–5.
8. American Society of Health-System Pharmacists. ASHP guidelines on the pharmacist's role in immunization. *Am J Health-Syst Pharm.* 2003; 60:1371–7.
9. American Society of Health-System Pharmacists. ASHP statement on the pharmacist's role in substance abuse prevention, education, and assistance. *Am J Health-Syst Pharm.* 2003; 60:1995–8.
10. American Society of Health-System Pharmacists. ASHP Residency Accreditation. www.ashp.org/menu/Accreditation/ResidencyAccreditation.aspx (accessed 10 Jan 2012).
11. American Society of Hospital Pharmacists. ASHP statement on continuing education. *Am J Hosp Pharm.* 1990; 47:1855.
12. American Society of Health-System Pharmacists. ASHP guidelines on the recruitment, selection, and retention of pharmacy personnel. *Am J Health-Syst Pharm.* 2003; 60:587–93.
13. American Pharmacists Association. Code of Ethics for Pharmacists. www.pharmacist.com/AM/Template.cfm?Section=Search1&template=/CM/HTMLDisplay.cfm&ContentID=2903 (accessed 10 Jan 2012).
14. American Society of Health-System Pharmacists. ASHP guidelines on quality assurance for pharmacy-prepared sterile products. *Am J Health-Syst Pharm.* 2000; 57:1150–69.
15. American Society of Hospital Pharmacists. ASHP technical assistance bulletin on single unit and unit dose packages of drugs. *Am J Hosp Pharm.* 1985; 42:378–9.
16. American Society of Hospital Pharmacists. ASHP technical assistance bulletin on compounding nonsterile products in pharmacies. *Am J Hosp Pharm.* 1994; 51:1441–8.
17. American Society of Health-System Pharmacists. ASHP guidelines on handling hazardous drugs. *Am J Health-Syst Pharm.* 2006; 63:1172–93.
18. American Society of Hospital Pharmacists. ASHP technical assistance bulletin on repackaging oral solids and liquids in single unit and unit dose packages. *Am J Hosp Pharm.* 1983; 40:451–2.
19. General chapter 797—pharmaceutical compounding: nonsterile preparations. Rockville, MD: United

States Pharmacopeial Convention; The United States pharmacopeia, 32nd rev., and The national formulary, 27th ed. Rockville, MD: United States Pharmacopeial Convention; 2009:318–54.

20. General chapter 795—pharmaceutical compounding: nonsterile preparations. The United States pharmacopeia, 35th rev., and The national formulary, 30th ed. Rockville, MD: United States Pharmacopeial Convention; 2011: 344–50.

21. American Society of Health-System Pharmacists. ASHP guidelines on pharmacist-conducted patient education and counseling. *Am J Health-Syst Pharm.* 1997; 54:431–4.

22. American Society of Health-System Pharmacists. ASHP guidelines on the safe use of automated compounding devices for the preparation of parenteral nutrition admixtures. *Am J Health-Syst Pharm.* 2000; 57:1343–8.

23. American Society of Health-System Pharmacists. ASHP guidelines on pharmacy planning for implementation of computerized provider order entry systems in hospitals and health systems. *Am J Health-Syst Pharm.* 2011; 68:e9–e31.

24. American Society of Health-System Pharmacists. ASHP statement on the pharmacist's role in antimicrobial stewardship and infection prevention and control. *Am J Health-Syst Pharm.* 2010; 67:575–7.

25. American Society of Health-System Pharmacists. ASHP statement on the pharmacist's role in informatics. *Am J Health-Syst Pharm.* 2007; 64:200–3.

26. American Society of Health-System Pharmacists. ASHP statement on the roles and responsibilities of the pharmacy executive. *Am J Health-Syst Pharm.* 2009; 66:499–502.

27. American Society of Health-System Pharmacists. ASHP guidelines on the pharmacist's role in the development, implementation, and assessment of critical pathways. *Am J Health-Syst Pharm.* 2004; 61:939–45.

28. American Society of Health-System Pharmacists. ASHP guidelines on the provision of medication information by pharmacists. *Am J Health-Syst Pharm.* 1996; 53:1843–5.

29. Office of the Law Revision Counsel, United States House of Representatives. USC*prelim.* 42 U.S.C. Sec. 299b-35(c), MTM services to eligible individuals. Available at: http://uscode.house.gov/lawrevision-counsel.shtml (accessed 24 Apr 2012).

30. American Society of Health-System Pharmacists. ASHP guidelines on documenting pharmaceutical care in patient medical records. *Am J Health-Syst Pharm.* 2003; 60:705–7.

31. American Society of Hospital Pharmacists. ASHP guidelines for selecting pharmaceutical manufacturers and suppliers. *Am J Hosp Pharm.* 1991; 48:523–4.

32. American Society of Health-System Pharmacists. ASHP guidelines on medication cost management strategies for hospitals and health systems. *Am J Health-Syst Pharm.* 2008; 65:1368–84.

33. American Society of Hospital Pharmacists. ASHP guidelines for pharmacists on the activities of vendors' representatives in organized health care systems. *Am J Hosp Pharm.* 1994; 51:520–1.

34. American Society of Health-System Pharmacists. ASHP Drug Shortages Resource Center. www.ashp.org/shortages (accessed 11 Jan 2012).

35. U.S. Food and Drug Administration. Drug shortages. www.fda.gov/cder/drug/shortages/ (accessed 11 Jan 2012).

36. American Society of Health-System Pharmacists. ASHP guidelines on managing drug product shortages in hospitals and health systems. *Am J Health-Syst Pharm.* 2009; 66:1399–406.

37. American Society of Health-System Pharmacists. ASHP guidelines on outsourcing sterile compounding services. *Am J Health-Syst Pharm.* 2010; 67:757–65.

38. American Society of Health-System Pharmacists. ASHP statement on bar-code-enabled medication administration technology. *Am J Health-Syst Pharm.* 2009; 66:588–90.

39. American Society of Health-System Pharmacists. ASHP statement on bar-code verification during inventory, preparation, and dispensing of medications. *Am J Health-Syst Pharm.* 2011; 68:442–5.

40. American Society of Health-System Pharmacists. ASHP guidelines on adverse drug reaction monitoring and reporting. *Am J Health-Syst Pharm.* 1995; 52:417–9.

41. American Society of Health-System Pharmacists. ASHP guidelines on medication-use evaluation. *Am J Health-Syst Pharm.* 1996; 53:1953–5.

42. Khatri N, Brown GD, Hicks LL. From a blame culture to a just culture in health care. *Health Care Manage Rev.* 2009; 34(4):312–22.

43. American Society of Hospital Pharmacists. ASHP guidelines on preventing medication errors in hospitals. *Am J Hosp Pharm.* 1993; 50:305–14.

44. American Society of Health-System Pharmacists. ASHP guidelines on clinical drug research. *Am J Health-Syst Pharm.* 1998; 55:369–76.

45. American Society of Hospital Pharmacists. ASHP guidelines for pharmaceutical research in organized health-care settings. *Am J Hosp Pharm.* 1989; 46:129–30.

Developed through the ASHP Council on Pharmacy Practice and approved by the ASHP Board of Directors on April 13, 2012.

ASHP gratefully acknowledges the contributions made by the following individuals to various drafts of these guidelines: Thomas S. Brenner, B.S.Pharm., FASHP; Harold N. Godwin, M.S., FASHP, FAPhA; William A. Gouveia, M.S., FASHP; Brian D. Hodgkins, Pharm.D., FCSHP, FASHP; Stanley S. Kent, M.S., FASHP; Patricia C. Kienle, M.P.A., FASHP; Harold J. Kornfuhrer, B.S.Pharm., FASHP; Emory S. Martin III, Pharm.D., BCPS; J. Russell May, Pharm.D., FASHP; Gerald E. Meyer, Pharm.D., M.B.A., FASHP; Thomas E. O'Brien, Pharm.D., M.S., FASHP; Sherri L. Ramsey, D.Ph., BCPS; Frank G. Saya, Pharm.D., FCSHP, FASHP; Donna L. Soflin, B.S.Pharm., FASHP; David K. Solomon, Pharm.D., FASHP; Kasey K. Thompson, Pharm.D., M.S.; and Billy W. Woodward, B.S.Pharm.

ASHP also gratefully acknowledges the following organizations and individuals for reviewing drafts of these guidelines (review does

not imply endorsement): American Nurses Association (ANA); Institute for Safe Medication Practices (ISMP); Rhode Island Society of Health-System Pharmacists (RISHP); South Carolina Society of Health-system Pharmacists (SCSHP); Wyoming Society of Health-Systems Pharmacy (WSHP); Tuesday Adams, RN-C, WCC; John A. Armitstead, M.S., FASHP; Phil Ayers, Pharm.D., BCNSP; Ronald Barnes, M.S.; Paul J. Barrett, Pharm.D. BCPS; Carol J. Bickford, Ph.D., RN-BC, CPHIMS (ANA); P. Justin Boyd, Pharm.D. BCPS, CDM; Tim Brown, Pharm.D., BCACP; Margaret Chrymko, Pharm.D.; Toby Clark, M.Sc., FASHP; Wayne F. Conrad, Pharm.D., FASHP; Gayle A. Cotchen, Pharm.D., M.B.A.; Debra Lynn Painter Cowan, Pharm.D., FASHP; Arash Dabestani, Pharm.D., M.H.A., FASHP, FABC; Denise F. Daly, Pharm.D., BCPS; Tina H. Denetclaw, Pharm.D., BCPS; Deanna Dossey, Pharm.D.; William L. Fritz, M.S., FASHP; Daphne Hsu Galang, RPhT, CPhT, B.S., M.H.A.; Michael A. Gillette, Pharm.D., BCPS, BCACP; Kathleen M. Gura, Pharm.D., BCNSP, FASHP, FPPAG; Reginald L. Hain, B.S.Pharm.; Thomas G. Hall, Pharm.D.; George Hatfield, Pharm.D.; Jesse Hogue, Pharm.D.; Andrew Jarrell, Pharm.D.; Jack G. Kitrenos, Pharm.D., FASHP; Jamie Kuo, Pharm.D.; Jim Lile, Pharm.D.; Charles "Kurt" Mahan, Pharm.D., Ph.C.; Linda Gore Martin, Pharm.D., M.B.A., BCPS (WSHP); Justine Medina, M.S., RN; Dayna Mitchell, Pharm.D., BCPS; Holly Monatt, Pharm.D., BCPS; Selma Morrison; Robert J. Moura, M.S.; Jonathan M. Mundy, M.B.A. (RISHP); Bruce A. Nelson, M.S.; Beth Norman, M.S., RN, CNS, ACNS-BC; Robert S. Oakley, M.S.; Fred J. Pane, B.S.Pharm., FASHP; Shreya Parekh, Pharm.D.; Jennifer Phillips, Pharm.D.; James Ponto, BCNP, FASHP; Curt W. Quap, M.S., FASHP; Todd Rowland, Pharm.D.; Renee B. Sager, Pharm.D.; Joseph Sceppa, M.S., M.B.A.; Nicole Shumiloff, Pharm.D.; Nancy R. Smestad, M.S.; Carolyn M. Smith, Pharm.D., M.B.A., BCPS (SCHSP); William E. Smith, Pharm.D., M.P.H., Ph.D., FASHP; Richard L. Stambaugh, Pharm.D., M.S., BCPS; Therese Staublin, Pharm.D.; Marc Stranz, Pharm.D.; Timothy P. Stratton, Ph.D.; Pamela Swarny, Pharm.D., J.D.; Jane Tennis, B.S.Pharm., M.B.A.; Sherry Umhoefer, M.B.A.; Allen J. Vaida, Pharm.D., FASHP (ISMP); Jody Jacobson Wedret, FASHP, FCSHP; Roger Woolf, Pharm.D.; and Kevin Zak, Pharm.D.

Note: These guidelines had not been published in the *American Journal of Health-System Pharmacy* (*AJHP*) when *Best Practices for Hospital & Health-System Pharmacy 2012–2013* went to press. Some minor editorial differences may exist between this document and the official one that will eventually appear in *AJHP* and subsequent editions of this publication.

ASHP Guidelines on Pharmaceutical Services in Correctional Facilities

Introduction

Pharmaceutical services in correctional facilities encompass many aspects of community, hospital, and consultant pharmacy practice. These guidelines are intended to address some of the unique aspects of pharmacy practice and services in correctional facilities. Some correctional facilities may not require, or be able to obtain, the services of a pharmacist. However, the concepts, principles, and recommendations contained in this standard are applicable to all correctional facilities, regardless of size or type. Thus, the part-time pharmacy director or consultant pharmacist has the same basic obligations and responsibilities as his or her fulltime counterpart in larger settings. This document should serve as a guide for the provision of pharmaceutical services in correctional institutions.

Administration

Pharmaceutical services are an integral part of health care provided in correctional institutions. The pharmacist is usually responsible for multiple tasks ranging from the management of the pharmacy to the direct provision of services to inmate-patients. Two primary management responsibilities pertain to human and fiscal resources.

Personnel[1]
- Sufficient support personnel should be available to maximize the use of pharmacists in tasks requiring professional judgment. Appropriate supervisory controls for support personnel should be maintained. The use of pharmacy technicians graduated from ASHP-accredited pharmacy technician training programs is recommended. Pharmacy technicians should be certified by the Pharmacy Technician Certification Board.
- All personnel should possess the education and training needed to carry out their responsibilities. The competence of all staff may be enhanced through relevant continuing education. Credentialing of eligible staff as Certified Correctional Health Professionals through the National Commission on Correctional Health Care is recommended.
- A pharmacist should be available, at a minimum, on a consulting basis; the pharmacist should visit each facility no less than monthly. If the only pharmaceutical services provided are those of a consultant pharmacist, the consultant pharmacist should assume the role of pharmacy director.
- If the pharmacist is an employee of a contract vendor, he or she should be designated as the pharmacy director and assume the associated obligations and responsibilities.
- Health care services should be available to inmate-patients 24 hours a day. Pharmacist services should also be available, at least on an "on call" basis.
- Other pertinent guidelines of the American Society of Health-System Pharmacists, the National Commission on Correctional Health Care, and the American

Correctional Association should be followed, and requirements set by federal, state, and local laws and regulations with respect to personnel should be met.

Fiscal Resources

Pharmacists serving correctional institutions should strive to manage expenses while providing optimal care to the inmate-patients. The pharmacist should

- Work with the administrators of the correctional institution to establish a budget for the operation of the pharmacy.
- Consider factors unique to each institution for the development of the budget (e.g., total inmate capacity, average daily inmate population, demographics of the inmate population).
- Make allowances for the disproportionate amount of chronic communicable disease in the prison population and the regional variability of diseases.
- Apply the ASHP Technical Assistance Bulletin on Assessing Cost-Containment Strategies for Pharmacies in Organized Health-Care Settings, as appropriate.[2]

Policies and Procedures

A policies and procedures manual specifically written to address aspects of pharmacy practice in the correctional facility should exist.

- All policies and procedures should conform to federal, state, and local laws and regulations.
- The pharmacy director should be familiar with the Standards for Health Services promulgated by the National Commission on Correctional Health Care and the standards of the American Correctional Association.
- The pharmacy director should be familiar with the constitutional rights of inmate-patients, current literature about inmates' rights, and court rulings affecting the practice of correctional health care in general and correctional pharmacy in particular. Attention to these concepts should be reflected in the manual.
- The pharmacy director should be familiar with current literature, laws, and regulations governing confidentiality, consent, and other areas of correctional health care that diverge from more traditional standards of pharmacy practice. Attention to these should be reflected in the manual.
- Transportation of inmate-patients' medications within and among facilities should be addressed.
- Security of drug products, entry into the pharmacy during the absence of a pharmacist, use of night cabinets, emergency supplies of medications, and disaster services should be addressed.
- Policies and procedures on the pharmacy's role in preparing lethal injections for capital punishment should exist.

Administrative Reports

Administrative reports generated by the pharmacy department will vary from facility to facility depending on the level of pharmaceutical services provided. Reports should include

- The amounts and cost of drugs and services furnished
- Destruction of unusable or outdated medications
- Inventory value and quantities
- Records of formal meetings with administrators, physicians, nurses, and other staff and any changes implemented as a result of those meetings
- Minutes of pharmacy and therapeutics committee meetings
- Medication administration records
- Reports of quality-control and quality-improvement activities
- Reports generated as required by applicable state laws regulating the practice of pharmacy. (While often not specifically written for the practice of correctional pharmacy, these laws are nonetheless usually pertinent to pharmacy practice within the correctional setting.)

Facilities

The pharmacy should be located within or in an area contiguous to the space provided for other health care services. Facilities should be adequate to accommodate appropriate security of all drug products, especially controlled substances.[3]

Purchasing, Distribution, and Control of Medications

Purchasing, distribution, and control of medications are essential elements of any pharmacy operation. Adequate methods to ensure that these responsibilities are met should exist.

Purchasing

- The pharmacy director should be responsible for choosing the sources from which to obtain drug products.[4]
- The pharmacy director should ensure that all medications meet applicable legal requirements. Guidance on the obligations of drug product suppliers and purchasers appears in the ASHP Guidelines for Selecting Pharmaceutical Manufacturers and Suppliers.[5]
- The pharmacy director should ensure that medications purchased from sources other than manufacturers or wholesalers (e.g., other pharmacies, contract providers) meet all applicable legal requirements. All suppliers should be able, at the request of the pharmacy director, to provide data on the quality of products.
- To the extent possible, all drug products should be contained in single-unit or unit dose packages.

Distribution

The pharmacist is responsible for the distribution and control of all drug products (including diagnostics and drug-related devices).

- A unit dose drug distribution and control system is recommended.

- The system employed should focus on patient safety and result in a minimal incidence of medication errors and adverse drug reactions. Ongoing processes for the monitoring and reporting of adverse drug reactions and the detection and prevention of medication errors should exist.
- The system employed should be cost-effective.
- The system employed should foster drug-control and drug-use monitoring.
- The system employed should foster patient compliance, recovery of drugs because of expired orders, and ultimate destruction of all unusable and outdated medications.
- Inmates should not be used in the distribution process.
- Patient confidentiality should be ensured in the distribution process (e.g., patients receiving medications for the treatment of AIDS).

Drug Storage

- The pharmacy director should ensure the proper security of medications stored in each location.
- The pharmacy director should ensure that drug products are stored in accordance with manufacturer or USP requirements.
- The pharmacy director should ensure that stored drug products are not expired.

Control

- A process for the recovery of medications dispensed to inmate-patients after the discontinuance of orders or in compliance with automatic stop orders should exist.
- A process for minimizing and eliminating unauthorized use of medications by anyone other than the intended patient (e.g., exchange of medications between inmates) should exist.
- A process for minimizing and eliminating pilferage should exist.
- A process for monitoring and preventing the dispensing of unusually large quantities of medications should exist.
- A process for preventing the dispensing of sufficient doses of any medication to enable potential suicide should exist. Individuals who are evaluated as high risks for suicide should be identified.
- A process for the security and dispensing of controlled substances should exist.
- The pharmacy director, in conjunction with the facility's medical staff and other responsible health authorities, should maintain policies and procedures for the routine review and renewal of medication orders and for any automatic discontinuance of orders.
- Access to patients' medication records should be limited to authorized personnel only. Complete access by the pharmacist should be ensured.
- A process for pharmacist review of medication orders to ensure patient safety and appropriateness of medication should exist. Medication orders (except in emergency situations) should be reviewed by the pharmacist before the first dose is dispensed.

Medication Administration

While medication administration is traditionally the responsibility of nurses, in the correctional setting some or all of this responsibility may be assigned to other personnel.

- The pharmacy director should be familiar with standards of the National Commission on Correctional Health Care with respect to medication administration by non-health-care personnel, and policies and procedures specifically addressing such administration should exist.
- The pharmacy director should participate in development of medication administration forms and ensure that all relevant information is incorporated into the forms.
- The pharmacy director should regularly educate all personnel involved in medication administration. These educational programs should include information on proper administration, indications, monitoring for adverse effects and allergic reactions, documentation, accountability, confidentiality, and the importance of compliance. Inmates who repeatedly refuse to take medications should be counseled by a pharmacist.
- Policies should be developed regarding the administration of medication to inmate-patients assigned to jobs or on work-release programs.
- Policies and procedures should be developed to ensure continuity of therapy upon release. Released inmates should have access to a limited supply of medications; either the drugs should be provided upon release or released inmates should have a prescription order transmitted to the pharmacy of their choice.

Documentation

- Medication administration records should be reviewed by the pharmacist at least monthly for proper documentation of medication administration.
- Review of the medication administration record should include assessments of documentation of medications administered, doses, frequency of administration, compliance, start and stop dates, and medication allergies.
- Pharmacist interventions should be documented in patients' medical records.
- The pharmacist should document refills in accordance with state laws and regulations.
- Policies and procedures should exist for documenting the transportation of medication among separate sites in correctional facilities, including accountability from pickup to drop off.
- A consistent pattern of refusal by an inmate-patient to take medication should be documented in the patient's medical record.
- Policies and procedures should exist for the proper documentation of the receipt, placement in inventory, dispensing, administration, and destruction of controlled substances.

Emergency Services

- A pharmacist should educate medical and correctional personnel on the proper use of medications stocked for emergency use.
- A pharmacist should be available on an on-call basis in case of emergencies.
- Policies and procedures for the use of emergency kits of medications in life-threatening situations should exist. These kits should be maintained by a pharmacist.

- The pharmacy director should maintain policies and procedures for accessibility of medications in case of riots or other emergency situations.
- The pharmacy director, in conjunction with the medical director or other responsible health authority and the correctional institution's administrator, should develop policies and the procedures that complement the standards of the National Commission on Correctional Health Care regarding emergency services.

Therapeutic Policies

- The pharmacy director should be a member of the pharmacy and therapeutics committee or its equivalent.
- A formulary should exist in accordance with the ASHP Statement on the Formulary System, the ASHP Guidelines on Formulary System Management, the ASHP Technical Assistance Bulletin on Drug Formularies, and the ASHP Technical Assistance Bulletin on the Evaluation of Drugs for Formularies.[6–9]
- Drug products selected for formulary inclusion should serve the needs of the inmate-patient population and at the same time be as cost-effective as possible. The pharmacy director should ensure that cost is not the only determinant for drug product selection.
- Procedures should exist for the provision of nonformulary medications when necessary.
- The pharmacy director should, in conjunction with the facility's medical staff, maintain policies and procedures for the use of investigational medications that ensure adherence to the rights of inmate-patients.
- The pharmacy director should, in conjunction with the facility's psychiatrist or medical director, maintain policies and procedures for the use of psychotropic medications.
- The pharmacy director should be familiar with laws and regulations governing the treatment of patients with AIDS and make appropriate procedural allowances for the treatment of these patients.
- The pharmacist should have input into decisions about infection control policies and procedures pertinent to medication use.

Quality Improvement

- The pharmacy director should encourage the development of and participate in an ongoing quality improvement process that includes drug-use evaluation and drug-regimen review.

Drug Information

- A program should exist for regular education of health care and pertinent non-health-care personnel with respect to medication use.
- An up-to-date resource library that includes current publications and those required by law and regulation should be maintained by the pharmacy.
- The pharmacist should provide drug consultations as required to nurses, physician assistants, physicians, and any others involved in initiating, executing, and monitoring medication therapy.
- The pharmacist should educate and counsel inmate-patients on the proper use of medications.

Research

- Policies and procedures for the use of investigational drugs within the correctional facility should exist. (Additional guidance on pertinent policies and procedures can be found in the ASHP Guidelines for the Use of Investigational Drugs in Organized Health-Care Settings.[10])
- The pharmacy director should adhere to the Federal Regulations on Medical Research in Correctional Facilities (45 C.F.R. 46, revised March 6, 1983) when devising policies and procedures for use of investigational drugs.
- Information on issues that affect pharmacy practice within the correctional environment (e.g., criminology, medical-legal issues, endemic patient population) should be maintained.

References

1. American Society of Hospital Pharmacists. ASHP guidelines: minimum standard for pharmacies in institutions. *Am J Hosp Pharm.* 1985; 42:372–5.
2. American Society of Hospital Pharmacists. ASHP technical assistance bulletin on assessing cost-containment strategies for pharmacies in organized health-care settings. *Am J Hosp Pharm.* 1992; 49:155–60.
3. American Society of Hospital Pharmacists. ASHP technical assistance bulletin on use of controlled substances in organized health-care settings. *Am J Hosp Pharm.* 1993; 50:155–501.
4. American Society of Hospital Pharmacists. ASHP technical assistance bulletin on drug distribution and control. *Am J Hosp Pharm.* 1980; 37:1097–103.
5. American Society of Hospital Pharmacists. ASHP guidelines for selecting pharmaceutical manufacturers and suppliers. *Am J Hosp Pharm.* 1991; 48:523–4.
6. American Society of Hospital Pharmacists. ASHP guidelines on formulary system management. *Am J Hosp Pharm.* 1992; 49:648–52.
7. American Society of Hospital Pharmacists. ASHP technical assistance bulletin on drug formularies. *Am J Hosp Pharm.* 1991; 48:791–3.
8. American Society of Hospital Pharmacists. ASHP technical assistance bulletin on the evaluation of drugs for formularies. *Am J Hosp Pharm.* 1988; 45:386–7.
9. American Society of Hospital Pharmacists. ASHP statement on the formulary system. *Am J Hosp Pharm.* 1983; 1384–5.
10. American Society of Hospital Pharmacists. ASHP guidelines for the use of investigational drugs in organized health-care settings. *Am J Hosp Pharm.* 1991; 48:315–9.

These guidelines were reviewed in 2008 by the Council on Pharmacy Practice and by the Board of Directors and were found to still be appropriate.

Approved by the ASHP Board of Directors, April 26, 1995. Developed by the Council on Professional Affairs. Drafted for council review by Ronald L. Rideman.

The bibliographic citation for this document is as follows: American Society of Health-System Pharmacists. ASHP guidelines on pharmaceutical services in correctional facilities. *Am J Health-Syst Pharm.* 1995; 52:1810–3.

ASHP Guidelines on the Pharmacist's Role in Home Care

Purpose

The purpose of these guidelines is to define the role of the pharmacist in providing pharmaceutical care to patients in the home[1] or alternate-site setting. In broad terms, home care is the provision of specialized, complex pharmaceutical products and clinical assessment and monitoring to patients in their homes. This generally includes home infusion therapy and other injectable drug therapy and parenteral and enteral nutrition therapy. These therapies require resources and support beyond those of the traditional orally and topically administered therapies. Specific pharmacist education and training, drug product admixtures and administration techniques, equipment operation and maintenance, and patient monitoring are required to ensure successful outcomes. These guidelines outline the pharmacist's role in providing these services and products. They are not intended to apply to home health services that do not involve the provision of pharmaceutical services.

Many of the activities included in these guidelines are the subjects of other ASHP policy and guidance documents, which should be referred to for additional information. Pharmacists practicing in home care should use professional judgment in assessing ASHP's policy and guidance documents and in adapting them to meet their health care organizations' and patients' needs and circumstances.

Background

Home care services are provided by a variety of organizations, including hospitals, community pharmacies, home health agencies, hospices, and specialized infusion companies. Patients receive care in noninpatient settings, such as their homes and ambulatory infusion centers, or in alternate-site settings, such as skilled-nursing facilities. These guidelines apply to the provision of home care services by pharmacists practicing in all health care settings. It should be noted that different aspects of home care can be provided by different organizations. When services are shared among providers, pharmacists have a professional responsibility to ensure that all patient care responsibilities are defined, understood, agreed upon, and documented in advance by all providers.

Pharmacists' Responsibilities

Preadmission Assessment. The pharmacist should ensure that each patient referred for home care is assessed for appropriateness on the basis of admission criteria, including the following:

- The patient, family, and caregiver agree with provision of care services in the home.
- The patient or caregiver is willing to be educated about the correct administration of medications.
- The home environment is conducive to the provision of home care services (e.g., electricity and running water are present, and the home is clean).
- The home care provider has reasonable geographic access to the patient.

- There is psychosocial and family support (e.g., caregiver requirements and financial concerns are manageable, and the family environment is suitable).
- There is ongoing prescriber involvement in the assessment and treatment of the patient.
- The medical condition and prescribed medication therapy are suitable for home care services, and there is a prognosis with clearly defined outcome goals.
- The indication, dosage, and route and method of administration of medications are appropriate.
- Appropriate laboratory tests are ordered for monitoring the patient's response to medications.

Using the information collected during the preadmission assessment, the pharmacist, in conjunction with the other health care providers involved in the patient's care and the patient or caregiver, will determine the patient's appropriateness for home infusion services. The conclusions of the assessment should be communicated to all parties and appropriately documented.

Before the start of home care services, patients should be informed of their rights and responsibilities, including financial obligations. These should be explained in detail; given to the patient, family member, or other caregiver in writing; and documented in the patient's record.

In cases in which the first dose of a medication is to be given at home, the pharmacist should use clinical judgment in determining, in conjunction with the prescriber, home care nurse, and patient or caregiver, if home administration of the first dose is appropriate. Policies and procedures should define factors to be used in making this decision and precautions necessary when first doses are administered at home (e.g., emergency medications, monitoring and observation, and presence of a health care provider).[2]

Once a patient is accepted for home care, the pharmacist should assess the patient's current status and develop a patient database for ongoing drug therapy monitoring and as an evaluation tool for measuring patient outcomes. In most home care practice sites, the pharmacist is responsible for obtaining the medication order from the prescriber. In addition, the pharmacist should assess the legality and appropriateness of the medication order.

Initial Patient Database and Assessment. The complete patient database should be documented in the patient's home care record. This database should include, at a minimum, the following:

- The patient's name, address, telephone number, and date of birth,
- The person to contact in the event of an emergency, including the legal guardian or representative, if applicable,
- Information on the existence, content, and intent of an advance directive, if applicable,
- The patient's height, weight, and sex,
- All diagnoses,
- The location and type of intravenous access and when it was placed, if applicable,
- Pertinent laboratory test results,

- Pertinent medical history and physical findings,
- Nutrition screening test results,
- An accurate history of allergies,
- Initial and ongoing pharmaceutical assessments,
- A detailed medication profile, including all medications (prescription and nonprescription), immunizations, home remedies, and investigational and nontraditional therapies,
- The prescriber's name, address, and telephone number and any other pertinent information (e.g., Drug Enforcement Administration number),
- Other agencies and individuals involved in the patient's care and directions for contacting them,
- A history of medication use,
- A care plan and a list of drug-related problems, if any,
- Treatment goals and the expected duration of therapy,
- Indicators of desired outcomes,
- Patient education previously provided,
- Any functional limitations of the patient, and
- Any pertinent social history (e.g., alcohol consumption and tobacco use).

To obtain this information, the pharmacist could use the medical record; laboratory test results; direct communication with the patient, caregiver, nurse, and prescriber; and direct observation. When the pharmacist cannot directly observe the patient, the patient's home care nurse or other appropriate health care provider could provide the results of direct observation and physical assessment. If a shared-service agreement exists among multiple providers, the pharmacist should ensure that this agreement specifies the responsibilities of each provider for obtaining and sharing pertinent patient information.

Selection of Products, Devices, and Ancillary Supplies. The pharmacist, in collaboration with other health care providers and the patient, is responsible for selecting infusion devices, ancillary drugs (e.g., heparin lock flush solution and 0.9% sodium chloride injection), and ancillary supplies (e.g., dressing kits, syringes, and administration sets).[3,4] Pharmacists should be thoroughly trained and knowledgeable in the selection, proper use, and maintenance of these devices, drugs, and supplies. Factors involved in the selection of devices and ancillary supplies may include the following:

- The stability and compatibility of prescribed medications in infusion device reservoirs,
- The ability of an infusion device to accommodate the appropriate volume of medication and diluent and to deliver the prescribed dose at the appropriate rate,
- The ability of the patient or caregiver to learn to operate an infusion device,
- The potential for patient complications and noncompliance,
- Patient convenience,
- Nursing or caregiver experience with therapies and selected devices,
- Prescriber preferences,
- Cost considerations, and
- The safety features of infusion devices.

The home care pharmacist, in consultation with the prescriber, should determine when emergency medications and supplies (e.g., anaphylaxis "kits") should be dispensed to home care patients. When standing orders for ancillary drugs or supplies or standardized treatment protocols are used, the pharmacist should review each protocol to determine its appropriateness for the patient.

Development of Care Plans. The pharmacist, in collaboration with the patient or caregiver and other health care providers, is responsible for developing an appropriate and individualized care plan for each patient. The pharmacist's contribution to the care plan should be based on information obtained from the initial pharmacy assessment and other relevant information obtained from the nurse, the prescriber, the patient, and the caregiver. At a minimum, the pharmacist's contribution to the care plan should include the following[5]:

- A description of actual or potential drug therapy problems and their proposed solutions,
- A description of desired outcomes of drug therapy provided,
- A proposal for patient education and counseling, and
- A plan specifying proactive objective and subjective monitoring (e.g., vital signs, laboratory tests, physical findings, patient response, toxicity, adverse reactions, and noncompliance) and the frequency with which monitoring is to occur.

The care plan should be developed at the start of therapy and regularly reviewed and updated. The degree of detail of the plan should be based on the complexity of drug therapy and the patient's condition.

The pharmacist is responsible for communicating care plan contributions to other health care providers involved in the patient's care, to the patient, and to the caregiver. Updates, as they occur, should be communicated to the appropriate persons. The care plan and updates should be a part of the patient's record.

Patient Education and Counseling. The pharmacist is responsible for ensuring that the patient or caregiver receives appropriate education and counseling about the patient's medication therapy. The pharmacist should verify that the patient or caregiver understands the therapy. Other health care providers may be involved. A home care pharmacist should be readily accessible if questions or problems arise. Supplementary written information should be provided to reinforce oral communications. Contingencies should be available to provide education, counseling, and written materials to patients who do not speak English. Depending on the need, this might require access to interpreters or bilingual pharmacists.

Professional judgment is required to determine what information should be included in patient education and counseling. The following should be considered:

- A description of medication therapy, including drug, dose, route of administration, dosage interval, and duration of therapy,
- The goals of medication therapy and indicators of progress toward those goals,
- Self-assessment techniques for monitoring the effectiveness of therapy,
- The importance of following the therapeutic plan,
- Proper aseptic technique,
- Proper care of the vascular-access device and site, if applicable,

- Precautions and directions for administering medications,
- Inspection of medications, containers, and supplies prior to use,
- Equipment use, maintenance, and troubleshooting,
- Home inventory management and procedures for securing additional supplies and medications when needed,
- Potential adverse effects, drug–drug interactions, drug–nutrient interactions, contraindications, and adverse reactions, and their management,
- Special precautions and directions for the preparation, storage, handling, and disposal of drugs, supplies, and biomedical waste,
- Information on contacting health care providers involved in the patient's care,
- Examples of situations that should be brought to the attention of the pharmacist or other health care providers involved in the patient's care (e.g., missed doses, doses not given at the proper time, and low supplies), and
- Emergency procedures.

Patient counseling and education should be performed in accordance with applicable state regulations and documented in the patient's home care record.

Clinical Monitoring. The pharmacist is responsible for ongoing clinical monitoring of the patient's drug therapy according to the care plan and for appropriately documenting and communicating the results of all pertinent monitoring activities to other health care providers involved in the patient's care. The pharmacist is also responsible for ensuring that relevant information is obtained from the patient, the caregiver, and other health care providers and for documenting this information in the patient's home care record.

Pharmacists may, in collaboration with prescribers and others, wish to develop clinical monitoring protocols for various therapies that could be individualized in specific care plans. Pharmacists may receive laboratory test results before other health care providers. In such cases, the pharmacist is responsible for communicating the test results to the prescriber and other health care providers. The pharmacist should provide an interpretive analysis of the information and recommendations for dosage adjustments and for continuation or discontinuation of drug therapy. The pharmacist should ensure that sufficient laboratory test results are readily available for monitoring the patient's therapy. In shared-service arrangements, clinical monitoring responsibilities should be delineated.

Effective communication with prescribers, nurses, and other health care providers. Effective communication among pharmacists, prescribers, nurses, and other health care providers is essential to ensuring continuous, coordinated care. The pharmacist should ensure that effective channels of communication about care are in place, including shared-service arrangements (e.g., regarding pain assessments and laboratory test data). Both oral and written communication methods can be used for communicating patient information. All relevant clinical communication should be documented in the patient's home care record. The pharmacist is responsible for protecting the patient's privacy and confidentiality while communicating this information to other health care providers. It is recommended that personnel involved in the care of the patient (e.g., nurses, pharmacists, dietitians, delivery representatives, and reimbursement coordinators)

meet regularly to discuss the clinical status of the patient and any operational issues related to the patient's care.

The patient, the family, the caregiver, and all health care providers involved in the patient's care should have access to a pharmacist 24 hours a day. The pharmacist is responsible for providing a summary of all relevant clinical information to another pharmacist providing coverage for that patient (e.g., an on-call pharmacist) before transferring patient care responsibilities.

Communication with the Patient and the Caregiver. The pharmacist providing home care services should establish free and open channels of communication with the patient or the caregiver. The pharmacist should contact the patient or the caregiver, as appropriate, to

- Obtain information needed for the initial pharmacy assessment,
- Provide supplemental patient education and counseling as needed,
- Assess compliance with drug therapy,
- Assess progress toward the goal of therapy,
- Inform the patient how to contact the pharmacist when needed, and
- Assess drug therapy problems (e.g., failure to respond to therapy and adverse drug events).

All contacts with the patient should be documented in the patient's home care record.

Coordination of Drug Preparation, Delivery, Storage, and Administration. The pharmacist is responsible for ensuring the proper acquisition, compounding, dispensing, storage, delivery, and administration of all medications and related equipment and supplies. Compounding of sterile products should comply with applicable practice standards, accreditation standards, and pertinent state and federal laws and regulations. If these services are being provided by another pharmacy, the pharmacist should have reasonable assurance that these standards are being met by the pharmacy providing the service. Pharmacists may administer medications to patients in the home setting unless prohibited by applicable laws and regulations.

The pharmacist should ensure that the delivery of medications and supplies to the patient occurs in a timely manner to avoid interruptions in drug therapy. Furthermore, the pharmacist should ensure that storage conditions during delivery and while in the patient's home are consistent with the recommendations for storing the product and beyond-use dating. The temperature of home refrigerators or freezers in which medications are stored should be within acceptable limits and should be monitored by the patient or caregiver. The pharmacist should ensure that an adequate inventory of medications and ancillary supplies is available in the patient's home. It may be appropriate to provide additional inventory for unforeseen circumstances in which extra doses or supplies may be required (e.g., waste, breakage, and emergencies).

Standard Precautions for Employee and Patient Safety. A home care organization is responsible for helping teach employees, patients, family members, and caregivers about standard safety precautions. The pharmacist should ensure

that the home care organization provides appropriate education for its employees and patients, including education about appropriate disposal and handling of medical waste, procedures for preventing and managing needle and sharps stick injuries, handling of cytotoxic and hazardous medications,[6] and material safety data sheets. The pharmacist should be a key resource in the development of such educational programs. The pharmacist should assume an active role in the home care organization's infection-control activities.

Documentation in the Home Care Record. A home care record should be developed and used for documenting the home care services provided to each patient. Written organizational policies and procedures should address the security of home care records and specify personnel authorized to review patient records and to make entries. The need to maintain confidentiality of patient information should be stressed to all personnel.

The pharmacist is responsible for documenting all pharmacy clinical activities in the patient's record in a timely manner. General clinician-oriented forms are preferred over specific nursing, pharmacy, and other health care professional forms to minimize duplication of information.

It may be advisable for organizations that provide multiple home care services (e.g., pharmacy, nursing, and respiratory therapy) to use a single home care record for documenting all clinical information regarding each patient. The patient's record should be accessible at all times to authorized personnel involved in the care of the patient, but confidentiality should be maintained.

Adverse Drug Event Reporting and Performance Improvement. The home care pharmacist should take a leadership role in the development of a program for reporting and monitoring all adverse drug events and device-related events, including adverse drug reactions and medication errors. The pharmacist should ensure that the prescriber is notified promptly of any suspected adverse drug events. Adverse drug events should serve as outcome indicators of quality, and the monitoring of adverse drug events should be a part of the organization's ongoing performance improvement program. Relevant trends should be integrated into staff development and inservice education programs for pharmacists and nurses to improve the quality of care and patient outcomes. Serious adverse drug reactions and device-related problems should be reported promptly to the manufacturer and to the Food and Drug Administration's MedWatch program. Medication errors should be reported to the USP Practitioner Reporting Program. Sentinel events should be reported to the Joint Commission on Accreditation of Healthcare Organizations.

Participation in Clinical Drug Research in the Home. The pharmacist should play a key role in the development of policies and procedures for handling investigational drugs and their protocols in the home care setting. When patient participation in clinical drug research is initiated in the institutional setting or another setting before the patient's transfer to the home care setting, it is important that the home care pharmacist obtain and keep on file sufficient information about the investigational drug protocol and drugs. If an investigational drug is dispensed or administered by the home care organization, a copy of the completed and signed informed consent should be placed in the patient's home care record. The home care pharmacist should review the protocol before the patient is admitted to the home

care service to determine whether it would be appropriate to treat the patient at home. When investigational drug inventories are maintained in the home care pharmacy, the pharmacist is responsible for accurate record keeping. The pharmacist should be an active participant in coordinating and monitoring clinical drug research in home care.

Participation in Performance Improvement Activities. Pharmacists should be active participants in performance improvement activities in their organizations. A performance improvement program for home care should monitor patient satisfaction and outcomes. Aspects of care that may be monitored include, but are not limited to, the following:

- Unscheduled inpatient admissions,
- Unexpected discontinuation of infusion therapy,
- Interruption of infusion therapy,
- Development of infections or complications,
- Reported adverse drug reactions and adverse device-related reactions,
- Medication errors, and
- Medication-related problems.

The performance improvement program should include appropriate quality control measures for compounding sterile products and other activities.

Policies and Procedures. The home care pharmacist should be an active participant in the development of organizational policies and procedures. The organization should maintain current policies and procedures for all aspects of patient care and quality assurance. Activities that should be addressed in policies and procedures include criteria for accepting patients into home care services, patient education and counseling, drug preparation and dispensing, equipment maintenance, quality assurance in sterile product compounding, infection control, and documentation.

Licensure. Pharmacists who provide home care services must have an active license to practice pharmacy issued by the applicable state board of pharmacy and other credentials as required by local, state, or federal laws and regulations. Some states require special licensure or training for preparing sterile products. Pharmacists dispensing medications to patients who reside in other states may also be subject to laws and regulations in those states; additional licensure may be required. The pharmacist should know about all applicable federal and state laws and regulations.

Training, Continuing Education, and Competence. Pharmacists should receive training as necessary to ensure that they possess the knowledge and skills required for the provision of home care services. They should participate in ongoing continuing-education activities to update and enhance their knowledge and skills related to home care. Pharmacists should participate in an ongoing competence assessment program as part of an overall staff development program. A valid assessment of competence should consider the pharmacist's responsibilities and the types and ages of patients. The assessment should be conducted and documented on an ongoing basis for all pharmacists. When appropriate, pharmacists should assist in training and in continuing-education programs for other home care providers Pharmacists should

provide, to the extent possible in their organizations, student clerkship, externship, and internship training, as well as postgraduate residency training.

References

1. Pelham LD, Norwood MR. Home health care services. In: Brown TR, ed. Handbook of institutional pharmacy practice. 3rd ed. Bethesda, MD: American Society of Hospital Pharmacists; 1992:357–66.

2. McNulty TJ. Initiation of antimicrobial therapy in the home. *Am J Hosp Pharm.* 1993; 50:773–4.

3. Kwan J. High-technology i.v. infusion devices. *Am J Hosp Pharm.* 1991; 48:536–51.

4. Bowles C, McKinnon BT. Selecting infusion devices. *Am J Hosp Pharm.* 1993; 50:1228–30.

5. Hepler CD, Strand LM. Opportunities and responsibilities in pharmaceutical care. *Am J Hosp Pharm.* 1990; 47:533–43.

6. Schaffner A. Safety precautions in home chemotherapy. *Am J Nurs.* 1984; 84:346–7.

Developed through the ASHP Council on Professional Affairs with the assistance of the Executive Committee and Professional Practice Committee of the ASHP Section of Home Care Practitioners and approved by the ASHP Board of Directors on April 27, 2000.

The bibliographic citation for this document is as follows: American Society of Health-System Pharmacists. ASHP guidelines on the pharmacist's role in home care. *Am J Health-Syst Pharm.* 2000; 57:1252–7.

Research

Research

Research on Drug Use in Obese Patients (1013)

Source: Council on Therapeutics

To encourage drug product manufacturers to conduct pharmacokinetic and pharmacodynamic research in obese patients to facilitate safe and effective dosing of medications in this patient population, especially for medications most likely to be affected by obesity; further,

To encourage manufacturers to include in the Food and Drug Administration (FDA)-approved labeling detailed information on characteristics of individuals enrolled in drug dosing studies; further,

To advocate that the FDA develop guidance for the design and reporting of studies that support dosing recommendations in obese patients; further,

To advocate for increased enrollment of obese patients in preapproval clinical trials of new medications; further,

To encourage independent research on the clinical significance of obesity on drug use, as well as the reporting and dissemination of this information via published literature, patient registries, and other mechanisms.

Institutional Review Boards and Investigational Use of Drugs (0711)

Source: Council on Pharmacy Practice

To support mandatory education and training on human subject protections and research bioethics for members of institutional review boards (IRBs), principal investigators, and all others involved in clinical research; further,

To advocate that principal investigators discuss their proposed clinical drug research with representatives of the pharmacy department before submitting a proposal to the IRB; further,

To advocate that IRBs include pharmacists as voting members; further,

To advocate that IRBs inform pharmacy of all approved clinical research involving drugs within the hospital or health system; further,

To advocate that pharmacists act as liaisons between IRBs and pharmacy and therapeutics committees in the management and conduct of clinical drug research studies; further,

To strongly support pharmacists' management of the control and distribution of drug products used in clinical research.

This policy was reviewed in 2011 by the Council on Therapeutics and by the Board of Directors and was found to still be appropriate.

Clinical Investigations of Drugs Used in Elderly and Pediatric Patients (0229)

Source: Council on Professional Affairs

To advocate increased enrollment of pediatric and geriatric patients in clinical trials of new medications; further,

To encourage pharmacodynamic and pharmacokinetic research in geriatric and pediatric patients to facilitate the safe and effective use of medications in these patient populations.

This policy was reviewed in 2011 by the Council on Therapeutics and by the Board of Directors and was found to still be appropriate.

ASHP Statement on Pharmaceutical Research in Organized Health-Care Settings

Pharmacy practice is grounded in the physicochemical, biological, and socioeconomic sciences. Hence, the continued and future success and self-esteem of the profession are dependent on the expanded knowledge base that can be produced through dynamic and rigorous scientific research and development. This research, to be meaningful and productive in terms of pharmacy's needs and goals in organized health-care settings, must include the participation of pharmacists practicing in those settings.

Pharmacists in organized health-care settings function in cooperation with other health-care professionals. They contribute a unique expertise to the drug-related aspects of patient care and take personal professional responsibility for the outcomes from the pharmaceutical care they provide to patients. Improvements in drug therapy depend on new knowledge generated by scientific research. Thus, pharmacists in organized health-care settings have a professional obligation to participate actively in and increase pharmacy-related and drug-related research efforts.[1,2]

Reflecting the collaborative nature of contemporary health care, this research should be multidisciplinary to be most beneficial. Thus, ASHP encourages pharmacists with a researchable idea or problem to seek the advice and active participation of people and organizations with scientific expertise such as

- College faculty (especially college of pharmacy faculty).
- Other staff and departments within the setting.
- Staff and departments in other health-care organizations.
- Industrial research personnel and laboratories.

It also is appropriate for pharmacists to function as principal investigators in research projects.

ASHP encourages pharmacists to increase their involvement in the following kinds of scientific research and development:

- Pharmaceutical research, including the development and testing of new drug dosage forms and drug preparation and administration methods and systems.

- Clinical research, such as the therapeutic characterization, evaluation, comparison, and outcomes of drug therapy and drug treatment regimens.
- Health services research and development, including behavioral and socioeconomic research such as research on cost–benefit issues in pharmaceutical care.
- Operations research, such as time and motion studies and evaluation of new and existing pharmacy programs and services.

This research will be a critical contribution of pharmacy to health care and must be fostered by all facets of the profession.

References

1. American Society of Hospital Pharmacists. ASHP guidelines for pharmaceutical research in organized healthcare settings. *Am J Hosp Pharm.* 1989; 46:129–30.
2. American Society of Hospital Pharmacists. ASHP guidelines for the use of investigational drugs in organized healthcare settings. *Am J Hosp Pharm.* 1991; 48:315–9.

Approved by the ASHP Board of Directors, November 14, 1990, and the ASHP House of Delegates, June 3, 1991. Revised by the ASHP Council on Professional Affairs. Supersedes a previous statement, "ASHP Statement on Institutional Pharmacy Research," approved by the ASHP House of Delegates on June 3, 1985, and the ASHP Board of Directors on November 14–15, 1984.

The bibliographic citation for this document is as follows: American Society of Hospital Pharmacists. ASHP statement on pharmaceutical research in organized health-care settings. *Am J Hosp Pharm.* 1991; 48:1781.

ASHP Guidelines on Clinical Drug Research

Purpose

The use of drug products to manage diseases and improve patients' quality of life is increasing as more effective and safer agents become available. Research to develop these agents is occurring in health system practice settings throughout the world. The credibility of this research and the protection of human subjects is a major responsibility of all health professionals involved.

ASHP believes pharmacists should play a pivotal role in the management of drugs used in the conduct of clinical research.[1-3] Pharmacists have become essential components of health system infrastructures supporting clinical research with both approved drugs and investigational drugs.[a,b] Pharmacists' roles in clinical research generally fall into one of two categories: (1) drug storage, preparation, and record keeping, frequently through an investigational drug service, and (2) serving as a principal investigator or a subinvestigator, manager, or coordinator within a research team that may include other health care professionals, research sponsors, monitors, contract research organizations, institutional review boards (IRBs), and institutional administrators.

The purposes of this document are to (1) outline the principles of clinical research, (2) describe the roles of participants in clinical research, (3) define pharmacists' roles in the use of drugs in clinical research, and (4) provide guidance to pharmacists and others responsible for the medication management component of clinical research. ASHP believes these guidelines are applicable to clinical research conducted in any health-system practice setting. These guidelines are an interpretation of federal laws, regulations, and standards for pharmacy practice in health systems. They should be used in conjunction with the applicable federal and state laws and regulations, not as a substitute for them. This document uses the term *shall* when the content is based on law or regulation and the term *should* for advice based on other guidelines, professional judgment, or expert opinion.

Background

The United States has benefited from a system for researching and marketing drug products that is codified in federal and state laws and regulations. The federal Food, Drug, and Cosmetic Act and its amendments[4] regulate drug product quality, safety, and effectiveness. The Food and Drug Administration (FDA) is the federal agency charged with enforcing the act and promulgating regulations for its implementation. FDA regulations concerning the conduct of clinical research with drug products of particular relevance for health-system pharmacists include Title 21 Code of Federal Regulations (CFR) Part 50, Protection of Human Subjects; Title 21 CFR Part 56, Institutional Review Boards; and Title 21 CFR Part 312, Investigational New Drug Application. Also applicable are the Department of Health and Human Services regulations in Title 45 CFR Part 46, Protection of Human Subjects. Requirements for and guidance on compliance with regulations are provided in FDA Information Sheets.

FDA has also published the Good Clinical Practice Consolidated Guideline[5] that was prepared under the auspices of the International Conference on Harmonisation of Technical Requirements for Registration of Pharmaceuticals for Human Use. The guideline offers a unified standard for designing, conducting, recording, and reporting trials that involve the participation of human subjects in the United States, Japan, and the European Union. In particular, the guideline provides a clearer understanding of behavioral and compliance standards for regulated drug research.

Basic Principles

The institutional components and practice settings of health systems participating in clinical drug research shall develop mechanisms, generally in the form of policies and procedures, for the approval, planning, and implementation of protocols. Good clinical practices, consistent with national and international standards, are the cornerstone of drug research in humans. Principles consistent with good clinical practices include the following:

1. An organization participating in human drug research studies shall ensure that such studies contain adequate safeguards for human subjects, its staff, and the scientific integrity of the study. There shall be written policies and procedures for the approval, management, and control of research involving investigational (not FDA-approved) drugs and post-marketing studies of FDA-approved drugs used in a research protocol. All research team members shall be fully informed about and comply with these policies and procedures.

2. The clinical trial shall have adequate prior information to justify use of human subjects, have a clearly defined protocol, and have received IRB approval before implementation.

3. All drug studies shall meet accepted ethical, legal, and scientific standards and be conducted by appropriately qualified investigators. Investigator qualifications, such as prior training and experience in research and with certain disease states, are required to be reviewed by IRBs, study sponsors, and FDA if the research will be submitted under an investigational new drug application (IND).

4. Every member of the research team shall be qualified by experience or training to perform his or her respective role.

5. All subjects must freely provide informed consent (documented in writing) before treatment with study drugs is begun. Accurate and complete information about the study's objectives, risks, and benefits must be provided before consent is obtained from the subject or his or her legally authorized representative. No unreasonable inducements (i.e., coercion or undue influence) shall be offered to subjects to encourage their participation in the study.

6. All clinical trial data shall be recorded and the records stored in such a way that the subject's rights of privacy and confidentiality are protected. All records shall be managed in a way that permits accurate reporting, verification, and retrieval after archiving.

7. Qualified pharmacists and other nonphysicians may serve as principal investigators as long as medical decisions made for the subjects are always the responsibility of a qualified physician or dentist.

Health-System Organization and Oversight

The health system should have processes for the administration of research that ensure that the aforementioned principles are upheld and the following responsibilities are met.

1. The health system shall be able to review and approve a protocol in the context of federal, state, and local laws and regulations. The health system should consider whether its own sponsored research or intellectual property development of drugs requires an IND for drugs not commercially available and approved drugs for unlabeled uses. An IND may be required if proposed research on the use of a marketed drug is intended to support the sponsor's change in drug labeling, advertising, or indications for use; a significant increase in risk; or a change in dosage level or route of administration. The health system should consult FDA for guidance.

2. The health system should have a mechanism for review and approval of the financial aspects of drug research, whether the study is sponsored by government agencies, foundations, or the pharmaceutical industry or is not sponsored.[6] Financial aspects may include contractual agreements stipulating cost recovery for resources, intellectual property agreements, insurance provisions, indemnification terms, and conflict-of-interest statements. Cost identification, allocation, and recovery mechanisms are imperative items for review and approval.

3. As required by federal regulation, clinical research shall be reviewed and approved by an IRB or equivalent committee (21 CFR 56.109). This committee shall evaluate each proposed clinical research study in terms of human subject protections and compliance with recognized ethical, legal, and scientific standards. No clinical study may be initiated unless approved in writing by the committee. Spoken IRB approval may be granted in emergency situations for a single subject's access to an investigational drug, but emergency use shall be reported to the IRB within five days; subsequent use requires full IRB review. Studies on the use of drugs in emergency or critical care settings do not in themselves qualify for single-subject approval and emergency exemption. Specific regulations govern research in the emergency setting and should be consulted in preparing protocols, IRB submissions, and consent procedures.[c,7]

 Treatment IND protocols are also subject to IRB review and approval. These protocols permit patient access to investigational drugs through a special program established by a sponsor. The physician and patient must agree that use of the agent may be in the patient's best interest and must document this agreement on a consent form.

 The IRB shall monitor approved studies to ensure that they are carried out appropriately and that the protocols are reassessed at least annually. Health system policies and procedures shall provide guidance on the conversion of human subjects to other therapies in the event that approval of an existing protocol is withdrawn by the IRB. The investigational-drug pharmacist, pharmacy director, or pharmacy director's designee should be a member of the IRB and should be consulted by the committee whenever drug studies are reviewed.

4. Investigational drugs shall be used only under the supervision of the principal investigator or authorized subinvestigators, all of whom shall be members of the professional staff. The determination of qualifications for investigators is the responsibility of the sponsor, IRB, and FDA when appropriate. Properly qualified pharmacists with experience and training in research may serve as principal investigators or subinvestigators.

5. The principal investigator or designee is responsible for obtaining informed consent from each subject who is eligible for participation in the study (i.e., meets inclusion and exclusion criteria).[c] The informed consent process shall conform to current federal and state regulations. IRB approval of the consent form (and assent form for minors) is required. Review by legal counsel may be desirable. The following points shall be included in the consent document and in an accompanying oral explanation by the investigator:

 a. That the trial involves research.

 b. The nature and purpose of the study and its expected benefits and foreseeable risks or discomforts. The name and telephone number of the principal investigator and persons to contact for questions about the study or drug.

 c. A balanced description of the alternative treatments available, including their respective risks and benefits.

 d. A general description of the study procedures, identification of any procedures that are experimental, expected length of therapy with the drug, and the subject's responsibilities. The name(s) of the investigational drug(s), including brand and generic names of commercial products.

 e. A statement that (1) participation is voluntary, (2) the subject may withdraw from the study at any time, (3) refusal to participate in or withdrawal from the study will involve no penalty or loss of benefits to which the subject is otherwise entitled, and (4) the principal investigator may remove the subject from the study if circumstances warrant. The investigator shall supply any new information that may affect a subject's desire to continue in a study.

 f. The name and signature of the subject (or his or her legally authorized representative), the name and signature of the principal investigator or subinvestigator, and the name and signature of the person presenting the consent form, with lines for each to personally date the signature.

 g. A statement of who will have access to any study records that contain subject identifiers, including monitoring personnel from the study sponsor or FDA who may inspect the records to assess compliance with the study protocol and all regulations, or institutional personnel auditing the quality of clinical research or financial transactions.

 h. Compensation or treatment available for a research-related injury.

 i. Anticipated payments to subjects, pro rata terms, or expenses subjects may incur. Any costs for which the subject will be responsible.

 The consent form shall be as detailed as is practical, with the goal of minimizing the amount of information that must be presented orally yet enabling

comprehension by most persons reading the form. For non-English-speaking subjects the consent form shall be in the subject's own language when feasible, or adequate interpretation shall be provided. For children able to read, an assent form shall be used to document their participation in the research process. The subject (or his or her representative) must have adequate time to read the consent form before signing it and shall receive a copy of the signed and dated form, along with any amendments to it. The subject shall retain a copy of the consent form. Additional copies of the consent form shall be kept on file as required by the sponsor, the IRB, the individual health system, and the medical records department.

Under certain protocols, patient drug or medical information may be collected from existing medical or pharmacy records. Pharmacists and investigators should consult the IRB to determine protocol-review and informed-consent requirements for any proposed studies.

6. The principal investigator is responsible for the proper maintenance of case report forms and all other study records required by the health system, the sponsor, and FDA.

7. The health system's medication-use system shall contain the following elements concerning drugs used in clinical research:

 a. Drugs shall be properly packaged in accordance with all applicable federal and state laws, regulations, and standards (e.g., FDA, *The United States Pharmacopeia and The National Formulary* [*USP–NF*], and the Poison Prevention Packaging Act).

 b. Drugs shall be labeled properly to ensure their safe use by the research and institutional staff and the subject.

 c. There shall be a mechanism to ensure that sufficient supplies of the drugs will be always available for the duration of the study.

 d. A mechanism shall be in place to allow the pharmacist or other designated health care provider, in a medical emergency during a randomized and blinded trial, to break the blinding code and reveal the identity of the study drug to other health care professionals. A reason to break the blind might be the need for a treatment decision that can be made only with knowledge of drug assignment.

 e. Nurses, pharmacists, physicians, and other health care practitioners (e.g., respiratory therapists, physician assistants) called on to administer or dispense investigational drugs should have adequate written information about (1) pharmacology (particularly adverse effects), (2) storage requirements, (3) method of dose preparation and administration, (4) disposal of unused drug, (5) precautions to be taken, including handling recommendations, (6) authorized prescribers, (7) human subject safety monitoring guidelines, and (8) any other material pertinent to safe and proper use of investigational drugs. These health care providers should be informed about the overall study objectives and procedures and shall have available a complete copy of the protocol for reference. Under all circumstances, investigational drugs shall be safely controlled, administered, and destroyed.

 f. Bulk supplies of the investigational drug shall be properly stored and adequately secured. When practical, all bulk supplies shall be stored in the pharmacy to ensure that storage, dispensing, accountability, and security are in compliance with federal and state laws and regulations and with standards used by the pharmacy department.

 g. There shall be a method for ensuring that only an authorized practitioner or designee prescribes the investigational drug.

 h. Records of the amount of investigational drug received from the sponsor and of its disposition (e.g., amounts dispensed to subjects or returned to sponsor) shall be maintained. These records shall be retained as required by regulation. Generally, records shall be maintained for at least two years after the date of an approved new-drug application (NDA) for the indication that is being investigated or, if the application is not approved or no application is filed, for at least two years after the investigation is discontinued and FDA is notified. Institutions should consider retaining records indefinitely. For studies involving international sites, records shall be maintained for 15 years after study closure. The sponsor may also request that records be stored longer than the minimum required time.

 i. If the subject is to receive the investigational drug at another facility, suitable arrangements shall be made for transfer of the drug. Sufficient information for safe use of the investigational drug, including copies of the subject's signed consent form, the study protocol, and the IRB approval letter, shall accompany the drug. The responsibilities of the facility to which the drug is transferred are based on whether that facility is providing care incidental to or as a participant in the research protocol.[8]

 j. The institution's records on investigational-drug studies should be designed so that various descriptive reports (e.g., names of all drugs under study, names of subjects who have received a given drug) can be generated conveniently and expeditiously. Once a study is closed, a copy of all pharmacy-related records should be provided to the principal investigator for storage. For its own records, the pharmacy should have a mechanism for long-term storage. The drug control responsibilities previously described shall be assigned to a pharmacist. If a pharmacist is not available, the investigator shall make arrangements to comply with these standards.

Pharmaceutical Services

A pharmacist should be responsible for ensuring that procedures for the control of drugs used in clinical research are developed and implemented. Each health system should develop a structure and procedures specific to its own needs and organization.

1. A copy of the IRB-approved research protocol and investigator's brochure or drug data sheet (see item 2 below), or both, and all amendments should be kept by a pharmacist.

2. Using the protocol and additional information (if needed) supplied by the principal investigator and sponsor, the pharmacist should prepare an investigational-drug data

sheet that concisely summarizes for the medical, nursing, and pharmacy staff's information pertinent to use of the drug. This communication should contain, at a minimum

a. Drug designation and common synonyms.
b. Dosage forms and strengths.
c. Usual dosage range, including dosage schedule and route of administration.
d. Indications pursued in this study.
e. Expected therapeutic effect to be studied.
f. Expected and potential adverse effects, including symptoms of toxicity and their treatment.
g. Drug–drug and drug–food interactions.
h. Contraindications.
i. Storage requirements.
j. Instructions for dosage preparation and administration, including stability and handling guidelines.
k. Instructions for disposition of unused doses.
l. Names and telephone numbers of principal and authorized subinvestigators and study coordinators.

Confidential copies should be distributed to the appropriate pharmacy staff and all areas within the health system where the investigational drug will be administered and the subjects monitored. Through the pharmacy or health-system computer system, this information can be made available to all staff members who need it. It is staff members' responsibility to become familiar with the information in these data sheets and to not share the information with persons who do not need it.

3. When it is practical, investigational-drug supplies should be stored in a pharmacy. When the drug is stored outside a pharmacy (e.g., small quantities in the investigator's office or in clinics where the drug is administered), methods used by the investigator responsible for the drug shall be audited by a pharmacist to ensure that storage, dispensing, accountability, and security comply with federal and state laws and regulations and with institutional policy.

4. The pharmacist shall maintain a perpetual inventory record for investigational drugs stored in the pharmacy. This record shall contain the drug's name, dosage form and strength, lot number, and expiration date; the name, address, and telephone number of the sponsor; the protocol number; and any other information needed for ordering the drug. Space shall be provided for recording data on the disposition of the drug (amounts received, transferred, wasted, or dispensed, with dates; the names of or codes for persons receiving the drug; and the names of prescribers), the amount currently on hand, the minimum reorder level, and the recorder's initials. The inventory record shall reflect drug doses that were dispensed but not administered and were returned to the pharmacist. These records are commonly audited by the sponsor, the sponsor's representatives, or FDA.[9,10]

5. The dispensing of investigational drugs should be integrated with the rest of the medication-use system, including, but not limited to, order review, profile maintenance, packaging, labeling, delivery, and quality-assurance procedures. However, prescription labels for investigational drugs shall be marked "investigational drug" or otherwise distinguished from other labels. The label should also include an alert to any possible hazards. There shall be a method for verifying that a valid, signed consent has been obtained. The investigational drug shall be dispensed only on the order of an authorized investigator or designee.

6. Educating patients and monitoring therapy (including adverse drug reaction monitoring) are two clinical functions that are particularly important and applicable to investigational drugs. The protocol should specify the provision of these functions by the pharmacists, the authorized investigator(s), and other members of the research team.

7. At the conclusion of the study, the pharmacist shall return, transfer, or dispose of all unused investigational drugs according to the specific instructions provided by the sponsor and in accordance with applicable regulations.

8. The pharmacist should prepare an annual or semiannual descriptive summary of investigational-drug use for the pharmacy director and pharmacy and therapeutics committee. This summary should include the number of studies in progress, a list of all drugs studied during the previous period, and a financial statement.

9. Drug costs and other expenses associated with drug studies (e.g., costs of record keeping and drug administration) should be properly allocated and reimbursed. Policies and procedures should address the role pharmacists play in billing sponsors, subjects, and third-party payers for services and goods related to research. In general, sponsors and health systems cannot charge subjects for an investigational drug. Sponsors may petition FDA for an exception. Health systems may charge subjects for drug preparation and other services necessary to deliver a final product, as is customary for delivery of services within the practice setting and when sponsors do not reimburse for this service. The anticipated costs of research should be described in the consent form. Subjects must be advised that they or their third-party payers are responsible for these charges and that a third-party payer may refuse to pay for charges related to research.

10. The investigational drugs shall be stored under appropriate environmental control in a limited-access area separate from routine drug stocks and shall be inventoried on a regular basis.

11. Pharmacists may be confronted with circumstances related to a patient who is receiving an investigational drug provided by an investigator at a nonaffiliated practice setting and is admitted to their own practice setting for care incidental to the research protocol. Pharmacists should have a policy for managing investigational drugs under those circumstances that meets FDA guidelines.[8]

12. Pharmacists must ensure the scientific integrity of drug studies by managing access to treatment-assignment records in blinded studies and by ensuring that the correct drug was dispensed. The pharmacist, investigator, and sponsor must agree on a procedure for unblinding treatment assignment in emergencies.

13. Pharmacists who are assigned to manage investigational drugs may at times have to delegate certain dispensing activities to other pharmacists within the health system. To ensure continuity of quality dispensing services, the responsible pharmacist should design and implement procedures for educating other members of the pharmacy

staff about the protocol and dispensing requirements. Often this can be accomplished by personal instruction and by preparing written directives and references for use by other pharmacists when they are called upon to dispense an investigational drug.

14. Pharmacists managing investigational drugs are in a unique position to monitor patient adherence to medication regimens. Because of the requirement that medication dispensed and returned be accounted for, pharmacists can readily surmise whether study patients are consuming the medication in the prescribed manner. At a minimum, pharmacists should counsel the investigator's research staff with regard to patient adherence. Pharmacists' skills in patient counseling should be used to support the investigators' efforts to encourage patients to adhere to their protocols.

Pharmaceutical Research Sponsors, Monitors, and Contract Research Organizations

The pharmaceutical company, or any study sponsor, that supports the use of investigational drugs in health systems should receive reliable and valid data. The following recommendations will serve as a guide to the pharmaceutical industry or other study sponsors to ensure that investigational drug use is managed appropriately and that studies are conducted effectively, efficiently, and safely.

1. Drugs shall be properly packaged in accordance with all applicable federal and state laws, regulations, and standards (e.g., FDA, *USP–NF*, and the Poison Prevention Packaging Act).
2. Drugs shall be properly labeled in accordance with applicable laws, regulations, and standards. If possible, ample space shall be left on the drug product container for further labeling by the pharmacist. Expiration dates and lot numbers should also be noted on the label.
3. A 24-hour telephone number should be available to study personnel, including the principal investigator and the pharmacy department. In the event of an emergency, information should be available pertaining to (1) adverse effects and their treatment, (2) emergency protocol management and dosing and administration guidelines, (3) the ability to break a "blinded code" to determine the treatment regimen, and (4) the mechanism for procuring a supply of medication under an emergency-use protocol.
4. Company representatives should be designated to handle routine requests, such as those for additional forms and resupply of investigational drugs. If possible, direct telephone or fax access should be available to expedite requests.
5. Investigational drugs should be shipped to the principal investigator in care of a pharmacist. The following information about procurement should also be supplied to the pharmacist:
 a. Name and telephone number of the sponsor's study monitor or field representative responsible for drug ordering.
 b. Estimated time for fulfillment of orders.
 c. Limits on quantities that can be ordered.
 d. Special ordering instructions.

 e. How the order is to be shipped (e.g., specific package-shipping firms).
 f. Disposition of invoice or drug receipt form once the drug is received.
6. The following information should be supplied by a sponsor or investigator to the pharmacist, preferably in an investigator's brochure, as applicable:
 a. Storage conditions required before and after preparation.
 b. Amounts and types of diluents for reconstitution and administration and the resulting final concentration of active drug.
 c. Stability of the prepared (i.e., ready-to-administer, reconstituted, or diluted) product and compatibility with drug delivery systems, diluents or i.v. fluids, containers, i.v. tubing, and filters.
 d. Known compatibility or incompatibility with other products.
 e. Light sensitivity.
 f. Filtration needs.
 g. Expiration dates or retest dates.
 h. Special instructions for preparation and administration.
 i. Acceptable and recommended routes and methods of administration, including rates of infusion for injectable products.
 j. Known adverse effects during or after administration (e.g., pain, phlebitis, and nausea) and how to avoid and treat them.
 k. Usual dosage regimens and highest dose tested for specific disease states, including dosage expressions for prescribing and labeling that could minimize misreading and misinterpretation.
 l. Contraindications.
 m. Drug interactions.
 n. Special precautions for storage, handling, and disposal of the drugs, including cytotoxic and hazardous drugs. For all hazardous drugs, the pharmacy department must be supplied with material safety data sheets.
 o. Pharmacology, including mechanism of action.
 p. Pharmacokinetic characteristics.
7. If all unused drugs are to be returned to the sponsor, information regarding storage and return procedures should be provided to the pharmacist. Drugs that are contaminated, outdated, or otherwise unsuitable should be returned to the sponsor or destroyed according to the institution's policies and procedures and applicable laws and regulations. These options should be agreed on beforehand by the sponsor and the pharmacist.
8. A complete current copy of the research protocol and investigator's brochure should be supplied to the pharmacist. Additional educational materials for use in informing pharmacists, physicians, and nurses about the investigational drug and research protocol should also be provided.
9. An appropriate allotment of research funds should be designated as reimbursement for
 a. Personnel.
 b. Storage facilities.
 c. Equipment.
 d. Ancillary products, such as diluents, syringes, and needles.
 e. Forms and miscellaneous clerical materials.

f. Computer and other data-processing costs.

g. Other expenses attributable to the pharmacist's involvement in the study.

h. Apportioned pharmacy overhead costs.

10. Sponsors should respond to requests for information from pharmacists involved in treating patients without formal research approval at that institution. This may occur, for example, when a patient is hospitalized (e.g., in an emergency) at a facility other than his or her usual care site.

11. When seeking marketing approval for an investigational drug, sponsors should consult pharmacists, physicians, and others involved in their investigational-drug studies for information. Because of their experience with the drug, these practitioners can supply valuable suggestions for labeling, packaging, palatability, routes of administration, and other dosage form characteristics, as well as information regarding patient monitoring and education.

12. The sponsor of an investigational drug study should provide final closure details within six months of trial completion. This includes prompt notification of closure, directions for drug disposition, and final audits of all study records.

13. These recommendations should also apply to the postmarketing approval of drugs under study for new indications or diseases.

References

1. Stolar MH, ed. Pharmacy-coordinated investigational drug services. Revised ed. Bethesda, MD: American Society of Hospital Pharmacists; 1986.

2. American Society of Health-System Pharmacists. ASHP guidelines: minimum standard for pharmacies in hospitals. *Am J Health-Syst Pharm.* 1995; 52:2711–7.

3. American Society of Hospital Pharmacists. ASHP statement on the use of medications for unlabeled uses. *Am J Hosp Pharm.* 1992; 49:2006–8.

4. Federal Food, Drug, and Cosmetic Act (21 U.S.C. 301 et seq.) 1938, as amended.

5. Food and Drug Administration, Department of Health and Human Services. International conference on harmonisation; good clinical practice consolidated guideline. *Fed Regist.* 1997; 62:25692–709.

6. Wermeling DP, Piecoro LT, Foster TS. Financial impact of clinical research on a health system. *Am J Health-Syst Pharm.* 1997; 54:1742–51.

7. Bailey EM, Habowski SR. How to apply for emergency use of an investigational agent. *Am J Health-Syst Pharm.* 1996; 53:208–10.

8. Food and Drug Administration. Use of investigational products when subjects enter a second institution. IRB operations and clinical investigation information sheet. http://www.fda.gov/oc/oha/useofinv.html (accessed August 25, 1997).

9. Food and Drug Administration. Institutional review board inspections. IRB operations and clinical investigation information sheet. http://www.fda.gov/oc/oha/institut.html (accessed August 25, 1997).

10. Food and Drug Administration. Inspections of clinical investigators. IRB operations and clinical investigation information sheet. http://www.fda.gov/oc/oha/inspect.html (accessed August 25, 1997).

Suggested Internet Source

Food and Drug Administration information for clinical investigators. http://www.fda.gov/cder/about/smallbiz/clinical_investigator.htm.

Glossary[d]

Adverse Drug Reaction (ADR): In preapproval clinical experience with a new medicinal product or its new usages, particularly since the therapeutic dose(s) may not be established, all noxious and unintended responses to a medicinal product related to any dose should be considered adverse drug reactions. "Responses to a medicinal product" means that a causal relationship between a medicinal product and an adverse event is at least a reasonable possibility (i.e., that the relationship cannot be ruled out).

An ADR to a marketed medicinal product is a response to a drug that is noxious and unintended and that occurs at doses normally used in humans for prophylaxis, diagnosis, or therapy of diseases or for modification of physiological function.

Adverse Event (AE): An AE is any untoward medical event that occurs in a patient or clinical investigation subject administered a pharmaceutical product and that does not necessarily have a causal relationship to this treatment. An AE can therefore be any unfavorable and unintended sign (including an abnormal laboratory finding), symptom, or disease temporally associated with the use of a medicinal (investigational) product, whether or not related to the medicinal (investigational) product.

Audit: A systematic and independent examination of trial-related activities and documents to determine whether the evaluated trial-related activities were conducted and the data were recorded, analyzed, and accurately reported according to the protocol, sponsor's standard operating procedures, good clinical practice, and the applicable regulatory requirements.

Audit Report: A written evaluation by the sponsor's auditor of the results of the audit.

Case Report Form: A printed, optical, or electronic document designed to record all of the protocol-required information to be reported to the sponsor on each trial subject.

Clinical Trial or Study: Any investigation in human subjects that is intended to discover or verify the clinical, pharmacologic, or other pharmacodynamic effects of an investigational product, to identify any adverse reactions to an investigational product, or to study absorption, distribution, metabolism, and excretion of an investigational product with the object of ascertaining its safety, efficacy, or both. (The terms clinical trial and clinical study are synonymous.)

Clinical Trial/Study Report: A written description of a trial or study of any therapeutic, prophylactic, or diagnostic agent conducted in humans, in which the clinical and statistical description, presentations, and analyses are fully integrated into a single report.

Contract Research Organization: A person or organization (commercial, academic, or other) contracted by the sponsor to perform one or more of a sponsor's trial-related duties and functions.

Direct Access: Permission to examine, analyze, verify, and reproduce any records and reports that are important

in the evaluation of a clinical trial. Any party (e.g., domestic and foreign regulatory authorities, sponsors, monitors, and auditors) with direct access should take all reasonable precautions within the constraints of the applicable regulatory requirements to maintain the confidentiality of subjects' identities and sponsors' proprietary information.

Documentation: All records, in any form (including but not limited to written, electronic, magnetic, and optical records and scans, roentgenograms, and electrocardiograms) that describe or record the methods, conduct, or results of a trial, the factors affecting a trial, and the actions taken.

Essential Documents: Documents that individually and collectively permit evaluation of the conduct of a study and the quality of the data produced.

Good Clinical Practice: A standard for the design, conduct, performance, monitoring, auditing, recording, analysis, and reporting of clinical trials that provides assurance that the data and reported results are credible and accurate and that the rights, integrity, and confidentiality of trial subjects are protected.

Independent Ethics Committee: An independent body (institutional, regional, national, or supranational review board or committee), constituted of medical or scientific professionals and nonmedical or nonscientific members, whose responsibility it is to ensure the protection of the rights, safety, and well-being of human subjects involved in a trial and to provide public assurance of that protection by, among other things, reviewing and approving or providing favorable opinion on the trial protocol and the suitability of the investigators, the facilities, and the methods and material to be used in obtaining and documenting informed consent of the trial subjects.

Informed Consent: A process by which a subject voluntarily confirms his or her willingness to participate in a particular trial, after having been informed of all aspects of the trial that are relevant to the decision to participate. Informed consent is documented by means of a written, signed, and dated form.

Investigator's Brochure: A compilation of clinical and nonclinical data on an investigational product that are relevant to the study of the product in human subjects.

Monitoring: Overseeing the progress of a clinical trial and ensuring that it is conducted, recorded, and reported in accordance with the protocol, standard operating procedures, good clinical practice, and the applicable regulatory requirements.

Monitoring Report: A written report from the monitor to the sponsor after each site visit or other trial-related communication, according to the sponsor's standard operating procedures.

Protocol: A document that describes the objectives, design, methods, statistical considerations, and organization of a trial. The protocol usually also gives the background and rationale for the trial, but these could be provided in other protocol-referenced documents. (Throughout the ICH GCP Guideline, the term protocol refers to protocol and protocol amendments.)

Serious Adverse Event or Serious Adverse Drug Reaction: Any untoward medical event that occurs in a patient or subject receiving a drug at any dose and results in death, is life-threatening, requires inpatient hospitalization or prolongation of existing hospitalization, results in persistent or significant disability or incapacity, or is a congenital anomaly or birth defect.

Source Data: All information in original records and certified copies of original records of clinical findings, observations, or other activities in a clinical trial that is necessary for the reconstruction and evaluation of the trial. Source data are contained in source documents (original records or certified copies).

Source Documents: Original documents, data, and records (e.g., hospital records, clinical and office charts, laboratory notes, memoranda, subjects' diaries or evaluation checklists, pharmacy dispensing records, recorded data from automated instruments, copies or transcriptions certified after verification as being accurate and complete, microfiches, photographic negatives, microfilm or magnetic media, roentgenograms, and subject files and records kept at the pharmacy, the laboratories, and the medicotechnical departments involved in the clinical trial).

Sponsor: An individual, a company, an institution, or an organization that takes responsibility for the initiation, management, or financing of a clinical trial.

Sponsor–Investigator: An individual who both initiates and conducts, alone or with others, a clinical trial, and under whose immediate direction the investigational product is administered to, dispensed to, or used by a subject. The term does not include any person other than an individual (e.g., it does not include a corporation or an agency). The obligations of a sponsor-investigator include both those of a sponsor and those of an investigator.

[a]In this document investigational drugs are defined as those that are being considered for but have not yet received marketing approval by FDA for human use and those that have FDA approval for at least one indication but are being studied for new indications, new routes of administration, or new dosage forms.

[b]The principles and procedures described here are applicable to all clinical drug studies, not just those involving investigational drugs.

[c]In certain emergency situations, prior consent may be waived (21 CFR 50.24).

[d]Definitions selected from reference 5.

These guidelines were reviewed in 2003 by the Council on Professional Affairs and by the Board of Directors and were found to still be appropriate.

Approved by the ASHP Board of Directors, November 15, 1997. Developed by the ASHP Council on Professional Affairs. Supersedes the ASHP Guidelines for the Use of Investigational Drugs in Organized Health-Care Settings, dated November 14, 1990.

The bibliographic citation for this document is as follows: American Society of Health-System Pharmacists. ASHP guidelines on clinical drug research. *Am J Health-Syst Pharm.* 1998; 55:369–76.

ASHP Guidelines for Pharmaceutical Research in Organized Health-Care Settings

The promotion of research in the health and pharmaceutical sciences and in pharmaceutical services is a purpose of the American Society of Hospital Pharmacists, as stated in its Charter.[1] In keeping with this purpose, pharmacists in organized health-care settings should understand the (1) basic need for research and systematic problem solving in pharmacy practice; (2) fundamental scientific approach; (3) basic components of a research plan; (4) process of documenting and reporting findings; and (5) responsibilities of investigators with respect to patients, employers, grantors, and science in general.

In its purest form, scientific research is the systematic, controlled, empirical, and critical investigation of hypothetical propositions (theories) about presumed relationships among natural phenomena.[2] Aspects of the research process (e.g., problem definition, systematic data gathering, interpretation, and reporting), however, are also applicable to resolving specific practice problems. Independent, intraprofessional, and interdisciplinary collaborative research and problem solving are encouraged.

Need

Since pharmacy is based on the theories of the pharmaceutical, medical, and social sciences, pharmacy's advancement is linked to advancement in those sciences. Scientific inquiry, through formal research and systematic problem solving, leads to an expansion of knowledge and thus to advancement. Both research and systematic problem solving in organized health-care settings are needed for developing knowledge in pharmaceutics and drug therapy and for evaluation, modification, and justification of specific practices. Therefore, an understanding of the research process is important to pharmacists in such settings.

Primary areas for research by pharmacists in organized health-care settings are those in which pharmacists possess special expertise or unique knowledge. These areas include drug therapy, pharmaceutics, bioavailability, pharmacy practice administration, sociobehavioral aspects of pharmaceutical service systems, and application of information handling and computer technology to pharmacy practice.

The Scientific Approach

Aspects of the scientific approach may be applied to formal research and systematic problem solving. The scientific approach consists of four basic steps:

1. *Problem—Obstacle—Idea.*[3] The scientist experiences an obstacle to understanding or curiosity as to why something is as it is. The scientist's first step is to express the idea in some reasonably manageable form, even if it is ill defined and tentative.
2. *Hypothesis.* The scientist looks back on experience for possible solutions—personal experience, the literature, and contacts with other scientists. A tentative proposition (hypothesis) is formulated about the relationship between two or more variables in the problem; for example, "If such and such occurs, then so and so results."

3. *Reasoning—Deduction.* The scientist deduces the consequences of the formulated hypothesis. The scientist may find that the deductions reveal a new problem that is quite different from the original one. On the other hand, deductions may lead to the conclusion that the problem cannot be solved with existing technical tools. Such reasoning can help lead to wider, more basic, and more significant problems as well as to more narrow (testable) implications of the original hypothesis.
4. *Observation—Test—Experiment.* If the problem has been well stated, the hypotheses have been adequately formulated, and the implications of the hypotheses have been carefully deduced, the next step is to test the relationships expressed by the hypotheses, that is, the relationships among the variables. All testing is for one purpose: putting the relationships among the variables to an empirical test. It is not the hypotheses that are tested but the deduced implications of the hypotheses. On the basis of the research evidence, each hypothesis is either accepted or rejected.

Components of a Research Plan

Formal research frequently requires the development of a written plan (protocol or proposal). In funded research, the plan may take the form of a grant application. A typical plan might include

1. A problem statement.
2. A review of available literature on the subject.
3. The objectives for the project, including the hypotheses and the to-be-tested relationships among variables.
4. A description of the methodology to be used.
5. A description of statistical analyses to be applied to the data collected.
6. A budget and time frame for the project (where applicable).
7. The expected applicability of the research findings.

Documentation and Reporting

The structure of a research report is similar to the structure of a research plan. A typical outline is as follows:

1. Problem.
 a. Theories, hypotheses, and definitions.
 b. Previous research: the literature.
2. Methodology.
 a. Sample and sampling method.
 b. Experimental procedures and instrumentation.
 c. Measurement of variables.
 d. Statistical methods of analysis.
 e. Pretesting and pilot studies.
3. Results, interpretation, and conclusions.

The statement of the problem sets the general stage for the reader and may be in question form. A common

practice is to state the broader, general problem and then to state the hypotheses, both general and specific. All important variables should be defined, both in general and in operational terms, giving a justification for the definitions used, if needed.

The general and research literature related to the problem is discussed to explain the theoretical rationale of the problem, to tell the reader what research has and has not been carried out on the problem, and to show that this particular investigation has not been conducted before (except in the case of validating research).

The methodology section should meticulously describe what was done so as to enable another investigator to reproduce the research, reanalyze the data, and arrive at unambiguous conclusions about the adequacy of the methods. This section should tell what samples were used, how they were selected, and why they were selected. The means of measurement of the variables should be described. The data analysis methods should be outlined and justified. Where pilot studies and pretesting were used, they should be described.

Results and data should be condensed and expressed in concise form. Limitations and weaknesses of the study should be discussed. The question of whether the data support the hypotheses must be foremost in the mind of the report writer. Everything written should relate the results and data to the problem and the hypotheses.

Investigators' Responsibilities

Investigators bear a general responsibility to be scientifically objective in their research inquiries, conclusions, and reports. They bear a responsibility for being methodical and meticulous in the gathering of research data. They also bear both a fiduciary and a reporting responsibility to employers and grantors. In general, employee investigators are at least partially responsible to their employer organizations in the choice of research topics. Research funded from sources outside an investigator's organization may impose additional contractual obligations on the investigator and the organization.

In research involving patients, investigators are responsible for protecting patients from harm while the patients are participating in the research. All research involving patients should be reviewed and approved, before initiation, by an institutional review board. Written, informed consent should be obtained from every patient participating in each research project.[4] Meticulous record-keeping is required regarding the clinical experience of patients participating in research projects.

Employee investigators bear responsibility for helping their organizations differentiate true, objective research from product marketing trials and promotions that may purport to be research projects. Grants for bona fide research typically bear a direct cost-recovery relationship to projects and typically involve the direct transfer of grant funds from grantors to the employee investigator's employer organization. Specific institutional policies vary widely, but employee investigators can generally better fulfill their fiduciary responsibilities when funds are not distributed directly from grantors to investigators. In keeping with their fiduciary responsibilities and their responsibility to be scientifically objective, investigators should be wary of arrangements in which prospective grantors offer inducements of value (gifts, trips, experiences, publicity, publications, etc.) to investigators, institutions, or patients before, during, or after the completion of proposed projects.

Investigators should make legitimate efforts to document publicly the findings of research in scientific, objectively refereed publications.

References

1. American Society of Hospital Pharmacists. Governing documents of the American Society of Hospital Pharmacists. Bethesda, MD: American Society of Hospital Pharmacists; 1984.
2. Kerlinger F. Foundations of behavioral research. New York: Holt, Rinehart and Winston; 1964:13.
3. Dewey J. How we think. Boston: Heath; 1933:106–18, as adapted to the scientific framework by Kerlinger, op cit., p 13–5.
4. American Society of Hospital Pharmacists. ASHP guidelines for the use of investigational drugs in institutions. *Am J Hosp Pharm.* 1983; 40:449–51.

Approved by the ASHP Board of Directors, September 30, 1988. Developed by the Council on Professional Affairs. Supersedes the "ASHP Guidelines for Scientific Research in Institutional Pharmacy" approved on November 15, 1977.

The bibliographic citation for this document is as follows: American Society of Hospital Pharmacists. ASHP guidelines for pharmaceutical research in organized health-care settings. *Am J Hosp Pharm.* 1989; 46:129–30.

ASHP
Therapeutic Position Statements

ASHP Therapeutic Position Statement on Antithrombotic Therapy in Chronic Atrial Fibrillation

Position

The American Society of Health-System Pharmacists (ASHP) supports the routine use of antithrombotic therapy (warfarin or aspirin) for stroke prevention in patients with chronic atrial fibrillation (AF). Antithrombotic therapy given to patients with AF for primary prevention (before the first stroke or episode of systemic embolism) or as a secondary intervention (after stroke or systemic embolism has occurred) unequivocally reduces the risk of stroke.[1] Warfarin is more effective than aspirin but carries a higher risk of bleeding and requires regular medical and therapeutic monitoring.

ASHP supports recommendations established by the American College of Chest Physicians (ACCP) (Table 1) for the use of antithrombotic therapy in patients with AF to reduce the morbidity and mortality associated with stroke.[1] ASHP encourages the use of war-farin, if it can be administered safely, in all patients with chronic AF who are younger than 75 years and have one or more clinical risk factors for stroke or who are older than 75 years. However, ASHP recognizes that for patients age 65–75 years without clinical risk factors, either warfarin or aspirin may be an option, depending on individual patient circumstances. Aspirin may be an appropriate choice for AF patients younger than 65 with no risk factors and for any patient with AF who is not a candidate for warfarin therapy. There is no evidence that the combination of warfarin and aspirin is superior to warfarin alone for stroke prevention in AF.[1]

Many patients who are eligible for antithrombotic therapy remain unprotected, possibly because of prescriber concerns about the potential for hemorrhagic complications and the difficulty of managing oral anticoagulation.[1] ASHP

believes that the safe and effective use of warfarin is dependent on adequate patient education and monitoring, which are services that can be efficiently provided by pharmacists. ASHP encourages pharmacists to work actively with other health care providers to optimize anticoagulant therapy through the provision of these services.

Background

AF is the most commonly encountered cardiac arrhythmia in clinical practice. It has been estimated that close to 2.5 million people in the United States currently have AF. By 2050, this number is expected to increase to more than 5.6 million.[2,3] The presence of AF is strongly related to age, occurring in 2.3% of people over age 40 years, 5% of people older than 65 years, and nearly 10% of individuals older than 80 years.[2-4] Given the predominance of AF among older patients and the aging of the U.S. population, the health care burden caused by AF is estimated to increase dramatically.[5] In fact, hospitalization rates attributable to AF have doubled to tripled in recent years.

AF is a strong independent risk factor for ischemic stroke.[6] Approximately 15% of all ischemic strokes in the United States can be attributed to AF.[1] The risk of stroke in patients with AF is four to five times higher than in an age-matched population without AF. This corresponds to an increased incidence of stroke of approximately 5% per year for primary events and 12% per year for secondary events.[1,7] As the risk of AF increases with advanced age, so does the risk of stroke attributable to AF. The frequency of stroke attributable to AF is 1.5% in patients age 50–59 years and 23.5% in patients 80–89 years.[6] Stroke caused by AF results in significant morbidity and mortality and poor quality of life in stroke survivors.[2,8] Worse outcomes with higher mortality and disability have been reported in patients with AF who have a stroke versus patients who have a stroke but do not have AF.[9,10]

For platelet-rich thrombi that form in high-flow arteries, antiplatelet agents such as aspirin are considered to be optimal therapy. Because patients with AF frequently have vascular disease, thrombi may arise in high-flow areas such as the carotid circulation and cardiac chambers, and antiplatelet therapy may protect some patients in whom thrombi develop in this manner.[7,11] However, patients with AF may also develop thrombi in the atria, especially the atrial appendages, because of stasis or turbulent blood flow. These cardiogenic emboli contain fewer platelets, are less responsive to antiplatelet therapy, and are best prevented by anticoagulant therapy.[1,7,11]

Most strokes in patients with AF appear to be the result of cardiogenic embolism.[1] Patients with cardioembolic stroke typically have an abrupt onset of symptoms and die suddenly or are left with major neurologic sequelae. While the benefits of antithrombotic therapy in preventing stroke are well established, only about 25–50% of patients with AF

Table 1.
Recommendations for the Use of Antithrombotic Therapy in Chronic Atrial Fibrillation[1]

Age (yr)	Risk Factors[a]	Recommendation[b]
>75	No	Warfarin
>75	Yes	Warfarin
65–75	No	Warfarin or aspirin 325 mg/day
65–75	Yes	Warfarin
<65	No	Aspirin 325 mg/day
<65	Yes	Warfarin

[a]The presence of one or more of the following risk factors is an indication for warfarin therapy: age > 75 years; prior ischemic stroke, transient ischemic attack, or systemic embolism; moderately or severely impaired left ventricular systolic function; congestive heart failure; hypertension; and diabetes mellitus.
[b]Target International Normalized Ratio for warfarin therapy is 2.5 (range, 2.0–3.0).

are receiving warfarin,[4,11-14] perhaps because of physician concerns about the small (1–3%) but important risk of serious hemorrhagic complications. It is therefore prudent that practitioners have a thorough understanding of the risks and benefits of this therapy

Definitions

This therapeutic position statement is an update of the 1998 ASHP Therapeutic Position Statement on Antithrombotic Therapy in Chronic Atrial Fibrillation.[15] AF can be categorized as initial or acute (onset detected within 48 hours), paroxysmal (intermittent or terminated spontaneously on at least one occasion), persistent (duration of >seven days and not terminated spontaneously), or permanent (resistant to pharmacologic or electrical cardioversion).[16] The chronic cardiac conditions most commonly associated with the development of AF are rheumatic mitral valve disease, coronary artery disease, congestive heart failure, and hypertension. Noncardiac etiologies, often reversible, include hyperthyroidism, hypoxic pulmonary conditions, surgery, and alcohol withdrawal. In up to a third of cases, no predisposing condition exists; this type of AF is called "lone AF." The most predominant form of AF is nonvalvular AF.[16] This document focuses on nonvalvular AF, or AF not associated with rheumatic mitral valve disease or prosthetic heart valves. Hereafter, AF refers to nonvalvular AF.

The benefit of antithrombotic therapy for the prevention of stroke in patients with AF has been well established. This benefit can be expressed as the absolute risk reduction $x-y$, where x is the risk in the control group and y is the risk in the treated group, or as the relative risk reduction ($[x-y]/x$) $\times$ 100%, where y and x are the percent reductions in risk in the treated and control groups, respectively. When comparing treatments, reporting only the relative risk ratio or the percent change in the event rate can be misleading. This is particularly true for antithrombotic therapy in AF, since the absolute risk of stroke varies widely, from about 1% with no risk factors to more than 15% with multiple risk factors.[17] A useful estimate of benefit can be calculated from the absolute risk reduction and expressed as the number needed to treat (NNT).[18] The NNT is defined as the number of persons who must be treated to prevent one event per year and is equal to 1/(treatment event rate − control event rate).

Risk Stratification

The risk of stroke varies greatly depending on age, the presence of coexisting cardiovascular disease, and the presence of additional risk factors. Therefore, antithrombotic therapy must be tailored based on each patient's age, comorbidities, contraindications, and stroke risk. Several risk-stratification models have been developed using data from pooled analyses of the original antithrombotic treatment trials and expert consensus (Table 2). The most commonly cited risk-stratification schemes have been derived from the Atrial Fibrillation Investigators (AFI),[19] two analyses from the Stroke Prevention in Atrial Fibrillation (SPAF) investigators,[20,21] the Framingham score,[22] the CHADS$_2$ (Congestive Heart Failure, Hypertension, Age, Diabetes, and Stroke-

Table 2.
Summary of the Main Stroke Risk-Stratification Schemes for Patients with Atrial Fibrillation[a]

Risk-Stratification Scheme	Risk Group[b]		
	High	Moderate	Low
ACCP[1]	Prior stroke, TIA, or systemic thromboembolism; age > 75 yr; hypertension; DM; moderate or severe LVSD and/or CHF	Age 65–75 yr with no other risk factors	Age < 65 yr with no other risk factors
ACC/AHA/ESC guidelines[16]	Prior stroke, TIA, embolism, mitral stenosis, prosthetic heart valve	Age ≥ 75 yr, hypertension, DM; CHF, LVSD (EF < 35%)	Age 65–74 yr, women, CAD, thyrotoxicosis
AFI[19]	Age ≥ 65 yr, history of hypertension, CAD, or DM	Age ≥ 65 yr, history of hypertension, CAD, or DM	Age < 65 yr, no high-risk features
SPAF[20,21]	Women age > 75 yr, SBP > 160 mm Hg, LVD	History of hypertension, no high-risk features	No history of hypertension, no high-risk features
Framingham[22]	…[c]	…	…
CHADS$_2$[23,d]	3–6	1–2	0

[a]Adapted from references 1, 7, and 16. ACCP = American College of Chest Physicians, TIA = transient ischemic attack, DM = diabetes mellitus, LVSD = left ventricular systolic dysfunction, CHF = coronary heart failure, ACC = American College of Cardiology, AHA = American Heart Association, ESC = European Society of Cardiology, EF = ejection fraction, CAD = coronary artery disease, AFI = Atrial Fibrillation Investigators, SPAF = Stroke Prevention in Atrial Fibrillation, SBP = systolic blood pressure, LVD = left ventricular dysfunction, CHADS$_2$ = Congestive Heart Failure, Hypertension, Age, Diabetes, and Stroke-doubled.
[b]The annual risk of stroke for the high-, moderate-, and low-risk groups is 8–12%, 4%, and 1%, respectively.
[c]Uses a weighted point scoring system, where the total score (maximum 31 points) corresponds to a predicted five-year stroke risk. Risk factors included older age, female sex, elevated blood pressure, and DM.
[d]Scheme assigns one point each for recent congestive heart failure, hypertension, age ≥ 75 years, and DM and two points for history of stroke or TIA.

doubled) score,[23] and the ACCP Consensus Guidelines on Antithrombotic and Thrombolytic Therapy.[1] Although there is some variation among the various risk-stratification models, the major risk factors tend to overlap. The most commonly identified risk factors for stroke include older age, history of previous systemic thromboembolism, hypertension, female sex, congestive heart failure or left ventricular systolic dysfunction, elevated systolic blood pressure, and diabetes (Table 3).[24]

When determining a patient's composite stroke risk, it is important to note that the presence of various risk factors is additive and not mutually exclusive.[21] Patients with one or more risk factors in the AFI and SPAF trials had higher annual stroke rates (4.3–8.1% and 2.6–7.1%, respectively), depending on the number and type of risk factors.[19,21] The CHADS$_2$ risk-scoring system integrates factors from the AFI and the SPAF I–II schemes. The risk of stroke is increased with higher CHADS$_2$ scores (Table 4).[23] In a recent study, the CHADS$_2$ risk-scoring system demonstrated greater predictive value for stroke than the AFI, SPAF, Framingham, or ACCP criteria.[25] Other recent efforts to compare the various risk-stratification schemes found that stroke rates varied among the schemes, with significant variation noted in the moderate-to-high-risk categories but more consistent rates in the low-risk categories.[26]

Evidence for Efficacy of Antithrombotic Therapy

Oral Anticoagulation—Warfarin. Five randomized controlled trials of oral vitamin K antagonist therapy for primary prevention of stroke and systemic embolism in AF[27-31] and one trial for secondary intervention[32,33] have been published (Table 5). Patients with chronic persistent AF and patients with paroxysmal AF were included in these trials. Warfarin was the oral anticoagulant used in the primary prevention trials and phenprocoumon or acenocoumarol was used in the secondary prevention trial. There was variation between the target intensity of anticoagulation in the six trials. Although the definition of primary outcome varied among the trials, all studies considered stroke a primary event. Due to the great benefit observed with oral anticoagulation, most of these trials were terminated early, and the numbers of events reported were fairly small. Compared with placebo, oral anticoagulation reduces the relative risk of stroke by nearly 70% when the International Normalized Ratio (INR) target range is 1.5–4.5 (Table 6).[19] If an efficacy analysis is used rather than an intent-to-treat analysis, the relative risk reduction is over 80%.[41]

The annual absolute reduction in stroke risk with warfarin was 2.5–4.7% in the primary prevention studies and 8.4% in the secondary intervention study (Table 5). This implies that 22–40 patients would need to be treated with warfarin to prevent one first-time stroke or systemic embolism per year. Prevention of one secondary event per year would require warfarin therapy in only 12 patients. Anticoagulation was found to be effective in preventing strokes of all severities. Reduction in disabling stroke by warfarin averaged 1.5% per year in unselected AF patients.[19] The beneficial effect of warfarin on outcomes was maintained across all patient subgroups, and most of the strokes in the warfarin group occurred in patients who had an INR below the target range or who had stopped therapy. In the five primary prevention studies, the all-cause mortality rate was lowered by 33% in the anticoagulation-treated patients.[19] Taken together, this evidence supports the efficacy of oral anticoagulation therapy with warfarin for stroke prevention in patients with AF.

Aspirin. Aspirin is much less effective than warfarin in preventing stroke (primarily cardioembolic stroke) (Tables 5 and 6).[1] Five studies have compared the efficacy of aspirin with placebo,[27,29,32,34-36] with the aspirin dosage ranging from 50 mg/day[34] to 325 mg/day[29] (Table 5). The only study that demonstrated a significant benefit from aspirin was the SPAF trial, in which a 42% relative risk reduction was reported.[29] Three trials found no significant benefit with aspirin versus placebo.[27,32,34,35] Another trial, Low-

Table 3.
Independent Predictors of Stroke for Patients with Atrial Fibrillation[a]

Risk Factor	AFI[19]	SPAF[20,21]	Framingham Study[22]
Older age	+	+	+
Female		+	+
Prior ischemic stroke or TIA	+	+	+
Prior CHF or LVSD		+	
Hypertension	+	+	
Elevated systolic blood pressure			+
Diabetes mellitus	+		+

[a]Adapted from reference 24, with permission. AFI = Atrial Fibrillation Investigators, SPAF = Stroke Prevention in Atrial Fibrillation, TIA = transient ischemic attack, CHF = congestive heart failure, LVSD = left ventricular systolic dysfunction.

Table 4.
Association between CHADS$_2$ Scores and Risk of Future Stroke[a]

CHADS$_2$ Score[b]	Adjusted Stroke Rate, %[c] (95% CI)
0	1.9 (1.2–3.0)
1	2.8 (2.0–3.8)
2	4.0 (3.1–5.1)
3	5.9 (4.6–7.3)
4	8.5 (6.3–11.1)
5	12.5 (8.2–17.5)
6	18.2 (10.5–27.4)

[a]Adapted from reference 23, with permission. CHADS$_2$ = Congestive Heart Failure, Hypertension, Age, Diabetes, and Stroke-doubled, CI = confidence interval.
[b]Scheme assigns one point each for recent congestive heart failure, hypertension, age ≥ 75 years, and diabetes mellitus and two points for history of stroke or transient ischemic attack.
[c]Per 100 patient-years.

Table 5.

Efficacy of Antithrombotic Therapy for Reducing Risk of Ischemic Stroke in Patients with Atrial Fibrillation: Summary of the Major Randomized Trials[a]

Study	n	INR Range	Daily Aspirin Dose (mg)	No. Events/yr/100 pts Group 1	No. Events/yr/100 pts Group 2	RRR[b] (%)	ARR (%)/ yr	p
OAC (group 1) vs. control (group 2)								
AFASAK I[27]	671	2.8–4.2	…[c]	2.7	6.2	56	3.5	<0.05
BAATAF[28]	420	1.5–2.7[d]	…	0.4	3.0	86	2.6	0.002
SPAF I[29]	421	2.0–4.5	…	2.3	7.4	67	5.1	0.01
SPINAF[30]	571	1.4–2.8	…	0.9	4.3	79	3.4	0.001
CAFA[31]	378	2.0–3.0	…	3.4	4.6	26	1.2	NS
EAFT[32]	439	2.5–4.0	…	8.5	16.5	47	8.0	0.001
Aspirin (group 1) vs. control (group 2)								
AFASAK I[27]	672	…	75	5.2	6.2	16	1.0	NS
SPAF I[29]	1120	…	325	3.6	6.3	42	2.7	0.02
EAFT[32]	782	…	300	15.5	19.0	17	3.5	0.12
ESPS II[34,35]	211	…	50	13.8	20.7	33	6.9	0.16
LASAF[36]	195	…	125	2.6	2.2	15	0.4	NS
	181	…	125 q.o.d.	0.7	2.2	68	1.5	0.05
OAC (group 1) vs. aspirin (group 2)								
AFASAK I[27]	671	2.8–4.2	75	2.7	5.2	48	2.5	<0.05
EAFT[32]	455	2.5–4.0	300	NA	NA	40	NA	0.008
SPAF II[37]								
Age ≤ 75 yr	715	2.0–4.5	325	1.3	1.9	33	0.6	0.24
Age > 75 yr	385	2.0–4.5	325	3.6	4.8	27	1.2	0.39
SPAF III[38]	1044	2.0–3.0	325	1.9	7.9	74	6.0	<0.001
AFASAK II[39]	339	2.0–3.0	300	3.4	2.7	21	0.7	NS
PATAF[40]	272	2.5–3.5	150	2.5	3.1	19	0.6	NS

[a]INR = International Normalized Ratio, RRR = relative risk reduction, ARR = absolute risk reduction, OAC = oral anticoagulation, AFASAK = Atrial Fibrillation Aspirin Study of Anticoagulation from Kopenhagen, BAATAF = Boston Area Anticoagulation Trial for Atrial Fibrillation, SPAF = Stroke Prevention in Atrial Fibrillation, SPINAF = Stroke Prevention in Nonrheumatic Atrial Fibrillation, CAFA = Canadian Atrial Fibrillation Anticoagulation, NS = not significant, EAFT = European Atrial Fibrillation Trial, ESPS = European Stroke Prevention Study, LASAF = Low-Dose Aspirin, Stroke and Atrial Fibrillation, PATAF = Primary Prevention of Arterial Thromboembolism in Nonrheumatic AF in Primary Care Trial.
[b]Reduction compared with control (active treatment or placebo) using intent-to-treat analysis.
[c]Not applicable.
[d]INR estimated for BAATAF, SPAF I, and SPINAF, which used prothrombin time ratios.
[e]Aspirin 325 mg/day plus warfarin given to achieve an INR of 1.2–1.5.

Dose Aspirin, Stroke, and Atrial Fibrillation (LASAF), found inconsistent effects of aspirin versus placebo, with significant benefit reported in patients receiving aspirin 125 mg every other day but no significant benefit in patients receiving aspirin 125 mg every day.[36] Pooled data from the three largest studies[27,29,32] resulted in a 21% relative risk reduction (95% confidence interval [CI], 0–38%) in favor of aspirin versus placebo[42] (Table 6). Another meta-analysis of aspirin versus placebo found similar results (22% risk reduction [95% CI, 2–38%).[43]

Oral Anticoagulation versus Aspirin. The effect of vitamin K antagonists was compared with that of aspirin in six studies (Table 5).[27,32,37–40] Three of the trials[27,32,38] found significant benefit in favor of adjusted-dose warfarin (INR, 2.0–3.0), with relative risk reductions in primary events of 48%,[27] 40%,[32] and 74%.[38] The remaining three studies[37,39,40] found no

significant difference between adjusted-dose oral anticoagulation and aspirin; however, one study[39] was stopped early in light of the results of SPAF III,[38] and another study[40] was limited by low event rates, which decreased the power of the analysis.

A meta-analysis found a benefit in favor of the vitamin K antagonists versus aspirin, with a relative risk reduction of 46% (95% CI, 29–57%) for all strokes and 52% (95% CI, 37–63%) for ischemic stroke (Table 6).[44] However, there was a 1.7-fold increase in major bleeding reported (95% CI for hazard ratio, 1.21–2.41). In balancing the efficacy and safety of oral anticoagulation, treating 1000 AF patients for one year with adjusted-dose warfarin, compared with aspirin, would prevent 23 ischemic strokes and cause 9 additional major bleeding events.[1] Another metaanalysis showed similar results, with a 36% relative risk reduction in all strokes (95% CI, 14–52%) and a 46% reduction in ischemic stroke

Table 6.
Efficacy of Antithrombotic Therapy in Atrial Fibrillation from Pooled Data of Randomized Trials[a]

Treatment Comparison	RRR, %[b] (95% Confidence Interval)
Adjusted-dose oral anticoagulation vs. no antithrombotic therapy	68 (50–79)
Aspirin vs. no antithrombotic therapy	21 (0–38)
Adjusted-dose oral anticoagulation vs. aspirin	52 (37–63)

[a]Adapted from reference 1, with permission. RRR = relative risk reduction.
[b]Reduction in risk of ischemic stroke demonstrated by the first treatment mentioned.

(95% CI, 27–60%) in favor of adjusted-dose warfarin versus aspirin.[42]

Overall, these data suggest that the benefit in stroke reduction in patients with AF is greater with warfarin than with aspirin (Table 6). While the benefit of aspirin diminishes as the stroke risk increases,[42] adjusted-dose warfarin is effective in preventing severe strokes and strokes of lesser severity.[44,45] It has been reported that strokes in patients with AF are more severe than strokes in non-AF patients.[46] However, warfarin therapy to achieve an INR of ≥ 2.0 is associated with better short-term survival if stroke occurs.[47]

Combined Therapy with Oral Anticoagulation and an Antiplatelet Agent. In a primary and secondary prevention trial, the efficacy of low-intensity, fixed-dose warfarin (INR target of 1.2–1.5) plus aspirin (325 mg/day) was compared with that of conventional adjusted-dose warfarin therapy (INR target of 2.0–3.0) in high-risk AF patients.[38] Patients given adjusted-dose warfarin had a significantly lower rate of stroke and systemic embolism than patients given aspirin in combination with low-intensity warfarin therapy (1.9% per year versus 7.9% per year, respectively)—an absolute reduction in risk of 6.0% per year. Thus, 17 high-risk AF patients must be treated with adjusted-dose warfarin therapy to prevent one stroke not prevented by aspirin plus low-intensity warfarin therapy.[38] No positive synergistic effect of the combination aspirin and low-intensity warfarin was observed in this study.[38] In another trial that combined low-intensity anticoagulation with aspirin, the combination regimen was also found ineffective in preventing strokes.[39] One additional study compared the combination of aspirin 100 mg/day and the anticoagulant fluindione (target INR of 2.0–2.6) with fluindione monotherapy (target INR of 2.0–2.6).[48] This study was stopped early due to increased bleeding complications in the group receiving combination therapy.

Optimal Intensity of Anticoagulation Therapy

The optimal intensity of anticoagulation to adequately prevent stroke and minimize bleeding risk may depend on the inherent stroke risk and bleeding risk. In two of the early primary prevention trials, the Boston Area Anticoagulation Trial for Atrial Fibrillation (BAATAF)[28] and Stroke Prevention in Nonrheumatic Atrial Fibrillation (SPINAF),[30] low-intensity anticoagulation (estimated INR target range of 1.5–2.8) was found effective for relatively low-risk AF patients. However, low-intensity anticoagulation (target INR of 1.2–1.5), even when given in combination with aspirin (325 mg/day), was

ineffective in high-risk AF patients in the SPAF III study.[38] Another trial found a higher INR intensity (INR goal 2.5–4.0) effective for secondary prevention in patients with a previous event, but a reduction in efficacy at INRs of <2.0 was also observed.[33]

In a meta-analysis of three AF stroke-prevention trials, adjusted-dose anticoagulation (INR goal of 2.0–3.0) was found to be more effective than fixed low-dose warfarin, with a relative risk reduction of 38% (95% CI, –20% to 68%).[42] In a case–control study, Hylek et al.[49] found that an INR of <2.0 was associated with an increased risk of ischemic stroke in patients with AF. The risk of stroke was two times higher at an INR of 1.7 and three times higher at an INR of 1.5 compared with the risk of stroke at an INR of 2.0. Event rates were even higher in patients with an INR of <1.5. These findings were confirmed in another case–control study in which AF patients with an INR of <2.0 had an increased risk of stroke.[50] In addition, INRs of <2.0 have been linked to an increased risk of severe or fatal stroke.[47] These findings are useful for establishing the lower end of an INR range that should provide appropriate protection against stroke and severe stroke.

Although data from randomized trials comparing an INR of 1.5–2.0 with an INR of 2.0–3.0 and without the addition of aspirin are lacking, using an INR target of 2.0–3.0 would seem a reasonable standard as large randomized trials have used this range successfully. Current evidence does not support lower INR targets in patients over age 75 years. As these patients have a higher risk of bleeding and stroke, careful monitoring and warfarin dosing to aim for strict INR control (goal of 2.5) are preferred. In patients deemed to have a higher risk of bleeding, aiming for the lower half of the target INR range of 2.0–3.0 may be a reasonable approach. The current ACCP recommended range of intensity of anticoagulation in patients with AF is an INR of 2.0–3.0.[1]

Safety of Antithrombotic Therapy

Bleeding is the major complication associated with oral anticoagulation therapy. Although the definition of major bleeding varied slightly among the studies, generally an event was classified as such if it resulted in transfusion or hospitalization, caused death or permanent disability, or occurred in a critical anatomical location. In the pooled analysis[19] of five primary prevention trials,[27-31] there was no significant difference in the annual rate of major bleeding complications in patients treated with adjusted-dose anticoagulation versus patients who received placebo (1.3% versus 1.0%, respectively). The annual rate of intracranial hemorrhage (ICH) was 0.3% in the group receiving an oral anticoagulant and 0.1% in the control group.[19] ICH is of major concern, as it can cause complications that are considered greater than the ischemic strokes that the antithrombotic therapy is intended to prevent.

ICH during warfarin therapy in carefully monitored clinical trials occurs at a rate of 0.3–1.5% per year.[19,51] Thus, according to NNT analysis, one intracranial hemorrhage

will occur per year for every 67–250 patients treated with warfarin. While the intracranial bleeding rate with warfarin is fairly low in low-risk patients, the absolute risk of ICH may approach the absolute reduction in the risk of stroke in warfarin-treated patients at high risk for bleeding. Knowledge of patient-specific risk factors for bleeding complications will help in balancing the risks and benefits of anticoagulation. These principles should help clinicians more clearly discern the risk:benefit ratio of anticoagulants in a given patient and dispel the reluctance to prescribe this therapy in patients who would clearly benefit.

The risk:benefit ratio of warfarin treatment for chronic AF established in large clinical trials may not always be generalizable to routine clinical practice because patients generally are more carefully selected and more intensively monitored in clinical trials.[19,52] Persons over age 75 years constitute the group of most concern.[53] Several studies have shown that older patients may require smaller dosages of warfarin than younger patients to maintain a given level of anticoagulation and that they may be at greater risk for major hemorrhage.[52,54–56] Fihn et al.[54] found that life-threatening and fatal complications were more common in patients 80 years of age or older (relative risk, 4.5; absolute event rate, 3.3% per year). Palareti et al.[55] also found that age was strongly correlated with the risk of major hemorrhage. The rate of major hemorrhage in patients over 70 years of age was four times that in patients age 50–69 years. High INR values are also linked to increased rates of ICH at any age. An annual rate of ICH of >3% was reported in patients treated with anticoagulants, and this was strongly related to INRs of >4.0.[57] In addition, two large observational studies confirmed a drastic increase in ICH rates at INRs of >4.0.[56,58] In contrast, other reports have not found an association between advanced age and increased bleeding complications.[59] These controversial findings may be explained by the wide range in the mean age of patients enrolled in the various studies. One study reported that insufficient education about oral anticoagulant therapy was a significant predictive factor for bleeding complications in older patients.[60] The safety of anticoagulants in clinical practice can be improved by the implementation of systematic monitoring and education programs, such as anticoagulation clinics and patient self-testing and management.[59] Recent data suggest that low rates of hemorrhage can be attained in clinical practice, even in elderly patients, if well-organized anticoagulation clinics are involved in the process of care for patients on warfarin.[61,62]

Recommendations for the Use of Antithrombotic Therapy in Patients with Chronic AF

Adjusted-dose oral anticoagulation therapy is an effective measure in decreasing the risk of ischemic stroke in patients with AF, and it is considerably more effective than aspirin. The risk of bleeding, including ICH, associated with oral anticoagulation is also higher than in patients treated with aspirin, and the management of patients taking warfarin therapy is more complex than it is for patients treated with aspirin. Patients at high risk of stroke gain a greater absolute benefit from warfarin therapy than patients with a lower risk. To this end, warfarin use has been recommended mainly for patients who have a moderate-to-high risk of stroke, where the ben-

efits of therapy clearly outweigh the risk of bleeding and the burden of monitoring. Therefore, when selecting the optimal antithrombotic agent, the risk of stroke and hemorrhage and the ability to comply with therapy need to be considered and balanced in each patient's case.

Guidelines issued by ACCP[1]; the American College of Cardiology, the American Heart Association, and the European Society of Cardiology (ACC/AHA/ESC)[16]; and the American Academy of Family Physicians and the American College of Physicians (AAFP/ACP)[63] recommend antithrombotic therapy based on various risk-stratification algorithms. Both the ACCP and ACC/AHA/ESC guidelines use an age-based, risk-stratification scheme and recommend either aspirin (81–325 mg) or warfarin, depending on the presence of additional risk factors (Tables 1 and 7). Although similar in some respects, the guidelines differ regarding (1) risk stratification and recommendations for moderate- and high-risk patients, (2) the INR target ranges for elderly patients (INR target of 2.0 [range, 1.6–2.5] recommended by the AHA guidelines in patients 75 years or older who have an increased risk of bleeding versus an INR target of 2.5 [range, 2.0–3.0]) recommended by ACCP for all patients who are candidates for warfarin therapy), and (3) the age threshold for patients at high risk of stroke (Tables 1, 2, and 7).[1,16] The AAFP/ACP guidelines recommend the use of adjusted-dose warfarin in all patients with AF unless they are at low risk of stroke or have a contraindication to therapy.[63] The differences in recommendations for antithrombotic therapy among these guidelines are mainly based on the variation in the available risk-stratification schemes. Opinion is especially divided on the use of oral anticoagulation for patients at moderate risk (3–5% per year) of stroke.

Emerging Treatment Options

There is a need for novel antithrombotic therapies that are effective and safe in preventing strokes in patients with AF and that are more convenient to use in the clinical setting (no need for dosage adjustment or monitoring, lack of drug or food interactions) compared with warfarin. One class of drugs in development that appears to have some of these beneficial features are the oral direct thrombin inhibitors.[64] The first agent of this class, ximelagatran, did not gain approved labeling by the Food and Drug Administration in the United States and was withdrawn from the markets in several European countries due to concerns of hepatotoxicity with the drug. However, other agents of this class, such as dabigatran, are in Phase III development and may prove to be potential alternatives to warfarin.

Other agents that may prove beneficial for stroke prevention in patients with AF are the factor Xa inhibitors. Idraparinux, an extended-release derivative of fondaparinux, is a long-acting indirect inhibitor of factor Xa. AMADEUS (Evaluating the Use of SR34006 Compared to Warfarin or Acenocoumarol in Patients with Atrial Fibrillation), compared a weekly subcutaneous dose of idraparinux with adjusted-dose warfarin.[65] The trial was stopped early because of major and clinically relevant bleeding in the group receiving idraparinux ($p < 0.0001$). Bleeding was more pronounced in the elderly and in patients with renal impairment. The primary efficacy endpoint (cumulative incidence of symptomatic thromboembolism) met the criteria for noninfe-

Table 7.
ACC/AHA/ESC Recommendations for the Use of Antithrombotic Therapy in Chronic Atrial Fibrillation[16,a]

No. and Level of Risk Factors[b]	Recommended Therapy	Target INR (Range)
0	Aspirin 81–325 mg daily	
1 Moderate	Aspirin 81–325 mg daily or warfarin	2.5 (2.0–3.0)
>1 Moderate or ≥1 high	Warfarin	2.5 (2.0–3.0)[c]

[a]ACC = American College of Cardiology, AHA = American Heart Association, ESC = European Society of Cardiology, INR = International Normalized Ratio.
[b]See Table 2 for risk factors and risk-scoring criteria.
[c]If patient has mechanical valve, target INR should be >2.5.

riority (0.9% per patient-year with idraparinux and 1.3% per patient-year with warfarin, $p = 0.007$).[66] The BOREALIS-AF study is now underway and will compare the neutralizable form of idraparinux (biotinylated idraparinux) to warfarin, with considerations for doing adjustments based on age and renal function. Various oral factor Xa inhibitors are also in development.

The combination of clopidogrel and aspirin has also been proposed as a potential treatment option, as this combination may allow for fixed-dose therapy without the need for therapeutic monitoring. This combination is currently being tested in ACTIVE (Atrial Fibrillation Clopidogrel Trial with Irbesartan for Prevention of Vascular Events).[67] This trial is designed to assess the efficacy of combined aspirin plus clopidogrel versus either warfarin (ACTIVE W) or aspirin (ACTIVE A). However, the ACTIVE W part of this trial was stopped early because oral anticoagulation was found superior to the combination antiplatelet therapy in preventing vascular events (3.93% versus 5.6% annual risk, respectively) ($p = 0.0003$).[68] The ACTIVE A part of the study is still in progress.

Cost-Effectiveness of Therapy

The economic burden associated with stroke in the United States is extraordinarily high, and, with the increasing number of elderly patients with AF, this burden is expected to grow in coming years. In the United States, the overall cost associated with strokes for 2006 was estimated by the AHA to be $57.9 billion.[69] The total direct cost of AF-related strokes has been reported to be around $8 billion.[70] The average cost of caring for a stroke patient in the first 12 weeks after an ischemic stroke is about $14,000.[71] A large percentage of hospitalized patients with AF do not receive warfarin, and only about one third of those who receive warfarin have an INR in target range.[72] In AFFIRM (Atrial Fibrillation Follow-up Investigation of Rhythm Management), 72% of patients who had an ischemic stroke had either discontinued anticoagulation or had an INR of <2.0.[73] A recently published economic model suggests a potential saving of $2.5 billion in the United States if half of all patients with AF receiving inappropriate or no anticoagulation were appropriately managed.[70]

The benefits, risks, and costs associated with antithrombotic therapy need to be carefully considered and balanced when selecting the most appropriate treatment option for patients with AF. Cost-effectiveness modeling can serve as a useful guide in such situations. Antithrombotic prophylaxis for AF is considered to be cost-effective if the rate of thromboembolism is high relative to the rate of major bleeding events.[74] Using direct costs, Gage et al.[75] found that for patients with AF and one additional risk factor, the cost of warfarin therapy was $8,000 per quality-adjusted life-year (QALY) saved. Patients with a low risk of stroke or with lone AF were more costly to treat; the estimated cost of warfarin therapy was about $370,000 per QALY saved. For patients who were not prescribed warfarin, aspirin was preferred to no therapy on the basis of both quality-adjusted survival and cost in all cases, regardless of the number of risk factors present. Other investigators have also concluded that warfarin is cost-effective in patients with a moderate-to-high risk of AF.[76–78]

Managing Anticoagulant Therapy

To optimize the safety and effectiveness of long-term oral anticoagulant therapy, the pharmacist should take an active role in educating and monitoring the patient. Patients should be adequately counseled on the full range of issues pertaining to anticoagulation, such as the indication for therapy, the laboratory test used to monitor anticoagulation, the need for close medical supervision, signs and symptoms of bleeding or thromboembolic complications, dietary interactions, drug interactions, alcohol consumption, and possible alterations in the response to warfarin in the presence of various underlying medical conditions.[79] The pharmacist should also take an active role in closely monitoring and reporting newly observed adverse drug reactions and interactions. Long-term oral anticoagulant therapy should be regularly monitored by prothrombin time (PT) test, with conversion of the PT into the INR.[59] ASHP has previously endorsed the routine use of the INR for monitoring warfarin therapy.[80]

Safe and effective therapy has been achieved through the establishment of specialty practice anticoagulation clinics, and there are numerous reports and trials that document the role of pharmacists in and the value of these clinics.[81–83] Clinics with personnel focused on anticoagulation therapy management are capable of reducing hemorrhagic complication rates and thromboembolism rates compared with routine medical care (RMC). Ansell and Hughes[84] summarized the literature relating to the outcomes in patients undergoing anticoagulation therapy who were seen during RMC and in anticoagulation clinics staffed by pharmacists and other health professionals. Their review found that the rate of thromboembolism was reduced from 16.2% per patient-year in RMC to 2.4% per patient-year in anticoagulation clinics and that major hemorrhage was reduced from 10.9% per patient-year with RMC to 2.8% per patient-year with anticoagulation clinics. Cost savings of $800–$1600 per patient-year were also noted with anticoagulation clinics. Other studies conducted in pharmacist-run clinics support these findings.[85,86]

Pharmacists may also contribute to positive patient outcomes by helping to identify candidates for antithrombotic prophylaxis who are not receiving any form of therapy. Inpatients can be identified case by case or through screening of electrocardiograms. Inpatients and outpatients could be identified through diagnosis-related group or International Classification of Diseases codes. Once patients are identified, pharmacists should encourage the appropriate use of warfarin and aspirin through one-on-one interactions and educational programs based on guidelines of ACCP[1] and this ASHP therapeutic position statement.

Summary

Stroke is a potentially catastrophic, but largely preventable, consequence of AF. ASHP supports recommendations established by ACCP (Table 1) for the use of antithrombotic therapy in appropriate patients to reduce the morbidity and mortality associated with stroke. The selection of warfarin versus aspirin should be based on the presence of clinical risk factors for stroke and the patient's ability to safely undergo anticoagulation therapy. Adequate patient education and monitoring are keys to the successful use of antithrombotic therapy, and ASHP believes that pharmacists play an important role in providing these services.

References

1. Singer DE, Albers GW, Dalen JE et al. Antithrombotic therapy in atrial fibrillation: the Seventh ACCP Conference on Antithrombotic and Thrombolytic Therapy. *Chest.* 2004; 126(3, suppl):429S–56S.
2. Go AS, Hylek EM, Phillips KA et al. Prevalence of diagnosed atrial fibrillation in adults: national implications for rhythm management and stroke prevention: the Anticoagulation and Risk Factors in Atrial Fibrillation (ATRIA) study. *JAMA.* 2001; 285:2370–5.
3. Feinberg WM, Blackshear JL, Laupacis A et al. Prevalence, age distribution, and gender of patients with atrial fibrillation. *Arch Intern Med.* 1995; 155:469–73.
4. Furberg CD, Psaty BM, Manolio TA et al. Prevalence of atrial fibrillation in elderly subjects (the Cardiovascular Health Study). *Am J Cardiol.* 1994; 74:236–41.
5. Wattigney WA, Mensah GA, Croft JB. Increasing trends in hospitalization for atrial fibrillation in the United States, 1985 through 1999: implications for primary prevention. *Circulation.* 2003; 108:711–6.
6. Wolf PA, Abbot RD, Kannel WB. Atrial fibrillation as an independent risk factor for stroke: the Framingham Study. *Stroke.* 1991; 22:983–8.
7. Lip GY, Boos CJ. Antithrombotic treatment in atrial fibrillation. *Heart.* 2006; 92:155–61.
8. Benjamin EJ, Wolf PA, D'Agostino RB et al. Impact of atrial fibrillation on the risk of death: the Framingham Heart Study. *Circulation.* 1998; 98:946–52.
9. Marini C, De Santis F, Sacco S et al. Contribution of atrial fibrillation to incidence and outcome of ischemic stroke: results from a population-based study. *Stroke.* 2005; 36:1115–9.
10. Paciaroni M, Agnelli G, Caso V et al. Atrial fibrillation in patients with first-ever stroke: frequency, antithrom-

botic treatment before the event and effect on clinical outcome. *J Thromb Haemost.* 2005; 3:1218–23.
11. Falk RH. Atrial fibrillation. *N Engl J Med.* 2001; 344:1067–78. [Erratum, *N Engl J Med.* 2001; 344:1876.]
12. Go AS, Hylek EM, Borowsky LH et al. Warfarin use among ambulatory patients with nonvalvular atrial fibrillation: the Anticoagulation and Risk Factors in Atrial Fibrillation (ATRIA) study. *Ann Intern Med.* 1999; 131:927–34.
13. Villa A, Bacchetta A, Omboni E. Underuse of antithrombotic therapy in stroke patients with chronic atrial fibrillation. *Stroke.* 2000; 31:2266–7.
14. Stafford RS, Radley DC. The underutilization of cardiac medications of proven benefit, 1990 to 2002. *J Am Coll Cardiol.* 2003; 41:56–61.
15. American Society of Health-System Pharmacists. ASHP therapeutic position statement on antithrombotic therapy in chronic atrial fibrillation. *Am J Health- Syst Pharm.* 1998; 55:376–81.
16. Fuster V, Ryden LE, Cannom DS et al. ACC/AHA/ESC 2006 guidelines for the management of patients with atrial fibrillation—executive summary. A report of the American College of Cardiology/American Heart Association Task Force on Practice Guidelines and the European Society of Cardiology Committee for Practice Guidelines. (Writing Committee to Revise the 2001 Guidelines for the Management of Patients With Atrial Fibrillation). *Circulation.* 2006; 114:700–52. [Erratum, *Circulation.* 2007; 116:e137.]
17. Stroke Prevention in Atrial Fibrillation Investigators. Predictors of thromboembolism in atrial fibrillation: II. Echocardiographic features of patients at risk. *Ann Intern Med.* 1992; 116:6–12.
18. Laupacis A, Sackett DL, Robert RS. An assessment of clinically useful measurements of the consequences of treatment. *N Engl J Med.* 1988; 318:1728–33.
19. Atrial Fibrillation Investigators. Risk factors for stroke and efficacy of antithrombotic therapy in atrial fibrillation: analysis of pooled data from five randomized controlled trials. *Arch Intern Med.* 1994; 154:1449–57.
20. Stroke Prevention in Atrial Fibrillation. Risk factors for thromboembolism during aspirin therapy in patients with atrial fibrillation: the Stroke Prevention in Atrial Fibrillation study. *J Stroke Cerebrovasc Dis.* 1995; 5:147–57.
21. Hart RG, Pearce LA, McBride R et al. Factors associated with ischemic stroke during aspirin therapy in atrial fibrillation: analysis of 2012 participants in the SPAF I-III clinical trials. *Stroke.* 1999; 30:1223–9.
22. Wang TJ, Massaro JM, Levy D et al. A risk score for predicting stroke or death in individuals with new-onset atrial fibrillation in the community: the Framingham Heart Study. *JAMA.* 2003; 290:1049–56.
23. Gage BF, Waterman AD, Shannon W et al. Validation of clinical classification-schemes for predicting stroke: results from the National Registry of Atrial Fibrillation. *JAMA.* 2001; 285:2864–70.
24. Go AS. Efficacy of anticoagulation for stroke prevention and risk stratification in atrial fibrillation: translating trials into clinical practice. *Am J Manag Care.* 2004; 10:S58–65.

25. Gage BF, van Walraven C, Pearce L et al. Selecting patients with atrial fibrillation for anticoagulation: stroke risk stratification in patients taking aspirin. *Circulation.* 2004; 110:2287–92.

26. Pearce LA, Hart RG, Halperin JL. Assessment of three schemes for stratifying stroke risk in patients with nonvalvular atrial fibrillation. *Am J Med.* 2000; 109:45–51.

27. Petersen P, Boysen G, Godtfredsen J et al. Placebo controlled, randomised trial of warfarin and aspirin for prevention of thromboembolic complications in chronic atrial fibrillation (AFASAK). *Lancet.* 1989; 1:175–9.

28. Boston Area Anticoagulation Trial for Atrial Fibrillation Investigators. The effect of low-dose warfarin on the risk of stroke in nonrheumatic atrial fibrillation. *N Engl J Med.* 1990; 323:1505–11.

29. The Stroke Prevention in Atrial Fibrillation Study. Final results. *Circulation.* 1991; 84:527–39.

30. Ezekowitz MD, Bridgers SL, James KE et al. Warfarin in the prevention of stroke associated with nonrheumatic atrial fibrillation. *N Engl J Med.* 1992; 327:1406–12. [Erratum, *N Engl J Med.* 1993; 328:148.]

31. Connolly SJ, Laupacis A, Gent M et al., for the CAFA Study Co-investigators. Canadian Atrial Fibrillation Anticoagulation (CAFA) study. *J Am Coll Cardiol.* 1991; 18:349–55.

32. European Atrial Fibrillation Trial Study Group. Secondary prevention in nonrheumatic atrial fibrillation after transient ischemic attack or minor stroke. *Lancet.* 1993; 342:1255–62.

33. European Atrial Fibrillation Trial Study Group. Optimal oral anticoagulant therapy in patients with nonrheumatic atrial fibrillation and recent cerebral ischemia. *N Engl J Med.* 1995; 333:5–10.

34. Diener HC, Cunha L, Forbes C et al. European Stroke Prevention Study. 2. Dipyridamole and acetylsalicylic acid in the prevention of stroke. *J Neurol Sci.* 1996; 143:1–13.

35. Diener HC, Lowenthal A. Reply. (Antiplatelet therapy to prevent stroke: risk of brain hemorrhage and efficacy in atrial fibrillation.) *J Neuorol Sci.* 1997; 153:112. Letter.

36. Posada IS, Barriales V. Alternate-day dosing of aspirin in atrial fibrillation. *Am Heart J.* 1999; 138:137–43.

37. Warfarin versus aspirin for prevention of thromboembolism in atrial fibrillation: Stroke Prevention in Atrial Fibrillation II Study. *Lancet.* 1994; 343:687–91.

38. Adjusted-dose warfarin versus low-intensity, fixed-dose warfarin plus aspirin for high-risk patients with atrial fibrillation: Stroke Prevention in Atrial Fibrillation III randomised clinical trial. *Lancet.* 1996; 348:633–8.

39. Gullov AL, Koefoed BG, Petersen P et al. Fixed mini-dose warfarin and aspirin alone and in combination versus adjusted-dose warfarin for stroke prevention in atrial fibrillation: Second Copenhagen Atrial Fibrillation, Aspirin, and Anticoagulation Study. *Arch Intern Med.* 1998; 158:1513–21.

40. Hellemons BS, Langenberg M, Lodder J et al. Primary prevention of arterial thromboembolism in non-rheumatic atrial fibrillation in primary care: randomized controlled trial comparing two intensities of coumarin with aspirin. *BMJ.* 1999; 318:958–64.

41. Hart RG, Talbert RL, Kadri K et al. Warfarin for stroke prevention: a clinical review. *Neurologist.* 1996; 2:319–41.

42. Atrial Fibrillation Investigators. The efficacy of aspirin in patients with atrial fibrillation: analysis of pooled data from 3 randomized trials. *Arch Intern Med.* 1997; 157:1237–40.

43. Hart RG, Benavente O, McBride R et al. Antithrombotic therapy to prevent stroke in patients with atrial fibrillation: a meta-analysis. *Ann Intern Med.* 1999; 131:492–501.

44. Van Walraven C, Hart RG, Singer DE et al. Oral anticoagulants vs aspirin in nonvalvular atrial fibrillation: an individual patient metaanalysis. *JAMA.* 2002; 288:2441–8.

45. Hart RG, Pearce LA, Miller VT et al. Cardioembolic versus noncardioembolic strokes in atrial fibrillation: frequency and effect of antithrombotic agents in stroke prevention in atrial fibrillation studies. *Cerebrovasc Dis.* 2000; 10:39–43.

46. Lin HJ, Wolf PA, Kelly-Hayes M et al. Stroke severity in atrial fibrillation: the Framingham Study. *Stroke.* 1996; 27:1760–4.

47. Hylek EM, Go AS, Chang Y et al. Impact of intensity of oral anticoagulation on stroke severity and stroke mortality in patients with non-valvular atrial fibrillation. *N Engl J Med.* 2003; 349:1019–26.

48. Lechat P, Lardoux H, Mallet A et al. Anticoagulant (fluindione)-aspirin combination in patients with high-risk atrial fibrillation. A randomized trial (Fluindione, Fibrillation Auriculaire, Aspirin et Contraste Spontane; FFAACS). *Cerebrovasc Dis.* 2001; 12:245–52.

49. Hylek EM, Skates SJ, Sheehan MA et al. An analysis of the lowest effective intensity of prophylactic anticoagulation for patients with nonrheumatic atrial fibrillation. *N Engl J Med.* 1996; 335:540–6.

50. Brass LM, Krumholz HM, Scinto JM et al. Warfarin use among patients with atrial fibrillation. *Stroke.* 1997; 28:2382–9.

51. Hart RG, Boop BS, Anderson DC. Oral anticoagulants and intracranial hemorrhage. Facts and hypotheses. *Stroke.* 1995; 26:1471–7.

52. Gottleib LK, Salem-Schatz S. Anticoagulation in atrial fibrillation. Does efficacy in clinical trials translate into effectiveness in practice? *Arch Intern Med.* 1994; 154:1945–53.

53. Stroke Prevention in Atrial Fibrillation Investigators. Bleeding during antithrombotic therapy in patients with atrial fibrillation. *Arch Intern Med.* 1996; 156:409–16.

54. Fihn SD, Callahan CM, Martin DC et al. The risk for and severity of bleeding complications in elderly patients treated with warfarin. *Ann Intern Med.* 1996; 124:970–9.

55. Palareti G, Leali N, Coccheri S et al. Bleeding complications of oral anticoagulant treatment: an inception cohort, prospective collaborative study. *Lancet.* 1996; 348:423–8.

56. Hylek EM, Singer DE. Risk factors for intracranial hemorrhage in outpatients taking warfarin. *Ann Intern Med.* 1994; 120:897–902.

57. Goerter JW. Major bleeding during anticoagulation after cerebral ischemia: patterns and risk factors. *Neurology.* 1999; 53:1319–27.

58. Cannegiter SC, Rosendaal FR, Wintzen AR et al. Optimal oral anticoagulant therapy in patients with mechanical heart valves. *N Engl J Med.* 1995; 333:11–7.

59. Ansell J, Hirsh J, Poller L et al. The pharmacology and management of the vitamin K antagonists: the Seventh ACCP Conference on Antithrombotic and Thrombolytic Therapy. *Chest.* 2004; 126:204S–233S.

60. Kagansky N, Knobler H, Rimon E et al. Safety of anticoagulation therapy in well-informed older patients. *Arch Intern Med.* 2004; 164:2044–50.

61. Go AS, Hylek EH, Chang Y et al. Anticoagulation for stroke prevention in atrial fibrillation: how well do randomized trials translate into clinical practice? *JAMA.* 2003; 290:2685–92.

62. Palareti G, Manotti C, D'Angelo A et al. Thrombotic events during anticoagulant treatment: results of the inception-cohort, prospective, collaborative ISCOAT study. *Thromb Haemost.* 1997; 78:1438–43.

63. Snow W, Weiss KB, LeFevre M et al. Management of newly detected atrial fibrillation: a clinical practice guideline from the American Academy of Family Physicians and the American College of Physicians. *Ann Intern Med.* 2003; 139:1009–17.

64. Nutescu EA, Shapiro NL, Chevalier A. New anticoagulant agents: direct thrombin inhibitors. *Clin Geriatr Med.* 2006; 22:33–56.

65. Idraparinux sodium: SANORG 34006, SR 34006. *Drugs R D.* 2004; 5:164–5.

66. Buller H. Once-weekly subcutaneous idraparinux (anti-XA) versus oral vitamin K antagonist therapy for the prevention of thromboembolic events in patients with atrial fibrillation (O-W-054). Paper presented at 21st Congress of the International Society on Thrombosis and Haemostasis. Geneva; 2007 Jul 11.

67. The Active Steering Committee. Rationale and design of ACTIVE: the Atrial Fibrillation Clopidogrel Trial with Irbesartan for Prevention of Vascular Events. *Am Heart J.* 2006; 151:1187–93.

68. ACTIVE Writing Group on behalf of the ACTIVE Investigators. Clopidogrel plus aspirin versus oral anticoagulation for atrial fibrillation in the Atrial Fibrillation Clopidogrel Trial with Irbesartan for prevention of Vascular Events (ACTIVE W): a randomised controlled trial. *Lancet.* 2006; 367:1903–12.

69. American Heart Association. Heart disease and stroke statistics—2006 update. www.americanheart.org/downloadable/heart/113535864858055-1026_HS_Stats06book.pdf (accessed 2006 Mar 1).

70. Caro JJ. An economic model of stroke in atrial fibrillation: the cost of suboptimal oral anticoagulation. *Am J Manag Care.* 2004; 10:S451–61.

71. Caro JJ, Huybrechts KF, Duchesne I, for the Stroke Economic Analysis Group. Management patterns and costs of acute ischemic stroke: an international study. *Stroke.* 2000; 31:582–90.

72. Bungard TJ, Ackman ML, Ho G et al. Adequacy of anticoagulation in patients with atrial fibrillation coming to a hospital. *Pharmacotherapy.* 2000; 20:1060–5.

73. Wyse DG, Waldo AL, DiMarco JP et al. A comparison of rate control and rhythm control in patients with atrial fibrillation. *N Engl J Med.* 2002; 347:1825–33.

74. Eckman MH, Falk RH, Pauker SG. Cost-effectiveness of therapies for patients with nonvalvular atrial fibrillation. *Arch Intern Med.* 1998; 158:1669–77.

75. Gage BF, Cardinalli AB, Albers GW et al. Cost-effectiveness of warfarin and aspirin for prophylaxis of stroke in patients with nonvalvular atrial fibrillation. *JAMA.* 1995; 274:1839–45.

76. Kan BD, Katz DA. Cost-effectiveness of stroke prophylaxis for nonvalvular atrial fibrillation. *JAMA.* 1996; 275:909. Letter.

77. Lightowlers S, McGuire A. Cost-effectiveness of anticoagulation in nonrheumatic atrial fibrillation in the primary prevention of ischemic stroke. *Stroke.* 1998; 29:1827–32.

78. Szucs TD, Bramkamp M. Pharmacoeconomics of anticoagulation therapy for stroke prevention in atrial fibrillation: a review. *J Thromb Haemost.* 2006; 4:1180–5.

79. Nutescu EA, Helgason CM. Concomitant drug, dietary, and lifestyle issues in patients with atrial fibrillation receiving anticoagulation therapy for stroke prophylaxis. *Curr Treat Options Cardiovasc Med.* 2005; 7:241–50.

80. American Society of Health-System Pharmacists. ASHP therapeutic position statement on the use of the International Normalized Ratio system to monitor oral anticoagulant therapy. *Am J Health-Syst Pharm.* 1995; 52:529–31.

81. Radley AS, Hall J, Farrow M et al. Evaluation of anticoagulant control in a pharmacist operated anticoagulant clinic. *J Clin Pathol.* 1995; 48:545–7.

82. Lee YP, Schommer JC. Effect of a pharmacist-managed anticoagulation clinic on warfarin-related hospital readmissions. *Am J Health-Syst Pharm.* 1996; 53:1580–3.

83. Witt DM, Sadler MA, Shanahan RL et al. Effect of a centralized clinical pharmacy anticoagulation service on the outcomes of anticoagulation therapy. *Chest.* 2005; 127:1515–22.

84. Ansell JE, Hughes R. Evolving models of warfarin management: anticoagulation clinics, patient self-monitoring, and patient self-management. *Am Heart J.* 1996; 132:1095–100.

85. Chiquette E, Amato MG, Bussey HI. Comparison of an anticoagulation clinic with usual medical care: anticoagulation control, patient outcomes, and health care costs. *Arch Intern Med.* 1998; 158:1641–7.

86. Wilt VM, Gums JG, Ahmed OI et al. Outcome analysis of a pharmacist-managed anticoagulation service. *Pharmacotherapy.* 1995; 15:732–9.

Approved by the ASHP Board of Directors on June 23, 2007. Developed through the ASHP Council on Therapeutics.

Edith Nutescu, Pharm.D., FCCP is gratefully acknowledged for authoring this therapeutic position statement.

The bibliographic citation for this document is as follows: American Society of Health-System Pharmacists. ASHP therapeutic position statement on antithrombotic therapy in chronic atrial fibrillation. *Am J Health-Syst Pharm.* 2007; 64:2281–91.

ASHP Therapeutic Position Statement on the Cessation of Tobacco Use

Position

The American Society of Health-System Pharmacists (ASHP) discourages all use of tobacco products and supports evidence-based tobacco-control policies and activities that reduce the prevalence of tobacco use. ASHP strongly encourages health care providers to take an active role in promoting the health of their patients by systematically integrating into routine patient care (a) the identification of tobacco users and (b) the delivery of evidence-based tobacco-cessation interventions. ASHP recommends behavioral and pharmacologic therapies for cessation, advocates their use for all patients attempting to quit smoking (except when medically contraindicated or in specific populations for which there is insufficient evidence of effectiveness), and advises that these therapeutic interventions be reimbursed under health insurance plans.

To enable more effective and consistent identification of tobacco use and drug interactions with smoking, ASHP urges that all patient records, including those in electronic medical records and pharmacy information technology systems, include a designated field for the collection of tobacco-use data and that this field be integrated within the system such that clinically significant drug interactions with tobacco products are identified. Schools that offer health professional degree programs are encouraged to integrate comprehensive tobacco-cessation training as part of their core curricula, and licensed clinicians are advised to participate in continuing-education programs as necessary to acquire and maintain tobacco-cessation counseling skills. Given the established dangers of secondhand smoke exposure, ASHP supports legislation promoting smoke-free environments for the employees and patrons of all workplaces and public venues. Furthermore, because the sale of tobacco products contradicts the clinician's role in promoting health, ASHP strongly opposes the sale or distribution of tobacco products in all establishments where health care services are rendered.

Epidemiology of Tobacco Use

As the former U.S. Surgeon General C. Everett Koop stated in 1982, "Cigarette smoking is the chief single, avoidable cause of death in our society and the most important public health issue of our time."[1] This statement remains true today, nearly three decades later. The Centers for Disease Control and Prevention (CDC) estimates that nearly 438,000 Americans die each year from smoking,[2] and approximately 50,000 persons die annually due to involuntary exposure to tobacco smoke.[3] Cigarettes are the only marketed consumable product that, when used as intended, will contribute to the death of half or more of its users.[4]

While cigarettes are, by far, the most frequently used form of tobacco in the United States, other forms of smoked tobacco (e.g., cigars, clove cigarettes [kreteks], pipe tobacco, bidis, hookah) and smokeless tobacco (e.g., chewing tobacco, snuff) can also lead to dependence and should be addressed by clinicians. Despite the proven negative health consequences of tobacco use and the fact that approximately 70% of smokers want to quit,[5] 20.8% of the U.S. adult population continues to smoke either every day (16.7%) or some days (4.1%).[6] In 2006, more men (23.9%) than women (18.0%) were smokers.[6] The prevalence of smoking also varied by race or ethnicity (non-Hispanic American Indian/Alaska Native, 32.4%; non-Hispanic white, 21.9%; non-Hispanic black, 23.0%; Hispanic, 15.2%; non-Hispanic Asian, 10.4%), education level (higher education is associated with a lower prevalence), and poverty level (20.4% of individuals living at or above the federal poverty level; 30.6% of individuals living below the poverty level).[6] An estimated 44.3% of cigarettes smoked in the United States are by persons with mental illness.[7]

Smoking prevalence varies across the nation. In 2006, the highest median prevalence of smoking was evident in Kentucky (28.6%) and the lowest was in Utah (9.8%).[8] Because most teens who smoke at least monthly continue to smoke in adulthood,[9] tobacco-use trends among youth are viewed as a key indicator of future national health trends.[10] In 2007, an estimated 21.6% of 12th graders (23.1% of males and 19.6% of females) had smoked one or more cigarettes in the past 30 days.[11] The prevalence of smoking has declined among adolescents over the past decade; however, the downward trend has largely diminished among 12th graders in recent years.

In the past decade, the prevalence of cigarette smoking has decreased while the per-capita consumption of cigars has increased.[12] However, beginning in 2005, there has been a slight trend toward decreased cigar use. In 2007, the prevalence of cigar smoking (one or more cigars in the past month) among persons 12 years or older was 5.4%.[13] Cigar weight and nicotine content vary widely, with most cigars ranging in weight from 1 to 22 g. In comparison, a typical U.S. cigarette weighs <1 g. The nicotine content in 10 commercially available cigars studied in 1996 ranged from 10 to 444 mg.[14] Cigarette brands sold by major manufacturers in the United States have a lower and less-variable total nicotine content, ranging from 11.9 to 14.5 mg of nicotine per cigarette.[15] As such, it is possible for one large cigar to contain as much tobacco as an entire pack of cigarettes and to deliver enough nicotine to establish and maintain dependence.[14]

In 2007, an estimated 8.1 million Americans 12 years of age or older (3.2%) had used smokeless tobacco in the past month; men (6.3%) were more likely than were women (0.4%) to be users.[13] The prevalence of smokeless tobacco use is highest among individuals ages 18–25 years and is substantially higher among American Indians, Alaskan Natives, and residents of the southern United States and rural areas.[13,16] While sales of most forms of smokeless tobacco (e.g., looseleaf, plug, twist) have declined since the mid-1980s, moist snuff sales have increased steadily since the late 1980s.[12]

An enormous economic burden accompanies tobacco use. Each pack of cigarettes smoked costs society $7.18 ($3.45 for associated medical care and $3.73 for productiv-

ity losses), for a total of $157 billion in annual health-related economic losses.[17] The lifelong smoker (e.g., one pack per day for 50 years) spends more than $100,000 on his or her smoking habit in addition to the associated medical care costs of tobacco use.

Extensive evidence implicates tobacco as the primary known preventable cause of death in the United States. As such, ASHP strongly supports evidence-based tobacco-control initiatives that aim to reduce the prevalence of tobacco use by (a) preventing the initiation of tobacco use and (b) promoting and maintaining cessation. Tobacco-control initiatives (e.g., those described in each state's comprehensive cancer control plan) should comply with recommendations set forth by CDC as delineated in the "Best Practices for Comprehensive Tobacco Control Programs"[18] and the "Guide to Community Preventive Services: Tobacco Use Prevention and Control."[19]

Nicotine Pharmacology

Tobacco products are carefully engineered formulations that optimize the delivery of nicotine, a chemical that meets established criteria for an addictive substance.[20] Once absorbed, nicotine induces a variety of central nervous system, cardiovascular, and metabolic effects. Within seconds after inhalation, nicotine reaches the brain and stimulates the release of various neurotransmitters including dopamine, which induces nearly immediate feelings of pleasure and relieves nicotine-withdrawal symptoms. This rapid dose response reinforces the need to repeat the administration of nicotine, thereby perpetuating smoking behavior.[21] The short half-life ($t_{1/2}$ = 2 hours) of nicotine generally necessitates frequent dosing throughout the day, and tobacco users become adept at titrating nicotine intake to maintain pleasure and arousal, modulate mood, and avoid withdrawal symptoms.[21]

When nicotine is discontinued, the following withdrawal symptoms may develop: irritability, impatience, anxiety, difficulty concentrating, restlessness, hunger, depression, insomnia, and cravings.[22-24] Most physical withdrawal symptoms generally manifest within 24–48 hours after quitting and gradually dissipate over two to four weeks[23]; however, strong cravings for tobacco can persist for months or even years.[25] The nicotine levels generated by smokeless tobacco are similar to those of smoking, although their onset of action is less rapid. Upon quitting, smokeless tobacco users experience withdrawal symptoms similar to those of smokers.[26] Although nicotine is the dependence-causing component of tobacco, it is not directly responsible for the myriad of negative health consequences of tobacco use.

Health Consequences of Tobacco Use and Exposure to Secondhand Smoke

Smoking. According to the 2004 Surgeon General's report on the health consequences of smoking,[27] smoking harms nearly every organ of the body, is causally associated with numerous diseases (Table 1), and reduces the health of smokers in general. In addition to contributing to the development of disease, smoking also can lead to exacerbation or reduced control of existing conditions such as hypertension, diabetes mellitus, and asthma. On average, men and

Table 1.
Diseases and Other Adverse Health Effects Caused by Smoking[27]

Cancers
 Acute myeloid leukemia
 Bladder
 Cervical
 Esophageal
 Gastric
 Kidney
 Laryngeal
 Lung
 Oral cavity and pharyngeal
 Pancreatic
Cardiovascular diseases
 Abdominal aortic aneurysm
 Coronary heart disease (angina pectoris, ischemic heart disease, myocardial infarction)
 Cerebrovascular disease (transient ischemic attacks, stroke)
 Peripheral arterial disease
Pulmonary diseases
 Acute respiratory illnesses
 Upper respiratory tract (rhinitis, sinusitis, laryngitis, pharyngitis)
 Lower respiratory tract (bronchitis, pneumonia)
 Chronic respiratory illnesses
 Chronic obstructive pulmonary disease
 Respiratory symptoms: cough, phlegm, wheezing, dyspnea
 Poor asthma control
 Reduced lung function in infants exposed in utero to maternal smoking
Reproductive effects
 Reduced fertility in women
 Pregnancy and pregnancy outcomes
 Preterm or premature rupture of membranes
 Placenta previa
 Placental abruption
 Preterm delivery
 Low infant birth weight
 Infant mortality (sudden infant death syndrome)
Other effects
 Cataract
 Osteoporosis (reduced bone density in postmenopausal women, increased risk of hip fracture)
 Periodontitis
 Peptic ulcer disease (in patients who are infected with *Helicobacter pylori*)
 Adverse surgical outcomes
 Poor wound healing
 Respiratory complications

women lose 13.2 and 14.5 years of life because of smoking, respectively.[17] Between 1997 and 2001, an estimated 437,902 annual U.S. deaths were attributable to smoking. Of these deaths, 158,529 (36.2%) were due to cancer, 137,979 (31.5%) to cardiovascular disease, and 101,454 (23.2%) to respiratory disease.[2]

Smokeless Tobacco. Users of smokeless forms of tobacco are often under the mistaken impression that these formulations are a "safe" alternative to smoking cigarettes. In addition to cosmetic effects such as halitosis and staining of the teeth, smokeless tobacco use is associated with serious

health effects, including cancer, soft tissue alterations (e.g., leukoplakia), and periodontal effects.[16] Smokeless tobacco contains high concentrations of carcinogens, which have direct contact with mucosal tissues over prolonged periods of time. The most serious consequence of smokeless tobacco use is an increased risk of developing oral and pharyngeal cancers, and the risk appears to be dose related, in that heavy, longtime users are more likely to develop oral cancer than are nonusers. The health effects of smokeless tobacco with regard to cardiovascular disease are not well understood, and published data are conflicting.[28-30] Although smokeless tobacco products do not confer many of the risks associated with the inhalation of combusted tobacco (e.g., pulmonary disease, lung cancer), these products do impose harm and should not be recommended as aids for smoking cessation, because safer, effective products (i.e., medications with FDA-approved labeling for use in smoking cessation) are available.[31]

Secondhand Smoke Exposure. Exposure to secondhand smoke results in an estimated 50,000 deaths annually, in addition to contributing to numerous diseases among nonsmoking children and adults.[3] Major conclusions of the Surgeon General's report "The Health Effects of Involuntary Exposure to Tobacco Smoke" included the following:

1. Many millions of Americans, both children and adults, are still exposed to secondhand smoke in their homes and workplaces despite substantial progress in tobacco control,
2. Secondhand smoke exposure causes disease and premature death in children and adults who do not smoke,
3. Children exposed to secondhand smoke are at an increased risk for sudden infant death syndrome (SIDS), acute respiratory infections, ear problems, and more severe asthma; smoking by parents causes respiratory symptoms and slows lung growth in their children,
4. Exposure of adults to secondhand smoke has immediate adverse effects on the cardiovascular system and causes coronary heart disease and lung cancer,
5. The scientific evidence indicates that there is no risk-free level of exposure to secondhand smoke, and
6. Eliminating smoking in indoor spaces fully protects nonsmokers from exposure to secondhand smoke; separating smokers from nonsmokers, cleaning the air, and ventilating buildings cannot eliminate exposures of nonsmokers to secondhand smoke.

Supplementing the evidence presented in the Surgeon General's report,[3] the California Environmental Protection Agency in January 2006 designated secondhand smoke as a "toxic air contaminant" and, in addition to noting the tobacco-related diseases described in the Surgeon General's report, specified that exposure to smoke is associated with breast cancer in younger, primarily premenopausal women.[32]

Drug Interactions with Tobacco Smoke. Various substances in tobacco interact with several commonly prescribed drugs.[33,34] It is widely recognized that polycyclic aromatic hydrocarbons (PAHs), the products of the incomplete combustion of tobacco, are largely responsible for the majority of drug interactions with smoking. PAHs are found in appreciably large quantities in tobacco smoke and are potent inducers of hepatic microsomal (cytochrome P-450) enzymes CYP1A1, CYP1A2, and possibly CYP2E1. Although other substances in tobacco smoke such as acetone, pyridines, benzene, nicotine, carbon monoxide, and heavy metals (e.g., cadmium) might also interact with hepatic enzymes, their effects appear to be less significant.[34] To enable more effective screening for tobacco use and drug interactions with smoking, all patient records, including those stored and accessed via medical records and pharmacy information technology systems, should include a designated field for collection of tobacco-use data. This field should be integrated into the system so that relevant drug interactions with tobacco smoke can be identified.

Health Benefits of Smoking Cessation

Quitting smoking produces immediate as well as long-term benefits, reducing the risk of developing diseases caused by smoking and improving health in general.[35] Some benefits are incurred almost immediately—within the first 24 hours—after quitting. Within two weeks to three months after quitting, circulation improves, walking becomes easier, and lung function increases up to 30%. Within 1 year, the excess risk of coronary heart disease is decreased to half that of a smoker, and after 5–15 years, stroke risk is reduced to a rate similar to that of people who have never smoked. Ten years after quitting, an individual's chance of dying of lung cancer is approximately half that of continuing smokers. In addition, the risk for mouth, throat, esophagus, bladder, kidney, or pancreatic cancer is decreased. Fifteen years after quitting, an individual's risk of coronary heart disease is reduced to a rate similar to that of people who have never smoked. Quitting at ages 30, 40, 50, and 60 has been shown to be associated with 10, 9, 6, and 3 years of life gained, respectively.[4] Thus, the benefits of quitting the use of tobacco are significant. It is never too late to quit to incur health benefits, but there are clear advantages to quitting earlier.

Strategies for Promoting Tobacco Cessation

Because of the immense societal burden that smoking imposes, tobacco use and dependence should be addressed during each clinical encounter. Routine screening for tobacco-use status enables clinicians to prevent the initiation of tobacco use among nonusers, facilitate cessation among current users, and promote continued abstinence among former users.

For most smokers, the quitting process is characterized by a series of quit attempts and subsequent relapses. On average, former smokers report 10.8 quit attempts over a period of 18.6 years before achieving long-term cessation.[36] Most quit attempts are undertaken without assistance, and approximately 95% of attempts end in relapse.[37]

Given the decades of strong, consistent findings in support of the efficacy and cost-effectiveness of both behavioral and pharmacologic interventions to facilitate tobacco cessation, ASHP recommends the use of evidenced-based behavioral and pharmacologic strategies for all patients attempting to quit smoking (except when medically contraindicated or in specific populations for which there is insufficient evidence of effectiveness [e.g., pregnant women, smokeless tobacco

users, light smokers, adolescents]). Treatment for tobacco dependence is highly cost-effective relative to other medical interventions (e.g., periodic mammography screening, treatment for hypertension and hyperlipidemia) and should be made available to all tobacco users.[37] In accordance with recommendations set forth in the 2008 clinical practice guideline, Treating Tobacco Use and Dependence,[37] ASHP recommends that (1) all insurance plans include counseling and evidence-based pharmacotherapy treatments as a reimbursable benefit and (2) clinicians be reimbursed for providing treatment for tobacco dependence, just as they are reimbursed for treatment of other chronic conditions.

Data consistently reveal that behavioral interventions (e.g., counseling from a health care provider) and pharmacotherapy, used either alone or in combination, increase patients' odds for quitting their use of tobacco.[37] In a meta-analysis of 29 studies, it was determined that patients who receive a tobacco-cessation intervention from a nonphysician clinician or a physician clinician are 1.7 and 2.2 times as likely to quit (for at least five months), respectively, compared with patients who do not receive an intervention from a clinician.[37] Estimates of the efficacy of various behavioral and pharmacotherapy treatment strategies are shown in Table 2.

As delineated in the clinical practice guideline, clinicians should routinely screen for tobacco use and apply appropriate interventions (Figure 1), addressing five key components for comprehensive tobacco-cessation counseling (the 5 A's): (1) asking patients about tobacco use, (2) advising tobacco users to quit, (3) assessing their willingness to make a quit attempt, (4) assisting patients with quitting, and (5) arranging follow-up care (Appendix A). To increase the odds for success, patients who are not ready to quit should receive tailored motivational interventions that address the 5 R's[37] (Appendix B). Patients who are ready to quit should be provided with a treatment plan that includes behavioral counseling plus pharmacotherapy (as appropriate) and follow-up counseling.

Clinicians should become familiar with local community-based resources for tobacco cessation, including group programs and telephone counseling.[37] When expertise, practice site logistics,

or time constraints do not afford an opportunity to provide comprehensive tobacco-cessation counseling, clinicians should apply a truncated 5 A's model whereby they *ask* about tobacco use, *advise* tobacco users to quit, and then *refer* patients to appropriate cessation providers or programs. With the October 2004 introduction of a national toll-free quit line number (1-800-QUIT-NOW), all residents of the United States can receive tobacco-cessation counseling at no cost. In clinical trials, telephone counseling services for smoking cessation have been shown to be effective among the patients

Table 2.
Efficacy of Treatment Methods for Tobacco Use and Dependence[a,b]

Treatment Method	Estimated Odds Ratio[c] (95% CI)	Estimated Abstinence[d] Rate (95% CI)
Behavioral interventions		
Advice to quit		
No advice to quit	1.0	7.9
Physician advice to quit	1.3 (1.1–1.6)	10.2 (8.5–12.0)
Clinician intervention		
No counseling by a clinician	1.0	10.2
Counseling by a nonphysician	1.7 (1.3–2.1)	15.8 (12.8–18.8)
Counseling by a physician	2.2 (1.5–3.2)	19.9 (13.7–26.2)
Format of smoking cessation counseling		
No format	1.0	10.8
Self-help	1.2 (1.0–1.3)	12.3 (10.9–13.6)
Proactive telephone counseling[e]	1.2 (1.1–1.4)	13.1 (11.4–14.8)
Group counseling	1.3 (1.1–1.6)	13.9 (11.6–16.1)
Individual counseling	1.7 (1.4–2.0)	16.8 (14.7–19.1)
Pharmacotherapy		
Placebo	1.0	13.8
First-line agents		
Bupropion SR	2.0 (1.8–2.2)	24.2 (22.2–26.4)
Nicotine gum (6–14 wk)	1.5 (1.2–1.7)	19.0 (16.5–21.9)
Nicotine inhaler	2.1 (1.5–2.9)	24.8 (19.1–31.6)
Nicotine lozenge (2 mg)	2.0 (1.4–2.8)	24.2[f]
Nicotine patch (6–14 wk)	1.9 (1.7–2.2)	23.4 (21.3–25.8)
Nicotine nasal spray	2.3 (1.7–3.0)	26.7 (21.5–32.7)
Varenicline (2 mg/day)	3.1 (2.5–3.8)	33.2 (28.9–37.8)
Second-line agents		
Clonidine	2.1 (1.2–3.7)	25.0 (15.7–37.3)
Nortriptyline	1.8 (1.3–2.6)	22.5 (16.8–29.4)
Combination therapy		
Patch (>14 weeks) + *ad lib* nicotine	3.6 (2.5–5.2)	36.5 (28.6–45.3)
Nicotine patch + bupropion SR	2.5 (1.9–3.4)	28.9 (23.5–35.1)
Nicotine patch + nortriptyline	2.3 (1.3–4.2)	27.3 (17.2–40.4)
Nicotine patch + nicotine inhaler	2.2 (1.2–3.6)	25.8 (17.4–36.5)

[a]Reprinted from reference 43, with permission.
[b]Data from reference 37.
[c]Estimated relative to referent group. CI = confidence interval.
[d]Abstinence percentages for specified treatment method.
[e]A quitline that responds to incoming calls and makes outbound follow-up calls. After an initial request by the smoker or via a fax-to-quit program, the clinician initiates telephone contact to counsel the patient.
[f]One qualifying randomized trial; 95% CI not reported.

Figure 1. Assessing readiness to quit.[38] Algorithm for treating tobacco use.

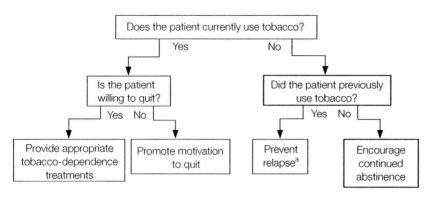

[a]Relapse-prevention interventions are not necessary for adults who have not used tobacco for many years.

who use them.[37-39] These positive results have been shown to translate into real-world effectiveness,[40] as evidenced in several meta-analytic reviews.[37,38,41,42]

Even the busiest of clinicians can serve an important role by spending approximately one minute per patient to identify tobacco users and to provide referrals to the quit line for more comprehensive counseling. When patients indicate a willingness to set a quit date in the next month, clinicians should consider a proactive approach whereby they obtain the patient's permission to contact the quit line directly on the patient's behalf as opposed to their providing a passive referral (by simply offering the patient contact information for the quit line).[38]

Pharmacotherapy for Cessation. All patients attempting to quit using tobacco should be encouraged to use effective pharmacotherapies (Table 3) for smoking cessation,[43] except when medically contraindicated or in specific populations in which there is insufficient evidence of effectiveness (e.g., pregnant women, smokeless tobacco users, light smokers, adolescents).[37] Currently, the agents with approved FDA labeling for smoking cessation include five nicotine-replacement therapy (NRT) dosage forms, sustained-release bupropion, and varenicline. Pharmacologic agents that have not received FDA approval for use in smoking cessation but have demonstrated efficacy are clonidine and nortriptyline.[37]

NRT. Formulations of NRT products currently available in the United States include nicotine gum, lozenge, transdermal patch, nasal spray, and oral inhaler (Table 3). These agents improve quit rates by reducing the symptoms of nicotine withdrawal, enabling the patient to focus on behavior modification and coping with the psychological aspects of quitting. In addition, because the onset of action with NRT is not as rapid as that of nicotine obtained through tobacco (Figure 2), patients become less accustomed to the nearly immediate, reinforcing effects of tobacco. Patients using NRT are approximately two times as likely to quit smoking than are those receiving placebo.[37]

For selected patients with cardiovascular disease,[37] NRT should be used with caution, because nicotine can increase the heart rate and blood pressure and also act as a coronary vasoconstrictor.[44] Despite these effects, randomized, controlled trials have found no significant increase in the in-

cidence of cardiovascular events or mortality among patients with cardiovascular disease receiving NRT when compared with that of patients receiving placebo.[45-47] However, because these studies specifically excluded patients with severe, underlying cardiac diseases, the clinical practice guideline[37] recommends that because of a lack of safety data in these higher-risk populations, NRT should be used with caution among patients who have experienced a myocardial infarction within the past two weeks and among those with serious arrhythmias or unstable angina.[37] A large observational study of more than 33,000 patients found that NRT use was not associated with an increased risk of myocardial infarction, stroke, or death.[48] Because the serum concentrations of nicotine achieved with the recommended dosages of NRT are generally much lower than those attained with smoking, most experts have concluded that the risks associated with NRT use in patients with cardiovascular disease are minimal relative to the risks of continued tobacco use.[44,49-52]

Other conditions for which NRT should be used with caution include active temporomandibular joint disease, pregnancy, and lactation. Patients with active temporomandibular joint disease should not use nicotine gum because doing so might exacerbate their condition. FDA classifies prescription formulations of nicotine as pregnancy category D, indicating that there is evidence of risk to the human fetus. Accordingly, none of the NRT formulations have received FDA approval for use during pregnancy. Although NRT may pose a risk to the developing fetus, it is arguably less than the risks associated with continued smoking.[53] However, because NRT has the potential to cause fetal harm and because of insufficient evidence supporting its efficacy in pregnant women, the 2008 clinical practice guideline does not recommend use during pregnancy.[37] Nicotine is secreted in breast milk[53] and, while the risk is slight, clinicians should be aware that the nursing infant is at risk for nicotine toxicity, especially if the mother concomitantly smokes and uses NRT.

Sustained-Release Bupropion. The first nonnicotine medication FDA approved for smoking cessation was sustained-release bupropion (Zyban, GlaxoSmithKline, Philadelphia). This agent, which was originally marketed as an antidepressant, is hypothesized to promote smoking cessation by inhibiting the reuptake of dopamine and norepinephrine in the central nervous system[54] and may function as a nicotinic acetylcholine-receptor antagonist.[55] The neurochemical effects are believed to modulate the dopamine reward pathway and reduce the cravings for nicotine and symptoms of withdrawal.[37] Bupropion is effective in smokers with or without a history of major depression,[56] suggesting that the mechanism of action is independent of the agent's antidepressant effects. Clinical trials involving almost 10,000 participants have confirmed the effectiveness of sustained-release bupropion as an aid to tobacco cessation; a recent meta-analysis of 31 trials concluded that the

odds of tobacco abstinence at six or more months was 1.9 (sustained-release bupropion relative to placebo, 95% CI, 1.7–2.2).[57] Patients receiving sustained-release bupropion are approximately two times more likely to quit smoking than are patients receiving placebo.[44]

Bupropion is contraindicated in patients (1) with a seizure disorder, (2) with a history of anorexia or bulimia nervosa, (3) who are using another formulation of bupropion (Wellbutrin, Wellbutrin SR, Wellbutrin XL), (4) who have used a monoamine oxidase inhibitor within the past 14 days, and (5) who are undergoing abrupt discontinuation of alcohol or sedatives (including benzodiazepines).[58] In clinical trials for smoking cessation, the frequency of seizures with bupropion was <0.1% (seven seizures among 8000 bupropion-treated patients).[57] This frequency is comparable to the report rate of seizures (0.1%) when sustained-release bupropion was used in the treatment of depression.[59] For this reason, bupropion should be used with extreme caution in patients with a history of seizures, those who have experienced cranial trauma, and those receiving medications known to lower the seizure threshold or those with underlying severe hepatic cirrhosis. In addition, caution should be exercised in patients with certain depressive or psychiatric disorders. FDA has recently reclassified bupropion as a pregnancy category C drug, meaning that either (1) animal studies have demonstrated that the drug exerts animal-teratogenic or embryocidal effects, but there are no controlled studies in women, or (2) no studies are available in either animals or women. The pregnancy category reclassification resulted after the reanalysis of preclinical animal data demonstrated an increased incidence of fetal malformations and skeletal variations in rabbits receiving dosages approximately twofold higher than the maximum recommended human dose (on a milligram per square meter basis) of bupropion. The manufacturer continues to recommend that bupropion be used during pregnancy only if clearly needed.[58]

Varenicline. A partial agonist selective for the $\alpha_4\beta_2$ nicotinic acetylcholine receptor, varenicline (Chantix, Pfizer, Inc., New York, NY) was approved in May 2006 for use as an aid to smoking cessation. The drug's efficacy in smoking cessation is believed to be the result of low-level agonist activity at the receptor site combined with the competitive inhibition of nicotine binding. The partial agonist activity induces modest receptor stimulation that attenuates the symptoms of nicotine withdrawal. In addition, by blocking the ability of nicotine to activate $\alpha_4\beta_2$ nicotinic acetylcholine receptors, varenicline inhibits the surges of dopamine release that are believed to be responsible for the reinforcement and reward associated with smoking.[60]

Data from meta-analyses suggest that the use of varenicline significantly increases long-term smoking-abstinence rates relative to placebo and sustained-release bupropion.[37,61] FDA has classified varenicline as a pregnancy category C drug. The manufacturer recommends varenicline use during pregnancy only if the potential benefit justifies the potential risk to the fetus.[62]

In February 2008, FDA issued a public health advisory to alert health care providers about reports of serious neuropsychiatric symptoms in patients attempting to quit smoking while using varenicline, including changes in behavior, depressed mood, agitation, and suicidal ideation and behavior. The warnings and precautions sections of the drug's prescribing information have been updated, and FDA recommends that (1) patients tell their health care providers about any history of psychiatric illness before starting varenicline and (2) clinicians and patients monitor for changes in mood and behavior during treatment with varenicline.[63]

Second-Line Agents. Second-line agents that have not received an FDA indication for smoking cessation include the prescription medications clonidine and nortriptyline.[37] Controlled trials suggest that these agents are effective in treating tobacco dependence (Table 2), but they have a greater incidence of adverse effects and should be reserved for patients unable to quit with medications approved for smoking cessation.[37]

Combination Therapy. Certain combinations of medications have been shown to be effective smoking-cessation treatments. In the previous guideline, combination therapy was recommended only for patients unable to quit after monotherapy with a first-line agent. Based on data from eight clinical trials, the 2008 clinical practice guideline recommends that clinicians consider using combinations of first-line agents for patients who are willing to quit.[37] Combination NRT involves the use of a long-acting formulation (e.g., nicotine patch) along with a short-acting formulation (i.e., gum, lozenge, inhaler, or nasal spray). The long-acting formulation, which delivers nicotine at relatively constant levels, is used to prevent the onset of severe withdrawal symptoms; the short-acting formulation, which delivers nicotine at a more rapid rate, is used as needed to control the withdrawal symptoms that may occur during potential relapse situations (e.g., after meals, during times of stress, when around other smokers).

Controlled trials suggest that the nicotine patch in combination with short-acting NRT formulations (i.e., gum, nasal spray, or inhaler) significantly increases quit rates relative to placebo.[37] Similar results have been observed in trials using combination therapy with sustained-release bupropion and the nicotine patch. Results from an open-label trial suggest that a more-aggressive approach consisting of triple agent NRT (e.g., inhaler, patch, and nasal spray) with or without sustained-release bupropion is safe and effective among highly dependent smokers.[64] Clinicians should be aware that while the combination of the nicotine patch and sustained-release bupropion has been approved by FDA, the concurrent use of two NRT products is not FDA-approved for tobacco cessation. Furthermore, the optimal combinations, dosages, and duration of dual NRTs are currently unknown. The safety and effectiveness of varenicline used with sustained-release bupropion or NRT have not been established. Pilot data suggest that patients receiving both varenicline and the nicotine patch are more likely to experience adverse effects (nausea, headache, vomiting, dizziness, dyspepsia, and fatigue) than are those receiving the patch alone.[62]

Smoke-Free Environments

Smoking initiation and cessation result from the interplay of numerous factors, including but not limited to environmental influences.[21] Smokers in one's environment can both promote initiation and inhibit cessation.

Data on state-specific trends in smoke-free working environments indicate that 73.4% of employees who work indoors were covered by a smoke-free workplace policy,

Table 3.

Medications with FDA-Approved Indications for Smoking Cessation [43,a]

Product Name and Availability	Precautions	Dosing	Administration and Pt Information
Nicorette gum, generic, nonprescription, 2 or 4 mg	Pregnancy[c] (Category D), breastfeeding, recent (≤2 wk) MI, serious underlying arrhythmia, serious or worsening angina pectoris, TMJ disease	≥25 cigarettes/day: 4 mg, <25 cigarettes/day: 2 mg Wk 1–6: 1 piece every 1–2 hr, wk 7–9: 1 piece every 2–4 hr, wk 10–12: 1 piece every 4–8 hr Maximum, 24 pieces/day Duration, up to 12 wk	Chew each piece slowly, park between cheek and gum when peppery or tingling sensation appears (~15–30 chews), resume chewing when taste or tingle fades, repeat chew/park steps until most of the nicotine is gone (taste or tingle does not return; generally 30 min), park in different areas of mouth, no food or beverages 15 min before or during use
Commit lozenges, generic nonprescription, 2 or 4 mg	Pregnancy[c] (Category D), breastfeeding, recent (≤2 wk) MI, serious underlying arrhythmia, serious or worsening angina pectoris	First cigarette ≤30 min after waking: 4 mg, first cigarette >30 min after waking: 2 mg Wk 1–6: 1 lozenge every 1–2 hr, wk 7–9: 1 lozenge every 2–4 hr, wk 10–12: 1 lozenge every 4–8 hr Maximum, 20 lozenges/day Duration, up to 12 wk	Allow to dissolve slowly (20-30 min), nicotine release may cause a warm, tingling sensation, do not chew or swallow, occasionally rotate to different areas of the mouth, no food or beverages 15 min before or during use
Nicoderm CQ transdermal patch, nonprescription, 24-hr release; 7,14, or 21 mg	Pregnancy[c] (Category D), breastfeeding, recent (≤2 wk) MI, serious underlying arrhythmia, serious or worsening angina pectoris	>10 cigarettes/day: 21 mg/day × 6 wk, 14 mg/day × 2 wk, 7 mg/day × 2 wk ≤10 cigarettes/day: 14 mg/day × 6 wk, 7 mg/day × 2 wk Duration: 8–10 wk	May wear patch for 16 hr if pt has sleep disturbances (remove at bedtime)
Generic patch (formerly Habitrol), prescription or nonprescription, 24-hour release; 7,14, or 21 mg	Pregnancy[c] (Category D), breastfeeding, recent (≤2 wk) MI, serious underlying arrhythmia, serious or worsening angina pectoris	>10 cigarettes/day: 21 mg/day × 4 wk, 14 mg/day × 2 wk, 7 mg/day × 2 wk ≤10 cigarettes/day: 14 mg/day x 6 wk, 7 mg/day × 2 wk Duration: 8–10 wk	May wear patch for 16 hr if pt has sleep disturbances (remove at bedtime)
Nicotrol NS, metered spray, prescription, 0.5 mg nicotine in 50 µL aqueous nicotine solution	Pregnancy[c] (Category D), breastfeeding, recent (≤2 wk) MI, serious underlying arrhythmia, serious or worsening angina pectoris, underlying chronic nasal disorders (rhinitis, nasal polyps, sinusitis), severe reactive airway disease	1–2 doses/hr (8–40 doses/day) 1 dose = 2 sprays (1 in each nostril); each spray delivers 0.5 mg of nicotine Maximum of 5 doses/hr or 40 doses/day Duration, 3–6 mo	For best results, initially use at least 8 doses/day; pts should not sniff, swallow, or inhale through nose as spray is administered

Adverse Effects	Advantages	Disadvantages	Cost/Day[b]
Mouth/jaw soreness, hiccups, dyspepsia, hypersalivation, effects associated with incorrect chewing technique (lightheadedness, nausea/vomiting, throat and mouth irritation)	Might satisfy oral cravings, may delay weight gain; pts can adjust therapy to manage withdrawal symptoms; available in a variety of flavors	Gum chewing may not be socially acceptable, might be problematic for patients with significant dental work; pts must use proper chewing technique to minimize adverse effects	2 mg: $3.28–$6.58 (9 pieces), 4 mg: $4.31–$6.58 (9 pieces)
Nausea, hiccups, cough, heartburn, headache, flatulence, insomnia	Might satisfy oral cravings, might delay weight gain, easy to use and conceal; pts can adjust therapy to manage withdrawal symptoms; available in a variety of flavors	Adverse gastrointestinal effects (nausea, hiccups, heartburn) might be bothersome; need for frequent dosing can compromise adherence	2 mg or 4 mg: $3.66–$5.26 (9 pieces)
Local skin reactions (erythema, pruritus, burning), headache, sleep disturbances (insomnia), abnormal or vivid dreams (associated with nocturnal nicotine absorption)	Provides consistent nicotine levels over 24 hr; easy to use and conceal; once-daily administration associated with fewer adherence problems	Pts cannot adjust dosage; allergic reactions to adhesive might occur, pts with dermatological conditions should not use patch	$1.90–$3.89 (1 patch)
Local skin reactions (erythema, pruritus, burning), headache, sleep disturbances (insomnia), abnormal or vivid dreams (associated with nocturnal nicotine absorption)	Provides consistent nicotine levels over 24 hr; easy to use and conceal; once-daily administration associated with fewer adherence problems	Pts cannot adjust dosage; allergic reactions to adhesive might occur, pts with dermatological conditions should not use patch	$1.90–$3.89 (1 patch)
Nasal or throat irritation (hot, peppery, or burning sensation), rhinitis, tearing, sneezing, cough, headache	Pts can adjust therapy to manage withdrawal symptoms	Nasal or throat irritation may be bothersome; dependence can result; pts must wait 5 min before driving or operating heavy machinery; pts with chronic nasal disorders or severe reactive airway disease should not use spray; need for frequent dosing can compromise adherence	$3.72 (8 doses)

Continued on next page

Table 3. *(continued)*
Medications with FDA-Approved Indications for Smoking Cessation [43,a]

Product Name and Availability	Precautions	Dosing	Administration and Pt Information
Nicotrol inhaler, prescription, 10-mg cartridge delivers 4 mg inhaled nicotine vapor	Pregnancy[c] (Category D), breastfeeding, recent (≤2 wk) MI, serious underlying arrhythmia, serious or worsening angina pectoris, bronchospastic disease	6–16 cartridges/day for up to 6 mo, individualized dosing Duration, 3–6 mo	Initially, use at least 6 cartridges/day; best effects with continuous puffing for 20 min; nicotine in cartridge depleted after 20 min of active puffing; pt should inhale into back of throat or puff in short breaths; do not inhale into lungs (like a cigarette) but "puff" as if lighting a pipe; open cartridge retains potency for 24 hr
Zyban (bupropion SR), generic and prescription, 150-mg sustained-release tablets	Pregnancy[c] (Category C), breastfeeding, concomitant therapy with medications or medical conditions known to lower the seizure threshold, severe hepatic cirrhosis *Contraindications:* Seizure disorder, concomitant bupropion (e.g., Wellbutrin) therapy, current or prior diagnosis of bulimia or anorexia nervosa, simultaneous abrupt discontinuation of alcohol or sedatives (including benzodiazepines), MAOI therapy in previous 14 days	150 mg p.o. every morning x 3 days, then increase to 150 mg p.o. twice daily; not to exceed 300 mg/day Duration: 7–12 wk, with maintenance up to 6 mo in selected patients	Treatment should be initiated while pt is still smoking; set quit date 1–2 wk after initiation of therapy; allow at least 8 hr between doses; avoid bedtime administration to minimize insomnia; dose tapering not necessary; can be used safely with NRT
Chantix (varenicline), prescription, 0.5- and 1-mg tablets	Pregnancy[c] (Category C), breastfeeding, severe renal impairment (dosage adjustment is necessary), safety and efficacy have not been established in patients with serious psychiatric illness	Days 1–3: 0.5 mg p.o. every morning, days 4–7: 0.5 mg p.o. twice daily, wk 2–12:1 mg p.o. twice daily Duration: 12 wks; an additional 12-wk course may be used in selected patients	Pts should begin therapy 1 wk before quit date; take dose after eating with full glass of water; dose tapering is not necessary; nausea and insomnia are side effects that are usually temporary

[a]Reprinted from reference 43, with permission. Copyright © 1999-2007 The Regents of the University of California, University of Southern California, and Western University of Health Sciences. All rights reserved. For complete prescribing information, please refer to the manufacturers' package inserts. FDA = Food and Drug Administration, MI = myocardial infarction, TMJ = temporomandibular joint, NRT = nicotine-replacement therapy, MAOI = monoamine oxidase inhibitor.

according to a survey of 14 states conducted in 2005.[65] Smoke-free workplaces have been shown to not only protect individuals from secondhand smoke but also to reduce the prevalence of smoking.[66] In a simulation study, smoke-free workplace policies were estimated to be approximately nine times more cost-effective per patient than are programs that provide NRT at no cost.[67]

Over the past few years, numerous cities and states have adopted clean indoor air laws in workplaces.[68] Nationally, the effects of transitioning all workplaces to smoke-free environments would yield an estimated 4.5% decrease in the overall prevalence of smoking.[66] In its first year of implementation, a nationwide smoke-free workplace policy would produce an estimated 1.3 million new quitters, 1500 fewer myocardial infarctions, 350 fewer strokes, and a direct saving of nearly $60 million in medical costs.[69] Given this substantial impact on public health, ASHP supports the implementation of smoke-free policies for the

employees and patrons of all workplaces and public venues, including but not limited to offices, restaurants, bars, bowling alleys, and casinos, and for establishments where health care services are rendered. ASHP also strongly supports smoke-free campuses for all health care institutions and facilities. In practice, clinicians should educate patients about the dangers of secondhand smoke and encourage patients who continue to smoke to do so outdoors.

The Clinician's Role

To ensure that all future clinicians have received adequate training for treating tobacco use and dependence, schools offering health-profession courses or degrees are advised to incorporate comprehensive tobacco-cessation training as part of the required curriculum for all students.[37] Licensed clinicians who have not received the formal training necessary to provide comprehensive tobacco-cessation counseling are encouraged

Adverse Effects	Advantages	Disadvantages	Cost/Day[b]
Mouth or throat irritation, unpleasant taste, cough, headache, rhinitis, dyspepsia, hiccups	Pts can adjust therapy to manage withdrawal symptoms; mimics hand-to-mouth ritual of smoking	Initial throat or mouth irritation can be bothersome; cartridges should not be stored in very warm conditions or used in very cold conditions; pts with underlying bronchospastic disease must use inhaler with caution; need for frequent dosing can compromise adherence	$5.29 (6 cartridges)
Insomnia, dry mouth, nervousness/difficulty concentrating, rash, constipation, seizures (risk is 1/1,000 [0.1%])	Easy to use; oral formulation might be associated with fewer compliance problems; can be used with NRT; might be beneficial in patients with depression	Seizure risk is increased; several contraindications and precautions can preclude use	$3.62–$7.40 (2 tablets)
Nausea, sleep disturbances (insomnia, abnormal dreams), constipation, flatulence, vomiting, neuropsychiatric symptoms (behavior changes, agitation, depressed mood, suicidal ideation or behavior)	Easy to use; oral formulation might be associated with fewer compliance problems; offers new mechanism of action for pts who have not succeeded with other agents	May induce nausea in up to one third of pts; postmarketing surveillance data indicate potential for neuropsychiatric symptoms	$4.49–$4.75 (2 tablets)

[b]Average wholesale price from Medi-Span Electronic Drug File. Indianapolis, IN; Wolters Kluwer Health, September 2008.
[c]The U.S. clinical practice guideline states that pregnant smokers should be encouraged to quit without medication based on insufficient evidence and hypothetical concerns with safety. Pregnant smokers should be offered cessation counseling interventions that exceed minimal advice to quit.[37]

to complete continuing-education programs. Furthermore, clinicians should systematically integrate the identification of tobacco users and the delivery of evidence-based tobacco-use cessation interventions into routine patient care. In the absence of time or expertise to provide comprehensive cessation counseling, clinicians should—at a minimum—ask patients about tobacco use, advise patients to quit, and refer these patients to external resources such as the toll-free quit line (1-800-QUIT-NOW) or a group program.[37] Because higher quit rates result when patients receive assistance from multiple health care providers,[37] clinicians are encouraged to work in tandem with other providers as part of a team approach to helping patients quit smoking. Table 4 provides useful online links to assist clinicians in tobacco-control initiatives.

Given that the sale of tobacco contradicts both the clinician's role in promoting health and the pharmacist's code of ethics,[70] ASHP strongly opposes the sale or distribution of tobacco products in all establishments where health care services are rendered (e.g., hospitals, clinics, retail chain and community pharmacies).[71] For more than three decades, the pharmacy profession has repeatedly voiced opposition to the sale of tobacco products in pharmacies,[72] including formal resolutions from state and national organizations. Notably, few licensed pharmacists (estimated at <2%)[73] and pharmacy students (3.5%)[74] are in favor of tobacco sales in pharmacies. Given this overwhelming lack of support, members of the profession are advised to insist that tobacco sales no longer occur in the environments where pharmaceutical care is rendered. Furthermore, in accordance with a 2003 resolution set forth by the American Association of Colleges of Pharmacy, ASHP encourages colleges and schools of pharmacy to give preference as clerkship sites to those pharmacies that choose not to sell tobacco products.[74]

Figure 2. Plasma nicotine concentrations for nicotine-containing products. Reprinted with permission from reference 43.

Conclusion

Given the extensive body of data implicating tobacco as the primary known preventable cause of death in the United States, ASHP strongly supports evidence-based tobacco-control initiatives that aim to reduce the prevalence of tobacco use. These efforts should address a continuum of services, activities, and policies ranging from the integration of tobacco-cessation counseling as a routine component of patient care to the adoption of clean indoor air laws. ASHP believes that the active involvement of health care providers is crucial to effective tobacco control at the population level and that the pharmacy profession—as a primary and accessible point of contact between the health care system and the public (including the medically underserved)—has a unique opportunity to serve as a cornerstone for the nation's tobacco-control efforts.

References

1. The health consequences of smoking: cancer. A report of the Surgeon General. http://profiles.nlm.nih.gov/NN/B/C/D/W/_/nnbcdw.pdf (accessed 2008 Jul 16).
2. Centers for Disease Control and Prevention. Annual smoking-attributable mortality, years of potential life lost, and productivity losses—United States, 1997-2001. *MMWR.* 2005; 54:625–8.
3. U.S. Department of Health and Human Services. 2006 Surgeon General's report: the health consequences of involuntary exposure to tobacco smoke. www.cdc.gov/tobacco/data_statistics/sgr/sgr_2006/index.htm (accessed 2008 Jul 16).
4. Doll R, Peto R, Boreham J et al. Mortality in relation to smoking: 50 years' observations on male British doctors. *BMJ.* 2004; 328:1519.
5. Centers for Disease Control and Prevention. Cigarette smoking among adults—United States, 2000. *MMWR.* 2002; 51:642–5.
6. Centers for Disease Control and Prevention. Cigarette smoking among adults—United States, 2006. *MMWR.* 2007; 56:1157–61.
7. Lasser K, Boyd JW, Woolhandler S et al. Smoking and mental illness: a population-based prevalence study. *JAMA.* 2000; 284:2606–10.
8. Centers for Disease Control and Prevention. State-specific prevalence of cigarette smoking among adults and quitting among persons aged 18-35 years—United States, 2006. *MMWR.* 2007; 56:993–6.
9. U.S. Department of Health and Human Services. 1994 Surgeon General's report—preventing tobacco use among young people. www.cdc.gov/tobacco/data_statistics/sgr/sgr_1994/index.htm (accessed 2008 Aug 13).
10. U.S. Department of Health and Human Services. Healthy People 2010. Vol. I and II. www.healthypeople.gov/publications/ (accessed 2008 Jul 16).
11. Johnston LD, O'Malley PM, Bachman JG et al. Teen smoking resumes decline. www.monitoringthefuture.org/data/07data.html#2007data-cigs (accessed 2008 May 21).
12. U.S. Department of Agriculture. Tobacco outlook. Report TBS-263. http://usda.mannlib.cornell.edu/usda/ers/TBS//2000s/2007/TBS-10-24-2007.pdf (accessed 2008 Aug 13).
13. Substance Abuse and Mental Health Services Administration Offices of Applied Studies (2008). Results from the 2007 National Survey on Drug Use and Health: National findings (DHHS publication no. SMA 08-4343). Rockville, MD.
14. Henningfield JE, Fant RV, Radzius A et al. Nicotine concentration, smoke pH and whole tobacco aqueous

Table 4.
Tobacco-Cessation Resources

Resource	Contact Information
Governmental agencies	
Centers for Disease Control and Prevention	www.cdc.gov
Environmental Protection Agency	www.epa.gov
Federal Trade Commission	www.ftc.gov
Office of the Surgeon General	www.surgeongeneral.gov
National Institutes of Health	www.nih.gov
National Cancer Institute	www.cancer.gov
National Heart, Lung, and Blood Institute	www.nhlbi.nih.gov
National Institute on Drug Abuse	www.nida.nih.gov
Organizations	
American Cancer Society	www.cancer.org
American Heart Association	www.americanheart.org
American Legacy Foundation	www.americanlegacy.org
American Lung Association	www.lungusa.org
American Society of Health-System Pharmacists	www.ashp.org/s_ashp/tobacco
Campaign for Tobacco-Free Kids	www.tobaccofreekids.org
Global Network of Pharmacists Against Tobacco	www.fip.org/pharmacistsagainsttobacco
North American Quitline Consortium	www.naquitline.org
Society for Research on Nicotine & Tobacco	www.srnt.org
University of California Smoking Cessation Leadership Center	smokingcessationleadership.ucsf.edu
University of California Tobacco-Related Disease Research Program	www.trdrp.org
World Health Organization	www.who.int
Documents	
Clinical Practice Guideline for Treating Tobacco Use and Dependence	www.surgeongeneral.gov/tobacco
Legacy Tobacco Industry Documents Archive	www.legacy.library.ucsf.edu
Pharmacologic aids for cessation—online support	
Committed Quitters Program	
Nicorette gum	www.nicorette.com
Nicoderm patch	www.nicodermcq.com
Commit lozenge	www.commitlozenge.com
GETQUIT Support Plan	
Chantix	www.chantix.com
Helping Hand Program	
Nicotrol nasal spray and inhaler	www.nicotrol.com
Smoke-Free Program	
Generic patch (formerly Habitrol)	www.habitrol.com
Nonpharmaceutical cessation support and programs	
QuitKey (handheld computer for scheduled gradual reduction of smoking)	www.quitkey.com
QuitNet (comprehensive online tobacco-cessation support program)	www.quitnet.com
Rx for Change: Clinician-Assisted Tobacco Cessation (evidence-based tobacco-cessation training materials for educating health professional students and licensed clinicians)	rxforchange.ucsf.edu
Tobacco-Free Nurses (national program focused on helping nurses and student nurses to stop smoking)	www.tobaccofreenurses.org
Toll-free quit lines (telephone counseling for cessation, available at no cost to all callers)	1-800-QUIT-NOW

pH of some cigar brands and types popular in the United States. *Nicotine Tob Res.* 1999; 1:163–8.

15. Connolly GN, Alpert HR, Wayne GF et al. Trends in nicotine yield in smoke and its relationship with design characteristics among popular US cigarette brands, 1997-2005. *Tob Control.* 2007; 16:e5.

16. Ebbert JO, Carr AB, Dale LC. Smokeless tobacco: an emerging addiction. *Med Clin North Am.* 2004; 88:1593–605.

17. Centers for Disease Control and Prevention. Annual smoking-attributable mortality, years of potential life lost, and economic costs—United States, 1995–1999. *MMWR.* 2002; 51:300–3.

18. Best practices for comprehensive tobacco control programs—2007. Atlanta: Centers for Disease Control and Prevention; 2007.

19. Task Force on Community Preventive Services. The guide to community preventive services: tobacco use prevention and control. *Am J Prev Med.* 2001; 20(suppl 2):1–88.

20. U.S. Department of Health and Human Services. The health consequences of smoking: nicotine addiction: a report of the Surgeon General. http://profiles.nlm.nih.gov/NN/B/B/Z/D/_/nnbbzd.pdf (accessed 2008 Jul 16).

21. Benowitz NL. Clinical pharmacology of nicotine: implications for understanding, preventing and treating tobacco addiction. *Clin Pharm Ther.* 2008; 83:531–41.

22. Hughes JR, Gust SW, Skoog K et al. Symptoms of tobacco withdrawal: a replication and extension. *Arch Gen Psychiatry.* 1991; 48:52–9.

23. Hughes JR. Effects of abstinence from tobacco: valid symptoms and time course. *Nicotine Tob Res.* 2007; 9:315–327.

24. American Psychiatric Association. Diagnostic and statistical manual of mental disorders, 4th edition. Washington, DC: American Psychiatric Publishing; 1994.

25. Benowitz NL. Cigarette smoking and nicotine addiction. *Med Clin North Am.* 1992; 76:415–37.

26. Hatsukami DK, Gust SW, Keenan RM. Physiologic and subjective changes from smokeless tobacco withdrawal. *Clin Pharmacol Ther.* 1987; 41:103–7.

27. Centers for Disease Control and Prevention. U.S. 2004 Surgeon General's report—the health consequences of smoking. www.cdc.gov/tobacco/data_statistics/sgr/sgr_2004/index.htm (accessed 2008 Jul 16).

28. Henley SJ, Thun MJ, Connell C et al. Two large prospective studies of mortality among men who use snuff or chewing tobacco (United States). *Cancer Causes Control.* 2005; 16:347–58.

29. Hergens MP, Ahlbom A, Andersson T et al. Swedish moist snuff and myocardial infarction among men. *Epidemiology.* 2005; 16:12–16.

30. Gupta R, Gurm H, Bartholomew JR. Smokeless tobacco and cardiovascular risk. *Arch Intern Med.* 2004; 164:1845–9.

31. Henley SJ, Connell CJ, Richter P et al. Tobacco-related disease mortality among men who switched from cigarettes to spit tobacco. *Tob Control.* 2007; 16:22–8.

32. California Environmental Protection Agency. Proposed identification of environmental tobacco smoke as a toxic air contaminant: executive summary. www.arb.ca.gov/regact/ets2006/ets2006.htm (accessed 2008 Oct 1).

33. Kroon LA. Drug interactions with smoking. *Am J Health-Syst Pharm.* 2007; 64:1917–21.

34. Zevin S, Benowitz NL. Drug interactions with tobacco smoking. *Clin Pharmacokinet.* 1999; 36:425–38.

35. U.S. Department of Health and Human Services. The benefits of smoking cessation. A report of the surgeon general (DHHS publication no. CDC 90-8416). U.S. Department of Health and Human Services, Public Health Service, Centers for Disease Control and Prevention and Health Promotion, Office on Smoking and Health. 1990.

36. Hazelden Foundation. Survey on current and former smokers—1998. www.hazelden.org/web/public/smokers1998.page (accessed 2008 Aug 13.).

37. Fiore MC, Jaen CR, Baker TB et al. Treating tobacco use and dependence—2008 update. Clinical practice guideline. www.surgeongeneral.gov/tobacco/treating_tobacco_use08.pdf (accessed 2008 Jul 16).

38. Stead L, Perera R, Lancaster T. Telephone counselling for smoking cessation. *Cochrane Database Syst Rev.* 2006; 3:CD002850.

39. Ossip-Klein DJ, McIntosh S. Quitlines in North America: evidence base and applications. *Am J Med Sci.* 2003; 326:201–5.

40. Zhu SH, Anderson CM, Tedeschi GJ et al. Evidence of real-world effectiveness of a telephone quitline for smokers. *N Engl J Med.* 2002; 347:1087–93.

41. Lichtenstein E, Glasgow RE, Lando HA et al. Telephone counseling for smoking cessation: rationales and meta-analytic review of evidence. *Health Educ Res.* 1996; 11:243–57.

42. Hopkins DP, Briss PA, Ricard CJ et al. Reviews of evidence regarding interventions to reduce tobacco use and exposure to environmental tobacco smoke. *Am J Prev Med.* 2001; 20(2, suppl):16–66.

43. Rx for Change: clinician-assisted tobacco cessation. http://rxforchange.ucsf.edu (accessed 2008 Oct 1).

44. Benowitz NL. Cigarette smoking and cardiovascular disease: pathophysiology and implications for treatment. *Prog Cardiovasc Dis.* 2003; 46:91–111.

45. Working Group for the Study of Transdermal Nicotine in Patients with Coronary Artery Disease. Nicotine replacement therapy for patients with coronary artery disease. *Arch Intern Med.* 1994; 154:989–95.

46. Joseph AM, Norman SM, Ferry LH et al. The safety of transdermal nicotine as an aid to smoking cessation in patients with cardiac disease. *N Engl J Med.* 1996; 335:1792–8.

47. Tzivoni D, Keren A, Meyler S et al. Cardiovascular safety of transdermal nicotine patches in patients with coronary artery disease who try to quit smoking. *Cardiovasc Drugs Ther.* 1998; 12:239–44.

48. Hubbard R, Lewis S, Smith C et al. Use of nicotine replacement therapy and the risk of acute myocardial infarction, stroke, and death. *Tob Control.* 2005; 14:416–21.

49. McRobbie H, Hajek P. Nicotine replacement therapy in patients with cardiovascular disease: guidelines for health professionals. *Addiction.* 2001; 96:1547–51.

50. Joseph AM, Fu SS. Safety issues in pharmacotherapy for smoking in patients with cardiovascular disease. *Prog Cardiovasc Dis.* 2003; 45:429–41.

51. Benowitz NL, Gourlay SG. Cardiovascular toxicity of nicotine: implications for nicotine replacement therapy. *J Am Coll Cardiol.* 1997; 29:1422–31.

52. Meine TJ, Patel MR, Washam JB et al. Safety and effectiveness of transdermal nicotine patch in smokers admitted with acute coronary syndromes. *Am J Cardiol.* 2005; 95:976–8.

53. Benowitz NL, Dempsey DA. Pharmacotherapy for smoking cessation during pregnancy. *Nicotine Tob Res.* 2004;6(Suppl 2):S189–202.

54. Ascher JA, Cole JO, Colin J et al. Bupropion: a review of its mechanism of antidepressant activity. *J Clin Psychiatry.* 1995; 56:395–401.

55. Slemmer JE, Martin BR, Damaj MI. Bupropion is a nicotinic antagonist. *J Pharmacol Exp Ther.* Oct 2000; 295:321–7.

56. Hayford KE, Patten CA, Rummans TA et al. Efficacy of bupropion for smoking cessation in smokers with a former history of major depression or alcoholism. *Br J Psychiatry.* 1999; 174:173–8.

57. Hughes J, Stead L, Lancaster T. Antidepressants for smoking cessation. *Cochrane Database Syst Rev.* 2007(1):CD000031.

58. Zyban (bupropion hydrochloride) package insert. Research Triangle Park, NC: GlaxoSmithKline, Inc.; 2007 Aug.

59. Dunner DL, Zisook S, Billow AA et al. A prospective safety surveillance study for bupropion sustained-release in the treatment of depression. *J Clin Psychiatry.* 1998; 59:366–73.

60. Foulds J. The neurobiological basis for partial agonist treatment of nicotine dependence: varenicline. *Int J Clin Pract.* May 2006; 60:571–6.

61. Cahill K, Stead LF, Lancaster T. Nicotine receptor partial agonists for smoking cessation. *Cochrane Database Syst Rev.* 2008(3):CD006103.

62. Chantix (varenicline) package insert. New York: Pfizer, Inc.; 2008 May.

63. Food and Drug Administration. Varenicline information. www.fda.gov/cder/drug/infopage/varenicline/default.htm (accessed 2008 May 22).

64. Bars MP, Banauch GI, Appel D et al. Tobacco Free With FDNY: the New York City Fire Department World Trade Center Tobacco Cessation Study. *Chest.* 2006; 129:979–87.

65. State-specific prevalence of current cigarette smoking among adults and second hand smoke rules and policies in homes and workplaces, United States, 2005. *MMWR.* 2006; 55:1148–51.

66. Fichtenberg CM, Glantz SA. Effect of smoke-free workplaces on smoking behaviour: systematic review. *BMJ.* 2002; 325:188.

67. Ong MK, Glantz SA. Free nicotine replacement therapy programs vs implementing smoke-free workplaces: a cost-effectiveness comparison. *Am J Public Health.* 2005; 95:969–75.

68. American Nonsmokers' Rights Foundation. States, commonwealths, and municipalities with 100% smokefree laws in workplaces, restaurants or bars. www.no-smoke.org/pdf/100ordlist.pdf (accessed 2008 Aug 13).

69. Ong MK, Glantz SA. Cardiovascular health and economic effects of smoke-free workplaces. *Am J Med.* 2004; 117:32–8.

70. American Pharmacists Association. Code of ethics for pharmacists. http://www.pharmacist.com/AM/Template.cfm?Section=Code_of_Ethics_for_Pharmacists&Template=/CM/HTMLDisplay.cfm&ContentID=5420 (accessed 2008 Aug 13).

71. American Society of Health-System Pharmacists. ASHP policy position 0713: tobacco and tobacco products. http://www.ashp.org/s_ashp/docs/files/BP07/HR_Positions.pdf (accessed 2008 Aug 13).

72. Davis RM. Tobacco sales in pharmacies: mixing good drugs and bad drugs. *Tob Control.* 1992; 1:84–96.

73. Hudmon KS, Prokhorov AV, Corelli RL. Tobacco cessation counseling: pharmacists' opinions and practices. *Patient Educ Couns.* 2006; 61:152–60.

74. Hudmon KS, Corelli RL, Fenlon CM et al. Pharmacy student perceptions of tobacco sales in pharmacies and suggested methods for promoting tobacco-free experiential sites. *Am J Pharm Educ.* 2006; 70:75.

Appendix A—The 5 A's of Tobacco Cessation Counseling[37]

Step	Action	Strategies for Implementation
Ask—Systematically identify all tobacco users at every visit	Implement a system that ensures that, for every patient at every clinic visit, tobacco use status is queried and documented.[a]	Expand the vital signs to include tobacco use, or use an alternative universal identification system.[b] VITAL SIGNS Blood Pressure: _____ Pulse: ___ Weight: _____ Temperature: _____ Respiratory Rate: _____ Tobacco Use (circle one): Current Former Never
Advise—Strongly urge all tobacco users to quit	In a clear, strong, and personalized manner, urge every tobacco user to quit.	Advice should be: • Clear—"It is important that you quit smoking (or using chewing tobacco) now, and I can help you." "Cutting down while you are ill is not enough." "Occasional or light smoking is still dangerous." • Strong—"As your clinician, I need you to know that quitting smoking is the most important thing you can do to protect your health now and in the future. The clinic staff and I will help you." • Personalized—Tie tobacco use to current symptoms and health concerns, and/or its social and economic costs, and/or the impact of tobacco use on children and others in the household. "Continuing to smoke makes your asthma worse, and quitting may dramatically improve your health." "Quitting smoking may reduce the number of ear infections your child has."

Continued on next page

Appendix A—The 5 A's of Tobacco Cessation Counseling[37] *(continued)*

Step	Action	Strategies for Implementation
Assess—Determine willingness to make a quit attempt	Assess every tobacco user's willingness to make a quit attempt at the time.	Assess patient's willingness to quit: "Are you willing to give quitting a try?" • If the patient is willing to make a quit attempt at the time, provide assistance. 　—If the patient will participate in an intensive treatment, deliver such a treatment or link/refer to an intensive intervention. 　—If the patient is a member of a special population (e.g., adolescent, pregnant smoker, racial/ethnic minority), consider providing additional information. • If the patient clearly states that he or she is unwilling to make a quit attempt at the time, provide an intervention shown to increase future quit attempts.
Assist—Aid the patient in quitting (provide counseling and medication)	Help the patient with a quit plan.	STAR: A patient's preparations for quitting: • **S**et a quit date. Ideally, the quit date should be within 2 weeks. • **T**ell family, friends, and coworkers about quitting, and request understanding and support. • **A**nticipate challenges to the upcoming quit attempt, particularly during the critical first few weeks. These include nicotine withdrawal symptoms. • **R**emove tobacco products from your environment. Prior to quitting, avoid smoking in places where you spend a lot of time (e.g., work, home, car). Make your home smoke-free.
	Recommend the use of approved medication, except when contraindicated or with specific populations for which there is insufficient evidence of effectiveness.	Recommend the use of medications found to be effective. Explain how these medications increase quitting success and reduce withdrawal symptoms. The first-line medications include: bupropion SR, nicotine gum, nicotine inhaler, nicotine lozenge, nicotine nasal spray, nicotine patch, and varenicline; second-line medications include: clonidine and nortriptyline. There is insufficient evidence to recommend medications for certain populations (e.g., pregnant women, smokeless tobacco users, light smokers, adolescents).
	Provide practical counseling (problem solving/skills training).	• Abstinence: Striving for total abstinence is essential. Not even a single puff after the quit date. • Past quit experience: Identify what helped and what hurt in previous quit attempts. Build on past success. • Anticipate triggers or challenges in the upcoming attempt. Discuss challenges/triggers and how the patient will successfully overcome them (e.g., avoid triggers, alter routines). • Alcohol: Because alcohol is associated with relapse, the patient should consider limiting/abstaining from alcohol while quitting. (Note that reducing alcohol intake could precipitate withdrawal in alcohol-dependent persons.) • Other smokers in the household: Quitting is more difficult when there is another smoker in the household. Patients should encourage housemates to quit with them or to not smoke in their presence.
	Provide intratreatment social support.	Provide a supportive clinical environment while encouraging the patient in his or her quit attempt. "My office staff and I are available to assist you." "I'm recommending treatment that can provide ongoing support."
	Provide supplementary materials, including information on quitlines.	• Sources: Federal agencies, nonprofit agencies, national quitline network (1-800-QUIT-NOW), or local/state/tribal health departments/quitlines. • Type: Culturally/racially/educationally/age-appropriate for the patient. • Location: Readily available at every clinician's workstation.
Arrange—Ensure follow-up contact	Arrange for follow-up contacts, either in person or via telephone.	• Timing: Follow-up contact should begin soon after the quit date, preferably during the first week. A second follow-up contact is recommended within the first month. Schedule further follow-up contacts as indicated. • Actions during followup contact: For all patients, identify problems already encountered and anticipate challenges in the immediate future. Assess medication use and problems. Remind patients of quitline support (1-800-QUIT-NOW). Address tobacco use at next clinical visit (treat tobacco use as a chronic disease). • For patients who are abstinent, congratulate them on their success. If tobacco use has occurred, review circumstances and elicit recommitment to total abstinence. Consider use of or link to more intensive treatment.

[a]Repeated assessment is not necessary in the case of the adult who has never used tobacco or has not used tobacco for many years and for whom this information is clearly documented in the medical record.
[b]Alternatives to expanding the vital signs include using tobacco use status stickers on all patient charts or indicating tobacco use status via electronic medical records or computerized reminder systems.

Appendix B—Enhancing Motivation to Quit: The 5 R's of Tobacco-Cessation Counseling[37]

Relevance

Encourage the patient to indicate why quitting is personally relevant, being as specific as possible. Motivational information has the greatest impact if it is relevant to a patient's disease status or risk, family or social situation (e.g., having children in the home), health concerns, age, gender, and other important patient characteristics (e.g., prior quitting experience, personal barriers to cessation).

Risks

The clinician should ask the patient to identify potential negative consequences of tobacco use. The clinician may suggest and highlight those that seem most relevant to the patient. The clinician should emphasize that smoking low-tar/low-nicotine cigarettes or use of other forms of tobacco (e.g., smokeless tobacco, cigars, and pipes) will not eliminate these risks. Examples of risks are:

- Acute risks: Shortness of breath, exacerbation of asthma, increased risk of respiratory infections, harm to pregnancy, impotence, infertility.
- Long-term risks: Heart attacks and strokes, lung and other cancers (e.g., larynx, oral cavity, pharynx, esophagus, pancreas, stomach, kidney, bladder, cervix, and acute myelocytic leukemia), chronic obstructive pulmonary diseases (chronic bronchitis and emphysema), osteoporosis, long-term disability, and need for extended care.
- Environmental risks: Increased risk of lung cancer and heart disease in spouses; increased risk for low birthweight, sudden infant death syndrome (SIDS), asthma, middle ear disease, and respiratory infections in children of smokers.

Rewards

The clinician should ask the patient to identify potential benefits of stopping tobacco use. The clinician may suggest and highlight those that seem most relevant to the patient. Examples of rewards include:

- Improved health
- Food will taste better
- Improved sense of smell
- Saving money
- Feeling better about oneself
- Home, car, clothing, breath will smell better
- Setting a good example for children and decreasing the likelihood that they will smoke
- Having healthier babies and children

- Feeling better physically
- Performing better in physical activities
- Improved appearance, including reduced wrinkling/aging of skin and whiter teeth

Roadblocks

The clinician should ask the patient to identify barriers or impediments to quitting and provide treatment (problem solving counseling, medication) that could address barriers. Typical barriers might include:

- Withdrawal symptoms
- Fear of failure
- Weight gain
- Lack of support
- Depression
- Enjoyment of tobacco
- Being around other tobacco users
- Limited knowledge of effective treatment options

Repetition

The motivational intervention should be repeated every time an unmotivated patient visits the clinic setting. Tobacco users who have failed in previous quit attempts should be told that most people make repeated quit attempts before they are successful.

Developed by the ASHP Council on Therapeutics and approved by the ASHP Board of Directors on June 30, 2008.

Karen Suchanek Hudmon, Dr.P.H., M.S., and Robin L. Corelli, Pharm.D., are gratefully acknowledged for authoring this therapeutic position statement. Dr. Suchanek Hudmon is Associate Professor, Department of Pharmacy Practice, Purdue University School of Pharmacy and Pharmaceutical Sciencs, West Lafayette, IN. Dr. Corelli is Professor of Clinical Pharmacy, Department of Clinical Pharmacy, University of California San Francisco, San Francisco.

The following individuals are acknowledged for reviewing draft versions of this statement: John R. Hughes, M.D., Connie C. Revell, M.A., Mary H. Zimmerman, BCPS, CACP, Thomas P. Houston, M.D., FAAFP, FACPM, Candice Garwood, Pharm.D., BCPS, Karen Gunning, Pharm.D., BCPS, Carol Southard, R.N., M.S.N., Frank Vitale, M.A., Alan J. Zillich, Pharm.D., Laura B. Hanson, Pharm.D., Daniel A. Hussar, Ph.D., and the American Nurses Association.

The bibliographic citation for this document is as follows: American Society of Health-System Pharmacists. ASHP therapeutic position statement on the cessation of tobacco use. *Am J Health-Syst Pharm.* 2008; 65:2055–72.

ASHP Therapeutic Position Statement on the Institutional Use of 0.9% Sodium Chloride Injection to Maintain Patency of Peripheral Indwelling Intermittent Infusion Devices

Statement of Position

0.9% Sodium chloride injection is a safe and effective indwelling solution for maintaining catheter patency of peripheral indwelling intermittent infusion devices (PIIIDs) in adults and children age one year or older. ASHP supports the use of 0.9% sodium chloride injection in preference to heparin-containing flush solutions (heparin flush) in the institutional setting, on the basis of clinical evidence indicating that 0.9% sodium chloride injection (1) is as effective as heparin flush in maintaining the patency of PIIIDs when blood is not aspirated into the device, (2) is safer to use than heparin flush because of a lower potential for adverse effects, (3) avoids drug incompatibilities associated with heparin flush, and (4) is a cost-effective alternative to heparin flush. Because of limited and conflicting available scientific evidence to date, this recommendation is not applicable to children under the age of one year or patients in the home or other outpatient settings. This document is not applicable to catheters used for central venous or arterial access (including peripherally inserted central catheters and midline catheters) and the maintenance of patency in indwelling venipuncture devices used to obtain blood samples. Further research on PIIID patency in the aforementioned patient populations and settings is warranted.

Background

PIIIDs, often referred to as "saline locks" and frequently and inappropriately called "heparin locks," are used to provide convenient i.v. access in patients who require intermittent i.v. administration of medications without a continuous infusion of i.v. fluids. The advantages of PIIIDs include patient mobility and comfort and reduced fluid load.[1-4] PIIIDs most commonly consist of an intravenously inserted catheter attached to a short external cannula with a resealable injection port that is designed to facilitate multiple needle entries; thus, these devices eliminate the unnecessary trauma of multiple venipunctures.[4] A problem frequently encountered with PIIIDs is the loss of patency because of clot formation within the catheter. To prevent clot formation, catheters are commonly flushed after each administration of i.v. medication and every 8–12 hours when the device is not in use.[5] Because of heparin's anticoagulant effects, diluted solutions of heparin in 0.9% sodium chloride injection (e.g., 10 or 100 units/mL) have traditionally been used to periodically flush and fill these devices and prevent the formation of clots. Diluted heparin solutions are used to maintain patency while avoiding the systemic effects associated with therapeutic doses of heparin.[6]

However, due to the aforementioned concerns regarding heparin administration and the potential for medication dose error, many clinicians preferentially began using sodium chloride for flushes even before evidence was available that supported the use of sodium chloride instead of heparin.

Efficacy

Studies have indicated that 0.9% sodium chloride injection alone is as effective as heparin-containing solutions in maintaining PIIID patency.[7-16] In several randomized, double-blind studies in which PIIIDs composed principally of fluoroethylene propylene (Teflon) were used, 0.9% sodium chloride injection for flushing was associated with patency rates similar to those achieved with flush solutions containing heparin sodium 10 or 100 units/mL.[10-12] The frequency of phlebitis associated with the use of these solutions was also similar.[7,8,17-19] The type of solution used to maintain PIIID patency may not be as important as the positive pressure maintained in the i.v. line by the capped (sealed) injection device, which appears to prevent blood reflux and clot formation in the devices.[8,19] Several studies provide a scientific basis for using heparin flush,[6,20,21] but most published research supports 0.9% sodium chloride injection as an effective alternative to heparin flush in maintaining the patency of PIIIDs. However, 0.9% sodium chloride or heparin flush may not be the appropriate flush solution when flushing drugs that may not be compatible with 0.9% sodium chloride or heparin. Specific examples of such drugs include liposomal amphotericin B, doxorubicin, and i.v. immune globulin.[22] These drugs may need to be "preflushed" with another compatible solution such as 5% dextrose injection before and after administering the incompatible drug. In addition, the size of the i.v. catheter in pediatric patients appears to be a contributing factor in determining success with 0.9% sodium chloride for maintaining the patency of PIIIDs. Evidence supports the use of 0.9% sodium chloride flushes over heparin in pediatric patients,[23-27] and 0.9% sodium chloride injection is the preferred solution mentioned in the available nursing guidelines on infusion standards.[28]

One survey found that in neonates, it was common practice to flush catheter devices with heparin 1–2 units/mL,[29] and the literature supports the use of heparin 0.5 unit/mL added to continuous infusions through peripheral lines.[30] Concentrations of heparinized 0.9% sodium chloride injection 1–10 units/mL for flushing have been studied in neonatal patients, with no significant difference in catheter life or patency between 0.9% sodium chloride injection and heparinized 0.9% sodium chloride injection.[31-33] A limitation of these studies is small sample size, indicating low statistical power. Despite the lack of evidence-based literature supporting the superiority of heparin over 0.9% sodium chloride injection or vice versa for neonatal peripheral i.v. flushes, current guidelines published by the National Association of Neonatal Nurses state that heparinized 0.9% sodium chlo-

ride 0.5 unit/mL should be used to flush peripheral i.v. catheters using 0.2–0.5 mL every three to four hours.[34] If using 0.9% sodium chloride injection in pediatric patients, avoid bacteriostatic 0.9% sodium chloride, especially in neonates.

One trial of pregnant women demonstrated significantly increased efficacy and decreased complication rates with heparin-infused catheters compared with those flushed with 0.9% sodium chloride.[35] A subsequent study of pregnant women found no significant differences in the number of patent catheters or in complications with catheters flushed with either heparin or 0.9% sodium chloride.[36] However, the authors from both studies noted that their sample sizes were small and not powered sufficiently to detect a significant difference in patency or complications, possibly affecting the true clinical significance of their results. While published data from pregnant patients are conflicting, common practice is to use 0.9% sodium chloride flushes for peripheral i.v. catheters in this patient population.

Adverse Effects of Heparin Flush

Heparin, even when used in small doses, may elicit adverse reactions in some patients. The potential for bleeding complications increases when patients receive multiple unmonitored heparin flushes.[37] Repeated injections of heparin, even in small doses, can alter activated partial thromboplastin time.[38] Allergic reactions are an inherent risk of using heparin. Although rare, heparin-flush-associated thrombocytopenia and hemorrhage have been reported.[37,39-41] The risks of these adverse effects may be avoided by using 0.9% sodium chloride injection instead of heparin flush. Heparin is incompatible with many anthracyclines, including daunorubicin and doxorubicin, as well as benzodiazepines such as diazepam and midazolam.[22]

Cost Implications

Enhanced quality of patient care should be the primary reason for deciding to use 0.9% sodium chloride injection for flushing. Secondarily, the choice of 0.9% sodium chloride injection may avoid substantial costs associated with drugs, related supplies, and staff time.[9]

Summary

Because current therapeutic evidence supports the efficacy of 0.9% sodium chloride injection in maintaining PIIID patency and due to the inherent risks associated with heparin, ASHP believes that the use of 0.9% sodium chloride injection is appropriate for maintaining the patency of PIIIDs in adults and children age one year or older in institutional settings. Because of limited and conflicting scientific evidence available to date, this recommendation is not applicable to neonates, patients in the home or other outpatient settings, catheters used for central venous or arterial access (including peripherally inserted central catheters and midline catheters), which was beyond the scope of this therapeutic position statement, and the maintenance of patency in indwelling venipuncture devices used to obtain blood samples.

References

1. Millam DA. Intermittent devices. *NITA.* 1981; 4:142–5.
2. Larkin M. Heparin locks. *NITA.* 1979; 2:18–9.
3. Thomas RB, Salter FJ. Heparin locks: their advantages and disadvantages. *Hosp Formul.* 1975; 10:536–8.
4. Deeb EN, Di Mattia PE. How much heparin in the lock? *Am J IV Ther.* 1976; 3:22–6.
5. Tuten SH, Gueldner SH. Efficacy of sodium chloride versus dilute heparin for maintenance of peripheral intermittent intravenous devices. *Appl Nurs Res.* 1991; 2:63–71.
6. Hanson RL, Grant AM, Majors KR. Heparin-lock maintenance with ten units of sodium heparin in one milliliter of normal saline solution. *Surg Gynecol Obstet.* 1976; 142:373–6.
7. Barrett PJ, Lester RL. Heparin versus saline flushing solutions in a small community hospital. *Hosp Pharm.* 1990; 25:115–8.
8. Dunn DL, Lenihan SF. The case for the saline flush. *Am J Nurs.* 1987; 87:798–9.
9. Fry B. Intermittent heparin flushing protocols. A standardization issue. *J Intraven Nurs.* 1992; 15:160–3.
10. Epperson EL. Efficacy of 0.9% sodium chloride injection with and without heparin for maintaining indwelling intermittent injection sites. *Clin Pharm.* 1984; 3:626–9.
11. Garrelts JC, LaRocca J, Ast D, et al. Comparison of heparin and 0.9% sodium chloride injection in the maintenance of indwelling intermittent i.v. devices. *Clin Pharm.* 1989; 8:34–9.
12. Hamilton RA, Plis JM, Clay C, et al. Heparin sodium versus 0.9% sodium chloride injection for maintaining patency of in-dwelling intermittent infusion devices. *Clin Pharm.* 1988; 7:439–43.
13. Shearer J. Normal saline versus dilute heparin flush: a study of peripheral intermittent i.v. devices. *NITA.* 1987; 10:425–7.
14. Miracle V, Fangman B, Kayrouz P, et al. Normal saline vs. heparin lock flush solution: one institution's findings. *Ky Nurse.* 1989; 37(Jul–Aug):1, 6–7.
15. Ashton J, Gibson V, Summers S. Effects of heparin versus saline solution on intermittent infusion device irrigation. *Heart Lung.* 1990; 19:608–12.
16. Hook ML, Ose P. Heparin vs. normal saline. *J Intraven Nurs.* 1990; 13:150–1. Letter.
17. Garrelts JC. White clot syndrome and thrombocytopenia: reasons to abandon heparin i.v. lock flush solution. *Clin Pharm.* 1992; 11:797–9.
18. Weber DR. Is heparin really necessary in the lock and, if so, how much? *DICP.* 1991; 25:399–407.
19. Goode CJ, Titler M, Rakel B, et al. A meta-analysis of effects of heparin flush and saline flush: quality and cost implications. *Nurs 2Res.* 1991; 40:324–30.
20. Cyganski JM, Donahue JM, Heaton JS. The case for the heparin flush. *Am J Nurs.* 1987; 87:796–7.
21. Holford NH, Vozeh S, Coates P, et al. More on heparin lock. *N Engl J Med.* 1977; 296:1300–1. Letter.
22. Trissel LA. Handbook on injectable drugs. 16th ed. Bethesda, MD: American Society of Health-System Pharmacists; 2011.

23. Mok E, Kwong TK, Chan MF. A randomized controlled trial for maintaining peripheral intravenous lock in children. *Int J Nurs Pract.* 2007; 13:33–45.

24. Hanrahan KS, Kleiber C, Fagan CL. Evaluation of saline for iv locks in children. *Pediatr Nurs.* 1994; 20:549–52.

25. Kleiber C, Hanrahan K, Fagan CL, et al. Heparin vs saline for peripheral i.v. locks in children. *Pediatr Nurs.* 1993; 19:405–9.

26. Danek G, Noris EM. Pediatric iv catheters: efficacy of saline flush. *Pediatr Nurs.* 1992; 18:111–3.

27. LeDuc K. Efficacy of normal saline solution versus heparin solution for maintaining patency of peripheral intravenous catheters in children. *J Emerg Nurs.* 1997; 23:306–9.

28. Intravenous Nurses Society. Infusion nursing standards of practice. *J Infus Nurs.* 2011; 34:37–72.

29. Romanowski GL, Zenk KE. Intravenous flush solutions for neonates. Paper presented at ASHP Midyear Clinical Meeting. New Orleans, LA; 1991 Dec 10.

30. Klenner AF, Fusch C, Rakow A, et al. Benefit and risk of heparin for maintaining peripheral venous catheters in neonates: a placebo-controlled trial. *J Pediatr.* 2003; 143:741–5.

31. Shah PS, Ng E, Sinha AK. Heparin for prolonging peripheral intravenous catheter use in neonates. *Cochrane Database Syst Rev.* 2005; 4:CD002774.

32. Goldberg M, Sankaran R, Givelichan L, et al. Maintaining patency of peripheral intermittent infusion devices with heparinized saline and saline. *Neonatal Intensive Care.* 1999; 12:18–22.

33. Heilskov J. A randomized trial of heparin and saline for maintaining intravenous locks in neonates. *J Soc Pediatr Nurs.* 1998; 3:111–6.

34. Altimier L, Brown B, Tedeschi L. NANN guidelines for neonatal nursing policies, procedures, competencies, and clinical pathways. 4th ed. Glenview, IL: National Association of Neonatal Nurses; 2006.

35. Meyer BA, Little CJ, Thorp JA, et al. Heparin versus normal saline as a peripheral line flush in maintenance of intermittent intravenous lines in obstetric patients. *Obstet Gynecol.* 1995; 85:433–6.

36. Niesen KM, Harris DY, Parkin LS, et al. The effects of heparin versus normal saline for maintenance of peripheral intravenous locks in pregnant women. *J Obstet Gynecol Neonatal Nurs.* 2003; 32:503–8.

37. Passannante A, Macik BG. The heparin flush syndrome: a cause of iatrogenic hemorrhage. *Am J Med Sci.* 1988; 296:71–3.

38. Heparin sodium monograph. In: McEvoy GK, ed. *AHFS Drug Information.* Bethesda, MD: American Society of Health-System Pharmacists; 2006:2616.

39. Heeger PS, Backstrom JT. Heparin flushes and thrombocytopenia. *Ann Intern Med.* 1986; 105:143. Letter.

40. Doty JR, Alving BM, McDonnell DE, et al. Heparin-associated thrombocytopenia in the neurosurgical patient. *Neurosurgery.* 1986; 19:69–72.

41. Cines DB, Tomaski A, Tannenbaum S. Immune endothelial-cell injury in heparin-associated thrombocytopenia. *N Engl J Med.* 1987; 316:581–9.

Approved by the ASHP Board of Directors on April 13, 2012. Developed through the Council on Therapeutics.

This document supersedes the ASHP therapeutic position statement on the institutional use of 0.9% sodium chloride injection to maintain patency of peripheral indwelling intermittent infusion devices approved by the ASHP Board of Directors on January 12, 2006.

Kim W. Benner, Pharm.D., BCPS, FASHP, and Amber J. Lucas, Pharm.D., BCPS, FASHP, are gratefully acknowledged for authoring this document.

The bibliographic citation for this document is as follows: American Society of Health-System Pharmacists. ASHP therapeutic position statement on the institutional use of 0.9% sodium chloride injection to maintain patency of peripheral indwelling intermittent infusion devices. *Am J Health-Syst Pharm.* 2012; 69:1252–4.

ASHP Therapeutic Position Statement on the Preferential Use of Metronidazole for the Treatment of *Clostridium difficile*-Associated Disease

Statement of Position

ASHP supports the use of oral metronidazole as the preferred antimicrobial agent for treating *Clostridium difficile*-associated disease (CDAD). Oral metronidazole and oral vancomycin appear to be equally efficacious for the treatment of CDAD in most situations. However, routine use of oral vancomycin may contribute to the emergence of vancomycin-resistant *Enterococcus* species, and oral vancomycin is more costly than oral metronidazole. Oral vancomycin should be reserved for the most severe, potentially life-threatening forms of the disorder, for cases that fail to respond to oral metronidazole, and for patients who are unable to tolerate oral metronidazole or to whom metronidazole should not be given. Mild cases of CDAD may respond to discontinuation of the inciting agent, making antimicrobial treatment unnecessary and reducing the possibility of CDAD relapse. Asymptomatic carriers of *C. difficile* should not be treated for CDAD.

Background

CDAD is an infectious disorder that can develop when toxin-producing *C. difficile* is acquired as a component of the colonic microflora. If an individual harboring the organism is subsequently exposed to certain antimicrobial agents, *C. difficile* is able to evade eradication by spore formation, while many of the bacteria that help maintain normal microbial ecology in the colon are destroyed. This selective advantage for replication can result in the uncontrolled overgrowth of *C. difficile* and production of bacterial exotoxins that cause inflammation and cellular damage.[1,2] When symptomatic disease ensues, its severity ranges from self-limiting diarrhea to life-threatening enterocolitis with toxic megacolon.[2,3]

CDAD is predominantly, but not exclusively, a nosocomial disease.[1] Epidemic outbreaks of CDAD may occur within institutions, with patterns of antimicrobial use contributing to the initiation of an outbreak as well as compromising the efficacy of infection control measures intended to limit it.[4] The frequency of community-acquired CDAD is less than one case per 10,000 antimicrobial prescriptions,[5] compared with as many as one case per 100 hospitalized adult patients treated with an antimicrobial agent.[2] However, CDAD will likely become more common in the community setting as outpatient antimicrobial treatment of serious infections increases.

Minimum criteria for diagnosis of CDAD consist of mild to moderate diarrhea accompanied either by a positive *C. difficile* cytotoxin (or toxin b) test result or by endoscopically observed pseudomembranes.[1] Concurrent or recent antimicrobial use is usually present but is not a criterion for definitive diagnosis.[1] However, a recent study indicated that hospitalized patients without antimicrobial exposure during the previous month and either significant diarrhea or abdominal pain are unlikely to have a positive *C. difficile* cytotoxin test result.[6]

Virtually all antimicrobial agents and certain antineoplastic agents with antimicrobial activity have been implicated in precipitating CDAD,[3] but data suggest that second- and third-generation cephalosporins play an increasingly important role.[7-9] Amoxicillin and amoxicillin–clavulanate are among the most frequently implicated antimicrobial agents in community-acquired CDAD.[10] Although the time of onset of CDAD ranges from within one to two days after the initiation of therapy to as long as 10 weeks after drug discontinuation, most cases occur after several days of treatment or within the first few weeks after discontinuation of therapy.[2,3]

Asymptomatic colonization by *C. difficile* can occur, especially in healthy neonates and infants. Long-term carriage of the organism has been documented.[1,2] A well-designed study showed that treatment of asymptomatic carriers of *C. difficile* with either metronidazole or vancomycin is of no clinical value[11]; more recent data substantiate this.[12]

The initial steps in the management of all cases of CDAD are discontinuation of the precipitating agent, if feasible, and restoration of fluids and electrolytes, if needed.[2,3] Antimicrobial treatment should be reserved for cases that fail to respond promptly to this initial therapy and for cases in which discontinuation of the precipitating agent is not a therapeutic option.[2,3] In mild cases of CDAD (diarrhea accompanied by minimal or no constitutional symptoms), particularly those in individuals who are not elderly or debilitated, the patient should be monitored for symptomatic improvement for 48 hours before oral antimicrobial treatment is instituted. If symptomatic deterioration occurs, appropriate antimicrobial therapy should be started promptly.

Relative Efficacy of Oral Metronidazole and Oral Vancomycin in the Treatment of CDAD

Oral vancomycin was first reported to be effective in the treatment of CDAD in 1978.[13] In 1983, a small but well-designed clinical trial showed oral metronidazole to be equivalent to oral vancomycin for the treatment of CDAD.[14] By then oral vancomycin was already established as the drug of choice for CDAD.

Prospective, randomized comparisons have shown no significant difference in initial response rates or relapse rates between oral metronidazole and oral vancomycin in the treatment of CDAD.[1,2,14-17] Therefore, oral metronidazole is now the preferred therapy for most patients with CDAD.[1,3,18,19] Oral vancomycin is considered appropriate only in cases of severe, potentially life-threatening CDAD, when oral metronidazole fails, or when oral metronidazole is not tolerated or cannot be used.[3,18]

Severe CDAD is not clearly defined in the literature. It has been generally characterized in terms of pseudomembrane formation, fever exceeding 40 °C (104 °F), marked abdominal tenderness, and pronounced leukocytosis.[2,3,14] The detection of fecal leukocytes by microscopy also

suggests more severe disease.[9] Even in these clinical circumstances, there is little objective evidence that oral vancomycin is superior to oral metronidazole.[14-16] In rare instances, ileus and toxic megacolon develop. These constitute potentially life-threatening conditions in which oral therapy is not feasible, but optimal drug therapy remains undefined.[2,7]

Role of Vancomycin in the Emergence of Vancomycin-Resistant Enterococci

Many studies have identified prior exposure to vancomycin as a risk factor for colonization and infection by vancomycin-resistant enterococci (VRE).[20] Although intravenous rather than oral vancomycin appears to be the most significant risk factor, oral vancomycin use has also been implicated.[20-23] An apparent association between CDAD and the acquisition of VRE has also been described.[20,24,25] In two European studies it was found that glycopeptide-resistant enterococci could be isolated readily from stool samples after oral administration of vancomycin to healthy adults.[26,27]

Concern over the probable role of indiscriminate use of vancomycin in the emergence of VRE culminated in the publication, by the Hospital Infection Control Practices Advisory Committee of the Centers for Disease Control and Prevention, of consensus guidelines for prudent vancomycin use.[18] The guidelines deem oral vancomycin "appropriate or acceptable . . . when antibiotic-associated colitis (AAC) fails to respond to metronidazole therapy or if AAC is severe and potentially life threatening" and state that its use for the "primary treatment of AAC" should be discouraged.

Vancomycin and Metronidazole Dosage Regimens

Since *C. difficile* usually does not escape the gastrointestinal tract, only antimicrobial levels within the intestinal lumen are of consequence. When vancomycin is administered orally, high fecal concentrations are obtained because of poor absorption. A regimen of vancomycin 125 mg (as the hydrochloride salt) four times daily provides the same clinical outcome as 500 mg four times daily because it yields a mean fecal vancomycin concentration well above the highest reported minimum inhibitory concentration for *C. difficile.*[28]

In contrast to oral vancomycin, oral metronidazole attains very low fecal concentrations because of nearly complete absorption. Although this has resulted in lingering concern about the efficacy of oral metronidazole in the treatment of serious cases of CDAD,[1] such concern seems unwarranted. Some unmetabolized metronidazole is eliminated in the feces via biliary excretion, and the drug appears to cross the intestinal wall into the lumen of the inflamed colon. Furthermore, successful treatment of CDAD with metronidazole is well documented.[1,14-16] Total daily dosages of oral metronidazole in the treatment of CDAD have ranged from 1000 to 2250 mg administered in three or four divided doses.[2] Of three major studies that found oral metronidazole and oral vancomycin to be therapeutically equivalent for CDAD, two used a daily metronidazole dosage of 1000 mg (250 mg four times daily),[7,14] and one used a daily dosage of 1500 mg (500 mg three times daily).[16] No direct comparisons of metronidazole dosages have been published.[2]

Ten days has been the usual duration of therapy when either oral agent is used for CDAD.[2] Symptomatic

improvement may be apparent within 48 hours, but treatment is most likely to be successful if carried out for the full 10 days.[1] A slow or delayed response to therapy with either metronidazole or vancomycin may occur in patients with a pre-existing intestinal disorder and associated diarrhea.[17] However, therapeutic failure of metronidazole should not be assumed until a minimum of six days of treatment have been completed without symptomatic improvement.[7,14,16] Therapeutic failure rates of 2–5% can be anticipated with either oral metronidazole or oral vancomycin.[7,17]

Oral therapy is always preferable for the treatment of CDAD, but the oral route is not always feasible because of gastrointestinal obstruction or other reasons (e.g., toxic megacolon).[3] Treatment approaches in patients unable to tolerate oral medications have included i.v. vancomycin, i.v. metronidazole, and rectal vancomycin alone and in various combinations, but no comparative studies have been performed.[29] Because treatment failures have been reported with either i.v. metronidazole or i.v. vancomycin given alone,[30,31] consideration should be given to the concurrent use of i.v. metronidazole and either i.v. or rectal vancomycin.[3] Several regimens for the rectal administration of vancomycin have been described.[3,29] Because the available efficacy data are exclusively anecdotal, no definitive recommendations can be made regarding the treatment of CDAD in the patient who cannot take oral medications.

Treatment of Relapse

Approximately 15–35% of patients treated for CDAD with either oral metronidazole or oral vancomycin relapse within two months after completing initial therapy.[3] Relapse is defined as a return of symptoms and positive diagnostic test results after discontinuation of successful antimicrobial therapy for CDAD.[3] Most patients relapse only once, although multiple relapses occur in a small subset of patients.[2,17] Relapse frequency is unrelated to the antimicrobial selected for initial treatment of CDAD,[3,17] but additional exposure to antimicrobials given to treat other types of infection appears to be a significant risk factor for recurrence of CDAD, and the frequency of recurrence increases with the number of antimicrobials administered.[17]

A multitude of protocols for treating CDAD relapse are described in the literature, but no comparative studies have been conducted.[2,3,17] More than 90% of patients with CDAD who relapse respond to a single repeated course of oral medication, either metronidazole or vancomycin.[7] Since relapse is usually unrelated to antimicrobial resistance, the same agent used to treat CDAD initially can be used to treat the relapse.[2,3] Thus, patients with a first relapse of CDAD who were treated with oral metronidazole initially should receive a second 10-day course of metronidazole.[1] No definitive therapeutic recommendation can be made for a patient with multiple relapses. Therapeutic options are discussed in detail elsewhere.[2,3,17]

Special Populations

Asymptomatic carriage of toxin-producing *C. difficile* is common in newborn infants and in children less than two years of age, but CDAD is rare. It is also rare in older children. However, certain subpopulations, such as children with gastrointestinal motility disorders like Hirschsprung's disease (congenital megacolon) and severely neutropenic children with leukemia, are at increased risk.[32] Comparative

studies of oral metronidazole and oral vancomycin for the treatment of CDAD have not been conducted in the pediatric population. Since the pharmacokinetic profile of oral metronidazole in children is similar to that in adults, there is no reason to consider oral metronidazole inferior to oral vancomycin for CDAD in pediatric patients. However, commercial oral vancomycin solution may prove more palatable than an extemporaneously prepared metronidazole suspension for children who are unable to swallow metronidazole tablets or for whom the available tablet formulation is not appropriate.[33]

Recommended dosages for the treatment of CDAD in children are oral metronidazole 30 mg/kg/day given in divided doses every six hours or oral vancomycin 40 mg/kg/day given in divided doses every six to eight hours.[19] The maximum dosage in pediatric patients should not exceed the adult dosage.

The risk of metronidazole therapy during the first trimester of pregnancy is uncertain, and metronidazole use during that trimester is controversial.[34] Metronidazole is excreted into breast milk. Oral vancomycin may therefore be the preferred agent for the treatment of CDAD during the first trimester and in nursing mothers.[3]

Therapeutic Alternatives

The use of an anion-exchange resin such as cholestyramine, with or without metronidazole or vancomycin therapy, offers no demonstrable benefit and should be discouraged.[2,3] Concomitant use of cholestyramine and oral vancomycin is particularly undesirable because of binding of vancomycin by cholestyramine. Antiperistaltic agents can cause retention of C. difficile toxins in the colon and should be avoided.[2,3] Oral bacitracin, which is expensive and less efficacious than metronidazole or vancomycin,[2] should generally not be used. Biotherapy, such as supplementation of the normal colonic microflora with Saccharomyces boulardii, may be a future approach to the prevention and treatment of CDAD.[35]

The Pharmacist's Role

Pharmacists should strive to optimize the treatment of CDAD by encouraging the preferential use of metronidazole when antimicrobial therapy is warranted. Currently, excessive use of oral vancomycin for CDAD is largely an institutional problem because CDAD is primarily a nosocomial disease. However, as CDAD becomes more common in the community setting, ambulatory care pharmacists too will have a responsibility for ensuring optimal treatment of this disease.

The availability of guidelines for vancomycin use alone may not result in major changes in prescribing behavior.[33,36–39] Additional strategies for influencing vancomycin prescribing may include tailored educational efforts and interventions that encourage physicians to prescribe oral metronidazole preferentially for the treatment of CDAD when antimicrobial therapy is indicated. In addition, pharmacists should become involved in implementing comprehensive antimicrobial management programs that can both help to prevent the development of bacterial resistance and reduce overall expenditures.[38]

Pharmacists should collaborate on studies designed to clarify the relationship between oral vancomycin use and the acquisition of vancomycin-resistant bacteria, participate in surveillance for vancomycin-resistant organisms, and contribute to infection-control measures directed against vancomycin-resistant pathogens.[40]

Finally, pharmacists can play a key role in communicating to patients the risks of resistance associated with the indiscriminate use of antimicrobial agents and the potential adverse effects of therapy. Improved patient understanding of these risks should result in better adherence to therapy.

Summary

ASHP supports preferential use of oral metronidazole for treating CDAD when antimicrobial therapy is indicated. Oral vancomycin should be reserved for severe, potentially life-threatening cases or when oral metronidazole cannot be used. Oral metronidazole is as safe and effective as oral vancomycin and is considerably less costly. In addition, preliminary data suggest that routine use of oral vancomycin for CDAD may contribute to the spread of VRE—emerging nosocomial pathogens that can be extraordinarily difficult to treat. Pharmacists should work to foster preferential prescribing of oral metronidazole for the treatment of CDAD. Pharmacists should also actively seek opportunities to educate health care providers and counsel patients about the risks associated with the indiscriminate use of vancomycin and other antimicrobial agents.

References

1. Gerding DDN, Johnson S, Peterson LR, et al. Clostridium difficile-associated diarrhea and colitis. Infect Control Hosp Epidemiol. 1995; 16:459–77.
2. Reinke CM, Messick CR. Update on Clostridium difficile-induced colitis, parts 1 and 2. Am J Hosp Pharm. 1994; 51:1771–81, 1892–901.
3. Fekety R. Guidelines for the diagnosis and management of Clostridium difficile-associated diarrhea and colitis. Am J Gastroenterol. 1997; 92:739–50.
4. Lai KK, Melvin ZS, Menard MJ, et al. Clostridium difficile-associated diarrhea: epidemiology, risk factors, and infection control. Infect Control Hosp Epidemiol. 1997; 18:628–32.
5. Hirschhorn LR, Trnka Y, Onderdonk A, et al. Epidemiology of community-acquired Clostridium difficile-associated diarrhea. J Infect Dis. 1994; 169:127–33.
6. Katz DA, Lynch ME, Littenberg B. Clinical prediction rates to optimize cytotoxin testing for Clostridium difficile in hospitalized patients with diarrhea. Am J Med. 1996; 100:487–95.
7. Olson MM, Shanholtzer CJ, Lee JT Jr, et al. Ten years of prospective Clostridium difficile-associated disease surveillance and treatment at the Minneapolis VA medical center, 1982–1991. Infect Control Hosp Epidemiol. 1994; 15:371–81.
8. Nelson DE, Auerbach SB, Baltch AL, et al. Epidemic Clostridium difficile-associated diarrhea: role of second- and third-generation cephalosporins. Infect Control Hosp Epidemiol. 1994; 15:88–94.
9. Manabe YC, Vinetz JM, Moore RD, et al. Clostridium difficile colitis: an efficient clinical approach to diagnosis. Ann Intern Med. 1995; 123:835–40.
10. Riley TV, Cooper M, Bell B, et al. Community-acquired Clostridium difficile-associated diarrhea. Clin Infect Dis. 1995; 20(suppl 2):S263–5.
11. Johnson S, Homann SR, Bettin KM, et al. Treatment of asymptomatic Clostridium difficile carriers (fecal excretors) with vancomycin or metronidazole: a

randomized, placebo-controlled trial. *Ann Intern Med.* 1992; 117:297–302.

12. Samore MH, DeGirolami PC, Tlucko A, et al. *Clostridium difficile* colonization and diarrhea at a tertiary care hospital. *Clin Infect Dis.* 1994; 18:181–7.

13. Tedesco F, Markham R, Gurwith M, et al. Oral vancomycin for antibiotic-associated pseudomembranous colitis. *Lancet.* 1978; 2:226–8.

14. Teasley DG, Olson MG, Gebhard RI, et al. Prospective randomized trial of metronidazole versus vancomycin for *Clostridium difficile*-associated diarrhea and colitis. *Lancet.* 1983; 2:1043–6.

15. Anand A, Bahey B, Mir T, et al. Epidemiology, clinical manifestations, and outcome of *Clostridium difficile*-associated diarrhea. *Am J Gastroenterol.* 1994; 89: 519–23.

16. Wenisch C, Parschalk B, Hasenhundl M, et al. Comparison of vancomycin, teicoplanin, metronidazole, and fusidic acid for the treatment of *Clostridium difficile*-associated diarrhea. *Clin Infect Dis.* 1996; 22:813–8.

17. Fekety R, McFarland LV, Surawicz CM, et al. Recurrent *Clostridium difficile* diarrhea: characteristics of and risk factors for patients enrolled in a prospective, randomized, double-blinded trial. *Clin Infect Dis.* 1997; 24:324–33.

18. Centers for Disease Control and Prevention Hospital Infection Control Practices Advisory Committee. Recommendations for preventing the spread of vancomycin resistance. *Infect Control Hosp Epidemiol.* 1995; 16:105–13.

19. *Clostridium difficile.* In: Peter G, ed. American Academy of Pediatrics 1997 red book: report of the Committee on Infectious Diseases. 24th ed. Elk Grove Village, IL: American Academy of Pediatrics; 1997:177–8.

20. Gerding DN. Is there a relationship between vancomycin-resistant enterococcal infection and *Clostridium difficile* infection? *Clin Infect Dis.* 1997; 25(suppl 2):S206–10.

21. Fraise AP. The treatment and control of vancomycin-resistant enterococci. *J Antimicrob Chemother.* 1996; 38:753–6.

22. Carr JR, Fitzpatrick PE, Cumbo TJ, et al. A reduction in oral vancomycin use and a concomitant reduction in vancomycin-resistant *Enterococcus. Infect Control Hosp Epidemiol.* 1996; 17(suppl):25. Abstract.

23. Rao GG, Ojo F, Kolokithas D. Vancomycin-resistant gram-positive cocci: risk factors for fecal carriage. *J Hosp Infect.* 1997; 35:63–9.

24. Rafferty ME, McCormick MI, Bopp LH, et al. Vancomycin-resistant enterococci in stool specimens submitted for *Clostridium difficile* cytotoxin assay. *Infect Control Hosp Epidemiol.* 1997; 18:342–4.

25. Lam S, Singer C, Tucci V, et al. The challenge of vanco-mycin-resistant enterococci: a clinical and epidemiologic study. *Am J Infect Control.* 1995; 23:170–80.

26. Van der Auwera P, Pensart N, Korten V, et al. Influence of oral glycopeptides on the fecal flora of human volunteers: selection of highly glycopeptide-resistant enterococci. *J Infect Dis.* 1996; 173:1129–36.

27. Edlund C, Barkholt L, Olsson-Liljequist B, et al. Effect of vancomycin on intestinal flora of patients who previously received antimicrobial therapy. *Clin Infect Dis.* 1997; 25:729–32.

28. Fekety R, Silva J, Kaufman C, et al. Treatment of antibiotic-associated *Clostridium difficile* colitis with

oral vancomycin: comparison of two dosage regimens. *Am J Med.* 1989; 86:15–9.

29. Bublin JG, Barton TL. Rectal use of vancomycin. *Ann Pharmacother.* 1994; 28:1357–8.

30. Oliva SL, Guglielmo BJ, Jacobs R, et al. Failure of intravenous vancomycin and intravenous metronidazole to prevent or treat antibiotic-associated pseudomembranous colitis. *J Infect Dis.* 1989; 159:1154–5. Letter.

31. Kleinfeld D, Donta ST. Reply. (Failure of intravenous vancomycin and intravenous metronidazole to prevent or treat antibiotic-associated pseudomembranous colitis.) *J Infect Dis.* 1989; 159:1155. Letter.

32. Zwiener BJ, Belknap WM, Quan R. Severe pseudomembranous enterocolitis in a child: case report and literature review. *Pediatr Infect Dis J.* 1989; 8:876–82.

33. Evans ME, Kortas KJ. Vancomycin use in a university medical center: comparison with Hospital Infection Control Practices Advisory Committee guidelines. *Infect Control Hosp Epidemiol.* 1996; 17:356–9.

34. Metronidazole. In: Briggs GG, Freeman RK, Yaffe SJ, eds. Drugs in pregnancy and lactation: a guide to fetal and neonatal risk. 4th ed. Baltimore: Williams & Wilkins; 1994:585–9.

35. Eddy JT, Stamatakis MK, Makela EH. *Saccharomyces boulardii* for the treatment of *Clostridium difficile*-associated colitis. *Ann Pharmacother.* 1997; 31:919–21.

36. Johnson SV, Hoey LL, Vance-Bryan K. Inappropriate vancomycin prescribing based on criteria from the Centers for Disease Control and Prevention. *Pharmacotherapy.* 1995; 15:579–85.

37. Watanakunakorn C. Prescribing pattern of vancomycin in a community teaching hospital with low prevalence of vancomycin-resistant enterococci. *Infect Control Hosp Epidemiol.* 1997; 18:767–9.

38. Carr JR, Fitzpatrick P, Izzo JL, et al. Changing the infection control paradigm from offline to real time: the experience at Millard Fillmore Health System. *Infect Control Hosp Epidemiol.* 1997; 18:255–9.

39. Beidas S, Khamesian M. Vancomycin use in a university medical center: comparison with Hospital Infection Control Practices Advisory Committee guidelines. *Infect Control Hosp Epidemiol.* 1996; 17:773–4. Letter.

40. Schlaes DM, Gerding DN, John JF Jr, et al. Society for Healthcare Epidemiology of America and Infectious Diseases Society of America Joint Committee on the Prevention of Antimicrobial Resistance: guidelines for the prevention of antimicrobial resistance in hospitals. *Infect Control Hosp Epidemiol.* 1997; 18:275–91.

This therapeutic position statement was reviewed in 2002 by the Commission on Therapeutics and by the Board of Directors and was found to still be appropriate.

Approved by the ASHP Board of Directors April 22, 1998. Developed by the ASHP Commission on Therapeutics.

The bibliographic citation for this document is as follows: American Society of Health-System Pharmacists. ASHP therapeutic position statement on the preferential use of metronidazole for the treatment of *Clostridium difficile*-associated disease. *Am J Health-Syst Pharm.* 1998; 55:1407–11.

ASHP Therapeutic Position Statement on the Prevention and Treatment of Osteoporosis in Adults

Position

Osteoporosis is a devastating disease that may lead to significant morbidity and mortality from resultant fractures.[1-3] The efficacy of medications as one method to prevent and treat osteoporosis and avert future fractures, particularly vertebral fractures, is well documented in large clinical trials. However, despite this evidence, many patients at risk for osteoporosis are not screened or treated.[4-8] Screening for osteoporosis is considered a quality-of-care indicator by the Centers for Medicare and Medicaid Services and the National Committee for Quality Assurance.[9,10] The American Society of Health-System Pharmacists (ASHP) believes that all women age 65 years or older, postmenopausal women younger than age 65 years who have an increased risk of developing osteoporosis, all adult women with a history of nontraumatic fracture, and men with a significant risk of fracture should be screened for osteoporosis and treated, if indicated.

ASHP believes that there is a gap between the evidence and practice of prevention and treatment of osteoporosis in adults. In addition, ASHP believes that prevention and treatment of osteoporosis can decrease the morbidity and mortality associated with this condition, consistent with the *Healthy People 2010* objectives of reducing the percentage of adults with osteoporosis and those hospitalized with vertebral fractures.[11] Calcium and vitamin D,[12-17] bisphosphonates (alendronate, ibandronate, risedronate, and zoledronic acid),[18-25] calcitonin,[26] estrogen (with or without a progestin),[27,28] raloxifene,[29] and teriparatide[30] have all been shown to decrease the risk of osteoporotic fractures, though differences exist in each drug's ability to reduce fractures at all sites. Therefore, each drug's place in therapy varies.

ASHP encourages health care professionals to educate patients about risk factors associated with osteoporosis. In addition, the Society encourages health care professionals to identify and triage at-risk patients for osteoporosis screening and diagnosis. ASHP believes that patients at risk for osteoporosis and medical complications related to osteoporosis should receive an assessment of bone mineral density (BMD) by central dual-energy x-ray absorptiometry (DEXA) and both nonpharmacologic and pharmacologic therapy to prevent further bone loss and promote increased bone quality. Pharmacists may be well suited to provide osteoporosis screenings using peripheral devices and offer patient education regarding osteoporosis prevention and treatment,[31-35] though central DEXA is required for diagnosis.[36]

Background

Osteoporosis is a disease characterized by low bone mass and structural deterioration of bone tissue. Low bone mass may be due to either increased loss of bone or failure to achieve sufficient peak bone mass.[37] A decline in bone mass due to advancing age, medications, or other risk factors increases bone fragility and susceptibility to fractures, especially at the hip, spine, forearm, and wrist.

The World Health Organization (WHO) defines osteoporosis as a BMD of 2.5 or more standard deviations below that of a normal young adult (t score of $\leq$–2.5) for postmenopausal women and men over age 50 years as measured by central DEXA.[3,38] Osteopenia is defined as a BMD between –1 and –2.5 standard deviations below the young adult mean; a normal BMD value is defined as within 1 standard deviation of the mean BMD for a young adult. Patients who have a t score of $\leq$–2.5 and have already had one or more fractures are classified as having severe or established osteoporosis. Figure 1 shows the distribution of BMD in healthy women age 30–40 years.[36]

Osteoporosis is a major public health problem in the United States. In 2002, over 10 million individuals had known osteoporosis, 80% of whom were women.[39,40] Approximately 44 million men and women over age 50 years have either os-

Figure 1. Distribution of bone mineral density in healthy women age 30–40 years. Reproduced from reference 36, with permission.

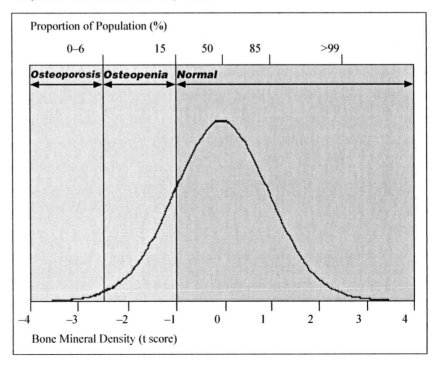

teoporosis or low BMD. If these trends continue, this figure may increase to over 61 million by 2020.[39]

Osteoporotic fractures are associated with significant morbidity and mortality. Patients who sustain a fracture are more likely to have lower health-related quality of life, depression, pain, disability, physical deconditioning due to inactivity, vertebral deformities with a resultant decrease in pulmonary function and increase in gastrointestinal complications (e.g., refractory reflux esophagitis), pressure ulcers, increased likelihood of nursing home placement, and changes in self-image.[41–51] Hip fractures, which are the most serious complication of osteoporosis, are associated with significant mortality.[52–55] Up to 38% of patients may die within one year after a hip fracture, and the risk of death is approximately double that of patients who do not sustain a hip fracture.[52,53,55]

The economic consequences of osteoporosis are enormous. In 1995, osteoporotic fractures were responsible for approximately 432,000 hospital admissions, 2.5 million physician's office visits, and 180,000 nursing home admissions.[1] Health care costs associated with osteoporotic fractures in 2001 were an estimated $17 billion. As the population of the United States continues to age, these costs will likely increase, with the number of hip fractures and associated costs possibly tripling by 2040.[1]

Despite the significant morbidity, mortality, and economic consequences of osteoporosis and resultant fractures, many patients are not screened or treated. In a study of 3812 women with an average age of 71 years who sustained a new fragility (i.e., minimal-trauma) fracture, only 11.7% had a diagnosis of osteoporosis before the index fracture, and only 46.4% were managed as specified by clinical guidelines.[5] In another study of patients who sustained a fragility fracture, few patients received densitometry testing either before (13%) or after (22.2%) the index fracture.[4] Only 18.5% were diagnosed with osteoporosis, and only 32.4% received calcium supplementation. Thus, significant improvements must be made in the diagnosis and treatment of osteoporosis.

Risk Assessment

Osteoporosis risk factor analysis is useful to identify patients at high risk of fractures, raise awareness of osteoporosis, promote strategies for prevention of fractures, and stimulate osteoporosis treatment (Table 1).[1,3,56] Prior fragility fracture as an adult and low BMD in patients with or without fractures are the two most important risk factors, both of which are clear indications for additional evaluation and possible therapeutic intervention.[3] Additional risk factors are listed in Table 1. ASHP encourages osteoporosis screening by all health care professionals, with specific attention to patients taking medications associated with decreased bone mass, including glucocortico-steroids, anticonvulsants (e.g., phenytoin, phenobarbital, carbamazepine), immunosuppressants, and excessive thyroid supplementation.[1]

ASHP believes health care professionals should conduct fall-risk assessment in conjunction with osteoporosis screening. All high-risk or elderly patients should be routinely asked about falls in the past year.[57] Older persons reporting a single fall should be assessed for balance and gait to detect balance problems.[57,58] Older persons who report recurrent falls or have gait or balance abnormalities will ben-

efit from a comprehensive fall evaluation.[57] Most patients demonstrate multiple risk factors for falls; common risk factors include muscle weakness, use of assistive devices, visual deficits, use of certain medications, arthritis, impaired activities of daily living, depression, cognitive impairment, and age greater than 80 years.[57] Three risk factors—hip weakness, unstable balance, and use of four or more medications—are highly predictive for one-year fall risk.[59] ASHP encourages a comprehensive drug regimen review to identify medications or drug-related problems that may increase fall risk. Medications commonly associated with increased falls include psychotropics, cardiovascular medications, and central nervous system agents.[57,60,61]

Evaluation

Patients at risk for osteoporosis and related fractures should receive BMD testing by central DEXA. These patients include women age 65 years or older (regardless of risk factors), postmenopausal women under age 65 years with risk factors (Table 1), and postmenopausal women with a history of non-traumatic fracture. In addition, testing should be considered for men age 70 years or older, for patients with diseases that may result in decreased bone strength, for patients taking long-term medications known to decrease BMD, and to assess response in patients receiving medications for the treatment of osteoporosis. These recommendations are consistent

Table 1.
Risk Factors for Osteoporosis and Related Fractures[1,3,57]

- Personal history of minimal-trauma fracture as an adult[a]
- History of fragility fracture in a first-degree relative[a]
- Low body weight (e.g., <127 lb)[a]
- Current smoking[a]
- Use of oral corticosteroid therapy for more than three months[a]
- Female sex
- Caucasian race
- Low physical activity
- Late menarche or early menopause
- Hypogonadism
- Low lifelong calcium intake
- Vitamin D deficiency
- Weight loss
- Impaired vision
- Dementia
- Poor health or frailty
- Recent falls
- Consumption of more than two alcoholic drinks per day
- Use of medications associated with falls (e.g., psychotropics, cardiovascular medications, central nervous system agents)
- Other medications with adverse bone effects (e.g., anticonvulsants, long-term heparin, immunosuppressants)
- Hyperthyroidism
- Hyperparathyroidism
- Renal hypercalciuria
- Chronic kidney or liver disease
- Gastrointestinal abnormalities (e.g., malnutrition, malabsorption, maldigestion)
- Rheumatoid arthritis
- Weightlessness

[a]Major risk factors in Caucasian postmenopausal women.[1]

with those of the National Osteoporosis Foundation (NOF), the American Association of Clinical Endocrinologists, and the U.S. Preventative Services Task Force.[1,3,62] While these recommendations may be considered broad, the use of validated risk assessments, such as SCORE (Simple Calculated Osteoporosis Risk Assessment) and ORAI (Osteoporosis Risk Assessment Instrument), may be useful in identifying women likely to have osteoporosis, thereby decreasing the number of women who undergo unnecessary central DEXA testing.[63–65] Further, a WHO working group in collaboration with the International Osteoporosis Foundation and NOF is developing and validating a new risk assessment tool.[66] This tool will use independent risk factors to calculate fracture probability, with or without the use of BMD, allowing treatment to be recommended for those with a fracture probability above the threshold for treatment.[67] A risk-assessment tool for use in men is discussed later in this document.

Currently, measurement of BMD by central DEXA is considered the gold standard for diagnosing osteoporosis, as it correlates significantly with the risk of fractures.[62,68,69] For each standard deviation decrease in femoral neck BMD, there is an approximate 2.5-fold increased risk of hip fracture.[70,71] Advantages of central DEXA include high sensitivity and specificity and the ability to measure BMD at numerous areas, including the hip, spine, and wrist. Disadvantages of central DEXA for mass screenings include equipment size and lack of portability, need for a dedicated room, expense, ionizing radiation, need for a radiation-certified and trained technician, lack of measurement of structure, and significant time required to screen and read the results.

Peripheral bone densitometers may be an ideal choice for mass screening and for assessing fracture risk.[68] These machines are generally much smaller and portable, require significantly less time to screen and read results, are available in models that use ultrasound rather than radiation, and have been shown to predict fracture risk.[72] Though useful in screening and identifying at-risk patients, peripheral bone densitometers should not be used as the primary tool for diagnosis or for monitoring treatment response due to their inability to measure BMD at all sites and the possibility of false-negative results.

Prevention and Treatment

Nonpharmacologic Therapies. Several nonpharmacologic interventions for the prevention of osteoporotic fractures should be considered for all patients. The attainment of high peak bone mass early in life is one of the most important protective factors against reduced BMD later in life.[2] In addition, strategies to maintain current bone mass for patients in later stages of life should be instituted. Thus, appropriate weight-bearing exercise, minimization or elimination of various modifiable risk factors (e.g., smoking, excessive alcohol intake, maintenance of euthyroid status), and maintenance of adequate calcium and vitamin D intake should be recommended for all patients.[1–3,37]

Adequate calcium and vitamin D intake is considered an essential component of osteoporosis prevention and treatment,[1–3,37] yet many men and women over age 65 years consume only 600 mg of calcium daily. However, there is controversy regarding calcium and vitamin D supplementation. There is no universal consensus for the most appropriate daily dose (Table 2), though all groups recommend at least 1000 mg, and data are lacking regarding the most effective calcium salt. In addition, questions have been raised about the efficacy of calcium and vitamin D for prevention of fractures.

Several randomized controlled trials found that supplemental calcium or vitamin D_3 or both were effective in decreasing the risk for fractures.[12–16] In a primary prevention study of 3270 healthy postmenopausal women (mean age, 84 years), 1200 mg of elemental calcium (as the tricalcium phosphate) plus 800 IU of vitamin D given daily for 18 months was associated with a 43% decrease in the risk of hip fractures (number needed to treat [NNT] = 56, p = 0.043) and a 32% decrease in nonvertebral fractures (NNT = 29, p = 0.015).[12] In a primary prevention study of 389 ambulatory men and women over age 65 years, 500 mg of calcium (as calcium citrate) plus 700 IU of vitamin D_3 given daily for three years decreased the risk of nonvertebral fractures by 50% (NNT = 14; 95% confidence interval [CI], 0.2–0.9; p = 0.02).[13]

However, two more recently published studies appear to contradict previous findings. In the Randomized

Table 2.
Recommended Daily Dietary Reference Intakes of Elemental Calcium and Vitamin D[a]

Supplement	National Academy of Sciences[73–75]	National Osteoporosis Foundation[1]	NIH Consensus Panel[76]
Elemental calcium	Age 31–50 yr: 1000 mg	Age <50 yr: 1000 mg	Age 25–65 yr and women >50 yr receiving estrogen: 1000 mg
	Age >50 yr: 1200 mg	Age ≥50 yr: 1200 mg	Age >65 yr and women >50 yr not receiving estrogen: 1500 mg
Vitamin D	Age 31–50 yr: 200 IU	Age <50 yr: 400–800 IU	. . .[b]
	Age 50–70 yr: 400 IU	Age ≥50 yr: 800–1000 IU	
	Age >70 yr: 600 IU		

[a]Recommendations are for both men and women unless otherwise stated. NIH = National Institutes of Health.
[b]The NIH consensus panel does not provide recommendations for vitamin D supplementation.

Evaluation of Calcium or Vitamin D (RECORD) secondary prevention study, 5,292 elderly patients (mean age, 77 years) who had a low-trauma, osteoporotic fracture in the previous 10 years were randomized to receive 1000 mg calcium (as the carbonate), 800 IU of vitamin D_3, the combination, or placebo.[77] After a median follow-up of 45 months, there was no significant difference in the rate of new low-trauma fractures ($p > 0.05$ for all active treatments versus placebo). A significant limitation of this study was a low adherence rate at 24 months based on mailed questionnaires (60% adherence based on returned questionnaires, 47% adherence assuming nonresponders were nonadherent). Likewise, in the Women's Health Initiative (WHI) Calcium with Vitamin D Trial, which evaluated the effect of calcium and vitamin D supplementation on the frequency of hip and other bone fractures, 1000 mg calcium (as the carbonate) plus 400 IU of vitamin D given daily failed to reduce the risk of hip fracture, clinical spine fracture, or total fracture in 36,282 healthy postmenopausal women over seven years of use and increased the risk of renal calculi (number needed to harm [NNH] = 273).[78] There are several possible explanations for this lack of benefit, including the relatively low daily dose of vitamin D used, the fact that most patients did not have low BMD at baseline (mean hip t score, −0.65 in subgroup for whom BMD was measured), and a possible lack of power attributable to a lower-than-expected hip fracture rate. In patients who adhered to therapy at least 80% of the time, fractures were reduced by 29%.

The results of a meta-analysis of double-blind, randomized controlled trials of patients over age 60 years suggest that vitamin D dosages of 700–800 IU daily with or without calcium reduced the risk for hip fracture and any nonvertebral fracture by 26% (NNT = 45) and 23% (NNT = 27), respectively, versus calcium alone or placebo.[79] However, no significant fracture reduction was seen with low daily doses (400 IU) of vitamin D.

In 2007, a large meta-analysis of more than 63,000 patients in 29 randomized trials found good evidence that the use of calcium, alone or in combination with vitamin D, prevented osteoporosis in women and men age 50 years and older.[17] This study also showed a 12% reduction in the risk of fractures, with treatment being more effective at higher doses of calcium (>1200 mg) and vitamin D (>800 IU).

Based on available evidence, NOF in July 2007 updated its recommendations for daily adequate calcium and vitamin D intake to provide 1000 mg of elemental calcium and 400–800 IU of vitamin D daily for adults under age 50 years and 1200 mg of elemental calcium and 800–1000 IU of vitamin D daily for adults age 50 years or older.[73] These recommended doses should be taken in two or three divided doses daily and used in addition to other nonpharmacologic modalities. Specific dosing recommendations provided by the National Academy of Sciences, NOF, and the National Institutes of Health Consensus Panel are outlined in Table 2. It is important to note that all studies assessing osteoporosis medications included calcium and vitamin D as background therapy. Thus, for patients with osteoporosis or who are at high risk of developing osteoporosis (e.g., patients with osteopenia; those with prior vertebral, nonvertebral, or hip fracture; patients with a history of long-term systemic corticosteroid use), use of an antiresorptive or anabolic agent in addition to nonpharmacologic modalities and calcium and vitamin D supplementation should be considered.

Pharmacologic Therapies. A wide range of medications are used in the prevention and treatment of osteoporosis (Table 3). In addition to bisphosphonates, which are the primary treatment approach, other therapies, such as calcitonin, estrogen-replacement therapies or estrogen-receptor modulators, and teriparatide, are approved by the Food and Drug Administration (FDA) for the prevention or treatment of osteoporosis. Several other therapies are currently under investigation (Table 4).

Bisphosphonates. The bisphosphonates alendronate, risedronate, ibandronate, and zoledronic acid are nitrogen-containing compounds that increase BMD by inhibiting osteoclast-mediated bone resorption.[76] They have been shown to increase BMD approximately 2–8%, depending upon the dose and site measured, and have demonstrated efficacy in primary and secondary prevention of osteoporotic fractures.[18-25]

In the Fracture Intervention Trials (FIT), the effects of alendronate in patients with and without vertebral fractures were evaluated. In the arm that included patients without vertebral fractures, 4432 women (mean age 68 years) who had low BMD (mean t score, −0.6) with no history of vertebral fracture were randomized to receive either alendronate 5 mg for two years followed by 10 mg for two years or placebo.[18] After a mean follow-up of 4.2 years, women treated with alendronate demonstrated a 14% decrease in the rate of new clinical fractures, but this decrease was not statistically significant (hazard ratio [HR] = 0.86; 95% CI, 0.73–1.01). However, in patients with a femoral t score of <−2.5, the rate of clinical fractures was reduced by 36% (NNT = 15; 95% CI, 0.50–0.82) and clinical vertebral fractures decreased by 50% (NNT = 34; 95% CI, 0.31–0.82). Of the women who had at least one vertebral fracture (n = 2027), alendronate decreased the rate of clinical fractures by 55% at the vertebrae (NNT = 37; 95% CI, 0.27–0.72), by 51% at the hip (NNT = 91; 95% CI, 0.23–0.99), and by 48% at the wrist (NNT = 53; 95% CI, 0.31–0.87).[19]

Risedronate has also been associated with a decreased risk of vertebral, nonvertebral, and hip fractures. In the Vertebral Efficacy with Risedronate Therapy in North America (VERT-NA) and Vertebral Efficacy with Risedronate Therapy—Multinational (VERT-MN) studies, risedronate sodium 2.5 and 5 mg daily were compared with placebo in ambulatory postmenopausal women with at least one vertebral fracture.[20,21] The 2.5-mg treatment option was discontinued after one year in the VERT-NA study and after two years in the VERT-MN study. After three years, the rate of new vertebral fractures decreased in risedronate-treated women by 41% in VERT-NA (NNT = 20; 95% CI, 0.18–0.58; p = 0.003) and by 49% in VERT-MN (NNT = 10; 95% CI, 0.66–0.73; p < 0.001); nonvertebral fractures decreased by 39% (NNT = 31; 95% CI, 0.06–0.61; p = 0.02) and 33% (95% CI, 0.44–1.04; p = 0.063) in the VERT-NA and VERT-MN studies, respectively. In another study specifically designed to assess hip-fracture prevention, women age 70–79 years with confirmed osteoporosis (mean femoral neck t score, −3.7) or women age 80 years or older with at least one clinical risk factor were randomized to receive either risedronate sodium 2.5 or 5 mg daily or placebo. After three years, risedronate decreased the overall risk of hip fracture by 30% (NNT = 91; 95% CI, 0.6–0.9; p = 0.02). However, this effect was limited only to women age 70–79 years who had confirmed osteoporosis (relative risk [RR] =

Table 3.
Medications Used in the Management of Postmenopausal Osteoporosis

Agent	Labeled Indications	Typical Dosage	Fracture Reduction Data Available		
			Vertebral	Nonvertebral	Hip
Bisphosphonates[a]					
Alendronate	Prevention and treatment[80]	10 mg p.o. daily or 70 mg p.o. weekly[b]	Yes[18,19]	Yes[19]	Yes[19]
Ibandronate	Prevention and treatment[81,82]	2.5 mg p.o. daily or 150 mg p.o. monthly	Yes[23]	No	No
		3 mg i.v. every 3 mo	No	No	No
Risedronate	Prevention and treatment[83]	5 mg p.o. daily, 35 mg p.o. weekly, or 75 mg p.o. given on two consecutive days monthly (2 tablets/mo)	Yes[20,21]	Yes[20]	Yes[20]
Zoledronic acid	Treatment[84]	5 mg i.v. once yearly	Yes[24,25]	Yes[24,25]	Yes[25]
Calcitonin	Treatment[85]	1 spray (200 IU) intranasally, alternating nostrils daily	Yes[26]	No	No
Estrogen-replacement therapy	Prevention[86]	0.625 mg conjugated estrogens p.o. daily	Yes[27,28]	Yes[27,28]	Yes[27,28]
Raloxifene	Prevention and treatment[87]	60 mg p.o. daily	Yes[29]	No	No
Teriparatide	Treatment in patients at high risk for fracture[88,c]	20 μg s.c. daily	Yes[30]	Yes[30]	No

[a]Alendronate and risedronate are approved for the treatment of osteoporosis in men, glucocorticoid-induced osteoporosis, and Paget's disease. Ibandronate and zoledronic acid injections are approved only for treatment in postmenopausal women.
[b]Dosage for treatment. May use 5 mg p.o. daily or 35 mg p.o. weekly for the prevention of osteoporosis.[80]
[c]Approved for the treatment of osteoporosis in men at high risk for fracture.

Table 4.
Investigational Agents for the Treatment of Osteoporosis

Agent	Typical Dosage	Fracture Reduction Data Available		
		Vertebral	Nonvertebral	Hip
Denosumab	30 mg s.c. every 3 mo or 60 mg s.c. every 6 mo[89]	No	No	No
Parathyroid hormone 1-84	100 μg s.c. daily	Yes[90]	No	No
Sodium fluoride, sustained release	25 mg p.o. b.i.d. for 12 mo, then 2-mo drug-free interval[91,92]	Yes[91–93]	No	No
Strontium ranelate	2 g p.o. daily[94,95]	Yes[94,95]	Yes[95]	Yes[95,a]

[a]Hip fracture reduction seen only in patients at high risk (age ≥74 years with femoral neck bone mineral density t score of ≤-3).

0.60; NNT = 77; 95% CI, 0.4–0.9; $p = 0.009$), not in women selected primarily on the basis of clinical risk factors (RR = 0.80; 95% CI, 0.6–1.2; $p = 0.35$).

Ibandronate is the newest oral bisphosphonate approved for the prevention and treatment of postmenopausal osteoporosis. In the Oral Ibandronate Osteoporosis Vertebral Fracture Trial in North America and Europe (BONE) of 2946 postmenopausal women (mean age, 69 years) with a BMD t score of –2.0 to –5.0 in at least one vertebra (L1–4), ibandronate sodium 2.5 mg daily or 20 mg every other day for 12 doses every three months for three years decreased the risk of new vertebral fractures by 62% (NNT = 20; 95% CI, 0.41–0.75; $p = 0.0001$) and 50% (NNT = 21; 95% CI, 0.22–0.66; $p = 0.0006$), respectively, compared with placebo.[23] There was no significant difference in the frequency of nonvertebral fractures (8.2%, 9.1%, and 8.9% for daily ibandronate, intermittent ibandronate, and placebo, respectively). However, baseline BMD at the proximal femur and femoral

neck was relatively high (mean t scores, –1.73 and –2.03, respectively) compared with that found in other studies.

The use of intermittent i.v. bisphosphonate infusions for osteoporosis has been investigated. Ibandronate sodium injection given as a 3-mg i.v. infusion once every three months was recently approved by FDA for the treatment of postmenopausal osteoporosis.[80] In the Phase III, randomized, double-dummy, Dosing Intravenous Administration (DIVA) study, ibandronate sodium injection given as a 3-mg i.v. infusion once every three months for one year to 1395 postmenopausal women (mean age, 66–67 years) increased BMD at the lumbar spine and total hip to a greater extent than did 2.5 mg given orally (4.8% versus 3.8% and 2.1% versus 1.5%, respectively) ($p < 0.05$ for both comparisons).[97]

Zoledronic acid has also been found to increase BMD in a similar manner when given as an intermittent i.v. infusion.[98] In August 2007, zoledronic acid became the first bisphosphonate to receive FDA-approved labeling for once-

yearly administration in the treatment of osteoporosis in postmenopausal women.[84] Results of the Health Outcomes and Reduced Incidence with Zoledronic Acid Once Yearly (HORIZON) Pivotal Fracture Trial (PFT) demonstrated that a 5-mg i.v. infusion given once yearly for three years was effective in reducing the risk of new vertebral fractures by 70% (NNT = 13, $p < 0.001$), hip fractures by 41% (NNT = 91, $p = 0.002$), and nonvertebral fractures by 25% (NNT = 37, $p < 0.001$).[25] While most adverse effects were similar between groups, atrial fibrillation was more common in those receiving zoledronic acid (20 versus 50 patients) (NNH = 125, $p < 0.001$).

The subsequent HORIZON Recurrent Fracture Study assessing the effect of once-yearly zoledronic acid i.v. within 90 days after surgical repair of a hip fracture reduced the risk of any new clinical fracture by 35% (NNT = 19, $p = 0.001$), new clinical vertebral fractures by 46% (NNT = 48, $p = 0.02$), and new nonvertebral fractures by 27% (NNT = 32, $p = 0.03$) compared to placebo.[24] There was no statistically significant reduction in hip fractures (2.0% versus 3.5%, $p = 0.18$). However, mortality was reduced by 28% (NNT = 27, $p = 0.01$). The rate of atrial fibrillation in the zoledronic acid group (1.1%) was similar to the placebo group (1.3%).

While administration of bisphosphonates for postmenopausal osteoporosis allows for intermittent dosing (i.e., 70 mg orally once weekly for alendronate, 35 mg orally once weekly or 75 mg orally given on two consecutive days once a month for risedronate, 150 mg orally every month or 3 mg i.v. every three months for ibandronate, and 5 mg i.v. once yearly for zoledronic acid), it is important to note that, with the exception of zoledronic acid, studies specifically designed to assess fracture equivalency are lacking. Data demonstrating equivalency of BMD effects for oral intermittent and daily dosing are available.[99–101] Thus, intermittent regimens may be advocated, as they are likely to have similar efficacy regarding fracture reduction and have the potential to increase adherence and improve gastrointestinal tolerability,[102,103] though future studies are needed to confirm these benefits. In addition, while other bisphosphonates with a variety of indications are available (e.g., etidronate, pamidronate, tiludronate), these agents lack data demonstrating fracture reduction in postmenopausal osteoporosis and should not be used as a first-line treatment for this indication.

The long-term bone safety of bisphosphonates has recently been questioned. Unusual fractures and delayed healing, possibly due to oversuppression of bone turnover, have been reported.[103,105] In addition, there have been highly publicized cases of osteonecrosis of the jaw.[106] However, it is important to note that the majority of cases have occurred with i.v. bisphosphonates in patients with multiple myeloma and metastatic cancer of the skeleton, where the dosages used are considerably higher than those used for osteoporosis.[106] Thus, it is not known whether patients using bisphosphonates for the prevention or treatment of osteoporosis are at significant increased risk. In addition, long-term studies of alendronate and risedronate have not demonstrated these adverse effects.[107,108] Considering the increasing use of these agents, continued monitoring for potential adverse bone effects should be advocated.

Calcitonin. Calcitonin is a 32-amino-acid peptide that inhibits osteoclast-mediated bone resorption.[109] The salmon form is approximately 40-fold more potent than the human form, due to conformational flexibility.[110] Data are available

that support the use of salmon calcitonin for treatment of vertebral fractures in women with osteoporosis, though nonvertebral fracture data are generally lacking. In the Prevent Recurrence of Osteoporotic Fractures (PROOF) study, intranasal salmon calcitonin (100, 200, or 400 IU daily) was compared with placebo in 1255 postmenopausal women with preexisting vertebral compression fractures.[26] After five years of follow-up, 200 IU of salmon calcitonin daily was associated with a 33% decrease in the rate of new vertebral fractures (NNT = 13; RR = 0.67; 95% CI, 0.47–0.97; $p = 0.03$). No significant differences in the rate of new vertebral fractures were demonstrated in patients taking 100 or 400 IU of salmon calcitonin. One factor that may have limited the findings of this study was the high dropout rate. Fifty-nine percent of patients withdrew from the study early, though rates of discontinuation were similar in all treatment groups. In addition to the ability to prevent future vertebral fractures, salmon calcitonin also appears to possess analgesic activity.[111,112] Thus, this agent may be useful in the treatment of acute vertebral fractures, in which back pain can be significant.

Estrogen. Although estrogen-replacement therapy (ERT) was used as an antiresorptive therapy for many years for the prevention or treatment of osteoporosis, there was a paucity of data from clinical trials demonstrating a reduction in the risk of fractures, particularly at the hip. Previous recommendations for routine use of estrogen were based on observational studies and meta-analyses that indicated an approximate 30–60% reduction in vertebral and nonvertebral fractures with five or more years of ERT use.[113–116]

With the publication of the results of the WHI study, guidelines for ERT have significantly changed, now recommending against the use of ERT solely to prevent osteoporosis and encouraging the use of alternative therapies first.[1,3] The WHI study was the largest randomized, prospective trial to evaluate the risks and benefits of estrogen with and without a progestin in healthy postmenopausal women. The estrogen plus progestin group included 16,608 women with an intact uterus who received either 0.625 mg of conjugated equine estrogen (CEE) plus 2.5 mg of medroxyprogesterone acetate or placebo.[27] The estrogen-only group included 10,739 women with a prior hysterectomy who received 0.625 mg of CEE daily or placebo.[28] After an average follow-up of 5.2 years, estrogen plus progestin was discontinued due to a slightly increased risk of breast cancer (NNH = 237). In addition, investigators found that these women had a small increase in the risk of coronary heart disease (CHD) (NNH = 237), pulmonary embolism (NNH = 227), stroke (NNH = 225), and deep venous thrombosis (NNH = 141). There was a slight decrease in the risk of hip fracture (NNT = 345), clinical vertebral fracture (NNT = 387), and lower arm or wrist fracture (NNT = 125).[117] Likewise, estrogen-only therapy was discontinued after a mean follow-up of 6.8 years due to lack of benefit for the primary outcome of CHD and an increased risk of stroke (NNH = 125). While the estrogen-only group did have an increased risk of deep venous thrombosis (NNH = 220), there was no increased risk of pulmonary embolism or breast cancer. CEE alone did decrease the risk of hip and vertebral fractures slightly (NNT = 216 and NNT = 225, respectively).

Based on the results of the WHI study, estrogen should not be used to prevent CHD or as first-line therapy for postmenopausal osteoporosis and should generally be used

at the lowest therapeutic dosage for the shortest time possible to control significant menopausal symptoms (e.g., hot flashes).[27,28,118] Strong consideration of other medications that have been shown to decrease the risk of fractures and weighing of the risks and benefits are recommended before using estrogen solely to prevent osteoporosis.

Raloxifene. Raloxifene is a selective estrogen receptor modulator that has estrogenic effects on some tissues (e.g., bone [≈2–3% increase in BMD depending on dosage and site measured], lipid metabolism, clotting cascade) while having antiestrogenic effects on others (e.g., uterine endometrium, breast tissue).[29,119] Data are available that support the use of raloxifene for the treatment of osteoporosis. In the Multiple Outcomes of Raloxifene Evaluation (MORE), 7705 postmenopausal women (mean age, 67 years) with osteoporosis were randomized to receive raloxifene 60 mg daily, raloxifene 120 mg daily, or placebo.[29] After 36 months, the use of raloxifene 60 and 120 mg daily was associated with a 30% and 50% decrease in the rate of new vertebral fractures, respectively (NNT = 29; 95% CI, 0.5–0.8 and NNT = 21; 95% CI, 0.4–0.7). There was no significant difference in the rate of nonvertebral fractures (RR = 0.9; 95% CI, 0.8–1.1). Importantly, raloxifene increased the rate of venous thromboembolism (NNH = 143; 95% CI, 1.5–6.2). Raloxifene was not associated with vaginal bleeding or breast pain, and patients who took the drug had a lower incidence of breast cancer than women who received placebo (RR = 0.3; 95% CI, 0.2–0.6). However, hot flashes were more common in the raloxifene group (9.7% and 11.7% for the 60- and 120-mg dosages, respectively, versus 6.5% for placebo).

The role of raloxifene in the management of osteoporosis may be further elucidated with the publication of two recent studies. The National Surgical Adjuvant Breast and Bowel Project Study of Tamoxifen and Raloxifene (STAR) P-2 study was a prospective, double-blind, randomized trial of 19,247 postmenopausal women (mean age, 58.5 years) with an increased risk of breast cancer (mean risk, 4.03%).[120] After a mean follow-up of 3.9 years, raloxifene 60 mg daily was shown to be as effective as tamoxifen in decreasing the risk of invasive breast cancer (168 cases with raloxifene versus 163 cases with tamoxifen) (RR = 1.02; 95% CI, 0.82–1.28). The Raloxifene for Use of the Heart (RUTH) study, a prospective, double-blind, randomized trial of 10,101 postmenopausal women (mean age, 67.5 years) with CHD or multiple risk factors for CHD, was designed to assess the effects of raloxifene 60 mg daily on cardiovascular disease.[121] After a median follow-up of 5.6 years, raloxifene did not decrease the risk of the primary outcome of death from coronary causes, myocardial infarction, or hospitalization for acute coronary syndrome (HR = 0.95; 95% CI, 0.84–1.07) or stroke (HR = 1.10; 95% CI, 0.92–1.32), though it did increase the risk of venous thromboembolism (NNH = 157) and fatal stroke (NNH = 251). Similar to other studies, raloxifene did decrease the risk of clinical vertebral fractures (NNT = 154), noninvasive breast cancer (NNT = 169), estrogen-receptor positive breast cancer (NNT = 169), and death from noncardiovascular and noncancer causes (NNT = 118 and NNT = 138, respectively).

The use of raloxifene for the management of osteoporosis should be based on a risk–benefit assessment. It may be an ideal choice for women who have contraindications to or do not tolerate a bisphosphonate, are not experiencing vasomotor symptoms, and do not have CHD or multiple risk factors for CHD. In addition, it may be particularly appealing for patients at high risk for breast cancer.

Teriparatide. Teriparatide, a recombinant form of parathyroid hormone (PTH 1-34), may increase or decrease BMD, depending on the route of administration. Given as an exogenous, intermittent injection, teriparatide increases BMD by stimulating bone formation.[122] The effects of teriparatide in postmenopausal women with prior vertebral fractures have been evaluated. In a placebo-controlled study of 1637 postmenopausal women (mean age, 69 years) with at least one prior vertebral fracture 20 and 40 μg of teriparatide given daily by subcutaneous injection decreased the rate of new vertebral fractures by 65% and 69%, respectively (NNT = 11 and NNT = 10).[30] In addition, new nonvertebral fragility fractures were decreased 53% and 54% for the 20- and 40-μg groups, respectively (NNT = 33 for both treatment groups).

Data from rat carcinogenicity studies have suggested a possible increased risk of osteosarcomas associated with the use of PTH 1–34 analogues.[122] Thus, teriparatide should not be used in patients who have an increased risk of developing osteosarcomas (e.g., those with Paget's disease of bone or unexplained elevations of alkaline phosphatase, open epiphyses, or prior external beam or implant radiation therapy involving the skeleton), and administration should be limited to two years' use.[88] In addition, due to significant costs (≈$850 per month[123]) and the need for daily injections, teriparatide should only be used in patients with established osteoporosis who have a high risk of future fractures or who are intolerant to or have contraindications to both bisphosphonates and raloxifene.

Combination therapies. There are limited data supporting the use of combination antiresorptive treatments for osteoporosis. While data are available demonstrating greater increases in BMD with the use of estrogen or raloxifene in combination with a bisphosphonate,[124-127] fracture data are lacking. In addition, the use of a bisphosphonate with PTH 1-84 or PTH 1-34 may result in attenuation of the anabolic effects of PTH,[128,129] though sequential treatment with a bisphosphonate after therapy with PTH 1-84 appears to maintain or increase BMD gains.[130] Thus, until fracture outcomes data are available, concurrent combination therapy should generally be avoided or used with caution by an osteoporosis specialist.

Investigational treatments. Denosumab is a monoclonal antibody to the receptor activator for nuclear factor-kappa B ligand (RANKL) that mimics osteoprotegerin and decreases bone resorption through inhibition of osteoclast differential, activation, and survival.[131] In a recent Phase II study, the safety and efficacy of denosumab were assessed in 412 postmenopausal women (mean age, 63 years) with low BMD (mean lumbar t score, −2.0 to −2.3; mean femoral neck t score, −1.7 to −2.0).[89] Patients were randomized to receive subcutaneous denosumab every 3 months (doses of 6, 14, or 30 mg), every 6 months (doses of 14, 16, or 30 mg), open-label alendronate sodium 70 mg p.o. weekly, or placebo. After 12 months of treatment, denosumab increased BMD at the lumbar spine by 3.0–6.7% (versus 4.8% with alendronate and −0.8% with placebo [p < 0.001 for comparison of denosumab with placebo]) and total hip by 1.9–3.6% (versus 2.1% with alendronate and −0.6% with placebo [p < 0.001 for comparison of denosumab with placebo]). Thus, denosumab holds promise as a future agent and may be particularly appealing from an adherence standpoint, though data regarding its ability to protect against fractures are needed.

PTH 1-84 is the full-length 84-amino acid PTH that was approved in April 2006 in the European Union for treatment of osteoporosis in postmenopausal women at high risk for fracture[132] and has received an approvable letter from FDA.[133] In the randomized, double-blind, placebo-controlled, Phase III Treatment of Osteoporosis with PTH (TOP) trial, 100 μg of PTH 1-84 was given subcutaneously once daily to 2532 postmenopausal women with osteoporosis (mean t score, -3.0), 19% of whom had experienced a prior vertebral fracture.[90] After a median of 18 months, PTH 1-84 decreased the risk of new vertebral fractures by 61% (NNT = 48, p = 0.001). There was no difference in the incidence of any nonvertebral fracture (5.52% for PTH 1-84 versus 5.86% for placebo).[134] In a recent international, multicenter, double-blind, randomized, parallel group trial of 2532 postmenopausal women with osteoporosis with and without prior fractures, 100 μg of PTH 1-84 given subcutaneously daily was compared with placebo.[135] After 18 months, PTH 1-84 decreased the risk of new or worsened vertebral fractures by 60% (NNT = 50, p = 0.001) in a modified intent-to-treat analysis, though this rate change was based on assumptions of fracture rates for those who withdrew early from the study. Adverse effects that were more common in the group treated with PTH 1-84 than in the placebo group included hypercalciuria (46.0% versus 22.3%, NNH = 4), hypercalcemia (27.8% versus 4.5%, NNH = 4), nausea (22.6% versus 9.2%, NNH = 7), and vomiting (7.7% versus 4.3%, NNH = 29). Thus, PTH 1-84 has potential as a future anabolic treatment for women at high risk for fracture, though comparative data with teriparatide (PTH 1-34) are needed to elucidate if any clinical differences in BMD or fracture efficacy exist between the full-length and shortened (i.e., PTH 1-34) versions.

Sodium fluoride is an anabolic agent that increases BMD by stimulating osteoblast activity.[136,137] While it has been available for many years and may be considered an alternative agent in Europe,[56] oral therapy has not been approved for use in the United States due to concerns regarding decreases in bone quality and strength, despite increases in BMD, and adverse effects such as gastrointestinal symptoms and lower-extremity pain.[138] These concerns may have been caused by higher doses and immediate-release formulations given on a continuous basis. While lower doses of a sustained-release formulation have been shown to increase BMD in vertebrae L2–L4 by 5.4% and decrease vertebral fractures by 68% (NNT = 8; 95% CI, 0.14–0.73; p = 0.007), with no additional increases in gastrointestinal and musculoskeletal adverse effects,[91] it is doubtful this agent will be approved for use in the United States.

Strontium ranelate is an orally active distrontium salt that has both anabolic and antiresorptive effects on bone.[139] It was approved in Europe in September 2004 for the treatment of postmenopausal osteoporosis[140] but is not yet approved for use in the United States. Strontium has been shown to decrease both vertebral and nonvertebral fractures. In a Phase III study of 1649 postmenopausal women with osteoporosis (mean age, 69 years) and at least one vertebral fracture, 2 g of strontium ranelate daily for three years decreased the rate of new vertebral fractures by 41% (NNT = 8; 95% CI, 0.48–0.73; p < 0.001).[94] In the Treatment of Peripheral Osteoporosis Study (TROPOS), strontium ranelate 2 g daily for three years in 5091 postmenopausal women with osteoporosis (mean age, 77 years) decreased the rate for all

nonvertebral fractures by 16% and decreased the rate of major fragility fractures (i.e., hip, wrist, pelvis, sacrum, ribs and sternum, clavicle, and humerus) by 19% (NNT = 59 for both fracture types) versus placebo.[95] There was no significant difference in hip fractures in the intent-to-treat population, but, for those in the high-risk subgroup (age ≥74 years with femoral neck BMD t score of ≤–3), there was a 36% reduction in fracture risk (NNT = 48; 95% CI, 0.412–0.997; p = 0.046). Strontium ranelate has potential as a future treatment in the United States for osteoporosis, though it remains to be seen if this agent will be brought to market.

Special Populations. *Nursing-home patients.* Approximately 80–85% of U.S. nursing-home residents suffer from osteoporosis.[141] Because nursing-home residents are often afflicted with multiple diseases, disabilities, and fragility, their fracture rates are much higher than the community-dwelling elderly. Other factors associated with the higher fracture rate among nursing-home residents include immobility, low body mass, difficulty transferring (e.g., moving from a bed to a wheelchair), falls, and multiple medications.[142] In addition, many nursing-home residents have inadequate nutritional status, including low intake of calcium and vitamin D as well as inadequate sunlight exposure.[142,143] Osteoporosis treatment for nursing-home residents ideally involves a multifactorial approach emphasizing fall prevention, adequate nutrition, strength and balance training, medication review, and environmental modifications (e.g., redesigning home environments, removal of floor rugs). While devices such as hip protectors have been shown to prevent fractures in patients at high risk,[144] more recent data indicated that these are ineffective interventions.[145] Underuse of osteoporosis diagnostic procedures in nursing-home residents is well documented.[146] Even when osteoporosis is diagnosed and documented in the medical record, few patients receive optimal therapy despite data demonstrating that screening and treatment are highly cost-effective.[147]

Calcium and vitamin D supplements are prescribed for approximately 60% of nursing-home residents with osteoporosis and only 25% of residents with hip fractures.[148] Similarly, bisphosphonate use among nursing-home residents with documented hip fractures approaches 25%.[149] Because the majority of nursing-home residents with osteoporosis receive inadequate drug therapy, ASHP urges interdisciplinary team approaches to detect and manage osteoporosis in this setting. osteoporosis guidelines are useful and may be cost-effective, with implementation dependent on cooperation from the facility medical director, attending physicians, the director of nursing, therapists, and the consultant pharmacist.[150]

Men. Two million American men have osteoporosis and another 12 million are at risk for developing osteoporosis.[151] Thirty percent of hip fractures occur in men, and one in eight men over age 50 years will have an osteoporosis-related fracture in his lifetime.[152] Hip fracture-related mortality and morbidity are significantly greater in men than in women, with one-year mortality after hip fracture approximately double that of women.[153] After sustaining a hip fracture, up to 50% of men require institutional care.

Despite the serious consequences of hip fracture for men, osteoporosis has only recently received attention as a major men's health issue. There remain significant barriers, particularly reimbursement for screening. Medicare

will only cover screening costs for "qualified individuals": estrogen-deficient women, individuals with vertebral abnormalities, those with known primary hyperparathyroidism, individuals receiving steroid therapy, and those receiving FDA-approved osteoporosis medications.[154] Risk factors associated with osteoporosis in men include hypogonadism associated with low testosterone and low estradiol, chronic diseases, chronic obstructive pulmonary disease, prolonged exposure to osteoporosis-inducing medications, Caucasian race, heredity, and advanced age.[151,155] Lifestyle may increase the risk of osteoporosis in men, including current smoking, excessive alcohol use, low calcium intake, and low physical activity. The Male Osteoporosis Risk Estimation Score, or MORES, has been developed as one approach to identify men age 60 years or older at risk for osteoporosis.[156] Those men found to be at risk should be referred for a DEXA scan. Osteoporosis treatment in men comprises calcium and vitamin D supplements; bisphosphonates; testosterone replacement, if indicated (i.e., hypogonadism); and teriparatide for men at high risk of fracture.[1,129,157]

Summary

ASHP believes that patients at risk for osteoporosis and related fractures (e.g., women age 65 years or older regardless of risk factors, postmenopausal women under age 65 years with risk factors, postmenopausal women with a history of nontraumatic fracture, men with a significant risk of fracture) should receive appropriate risk assessment and evaluation of BMD using central DEXA. Patients with confirmed low BMD who are at risk for fractures should receive treatment. ASHP believes that medications shown to reduce the risk of fractures should be used. These include calcium and vitamin D for all patients, bisphosphonates, raloxifene, calcitonin, estrogen, and teriparatide. ASHP acknowledges that the choice of agent will depend on its ability to increase BMD and decrease fractures, as well as various patient-specific criteria (e.g., medical history, contraindications, patient beliefs or preferences, finances). In general, agents that have been shown to decrease vertebral, nonvertebral, and hip fractures should be used preferentially.

ASHP believes that clinicians need to be actively involved in educating both patients and collaborative health care professionals regarding risk factors associated with osteoporosis and fractures. Efforts should include recommendations for appropriate weight-bearing exercise, identification of agents that may decrease BMD (e.g., corticosteroids) or increase the risk for falls (e.g., long-acting benzodiazepines), and appropriate calcium and vitamin D intake. Well-designed clinical trials are needed to better assess who should be screened, compare various medications' effects on fracture rates, and better identify patients who should receive treatment with antiresorptives, anabolic agents, or combination therapy.

References

1. National Osteoporosis Foundation. Physician's guide to prevention and treatment of osteoporosis. www.nof.org/physguide/index.htm (accessed 2005 Mar 23).
2. NIH Consensus Development Panel on Osteoporosis Prevention, Diagnosis, and Therapy. Osteoporosis prevention, diagnosis, and therapy. *JAMA.* 2001; 285:785–95.
3. Hodgson SF, Watts NB, Bilezikian JP et al. American Association of Clinical Endocrinologists medical guidelines for clinical practice for the prevention and treatment of postmenopausal osteoporosis: 2001 edition, with selected updates for 2003. *Endocr Pract.* 2003; 9:544–64. [Erratum, *Endocr Pract.* 2004; 10:90.]
4. Hajcsar EE, Hawker G, Bogoch ER. Investigation and treatment of osteoporosis in patients with fragility fractures. *CMAJ.* 2000; 163:819–22.
5. Feldstein AC, Nichols GA, Elmer PJ et al. Older women with fractures: patients falling through the cracks of guideline-recommended osteoporosis screening and treatment. *J Bone Joint Surg Am.* 2003; 85-A:2294–302.
6. Andrade SE, Majumdar SR, Chan KA et al. Low frequency of treatment of osteoporosis among postmenopausal women following a fracture. *Arch Intern Med.* 2003; 163:2052–7.
7. Harrington JT, Broy SB, Derosa AM et al. Hip fracture patients are not treated for osteoporosis: a call to action. *Arthritis Rheum.* 2002; 47:651–4.
8. Solomon DH, Finkelstein JS, Katz JN et al. Underuse of osteoporosis medications in elderly patients with fractures. *Am J Med.* 2003; 115:398–400.
9. Adler GS, Shatto A. Screening for osteoporosis and colon cancer under Medicare. *Health Care Financ Rev.* 2002; 23:189–200.
10. National Committee for Quality Assurance. Osteoporosis management in women who had a fracture. In: The state of health care quality, 2005. www.ncqa.org/Docs/SOHCQ_2005.pdf (accessed 2007 Nov 27).
11. Centers for Disease Control and Prevention and National Institutes of Health. Healthy People 2010: arthritis, osteoporosis, and chronic back conditions. www.healthypeople.gov/Document/HTML/Volume1/02Arthritis.htm (accessed 2006 Jul 11).
12. Chapuy MC, Arlot ME, Duboeuf F et al. Vitamin D3 and calcium to prevent hip fractures in the elderly women. *N Engl J Med.* 1992; 327:1637–42.
13. Dawson-Hughes B, Harris SS, Krall EA et al. Effect of calcium and vitamin D supplementation on bone density in men and women 65 years of age or older. *N Engl J Med.* 1997; 337:670–6.
14. Larsen ER, Mosekilde L, Foldspang A. Vitamin D and calcium supplementation prevents osteoporotic fractures in elderly community dwelling residents: a pragmatic population-based 3-year intervention study. *J Bone Miner Res.* 2004; 19:370–8.
15. Trivedi DP, Doll R, Khaw KT. Effect of four monthly oral vitamin D3 (cholecalciferol) supplementation on fractures and mortality in men and women living in the community: randomised double blind controlled trial. *BMJ.* 2003; 326:469.
16. Tilyard MW, Spears GF, Thomson J et al. Treatment of postmenopausal osteoporosis with calcitriol or calcium. *N Engl J Med.* 1992; 326:357–62.
17. Tang BM, Eslick GD, Nowson C et al. Use of calcium or calcium in combination with vitamin D supplementation to prevent fractures and bone loss in people aged

50 years and older: a meta-analysis. *Lancet.* 2007; 370:657–66.

18. Cummings SR, Black DM, Thompson DE et al. Effect of alendronate on risk of fracture in women with low bone density but without vertebral fractures: results from the Fracture Intervention Trial. *JAMA.* 1998; 280:2077–82.

19. Black DM, Cummings SR, Karpf DB et al. Randomised trial of effect of alendronate on risk of fracture in women with existing vertebral fractures. *Lancet.* 1996; 348:1535–41.

20. Harris ST, Watts NB, Genant HK et al. Effects of risedronate treatment on vertebral and nonvertebral fractures in women with postmenopausal osteoporosis: a randomized controlled trial. *JAMA.* 1999; 282:1344–52.

21. Reginster J, Minne HW, Sorensen OH et al. Randomized trial of the effects of risedronate on vertebral fractures in women with established postmenopausal osteoporosis. *Osteoporos Int.* 2000; 11:83–91.

22. McClung MR, Geusens P, Miller PD et al. Effect of risedronate on the risk of hip fracture in elderly women. *N Engl J Med.* 2001; 344:333–40.

23. Chesnut IC, Skag A, Christiansen C et al. Effects of oral ibandronate administered daily or intermittently on fracture risk in postmenopausal osteoporosis. *J Bone Miner Res.* 2004; 19:1241–9.

24. Lyles KW, Colón-Emeric CS, Magaziner JS et al. Zoledronic acid and clinical fractures and mortality after hip fracture. *N Engl J Med.* 2007; 357:1799–809.

25. Black DM, Delmas PD, Eastell R et al. Once-yearly zoledronic acid for treatment of postmenopausal osteoporosis. *N Engl J Med.* 2007; 356:1809–22.

26. Chesnut CH 3rd, Silverman S, Andriano K et al. A randomized trial of nasal spray salmon calcitonin in postmenopausal women with established osteoporosis: the Prevent Recurrence Of Osteoporotic Fractures Study. *Am J Med.* 2000; 109:267–76.

27. Writing Group for the Women's Health Initiative Investigators. Risks and benefits of estrogen plus progestin in healthy postmenopausal women: principal results from the Women's Health Initiative randomized controlled trial. *JAMA.* 2002; 288:321–33.

28. The Women's Health Initiative Steering Committee. Effects of conjugated equine estrogen in postmenopausal women with hysterectomy: the Women's Health Initiative randomized controlled trial. *JAMA.* 2004; 291:1701–12.

29. Ettinger B, Black DM, Mitlak BH et al. Reduction of vertebral fracture risk in postmenopausal women with osteoporosis treated with raloxifene: results from a 3-year randomized clinical trial. *JAMA.* 1999; 282:637–45.

30. Neer RM, Arnaud CD, Zanchetta JR et al. Effect of parathyroid hormone (1-34) on fractures and bone mineral density in postmenopausal women with osteoporosis. *N Engl J Med.* 2001; 344:1434–41.

31. MacLaughlin EJ, MacLaughlin AA, Snella KA et al. Osteoporosis screening and education in community pharmacies using a team approach. *Pharmacotherapy.* 2005; 25:379–86.

32. Goode JV, Swiger K, Bluml BM. Regional osteoporosis screening, referral, and monitoring program in community pharmacies: findings from Project ImPACT: Osteoporosis. *J Am Pharm Assoc.* 2004; 44:152–60.

33. Elliott ME, Meek PD, Kanous NL et al. Osteoporosis screening by community pharmacists: use of National Osteoporosis Foundation resources. *J Am Pharm Assoc.* 2002; 42:101–10.

34. Lata PF, Binkley NC, Elliott ME. Acceptability of pharmacy-based bone density measurement by women and primary healthcare providers. *Menopause.* 2002; 9:449–55.

35. Cerulli J, Zeolla MM. Impact and feasibility of a community pharmacy bone mineral density screening and education program. *J Am Pharm Assoc.* 2004; 44:161–7.

36. Kanis JA. Diagnosis of osteoporosis and assessment of fracture risk. *Lancet.* 2002; 359:1929–36.

37. World Health Organization. Diet, nutrition and the prevention of chronic diseases: report of a joint WHO/FAO Expert Consultation. WHO technical report series no. 916. http://whqlibdoc.who.int/trs/WHO_TRS_916.pdf (accessed 2007 Nov 1).

38. Kanis JA, Gluer CC. An update on the diagnosis and assessment of osteoporosis with densitometry. *Osteoporos Int.* 2000; 11:192–202.

39. National Osteoporosis Foundation. America's bone health: the state of osteoporosis and low bone mass, 2005. www.nof.org/advocacy/prevalence/index.htm (accessed 2007 Nov 28).

40. National Osteoporosis Foundation. Fast facts. www.nof.org/osteoporosis/diseasefacts.htm (accessed 2005 Apr 22).

41. Lips P, Cooper C, Agnusdei D et al. Quality of life in patients with vertebral fractures: validation of the Quality of Life Questionnaire of the European Foundation for Osteoporosis (QUALEFFO). *Osteoporos Int.* 1999; 10:150–60.

42. Gold DT, Shipp KM, Lyles KW. Managing patients with complications of osteoporosis. *Endocrinol Metab Clin North Am.* 1998; 27:485–96.

43. Yamaguchi T, Sugimoto T, Yamauchi M et al. Multiple vertebral fractures are associated with refractory reflux esophagitis in postmenopausal women. *J Bone Miner Metab.* 2005; 23:36–40.

44. Hallberg I, Rosenqvist AM, Kartous L et al. Health-related quality of life after osteoporotic fractures. *Osteoporos Int.* 2004; 15:834–41.

45. Nevitt MC, Ettinger B, Black DM et al. The association of radiographically detected vertebral fractures with back pain and function: a prospective study. *Ann Intern Med.* 1998; 128:793–800.

46. Fink HA, Ensrud KE, Nelson DB et al. Disability after clinical fracture in postmenopausal women with low bone density: the Fracture Intervention Trial (FIT). *Osteoporos Int.* 2003; 14:69–76.

47. Ensrud KE, Thompson DE, Cauley JA et al. Prevalent vertebral deformities predict mortality and hospitalization in older women with low bone mass. *J Am Geriatr Soc.* 2000; 48:241–9.

48. Margolis DJ, Knauss J, Bilker W et al. Medical conditions as risk factors for pressure ulcers in an outpatient setting. *Age Ageing.* 2003; 32:259–64.

49. Melton LJ 3rd. Adverse outcomes of osteoporotic fractures in the general population. *J Bone Miner Res.* 2003; 18:1139–41.

50. Schlaich C, Minne HW, Bruckner T et al. Reduced pulmonary function in patients with spinal osteoporotic fractures. *Osteoporos Int.* 1998; 8:261–7.

51. Adachi JD, Ioannidis G, Olszynski WP et al. The impact of incident vertebral and non-vertebral fractures on health related quality of life in postmenopausal women. *BMC Musculoskelet Disord.* 2002; 3:11.

52. Empana JP, Dargent-Molina P, Breart G. Effect of hip fracture on mortality in elderly women: the EPIDOS prospective study. *J Am Geriatr Soc.* 2004; 52:685–90.

53. Center JR, Nguyen TV, Schneider D et al. Mortality after all major types of osteoporotic fracture in men and women: an observational study. *Lancet.* 1999; 353:878–82.

54. Cauley JA, Thompson DE, Ensrud KC et al. Risk of mortality following clinical fractures. *Osteoporos Int.* 2000; 11:556–61.

55. Keene GS, Parker MJ, Pryor GA. Mortality and morbidity after hip fractures. *BMJ.* 1993; 307:1248–50.

56. New Europe Consensus on Osteoporosis. 2nd Central and Eastern European Regional Osteoporosis Meeting. www.iofbonehealth.org/download/osteofound/filemanager/policy_advocacy/pdf/lacrima.pdf (accessed 2007 Nov 27).

57. American Geriatrics Society, British Geriatrics Society, and American Academy of Orthopaedic Surgeons Panel on Falls Prevention. Guideline for the prevention of falls in older persons. *J Am Geriatr Soc.* 2001; 49:664–72.

58. Podsiadlo D, Richardson S. The timed "up & go": a test of basic functional mobility for frail elderly persons. *J Am Geriatr Soc.* 1991; 39:142–8.

59. Robbins AS, Rubenstein LZ, Josephson KR et al. Predictors of falls among elderly people. Results of two population-based studies. *Arch Intern Med.* 1989; 149:1628–33.

60. Fick DM, Cooper JW, Wade WE et al. Updating the Beers criteria for potentially inappropriate medication use in older adults: results of a US consensus panel of experts. *Arch Intern Med.* 2003; 163:2716–24.

61. Sleeper RB, Bond C, Rojas-Fernandez C. Psychotropic drugs and falls: new evidence pertaining to SSRIs. *Pharmacotherapy.* 2000; 20:308–17.

62. Agency for Healthcare Research and Quality. Screening for osteoporosis in postmenopausal women: recommendations and rationale. www.ahrq.gov/clinic/3rduspstf/osteoporosis/osteorr.htm (accessed 2005 Apr 21).

63. Lydick E, Cook K, Turpin J et al. Development and validation of a simple questionnaire to facilitate identification of women likely to have low bone density. *Am J Manag Care.* 1998; 4:37–48.

64. Cadarette SM, Jaglal SB, Kreiger N et al. Development and validation of the Osteoporosis Risk Assessment Instrument to facilitate selection of women for bone densitometry. *CMAJ.* 2000; 162:1289–94.

65. Cadarette SM, Jaglal SB, Murray TM et al. Evaluation of decision rules for referring women for bone densitometry by dual-energy x-ray absorptiometry. *JAMA.* 2001; 286:57–63.

66. International Osteoporosis Foundation. WHO Working Group on Fracture Risk Assessment. www.iofbonehealth.org/about-iof/partnerships/who.html (accessed 2006 Jul 20).

67. Kanis JA, Borgstrom F, De Laet C et al. Assessment of fracture risk. *Osteoporos Int.* 2005; 16:581–9.

68. Lewiecki EM, Watts NB, McClung MR et al. Official positions of the International Society for Clinical Densitometry. *J Clin Endocrinol Metab.* 2004; 89: 3651–5.

69. Cummings SR, Bates D, Black DM. Clinical use of bone densitometry: scientific review. *JAMA.* 2002; 288:1889–97.

70. Cummings SR, Black DM, Nevitt MC et al. Bone density at various sites for prediction of hip fractures. *Lancet.* 1993; 341:72–5.

71. Marshall D, Johnell O, Wedel H. Meta-analysis of how well measures of bone mineral density predict occurrence of osteoporotic fractures. *BMJ.* 1996; 312:1254–9.

72. Siris ES, Miller PD, Barrett-Connor E et al. Identification and fracture outcomes of undiagnosed low bone mineral density in postmenopausal women: results from the National Osteoporosis Risk Assessment. *JAMA.* 2001; 286:2815–22.

73. National Osteoporosis Foundation. National Osteoporosis Foundation's updated recommendations for calcium and vitamin D intake. www.nof.org/prevention/calcium_and_VitaminD.htm (accessed 2007 Jul 31).

74. Institute of Medicine. Dietary reference intake tables: elements. www.iom.edu/Object.File/Master/7/294/0.pdf (accessed 2005 May 3).

75. Institute of Medicine. Dietary reference intake tables: vitamins. www.iom.edu/Object.File/Master/7/296/0.pdf (accessed 2005 May 3).

76. NIH Consensus Conference. Optimal calcium intake. NIH Consensus Development Panel on Optimal Calcium Intake. *JAMA.* 1994; 272:1942–8.

77. Grant AM, Avenell A, Campbell MK et al. Oral vitamin D3 and calcium for secondary prevention of low-trauma fractures in elderly people (Randomised Evaluation of Calcium Or vitamin D, RECORD): a randomised placebo-controlled trial. *Lancet.* 2005; 365:1621–8.

78. Jackson RD, LaCroix AZ, Gass M et al. Calcium plus vitamin D supplementation and the risk of fractures. *N Engl J Med.* 2006; 354:669–83.

79. Bischoff-Ferrari HA, Willett WC, Wong JB et al. Fracture prevention with vitamin D supplementation: a meta-analysis of randomized controlled trials. *JAMA.* 2005; 293:2257–64.

80. Fosamax (alendronate) package insert. Whitehouse Station, NJ: Merck; 2004.

81. Boniva (ibandronate sodium) injection package insert. Nutley, NJ: Roche Laboratories; 2006.

82. Boniva (ibandronate sodium) package insert. Nutley, NJ: Roche Laboratories; 2005.

83. Actonel (risedronate) package insert. Cincinnati: Procter & Gamble Pharmaceuticals; 2007.

84. Reclast (zoledronic acid) injection package insert. East Hanover, NJ: Novartis Pharmaceuticals Corporation; 2007 Aug.

85. Miacalcin (calcitonin-salmon) package insert. East Hanover, NJ: Novartis; 2003.

86. Premarin (Conjugated Estrogens Tablets, USP) package insert. Philadelphia: Wyeth; 2005.

87. Evista (raloxifene) package insert. Indianapolis: Eli Lilly and Company; 2003.

88. Forteo (teriparatide [rDNA origin] injection) package insert. Indianapolis: Eli Lilly and Company; 2004.

89. McClung MR, Lewiecki EM, Cohen SB et al. Denosumab in postmenopausal women with low bone mineral density. N Engl J Med. 2006; 354:821–31.

90. Greenspan SL, Bone HG, Marriott TB et al. Preventing the first vertebral fracture in postmenopausal women with low bone mass using PTH (1-84): results from the TOP study. J Bone Miner Res. 2005; 05-A-1321-ASBMR. Abstract.

91. Rubin CD, Pak CY, Adams-Huet B et al. Sustained-release sodium fluoride in the treatment of the elderly with established osteoporosis. Arch Intern Med. 2001; 161:2325–33.

92. Pak CY, Sakhaee K, Adams-Huet B et al. Treatment of postmenopausal osteoporosis with slow-release sodium fluoride. Final report of a randomized controlled trial. Ann Intern Med. 1995; 123:401–8.

93. Reginster JY, Meurmans L, Zegels B et al. The effect of sodium monofluorophosphate plus calcium on vertebral fracture rate in postmenopausal women with moderate osteoporosis. A randomized, controlled trial. Ann Intern Med. 1998; 129:1–8.

94. Meunier PJ, Roux C, Seeman E et al. The effects of strontium ranelate on the risk of vertebral fracture in women with postmenopausal osteoporosis. N Engl J Med. 2004; 350:459–68.

95. Reginster JY, Seeman E, De Vernejoul MC et al. Strontium ranelate reduces the risk of nonvertebral fractures in postmenopausal women with osteoporosis: Treatment of Peripheral Osteoporosis Study (TROPOS). J Clin Endocrinol Metab. 2005; 90:2816–22.

96. Licata AA. Discovery, clinical development, and therapeutic uses of bisphosphonates. Ann Pharmacother. 2005; 39:668–77.

97. Delmas PD, Adami S, Strugala C et al. Intravenous ibandronate injections in postmenopausal women with osteoporosis: one-year results from the dosing intravenous administration study. Arthritis Rheum. 2006; 54:1838–46.

98. Reid IR, Brown JP, Burckhardt P et al. Intravenous zoledronic acid in postmenopausal women with low bone mineral density. N Engl J Med. 2002; 346:653–61.

99. Rizzoli R, Greenspan SL, Bone G III et al. Two-year results of once-weekly administration of alendronate 70 mg for the treatment of postmenopausal osteoporosis. J Bone Miner Res. 2002; 17:1988–96.

100. Brown JP, Kendler DL, McClung MR et al. The efficacy and tolerability of risedronate once a week for the treatment of postmenopausal osteoporosis. Calcif Tissue Int. 2002; 71:103–11.

101. Miller PD, McClung MR, Macovei L et al. Monthly oral ibandronate therapy in postmenopausal osteoporosis: 1-year results from the MOBILE study. J Bone Miner Res. 2005; 20:1315–22.

102. Tsun EC, Heck AM. Intermittent dosing of alendronate. Ann Pharmacother. 2001; 35:1471–5.

103. Bauss F, Russell RG. Ibandronate in osteoporosis: preclinical data and rationale for intermittent dosing. Osteoporos Int. 2004; 15:423–33.

104. Odvina CV, Zerwekh JE, Rao DS et al. Severely suppressed bone turnover: a potential complication of alendronate therapy. J Clin Endocrinol Metab. 2005; 90:1294–301.

105. Ott SM. Long-term safety of bisphosphonates. J Clin Endocrinol Metab. 2005; 90:1897–9.

106. Woo SB, Hellstein JW, Kalmar JR. Systematic review: bisphosphonates and osteonecrosis of the jaws. Ann Intern Med. 2006; 144:753–61.

107. Ensrud KE, Barrett-Connor EL, Schwartz A et al. Randomized trial of effect of alendronate continuation versus discontinuation in women with low BMD: results from the Fracture Intervention Trial long-term extension. J Bone Miner Res. 2004; 19:1259–69.

108. Ste-Marie LG, Sod E, Johnson T et al. Five years of treatment with risedronate and its effects on bone safety in women with postmenopausal osteoporosis. Calcif Tissue Int. 2004; 75:469–76.

109. Pondel M. Calcitonin and calcitonin receptors: bone and beyond. Int J Exp Pathol. 2000; 81:405–22.

110. Zaidi M, Moonga BS, Abe E. Calcitonin and bone formation: a knockout full of surprises. J Clin Invest. 2002; 110:1769–71.

111. Lyritis GP, Paspati I, Karachalios T et al. Pain relief from nasal salmon calcitonin in osteoporotic vertebral crush fractures. A double blind, placebo-controlled clinical study. Acta Orthop Scand Suppl. 1997; 275:112–4.

112. Lyritis GP, Tsakalakos N, Magiasis B et al. Analgesic effect of salmon calcitonin in osteoporotic vertebral fractures: a double-blind placebo-controlled clinical study. Calcif Tissue Int. 1991; 49:369–72.

113. Naessen T, Persson I, Adami HO et al. Hormone replacement therapy and the risk for first hip fracture. A prospective, population-based cohort study. Ann Intern Med. 1990; 113:95–103.

114. Torgerson DJ, Bell-Syer SE. Hormone replacement therapy and prevention of nonvertebral fractures: a meta-analysis of randomized trials. JAMA. 2001; 285:2891–7.

115. Torgerson DJ, Bell-Syer SE. Hormone replacement therapy and prevention of vertebral fractures: a meta-analysis of randomised trials. BMC Musculoskelet Disord. 2001; 2:7.

116. Weiss NS, Ure CL, Ballard JH et al. Decreased risk of fractures of the hip and lower forearm with postmenopausal use of estrogen. N Engl J Med. 1980; 303:1195–8.

117. Cauley JA, Robbins J, Chen Z et al. Effects of estrogen plus progestin on risk of fracture and bone mineral density: the Women's Health Initiative randomized trial. JAMA. 2003; 290:1729–38.

118. National Heart, Lung, and Blood Institute. Facts about postmenopausal hormone therapy. www.nhlbi.nih.gov/health/women/pht_facts.htm (accessed 2005 May 6).

119. Delmas PD, Bjarnason NH, Mitlak BH et al. Effects of raloxifene on bone mineral density, serum cholesterol concentrations, and uterine endometrium in postmenopausal women. N Engl J Med. 1997; 337:1641–7.

120. Vogel VG, Costantino JP, Wickerham DL et al. Effects of tamoxifen vs raloxifene on the risk of developing invasive breast cancer and other disease outcomes: the

NSABP Study of Tamoxifen and Raloxifene (STAR) P-2 trial. *JAMA.* 2006; 295:2727–41.

121. Barrett-Connor E, Mosca L, Collins P et al. Effects of raloxifene on cardiovascular events and breast cancer in postmenopausal women. *N Engl J Med.* 2006; 355:125–37.

122. Hodsman AB, Bauer DC, Dempster D et al. Parathyroid hormone and teriparatide for the treatment of osteoporosis: a review of the evidence and suggested guidelines for its use. *Endocr Rev.* 2005; 26:688–703.

123. DrugStore.com. Drug prices and information: Forteo. www.drugstore.com/pharmacy/prices/drugprice.asp?ndc=00002897101&trx=1Z5066#info (accessed 2007 Nov 29).

124. Bone HG, Greenspan SL, McKeever C et al. Alendronate and estrogen effects in postmenopausal women with low bone mineral density. *J Clin Endocrinol Metab.* 2000; 85:720–6.

125. Greenspan SL, Resnick NM, Parker RA. Combination therapy with hormone replacement and alendronate for prevention of bone loss in elderly women: a randomized controlled trial. *JAMA.* 2003; 289:2525–33.

126. Harris ST, Eriksen EF, Davidson M et al. Effect of combined risedronate and hormone replacement therapies on bone mineral density in postmenopausal women. *J Clin Endocrinol Metab.* 2001; 86:1890–7.

127. Johnell O, Scheele WH, Lu Y et al. Additive effects of raloxifene and alendronate on bone density and biochemical markers of bone remodeling in postmenopausal women with osteoporosis. *J Clin Endocrinol Metab.* 2002; 87:985–92.

128. Black DM, Greenspan SL, Ensrud KE et al. The effects of parathyroid hormone and alendronate alone or in combination in postmenopausal osteoporosis. *N Engl J Med.* 2003; 349:1207–15.

129. Finkelstein JS, Hayes A, Hunzelman JL et al. The effects of parathyroid hormone, alendronate, or both in men with osteoporosis. *N Engl J Med.* 2003; 349:1216–26.

130. Black DM, Bilezikian JP, Ensrud KE et al. One year of alendronate after one year of parathyroid hormone (1-84) for osteoporosis. *N Engl J Med.* 2005; 353:555–65.

131. Whyte MP. The long and the short of bone therapy. *N Engl J Med.* 2006; 354:860–3.

132. European Medicines Agency. Preotact: European public assessment report. www.emea.eu.int/humandocs/Humans/EPAR/preotact/preotact.htm (accessed 2007 Jul 26).

133. NPS Pharmaceuticals, Inc. Preos: NPS updates status of Preos NDA. www.drugs.com/nda/preos_060329.html (accessed 2006 Jul 27).

134. Preotact (parathyroid horomone 1-84) package insert. Rosklide, Denmark: Nycomed Danmark ApS; 2006.

135. Greenspan SL, Bone HG, Ettinger MP et al. Effect of recombinant human parathyroid hormone (1-84) on vertebral fracture and bone mineral density in postmenopausal women with osteoporosis. *Ann Intern Med.* 2007; 146:326–39.

136. Farley JR, Wergedal JE, Baylink DJ. Fluoride directly stimulates proliferation and alkaline phosphatase activity of bone-forming cells. *Science.* 1983; 222:330–2.

137. Kanis JA. Treatment of symptomatic osteoporosis with fluoride. *Am J Med.* 1993; 95:53S–61S.

138. Riggs BL, Hodgson SF, O'Fallon WM et al. Effect of fluoride treatment on the fracture rate in postmenopausal women with osteoporosis. *N Engl J Med.* 1990; 322:802–9.

139. Marie PJ. Optimizing bone metabolism in osteoporosis: insight into the pharmacologic profile of strontium ranelate. *Osteoporos Int.* 2003; 14(suppl 3):S9–12.

140. Protelos (strontium ranelate) package insert. Neuilly sur Seine, France: Les Laboratoires Servier; 2004.

141. Zimmerman SI, Girman CJ, Buie VC et al. The prevalence of osteoporosis in nursing home residents. *Osteoporos Int.* 1999; 9:151–7.

142. Wallace RB. Bone health in nursing home residents. *JAMA.* 2000; 284:1018–9.

143. Gaugris S, Heaney RP, Boonen S et al. Vitamin D inadequacy among post-menopausal women: a systematic review. *QJM.* 2005; 98:667–76.

144. Parker MJ, Gillespie LD, Gillespie WJ. Hip protectors for preventing hip fractures in the elderly. *Cochrane Database Syst Rev.* 2000; 4:CD001255.

145. Parker MJ, Gillespie WJ, Gillespie LD. Effectiveness of hip protectors for preventing hip fractures in elderly people: systematic review. *BMJ.* 2006; 332:571–4.

146. Gupta G, Aronow WS. Underuse of procedures for diagnosing osteoporosis and of therapies for osteoporosis in older nursing home residents. *J Am Med Dir Assoc.* 2003; 4:200–2.

147. Schousboe JT, Ensrud KE, Nyman JA et al. Universal bone densitometry screening combined with alendronate therapy for those diagnosed with osteoporosis is highly cost-effective for elderly women. *J Am Geriatr Soc.* 2005; 53:1697–1704.

148. Kamel HK. Underutilization of calcium and vitamin D supplements in an academic long-term care facility. *J Am Med Dir Assoc.* 2004; 5:98–100.

149. Rojas-Fernandez C, Lapane KL, MacKnight C et al. Undertreatment of osteoporosis in residents of nursing homes: population-based study with use of the Systematic Assessment of Geriatric Drug Use via Epidemiology (SAGE) database. *Endocr Pract.* 2002; 8:335–42.

150. Colon-Emeric CS, Casebeer L, Saag K et al. Barriers to providing osteoporosis care in skilled nursing facilities: perceptions of medical directors and directors of nursing. *J Am Med Dir Assoc.* 2004; 5:361–6.

151. Amin S, Felson DT. Osteoporosis in men. *Rheum Dis Clin North Am.* 2001; 27:19–47.

152. National Osteoporosis Foundation. Osteoporosis: men. www.nof.org/men/index.htm (accessed 2005 Mar 23).

153. Olszynski WP, Shawn Davison K, Adachi JD et al. Osteoporosis in men: epidemiology, diagnosis, prevention, and treatment. *Clin Ther.* 2004; 26:15–28.

154. Centers for Medicare and Medicaid Services. Bone mass measurement. www.cms.hhs.gov/BoneMassMeasurement/ (accessed 2006 Jul 14).

155. Biskobing DM. COPD and osteoporosis. *Chest.* 2002; 121:609–20.

156. Shephard AJ, Cass AR, Carlson CA et al. Development and internal validation of the male osteoporosis risk estimation score. *Ann Fam Med.* 2007; 5:540–6.

157. Orwoll E, Ettinger M, Weiss S et al. Alendronate for the treatment of osteoporosis in men. *N Engl J Med.* 2000; 343:604–10.

Approved by the ASHP Board of Directors on June 23, 2007. Developed through the ASHP Council on Therapeutics.

Eric J. MacLaughlin, Pharm.D., BCPS, and Cynthia L. Raehl, Pharm.D., FASHP, FCCP are gratefully acknowledged for authoring this therapeutic position statement.

The bibliographic citation for this document is as follows: American Society of Health-System Pharmacists. ASHP therapeutic position statement on the prevention and treatment of osteoporosis in adults. *Am J Health-Syst Pharm.* 2008; 65:343–57.

ASHP Therapeutic Position Statement on Strategies for Identifying and Preventing Pneumococcal Resistance

Statement of Position

The American Society of Health-System Pharmacists (ASHP) supports the establishment of state and national surveillance systems to track the prevalence of drug-resistant *Streptococcus pneumoniae* so that appropriate antimicrobial regimens can be used to treat infections caused by this common community-acquired pathogen.

ASHP supports continued educational efforts to promote the rational use of antimicrobials as a strategy for preventing the development of drug-resistant bacteria.

ASHP supports the vaccination of all persons at risk for acquiring pneumococcal disease. Use of pneumococcal vaccines is a reliable strategy to decrease the morbidity and mortality associated with invasive infections due to *S. pneumoniae*.

Background

S. pneumoniae, also known as pneumococcus, is the most common cause of community-acquired bacterial respiratory-tract infections. It is a frequent cause of meningitis, bacteremia, otitis media, and community-acquired pneumonia. Infections caused by *S. pneumoniae* have been associated with increased morbidity and mortality, especially in children under two years of age and elderly adults. Infections caused by *S. pneumoniae* have typically been successfully treated with a variety of antimicrobials, including penicillin, cephalosporins, and erythromycin. In the early 1990s the first reports of penicillin nonsusceptible *S. pneumoniae* (PNSP) began to appear in the United States; penicillin nonsusceptible strains include both intermediately resistant and resistant strains of *S. pneumoniae*. During the past decade the reports of increasing resistance of *S. pneumoniae* to penicillin and cephalosporins continued, and in the late 1990s reports of increasing resistance to trimethoprim–sulfamethoxazole, macrolides, and fluoroquinolones began to appear. Many isolates developed resistance to multiple classes of drugs and became known as multi-drug resistant *S. pneumoniae* (MDRSP). The increasing prevalence of MDRSP is creating a challenge for health care providers in treating this common community-acquired pathogen.

The clinical significance of drug-resistant *S. pneumoniae* on treatment outcomes is unclear. Most of the available data on clinical outcomes are from retrospective reviews, case–control studies, and case reports. There is evidence that meningitis due to PNSP does not respond to treatment with either penicillin or standard doses of cephalosporins, leading to poor clinical outcomes.[1] In contrast, there does not appear to be a significant difference in clinical outcome, primarily mortality, when pneumonia or other nonmeningeal infections due to PNSP are treated with penicillin or cephalosporins. On the contrary, macrolides and fluoroquinolones with poor in vitro activity against *S. pneumoniae* have been associated with poor clinical outcomes and even treatment failures. It is likely that clinical outcomes be depend on the mechanism and degree of resistance, the site of infection, and the pharmacokinetic and pharmacodynamic characteristics of the antimicrobial agents used in treatment.

Definitions. NCCLS, previously known as the National Committee for Clinical Laboratory Standards, revised the definitions of *S. pneumoniae* susceptibility to several antimicrobials in its 2002 standards. *S. pneumoniae* resistant to penicillin is defined in terms of the minimum inhibitory con-centration (MIC) of penicillin. Strains may be distinguished as susceptible (MIC < 0.06 µg/mL), intermediately resistant (MIC 0.12–1.0 µg/mL), or highly resistant (MIC $\geq$ 2 µg/mL).[2] The most notable change in 2002 was the increase in breakpoint values for susceptibility of nonmeningitis isolates of *S. pneumoniae*. NCCLS took into account the pharmacokinetic and pharmacodynamic factors of a drug in redefining susceptibility breakpoints. The definition of multidrug-resistant *S. pneumoniae* is a strain resistant to three or more classes of antimicrobials.

Epidemiology. Numerous national and international surveillance studies have been conducted to determine the prevalence of *S. pneumoniae* resistance.[3-7] These networks used similar methodologies and specimens: clinical isolates of *S. pneumoniae* from sterile body sites or the respiratory tract, with susceptibility testing in accordance with NCCLS standards. Although these studies showed differing resistance rates to the antimicrobials tested, some common

Table 1.
Susceptibility of *Streptococcus pneumoniae* Isolates to Commonly Used Antimicrobials

Ref.	*n*	% Resistant Isolates					
		IR Penicillin	Resistant Penicillin	Ceftriaxone[a]	Erythromycin	Trimethoprim– Sulfamethoxazole	Levofloxacin
3	3,447	9.6	15.5	NA[b]	19.2	24.0	0.7
4[c]	2,432	12.0	25.0	4.3	28.8	37.5	NA
5	10,012	14.2	21.2	NA	27.9	NA	1.0
6	1,531	12.7	21.5	NA	25.7	30.3	0.3
7	7,671	15.5	18.4	1.7	NA	26.0	0.9

[a]NCCLS nonmeningitis breakpoints.
[b]NA = not applicable.
[c]U.S. data only.

trends emerged (Table 1). The incidence of strains highly resistant to penicillin has surpassed that of intermediately resistant strains. The rates of resistance to non-β-lactams have also increased: the prevalence of macrolide resistance is 20–30%, and trimethoprim–sulfamethoxazole resistance ranges between 24% and 38%. *S. pneumoniae* resistance to levofloxacin is hovering around 1%. However, there have been reports from Canada[8] and the Centers for Disease Control and Prevention (CDC)[9] of increasing resistance of *S. pneumoniae* to fluoroquinolones. Most fluoroquinolone-resistant isolates are resistant to other antimicrobials. Fluoroquinolone-resistant organisms are more likely to be found in persons over 65 years of age, the population with the highest use of fluoroquinolones.

Persons at Risk. The greatest risk factor for becoming infected with a drug-resistant strain of *S. pneumoniae* is prior antimicrobial use. Other risk factors include carriage of *S. pneumoniae*, daycare attendance, exposure to children who attend daycare, severe medical comorbidities, immunosuppression, and high alcohol intake.[1] Smoking has been identified as a risk factor for developing invasive *S. pneumoniae* infections.[10] The risk of invasive *S. pneumoniae* infections is 4-fold if the patient is a smoker and 2.5-fold if the patient is exposed to secondhand smoke. The risk of invasive disease declines over time for persons who have stopped smoking.

Mechanisms of Resistance. Resistance of *S. pneumoniae* to β-lactams is due to genetic mutations leading to alterations in three or four of the five high-molecular-weight penicillin-binding proteins (PBPs).[11] The degree of *S. pneumoniae* resistance is dependent on which PBPs are involved and the affinity of the β-lactam agent to the PBP. The differences in expression of these PBPs explain the differences in susceptibility to a variety of β-lactams.

S. pneumoniae resistance to macrolides occurs primarily through two mechanisms: active drug efflux (M phenotype) or ribosomal modification (MLS$_\beta$ phenotype).[12] Active drug efflux confers resistance to all agents within the class, whereas ribosomal modification confers resistance not only to the macrolides but also to clindamycin and streptogramins. Approximately 75% of macrolide-resistant *S. pneumoniae* found in the United States is attributable to active drug efflux.

Resistance of *S. pneumoniae* to fluoroquinolones is primarily a result of mutations of the *parC* and *gyrA* genes, although efflux pumps may also play a role.[13] Alterations in the parC subunit of topoisomerase IV result in the reduced susceptibility of *S. pneumoniae* to gatifloxacin, levofloxacin, and moxifloxacin. This single-step mutation is difficult to detect clinically because isolates with a *parC* mutation are reported as susceptible using standard laboratory testing. This is concerning because isolates with single-step mutations are the progenitors for fully drug-resistant strains of *S. pneumoniae*, which have additional mutations in the gyrA subunit of DNA gyrase.

Establishment of Surveillance Systems

Surveillance systems are an integral component of combating bacterial resistance. The data gathered from surveillance systems can be used for many purposes, such as identifying and tracking global outbreaks, setting public health policy, determining appropriate treatments for different infections, and heightening awareness of health care providers to local resistance trends that may affect the routine care of patients.

Health systems should develop a mechanism for the surveillance of bacterial resistance. Ideally, the surveillance system should identify trends in bacterial susceptibility patterns and correlate this with antimicrobial use in both health systems and communities.[14] The clinical microbiology laboratory, pharmacy, information systems, and infection control departments play important roles in maintaining an active surveillance system. Surveillance systems for tracking the prevalence of *S. pneumoniae* include two approaches, each providing differing types of information. The more common system uses culture data from clinical isolates causing invasive disease, which give an indication of the resistance patterns of strains actually causing clinical infection. The other approach determines the community *S. pneumoniae* carriage rate by testing nasopharyngeal swabs from individuals without clinical illness, demonstrating which strains could cause clinical infection. However, one study found that nasopharyngeal swabs overestimate the rate of *S. pneumoniae* colonization because of misidentification of oral streptococci as *S. pneumoniae*.[15] The importance of accurately identifying *S. pneumoniae* and determining susceptibility cannot be overstated.

Guidelines for the treatment of common community-acquired infections developed by various national organizations can be found in the appendix. These guidelines incorporate data from large surveillance studies of microbial resistance to make recommendations for initial treatment regimens. Local surveillance data can be used to tailor national guidelines when developing local recommendations for empirical treatments.

Participation in an active surveillance system should not be limited to individual institutions. Health systems should actively participate in state and national surveillance initiatives. Sentinel surveillance, which incorporates data from a small number of laboratories to determine trends for a much larger area, can accurately detect large changes in the susceptibility of *S. pneumoniae*, but it infrequently detects emerging resistance profiles, such as the fluoroquinolone resistance of *S. pneumoniae*.[16] Sentinel surveillance is also useful in showing trends in susceptibility over time. CDC, the Food and Drug Administration, and the National Institutes of Health have launched an action plan to combat antimicrobial resistance.[17] One of the four major components of this plan is the enhancement of surveillance systems. CDC will coordinate efforts with state and local health departments to develop national, regional, state, and local surveillance networks. The data gained from this initiative can be used to target areas with a high prevalence of PNSP for pneumococcal vaccination programs and efforts to promote the judicious use of antimicrobials.

Rational Use of Antimicrobials

There is an abundance of literature showing the relationship between antimicrobial-use patterns and the development of resistance. However, the bulk of this literature has been generated from hospital or institutional studies and has little bearing on PNSP. Since *S. pneumoniae* is primarily a community-acquired pathogen, antimicrobial use in the outpatient setting has the greatest influence on the susceptibility profile of *S. pneumoniae*. Few studies have shown a relationship between outpatient prescription use and *S. pneumoniae* susceptibility patterns. In the United States, Diekema and colleagues[18] found a positive correlation between high usage rates of outpatient

β-lactam agents and the decreased penicillin susceptibility of *S. pneumoniae*. No correlation was found between the use of other antimicrobial classes (e.g., macrolides, tetracyclines, and fluoroquinolones) and the decreased penicillin susceptibility of *S. pneumoniae*. Bronzwaer et al.[19] found a relationship between high outpatient use of β-lactam agents and macrolides and the decreased penicillin susceptibility of *S. pneumoniae* in Europe. A major limitation of both of these studies was the failure to track patient adherence to prescribed regimens; however, these studies demonstrated that the community burden of high antimicrobial use is substantial and plays a role in the development of microbial resistance.

Several national organizations,[14] CDC, and the World Health Organization have advocated judicious antimicrobial-use stewardship as a mechanism to limit the development of bacterial resistance. One of the cornerstones of antimicrobial-use stewardship is the appropriate use of antimicrobials. Approximately 50% of adults,[20] and over 20% of children's[21] prescriptions for antibacterials are unnecessary. These agents were usually prescribed for treatment of the common cold, upper-respiratory-tract infections, and bronchitis, ailments often caused by viruses that do not respond to antibacterials.

Hennessy et al.[22] attempted to demonstrate that decreased outpatient antimicrobial use could reduce the carriage of PNSP. In a controlled intervention trial in rural Alaska, investigators provided extensive education to the health care providers and the public on the management of respiratory-tract infections and the appropriate use of antimicrobials. They tracked the nasal carriage of penicillin-susceptible *S. pneumoniae* and PNSP, as well as antimicrobial use in the region for a three-year period. During the first year they found a significant decrease in the nasal carriage of PNSP and antimicrobial use. However, the carriage of PNSP increased to almost preintervention levels in the following two years of the study, despite the continued low rate of antimicrobial use. This suggests that changing antimicrobial-use patterns is only one part of solving a complex problem. Such changes will likely need to be coupled with other programs, including aggressive vaccination, to show a significant effect on decreasing the carriage of *S. pneumoniae*.

Education of health care providers and the public is essential for ensuring the rational use of antimicrobials. Pharmacists can play a significant role in educating both groups,[23] assuming roles as educators to assist in disseminating vital information that encourages the rational use of antimicrobials.

Educating the public about antimicrobial use and misuse is essential because consumers play a key role in drug utilization. In focus groups, patients have indicated that if physicians explain why an antimicrobial was not needed, they would be satisfied with not receiving a prescription for one.[24] For many reasons, most health care providers cannot or do not spend the time necessary to adequately educate their patients or patients' caregivers on the potential dangers of the inappropriate use of antimicrobials. Pharmacists are encouraged to assume responsibility for educating patients about these dangers. A mass media campaign geared to the public on the dangers of emerging infectious diseases has been underway for several years.[25] This campaign should be tailored for the needs of individual communities.

Vaccination

Infections caused by *S. pneumoniae* continue to cause significant morbidity and mortality despite the availability of effective vaccines. Both the 23-valent pneumococcal polysaccharide vaccine (PPV) and the 7-valent pneumococcal conjugate vaccine (PCV7) have been shown to be highly effective in providing protection against the most commonly isolated pneumococcal serotypes that cause human disease, including those serotypes known to be antimicrobial resistant. While the use of these vaccines will not prevent the development of drug-resistant *S. pneumoniae*, they will likely prevent invasive infection caused by a drug-resistant organism. PPV is recommended for all adults aged 65 years or older.[26] It may also be given to select groups of high-risk patients over 2 years of age. This vaccine does not produce an adequate immunological response in children under 2 years old and should not be used in that population. PCV7 was added to the standard recommended pediatric vaccines in October 2000.[27] The PCV7 series should be given to all children beginning at age 2 months. The CDC National Immunization Program has established current recommendations for pneumococcal vaccine administration.[28]

PPV was licensed in the early 1980s and has demonstrated good immunogenicity in both young and older adults; however, an individual will not develop an immune response to all 23 pneumococcal serotypes.[29] The reason for this is unclear. Despite the vaccine's long-standing availability and documented effectiveness, less than 60% of eligible persons actually receive it.[30] One of the Healthy People 2010 goals is for 90% of eligible adults to receive pneumococcal vaccine.[30] This is an excellent opportunity for pharmacists to improve the vaccination rate of older adult patients and help promote national health care goals.

Revaccination with PPV is recommended for adults over age 65 years if the first dose was administered when he or she was under 65 years old at the time of vaccination and at least five years have elapsed since the first dose.[26] In addition, persons younger than 65 years with immunocompromising conditions may receive a one-time revaccination if five years have elapsed since the first dose of PPV. Revaccination with PPV results in a somewhat blunted immune response and is associated with increased injection-site reactions.[29]

PCV7 for children has been available since February 2000. Use of this vaccine has been shown to decrease the carriage rate of *S. pneumoniae* and the incidence of invasive pneumococcal disease, acute otitis media, and pneumonia in vaccinated populations.[31,32] The rate of vaccine-specific serotype *S. pneumoniae* carriage in vaccinated children remains below the rate for nonvaccinated children over prolonged periods of time. Widespread vaccination of children with PCV7 has shown a "herd effect" in decreasing the carriage rate of *S. pneumoniae* in children, who are an important vector for the transmission of *S. pneumoniae* to other children and adults.[31] This indirect effect was recently documented by the CDC Active Bacterial Core Surveillance Network, which found a decrease of 32% in invasive disease in adults age 20–39 years, 8% for those 40–64 years of age, and 18% for those 65 years or older.[32] This is similar to what was seen with widespread use of the *Haemophilus influenzae* type B vaccine and the marked decrease in *H. influenzae*-related infections.

Most people who succumb to preventable infections had visited a health care provider in the preceding year but were not vaccinated.[33–37] Clinicians need to ensure that people receive proper immunizations[38,39] and pharmacists can promote vaccination efforts by serving as educators, facilitators, and vaccinators. Although vaccinations are typi-

cally administered in the ambulatory care setting, clinicians seize opportunities to vaccinate hospitalized patients as well. Pharmacists have demonstrated that they can increase the number of persons receiving needed vaccines in both inpatient and ambulatory care settings.[40]

Summary

The incidence of drug-resistant *S. pneumoniae* continues to increase, causing significant morbidity and mortality. Health care providers should seize the opportunity to promote the judicious use of antimicrobials and aggressive vaccination with the pneumococcal vaccines as a means to lessen this significant health problem.

References

1. Pallares R, Fenoll A, Linares J et al. The epidemiology of antibiotic resistance in *Streptococcus pneumoniae* and the clinical relevance of resistance to cephalosporins, macrolides and quinolones. *Int J Antimicrob Agents.* 2003; 22(suppl 1):S15–24.
2. Performance standards for antimicrobial susceptibility testing; 12th informational supplement. Wayne, PA: NCCLS; 2002. NCCLS document M100–S12.
3. Centers for Disease Control and Prevention. Active bacterial core surveillance report, emerging infections program network, *Streptococcus pneumoniae*, 2001. www.cdc.gov/ncidod/dbmd/survreports/spneu01.pdf (accessed 2004 Jul 30).
4. Jacobs MR, Felmingham D, Appelbaum PC et al. The Alexander Project 1998–2000: susceptibility of pathogens isolated from community-acquired respiratory tract infection to commonly used antimicrobial agents. *J Antimicrob Chemother.* 2003; 52:229–46.
5. Doern G, Rybak MJ. Activity of telithromycin against *Streptococcus pneumoniae* resistant to penicillin, macrolides and fluoroquinolones isolated from respiratory tract infections: PROTEK US year 2 (2001–2002). Paper presented at the 43rd Annual Interscience Conference on Antimicrobial Agents and Chemotherapy. Chicago, IL; 2003 Sept 16.
6. Doern GV, Heilmann KP, Huynh HK et al. Antimicrobial resistance among clinical isolates of *Streptococcus pneumoniae* in the United States during 1999–2000, including a comparison of resistance rates since 1994–1995. *Antimicrob Agents Chemother.* 2001; 45:1721–9.
7. Karlowsky JA, Thornsberry C, Jones ME et al. Factors associated with relative rates of antimicrobial resistance among *Streptococcus pneumoniae* in the United States: results from the TRUST surveillance program (1998–2002). Clin Infect Dis. 2003; 36:963–70.
8. Chen DK, McGeer A, de Azavedo JC et al. Decreased susceptibility of *Streptococcus pneumoniae* to fluoroquinolones in Canada. *N Engl J Med.* 1999; 341:233–9.
9. Centers for Disease Control and Prevention. Resistance of *Streptococcus pneumoniae* to fluoroquinolones— United States, 1995–1999. *MMWR.* 2001; 50:800–4.
10. Nuorti JP, Butler JC, Farley MM et al. Cigarette smoking and invasive pneumococcal disease. *N Engl J Med.* 2000; 342:681–9.
11. Appelbaum PC. Resistance among *Streptococcus pneumoniae*: implications for drug selection. *Clin Infect Dis.* 2002; 34:1613–20.
12. Lynch JP, Martinez FJ. Clinical relevance of macrolide-resistant *Streptococcus pneumoniae* for community-acquired pneumonia. *Clin Infect Dis.* 2002; 34 (suppl 1):S27–46.
13. Hooper DC. Fluoroquinolone resistance among gram-positive cocci. *Lancet Infect Dis.* 2002; 2:530–8.
14. Shlaes DM, Gerding DN, John JF Jr et al. Society for Healthcare Epidemiology of American and Infectious Diseases Society of America Joint Committee on Prevention of Antimicrobial Resistance: guidelines for the prevention of antimicrobial resistance in hospitals. *Clin Infect Dis.* 1997; 25:584–99.
15. Wester CW, Ariga D, Nathan C et al. Possible overestimation of penicillin resistant *Streptococcus pneumoniae* colonization rates due to misidentification of oropharyngeal streptococci. *Diagn Microbiol Infect Dis.* 2002; 42:263–8.
16. Schrag SJ, Zell ER, Schuchat A et al. Sentinel surveillance: a reliable way to track antibiotic resistance in communities? *Emerg Infect Dis.* 2002; 8:496–502.
17. Centers for Disease Control and Prevention. National Center for Infectious Diseases: antimicrobial resistance. www.cdc.gov/drugresistance/ (accessed 2004 Aug 1).
18. Diekema DJ, Brueggemann AB, Doern GV. Antimicrobial-drug use and changes in resistance in *Streptococcus pneumoniae*. *Emerg Infect Dis.* 2000; 6:552–6.
19. Bronzwaer SL, Cars O, Buchholz U et al. A European study on the relationship between antimicrobial use and antimicrobial resistance. *Emerg Infect Dis.* 2002; 8:278–82.
20. Gonzales R, Steiner JF, Sande MA. Antibiotic prescribing for adults with colds, upper respiratory tract infections, and bronchitis by ambulatory care physicians. *JAMA.* 1997; 278:901–4.
21. Nyquist AC, Gonzales R, Steiner JF et al. Antibiotic prescribing for children with colds, upper respiratory tract infections, and bronchitis. *JAMA.* 1998; 279:875–7. [Erratum, *JAMA.* 1998; 279:1702.]
22. Hennessy TW, Petersen KM, Bruden D et al. Changes in antibiotic-prescribing practices and carriage of penicillin-resistant *Streptococcus pneumoniae*: a controlled intervention trial in rural Alaska. *Clin Infect Dis.* 2002; 34:1543–50.
23. Dickerson LM, Mainous AG III, Carek PJ. The pharmacist's role in promoting optimal antimicrobial use. *Pharmacotherapy.* 2000; 20:711–23.
24. Avorn J, Solomon DH. Cultural and economic factors that (mis)shape antibiotic use: the nonpharmacologic basis of therapeutics. *Ann Intern Med.* 2000; 133:128–35.
25. Freimuth V, Linnan HW, Potter P. Communicating the threat of emerging infections to the public. *Emerg Infect Dis.* 2000; 6:337–47.
26. Centers for Disease Control and Prevention. Prevention of pneumococcal diseases: recommendations of the Advisory Committee on Immunization Practices. *MMWR.* 1997; 46(RR-8):1–24.
27. Centers for Disease Control and Prevention. Preventing pneumococcal disease among infants and young children: recommendations of the Advisory Committee on Immunization Practices. *MMWR.* 2000; 49 (RR-9):1–35.

28. Centers for Disease Control and Prevention. National Immunization Program. www.cdc.gov/nip/ (accessed 2004 Aug 1).

29. Artz AS, Ershler WB, Longo DL. Pneumococcal vaccination and revaccination of older adults. *Clin Microbiol Rev.* 2003; 16:308–18.

30. Office of Disease Prevention and Health Promotion, Department of Health and Human Services. Healthy people 2010. www.healthypeople.gov (accessed 2004 Aug 1).

31. Dagan R, Fraser D. Conjugate pneumococcal vaccine and antibiotic-resistant *Streptococcus pneumoniae*: herd immunity and reduction of otitis morbidity. *Pediatr Infect Dis J.* 2000; 19:S79–88.

32. Whitney CG, Farley MM, Hadler J et al. Decline in invasive pneumococcal disease after the introduction of protein-polysaccharide conjugate vaccine. *N Engl J Med.* 2003; 348:1737–46.

33. Williams WW, Hickson MA, Kane MA et al. Immunization policies and vaccine coverage among adults. The risk for missed opportunities. *Ann Intern Med.* 1988; 108:616–25. [Erratum, *Ann Intern Med.* 1988; 109:348.]

34. Fedson DS, Harward MP, Reid RA et al. Hospital-based pneumococcal immunization. Epidemiologic rationale from the Shenandoah study. *JAMA.* 1990; 264:1117–22.

35. Fedson DS. Influenza and pneumococcal immunization strategies for physicians. *Chest.* 1987; 91:436–43.

36. Magnussen CR, Valenti WM, Mushlin AI. Pneumococcal vaccine strategy. Feasibility of a vaccination program directed at hospitalized and ambulatory patients. *Arch Intern Med.* 1984; 144:1755–7.

37. Vondracek TG, Pham TP, Huycke MM. A hospital-based pharmacy intervention program for pneumococcal vaccination. *Arch Intern Med.* 1998; 158:1543–7.

38. American Society of Health-System Pharmacists. ASHP guidelines on the pharmacist's role in immunization. *Am J Health-Syst Pharm.* 2003; 60:1371–7.

39. Grabenstein JD, Bonasso J. Health-system pharmacists' role in immunizing adults against pneumococcal disease and influenza. *Am J Health-Syst Pharm.* 1999; 56(suppl 2):S2–25.

40. Noped JC, Schomberg R. Implementing an inpatient pharmacy-based pneumococcal vaccination program. *Am J Health-Syst Pharm.* 2001; 58:1852–5.

Appendix—Selected Guidelines for the Treatment of Common Community-Acquired Respiratory-Tract Infections

Bronchitis
Snow V, Mottur-Pilson C, Hickner JM et al. for the American College of Physicians–American Society of Internal Medicine. Principles of appropriate antibiotic use for treatment of acute bronchitis in adults. *Ann Intern Med.* 2001; 134:518–20.

Community-Acquired Pneumonia
Mandell LA, Bartlett JG, Dowell SF et al. Update of practice guidelines for the management of community-acquired pneumonia in immunocompetent adults. *Clin Infect Dis.* 2003; 37:1405–33.

Otitis Media
American Academy of Pediatrics Subcommittee on Diagnosis and Management of Acute Otitis Media. Diagnosis and management of acute otitis media. *Pediatrics.* 2004; 113:1451–65.

American Academy of Family Physicians, American Academy of Otolaryngology-Head and Neck Surgery, American Academy of Pediatrics. Subcommittee on Diagnosis and Management of Otitis Media with Effusion. Otitis media with effusion. *Pediatrics.* 2004; 113:1412–29.

Sinusitis
American Academy of Pediatrics. Subcommittee on Management of Sinusitis and Committee on Quality Improvement. Clinical practice guideline: management of sinusitis. *Pediatrics.* 2001; 108:798–808.

Snow V, Mottur-Pilson C, Hickner JM, for the American College of Physicians–American Society of Internal Medicine. Principles of appropriate antibiotic use for acute sinusitis in adults. *Ann Intern Med.* 2001; 134:495–7.

Approved by the ASHP Board of Directors on April 15, 2004. Developed through the ASHP Commission on Therapeutics.

The bibliographic citation for this document is as follows: American Society of Health-System Pharmacists. ASHP therapeutic position statement on strategies for identifying and preventing pneumococcal resistance. *Am J Health-Syst Pharm.* 2004; 61:2430–5.

Therapeutic Monitoring of Vancomycin in Adult Patients: A Consensus Review of the American Society of Health-System Pharmacists, the Infectious Diseases Society of America, and the Society of Infectious Diseases Pharmacists

Vancomycin is a glycopeptide antibiotic that has been in clinical use for nearly 50 years as a penicillin alternative to treat penicillinase-producing strains of *Staphylococcus aureus*. It is one of the most widely used antibiotics in the United States for the treatment of serious gram-positive infections involving methicillin-resistant *S. aureus* (MRSA).[1] Early use of vancomycin was associated with a number of adverse effects, including infusion-related toxicities, nephrotoxicity, and possible ototoxicity. Upon further investigation, it appears that the impurities in early formulations of vancomycin caused many of these adverse events.[1-4] Its overall use was curtailed significantly with the development of semisynthetic penicillins (e.g., methicillin, oxacillin, nafcillin) that were considered less toxic.[1-4] However, the steady rise in the number of MRSA infections since the early 1980s has once again brought vancomycin into the forefront as the primary treatment for infections caused by this organism.

Over the years, vancomycin has been one of the most studied antibiotics. Extensive pharmacokinetic studies in a variety of patient populations and the availability of commercial drug assays have allowed clinicians to target serum vancomycin concentrations precisely in a relatively narrow range. This approach has been advocated to lessen the potential for nephrotoxicity and ototoxicity and to achieve therapeutic concentrations. However, it should be noted that the practice of routine monitoring and adjusting of serum vancomycin drug concentrations has been the subject of intense debate for many years.[5-9] The controversy has resulted from conflicting evidence regarding the use of serum vancomycin concentrations to predict and prevent drug-induced toxicity and as a measure of effectiveness in treating infections. Further, data derived from more recent studies appear to suggest that vancomycin has little potential for nephrotoxicity or ototoxicity when used at conventional dosages (e.g., 1 g every 12 hours [15 mg/kg every 12 hours]), unless it is used concomitantly with known nephrotoxic drugs or at very high dosages.[10-12] This consensus review evaluates the scientific data and controversies associated with serum vancomycin monitoring and provides recommendations based on the available evidence.

This is a consensus statement of the American Society of Health-System Pharmacists (ASHP), the Infectious Diseases Society of America (IDSA), and the Society of Infectious Diseases Pharmacists (SIDP). Consensus committee members were assigned key topics regarding vancomycin that contribute to current knowledge about patient monitoring. A draft document addressing these areas that included specific recommendations was reviewed by all committee members. After peer review by members of ASHP, IDSA, and SIDP, the committee met to review the submitted comments and recommendations. After careful discussion and consideration of these suggestions, the document was revised and circulated among the committee and supporting organizations for final comment. This consensus review represents the opinion of the majority of committee members.

A search of PubMed was conducted using the following search terms: vancomycin pharmacokinetics, pharmacodynamics, efficacy, resistance, and toxicity. All relevant and available peer-reviewed studies in the English language published between 1958 and 2008 were considered. Studies were rated by their quality of evidence, and the subsequent recommendations were graded using the classification schemata of the Canadian Medical Association (Table 1).[13] Recommendations of the expert panel are presented in Table 2.

Potential limitations of this review include the facts that few prospective or randomized trials of vancomycin monitoring were available and that most of the published literature regarding vancomycin monitoring described observational studies in patients with *S. aureus* infection. Vancomycin monitoring in pediatric patients is beyond the scope of this review.

Table 1.
Definitions of Levels and Grades for Recommendations[13]

Quality Indicator	Type of Evidence
Level of evidence	
I	Evidence from at least one properly randomized, controlled trial
II	Evidence from at least one well-designed clinical trial, without randomization; from cohort or case-controlled analytic studies (preferably from more than one center); from multiple time series; or from dramatic results from uncontrolled experiments
III	Evidence from opinions of respected authorities, based on clinical experience, descriptive studies, or reports of expert committees
Grade of recommendation	
A	Good evidence to support a recommendation for use
B	Moderate evidence to support a recommendation for use
C	Poor evidence to support a recommendation for use

Overview of Vancomycin Pharmacokinetic and Pharmacodynamic Properties

Sophisticated pharmacokinetic techniques such as Bayesian and noncompartmental modeling have been used to derive pharmacokinetic parameters for vancomycin. The serum vancomycin concentration–time profile is complex and has been characterized as one-, two-, and three-compartment pharmacokinetic models. In patients with normal renal function, the α-distribution phase ranges from 30 minutes to 1 hour, and the β-elimination half-life ranges from 6 to 12 hours. The volume of distribution is 0.4–1 L/kg.[14-18]

While reports of the degree of vancomycin protein binding have varied, a level of 50–55% is most often stated.[19,20] Penetration of vancomycin into tissues is variable and can be affected by inflammation and disease state. For example, with uninflamed meninges, cerebral spinal fluid vancomycin concentrations ranging from 0 to approximately 4 mg/L have been reported, whereas concentrations of 6.4–11.1 mg/L have been reported in the presence of inflammation.[21] Penetration into skin tissue is significantly lower for patients with diabetes (median, 0.1 mg/L; range, 0.01–0.45 mg/L) compared with nondiabetic patients based on the median ratio of tissue vancomycin to plasma vancomycin concentrations (median, 0.3 mg/L; range, 0.46–0.94 mg/L).[21] Vancomycin concentrations in lung tissue ranging from 5% to 41% of serum vancomycin concentrations have been reported in studies of healthy volunteers and patients.[5,6,22,23] Epithelial lining fluid (ELF) penetration in critically injured patients is highly variable, with an overall blood:ELF penetration ratio of 6:1.[23,24]

Selection of Pharmacokinetic and Pharmacodynamic Monitoring Parameters

A variety of pharmacokinetic and pharmacodynamic monitoring parameters have been proposed for vancomycin, including time (t) the concentration of vancomycin remains above the minimum inhibitory concentration (MIC), the ratio of the area under the serum drug concentration-versus-time curve and the MIC, and the ratio of the maximum serum drug concentration (C_{max}) and the MIC. These parameters are abbreviated t>MIC, AUC/MIC, and C_{max}/MIC, respectively. Reviews of pharmacokinetics and pharmacodynamics have recommended the AUC/MIC as the preferred parameter based in part on data from animal models, in vitro studies, and limited human studies.[6,25-28] Studies by Ackerman et al.,[29] Löwdin et al.,[30] and Larsson et al.[31] demonstrated that vancomycin kills S. aureus and Staphylococcus epidermidis in a concentration-independent fashion. By simulating free vancomycin peak concentrations of 40, 20, 10, and 5 mg/L in an in vitro chemostat model with a normal vancomycin terminal half-life of six hours, Larsson et al.[31] found no difference in the corresponding bacterial kill curves for S. aureus.

Using neutropenic mouse models, investigators have concluded that the AUC/MIC is the pharmacodynamically linked parameter for measuring vancomycin's effectiveness in treating S. aureus, including methicillin-susceptible S. aureus (MSSA), MRSA, and vancomycin-intermediate S. aureus (VISA) strains.[6,25] (Note: The total AUC/MIC and the free vancomycin AUC/MIC [AUC × 50% protein binding/MIC] have been interchangeably reported for vancomycin. Unless designated fAUC/MIC, this consensus review refers to total AUC/MIC.)

Craig and Andes[32] recently evaluated the use of free vancomycin AUC_{0-24hr}/MIC (fAUC/MIC) as the primary parameter for predicting vancomycin activity against VISA, heteroresistant VISA (hVISA), and MSSA in the murine neutropenic mouse model. They found that the fAUC/MIC requirement varied depending on the vancomycin MIC and was a function of bacterial density at the site of infection, with a lower fAUC/MIC needed for a lower bacterial inoculum. Of interest, the dose required for a 2 log colony-forming unit/g kill was 2.5 times higher for hVISA strains than for VISA and vancomycin-susceptible S. aureus strains. The researchers concluded that vancomycin dosages of 500 mg every 6 hours or 1 g every 12 hours provide fAUC/MIC values of 100–250 and suggested that values around 500 may enhance the therapeutic effectiveness of vancomycin in humans.

Moise-Broder et al.[33] explored the use of AUC/MIC in predicting clinical and microbiological success in treating ventilator-associated S. aureus pneumonia. These investigators suggested an average AUC/MIC of 345 for a successful clinical outcome and a ratio of 850 for a successful microbiological outcome. For pathogens with an MIC of 1 mg/L, an AUC/MIC of approximately 250 can be achieved in most patients with 1 g every 12 hours based on a patient with an actual body weight (ABW) of 80 kg and normal renal function (i.e., creatinine clearance [CL_{cr}] = 100 mL/min), but obtaining a target AUC/MIC of 850 would require much higher dosages for most patients.

Summary: *Based on these study results, an AUC/MIC ratio of ≥400 has been advocated as a target to achieve clinical effectiveness with vancomycin. Animal studies and limited human data appear to demonstrate that vancomycin is not concentration dependent and that the AUC/MIC is a predictive pharmacokinetic parameter for vancomycin.*

Impact of Dosing Strategies on Pharmacokinetic and Pharmacodynamic Parameters

The initial clinical dosing strategies for vancomycin were developed in the late 1950s before the emergence of antibiotic pharmacodynamics.[34] Published data on the pharmacodynamics of vancomycin against specific bacterial pathogens or infections are very limited, with much of the available data generated from in vitro or animal models. This is partly due to the drug's generic status, which discourages manufacturers from conducting well-controlled scientific investigations that would provide additional and clarifying pharmacodynamic data. It is recommended that dosages be calculated based on ABW. There are limited data on dosing in obese patients; however, initial dosages should be based on ABW and adjusted based on serum vancomycin concentrations to achieve therapeutic levels.[17]

Vancomycin is ideally suited from a pharmacokinetic and pharmacodynamic perspective for intermittent administration based on the usual susceptibility of staphylococci and streptococci (MIC values of ≤1 mg/L), the most commonly used dosage regimen for vancomycin (1 g every 12 hours), and the concentration-independent nature of the drug. As a

Table 2.

Summary of Expert Panel Recommendations for Vancomycin Therapeutic Drug Monitoring (TDM)[a]

Variable	Recommendation	Level of Evidence and Grade of Recommendation	Section of Consensus Review
Recommended TDM Parameters			
Optimal monitoring parameter	Trough serum vancomycin concentrations are the most accurate and practical method for monitoring efficacy.	IIB	Therapeutic vancomycin drug monitoring, Peak versus trough concentrations
Timing of monitoring	Troughs should be obtained just prior to the next dose at steady-state conditions (just before the fourth dose).	IIB	Therapeutic vancomycin drug monitoring, Peak versus trough concentrations
Optimal trough concentration (see also Optimal trough concentration—complicated infections)	Minimum serum vancomycin trough concentrations should always be maintained above 10 mg/L to avoid development of resistance. For a pathogen with an MIC of 1 mg/L, the minimum trough concentration would have to be at least 15 mg/L to generate the target AUC:MIC of 400.	IIIB	Therapeutic vancomycin drug monitoring, Optimal trough concentrations
Optimal trough concentration—complicated infections (bacteremia, endocarditis, osteo-myelitis, meningitis, and hospital-acquired pneumonia caused by *Staphylococcus aureus*)	Vancomycin serum trough concentrations of 15–20 mg/L are recommended to improve penetration, increase the probability of obtaining optimal target serum concentrations, and improve clinical outcomes.	IIIB	Therapeutic vancomycin drug monitoring, Optimal trough concentrations
Dosing Regimen			
Dosing to achieve optimal trough concentrations	Doses of 15–20 mg/kg (as actual body weight) given every 8–12 hr are recommended for most patients with normal renal function to achieve the suggested serum concentrations when the MIC is ≤1 mg/L. In patients with normal renal function, the targeted AUC:MIC of >400 is not achievable with conventional dosing methods if the MIC is ≥2 mg/L in a patient with normal renal function.	IIIB	Therapeutic vancomycin drug monitoring, Optimal trough concentrations
Loading doses—complicated infections	In seriously ill patients, a loading dose of 25–30 mg/kg (based on actual body weight) can be used to facilitate rapid attainment of target trough serum vancomycin concentration.	IIIB	Therapeutic vancomycin drug monitoring, Optimal trough concentrations
Continuous vs. intermittent dosing	Continuous infusion regimens are unlikely to substantially improve patient outcome when compared to intermittent dosing.	IIA	Impact of dosing strategies on pharmacokinetic and pharmacodynamic parameters
TDM for Vancomycin-Induced Nephrotoxicity			
Definition	A minimum of two or three consecutive documented increases in serum creatinine concentrations (defined as an increase of 0.5 mg/dL or a ≥50% increase from baseline, whichever is greater) after several days of vancomycin therapy.	IIB	Vancomycin toxicity; Incidence, mechanism, and definition of nephrotoxicity

Continued on next page

Table 2. *(continued)*

Summary of Expert Panel Recommendations for Vancomycin Therapeutic Drug Monitoring (TDM)[a]

Variable	Recommendation	Level of Evidence and Grade of Recommendation	Section of Consensus Review
Criteria for monitoring	Data do not support using peak serum vancomycin concentrations to monitor for nephrotoxicity.	IIB	Vancomycin toxicity, Role of therapeutic drug monitoring in preventing nephrotoxicity
	Trough monitoring is recommended for patients receiving aggressive dosing (i.e., to achieve sustained trough levels of 15–20 mg/L) and all patients at high risk of nephrotoxicity (e.g., patients receiving concurrent nephrotoxins).	IIIB	Vancomycin toxicity, Role of therapeutic drug monitoring in preventing nephrotoxicity
	Monitoring is also recommended for patients with unstable (i.e., deteriorating or significantly improving) renal function and those receiving prolonged courses of therapy (more than three to five days).	IIB	Vancomycin toxicity, Role of therapeutic drug monitoring in preventing nephrotoxicity
Frequency of monitoring	Frequent monitoring (more than one trough before the fourth dose) for short course or lower intensity dosing (to attain target trough concentrations below 15 mg/L) is not recommended.	IIB	Vancomycin toxicity, Role of therapeutic drug monitoring in preventing nephrotoxicity
	All patients on prolonged courses of vancomycin (exceeding three to five days) should have at least one steady-state trough concentration obtained no earlier than at steady state (just before the fourth dose) and then repeated as deemed clinically appropriate.	IIB	Vancomycin toxicity, Role of therapeutic drug monitoring in preventing nephrotoxicity
	There are limited data supporting the safety of sustained trough concentrations of 15–20 mg/L. Clinical judgment should guide the frequency of trough monitoring when the target trough is in this range. Once-weekly monitoring is recommended for hemodynamically stable patients. More frequent or daily trough monitoring is advisable in patients who are hemodynamically unstable.	IIIB	Vancomycin toxicity, Role of therapeutic drug monitoring in preventing nephrotoxicity

TDM for Vancomycin-Induced Ototoxicity

Variable	Recommendation	Level of Evidence and Grade of Recommendation	Section of Consensus Review
Criteria for monitoring	Monitoring for ototoxicity is not recommended for patients receiving vancomycin monotherapy.	IIIB	Vancomycin toxicity, Incidence of ototoxicity and role of therapeutic drug monitoring for prevention of vancomycin-induced hearing loss
	Monitoring should be considered for patients receiving additional ototoxic agents, such as aminoglycosides.	IIIB	Vancomycin toxicity, Incidence of ototoxicity and role of therapeutic drug monitoring for prevention of vancomycin-induced hearing loss

[a]MIC = minimum inhibitory concentration, AUC = area under the concentration-versus-time curve.

result, the likelihood of maintaining free or unbound serum vancomycin concentrations in excess of the bacterial MIC for the entire dosing interval is usually 100% with standard intermittent i.v. infusions for typical staphylococci and streptococci.

Despite the absence of clinical data supporting t>MIC as a predictive parameter for clinical effectiveness, continuous-infusion strategies have been suggested as a possible means to optimize the serum vancomycin concentration and improve effectiveness. Using a randomized crossover study design in intensive care unit (ICU) patients, James et al.[35] found no significant difference between intermittent and continuous administrations when measuring killing activity in vitro, although the ability to maintain serum bactericidal titers above 1:8 was better with a continuous infusion. In a similarly designed study in healthy subjects, Lacy et al.[36] found virtually no difference in activity as measured by bactericidal titers between continuous and intermittent infusions. Further, in a randomized study, Wysocki et al.[37,38] evaluated 160 patients with severe staphylococcal infections. No difference in patient outcome was observed between those receiving intermittent or continuous infusion vancomycin. Vancomycin differs from β-lactam antibiotics, which typically have short half-lives and often require shorter dosage intervals or continuous infusion to optimize therapy. Therefore, based on the available evidence, there does not appear to be any difference in patient outcomes between vancomycin administered by continuous infusion or by intermittent administration.

Summary and recommendations: *Vancomycin dosages should be calculated on ABW. For obese patients, initial dosing can be based on ABW and then adjusted based on serum vancomycin concentrations to achieve therapeutic levels. Continuous infusion regimens are unlikely to substantially improve patient outcome when compared with intermittent dosing. (Level of evidence = II, grade of recommendation = A.)*

Therapeutic Vancomycin Drug Monitoring

Peak versus Trough Concentrations. Over the years, serum vancomycin concentration monitoring practices have varied. Early suggestions, such as those of Geraci,[39] who recommended peak serum vancomycin concentrations of 30–40 mg/L and trough concentrations of 5–10 mg/L, likely did not appreciate the multiexponential decline in the serum vancomycin concentration-versus-time curve.

How Geraci defined peak concentration is unclear. In addition, the pharmacodynamic properties of vancomycin had not been evaluated at the time these recommendations were made. Because the AUC/MIC has been found to correlate with efficacy in experiments conducted with in vitro or animal models, this evidence has led some clinicians to question the relevance of monitoring peak serum vancomycin concentrations.[6] Consequently, some clinicians have decreased the extent of pharmacokinetic monitoring for this antibiotic.[40] However, because it can be difficult in the clinical setting to obtain multiple serum vancomycin concentrations to determine the AUC and subsequently calculate the AUC/MIC, trough serum concentration monitoring, which can be used as a surrogate marker for AUC, is recommended as the most accurate and practical method to monitor vancomycin.

Summary and recommendation: *Trough serum vancomycin concentrations are the most accurate and practical method for monitoring vancomycin effectiveness. Trough concentrations should be obtained just before the next dose at steady-state conditions. (Level of evidence = II, grade of recommendation = B.) (Note: Steady-state achievement is variable and dependent on multiple factors. Trough samples should be obtained just before the fourth dose in patients with normal renal function to ensure that target concentrations are attained.)*

Optimal Trough Concentrations. While Geraci's[39] recommendation for trough concentration was not based on prospective clinical trial data, the benchmark total drug concentration of 5–10 mg/L is likely to fall short of achieving the desired overall vancomycin exposure in many types of infection and isolates with higher (but susceptible) MICs. Therefore, targeting higher trough serum vancomycin concentrations should increase the likelihood of achieving more effective overall antibiotic exposures (i.e., AUC/MIC) and assist in addressing the trend of higher vancomycin MIC values in these organisms.

In recently published guidelines for hospital-acquired, ventilator-associated, and health-care-associated pneumonia, the American Thoracic Society (ATS) suggested an initial vancomycin dosage of 15 mg/kg every 12 hours in adults with normal renal function.[41] ATS acknowledged that vancomycin was a concentration-independent (time-dependent) killer of gram-positive pathogens but had lower penetration into the ELF and respiratory secretions. ATS further recommended that trough serum vancomycin concentrations be maintained at 15–20 mg/L. However, based on pharmacokinetic dosing principles for patients with a normal body weight and normal renal function, it is unlikely that vancomycin 15 mg/kg every 12 hours will produce trough concentrations of 15–20 mg/L. Furthermore, there are no data indicating that achieving these trough concentrations over time is well tolerated and safe.

In an attempt to evaluate the use of targeted trough concentrations of 15–20 mg/L, Jeffres et al.[42] retrospectively evaluated 102 patients with health-care-associated MRSA pneumonia. Overall mortality was 31% (32 patients). There were no significant differences in mean ± S.D. calculated trough serum vancomycin concentrations (13.6 ± 5.9 mg/L versus 13.9 ± 6.7 mg/L) or mean ± S.D. calculated AUC (351 ± 143 mg · hr/L versus 354 ± 109 mg · hr/L) between survivors and nonsurvivors. In addition, no relationship was found between trough serum vancomycin concentrations or AUC and hospital mortality. Although no significant differences were found between survivors and nonsurvivors in terms of trough serum vancomycin concentrations and AUCs, several factors should be noted. For instance, a sample size calculation was not predetermined; therefore, the potential for a Type II error is possible. There was also large variability in both vancomycin trough concentrations (range, 4.2–29.8 mg/L) and AUCs (range, 119–897 mg · hr/L), which may account for the lack of significant findings. Time to achieve targeted serum vancomycin concentrations was not measured and may be a critical factor in determining patient outcome. In addition, because a disk-diffusion method was used for susceptibility testing, organism MIC could not be determined. Therefore, only the AUC, not the AUC/MIC, was evaluated as a potential predictor of success or failure.

Although the results of this study are of interest, additional prospective studies are needed to confirm these data.

Relationship between trough vancomycin concentrations, resistance, and therapeutic failure. While vancomycin is considered a bactericidal antibiotic, the rate of bacterial kill is slow when compared with that of β-lactams, and vancomycin's activity is affected by the bacterial inoculum. Large bacterial burdens in the stationary growth phase or in an anaerobic environment pose a significant challenge to the speed and extent of vancomycin's bactericidal activity.[43-46]

In recent years, VISA or glycopeptide-intermediate susceptible *S. aureus* (GISA) and vancomycin-resistant *S. aureus* (VRSA) have appeared and raised questions about the overall utility of this antibiotic. (Note: The terms VISA and GISA are often used interchangeably. For the purpose of this consensus review, VISA will be used throughout.) Although infection with these organisms is infrequent, there is fear that the organisms could become more prevalent if the high rate of use and exposure pressure of vancomycin continues.[47] The discovery of inducible hVISA (i.e., strains with MIC values in the susceptible range of 0.5–2 mg/L in patients whose therapy with standard dosages of vancomycin has failed) raises further questions regarding current dosing guidelines and the overall use of this antibiotic. Concerns are related to treatment failures and the inability to easily detect hVISA isolates in clinical settings.[48-50]

In 2006, the Clinical and Laboratory Standards Institute (CLSI) lowered the susceptibility and resistance breakpoints for the MIC of vancomycin from ≤4 to ≤2 mg/L for "susceptible," from 8–16 to 4–8 mg/L for "intermediate," and from ≥32 to ≥16 mg/L for "resistant."[51] The decision to move the breakpoints was primarily based on clinical data indicating that patients were less likely to be successfully treated with vancomycin if the *S. aureus* MIC was ≤4 mg/L.[51] Despite the change in susceptibility and resistance breakpoints, two reports have suggested that patients with *S. aureus* isolates having vancomycin MICs of 1–2 mg/L are less likely to be successfully treated with vancomycin compared with patients with *S. aureus* isolates that demonstrate greater susceptibility.[52,53] However, this information alone does not address whether the use of higher concentrations of vancomycin would improve overall effectiveness. Low serum vancomycin concentrations may also create problems, as there appears to be a direct correlation between low serum vancomycin levels and the emergence of hVISA, VISA, or both, at least with certain genotypes of MRSA.[54] In addition, studies have suggested that trough serum vancomycin concentrations of <10 mg/L may predict therapeutic failure and the potential for the emergence of VISA or VRSA.[54,55]

Studies of MRSA and hVISA bacteremia have revealed significantly higher rates of morbidity in patients infected with hVISA.[50,55,56] These patients were more likely to have high bacterial load infections, low initial trough serum vancomycin concentrations, and treatment failure.[56] Jones[57] recently reported that approximately 74% of hVISA strains and 15% of wild-type *S. aureus* strains were tolerant (minimum bactericidal concentration of ≥32 mg/L) to the effects of vancomycin, which contributes to a low probability of success in patients harboring these organisms.

Sakoulas et al.[52] reported a significant correlation between vancomycin susceptibilities and patient outcome. Treatment of bloodstream infections caused by MRSA strains having a vancomycin MIC of ≤0.5 mg/L had an overall suc-

cess rate of 55.6%, while treatment of patients infected with MRSA strains having a vancomycin MIC of 1–2 mg/L had a success rate of only 9.5% (*p* = 0.03). (Treatment failure was defined as persistent signs or symptoms of infection [e.g., fever, leukocytosis], new signs or symptoms of infection, or worsening of signs or symptoms of infection in patients receiving at least five days of therapy with targeted trough serum vancomycin concentrations of 10–15 mg/L). However, this was a relatively small study (*n* = 30) of MRSA bacteremic patients who were refractory to vancomycin therapy and were enrolled in compassionate-use drug trials. In a more recent study of patients with MRSA bacteremia (*n* = 34), Moise et al.[58] demonstrated that patients with MRSA isolates with a vancomycin MIC of 2 mg/L had significantly higher median days to organism eradication, longer treatment with vancomycin, and a significantly lower overall likelihood of organism eradication. Hidayat et al.[53] evaluated the use of high-dosage vancomycin intended to achieve unbound trough serum vancomycin concentrations of at least four times the MIC in patients with MRSA infections. Of the 95 patients evaluated with MRSA pneumonia or bacteremia, or both, 51 (54%) had vancomycin MIC values of 1.5 or 2 mg/L. Although an initial response of 74% was demonstrated in patients achieving the desired target MIC, a high percentage of patients infected with strains having an MIC of 1.5 or 2 mg/L had a poorer response (62% versus 85%) and significantly higher infection-related mortality (24% versus 10%) compared with patients infected with low-MIC strains (0.5, 0.75, or 1 mg/L), despite achieving target trough serum vancomycin concentrations of 15–20 mg/L. The data from these two studies suggest that *S. aureus* isolates with MICs of 1–2 mg/L that are still within the susceptible range may be less responsive to vancomycin therapy. Soriano et al.[59] evaluated the influence of vancomycin MIC on outcome in a total of 414 episodes of MRSA bacteremic patients. MIC evaluations were determined by Etest methodology. Among several factors that predicted poor outcome, *S. aureus* isolates with an MIC of 2 mg/L were significantly associated with increased mortality. Based on the low probability of achieving an appropriate targeted vancomycin concentration exposure (AUC/MIC), the authors suggested that vancomycin should not be considered an optimal treatment approach for infection due to strains with a vancomycin MIC of >1 mg/L when using trough serum vancomycin concentrations of >10 mg/L as a target.

Lodise et al.[60] evaluated the relationship between vancomycin MIC and treatment failure among 92 adult nonneutropenic patients with MRSA bloodstream infections. Vancomycin failure was defined as 30-day mortality, 10 or more days of bacteremia on vancomycin therapy, or recurrence of MRSA bacteremia within 60 days of vancomycin discontinuation. Classification and regression tree analysis found that a vancomycin MIC breakpoint of ≥1.5 mg/L was associated with an increased probability of treatment failure. The 66 patients with a vancomycin MIC of ≥1.5 mg/L had a 2.4-fold higher rate of treatment failure compared with patients with a vancomycin MIC of ≤1 mg/L (36.4% versus 15.4%, respectively; *p* = 0.049). Poisson regression analysis determined that a vancomycin MIC of ≥1.5 mg/L was independently associated with treatment failure (*p* = 0.01). Based on these findings, the investigators suggested that an alternative therapy should be considered.

An analysis of a large surveillance database of 35,458 *S. aureus* strains by Jones[57] found that the MIC required to

inhibit the growth of 50% of organisms or the MIC required to inhibit the growth of 90% of organisms (MIC90) for vancomycin is 1 mg/L.[57] The Centers for Disease Control and Prevention 2005 U.S. Surveillance Network data of vancomycin susceptibility reported that 16.2% of 241,605 S. aureus isolates had an MIC of 2 mg/L.[51] Regional variability exists, and an MIC90 of 2 mg/L has recently been reported by several institutions. For example, Mohr and Murray[61] reported that as many as 30% of 116 MRSA blood culture isolates collected from the Texas Medical Center over a one-year period had a vancomycin MIC of 2 mg/L. There have been recent reports of significant shifts in bacterial susceptibility to vancomycin over a five-year surveillance period.[62-64] Increasing S. aureus MIC values, coupled with reports of failure rates associated with a vancomycin MIC of 2 mg/L, have raised the question of whether the breakpoint for vancomycin resistance should be lowered even further.[65]

New information is emerging regarding the importance of the accessory gene regulator (agr), a global quorum-sensing regulator in S. aureus that is responsible for orchestrating the expression of adherence factors, biofilm production, tolerance to vancomycin, and virulence factors.[66] The agr locus has been a subject of intense study because there appears to be a relationship between polymorphism in this gene cluster and patient response to vancomycin therapy. Several studies have determined that all VISA strains reported to date from the United States belong to agr group II. The agr group II includes the USA 100 MRSA clones that are predominately associated with nosocomial infections, and these strains have been associated with vancomycin treatment failure.[33,67] Sakoulas et al.[67,68] have determined in in vitro studies that the emergence of hVISA or VISA may occur when S. aureus isolates with a down-regulated or defective agr locus are exposed to suboptimal vancomycin concentrations. In a series of in vitro experiments, MRSA belonging to agr group II with a defective agr locus exposed to vancomycin concentrations of <10 mg/L produced heteroresistant-like characteristics similar to VISA strains with subsequent MIC increases from 1 to 8 mg/L.[67] This phenomenon was recently demonstrated in a patient with chronic renal failure undergoing hemodialysis who experienced recurrent MRSA bacteremia over a 30-month period.[54] The patient was treated repeatedly with vancomycin at trough serum concentrations that always exceeded 10 mg/L. Despite frequent recurrences of bacteremia with the same isolate, the isolate remained susceptible to vancomycin. The genetic background of this organism was found to be similar to other VISA strains belonging to agr group II. When the isolate was subjected to vancomycin concentrations of <10 mg/L under laboratory conditions, it quickly demonstrated characteristics similar to VISA strains with a subsequent increased MIC.

Tsuji et al.[69] used an in vitro pharmacodynamic model to evaluate S. aureus agr groups I–IV exposed to optimal and suboptimal vancomycin doses over a three-day period. In this study, low vancomycin exposures equivalent to total trough serum vancomycin concentrations of 1.5–10 mg/L and an AUC/MIC of 31–264 produced increases in the MIC to the range considered to be VISA by the current CLSI vancomycin breakpoints. Although resistance was produced in both agr functional and defective strains, the likelihood of resistance was fourfold to fivefold higher in agr-defective isolates. Subsequently, the investigators determined that as many as 48% of hospital-associated MRSA had a dysfunc-

tional agr locus, making this finding potentially clinically relevant and warranting further evaluation.[70]

Summary and recommendation: *Based on evidence suggesting that* S. aureus *exposure to trough serum vancomycin concentrations of <10 mg/L can produce strains with VISA-like characteristics, it is recommended that trough serum vancomycin concentrations always be maintained above 10 mg/L to avoid development of resistance. (Level of evidence = III, grade of recommendation = B.)*

Correlating dosing with optimal AUC/MIC and trough concentrations. As mentioned previously, an isolate's vancomycin MIC is an important parameter for determining the potential success of a given dosage regimen. Therefore, an actual vancomycin MIC value should ideally be obtained from the clinical microbiology laboratory. Currently, some clinical microbiology laboratories may be limited in their ability to report vancomycin MIC values, depending on the methodology (disk diffusion or automated microdilution) used to determine antimicrobial susceptibility. In some instances, supplemental Etest methods may be used to obtain this information.

As previously stated, an AUC/MIC of ≥400 has been promoted as the target predictive of successful therapy (i.e., organism eradication). Based on this information, a simple evaluation of standard dosing practices (e.g., 1 g every 12 hours) for an individual with normal renal function (CLcr of ≥100 mL/min) and average weight (80 kg) would only yield a 24-hour drug AUC of approximately 250 mg · hr/L. Unless the pathogen had a vancomycin MIC of ≤0.5 mg/L, this dosage regimen would not generate the targeted AUC/MIC of ≥400. For a pathogen with an MIC of 1 mg/L, the minimum trough serum vancomycin concentration would have to be at least 15 mg/L to obtain the target AUC/MIC. Using the vancomycin pharmacokinetic data generated by Jeffres et al.[42] in patients receiving vancomycin for the treatment of MRSA pneumonia, Mohr and Murray[61] determined by Monte Carlo simulation that the probability of achieving an AUC/MIC of ≥400 would be 100% if the S. aureus MIC for vancomycin was 0.5 mg/L but 0% if the MIC was 2 mg/L. Using a similar one-compartment model of vancomycin and a Monte Carlo simulation integrating S. aureus MIC values, del Mar Fernández de Gatta Garcia et al.[71] reported that a daily dosage of 3–4 g of vancomycin would be required to provide 90% probability of attaining a target AUC/MIC of 400 with an MIC of 1 mg/L. For VISA strains, a vancomycin daily dose of ≥5 g would be required to provide a high probability of target AUC/MIC attainment for this pathogen. For susceptible S. aureus, total daily doses of ≥40 mg/kg would likely be required for typical patients. Use of these larger dosages of vancomycin should be carefully monitored for the desired clinical outcome and the absence of drug-induced toxicity. The use of a nomogram is an alternative method for dosage adjustments; however, the majority of published nomograms in clinical use have been proven to be inaccurate, and most have not been clinically validated.[72] In addition, no published nomogram to date has been constructed to achieve trough serum vancomycin concentrations of 15–20 mg/L.

Loading doses have also been suggested for critically ill patients to attain target trough serum vancomycin levels earlier. In a small study of critically ill patients with seri-

ous *S. aureus* infections, a vancomycin loading dose of 25 mg/kg infused at a rate of 500 mg/hr was found to be safe without producing toxic peak serum drug levels.[73] While this approach is not currently supported by evidence from large randomized clinical trials, vancomycin loading doses can be considered in the treatment of serious MRSA infections.[63,74]

Summary and recommendations: *Based on the potential to improve penetration, increase the probability of optimal target serum vancomycin concentrations, and improve clinical outcomes for complicated infections such as bacteremia, endocarditis, osteomyelitis, meningitis, and hospital-acquired pneumonia caused by* S. aureus, *total trough serum vancomycin concentrations of 15–20 mg/L are recommended. Trough serum vancomycin concentrations in that range should achieve an AUC/MIC of ≥400 in most patients if the MIC is ≤1 mg/L. (Level of evidence = III, grade of recommendation = B.)*

In order to achieve rapid attainment of this target concentration for seriously ill patients, a loading dose of 25–30 mg/kg (based on ABW) can be considered. (Level of evidence = III, grade of recommendation = B.)

A targeted AUC/MIC of ≥400 is not achievable with conventional dosing methods if the vancomycin MIC is ≥2 mg/L in a patient with normal renal function (i.e., CL_{cr} of 70–100 mL/min). Therefore, alternative therapies should be considered.

Vancomycin dosages of 15–20 mg/kg (based on ABW) given every 8–12 hours are required for most patients with normal renal function to achieve the suggested serum concentrations when the MIC is ≤1 mg/L. It should be noted that currently available nomograms were not developed to achieve these targeted endpoints. Individual pharmacokinetic adjustments and verification of serum target achievement are recommended. When individual doses exceed 1 g (i.e., 1.5 and 2 g), the infusion period should be extended to 1.5–2 hours. (Level of evidence = III, grade of recommendation = B.)

Vancomycin Toxicity

Vancomycin was initially dubbed "Mississippi mud" because of the brown color of early formulations, which were about 70% pure. The impurities are thought to have contributed to the incidence of adverse reactions.[7,75,76] In the 1960s, purity increased to 75% and in 1985 to 92–95% for Eli Lilly's vancomycin product.[74] Concurrently, a decrease in the reporting of serious adverse events occurred.

The most common vancomycin adverse effects are unrelated to serum drug concentration and include fever, chills, and phlebitis.[7] Red man syndrome may be associated with histamine release and manifests as tingling and flushing of the face, neck, and upper torso. It is most likely to occur when larger dosages are infused too rapidly (>500 mg over ≤30 minutes).[7,77,78] Vancomycin should be administered intravenously over an infusion period of at least 1 hour to minimize infusion-related adverse effects. For higher dosages (e.g., 2 g), the infusion time should be extended to 1.5–2 hours. Less frequent adverse events, such as neutropenia, also appear unrelated to serum drug concentrations.[79,80]

Vancomycin has long been considered a nephrotoxic and ototoxic agent. Excessive serum drug concentrations

have been implicated, and it was assumed that monitoring of serum concentrations would allow interventions that decrease toxicity.

Incidence, Mechanism, and Definition of Nephrotoxicity. A review of the literature published from 1956 through 1986 identified 57 cases of vancomycin-associated nephrotoxicity, with over 50% of those cases identified within the first six years of vancomycin use when the product was relatively impure.[75] The rate of nephrotoxicity attributable to vancomycin monotherapy varied from 0% to 17% and from 7% to 35% with concurrent administration of aminoglycosides.[81-85] A review of the literature available through 1993, conducted by Cantu et al.,[8] identified 167 cases of vancomycin-related nephrotoxicity. However, the lack of clear-cut examples of vancomycin-induced nephrotoxicity (when the drug was used alone) was striking. The researchers determined that the frequency of nephrotoxicity due to vancomycin monotherapy was 5–7%. No evidence supported maintaining serum vancomycin concentrations within a given range to prevent nephrotoxicity. However, another study identified older age, longer treatment courses, and higher trough serum vancomycin concentrations (30–65 mg/L) as risk factors for vancomycin-induced nephrotoxicity.[81] Although the definition of vancomycin-induced nephrotoxicity has varied, a reasonable composite from the literature defines this adverse effect as an increase of >0.5 mg/dL (or a ≥50% increase) in serum creatinine over baseline in consecutively obtained daily serum creatinine values or a drop in calculated CL_{cr} of 50% from baseline on two consecutive days in the absence of an alternative explanation.[10,12,53,86-88]

The exact mechanism and incidence of vancomycin nephrotoxicity have been investigated in animals and humans. The filtration and energy-dependent transport mechanisms found in the proximal tubular epithelium render the kidneys susceptible to toxicant-induced injury.[89] Vancomycin exposure in renal proximal tubule epithelial cells results in increased cell proliferation. The stimulation of oxygen consumption and the increase in ATP concentrations support the role of vancomycin as a stimulant of oxidative phosphorylation.[89] In rats, antioxidants protect kidneys against vancomycin-induced injury, in theory, by inhibiting free oxygen radical production.[90] Human data suggest toxicity from vancomycin (or aminoglycosides) is not confined to the proximal tubule but may also involve the medullary region (loop of Henle and collecting duct) of the nephron.[91] Vancomycin destruction of glomeruli and necrosis of the proximal tubule are thought to be due to oxidative stress.[92]

In humans, nephrotoxicity due to vancomycin monotherapy with typical dosage regimens is uncommon, is usually reversible, and occurs with an incidence only slightly above what is reported with other antimicrobials not considered to be nephrotoxic.[11,83,93-96] Investigators have administered a wide dosing range of vancomycin monotherapy to rats without appreciable renal injury.[97,98] Renal impairment in rats was observed when concurrent aminoglycosides were administered[97-99] or if very high dosages of vancomycin were used (350 mg/kg twice daily for four days).[98] Wood et al.[100] investigated the influence of vancomycin on tobramycin-induced nephrotoxicity in rats and found that toxicity occurred earlier and was more severe with concurrent aminoglycoside and vancomycin therapy. Histological evidence of tubular necrosis occurred earlier and the percentage of

necrotic cells was higher in rats receiving combination therapy compared with animals administered tobramycin alone. Indeed, animals receiving vancomycin alone lacked evidence of nephrotoxicity. Enhanced renal accumulation of tobramycin was not evident in animals receiving both vancomycin and tobramycin. In fact, animals receiving the combination had lower renal tobramycin concentrations than did animals receiving tobramycin alone. Increased enzymuria and crystalluria were seen in rats and may suggest toxicity after vancomycin administration.[101-104] However, these markers are very sensitive and could reflect transient hypotension due to rapid administration rather than toxicity.[8] Enzymuria in humans was minimally affected during five days of vancomycin therapy.[105]

Data regarding concurrent vancomycin and aminoglycoside administration in humans provide conflicting information, with some reports indicating that the combination augments aminoglycoside-induced nephrotoxicity,[11,76,81,83,91,94,106,107] and others indicating no effect.[81,83,85,86,96,108-111] Rybak et al.[10] found that patients given vancomycin and an aminoglycoside were 6.7-fold more likely to develop nephrotoxicity than those receiving vancomycin alone. Vancomycin administration for more than 21 days was an additional risk factor ($p = 0.007$). Bertino et al.[107] found vancomycin to be an independent risk factor for aminoglycoside nephrotoxicity in a review of 1489 patients who prospectively received individualized pharmacokinetic monitoring. However, vancomycin use was not associated with increased risk when assessed in a multivariate model in this study. Most of the available data suggest a 3- to 4-fold increase in nephrotoxicity when aminoglycosides are combined with vancomycin.[81,83,93,94] Synergistic toxicity may also occur when vancomycin is used with other nephrotoxic agents (e.g., amphotericin B, certain chemotherapy agents) or used to treat certain diseases (e.g., sepsis, liver disease, obstructive uropathy, pancreatitis).[40,86,93]

Vancomycin administered either as a single, large, 30-mg/kg once-daily dose or in two divided doses did not influence nephrotoxicity significantly ($p = 0.71$).[112] However, "high-dose" (defined as a total daily dose of 40 mg/kg, either as a continuous infusion or divided every 12 hours, resulting in a mean ± S.D. concentration of 24.4 ± 7.8 mg/L) was found to be less nephrotoxic than "standard-dose" intermittent therapy (defined as 10 mg/kg every 12 hours, resulting in a mean ± S.D. trough serum vancomycin concentration of 10.0 ± 5.3 mg/L) ($p = 0.007$) by other investigators.[113] It should be noted that the average age of patients in this later investigation was 60 years; their average weight was not provided.

Human trials have suggested that trough serum vancomycin concentrations of >10 mg/L are associated with an increased risk of nephrotoxicity.[10,76,83,85,86] No correlation has been observed between peak vancomycin concentrations and nephrotoxicity.[10] Zimmermann et al.[114] found no correlation between nephrotoxicity and initial serum creatinine concentration, length of hospital stay, or duration of vancomycin therapy. However, the researchers did find that serum vancomycin concentrations were significantly higher in those patients who eventually developed nephrotoxicity. In that study, no patient who maintained trough serum vancomycin concentrations of <20 mg/L developed nephrotoxicity. It is noteworthy that 21 (57%) of 37 patients consistently had trough serum vancomycin concentrations of >20 mg/L and yet did not develop nephrotoxicity. Recent guidelines have

recommended target trough serum vancomycin concentrations of 15–20 mg/L.[41] However, the safety of higher trough vancomycin concentrations over a prolonged period has not been sufficiently studied.

Lee-Such et al.[115] conducted a retrospective chart review of patients over age 18 years who received vancomycin for at least 14 days and had an available baseline serum creatinine concentration and a CL_{cr} of >30 mL/min (calculated by Cockroft-Gault equation). Patients were categorized by trough serum vancomycin concentrations (≤15 mg/L [$n = 19$] or ≥15.1 mg/L [$n = 40$]). Nephrotoxicity was defined as a rise in serum creatinine of ≥0.5 mg/dL above baseline. The median maximum serum creatinine percentage increase was 0.0% (range, –31.3 to 30.0) in the low-trough-concentration group and 17.2% (range, –36.4 to 133) in the high-concentration group ($p = 0.0045$). There were no significant correlations between percent change in serum creatinine and duration of vancomycin therapy, highest trough concentration, or average daily dose. The frequency of nephrotoxicity was 0% in the low-trough-concentration group and 15% in the high-trough-concentration group. The investigators could not discern if higher vancomycin levels were a cause or an indicator of worsening renal function. In addition, a single trough vancomycin concentration of >15 mg/L placed a patient in the high-concentration group, but such a level could be due to a variety of clinical or operational factors not related to vancomycin-induced toxicity. Finally, the use of pressors and concurrent nephrotoxins was poorly described but could provide additional concurrent risk for renal dysfunction. Further details are lacking, as the data are currently available only in abstract form.

Jeffres et al.[87] conducted a similar but prospective investigation of 94 patients with health-care-associated pneumonia. Nephrotoxicity was defined as a 0.5-mg/dL increase from baseline in serum creatinine or an increase of ≥50% in serum creatinine from baseline during vancomycin therapy. Patients were stratified based on vancomycin trough concentrations of <15 mg/L ($n = 43$) or ≥15 mg/L ($n = 51$). Overall, 40 patients (42.6%) met the criteria for nephrotoxicity. The maximal serum creatinine concentration observed occurred after the maximum serum vancomycin concentration by at least 24 hours in 34 patients (85.0%). Patients who developed nephrotoxicity were more likely to have higher steady-state mean trough serum vancomycin concentrations (20.8 mg/L versus 14.3 mg/L, respectively; $p < 0.001$), trough serum vancomycin concentrations of >15 mg/L (67.5% versus 40.7%, $p = 0.01$), and a longer duration (≥14 days) of vancomycin therapy (45.0% versus 20.4%, $p = 0.011$) than those who did not develop nephrotoxicity.

Hidayat et al.[53] prospectively investigated the efficacy and toxicity of adjusting vancomycin troughs to achieve an unbound concentration of at least four times the MIC. Patients received vancomycin for 72 hours or more. Nephrotoxicity was defined as a 0.5-mg/dL or ≥50% increase from the baseline serum creatinine concentration in two consecutive laboratory analyses. For nephrotoxicity analysis, groups were divided based on trough serum vancomycin concentrations (<15 or ≥15 mg/L). Nephrotoxicity occurred only in the ≥15-mg/L group (11 of 63 patients [12%] versus 0 of 24 patients in the <15-mg/L group [$p = 0.01$]) and was predicted by the use of concurrent nephrotoxic agents ($p < 0.001$). By controlling for age, admission to ICUs, Acute Physiology and Chronic Evaluation II score, trough serum vancomycin level, and duration of therapy, multivariate analysis demonstrated

concurrent nephrotoxins to be the strongest predictor of vancomycin nephrotoxicity. Without concurrent nephrotoxins, nephrotoxicity occurred in only 1 (2%) of 44 patients with a trough concentration of ≥15 mg/L versus 0 of 24 patients in the <15-mg/L group.[12]

Lodise et al.[12] retrospectively examined the relationship between vancomycin dosage and rate of nephrotoxicity at a single institution. Nephrotoxicity was defined as an increase in serum creatinine of 0.5 mg/dL or an increase of 50%, whichever was greater, on at least two consecutive days during the period from initiation of vancomycin or linezolid therapy to 72 hours after completion of therapy. Linezolid usage was also included as a nonvancomycin comparator group. A significant difference in nephrotoxicity was noted among patients receiving vancomycin ≥4 g/day (34.6%), vancomycin <4 g/day (10.9%), and linezolid (6.7%) ($p = 0.001$). The relationship between high-dosage vancomycin and nephrotoxicity persisted in the multivariate analyses that controlled for potential confounding covariates. The multivariate analyses also demonstrated that patient total weight of ≥101.4 kg, estimated CL_{cr} of ≤86.6 mL/min, and ICU residence at the start of therapy each independently influenced the time to nephrotoxicity. In a secondary analysis, a significant relationship was found between the vancomycin AUC and nephrotoxicity. Specifically, a vancomycin AUC of ≥952 mg · L/hr was associated with a higher probability of vancomycin-related nephrotoxicity.

Nguyen et al.[88] retrospectively investigated patients receiving vancomycin between January and December 2006 at a single institution. Patients included were age ≥18 years, receiving vancomycin for at least 72 hours, and had at least one serum vancomycin value obtained. Hemodialysis patients were excluded. Nephrotoxicity was defined as an increase of >0.5 mg/dL over baseline in serum creatinine for two consecutive assays. Creatinine levels were followed until patient discharge. Patients were divided based on trough serum vancomycin concentration attainment of 5–15 mg/L ($n = 130$) or >15 mg/L ($n = 88$). The rate of nephrotoxicity was 6.2% in the lower-trough group and 18.2% in the higher-trough group ($p < 0.01$). Multivariate analysis indicated that the main predictors of nephrotoxicity were an elevated overall average trough concentration and duration of therapy.

Investigations, such as those described herein, are intriguing but often limited by small sample size, retrospective design, and questionable methodology. Additional data are needed, including the timing of the relationship between high vancomycin levels and nephrotoxicity (i.e., which one precedes the other). In addition, while statistically relevant, the clinical significance of minor and transient changes in creatinine or CL_{cr} can be debated. The effect of a 0.5-mg/dL increase in serum creatinine concentration would be greater in a patient with a lower initial CL_{cr} value than in one with a higher baseline CL_{cr} value.

Summary and recommendation: *There are limited data suggesting a direct causal relationship between toxicity and specific serum vancomycin concentrations. In addition, data are conflicting and characterized by the presence of confounding nephrotoxic agents, inconsistent and highly variable definitions of toxicity, and the inability to examine the time sequence of events surrounding changes in renal function secondary to vancomycin exposure.*

A patient should be identified as having experienced vancomycin-induced nephrotoxicity if multiple (at least two or three consecutive) high serum creatinine concentrations (increase of 0.5 mg/dL or ≥50% increase from baseline, whichever is greater) are documented after several days of vancomycin therapy in the absence of an alternative explanation. (Level of evidence = II, grade of recommendation = B.)

Role of Therapeutic Drug Monitoring in Preventing Nephrotoxicity. Because vancomycin is eliminated via glomerular filtration, a decrease in the glomerular filtration rate from any cause will increase the serum vancomycin concentration and make the association between renal dysfunction and trough concentrations difficult to assess.[8]

Some investigators have found vancomycin therapeutic drug monitoring to be associated with decreased nephrotoxicity. Other factors associated with decreased toxicity include shorter courses of therapy, less total dosage in grams of the drug, and a decreased length of hospital stay.[7,12,116,117] However, Darko et al.[7] found therapeutic drug monitoring to be cost-effective only in patients in ICUs, those receiving other nephrotoxins, and, possibly, oncology patients.

Summary and recommendations: *Available evidence does not support monitoring peak serum vancomycin concentrations to decrease the frequency of nephrotoxicity. (Level of evidence = I, grade of recommendation = A.)*

Monitoring of trough serum vancomycin concentrations to reduce nephrotoxicity is best suited to patients receiving aggressive dosing targeted to produce sustained trough drug concentrations of 15–20 mg/L or who are at high risk of toxicity, such as patients receiving concurrent nephrotoxins. (Level of evidence = III, grade of recommendation = B.)

Monitoring is also recommended for patients with unstable renal function (either deteriorating or significantly improving) and those receiving prolonged courses of therapy (over three to five days). (Level of evidence = II, grade of recommendation = B.)

All patients receiving prolonged courses of vancomycin should have at least one steady-state trough concentration obtained (just before the fourth dose). Frequent monitoring (more than a single trough concentration before the fourth dose) for short-course therapy (less than five days) or for lower-intensity dosing (targeted to attain trough serum vancomycin concentrations below 15 mg/L) is not recommended. (Level of evidence = II, grade of recommendation = B.)

There are limited data to support the safety of sustained trough serum vancomycin concentrations of 15–20 mg/L. When this target range is desired, obtaining once-weekly trough concentrations in hemodynamically stable patients is recommended. Frequent (in some instances daily) trough concentration monitoring is advisable to prevent toxicity in hemodynamically unstable patients. The exact frequency of monitoring is often a matter of clinical judgment. (Level of evidence = III, grade of recommendation = B.)

Data on comparative vancomycin toxicity using continuous versus intermittent administration are conflicting and no recommendation can be made.

Incidence of Ototoxicity and Role of Therapeutic Drug Monitoring for Prevention of Vancomycin-Induced Hearing Loss. Vancomycin-induced hearing loss is controversial. Vancomycin has not been found to be ototoxic in animal models.[97,98,100,118,119] Early literature attributed ototoxic events to impurities or to concurrent ototoxic agents.[119] Early studies indicated that other ototoxic agents, such as the aminoglycosides kanamycin and streptomycin, may have additive or synergistic toxicity when used in combination with vancomycin.[120] The frequency of ototoxicity in humans has been reported to range from 1% to 9%[3,8,48,121-124] and to be associated with serum vancomycin concentrations above 40 mg/L.[7,125] This most likely represents an inflated occurrence rate due to impurities associated with the older formulation or poor documentation of cause and effect as they relate to serum concentrations. The true risk of ototoxicity from vancomycin monotherapy is low without concurrent therapy with ototoxic agents.[77]

Severe ototoxicity induced by vancomycin is rare and characterized as damage to the auditory nerve that initially affects high-frequency sensory hairs in the cochlea, then the middle- and low-frequency hairs, and eventually can lead to total hearing loss.[75] High-tone deafness occurs before low-tone deafness at all frequencies and is permanent. Inability to hear high-frequency sounds and tinnitus are ominous signs that should result in discontinuation of vancomycin.[126,127] Also rare is reversible ototoxicity such as tinnitus, which can occur with or without high-tone deafness.[33,120,127] Investigation of pediatric pneumococcal meningitis noted that early vancomycin administration (relative to ceftriaxone administration) was associated with a substantially increased risk of hearing loss due to the effects of rapid bacterial killing by both antimicrobials and the resultant host inflammatory response.[128] However, toxicity did not correlate with vancomycin concentrations.

In 1958, Geraci et al.[129] described hearing loss in two patients with serum vancomycin concentrations of 80–100 mg/L. That report generated an impetus to monitor peak serum concentrations. However, Cantu et al.[8] reviewed 53 published cases of vancomycin-attributed ototoxicity and concluded that vancomycin was rarely ototoxic as a single agent. In addition, ototoxicity was fully reversible when other ototoxic agents were not involved.

Bailie and Neal[75] reviewed 28 cases of ototoxicity reported between 1956 and 1986, most of which involved vancomycin preparations with higher levels of impurities. Patients with severe renal dysfunction were found to be more susceptible to developing ototoxicity when their dosage regimen was not adjusted. The researchers were unable to correlate mild ototoxicity with excessive peak or trough serum vancomycin concentrations or prevention of ototoxicity by monitoring serum concentrations.

A lack of correlation between serum vancomycin levels and the development of ototoxicity has also been observed in cancer patients.[75] Of 742 patients analyzed, ototoxicity occurred in 18 (6%) of 319 patients (95% CI, 4–9%) who were receiving concurrent ototoxic agents (including aminoglycosides, cisplatin, loop diuretics, aspirin, and nonsteroidal antiinflammatory agents) and in 12 (3%) of 423 patients (95% CI, 2–5%) not treated with other ototoxic agents. All clinical ototoxicity resolved within three weeks after vancomycin discontinuation.

Summary and recommendation: *Monitoring serum vancomycin levels to prevent ototoxicity is not recommended* because this toxicity is rarely associated with monotherapy and does not correlate with serum vancomycin concentrations. Monitoring may be more important when other ototoxic agents, such as aminoglycosides, are administered. (Level of evidence = III, grade of recommendation = B.)

Summary

In general, pharmacodynamic dosing of antibiotics may significantly augment antibiotic performance. There seems to be little difference in the pharmacodynamics of intermittently or continuously dosed vancomycin. This consensus panel review supports that vancomycin is a concentration-independent killer of gram-positive pathogens and that the AUC/MIC is likely the most useful pharmacodynamic parameter to predict effectiveness. In many clinical settings where it may be difficult to obtain multiple serum vancomycin concentrations to determine the AUC and subsequently the AUC/MIC, trough serum vancomycin concentration monitoring can be recommended as the most accurate and practical method to monitor serum vancomycin levels. Increasing trough serum vancomycin concentrations to 15–20 mg/L to obtain an increased AUC/MIC of ≥400 may be desirable but is currently not supported by clinical trial data. Target attainment of an AUC/MIC of ≥400 is not likely in patients with *S. aureus* infections who have an MIC of ≥2 mg/L; therefore, treatment with alternative agents should be considered. Higher trough serum vancomycin levels may also increase the potential for toxicity, but additional clinical experience will be required to determine the extent of this potential.

References

1. Moellering RC Jr. Vancomycin: a 50-year reassessment. *Clin Infect Dis.* 2006; 42(suppl 1):S3–4.
2. Levine DP. Vancomycin: a history. *Clin Infect Dis.* 2006; 42(suppl 1):S5–12.
3. Murray BE, Nannini EC. Glycopeptides (vancomycin and teicoplanin), streptogramins (quinupristin-dalfopristin), and lipopeptides (daptomycin). In: Mandell GL, Bennett JE, Dolin R, eds. Mandell, Douglas and Bennett's principles and practice of infectious diseases. 6th ed. Oxford: Churchill Livingstone; 2005:417–40.
4. Virgincar N, MacGowan A. Glycopeptides (dalbavancin, oritavancin, teicoplanin, vancomycin). In: Yu VL, Edwards G, McKinnon PS et al., eds. Antimicrobial therapy and vaccines. Volume II: antimicrobial agents. 2nd ed. Pittsburgh: ESun Technologies; 2004:181–99.
5. Stevens DL. The role of vancomycin in the treatment paradigm. *Clin Infect Dis.* 2006; 42(suppl 1):S51–7.
6. Rybak MJ. The pharmacokinetic and pharmacodynamic properties of vancomycin. *Clin Infect Dis.* 2006; 42(suppl 1):S35–9.
7. Darko W, Medicis JJ, Smith A. Mississippi mud no more: cost-effectiveness of pharmacokinetic dosage adjustment of vancomycin to prevent nephrotoxicity. *Pharmacotherapy.* 2003; 23:643–50.
8. Cantu TG, Yamanaka-Yuen NA, Leitman PS. Serum vancomycin concentrations: reappraisal of their clinical value. *Clin Infect Dis.* 1994; 18:533–43.
9. Moellering RC Jr. Monitoring serum vancomycin levels: climbing the mountain because it is there? *Clin Infect Dis.* 1994; 18:544–6.

10. Rybak MJ, Albrecht LM, Boike SC et al. Nephrotoxicity of vancomycin alone and with an aminoglycoside. *J Antimicrob Chemother.* 1990; 25:679–87.

11. Rybak MJ, Abate BJ, Kang SL et al. Prospective evaluation of the effect of an aminoglycoside dosing regimen on rates of observed nephrotoxicity and ototoxicity. *Antimicrob Agents Chemother.* 1999; 43:1549–55.

12. Lodise TP, Lomaestro B, Graves J et al. Larger vancomycin doses (≥4 grams/day) are associated with an increased incidence of nephrotoxicity. *Antimicrob Agents Chemother.* 2008; 52:1330–6.

13. Canadian Task Force on the Periodic Health Examination. The periodic health examination. *Can Med Assoc J.* 1979; 121:1193–254.

14. Rodvold KA, Blum RA, Fischer JH et al. Vancomycin pharmacokinetics in patients with various degrees of renal function. *Antimicrob Agents Chemother.* 1988; 32:848–52.

15. Matzke GR, McGory RW, Halstenson CE et al. Pharmacokinetics of vancomycin in patients with various degrees of renal function. *Antimicrob Agents Chemother.* 1984; 25:433–7.

16. Rotschafer JC, Crossley K, Zaske DE et al. Pharmacokinetics of vancomycin: observations in 28 patients and dosage recommendations. *Antimicrob Agents Chemother.* 1982; 22:391–4.

17. Blouin RA, Bauer LA, Miller DD et al. Vancomycin pharmacokinetics in normal and morbidly obese subjects. *Antimicrob Agents Chemother.* 1982; 21:575–80.

18. Golper TA, Noonan HM, Elzinga L et al. Vancomycin pharmacokinetics, renal handling, and nonrenal clearances in normal human subjects. *Clin Pharmacol Ther.* 1988; 43:565–70.

19. Ackerman BH, Taylor EH, Olsen KM et al. Vancomycin serum protein binding determination by ultrafiltration. *Drug Intell Clin Pharm.* 1988; 22:300–3.

20. Albrecht LM, Rybak MJ, Warbasse LH et al. Vancomycin protein binding in patients with infections caused by *Staphylococcus aureus.* DICP. 1991; 25:713–5.

21. Skhirtladze K, Hutschala D, Fleck T et al. Impaired target site penetration of vancomycin in diabetic patients following cardiac surgery. *Antimicrob Agents Chemother.* 2006; 50:1372–5.

22. Cruciani M, Gatti G, Lazzarini L et al. Penetration of vancomycin into human lung tissue. *J Antimicrob Chemother.* 1996; 38:865–9.

23. Georges H, Leroy O, Alfandari S et al. Pulmonary disposition of vancomycin in critically ill patients. *Eur J Clin Microbiol Infect Dis.* 1997; 16:385–8.

24. Lamer C, de Beco V, Soler P et al. Analysis of vancomycin entry into pulmonary lining fluid by bronchoalveolar lavage in critical ill patients. *Antimicrob Agents Chemother.* 1993; 37:281–6.

25. Craig WA. Basic pharmacodynamics of antibacterials with clinical applications to the use of beta-lactams, glycopeptides, and linezolid. *Infect Dis Clin North Am.* 2003; 17:479–501.

26. Craig WA. Pharmacokinetic/pharmacodynamic parameters: rationale for antimicrobial dosing of mice and men. *Clin Infect Dis.* 1998; 26:1–10.

27. Drusano GL. Antimicrobial pharmacodynamics: critical interactions of bug and drug. *Nature Rev Microbiol.* 2004; 2:289–300.

28. Rybak MJ. Pharmacodynamics: relation to antimicrobial resistance. *Am J Med.* 2006; 119(6, suppl 1):S37–44.

29. Ackerman BH, Vannier AM, Eudy EB. Analysis of vancomycin time-kill studies with *Staphylococcus* species by using a curve stripping program to describe the relationship between concentration and pharmacodynamic response. *Antimicrob Agents Chemother.* 1992; 36:1766–9.

30. Löwdin E, Odenholt I, Cars O. In vitro studies of pharmacodynamic properties of vancomycin against *Staphylococcus aureus* and *Staphylococcus epidermidis. Antimicrob Agents Chemother.* 1998; 42:2739–44.

31. Larsson AJ, Walker KJ, Raddatz JK et al. The concentration-independent effect of monoexponential and biexponential decay in vancomycin concentrations on the killing of *Staphylococcus aureus* under aerobic and anaerobic conditions. *J Antimicrob Chemother.* 1996; 38:589–97.

32. Craig WA, Andes DR. In vivo pharmacodynamics of vancomycin against VISA, heteroresistant VISA (hVISA) and VSSA in the neutropenic murine thigh-infection model. Paper presented at 46th Interscience Conference on Antimicrobial Agents and Chemotherapy. San Francisco, CA: 2006 Sep.

33. Moise-Broder PA, Sakoulas G, Eliopoulos GM et al. Accessory gene regulator group II polymorphism in methicillin-resistant *Staphylococcus aureus* is predictive of failure of vancomycin therapy. *Clin Infect Dis.* 2004; 38:1700–5.

34. The development of vancomycin. In: Cooper GL, Given DB. Vancomycin: a comprehensive review of 30 years of clinical experience. New York: Park Row; 1986:1–6.

35. James JK, Palmer SM, Levine DP et al. Comparison of conventional dosing versus continuous-infusion vancomycin therapy for patients with suspected or documented gram-positive infections. *Antimicrob Agents Chemother.* 1996; 40:696–700.

36. Lacy MK, Tessier PR, Nicolau DP et al. Comparison of vancomycin pharmacodynamics (1 g every 12 or 24 h) against methicillin-resistant staphylococci. *Int J Antimicrob Agents.* 2000; 15:25–30.

37. Wysocki M, Thomas F, Wolff MA et al. Comparison of continuous with discontinuous intravenous infusion of vancomycin in severe MRSA infections. *J Antimicrob Chemother.* 1995; 35:352–4.

38. Wysocki M, Delatour F, Faurisson F et al. Continuous versus intermittent infusion of vancomycin in severe staphylococcal infections: prospective multicenter randomized study. *Antimicrob Agents Chemother.* 2001; 45:2460–7.

39. Geraci J. Vancomycin. *Mayo Clin Proc.* 1977; 52:631–4.

40. Karam CM, McKinnon PS, Neuhauser MM et al. Outcome assessment of minimizing vancomycin monitoring and dosing adjustments. *Pharmacotherapy.* 1999; 19:257–66.

41. American Thoracic Society, Infectious Diseases Society of America. Guidelines for the management of adults with hospital-acquired, ventilator-associated, and healthcare-associated pneumonia. *Am J Respir Crit Care Med.* 2005; 171:388–416.

42. Jeffres MN, Isakow W, Doherty JA et al. Predictors of mortality for methicillin-resistant *Staphylococcus aureus* health-care-associated pneumonia: specific evaluation of vancomycin pharmacokinetic indices. *Chest.* 2006; 130:947–55.

43. LaPlante KL, Rybak MJ. Impact of high-inoculum *Staphylococcus aureus* on the activities of nafcillin, vancomycin, linezolid, and daptomycin, alone and in combination with gentamicin, in an in vitro pharmacodynamic model. *Antimicrob Agents Chemother.* 2004; 48:4665–72.

44. Lamp KC, Rybak MJ, Bailey EM et al. In vitro pharmacodynamic effects of concentration, pH, and growth phase on serum bactericidal activities of daptomycin and vancomycin. *Antimicrob Agents Chemother.* 1992; 36:2709–14.

45. Peetermans WE, Hoogeterp JJ, Hazekamp-van Dokkum AM et al. Antistaphylococcal activities of teicoplanin and vancomycin in vitro and in an experimental infection. *Antimicrob Agents Chemother.* 1990; 34:1869–74.

46. Svensson E, Hanberger H, Nilsson LE. Pharmacodynamic effects of antibiotics and antibiotic combinations on growing and nongrowing *Staphylococcus epidermidis* cells. *Antimicrob Agents Chemother.* 1997; 41:107–11.

47. Cosgrove SE, Carroll KC, Perl TM. *Staphylococcus aureus* with reduced susceptibility to vancomycin. *Clin Infect Dis.* 2004; 39:539–45.

48. Liu C, Chambers HF. *Staphylococcus aureus* with heterogeneous resistance to vancomycin: epidemiology, clinical significance, and critical assessment of diagnostic methods. *Antimicrob Agents Chemother.* 2003; 47:3040–5.

49. Moore MR, Perdreau-Remington F, Chambers HF. Vancomycin treatment failure associated with heterogeneous vancomycin-intermediate *Staphylococcus aureus* in a patient with endocarditis and in the rabbit model of endocarditis. *Antimicrob Agents Chemother.* 2003; 47:1262–6.

50. Howden BP, Johnson PD, Ward PB et al. Isolates with low-level vancomycin resistance associated with persistent methicillin-resistant *Staphylococcus aureus* bacteremia. *Antimicrob Agents Chemother.* 2006; 50:3039–47.

51. Tenover FC, Moellering RC Jr. The rationale for revising the Clinical and Laboratory Standards Institute vancomycin minimal inhibitory concentration interpretive criteria for *Staphylococcus aureus. Clin Infect Dis.* 2007; 44:1208–15.

52. Sakoulas G, Moise-Broder PA, Schentag J et al. Relationship of MIC and bactericidal activity to efficacy of vancomycin for treatment of methicillin-resistant *Staphylococcus aureus* bacteremia. *J Clin Microbiol.* 2004; 42:2398–402.

53. Hidayat LK, Hsu DI, Quist R et al. High-dose vancomycin therapy for methicillin-resistant *Staphylococcus aureus* infections: efficacy and toxicity. *Arch Intern Med.* 2006; 166:2138–44.

54. Sakoulas G, Gold HS, Cohen RA et al. Effects of prolonged vancomycin administration on methicillin-resistant *Staphylococcus aureus* (MRSA) in a patient with recurrent bacteraemia. *J Antimicrob Chemother.* 2006; 57:699–704.

55. Howden BP, Ward PB, Charles PG et al. Treatment outcomes for serious infections caused by methicillin-resistant *Staphylococcus aureus* with reduced vancomycin susceptibility. *Clin Infect Dis.* 2004; 38:521–8.

56. Charles PG, Ward PB, Johnson PD et al. Clinical features associated with bacteremia due to heterogeneous vancomycin-intermediate *Staphylococcus aureus. Clin Infect Dis.* 2004; 38:448–51.

57. Jones RN. Microbiological features of vancomycin in the 21st century: minimum inhibitory concentration creep, bactericidal/static activity, and applied breakpoints to predict clinical outcomes or detect resistant strains. *Clin Infect Dis.* 2006; 42(suppl 1):S13–24.

58. Moise PA, Sakoulas G, Forrest A et al. Vancomycin in vitro bactericidal activity and its relationship to efficacy in clearance of methicillin-resistant *Staphylococcus aureus* bacteremia. *Antimicrob Agents Chemother.* 2007; 51:2582–8.

59. Soriano A, Marco F, Martinez JA et al. Influence of vancomycin minimum inhibitory concentration on the treatment of methicillin-resistant *Staphylococcus aureus* bacteremia. *Clin Infect Dis.* 2008; 46:193–200.

60. Lodise TP, Graves J, Graffunder E et al. Relationship between vancomycin MIC and failure among patients with methicillin-resistant *Staphylococcus aureus* bacteremia treated with vancomycin. *Antimicrob Agents Chemother.* 2008; 52:3315–20.

61. Mohr JF, Murray BE. Point: vancomycin is not obsolete for the treatment of infection caused by methicillin-resistant *Staphylococcus aureus. Clin Infect Dis.* 2007; 44:1536–42.

62. Rhee KY, Gardiner DF, Charles M. Decreasing in vitro susceptibility of clinical *Staphylococcus aureus* isolates to vancomycin at the New York Hospital: quantitative testing redux. *Clin Infect Dis.* 2005; 40:1705–6.

63. Wang G, Hindler JF, Ward KW et al. Increased vancomycin MICs for *Staphylococcus aureus* clinical isolates from a university hospital during a 5-year period. *J Clin Microbiol.* 2006; 44:3883–6.

64. Steinkraus G, White R, Friedrich L. Vancomycin MIC creep in non-vancomycin-intermediate *Staphylococcus aureus* (VISA), vancomycin-susceptible clinical methicillin-resistant *S. aureus* (MRSA) blood isolates from 2001-05. *J Antimicrob Chemother.* 2007; 60:788–94.

65. Deresinski S. Counterpoint: vancomycin and *Staphylococcus aureus*—an antibiotic enters obsolescence. *Clin Infect Dis.* 2007; 44:1543–8.

66. Novick RP. Autoinduction and signal transduction in the regulation of staphylococcal virulence. *Mol Microbiol.* 2003; 48:1429–49.

67. Sakoulas G, Eliopoulos GM, Moellering RC Jr et al. *Staphylococcus aureus* accessory gene regulator (agr) group II: is there a relationship to the development of intermediate-level glycopeptide resistance? *J Infect Dis.* 2003; 187:929–38.

68. Sakoulas G, Eliopoulos GM, Fowler VG Jr et al. Reduced susceptibility of *Staphylococcus aureus* to vancomycin and platelet microbicidal protein correlates with defective autolysis and loss of accessory gene regulator (agr) function. *Antimicrob Agents Chemother.* 2005; 49:2687–92.

69. Tsuji BT, Rybak MJ, Lau KL et al. Evaluation of accessory gene regulator (agr) group and function in the

proclivity towards vancomycin intermediate resistance in *Staphylococcus aureus*. *Antimicrob Agents Chemother.* 2007; 51:1089–91.

70. Tsuji BT, Rybak MJ, Cheung CM et al. Community- and health care-associated methicillin-resistant *Staphylococcus aureus*: a comparison of molecular epidemiology and antimicrobial activities of various agents. *Diagn Microbiol Infect Dis.* 2007; 58:41–7.

71. Del Mar Fernández de Gatta Garcia M, Revilla N, Calvo MV et al. Pharmacokinetic/pharmacodynamic analysis of vancomycin in ICU patients. *Intensive Care Med.* 2006; 33:279–85.

72. Murphy JE, Gillespie DE, Bateman CV. Predictability of vancomycin trough concentrations using seven approaches for estimating pharmacokinetic parameters. *Am J Health-Syst Pharm.* 2006; 63:2365–70.

73. Wang JT, Fang CT, Chen YC et al. Necessity of a loading dose when using vancomycin in critically ill patients. *J Antimicrob Chemother.* 2001; 47:246. Letter.

74. Mohammedi I, Descloux E, Argaud L et al. Loading dose of vancomycin in critically ill patients: 15 mg/kg is a better choice than 500 mg. *Int J Antimicrob Agents.* 2006; 27:259–62.

75. Bailie GR, Neal D. Vancomycin ototoxicity and nephrotoxicity. A review. *Med Toxicol Adverse Drug Exp.* 1988; 3:376–86.

76. Elting LS, Rubenstein EB, Kurtin D et al. Mississippi mud in the 1990s: risks and outcomes of vancomycin-associated toxicity in general oncology practice. *Cancer.* 1998; 83:2597–607.

77. Wilhelm MP, Estes L. Symposium on antimicrobial agents—part XII. *Vancomycin. Mayo Clinic Proc.* 1999; 74:928–35.

78. Rybak MJ, Boike SC. Monitoring vancomycin therapy. *Drug Intell Clin Pharm.* 1986; 20:757–61.

79. Henry K, Steinberg I, Crossley KB. Vancomycin-induced neutropenia during treatment of osteomyelitis in an outpatient. *Drug Intell Clin Pharm.* 1986; 20:783–5.

80. Koo KB, Bachand RL, Chow AW. Vancomycin-induced neutropenia. *Drug Intell Clin Pharm.* 1986; 20:780–2.

81. Farber BF, Moellering RC Jr. Retrospective study of the toxicity of preparations of vancomycin from 1974 to 1981. *Antimicrob Agents Chemother.* 1983; 23:138–41.

82. Mellor JA, Kingdom J, Cafferkey M et al. Vancomycin toxicity: a prospective study. *J Antimicrob Chemother.* 1985; 15:773–80.

83. Sorrell TC, Collignon PJ. A prospective study of adverse reactions associated with vancomycin therapy. *J Antimicrob Chemother.* 1985; 16:235–41.

84. Cimino MA, Rotstein C, Slaughter RL et al. Relationship of serum antibiotic concentrations to nephrotoxicity in cancer patients receiving concurrent aminoglycoside and vancomycin therapy. *Am J Med.* 1987; 83:1091–7.

85. Downs NJ, Neihart RE, Dolezal JM et al. Mild nephrotoxicity associated with vancomycin use. *Arch Intern Med.* 1989; 149:1777–81.

86. Pauly DJ, Musa DM, Lestico MR et al. Risk of nephrotoxicity with combination vancomycin-aminoglycoside antibiotic therapy. *Pharmacotherapy.* 1990; 10:378–82.

87. Jeffres MN, Isakow W, Doherty JA et al. A retrospective analysis of possible renal toxicity associated with vancomycin in patients with health care-associated methicillin-resistant *Staphylococcus aureus* pneumonia. *Clin Ther.* 2007; 29:1107–15.

88. Nguyen M, Wong J, Lee C et al. Nephrotoxicity associated with high dose vs standard dose vancomycin therapy. Paper presented at 47th Interscience Conference on Antimicrobial Agents and Chemotherapy. Chicago, IL; 2007 Sep.

89. King DW, Smith MA. Proliferative responses observed following vancomycin treatment in renal proximal tubule epithelial cells. *Toxicol In Vitro.* 2004; 18:797–803.

90. Celik I, Cihangiroglu M, Ilhan N et al. Protective effects of different antioxidants and amrinone on vancomycin-induced nephrotoxicity. *Basic Clin Pharmacol Toxicol.* 2005; 97:325–32.

91. Le Moyec L, Racine S, Le Toumelin P et al. Aminoglycoside and glycopeptide renal toxicity in intensive care patients studied by proton magnetic resonance spectroscopy of urine. *Crit Care Med.* 2002; 30:1242–5.

92. Nishino Y, Takemura S, Minamiyama Y et al. Inhibition of vancomycin-induced nephrotoxicity by targeting superoxide dismutase to renal proximal tubule cells in the rat. *Redox Rep.* 2002; 7:317–9.

93. Hailemeskel B, Namanny M, Wutoh A. Frequency of nephrotoxicity with vancomycin and aminoglycoside therapy. *Hosp Pharm.* 1999; 12:1417–20.

94. Salama SE, Rotstein C. Prospective assessment of nephrotoxicity with concomitant aminoglycoside and vancomycin therapy. *Can J Hosp Pharm.* 1993; 46:53–9.

95. Malacarne P, Bergamasco S, Donadio C. Nephrotoxicity due to combination antibiotic therapy with vancomycin and aminoglycosides in septic critically ill patients. *Chemotherapy.* 2006; 52:178–84.

96. Cunha BA, Mohan SS, Hamid N et al. Cost-ineffectiveness of serum vancomycin levels. *Eur J Clin Microbiol Infect Dis.* 2007; 26:509–11.

97. Wold JS, Turnipseed SA. Toxicity of vancomycin in laboratory animals. *Rev Infect Dis.* 1981; 3(suppl):S224–9.

98. Aronoff GR, Sloan RS, Dinwiddie CB Jr et al. Effects of vancomycin on renal function in rats. *Antimicrob Agents Chemother.* 1981; 19:306–8.

99. Beauchamp D, Pellerin M, Gourde P et al. Effects of daptomycin and vancomycin on tobramycin nephrotoxicity in rats. *Antimicrob Agents Chemother.* 1990; 34:139–47.

100. Wood CA, Kohlhepp SJ, Kohnen PW et al. Vancomycin enhancement of experimental tobramycin nephrotoxicity. *Antimicrob Agents Chemother.* 1986; 30:20–4.

101. Marre R, Schulz E, Anders T et al. Renal tolerance and pharmacokinetics of vancomycin in rats. *J Antimicrob Chemother.* 1984; 14:253–60.

102. Fauconneau B, De Lemos E, Pariat C et al. Chrono-nephrotoxicity in rat of a vancomycin and gentamicin combination. *Pharmacol Toxicol.* 1992; 71:31–6.

103. Marre R, Schulz E, Hedtke D et al. Influence of fosfomycin and tobramycin on vancomycin-induced nephrotoxicity. *Infection.* 1985; 13:190–2.

104. Kacew S, Hewitt WR, Hook JB. Gentamicin-induced renal metabolic alterations in newborn rat kidney: lack of potentiation by vancomycin. *Toxicol Appl Pharmacol.* 1989; 99:61–71.

105. Rybak MJ, Frankowski JJ, Edwards DJ et al. Alanine aminopeptidase and beta 2-microglobulin excretion in patients receiving vancomycin and gentamicin. *Antimicrob Agents Chemother.* 1987; 31:1461–4.

106. European Organization for Research and Treatment of Cancer (EORTC) International Antimicrobial Therapy Cooperative Group and the National Cancer Institute of Canada-Clinical Trials Group. Vancomycin added to empirical combination antibiotic therapy for fever in granulocytopenic cancer patients. *J Infect Dis.* 1991; 163:951–8. [Erratum, *J Infect Dis.* 1991; 164:832.]

107. Bertino JS Jr, Booker LA, Franck PA et al. Incidence of and significant risk factors for aminoglycoside-associated nephrotoxicity in patients dosed by using individualized pharmacokinetic monitoring. *J Infect Dis.* 1993; 167:173–9.

108. Karp JE, Dick JD, Angelopulos C et al. Empiric use of vancomycin during prolonged treatment-induced granulocytopenia: randomized, double-blind, placebo-controlled clinical trial in patients with acute leukemia. *Am J Med.* 1986; 81:237–42.

109. Goren MP, Baker DK Jr, Shenep JL. Vancomycin does not enhance amikacin-induced tubular nephrotoxicity in children. *Pediatr Infect Dis J.* 1989; 8:278–82.

110. Nahata MC. Lack of nephrotoxicity in pediatric patients receiving concurrent vancomycin and aminoglycoside therapy. *Chemotherapy.* 1987; 33:302–4.

111. Goetz MB, Sayers J. Nephrotoxicity of vancomycin and aminoglycoside therapy separately and in combination. *J Antimicrob Chemother.* 1993; 32:325–34.

112. Cohen E, Dadashev A, Drucker M et al. Once-daily versus twice-daily intravenous administration of vancomycin for infections in hospitalized patients. *J Antimicrob Chemother.* 2002; 49:155–60.

113. Boffi El Amari E, Vuagnat A, Stern R et al. High versus standard dose vancomycin for osteomyelitis. *Scand J Infect Dis.* 2004; 36:712–7.

114. Zimmermann AE, Katona BG, Plaisance KI. Association of vancomycin serum concentrations with outcomes in patients with gram-positive bacteremia. *Pharmacotherapy.* 1995; 15:85–91.

115. Lee-Such SC, Overholser BR, Munoz-Price LS. Nephrotoxicity associated with aggressive vancomycin therapy. Paper presented at 46th Interscience Conference on Antimicrobial Agents and Chemotherapy. San Francisco, CA; 2006 Sep.

116. Welty TE, Copa AK. Impact of vancomycin therapeutic drug monitoring on patient care. *Ann Pharmacother.* 1994; 28:1335–9.

117. Iwamoto T, Kagawa Y, Kojima M. Clinical efficacy of therapeutic drug monitoring in patients receiving vancomycin. *Biol Pharm Bull.* 2003; 26:876–9.

118. Davis RR, Brummett RE, Bendrick TW et al. The ototoxic interaction of viomycin, capreomycin and polymyxin B with ethacrynic acid. *Acta Otolaryngol.* 1982; 93:211–7.

119. Tange RA, Kieviet HL, von Marle J et al. An experimental study of vancomycin-induced cochlear damage. *Arch Otorhinolaryngol.* 1989; 246:67–70.

120. Traber PG, Levine DP. Vancomycin ototoxicity in a patient with normal renal function. *Ann Intern Med.* 1991; 95:458–60.

121. Brummett RE, Fox KE. Vancomycin- and erythromycin-induced hearing loss in humans. *Antimicrob Agents Chemother.* 1989; 33:791–6.

122. Dangerfield HG, Hewit WL, Monzon OT et al. Clinical use of vancomycin. *Antimicrob Agents Chemother.* 1960; 61:428–37.

123. Kirby WM, Perry DM, Bauer AW. Treatment of staphylococcal septicemia with vancomycin: report of thirty-three cases. *N Engl J Med.* 1960; 262:49–55.

124. Waisbren BA, Kleinerman L, Skemp J et al. Comparative clinical effectiveness and toxicity of vancomycin, ristocetin, and kanamycin. *Arch Intern Med.* 1960; 106:179–93.

125. Saunders NJ. Why monitor peak vancomycin concentrations? *Lancet.* 1994; 344:1748–50.

126. Fekety R. Vancomycin. *Med Clin North Amer.* 1982; 66:175–81.

127. Reynolds JE, ed. Martindale, the extra pharmacopoeia. 28th ed. London: Pharmaceutical Press; 1982.

128. Buckingham SC, McCullers JA, Lujan-Zilbermann J et al. Early vancomycin therapy and adverse outcomes in children with pneumococcal meningitis. *Pediatrics.* 2006; 117:1688–94.

129. Geraci JE, Heilman FR, Nichols DR et al. Antibiotic therapy of bacterial endocarditis. VII. Vancomycin for acute micrococcal endocarditis; preliminary report. *Proc Staff Meet Mayo Clin.* 1958; 33:172–81.

Developed through the ASHP Council on Therapeutics and approved by the ASHP Board of Directors on June 26, 2008, the Infectious Diseases Society of America's Board of Directors on June 16, 2008, and the Society of Infectious Diseases Pharmacists' Board of Directors on June 25, 2008.

Michael Rybak, Pharm.D., M.P.H. is Professor of Pharmacy and Medicine, and Director, Anti-Infective Research Laboratory, Eugene Applebaum College of Pharmacy and Health Science, Wayne State University (WSU), Detroit, MI. Ben Lomaestro, Pharm.D., is Senior Clinical Pharmacy Specialist in Infectious Diseases, Albany Medical Center, Albany, NY. John C. Rotschafer, Pharm.D., is Professor, Department of Experimental and Clinical Pharmacology, College of Pharmacy, University of Minnesota, Minneapolis. Robert Moellering Jr., M.D., is Shields Warren-Mallinckrodt Professor of Medical Research, Harvard Medical School, and Physician, Department of Medicine, Beth Israel Deaconess Medical Center, Boston, MA. William Craig, M.D., is Professor Emeritus, University of Wisconsin School of Medicine and Public Health, School of Medicine and Public Health, University of Wisconsin, Madison. Marianne Billeter, Pharm.D., BCPS, is Manager of Clinical Pharmacy Services at Ochsner Medical Center, New Orleans, LA. Joseph R. Dalovisio, M.D., is Chairman, Department of Infectious Diseases, Ochsner Health System, New Orleans. Donald P. Levine, M.D., is Professor of Medicine and Chief, Division of General Internal Medicine, WSU.

The following individuals are acknowledged for reviewing draft versions of this statement: Diane M. Cappelletty, Pharm.D.; Douglas N. Fish, Pharm.D., FCCP, FCCM, BCPS; William L. Greene, B.S., Pharm.D., BCPS, FASHP; David J. Ritchie, Pharm.D., FCCP,

BCPS; Annette M. Rowden, Pharm.D., BCPS; and Lynda J. Thompson, Pharm.D.

The bibliographic citation for this document is as follows: American Society of Health-System Pharmacists. Therapeutic monitoring of vancomycin in adult patients: A consensus review of the American Society of Health-System Pharmacists, the Infectious Diseases Society of America, and the Society of Infectious Diseases Pharmacists. *Am J Health-Syst Pharm.* 2009; 66:82–98.

ASHP Therapeutic Position Statement on the Use of Second-Generation Antipsychotic Medications in the Treatment of Adults with Psychotic Disorders

Position

The American Society of Health-System Pharmacists (ASHP) recognizes that schizophrenia, schizoaffective disorder, and other psychotic disorders are serious mental illnesses that can significantly affect an individual's perceptual, behavioral, affective, and cognitive functions. These conditions are usually chronic and recurrent, necessitating continuous treatment over the patient's lifetime. Individuals with these disorders frequently require lengthy and expensive hospitalizations, as well as a variety of ongoing rehabilitative and supportive services that can impose a significant burden on society. In addition, high rates of suicidal behavior and completed suicides have been observed in patients with psychotic disorders. The management of these disorders typically requires long-term treatment with antipsychotic medications, the use of adjunctive pharmacologic treatments, and ongoing psychosocial and supportive interventions to reduce morbidity and mortality.

ASHP encourages health professionals to consider the use of second-generation ("atypical" or "novel") antipsychotics as first-line drug treatments for individuals with psychotic disorders. Second-generation antipsychotics share the common pharmacologic action of dual serotonin–dopamine antagonism. While the acquisition costs of these agents are greater than those of older drugs, randomized controlled trials and naturalistic studies have demonstrated that second-generation antipsychotics effectively treat the symptoms of psychotic disorders while providing a tolerability profile that improves treatment adherence and reduces the severity of short- and long-term adverse motor effects. Second-generation antipsychotics have also been found to have improved profiles for cognitive impairments in schizophrenia, relative to older agents, allowing for opportunities toward psychosocial rehabilitation. There is also evidence that the use of these agents improves outcomes in patients with chronic psychotic disorders compared with older antipsychotics, specifically reducing the rates of symptom relapse and inpatient rehospitalization. However, it should be noted that second-generation antipsychotics are associated with significant treatment risks, such as adverse cardiovascular and metabolic effects, that should be carefully considered during treatment initiation and throughout the course of therapy.

Background

Schizophrenia and schizoaffective disorder are serious, chronic mental illnesses that affect perceptual, behavioral, and cognitive functioning. The *DSM-IV-TR* established criteria for five main subtypes of schizophrenia and for schizoaffective disorder.[1]

Individuals with schizophrenia generally exhibit a mixture of positive, negative, and cognitive symptoms with varying intensity throughout the course of their illness (Table 1). Schizoaffective disorder differs from schizophrenia in that recurrent mood episodes (mania or depression) occur over a substantial period of time over the course of the illness in addition to chronic psychotic symptoms. These two disorders have been studied together in many clinical trials and will be considered together for the purpose of this document.

It has been estimated that the worldwide lifetime frequency of psychotic disorders is about 1%.[2,3] Onset of the first severe psychotic symptoms in a patient with schizophrenia usually occurs between the late teens and mid-30s, with onset in males peaking between ages 15 and 30 and females exhibiting a later onset, between ages 20 and 35.[4,5] Late-onset schizophrenia, occurring after 40 years of age, may have an otherwise similar course to typical adult-onset schizophrenia. Prodromal symptoms of psychosis occurring in children and adolescents (e.g., apathy, social withdrawal) may be present before the first psychotic break, but the full symptoms of these disorders are rare in this population. Because these illnesses frequently have their symptom onset in early adulthood and are characterized by a wide range of symptoms, they usually cause significant, progressive impairment in the social, occupational, and academic functioning of affected individuals.

Pharmacologic Characteristics of Antipsychotic Drugs

The effectiveness of first-generation antipsychotic agents, whose primary mechanism of action was blockade of postsynaptic dopamine type 2 (D_2) receptors in the brain, led to the initial hypothesis regarding dopamine's role in schizophrenia. While it is apparent that increased dopamine in the mesolimbic pathway is responsible for the positive symptoms of schizophrenia, it is now understood that psychotic disorders frequently involve numerous neurochemical abnormalities. Psychosis has been observed in individuals with idiopathic[6] and drug-induced[7] hypofunction of the glutamate

Table 1.
Positive, Negative, and Cognitive Symptoms of Schizophrenia

Positive Symptoms	Negative Symptoms	Cognitive Symptoms
Hostility	Emotional withdrawal	Impaired attention
Excitement	Uncooperativeness	Impaired short-term memory
Hallucinations	Blunted affect	
Delusions	Inappropriate affect	Impaired executive functioning
Suspiciousness	Poverty of thought	
Grandiosity	Social withdrawal	Impaired verbal fluency
Conceptual disorganization	Lack of spontaneity	
	Poor abstract thinking	

system. In addition, the high rate of nicotine dependence in individuals with psychotic disorders–up to 88% in one study[8]—has led to the identification and study of acetyl-choline-receptor abnormalities in the patho-physiology of schizophrenia.[9]

The ideal drug for the treatment of psychotic disorders would have several important characteristics. It would provide effective relief and prevention of acute positive symptoms of schizophrenia. Other ideal characteristics would include effective relief of affective, cognitive, and negative symptoms; minimal short- and long-term adverse effects; few drug interactions; and low acquisition cost. Although no antipsychotic agent currently available completely fits all these criteria, second-generation antipsychotics offer many benefits not achieved with traditional antipsychotics.

First-generation antipsychotic agents primarily exert their therapeutic effects through the blockade of postsynaptic D_2 receptors in the mesolimbic pathway, thereby reducing positive symptoms over time. However, these drugs are not selective in their activity. Blockade of dopamine in other areas of the brain often leads to acute extrapyramidal motor effects (e.g., dystonias, parkinsonism), tardive dyskinesia, increased levels of serum prolactin, and exacerbation of negative symptoms. Although occurring infrequently at standard doses, an array of adverse neurologic, cardiovascular, and dermatologic effects are associated with these agents.

Second-generation antipsychotic drugs share the common pharmacologic action of dual serotonin–dopamine antagonism (Table 2). Aripiprazole differs slightly in that it functions as a partial agonist at dopamine receptors, reducing dopamine activity in the mesolimbic pathway.[10,11] Antagonism of serotonin type 2 (5-HT$_2$) receptors increases the release of endogenous dopamine.[12] This increase in dopamine decreases the likelihood of extrapyramidal motor symptoms and elevated prolactin levels without significantly reducing the beneficial effects against positive symptoms of psychosis. Theoretically, this property of the newer drugs may also help to improve the negative symptoms of schizophrenia.

Efficacy for Psychotic Symptoms

Second-generation antipsychotic agents have been demonstrated to be at least as effective as the traditional antipsychotic agents in the treatment of positive symptoms of schizophrenia when used in appropriate therapeutic doses. The newer antipsychotics also demonstrate benefits for affective symptoms, cognition, and psychosocial functioning not seen with the older agents.

Clozapine, the first second-generation antipsychotic introduced in the United States, has an established level of efficacy for use in individuals with psychotic disorders resistant to treatment with other antipsychotics. Kane et al.[13] conducted the landmark trial that demonstrated the superior efficacy of clozapine in individuals with treatment-resistant psychosis. This trial enrolled only patients whose psychosis was treatment resistant, defined as not responding to at least three periods of treatment in the preceding five years with antipsychotic agents from two different chemical classes at dosages equivalent to 1000 mg/day of chlorpromazine for six weeks. The previous antipsychotic trials must have failed to provide periods of good functioning or significant symptomatic relief. A six-week trial of haloperidol (mean dosage, 61 mg/day) and benztropine followed to confirm lack of drug response. Participants whose psychosis did not respond to haloperidol were randomized to receive clozapine (up to 900 mg/day) or chlorpromazine (up to 1800 mg/day) with benztropine. Using a priori criteria, response rates were 30% for patients treated with clozapine versus 4% for the chlorpromazine group. The authors found that improvements in the Brief Psychiatric Rating Scale total scores and clinical global impression (CGI) were three times greater in patients treated with clozapine.

The landmark clinical studies used in the evaluation of second-generation antipsychotics are summarized in Table 3. In general, these trials lasted four to six weeks and assessed the efficacy of these agents in the treatment of acute psychotic disorders. Because of the study designs employed, no assumptions can be made regarding the efficacy of these agents for long-term prevention of psychotic relapse, for comorbid substance abuse or mood disorders, or in other complex clinical situations. The medical literature suggests that all currently available second-generation antipsychotic agents are superior to placebo and at least as effective as the traditional antipsychotics in the reduction of positive symptoms of schizophrenia. With long-term therapy, second-generation antipsychotics may also have beneficial effects on negative symptoms; however, these benefits have not been consistently demonstrated in the four- to six-week clinical trials.

The Clinical Antipsychotic Trials of Intervention Effectiveness (CATIE) was a multicenter clinical study sponsored by the National Institute of Mental Health.[25] The first phase of this study, conducted between January 2001 and December 2004, involved 1460 patients with chronic schizophrenia age 18–65 years. Patients were randomized to treatment for up to 18 months with one of four available second-generation antipsychotics (olanzapine, quetiapine, risperidone, or ziprasidone) or perphenazine, a traditional antipsychotic. The primary outcome measured was time to discontinuation of treatment for any cause, including lack of efficacy, intolerable adverse effects, or patient's decision to end treatment. Treatment with olanzapine at a mean modal dosage (MMD) of 20.1 mg/day was associated with a significantly longer median duration of treatment (9.2 months) compared with quetiapine (4.6 months; MMD, 543.4 mg/day), risperidone

Table 2.
Second-Generation Antipsychotics Currently Available in the United States

Drug (Trade Name)	Manufacturer	Year Approved
Clozapine (Clozaril)	Novartis	1989
Risperidone (Risperdal)	Janssen Pharmaceutica	1993
Olanzapine (Zyprexa)	Eli Lilly	1996
Quetiapine (Seroquel)	AstraZeneca	1997
Ziprasidone (Geodon)	Pfizer	2001
Aripiprazole (Abilify)	Bristol-Myers Squibb	2002
Paliperidone (Invega)	Janssen Pharmaceutica	2006

Table 3.
Major Efficacy Trials of Second-Generation Antipsychotics[13-24]

Ref.	Patient Population	Treatment	Duration (wk)	Results[a]
13	268 inpatients with schizophrenia refractory to treatment with adequate trials with at least three agents from two different chemical classes, after nonresponse to 6-wk trial of haloperidol	Clozapine 500–900 mg/day vs. chlorpromazine 1000–1800 mg/day + benztropine (up to 6 mg/day)	6	BPRS total, CGI: Improvement with clozapine 3 times greater than with chlorpromazine ($p < 0.001$). Patient improvement (20% reduction in BPRS and either CGI of ≤3 or BPRS total of ≤35: Clozapine, 30%; chlorpromazine, 4% ($p < 0.001$).
14	39 outpatients with schizophrenia with history of residual symptoms after at least two 6-wk trials of neuroleptics from different classes, after nonresponse to 6-wk trial of fluphenazine	Clozapine 200–600 mg/day vs. haloperidol 10–30 mg/day + benztropine (up to 4 mg/day)	10	BPRS positive symptoms: Improvement with clozapine greater than with haloperidol ($p = 0.05$). SANS: Improvement with clozapine, worsening with haloperidol ($p = 0.04$). Clinical response rate: Clozapine, 44.4%; haloperidol, 5.5% ($p = 0.017$).
15	388 inpatients with schizophrenia	Risperidone 2, 6, 10, and 16 mg/day; haloperidol 20 mg/day; placebo	8	Clinical improvement (20% reduction in PANSS): Greater improvement in patients receiving risperidone 6 and 16 mg vs. haloperidol. Clinical improvement (Kane et al. criteria): Risperidone 6, 10, and 16 mg superior to placebo ($p < 0.05$).
16	135 patients with schizophrenia	Risperidone 2, 6, 10, and 16 mg/day; haloperidol 20 mg/day; placebo	8	Clinical improvement (20% reduction in PANSS): Greater improvement in patients receiving risperidone 2, 6, 10, and 16 mg and haloperidol recipients vs. placebo. PANSS—negative subscale: Only risperidone 6 mg superior to placebo.
17	400 patients with schizophrenia	Risperidone long-acting injection 25, 50, and 75 mg every 2 wk vs. placebo	12	Improvement in PANSS and CGI (LOCF) significant for all groups vs. placebo.
18	335 patients with schizophrenia	Olanzapine-L (2.5–7.5 mg/day), olanzapine-M (7.5–12.5 mg/day), olanzapine-H (12.5–17.5 mg/day), haloperidol 10–20 mg/day, placebo	6	CGI, BPRS: Olanzapine-M, olanzapine-H, and haloperidol groups significantly improved vs. placebo. SANS: Olanzapine-H group demonstrated significant improvement vs. haloperidol.
19	152 inpatients with schizophrenia	Olanzapine 1 and 10 mg/day vs. placebo	6	BPRS total, PANSS-negative score: Olanzapine 10-mg group superior to placebo. Olanzapine 1-mg group showed no improvement over placebo for any efficacy measure.
20	361 hospitalized patients with schizophrenia	Quetiapine 75, 150, 300, 600, and 750 mg/day; haloperidol 12 mg/day; placebo	6	BPRS total: Significant improvement from baseline vs. placebo noted in all treatment groups except quetiapine 75 mg. SANS: Significant improvement vs. placebo noted in quetiapine 300 mg and haloperidol groups.

(Continued on next page)

Table 3 *(continued)*

Ref.	Patient Population	Treatment	Duration (wk)	Results[a]
21	286 hospitalized patients with schizophrenia	Quetiapine-H (up to 750 mg/day), quetiapine-L (up to 250 mg/day), placebo	6	BPRS total, CGI, SANS: Quetiapine-H demonstrated significant improvement over placebo. Quetiapine-L group did not show superiority to placebo for any efficacy measure.
22	302 patients with schizophrenia or schizoaffective disorder	Ziprasidone 80 mg/day(40 mg b.i.d.) and 160 mg/day (80 mg b.i.d.), placebo	6	BPRS, PANSS, CGI: Both active treatment groups demonstrated significant improvement over placebo. MADRS: Subset of ziprasidone 160-mg group with depressive symptomatology demonstrated improvement vs. placebo.
23	139 patients with schizophrenia or schizoaffective disorder	Ziprasidone 40 and 120 mg/day, placebo	4	BPRS total, CGI: Ziprasidone 120-mg group demonstrated significant improvement.
24	414 patients with schizophrenia or schizoaffective disorder	Aripiprazole 15 and 30 mg/day, haloperidol 10 mg/day, placebo	4	PANSS total: Significant improvement with all active treatment groups at 2 wk. CGI: Scores in LOCF analysis superior to placebo for all active treatment groups.

[a]BPRS = Brief Psychiatric Rating Scale, CGI = clinical global impression, SANS = Schedule for the Assessment of Negative Symptoms, PANSS = Positive and Negative Syndrome Scale, MADRS = Montgomery–Asberg Depression Rating Scale, LOCF = last observation carried forward.

(4.8 months; MMD, 3.9 mg/day), perphenazine (5.6 months; MMD, 20.8 mg/day), and ziprasidone (3.5 months; MMD, 112.8 mg/day). For patients remaining on the assigned treatment over the course of the study, overall psychopathology as assessed by the Positive and Negative Syndrome Scale and the CGI showed improvement over time. Notably, the traditional antipsychotic perphenazine demonstrated comparable efficacy to the second-generation comparators across all measures.

There are several concerns that need to be considered regarding CATIE. First, within the 18-month study period, 74% of the patients discontinued their initial assigned drug therapy. Second, patients with preexisting tardive dyskinesia were not assigned to perphenazine and may have been less likely to exhibit adverse motor effects during the study. Finally, 30% of the patients receiving olanzapine experienced weight gain and adverse metabolic effects, including elevated blood glucose, cholesterol, triglyceride, and glycosylated hemoglobin levels. CATIE compared a single traditional antipsychotic, perphenazine, given at a low dosage to several second-generation antipsychotics. While the data generated from this study are helpful for determining differences in effectiveness between the assigned regimens and comparing important adverse effect issues, they support the widely held notion that the selection of antipsychotic drugs should be an individualized process.

Neurocognitive Effects

Impaired cognitive functioning has long been observed as a core feature of psychotic disorders. These impairments are relatively stable over the natural course of the illness, regardless of the frequency of acute exacerbations of psychotic symptoms.[26] Furthermore, cognitive impairment may have a greater impact on psychosocial functioning than any other feature of schizophrenia.[27,28]

Many domains of cognition, including attention, short-term memory, and executive function, are affected by schizophrenia.[26] Treatment with traditional antipsychotic drugs, while relieving positive symptoms of psychosis, do little to improve cognitive functioning. The concomitant use of anticholinergic drugs intended to prevent or treat extrapyramidal symptoms that accompany antipsychotic therapy may actually worsen some cognitive functions.[29]

Second-generation antipsychotics can play an important role in facilitating the psychosocial rehabilitation of individuals with psychotic disorders by improving cognition. These agents have been shown to improve scores on assessments representing a broad range of cognitive functions. A lower degree of binding to dopamine-D_2 receptors, as well as $5\text{-}HT_2$ antagonism, in the mesocortical pathway may contribute to the beneficial effects on cognition. The individualized receptor-binding properties of second-generation antipsychotics may contribute to differential improvements in various cognitive domains in individuals with psychotic disorders.

In a 14-week study of individuals with treatment-resistant schizophrenia, risperidone and olanzapine improved executive function, declarative memory, and attention.[30] Clozapine has been shown to positively affect executive function and working memory in numerous studies.[31-33] In an open-label study of 255 clinically stable patients, ar-

ipiprazole and olanzapine improved working memory from baseline after eight weeks of treatment, while aripiprazole showed a greater improvement than olanzapine in verbal learning at weeks 8 and 26.[34]

Adverse Effects

One of the primary advantages of second-generation antipsychotics in the chronic treatment of psychotic disorders is the improved tolerability profile over older antipsychotics. Adverse effects related to dopamine blockade in the central nervous system tend to occur less frequently in individuals treated with second-generation antipsychotics compared with those receiving traditional antipsychotics. However, the newer drugs have been associated with different problems that can affect drug therapy.

Motor Symptoms. Treatment with conventional antipsychotics has long been associated with both acute and chronic adverse motor effects. Acute extrapyramidal symptoms— dystonia, pseudoparkinsonism, and akathisia (a syndrome of subjective anxiety and restlessness)—are thought to be related to drug-induced blockade of dopamine receptors in the nigrostriatal pathway in the brain. Second-generation antipsychotics, possibly through a combination of $5-HT_2$-receptor antagonism and rapid dissociation from D_2 receptors,[35] produce antipsychotic effects with a lower likelihood of acute extrapyramidal symptoms.[36]

Tardive dyskinesia, a potentially irreversible chronic motor disorder caused by long-term exposure to dopamine antagonists, has been another serious concern with conventional antipsychotics. Though not completely eliminating the risk, second-generation antipsychotics have been shown to have a lower risk of treatment-emergent tardive dyskinesia with maintenance treatment. Using data pooled from three controlled comparative studies, Tollefson et al.[37] reported that 50 (7.1%) of 707 olanzapine-treated patients manifested symptoms of tardive dyskinesia during the trials, compared with 32 (16.2%) of 197 individuals treated with haloperidol ($p < 0.001$). In a nine-month prospective study of outpatients age 45 years or older, the risk of developing tardive dyskinesia was over four times greater for patients treated with haloperidol than for those receiving risperidone ($p = 0.045$).[38] Similar results have been found in other controlled and noncontrolled studies of risperidone, olanzapine, and quetiapine.[39-41]

Clozapine appears to have an especially favorable profile for the prevention and management of antipsychotic-induced movement disorders. In comparative trials, clozapine exhibited little to no evidence of inducing treatment-emergent extrapyramidal symptoms.[13,42,43] The risk of tardive dyskinesia associated with clozapine treatment also appears to be minimal.[44] In fact, clozapine has been used to successfully treat preexisting tardive dyskinesia. Remission of symptoms has been reported in some, but not all, cases of preexisting tardive dyskinesia treated with clozapine.[45-47] In addition, withdrawal of clozapine in patients with tardive dyskinesia has resulted in either maintenance of reduced movements[46] or worsening of dyskinesias. The inconsistent nature of tardive dyskinesia treatment makes prevention of this syndrome a very important consideration in the pharmacotherapy of psychotic disorders.[48]

Prolactin Elevation. Dopamine antagonists may elevate serum prolactin levels by decreasing the prolactin inhibitory effects of dopamine in the hypothalamus. Prolactin elevation has been reported to cause an irregular or suppressed menstrual cycle,[49] galactorrhea,[50] gynecomastia, and sexual dysfunction[51] in the short term. With long-term elevation of plasma prolactin levels, suppression of estrogen and testosterone may occur. These effects may lead to a decrease in bone mineral density and to osteoporosis.[52]

The degree of prolactin elevation that an antipsychotic agent may exert appears to be related to its dopamine- and serotonin-binding properties. Significant prolactin elevation and its associated adverse effects can occur with moderate-to-high doses of the traditional antipsychotics and risperidone.[52] Risperidone has been consistently associated with the greatest degree of prolactin elevation among the second-generation antipsychotics.[53,54] In a prospective trial, olanzapine was found to cause a low and transient increase in prolactin levels across its dosage range, compared with the significant, persistent hyperprolactinemia associated with haloperidol.[55] The effect of quetiapine treatment across its dosage range on plasma prolactin levels was comparable to placebo, while significant elevations were associated with haloperidol.[20] Similarly, aripiprazole has been shown to be comparable to placebo for prolactin elevation.[24] Antipsychotic-associated prolactin elevation has been successfully managed by switching to an antipsychotic agent with a lower propensity toward increasing prolactin.[56,57]

Weight Gain. The metabolic effects of antipsychotic drug therapy have become a source of concern for clinicians and patients. Psychotic disorders and antipsychotic drug treatment have long been associated with comorbid obesity[58] and its related conditions: type 2 diabetes mellitus[59,60] and cardiovascular disease.[61] In addition, drug treatments[62] and lifestyle changes[63,64] aimed at weight reduction may be ineffective or difficult to implement in this population.

Varying degrees of weight gain have been reported with chronic use of traditional and second-generation antipsychotics. Among the traditional antipsychotics, loxapine[65] and molindone[66,67] are notable for weight-loss or weight-neutral profiles. Of the second-generation antipsychotics, ziprasidone and aripiprazole have been associated with the lowest likelihood for causing weight gain. A large meta-analysis by Allison et al.[68] was conducted to compare the weight gain associated with the use of various antipsychotic drugs that were approved or under investigation in the United States. Table 4 lists estimated weight gain after 10 weeks of treatment on drugs for which sufficient data are available. Clozapine and olanzapine were associated with more weight gain than all other agents included in this review. The small weight loss associated with placebo may have been due to discontinuation of antipsychotic therapy as the subjects entered the studies.

The antipsychotic agents also appear to differ in the duration and rate of weight changes. In one study, weight increases with continuous clozapine treatment occurred until about 46 months of treatment, with the greatest amount of weight being gained during the first 12 months.[69] Weight gain with olanzapine may plateau after 4-5 months.[70]

Table 4.
Estimated Body Weight Changes at 10 Weeks in Patients Receiving Antipsychotics[68]

Treatment	Weight Gain (kg)
Placebo	-0.74
Molindone	-0.39
Ziprasidone	0.04
Fluphenazine	0.43
Haloperidol	1.08
Risperidone	2.10
Chlorpromazine	2.58
Thioridazine-mesoridazine	3.19
Olanzapine	4.15
Clozapine	4.45

Diabetes Mellitus. New-onset hyperglycemia and diabetes mellitus have also been observed with antipsychotic treatment. In some instances, the initial presentation consists of life-threatening diabetic ketoacidosis or hyperosmolar coma.[71] Frequently, clinically significant weight gain does not occur before the diagnosis of diabetes.[72] Koller et al.[73] reviewed cases of hyperglycemic episodes associated with risperidone and haloperidol reported to the Food and Drug Administration's (FDA's) MedWatch surveillance program. Of the 131 cases of hyperglycemia associated with antipsychotic monotherapy with risperidone, 78 were clearly identified as newly diagnosed hyperglycemia. In the cases for which adequate data were available, 71% of cases with preexisting hyperglycemia and 48% of cases of new-onset hyperglycemia occurred within the first three months of risperidone monotherapy.

Sernyak et al.[74] conducted a large analysis of a national sample of patients treated for schizophrenia in Veterans Affairs medical centers to investigate a possible association between the use of antipsychotic medications and development of diabetes mellitus. Patients were identified as being treated with clozapine, olanzapine, quetiapine, risperidone, or traditional antipsychotics. When the patients were stratified by age, significantly higher rates of comorbid diabetes were found in patients treated with second-generation antipsychotics. Overall, clozapine, olanzapine, and quetiapine were most frequently implicated. The strongest relationships were found in individuals less than 40 years of age.

Plasma glucose regulation in individuals receiving antipsychotics and in healthy controls was assessed using oral glucose tolerance tests.[75] Olanzapine-treated patients demonstrated significantly elevated plasma glucose levels while fasting and at 15, 45, and 75 minutes postload compared with controls and patients treated with traditional antipsychotics. Clozapine-treated patients had significant elevations while fasting and at 75 minutes postload compared with controls and patients receiving traditional antipsychotics. With risperidone, the elevations in plasma glucose were seen in the fasting state and at 45 and 75 minutes postload and were significantly higher compared with healthy controls.

Dyslipidemias. Hyperlipidemia is another significant cardiac risk associated with second-generation antipsychotic treatment. Increases in serum triglycerides and low-density lipoproteins with second-generation antipsychotics have not always correlated with significant weight gain.[76]

A retrospective analysis of long-term inpatients treated with risperidone and olanzapine was conducted to determine trends of various metabolic values.[77] The investigator reported that the average increase in triglyceride concentrations was 104.8 mg/dL with olanzapine versus 31.7 mg/dL with risperidone after one year. Total cholesterol increased by 30.7 mg/dL with olanzapine and 7.2 mg/dL with risperidone. A naturalistic study of clozapine treatment revealed a significant increase in serum triglyceride level over five years of treatment.[69] In CATIE, olanzapine was associated with the greatest exposure-adjusted increases in serum cholesterol and triglycerides.[25]

In November 2003, a consensus panel that included experts from the American Diabetes Association, American Psychiatric Association, American Association of Clinical Endocrinologists, and the North American Association for the Study of Obesity was convened. Using data collected during a comprehensive literature review and presentations from representatives from the pharmaceutical industry and FDA, the consensus panel developed a statement outlining the metabolic risks of treatment with second-generation antipsychotics.[78] The panel recommended careful consideration of metabolic risks whenever second-generation antipsychotics are initiated, especially in high-risk patients. The panel also recommended considering switching antipsychotics in patients who gain 5% or more of their initial weight, experience worsening hyperglycemia, or develop worsening hyperlipidemia.

Cardiac Toxicity. Certain traditional and second-generation antipsychotics have been associated with clinically significant prolongation of the corrected Q-T (Q-Tc) interval, which may lead to torsades de pointes, a fatal ventricular arrhythmia. The risk of cardiac mortality associated with psychotropic drug treatment is particularly troublesome because of its spontaneous and unpredictable nature.

The traditional antipsychotics thioridazine, mesoridazine, pimozide, and droperidol have been implicated in numerous cases of sudden unexpected death.[79] Electrocardiographic data have revealed that patients receiving droperidol and thioridazine are more likely to have an abnormally long Q-Tc interval.[80] Numerous reports of patient fatalities and the availability of safer alternatives have prompted FDA to recommend that thioridazine, mesoridazine, pimozide, and droperidol only be used as alternative agents with extreme caution.

Although regulatory scrutiny for cardiac assessment heightened during the development of second-generation antipsychotics, these agents are generally associated with a low risk of electrocardiographic abnormalities. Ziprasidone was found to be associated with modest Q-Tc prolongation during its premarketing studies. A comparative study that sought to determine the extent of Q-Tc prolongation seen with the target therapeutic dosages of haloperidol, risperidone, olanzapine, quetiapine, and ziprasidone was later presented to FDA.[81] Thioridazine was also assessed in this study at half its maximum recommended dosage. Thioridazine was associated with an average Q-Tc-interval increase of 35.6 milliseconds. Of the second-generation agents included in this study, ziprasidone was associated with the greatest mean increase in the Q-Tc interval—20.3

milliseconds. Haloperidol-treated subjects had an average Q-Tc-interval increase of 4.7 seconds, the smallest change observed in this study. Coadministration of other interacting drugs (e.g., cytochrome P-450 isoenzyme inhibitors) did not lead to significant changes in Q-Tc measurement. Ziprasidone's labeling warned of its greater potential of Q-Tc-interval prolongation and discouraged use in patients with electrolyte abnormalities, cardiac comorbidity, or concomitant use of metabolic inhibitors.[82]

Clozapine has been associated with treatment-emergent myocarditis and cardiomyopathy. Myocarditis associated with clozapine treatment presents as an acute inflammation of the myocardium, which may lead to congestive heart failure.[83] With over 180,000 patient exposures to clozapine during the first 10 years of its clinical use in the United States, FDA received 28 reports of myocarditis, including 18 deaths.[84] The greatest risk of fatal events appears to exist during the first month of therapy. Cardiomyopathy associated with clozapine is an insidious process characterized by ventricular dilatation, impaired contraction, and symptoms of congestive heart failure.[83] A total of 41 cases of cardiomyopathy, including 10 deaths, were reported to FDA between 1989 and 1999.[84]

Cerebrovascular Events. The use of second-generation antipsychotics for the treatment of dementia-related agitation and psychosis in elderly patients is an unlabeled use that is generally supported by efficacy data in published controlled clinical trials.[85] However, post hoc analyses of the safety data for these trials revealed an elevated risk of cerebrovascular adverse events (CVAEs), including stroke and transient ischemic attacks, among patients treated with second-generation antipsychotics. These data led FDA to issue a public health advisory warning of the potential for fatal CVAEs in patients with dementia being treated with second-generation antipsychotics. The manufacturers of second-generation antipsychotic agents were also requested to place a black-box warning describing this treatment risk on the labeling of these products.

A closer look at the applicable safety data reveals that the patients in the dementia trials were often at elevated risk for CVAEs because of advanced age, poor control of chronic cardiovascular disease, and the underlying etiology of the dementia.[86] Cases of CVAEs included nonspecific events, such as hypotensive episodes, periods of unresponsiveness, and slurred speech. For example, the pooled results of six placebo-controlled randomized studies of risperidone for the treatment of behavioral disturbances in patients with dementia revealed 33 CVAEs (3.3%) in 1009 subjects receiving the drug. The frequency of CVAEs was 1.1% (8 of 712) among placebo-treated patients ($p = 0.004$). However, serious CVAEs (fatal events, life-threatening events, or CVAEs associated with hospitalization or disability) occurred in 15 (1.5%) of 1009 patients treated with risperidone and 4 (0.6%) of 712 patients treated with placebo, a difference that failed to reach statistical significance. Furthermore, most patients experiencing stroke had risk factors, including hypertension, atrial fibrillation, and previous strokes.[86]

The nature of this type of safety data makes it difficult to determine causality. It has been postulated that the adverse effects of sedation, hypotension, pseudoparkinsonism, and enhanced platelet aggregation may contribute to the observed increase in CVAEs.[86] In addition, these findings have

not been widely observed among patients with psychotic disorders. It would therefore be advisable to consider stroke prophylaxis in all elderly patients receiving antipsychotic drugs, particularly high-risk patients.

Hematologic Toxicity, Respiratory Depression, and Seizures. Despite its superior efficacy for treatment-resistant psychotic disorders, the use of clozapine has remained restricted due to the potential of severe adverse effects not commonly seen with other antipsychotics. Agranulocytosis has been estimated to occur in 1–2% of patients treated with clozapine.[87] Episodes tend to occur between two and six months after initiation of treatment.[88] Fatal infectious complications may occur as a result of reduced white blood cell count. Clozapine-induced agranulocytosis can be reversed with the prompt discontinuation of treatment.

In the United States, clozapine is available only under the surveillance of one of the national manufacturer-operated registries that monitor weekly complete blood counts from individuals taking this agent. Consistent monitoring has resulted in a markedly reduced rate of agranulocytosis and mortality associated with clozapine-induced agranulocytosis.[89] Furthermore, the continual monitoring mandated by the clozapine registry programs likely allows for improved treatment adherence and outcomes.[90]

Other toxicities that are more common with clozapine than with other second-generation antipsychotics are respiratory depression and seizures. Respiratory collapse has been associated with rapid dosage adjustment and concomitant benzodiazepine use. It is therefore recommended that clozapine dosage be gradually adjusted from the starting dose if the patient is new to clozapine treatment or if two or more days have elapsed since the last dose. A dose-related reduction of the seizure threshold has been observed with clozapine.[91] Precautions should be taken for patients with seizure disorders receiving clozapine treatment.

Drug Selection and Dosing Considerations

With the notable exception of clozapine, the principal differences among the available second-generation antipsychotics lie in their adverse-effect profiles and dosage forms. Selection of an initial treatment for a patient whose psychosis is not considered to be treatment resistant should be individualized based on the patient's specific tolerability and compliance concerns.[92] Individuals with a sensitivity to extrapyramidal symptoms may benefit from quetiapine or aripiprazole. Patients with preexisting obesity or diabetes mellitus may benefit from an initial trial with ziprasidone or aripiprazole. The availability of orally disintegrating formulations of olanzapine, risperidone, and aripiprazole; liquid formulations of risperidone and aripiprazole; and a long-acting injectable formulation of risperidone provides options for patients with a history of poor treatment adherence or who have difficulty taking standard oral tablets or capsules. The traditional antipsychotics may be an initial choice for those who are at low risk for movement disorders[25] or for whom the newer drugs may be cost-prohibitive.

The importance of appropriate dosing of second-generation antipsychotics was highlighted in an analysis conducted by Love et al.[93] Results of the premarketing studies for

risperidone suggested that the dose–efficacy curve peaked at 6 mg/day, leading to the recommendation on the product labeling that risperidone be adjusted to this dosage over the first three days of treatment. After the introduction of risperidone to the mass market, numerous reports[94–96] demonstrated that the optimal dosage of risperidone for efficacy was between 4 and 6 mg/day, a dosage range not assessed in the original large efficacy studies. Aggregate computerized pharmacy records from state inpatient psychiatry facilities in Maryland revealed significantly higher discharge rates for patients receiving 2–4 mg/day than for those receiving 6 mg/day. It is now recommended that clinicians attempt to stabilize patients on risperidone 2–4 mg/day before initiating a trial at higher dosages.[93]

In general, clinical studies suggest that for most of the other second-generation antipsychotics indicated for first-line treatment, a more linear dose–response curve is applicable. Patients may require dosage adjustment to 10–20 mg/day of olanzapine, 300–800 mg/day of quetiapine, 80–160 mg/day of ziprasidone, or 10–30 mg/day of aripiprazole for control of acute psychotic symptoms.[13–24] Maintenance therapy can frequently be achieved with lower dosages, thereby reducing toxicity. Special populations, such as the elderly or individuals with hepatic impairment, may require lower doses due to increased sensitivity to adverse effects. In some individuals with a history of suboptimal response to antipsychotic treatment, additional benefit has been gained using second-generation antipsychotics with doses higher than the maximum recommended in the product labeling.[97]

In the event of nonresponse to an initial trial of antipsychotic medication, most treatment guidelines recommend sequential trials of second-generation antipsychotics with a minimum of three weeks duration at therapeutic doses.[98–100] A trial of clozapine is generally warranted for patients who demonstrate a suboptimal response to two or more trials with first-line antipsychotic agents. Traditional antipsychotics may also have a role for patients who fail treatment with second-generation antipsychotics. In addition, the adjunctive use of antidepressants, mood stabilizers, or anxiolytics may be beneficial in selected patients. The combined use of more than one antipsychotic drug is a controversial and costly practice.[101] Very little published evidence supports the use of multiple oral antipsychotics, except when attempting to transition a patient from one agent to another.[102]

Patient Monitoring

Frequent and continuous monitoring is necessary for individuals treated with antipsychotics in order to assess for therapeutic response and adverse effects. For the second-generation antipsychotics intended for first-line use, the recommended minimum trial duration is three weeks after adjustment to a recommended therapeutic dose. A longer trial is generally warranted for clozapine. Gradual reductions in the severity of psychotic symptoms (e.g., suspiciousness, hallucinations) are expected with adequate treatment.

Monitoring for metabolic adverse effects of second-generation antipsychotic therapy should consist of regular assessments of body weight, glucose levels, and lipid values (Table 5).[103] Treatment with clozapine requires weekly assessments of complete blood count and absolute neutrophil count for the first six months. If no evidence of neutropenia or granulocytopenia is found, the monitoring frequency can be reduced to every two weeks for the next six months and then every four weeks thereafter.

Despite the lower propensity for causing adverse motor effects, all patients receiving second-generation antipsychotics should be monitored for symptoms of dystonia, parkinsonism, akathisia, and tardive dyskinesia.[103] Patients should be evaluated for acute extrapyramidal symptoms weekly until two weeks after dose stabilization when antipsychotics are initiated or adjusted. Assessments for tardive dyskinesia should be conducted at least once yearly for individuals receiving continuous treatment with antipsychotics.[103]

Measurement of antipsychotic plasma levels is not clinically indicated, except to assess for treatment adherence or suspected drug interactions. However, a minimum plasma clozapine concentration of 350 ng/mL has been correlated with treatment response among patients whose psychosis has been identified as treatment resistant.[104,105] In a study of the use of therapeutic drug monitoring in long-term treatment with clozapine, relapse was more frequently associated with a decrease from a stable drug level than maintenance of a threshold minimum concentration.[106]

Treatment Outcomes

Schizophrenia and related disorders are characterized by chronic courses and periodic exacerbations. Exacerbations in the positive symptoms of schizophrenia may precipitate costly hospitalizations and may result in encounters with the legal system, while the negative and cognitive symptoms affect independent functioning, employment, and quality of life. Hospitalizations in specialty psychiatric facilities may

Table 5.
Monitoring Guidelines for Patients Treated with Second-Generation Antipsychotics

Assessment	Monitoring Frequency
Fasting blood glucose	All drugs: Baseline, then monthly for the first 3 mo and every 6 mo thereafter. More frequent assessments are indicated for individuals noted to be gaining weight.
Weight assessment	All drugs: Baseline and monthly thereafter. (Self-monitoring of weight should be encouraged.)
Electrocardiogram	Clozapine and ziprasidone: Baseline and annually thereafter. More frequent assessments may be indicated in patients over age 50 yr and in patients with a history of cardiac arrhythmias.
Complete blood count with differential	Clozapine: Weekly for the first 6 mo. Every other wk for the next 6 mo, and every 4 wk thereafter if no abnormalities are noted.
Fasting total cholesterol, low- and high-density lipoproteins, and triglycerides	All drugs: Baseline and every 2 yr thereafter if no abnormalities are noted. Every 6 mo for individuals noted to have hyperlipidemia or receiving lipid-lowering therapy.

result in lengths of stay measured in months or years. Thus, the single greatest component of the cost of schizophrenia is the cost of hospital stay. In contrast, drugs are thought to account for less than 10% of the direct costs of treating these illnesses.

Studies addressing the effect of second-generation antipsychotics on hospitalization have repeatedly found that these agents reduce the length of stay and readmission rate compared with conventional antipsychotics. Rabinowitz et al.[107] calculated a two-year rehospitalization rate of 31–33% for patients discharged from inpatient psychiatric hospitalization receiving olanzapine or risperidone, compared with a 48% rate for patients discharged on conventional antipsychotics ($p = 0.02$). In a landmark double-blind trial of risperidone versus haloperidol, Csernansky et al.[108] measured relapse by examining rehospitalization, signs of clinical decompensation, and increasing requirements for supervision. They found significantly lower relapse rates at one year and longer times to relapse with risperidone treatment. FDA accepted this trial as sufficient evidence to allow the manufacturer to indicate in the product labeling the drug's efficacy in delaying relapse.

A variety of studies have focused on the cost of second-generation antipsychotics in comparison with each other[109,110] and conventional agents.[111] In general, the generically available first-generation antipsychotics are less expensive than the newer second-generation agents. However, when overall costs of care are calculated, second-generation antipsychotics often demonstrate lower hospital utilization, improved symptomatic control, and fewer adverse effects, resulting in lower or equal total costs for the second-generation agents versus first-generation antipsychotics.[112]

While most studies examining outcomes with second-generation antipsychotics have focused on cost, hospitalization, and relapse, fewer have examined issues related to quality of life. Chouinard and Albright[113] addressed these issues by conducting a cost–utility analysis of risperidone versus haloperidol in association with a randomized clinical trial. Patients taking risperidone gained almost three quality-adjusted life years over those who received haloperidol. Franz et al.[114] conducted quality-of-life interviews with patients receiving conventional antipsychotics, clozapine, risperidone, or zotepine (not available in the United States). Patients receiving second-generation antipsychotics had a significantly higher total quality of life than those receiving conventional agents. They also demonstrated significantly superior ratings in the domains of physical well-being, social life, and everyday life.

Secondary depression is also a major problem in schizophrenia, and suicide is a leading cause of death in this population.[115] It has been estimated that about 10% of patients with psychotic disorders die by suicide.[116,117] In addition to having favorable effects on mood symptoms, there are indications that second-generation antipsychotics may also reduce suicide rates in some populations, with clozapine demonstrating a particular benefit in this regard.[118] In a study of 980 patients with schizophrenia or schizoaffective disorder at high risk for suicide, treatment with clozapine was associated with a significantly lower rate of suicide attempts and hospitalizations to prevent suicide compared with olanzapine (20.8% versus 28.8%, $p < 0.005$).[119]

Second-generation antipsychotics likely produce beneficial outcomes through a variety of effects. Compared with conventional antipsychotics and placebo, second-generation antipsychotics demonstrate improved efficacy for psychotic and cognitive symptoms. In controlled trials, these agents produce fewer disabling extrapyramidal adverse effects, such as akathisia and parkinsonism. These effects result in improved adherence to prescribed regiments, less interference with socialization and occupational function, and a feeling of improved well-being compared with the effects of conventional antipsychotics.

Summary

Psychotic disorders are chronic illnesses that impart a considerable burden on patients, families, and society. Although no known drug therapies can cure these illnesses, antipsychotic agents are a mainstay for the management of acute illness and prevention of relapse. The second-generation antipsychotics—risperidone, olanzapine, quetiapine, ziprasidone, aripiprazole, and paliperidone—offer numerous advantages over the older agents, including a lower risk of extrapyramidal motor symptoms and elevated serum prolactin levels, as well as improvements in cognitive symptoms. These advantages have led to improved long-term outcomes and cost-effectiveness, despite the higher acquisition costs of these drugs. Clozapine has demonstrated a unique level of efficacy for individuals with treatment-resistant psychotic disorders and for individuals at high risk for suicide and is very valuable in these subgroups, despite the additional adverse hematologic and cardiovascular effects. Metabolic adverse effects, including weight gain, glucose abnormalities, and hyperlipidemias, cause significant concern for patients receiving second-generation antipsychotics and must be managed proactively by clinicians. Health care professionals in all settings should play an active role in assisting in the selection of an appropriate antipsychotic agent, ensuring appropriate monitoring, and providing counseling to ensure that patients remain compliant with treatment. Additional readings and resources are listed in the appendix.

References

1. Schizophrenia and other psychotic disorders. In: American Psychiatric Association. DSM-IV-TR: diagnostic and statistical manual of mental disorders, 4th ed., text revision. Washington, DC: American Psychiatric Press; 2000.

2. Keith SJ, Regier DA, Rae DS. Schizophrenic disorders. In: Robins LN, Regier DA, eds. Psychiatric disorders in America: the Epidemiologic Catchment Area Study. New York: Free Press; 1991: 33–52.

3. Kessler RC, McGonagle KA, Zhao S et al. Lifetime and 12-month prevalence of DSM-III-R psychiatric disorders in the United States: results from the National Comorbidity Survey. *Arch Gen Psychiatry.* 1994; 52:8–19.

4. Loranger AW. Sex differences in age at onset of schizophrenia. *Arch Gen Psychiatry.* 1984; 41:157–61.

5. Hafner H, Maurer K, Loeffler W et al. The influence of age and sex on the onset and early course of schizophrenia. *Br J Psychiatry.* 1993; 162:80–6.

6. Kim JS, Kornhuber HH, Schmid-Burgk W et al. Low cerebrospinal fluid glutamate in schizophrenia patients

and a new hypothesis on schizophrenia. *Neurosci Lett.* 1980; 20:379–82.

7. Krystal JH, Karper LP, Seibyl JP et al. Subanesthetic effects of the noncompetitive NMDA antagonist, ketamine, in humans: psychotomimetic, perceptual, cognitive, and neuroendocrine responses. *Arch Gen Psychiatry.* 1994; 51:199–214.

8. Hughes JR, Hatsukami DK, Mitchell JE et al. Prevalence of smoking among psychiatric outpatients. *Am J Psychiatry.* 1986; 143:993–7.

9. Dalack GW, Healy DJ, Meador-Woodruff JH. Nicotine dependence in schizophrenia: clinical phenomena and laboratory findings. *Am J Psychiatry.* 1998; 155:1490–501.

10. Stahl SM. Dopamine system stabilizers, aripiprazole, and the next generation of antipsychotics, part I: "Goldilocks" actions at dopamine receptors. *J Clin Psychiatry.* 2001; 62:841–2.

11. Stahl SM. Dopamine system stabilizers, aripiprazole, and the next generation of antipsychotics, part II: illustrating their mechanism of action. *J Clin Psychiatry.* 2001; 62:923–4.

12. Kapur S, Remington G. Serotonin–dopamine interaction and its relevance to schizophrenia. *Am J Psychiatry.* 1996; 153:466–76.

13. Kane J, Honigfeld G, Singer J et al. Clozapine for the treatment-resistant schizophrenic, a double-blind comparison with chlorpromazine. *Arch Gen Psychiatry.* 1988; 45:789–96.

14. Breier A, Buchanan RW, Kirkpatrick B et al. Effects of clozapine on positive and negative symptoms in outpatients with schizophrenia. *Am J Psychiatry.* 1994; 152:20–6.

15. Marder SR, Meibach RC. Risperidone in the treatment of schizophrenia. *Am J Psychiatry.* 1994; 151:825–35.

16. Chouinard G, Jones B, Remington G et al. A Canadian multi-center placebo-controlled study of fixed doses of risperidone and haloperidol in the treatment of chronic schizophrenic patients. *J Clin Psychopharmacol.* 1993; 13:25–40.

17. Kane JM, Eerdekens M, Lindenmayer JP et al. Long-acting injectable risperidone: efficacy and safety of the first long-acting atypical antipsychotic. *Am J Psychiatry.* 2003; 160:1125–32.

18. Beasley CM, Tollfeson G, Tran P et al. Olanzapine versus placebo and haloperidol: acute phase results of the North American double-blind olanzapine trial. *Neuropsychopharmacology.* 1996; 14:111–23.

19. Beasley CM, Sanger T, Satterlee W et al. Olanzapine vs placebo: results of a double-blind, fixed-dose olanzapine trial. *Psychopharmacology.* 1996; 124:159–67.

20. Arvanitis LA, Miller BG. Multiple fixed doses of "Seroquel" (quetiapine) in patients with acute exacerbation of schizophrenia: a comparison with haloperidol and placebo. *Biol Psychiatry.* 1997; 42:233–46.

21. Small JG, Hirsch SR, Arvanitis LA et al. Quetiapine in patients with schizophrenia: a high- and low-dose double-blind comparison with placebo. *Arch Gen Psychiatry.* 1997; 54:549–57.

22. Daniel DG, Zimbroff DL, Potkin SG et al. Ziprasidone 80 mg/day and 160 mg/day in the acute exacerbation of schizophrenia and schizoaffective disorder: a 6-week placebo-controlled trial. *Neuropsychopharmacology.* 1999; 20:491–505.

23. Keck P Jr, Buffenstein A, Ferguson J et al. Ziprasidone 40 and 120 mg/day in the acute exacerbation of schizophrenia and schizoaffective disorder: a 4-week placebo-controlled trial. *Psychopharmacology.* 1998; 140:173–84.

24. Kane JM, Carson WH, Saha AR et al. Efficacy and safety of aripiprazole and haloperidol versus placebo in patients with schizophrenia and schizoaffective disorder. *J Clin Psychiatry.* 2002; 63:763–71.

25. Lieberman JA, Stroup TS, McEvoy JP et al. Effectiveness of antipsychotic drugs in patients with chronic schizophrenia. *N Engl J Med.* 2005; 353:1209–23.

26. Sharma T, Antonova L. Cognitive function in schizophrenia: deficits, functional consequences, and future treatment. *Psychiatr Clin North Am.* 2003; 26:25–40.

27. Green MF. What are the functional consequences of neurocognitive deficits of schizophrenia? *Am J Psychiatry.* 1996; 153:321–30.

28. Liddle PF. Cognitive impairment in schizophrenia: its impact on social functioning. *Acta Psychiatr Scand Suppl.* 2000; 400:11–6.

29. Spohn HE, Strauss ME. Relation of neuroleptic and anticholinergic medication to cognitive functions in schizophrenia. *J Abnorm Psychol.* 1989; 98:367–80.

30. Bilder RM, Goldman RS, Volavka J et al. Neurocognitive effects of clozapine, olanzapine, risperidone, and haloperidol in patients with chronic schizophrenia or schizoaffective disorder. *Am J Psychiatry.* 2002; 159:1018–28.

31. Hagger C, Buckley P, Kenny JT et al. Improvement in cognitive functions and psychiatric symptoms in treatment-refractory schizophrenic patients receiving clozapine. *Biol Psychiatry.* 1993; 34:702–12.

32. Grace J, Bellus SB, Raulin ML et al. Long-term impact of clozapine and psychosocial treatment on psychiatric symptoms and cognitive functioning. *Psychiatr Serv.* 1996; 47:41–5.

33. Buchanan RW, Holstein C, Breier A. The comparative efficacy and long-term effect of clozapine on neuropsychological test performance. *Biol Psychiatry.* 1994; 36:717–25.

34. Cornblatt B, Kern RS, Carson WH et al. Neurocognitive effects of aripiprazole versus olanzapine in stable psychosis. Presented at 23rd Collegium Internationale Neuropsychopharmacologicum Congress. Montreal, Canada; 2002 Jun.

35. Stahl SM. "Hit-and-run" actions at dopamine receptors, part 1: mechanism of action of second-generation antipsychotics. *J Clin Psychiatry.* 2001; 62:670–1.

36. Leucht S, Pitschel-Walz G, Abraham D et al. Efficacy and extrapyramidal side-effects of the new antipsychotics olanzapine, quetiapine, risperidone, and sertindole compared to conventional antipsychotics and placebo: a meta-analysis of randomized controlled trials. *Schizophr Res.* 1999; 35:51–68.

37. Tollefson GD, Beasley CM, Tamura RN et al. Blind, controlled, long-term study of the comparative incidence of treatment-emergent tardive dyskinesia with olanzapine or haloperidol. *Am J Psychiatry.* 1997; 154:1248–54.

38. Jeste DV, Lacro JP, Bailey A et al. Lower incidence of tardive dyskinesia with risperidone compared with haloperidol in older patients. *J Am Geriatr Soc.* 1999; 47:716–9.

39. Jeste DV, Okamoto A, Napolitano J et al. Low incidence of persistent tardive dyskinesia in elderly patients with dementia treated with risperidone. *Am J Psychiatry.* 2000; 157:1150–5.

40. Beasley CM, Dellva MA, Tamura RN et al. Randomised double-blind comparison of the incidence of tardive dyskinesia in patients with schizophrenia during long-term treatment with olanzapine or haloperidol. *Br J Psychiatry.* 1999; 174:23–30.

41. Farah A. Reduction of tardive dyskinesia with quetiapine. *Schizophr Res.* 2001; 47:309–10. Letter.

42. Povlssen UJ, Noring U, Fog R et al. Tolerability and therapeutic effect of clozapine: a retrospective investigation of 216 patients treated with clozapine for up to 12 years. *Acta Psychiatr Scand.* 1985; 71:176–85.

43. Kurz M, Hummer M, Oberbauer H et al. Extrapyramidal side effects of clozapine and haloperidol. *Psychopharmacology.* 1995; 118:52–6.

44. Casey DE. Clozapine: neuroleptic-induced EPS and tardive dyskinesia. *Psychopharmacology.* 1989; 99: S47–53.

45. Lieberman JA, Saltz BL, Johns CA et al. The effects of clozapine on tardive dyskinesia. *Br J Psychiatry.* 1991; 158:503–10.

46. Spivak B, Mester R, Abesgaus J et al. Clozapine treatment for neuroleptic-induced tardive dyskinesia, parkinsonism, and chronic akathisia in schizophrenic patients. *J Clin Psychiatry.* 1997; 58:318–22.

47. Tamminga CA, Thaker GK, Moran M et al. Clozapine in tardive dyskinesia: observations from human and animal model studies. *J Clin Psychiatry.* 1994; 55(suppl B):102–6.

48. Ahmed S, Chengappa KN, Naidu VR et al. Clozapine withdrawal-emergent dystonias and dyskinesias: a case series. *J Clin Psychiatry.* 1998; 59:472–7.

49. Dickson RA, Seeman MV, Corenblum B. Hormonal side effects in women: typical versus second-generation antipsychotic treatment. *J Clin Psychiatry.* 2000; 61(suppl 3):10–5.

50. Windgassen K, Wesselman U, Schulze-Monking H. Galactorrhea and hyper-prolactinemia in schizophrenic patients on neuroleptics: frequency and etiology. *Neuropsychobiology.* 1996; 33:142–6.

51. Arana GW. An overview of side effects caused by typical antipsychotics. *J Clin Psychiatry.* 2000; 61(suppl 8):5–11.

52. Petty RG. Prolactin and antipsychotic medications: mechanisms of action. *Schizophr Res.* 1999; 35(suppl): S67–73.

53. Volavka J, Czobor P, Cooper TB et al. Prolactin levels in schizophrenia and schizoaffective disorder patients treated with clozapine, olanzapine, risperidone, or haloperidol. *J Clin Psychiatry.* 2004; 65:57–61.

54. Breier AF, Malhotra AK, Su T et al. Clozapine and risperidone in chronic schizophrenia: effects on symptoms, parkinsonian side effects, and neuroendocrine response. *Am J Psychiatry.* 1999; 156:294–8.

55. Crawford AM, Beasley CM, Tollefson GD. The acute and long-term effect of olanzapine compared with placebo and haloperidol on serum prolactin concentrations. *Schizophr Res.* 1997; 26:41–54.

56. David SR, Taylor CC, Kinon BJ et al. The effects of olanzapine, risperidone, and haloperidol on plasma prolactin levels in patients with schizophrenia. *Clin Ther.* 2000; 22:1085–96.

57. Bunker MT, Marken PA, Schneiderhan ME et al. Attenuation of antipsychotic-induced hyperprolactinemia with clozapine. *J Child Adolesc Psychopharmacol.* 1997; 7:65–9.

58. Allison DB, Fontaine KR, Heo M et al. The distribution of body mass index among individuals with and without schizophrenia. *J Clin Psychiatry.* 1999; 60:215–20.

59. Mukherjee S, Decina P, Bocola V et al. Diabetes mellitus in schizophrenic patients. *Compr Psychiatry.* 1996; 37:68–73.

60. Brambilla F, Guastalla A, Guerrini A et al. Glucose-insulin metabolism in chronic schizophrenia. *Dis Nerv Syst.* 1976; 37:98–103.

61. Tsuang MT, Perkins K, Simpson JC. Physical diseases in schizophrenia and affective disorder. *J Clin Psychiatry.* 1983; 44:42–6.

62. Borovicka MC, Fuller MA, Konicki PE et al. Phenylpropanolamine appears not to promote weight loss in patients with schizophrenia who have gained weight during clozapine treatment. *J Clin Psychiatry.* 2002; 63:345–8.

63. Ball MP, Coons VB, Buchanan RW. A program for treating olanzapine-related weight gain. *Psychiatr Serv.* 2001; 52:967–9.

64. Green AI, Patel JK, Goisman RM et al. Weight gain from novel antipsychotic drugs: need for action. *Gen Hosp Psychiatry.* 2000; 22:224–35.

65. Doss FW. The effect of antipsychotic drugs on body weight: a retrospective review. *J Clin Psychiatry.* 1979; 40:528–30.

66. Parent MM, Roy S, Sramek J et al. Effect of molindone on weight change in hospitalized schizophrenic patients. *Drug Intell Clin Pharm.* 1986; 20:873–5.

67. Gardos G, Cole JO. Weight reduction in schizophrenics by molindone. *Am J Psychiatry.* 1977; 134:302–4.

68. Allison DB, Mentore JL, Heo M et al. Antipsychotic-induced weight gain: a comprehensive research synthesis. *Am J Psychiatry.* 1999; 156:1686–96.

69. Henderson DC, Cagliero E, Gray C et al. Clozapine, diabetes mellitus, weight gain, and lipid abnormalities: a five-year naturalistic study. *Am J Psychiatry.* 2000; 157:975–81.

70. Beasley CM, Tollefson GD, Tran PV. Safety of olanzapine. *J Clin Psychiatry.* 1997; 58(suppl 10):13–7,19–21.

71. Muench J, Carey M. Diabetes mellitus associated with second-generation antipsychotic medications: new case report and review of the literature. *J Am Board Fam Pract.* 2001; 14:278–82.

72. Jin H, Meyer JM, Jeste DV. Phenomenology of and risk factors for new onset diabetes mellitus associated with second-generation antipsychotics: an analysis of 45 published cases. *Ann Clin Psychiatry.* 2002; 14:59–64.

73. Koller EA, Cross JT, Doraiswamy PM et al. Risperidone-associated diabetes mellitus: a pharmacovigilance study. *Pharmacotherapy.* 2003; 23:735–44.

74. Sernyak MJ, Leslie DL, Alarcon RD. Association of diabetes mellitus with use of second-generation neuroleptics in the treatment of schizophrenia. *Am J Psychiatry.* 2002; 159:561–6.

75. Newcomer JW, Haupt DW, Fucetola R. Abnormalities in glucose regulation during antipsychotic treatment of schizophrenia. *Arch Gen Psychiatry.* 2002; 59:337–45.

76. Meyer JM. Novel antipsychotics and severe hyperlipidemia. *J Clin Psychopharm.* 2001; 21:369–74.

77. Meyer JM. A retrospective comparison of weight, lipid, and glucose changes between risperidone- and olanzapine-treated inpatients: metabolic outcomes after 1 year. *J Clin Psychiatry.* 2002; 63:425–33.

78. American Diabetes Association, American Psychiatric Association, American Association of Clinical Endocrinologists et al. Consensus development conference on antipsychotic drugs and obesity and diabetes. *Diabetes Care.* 2004; 27:596–601.

79. Mehtonen OP, Aranko K, Malkonen L et al. A survey of sudden death associated with the use of antipsychotic or antidepressant drugs: 49 cases in Finland. *Acta Psychiatr Scand.* 1991; 84:58–64.

80. Reilly JG, Ayis SA, Ferrier IN et al. QTc-interval abnormalities and psychotropic drug therapy in psychiatric patients. *Lancet.* 2000; 355:1048–52.

81. Food and Drug Administration. Briefing document for Zeldox capsules (ziprasidone HCl). www.fda.gov/ohrms/dockets/ac/00/backgrd/3619b1a.pdf (accessed 2007 Jan 16).

82. Geodon (ziprasidone hydrochloride) prescribing information. New York: Pfizer Inc.; 2006 Nov.

83. Merrill DB, Dec GW, Goff DC. Adverse cardiac effects associated with clozapine. *J Clin Psychopharmacol.* 2005; 25:32–41.

84. La Grenade L, Graham D, Trontell A. Myocarditis and cardiomyopathy associated with clozapine use in the United States. *N Engl J Med.* 2001; 345:224–5.

85. Sink KM, Holden KF, Yaffe K. Pharmacological treatment of neuropsychiatric symptoms of dementia: a review of the evidence. *JAMA.* 2005; 293:596–608.

86. Herrmann N, Lanctot KL. Do atypical antipsychotics cause stroke? *CNS Drugs.* 2005; 19:91–103.

87. Lieberman JA, Johns CA, Kane JM et al. Clozapine-induced agranulocytosis: non-cross-reactivity with other psychotropic drugs. *J Clin Psychiatry.* 1988; 49:271–7.

88. Alvir JJ, Lieberman JA, Safferman AZ et al. Clozapine-induced agranulocytosis—incidence and risk factors in the United States. *N Engl J Med.* 1993; 329:162–7.

89. Honigfeld G, Arellano F, Sethi J et al. Reducing clozapine-related morbidity and mortality: 5 years of experience with the Clozaril National Registry. *J Clin Psychiatry.* 1998; 59(suppl 3):3–7.

90. Munro J, O'Sullivan D, Andrews C et al. Active monitoring of 12,760 clozapine recipients in the UK and Ireland: beyond pharmacovigilance. *Br J Psychiatry.* 1999; 175:576–80.

91. Silvestri RC, Bromfield EB, Khoshbin S. Clozapine-induced seizures and EEG abnormalities in ambulatory psychiatric patients. *Ann Pharmacother.* 1998; 32:1147–51.

92. Sprague DA, Loewen PS, Raymond CB. Selection of atypical antipsychotics for the management of schizophrenia. *Ann Pharmacother.* 2004; 38:313–9.

93. Love RC, Conley RR, Kelly DL et al. A dose-outcome analysis of risperidone. *J Clin Psychiatry.* 1999; 60:771–5.

94. Moller HJ, Bauml J, Ferrero F et al. Risperidone in the treatment of schizophrenia: results of a study of patients from Germany, Austria and Switzerland. *Eur Arch Psychiatry Clin Neurosci.* 1997; 246:291–6.

95. Philipo M. Neuroleptic treatment long term: results with risperidone. Presented at 21st Collegium Internationale Neuro Psychopharmacologicum Congress. Glasgow, Scotland; 1998 Jul.

96. Sajatovic M, Ramirez LF, Belton J et al. Health resource utilization and risperidone therapy in patients with serious mental illness. Presented at 21st Collegium Internationale Neuro-Psychopharmacologicum Congress. Glasgow, Scotland; 1998 Jul.

97. Volavka J, Czobor P, Sheitman B et al. Clozapine, olanzapine, risperidone, and haloperidol in the treatment of patients with chronic schizophrenia and schizoaffective disorder. *Am J Psychiatry.* 2002; 159:255–62.

98. Miller AL, Hall CS, Buchanan RW et al. The Texas medication algorithm project—antipsychotic algorithm for schizophrenia: 2003 update. *J Clin Psychiatry.* 2004; 65:500–8.

99. Lehman AF, Lieberman JA, Dixon LB et al. Practice guideline for the treatment of patients with schizophrenia, second edition. *Am J Psychiatry.* 2004; 161(2 suppl):1–56.

100. Lehman AF, Steinwachs DM. Translating research into practice: the schizophrenia patient outcomes research team (PORT) treatment recommendations. *Schizophr Bull.* 1998; 24:1–10.

101. Stahl SM. Antipsychotic polypharmacy: squandering precious resources? *J Clin Psychiatry.* 2002; 63:93–4.

102. Casey DE, Saha AR, Ali MW et al. Switching to aripiprazole monotherapy. Presented at 23rd Collegium Internationale Neuropsycholpharmacologicum Congress. Montreal, Canada. 2002 Jun.

103. Marder SR, Essock SM, Miller AL et al. Physical health monitoring of patients with schizophrenia. *Am J Psychiatry.* 2004; 161:1334–49.

104. Perry PJ, Miller DD, Arndt SV et al. Clozapine and norclozapine plasma concentrations and clinical response of treatment refractory schizophrenic patients. *Am J Psychiatry.* 1991; 148:231–5.

105. Kronig MH, Munne RA, Szymanski S et al. Plasma clozapine levels and clinical response for treatment refractory schizophrenic patients. *Am J Psychiatry.* 1995; 152:179–82.

106. Gaertner I, Gaertner HJ, Vonthein R et al. Therapeutic drug monitoring of clozapine in relapse prevention: a five-year prospective study. *J Clin Psychopharmacol.* 2001; 21:305–10.

107. Rabinowitz J, Lichtenberg P, Kaplan Z et al. Rehospitalization rates of chronically ill schizophrenic patients discharged on a regimen of risperidone, olanzapine, or conventional antipsychotics. *Am J Psychiatry.* 2001; 158:266–9.

108. Csernansky JG, Mahmoud R, Brenner R. A comparison of risperidone and haloperidol for the prevention of relapse in patients with schizophrenia. *N Engl J Med.* 2002; 346:16–22.

109. Barbui C, Lintas C, Percudani M. Head-to-head comparison of the costs of atypical antipsychotics: a systematic review. *CNS Drugs.* 2005; 19:935–50.

110. Mladsi DM, Grogg AL, Irish WD et al. Pharmacy cost evaluation of risperidone, olanzapine, and quetiapine for the treatment of schizophrenia in acute care inpatient settings. *Curr Med Res Opin.* 2004; 20:1883–93.

111. Coley KC, Carter CS, DaPos SV et al. Effectiveness of antipsychotic therapy in a naturalistic setting: a comparison between risperidone, perphenazine, and haloperidol. *J Clin Psychiatry.* 1999; 60:850–6.

112. Rosenheck R, Cramer J, Allan E et al. Cost-effectiveness of clozapine in patients with high and low levels of hospital use. *Arch Gen Psychiatry.* 1999; 56:565–72.

113. Chouinard G, Albright PS. Economic and health state utility determinations for schizophrenic patients treated with risperidone or haloperidol. *J Clin Psychopharmacol.* 1997; 17:298–307.

114. Franz M, Lis S, Pluddemann K et al. Conventional versus second-generation neuroleptics: subjective quality of life in schizophrenic patients. *Br J Psychiatry.* 1997; 170:422–5.

115. Roy A. Depression, attempted suicide, and suicide in patients with chronic schizophrenia. *Psychiatr Clin North Am.* 1986; 9:193–206.

116. Radomsky ED, Haas GL, Mann JJ et al. Suicidal behavior in patients with schizophrenia and other psychotic disorders. *Am J Psychiatry.* 1999; 156:1590–5.

117. Cohen LJ, Test MA, Brown RL. Suicide and schizophrenia: data from a prospective community treatment study. *Am J Psychiatry.* 1990; 147:602–7.

118. Meltzer HY, Okayli G. Reduction of suicidality during clozapine treatment of neuroleptic-resistant schizophrenia: impact on risk-benefit assessment. *Am J Psychiatry.* 1995; 152:183–90.

119. Meltzer HY, Alphs L, Green AI et al. Clozapine treatment for suicidality in schizophrenia: International Suicide Prevention Trial (InterSEPT). *Arch Gen Psychiatry.* 2003; 60:82–91.

Appendix—Additional Readings and Resources

Andreasen NC. Scale for the assessment of negative symptoms (SANS). *Br J Psychiatry.* 1989; 155(suppl 7):53–8.

Barnes TR. A rating scale for drug-induced akathisia. *Br J Psychiatry.* 1989; 154:672–6.

Kay SR, Fiszbein A, Opler LA. The positive and negative syndrome scale (PANSS) for schizophrenia. *Schizophr Bull.* 1987; 13:261–76.

Lane RD, Glazer WM, Hansen TE et al. Assessment of tardive dyskinesia using the Abnormal Involuntary Movements Scale. *J Nerv Ment Dis.* 1985; 173:353–7.

Lehman AF, Kreyenbuhl J, Buchanan RW et al. The Schizophrenia Patient Outcomes Research Team (PORT): updated treatment recommendations 2003. *Schizophr Bull.* 2004; 30:193–217.

Montgomery SA, Asberg M. A new depression scale designed to be sensitive to change. *Br J Psychiatry.* 1979; 134:382–9.

CGI: clinical global impressions. In: Guy W, Bonato RR, eds. Manual for the ECDEU assessment battery. 2nd ed. Chevy Chase, MD: National Institute of Mental Health; 1970:12-1–12-6.

Overall JE, Gorham DR. The Brief Psychiatric Rating Scale. *Psychol Rep.* 1962; 10:799–812.

Simpson GN, Angus JW. A rating scale for extrapyramidal side effects. *Acta Psychiatr Scand Suppl.* 1970; 212:11–9.

Approved by the ASHP Board of Directors on June 24, 2006. Developed through the ASHP Council on Therapeutics.

Jason M. Noel, Pharm.D., BCPP, is gratefully acknowledged for authoring this therapeutic position statement. At the time of publication, Dr. Noel was Assistant Professor, University of Maryland School of Pharmacy, Baltimore, and Director of Clinical Pharmacy Services, Rosewood Center, Owings Mills, MD.

Marshall E. Cates, Pharm.D., BCPP, FASHP; Beth Dubisar, Pharm.D.; Julie A. Dopheide, Pharm.D., BCPP; W. Kennedy Klugh, Pharm.D.; Dan LeGrady, Pharm.D., FNIH; Rex S. Lott, Pharm.D.; Lisa Mican, Pharm.D.; Virginia Stauffer, Pharm.D.; and the American Academy of Nurse Practitioners are acknowledged for reviewing drafts of this document.

The bibliographic citation for this document is as follows: Noel JM. ASHP therapeutic position statement on the use of second-generation antipsychotic medications in the treatment of adults with psychotic disorders. *Am J Health-Syst Pharm.* 2007; 64:863–76.

ASHP
Therapeutic Guidelines

ASHP Therapeutic Guidelines on
Antimicrobial Prophylaxis in Surgery

The ASHP Therapeutic Guidelines on Antimicrobial Prophylaxis in Surgery,[1] which have provided practitioners with standardized effective regimens for the rational use of prophylactic antimicrobials, have been revised as described in this document on the basis of new clinical evidence and additional concerns. Recommendations are provided for adult and pediatric patients (1 to 21 years of age), including infants (one month to 2 years of age). Geriatric patients, newborns (premature and full-term), and patients with renal or hepatic dysfunction are not specifically addressed. Therefore, the guidelines may not be applicable to these patients, or certain adjustments to the recommendations may be necessary. The higher occurrence of resistant organisms and the importance of controlling health care costs are also considered.

Prophylaxis refers to the prevention of an infection and can be characterized as primary prophylaxis, secondary prophylaxis (suppression), or eradication. Primary prophylaxis refers to the prevention of an initial infection. Secondary prophylaxis refers to the prevention of recurrence or reactivation of a preexisting infection (e.g., prevention of the recurrence of a latent herpes simplex virus infection). Eradication refers to the elimination of a colonized organism to prevent the development of an infection (e.g., eliminating methicillin-resistant *Staphylococcus aureus* [MRSA] from the nares of health care workers). These guidelines focus on primary prophylaxis. Secondary prophylaxis and eradication are not addressed.

Guideline Development and Use

These guidelines were prepared by the Rocky Mountain Poison and Drug Center under contract to ASHP. The project was coordinated by a drug information pharmacist who worked with a multidisciplinary consortium of writers and consulted with six physicians on staff at the University of Colorado Health Sciences Center. The project coordinator worked in conjunction with an independent panel of eight clinical pharmacy specialists with expertise in either adult or pediatric infectious disease. The panel was appointed by ASHP. Panel members and contractors were required to disclose any possible conflicts of interest before their appointment. The guidelines underwent multidisciplinary field review to evaluate their validity, reliability, and utility in clinical practice. The final document was approved by the ASHP Commission on Therapeutics and the ASHP Board of Directors.

The recommendations in this document may not be appropriate for use in all clinical situations. Decisions to follow these recommendations must be based on the professional judgment of the clinician and consideration of individual patient circumstances and available resources.

These guidelines reflect current knowledge (at the time of publication) on antimicrobial prophylaxis in surgery. Given the dynamic nature of scientific information and technology, periodic review, updating, and revision are to be expected.

Strength of Evidence for Recommendations. The primary literature from the previous ASHP Therapeutic Guidelines on Antimicrobial Prophylaxis in Surgery[1] was reviewed together with the primary literature between the date of the previous guidelines and August 1997, identified by a MEDLINE search. Particular attention was paid to study design, with greatest credence given to randomized, controlled, double-blind studies. Established recommendations by experts in the area (i.e., Centers for Disease Control and Prevention [CDC], American College of Obstetricians and Gynecologists [ACOG]) were also considered.

Guideline development included consideration of the following characteristics: validity, reliability, clinical applicability, flexibility, clarity, and a multidisciplinary nature as consistent with ASHP's philosophy on therapeutic guidelines.[2] Recommendations on the use of an antimicrobial are substantiated by the strength of evidence that supports the recommendation. The strength of evidence represents only support for or against prophylaxis and does not apply to the antimicrobial choice, dose, or dosage regimen. Studies supporting the recommendations for the use of an antimicrobial were classified as follows:

Level I: (evidence from large, well-conducted randomized, controlled clinical trials or a meta-analysis)
Level II: (evidence from small, well-conducted randomized, controlled clinical trials)
Level III: (evidence from well-conducted cohort studies)
Level IV: (evidence from well-conducted case–control studies)
Level V: (evidence from uncontrolled studies that were not well conducted)
Level VI: (conflicting evidence that tends to favor the recommendation)
Level VII: (expert opinion)

This system has been used by the Agency for Health Care Policy and Research, and ASHP supports it as an acceptable method for organizing strength of evidence for a variety of therapeutic or diagnostic recommendations.[2] Each recommendation was assigned a category corresponding to the strength of evidence that supports the use or nonuse of antimicrobial prophylaxis:

Category A: (levels I–III)
Category B: (levels IV–VI)
Category C: (level VII)

A category C recommendation represents a consensus of the expert panel based on the clinical experience of individual panel members and a paucity of quality supporting literature. In cases for which opinions were markedly divided, the recommendations indicate that a substantial number of panel members supported an alternative approach.

Pediatrics. Pediatric patients are subject to many prophylaxis opportunities that are similar to those for adults. Although pediatric-specific prophylaxis data are sparse, available data have been evaluated and are presented in this document. However, in most cases, the pediatric recommendations, including recommendations for infants, have been extrapolated from adult data.

Clinical studies to determine the optimal dosages of antimicrobials used for pediatric prophylaxis are essentially nonexistent. In contrast, there are sufficient pharmacokinetic studies for most agents used that appropriate pediatric dosages can be estimated that provide systemic exposure, and presumably efficacy, similar to that demonstrated in the adult efficacy trials. It is also common clinical practice to use antimicrobial prophylaxis in pediatric patients in a manner that is similar, if not identical, to that used in adults. Therefore, the pediatric dosages provided in these guidelines are based largely on pharmacokinetic equivalence and the generalization of the adult efficacy data to pediatric patients.[3,4] Because pediatric trials have generally not been conducted, a strength of evidence has not been applied to these recommendations. With few exceptions (e.g., aminoglycoside dosages), pediatric dosages should not exceed the maximum adult recommended dosages. If dosages are calculated on a milligram-per-kilogram basis for children weighing more than 40–50 kg, the calculated dosage will exceed the maximum recommended dosage for adults; thus adult dosages should be used.

Resistance. The basis for guideline development was to recommend an effective antimicrobial with the narrowest spectrum of activity. Alternative antimicrobials were included on the basis of documented efficacy. Individual health systems must consider specific resistance patterns at their practice site when adopting these recommendations.

When considering the use of antimicrobials for prophylaxis, one must also take into account the risks of contributing to the development of antimicrobial resistance. In numerous studies of prophylaxis, both surgical[5,6] and nonsurgical,[7–16] attempts have been made to evaluate the impact of antimicrobial prophylaxis on the development of resistance. Numerous studies[5,7–13] demonstrated an increase in resistance, yet other studies[6,14–16] failed to demonstrate the emergence of resistance. Most of the studies demonstrating the development of resistance involved the use of broad-spectrum antimicrobials.[5,7–13] Thus, currently recommended practice is to use narrow-spectrum antimicrobials for the shortest duration to reduce the likelihood of the development of antimicrobial resistance.

The frequency with which MRSA has been recovered from various infection sites has increased steadily throughout the United States.[17–19] The frequency of methicillin resistance among staphylococcal strains rose from 2.4% in 1975 to 29% in 1991.[19] CDC's National Nosocomial Infections Surveillance identified a rapid increase in vancomycin-resistant enterococci (VRE) from 0.3% in 1989 to 7.9% in 1993. The rate of high-level enterococcal resistance to penicillin and aminoglycosides increased simultaneously. The use of vancomycin has been reported consistently as a risk factor for infection and colonization with VRE and may increase the possibility of the emergence of vancomycin-resistant *S. aureus* or vancomycin-resistant *Staphylococcus epidermidis.*[20] In response, the Hospital Infection Control Practices Advisory Committee (HICPAC), with the support of other major organizations, developed measures for preventing and controlling vancomycin resistance.[21] The ASHP guidelines are consistent with the HICPAC recommendations. The following situations are appropriate or acceptable for use of vancomycin: prophylaxis of endocarditis (as recommended by the American Heart Association [AHA]) before certain procedures and for major surgical procedures involving implantation of prosthetic materials or devices (e.g., cardiac and vascular procedures, total hip replacement) at institutions with a high rate of infections due to MRSA or methicillin-resistant *S. epidermidis* (MRSE). Use of vancomycin for routine surgical prophylaxis should be discouraged (other than in a patient with a life-threatening allergy to β-lactam antimicrobials).

Cost. Pharmacoeconomic studies have been lacking or inadequate with regard to the prophylactic use of antimicrobials; therefore, a cost-minimization approach was employed in developing these guidelines. When antimicrobials have been shown to be equally efficacious and safe, the recommendation is based on the least expensive agent (on the basis of average wholesale price). The other antimicrobials are considered to be alternative agents. The recommendation of an antimicrobial is determined primarily by efficacy and secondarily by cost. Because of variations in cost from one health system to another, health systems must tailor the choice of antimicrobials to their individual acquisition costs.

Goals of Surgical Prophylaxis

Ideally, an anti-infective drug for surgical prophylaxis should achieve the following goals: (1) prevent postoperative infection of the surgical site, (2) prevent postoperative infectious morbidity and mortality, (3) reduce the duration and cost of health care (when the costs associated with the management of postoperative infection are considered, the cost-effectiveness of prophylaxis becomes evident),[22,23] (4) produce no adverse effects, and (5) have no adverse consequences for the microbial flora of the patient or the hospital.[24] To achieve these goals, an anti-infective drug should be (1) active against the pathogens most likely to contaminate the wound, (2) given in an appropriate dosage and at a time that ensures adequate concentrations at the incision site during the period of potential contamination, (3) safe, and (4) administered for the shortest effective period to minimize adverse effects, development of resistance, and cost.[24] The benefits of preventing postoperative infection pertain to both outpatient and inpatient surgeries. Other guidelines on antimicrobial prophylaxis in surgery have been published.[25]

Although prophylactic antimicrobials play an important part in reducing the rate of postoperative wound infection, other factors, such as the surgeon's experience, the length of the procedure, hospital and operating-room environments, and the underlying medical condition of the patient, have a strong impact on wound infection rates. Medical conditions associated with an increased risk of postoperative infection include extremes of age, undernutrition, obesity, diabetes, hypoxemia, remote infection, corticosteroid therapy, recent operation, chronic inflammation, and prior site irradiation.[26] Antimicrobial prophylaxis may be justified for any procedure if the patient has an underlying medical condition associated with a risk of wound infection or if the patient is immunocompromised (e.g., malnourished, neutropenic, receiving immunosuppressive agents). These variables should be considered in evaluations of infection-control problems.

Antimicrobial prophylaxis is beneficial in surgical procedures associated with a high rate of infection (clean-contaminated or contaminated operations), for implantation of prosthetic materials, and in any procedure in which postoperative infection, however unlikely, may have severe consequences. Other clean procedures that may warrant prophylaxis are breast procedures[27,28] and hernia procedures,[27] although more data are needed.

The modified National Research Council wound classification criteria are as follow[28,29]:

- Clean surgical procedures (primarily closed, elective procedures involving no acute inflammation, no break in technique, and no transection of gastrointestinal [GI], oropharyngeal, genitourinary [GU], biliary, or tracheobronchial tracts)
- Clean-contaminated procedures (procedures involving transection of GI, oropharyngeal, GU, biliary, or tracheobronchial tracts with minimal spillage or with minor breaks in technique; clean procedures performed emergently or with major breaks in technique; reoperation of clean surgery within seven days; or procedures following blunt trauma)
- Contaminated procedures (clean-contaminated procedures during which acute, nonpurulent inflammation is encountered or major spillage or technique break occurs; procedures performed within four hours of penetrating trauma or involving a chronic open wound)
- Dirty procedures (procedures performed when there is obvious preexisting infection [abscess, pus, necrotic tissue present]; preoperative perforation of GI, oropharyngeal, biliary, or tracheobronchial tracts; or penetrating trauma greater than four hours old)

Typically, prophylactic antimicrobials are not indicated for clean surgical procedures. However, prophylaxis is justified for procedures involving prosthetic placement because of the potential for severe complications if postoperative infections involve the prosthesis. Antimicrobial prophylaxis is justified for the following types of surgical procedures: cardiothoracic, GI tract (e.g., colorectal and biliary tract operations), head and neck (except clean procedures), neurosurgical, obstetric or gynecologic, orthopedic (except clean procedures), urologic, and vascular. The use of antimicrobials for dirty and contaminated procedures is not classified as prophylaxis but as treatment for a presumed infection; therefore, dirty and contaminated procedures are not discussed in these guidelines.[30]

It is difficult to establish significant differences in efficacy between prophylactic antimicrobials and placebo when infection rates are low. A small sample size increases the likelihood of Type II error; therefore, there may be no apparent difference between the antimicrobial and placebo when in fact the antimicrobial has a beneficial effect.[31] A valid study would be placebo controlled and randomized with a large enough sample in each group to avoid Type II error. A large sample is rarely achieved in well-controlled studies of surgical prophylaxis. Thus, some of the surgical prophylaxis efficacy data are at risk for Type II error. Because of this obstacle, prophylaxis is recommended in some cases because the complications of postoperative infection (e.g., removal of an infected device) necessitate precautionary measures despite the lack of statistical support.

Selection of Antimicrobial Agents

The selection of an appropriate antimicrobial agent for specific patients should take into account not only comparative efficacy but also adverse-effect profiles and patient drug allergies. A discussion of adverse-effect profiles of the antimicrobials is beyond the scope of these guidelines. There is little evidence to suggest that the newer antimicrobials, with broader antibacterial activity in vitro, result in lower rates of postoperative wound infection than older drugs whose spectrum of activity is narrower. Because most comparative studies have a small number of patients, a significant difference between antimicrobials cannot be detected; therefore, antimicrobial selection is based on cost, adverse-effect profile, ease of administration, pharmacokinetic profile, and antibacterial activity. The agent chosen should have activity against the most common surgical wound pathogens. For clean-contaminated operations, the agent of choice should be effective against common pathogens found in the GI and GU tracts. In clean operations, the gram-positive cocci—*S. aureus* and *S. epidermidis*—predominate. For most procedures, cefazolin should be the agent of choice because of its relatively long duration of action, its effectiveness against the organisms most commonly encountered in surgery, and its relatively low cost.

Specific recommendations for the selection of prophylactic antimicrobials for various surgical procedures are provided in Table 1. Equivalent pediatric dosages have been included in Table 2; however, these recommendations are based on data derived primarily from adult patients and from tertiary references.[3,4,35] Neonatal (full-term and preterm) dosages are not provided. The reader is referred to Neofax for neonatal dosages.[36] There are few data on the use of surgical antimicrobial prophylaxis in the pediatric population. Available pediatric clinical data were evaluated and are presented in the efficacy section after the adult data.

Development of Colonization or Resistance. One factor that may influence the selection of cefazolin is the occurrence of surgical wound infections despite prophylaxis with cefazolin. An infection-control surveillance study of surgical wound infections implicated β-lactamase production as a possible cause of cefazolin and cefamandole failure.[39] β-lactamase-producing *S. aureus* isolates associated with the wound infections rapidly hydrolyzed cefamandole and cefazolin. Isolates of *S. aureus* taken from patients who had received cefazolin were more resistant than isolates taken from patients who had received cefamandole, and the cefazolin-associated isolates were capable of hydrolyzing cefazolin more rapidly. These findings may have important implications for the use of first-generation cephalosporins, particularly cefazolin, for surgical prophylaxis. However, the overall frequency of cefazolin failure as a result of resistance is low, and cefazolin continues to be the drug of choice. New studies comparing cefazolin with agents that are more resistant to β-lactamase, such as cefamandole and cefuroxime, may be needed.

A second factor that may discourage the selection of cefazolin is the recognition that MRSA and methicillin-resistant, coagulase-negative staphylococci are resistant to all cephalosporins. These organisms have been associated with infection after cardiothoracic, orthopedic, vascular, and cerebrospinal shunting procedures. This resistance pattern may influence drug selection in hospitals with a high frequency of such isolates. However, vancomycin use should be restricted because of the increase in vancomycin-resistant enterococci.

Table 1.

Recommendations for Surgical Antimicrobial Prophylaxis in Adults

Type of Surgery	Recommended Regimen[a]	Alternative Regimens[a]	Strength of Evidence[b]
Cardiothoracic	Cefazolin 1 g i.v. at induction of anesthesia and q 8 hr for up to 72 hr[c,d]	Cefuroxime 1.5 g i.v. at induction of anesthesia and q 12 hrfor up to 72 hr, cefamandole 1 g i.v. at induction of anesthesia and q 6 hr for up to 72 hr, vancomycin 1 g i.v. with or without gentamicin 2 mg/kg i.v.[e]	A
Gastrointestinal			
Gastroduodenal			
Procedures involving entry into the lumen of the gastrointestinal tract	Cefazolin 1 g i.v. at induction of anesthesia		A
Highly selective vagotomy, Nissen's fundoplication, and Whipple's procedure	Cefazolin 1 g i.v. at induction of anesthesia		C
Biliary tract			
Open procedure	Cefazolin 1 g i.v. at induction of anesthesia		A
Laparoscopic procedure	None		B
Appendectomy for uncomplicated appendicitis	Cefoxitin, cefotetan, or cefmetazole 1–2 g i.v. at induction of anesthesia	Piperacillin 2 g i.v. at induction of anesthesia; if patient is allergic to penicillin, metronidazole 500 mg i.v. plus gentamicin 2 mg/kg i.v. at induction of anesthesia	A
Colorectal	Neomycin sulfate 1 g plus erythromycin base 1 g p.o. (after mechanical bowel preparation is completed[f]) at 19, 18, and 9 hr before surgery; if oral route is contraindicated, cefoxitin, cefotetan, or cefmetazole 2 g i.v. at induction of anesthesia; for patients undergoing high-risk surgery (e.g., rectal resection), oral neomycin and erythromycin plus an i.v. cephalosporin		A
Head and neck			
Clean	None		B
With placement of prosthesis	Cefazolin 1 g i.v. at induction of anesthesia		C
Clean-contaminated	Cefazolin 2 g i.v. at induction of anesthesia and q 8 hr for 24 hr or clindamycin 600 mg i.v. at induction of anesthesia and q 8 hr for 24 hr	Addition of gentamicin 1.7 mg/kg i.v. to clindamycin regimen or of metronidazole 500 mg i.v. q 8 hr to cefazolin regimen is controversial; single-dose regimens might be preferable, but this approach is controversial	A
Elective craniotomy or cerebrospinal fluid shunting	Cefazolin 1 g i.v. at induction of anesthesia	Oxacillin 1 g or nafcillin 1 g i.v. at induction of anesthesia; vancomycin 1 g i.v.[g]	A
Obstetric or gynecologic			
Cesarean delivery[h]	Cefazolin 2 g i.v. immediately after clamping of umbilical cord		B (low risk), A (high risk)
Hysterectomy (vaginal, abdominal, or radical)[i]	Cefazolin 1 g i.v. or cefotetan 1 g i.v. at induction of anesthesia	Cefoxitin 1 g i.v. at induction of anesthesia	A
Ophthalmic	Topical neomycin–polymyxin B–gramicidin 1–2 drops or tobramycin 0.3% or gentamicin 0.3% 2 drops instilled before procedure[j]	Addition of tobramycin 20 mg by subconjunctival injection is optional	C
Orthopedic			
Clean, not involving implantation of foreign materials[k]	None		C
Hip fracture repair[l]	Cefazolin 1 g i.v. at induction of anesthesia and q 8 hr for 24 hr	Vancomycin 1 g i.v.[g]	A
Implantation of internal fixation devices[l]	Cefazolin 1 g i.v. at induction of anesthesia and q 8 hr for 24 hr	Vancomycin 1 g i.v.[g]	C
Total joint replacement	Cefazolin 1 g i.v. at induction of anesthesia and q 8 hr for 24 hr	Vancomycin 1 g i.v.[g]	A

Continued on next page

Table 1. (*continued*)
Recommendations for Surgical Antimicrobial Prophylaxis in Adults

Type of Surgery	Recommended Regimen[a]	Alternative Regimens[a]	Strength of Evidence[b]
Urologic (high-risk patients only[m])	Trimethoprim 160 mg with sulfamethoxazole 800 mg p.o. or lomefloxacin 400 mg p.o. 2 hr before surgery (if oral agents used) or cefazolin 1 g i.v. at induction of anesthesia (if injection preferred)		A
Vascular[n]	Cefazolin 1 g i.v. at induction of anesthesia and q 8hrfor 24 hr	Vancomycin 1 g i.v with or without gentamicin 2 mg/kg i.v.[g]	A
Transplantation			
Heart	Cefazolin 1 g i.v. at induction of anesthesia and q 8 hr for 48–72 hr[d]	Cefuroxime 1.5 g i.v. at induction of anesthesia and q 12 hr for 48–72 hr, cefamandole 1 g i.v. at induction of anesthesia and q 6 hr for 48–72 hr, or vancomycin 1 g i.v. with or without gentamicin 2 mg/kg i.v.[e]	A
Lung and heart–lung,[o,p]	Cefazolin 1 g i.v. at induction of anesthesia and q 8 hr for 48–72 hr	Cefuroxime 1.5 g i.v. at induction of anesthesia and q 12 hr for 48–72 hr, cefamandole 1 g i.v. at induction of anesthesia and q 6 hr for 48–72 hr, or vancomycin 1 g i.v.[g]	B
Liver	Cefotaxime 1 g i.v. plus ampicillin 1 g i.v. at induction of anesthesia and q 6 hr during procedure and for 48 hr beyond final surgical closure	Antimicrobials that provide adequate coverage against gram-negative aerobic bacilli, staphylococci, and enterococci may be appropriate	B
Pancreas and pancreas–kidney	Cefazolin 1 g i.v. at induction of anesthesia		B
Kidney	Cefazolin 1 g i.v. at induction of anesthesia		A

[a]If a short-acting agent is used, it should be readministered if the operation takes more than three hours. If an operation is expected to last more than six to eight hours, it would be reasonable to administer an agent with a longer half-life and duration of action or to administer a short-acting agent at three-hour intervals during the procedure. Readministration may also be warranted if prolonged or excessive bleeding occurs or there are factors that may shorten the half-life (e.g., extensive burns). Readministration may not be warranted in patients in whom the half-life is prolonged (e.g., patients with renal insufficiency or failure).

[b]Strength of evidence that supports the use or nonuse of prophylaxis is classified as A (levels I–III), B (levels IV–VI), or C (level VII). Level I evidence is from large, well-conducted randomized, controlled clinical trials. Level II evidence is from small, well-conducted randomized, controlled clinical trials. Level III evidence is from well-conducted cohort studies. Level IV evidence is from well-conducted case–control studies. Level V evidence is from uncontrolled studies that were not well conducted. Level VI evidence is conflicting evidence that tends to favor the recommendation. Level VII evidence is expert opinion.

[c]Duration is based on expert panel consensus. Prophylaxis for 24 hours or less may be appropriate.

[d]There is currently no evidence to support continuing antimicrobial prophylaxis until chest and mediastinal drainage tubes are removed.

[e]According to Hospital Infection Control Practices Advisory Committee guidelines[21] or American Heart Association recommendations for penicillin-allergic patients at high risk for endocarditis.[32]

[f]Mechanical bowel preparation is required for nonobstructed patients undergoing elective operations.

[g]According to Hospital Infection Control Practices Advisory Committee guidelines.[21]

[h]The American College of Obstetricians and Gynecologists (ACOG) considers the use of prophylaxis controversial in low-risk patients.[33] ACOG does not routinely recommend prophylaxis in low-risk patients because of concerns about adverse effects, development of resistant organisms, and relaxation of standard infection-control measures and proper operative technique.

[i]According to ACOG guidelines, first-, second-, and third-generation cephalosporins can be used for vaginal, abdominal, and radical hysterectomies.[34]

[j]The necessity of continuing topical antimicrobials postoperatively has not been established by data.

[k]Laminectomy and knee, hand, and foot surgeries. The evaluated studies did not include arthroscopy and did not identify specific procedures, like carpal tunnel release; however, arthroscopy and other procedures not involving implantation are similar enough to be included with clean orthopedic procedures not involving implantation.

[l]Procedures involving internal fixation devices (e.g., nails, screws, plates, wires).

[m]High risk is defined as prolonged postoperative catheterization, positive urine cultures, or hospital infection rate of greater than 20%.

[n]Prophylaxis is not indicated for brachiocephalic procedures. Although there are no data, patients undergoing brachiocephalic procedures involving vascular prostheses or patch implantation (e.g., carotid endartectomy) may benefit from prophylaxis.

[o]Patients undergoing lung transplantation with negative pretransplant cultures should receive antimicrobial prophylaxis as appropriate for other types of cardiothoracic surgeries.

[p]Patients undergoing lung transplantation for cystic fibrosis should receive 7–14 days of prophylaxis with antimicrobials selected according to pretransplant culture and susceptibility results. This may include additional antibacterial agents or antifungal agents.

Table 2.
Antimicrobial Regimens for Surgical Prophylaxis in Pediatric Patients[a]

Type of Surgery	Preferred Regimen[b]	Alternative Regimens[b]
Cardiothoracic	Cefazolin 20–30 mg/kg i.v. at induction of anesthesia and q 8 hr for upto 72 hr[c,d]	Cefuroxime 50 mg/kg i.v. at induction of anesthesia and q 8 hr for up to 72 hr,[c,d] vancomycin 15 mg/kg i.v. with or without gentamicin 2 mg/kg i.v.[e]
Gastrointestinal		
Gastroduodenal (procedures involving entry into the lumen of the gastrointestinal tract, highly selective vagotomy, Nissen's fundoplication, and Whipple's procedure)	Cefazolin 20–30 mg/kg i.v. at induction of anesthesia	
Biliary tract		
Open procedures	Cefazolin 20–30 mg/kg i.v. at induction of anesthesia	
Laparoscopic procedures	None	
Appendectomy for uncomplicated appendicitis	Cefoxitin 20–40 mg/kg i.v., cefotetan 20–40 mg/kg i.v., cefotaxime 25–50 mg/kg i.v., or ceftizoxime 25–50 mg/kg i.v. at induction of anesthesia	Piperacillin 50 mg/kg i.v. at induction of anesthesia; if patient is allergic to penicillin, metronidazole 10 mg/kg i.v. plus gentamicin 2 mg/kg i.v. at induction of anesthesia
Colorectal	Neomycin sulfate 20 mg/kg plus erythromycin base 10 mg/kg p.o. (after mechanical bowel preparation is completed) at 19, 18, and 9 hr before surgery; if oral route is contraindicated, cefoxitin or cefotetan 30–40 mg/kg i.v. at induction of anesthesia; for patients undergoing high-risk surgery (e.g., rectal resection), oral neomycin and erythromycin plus an i.v. cephalosporin	
Head and neck		
Clean	None	
With placement of prosthesis	Cefazolin 20–30 mg/kg i.v at induction of anesthesia	
Clean-contaminated	Cefazolin 30–40 mg/kg i.v. at induction of anesthesia and q 8 hr for 24 hr or clindamycin 15 mg/kg i.v. at induction of anesthesia and q 8 hr for 24 hr	Addition of gentamicin 2.5 mg/kg i.v. to clindamycin regimen or of metronidazole 10 mg/kg i.v. q 8 hr to cefazolin regimen is controversial; single-dose regimens might be preferable, but this approach is controversial
Elective craniotomy or cerebro-spinal-fluid shunting	Cefazolin 20–30 mg/kg i.v. at induction of anesthesia	Vancomycin 15 mg/kg i.v.[f]
Obstetric or gynecologic		
Cesarean delivery[g]	Cefazolin 2 g i.v. immediately after clamping of umbilical cord	
Hysterectomy (vaginal, abdominal, or radical)[h]	Cefazolin 1 g i.v. or cefotetan 1 g i.v. at induction of anesthesia	Cefoxitin 1 g i.v. at induction of anesthesia
Ophthalmic	Topical neomycin–polymyxin B–gramicidin 1–2 drops or tobramycin 0.3% or gentamicin 0.3% 2 drops instilled before procedure[i]	
Orthopedic		
Clean, not involving implanta-tion of foreign materials[j]	None	
Hip fracture repair,[k] implantation of internal fixation devices,[k] total joint replacement	Cefazolin 20–30 mg/kg i.v. at induction of anesthesia and q 8 hr for 24 hr	Vancomycin 15 mg/kg i.v.[f]
Urologic procedures (high-risk patients only[l])	Trimethoprim 6–10 mg/kg plus sulfamethoxazole 30–50 mg/kg p.o. 2 hr before surgery (if oral agents used) or cefazolin 20–30 mg/kg i.v. at induction of anesthesia (if injection preferred)	
Vascular procedures[m]	Cefazolin 20–30 mg/kg i.v. at induction of anesthesia and q 8 hr for 24 hr	Vancomycin 15 mg/kg i.v. with or without gentamicin 2 mg/kg i.v.[f]
Transplantation		
Heart	Cefazolin 20–30 mg/kg i.v. at induction of anesthesia and q 8 hr for 48–72 hr[d]	Cefuroxime 50 mg/kg i.v. at induction of anesthesia and q 8 hr for 48–72 hr,[c,d] vancomycin 15 mg/kg with or without gentamicin 2 mg/kg i.v.[e]

Continued on next page

Table 2. (*continued*)
Antimicrobial Regimens for Surgical Prophylaxis in Pediatric Patients[a]

Type of Surgery	Preferred Regimen[b]	Alternative Regimens[b]
Transplantation		
Lung and heart–lung[n,o]	Cefazolin 20–30 mg/kg i.v. at induction of anesthesia and q 8 hr for 48–72hr[d]	Cefuroxime 50 mg/kg i.v. at induction of anesthesia and q 8 hr for 48–72 hr,[d] vancomycin 15 mg/kg i.v.[f]
Liver	Cefotaxime 50 mg/kg i.v. plus ampicillin 50 mg/kg i.v. at induction of anesthesia and q 6 hr for 48 hr beyond final surgical closure	Antimicrobials that provide adequate coverage against gram-negative aerobic bacilli, staphylococci, and enterococci may be appropriate
Pancreas and pancreas–kidney	Cefazolin 20 mg/kg i.v. at induction of anesthesia	
Kidney	Cefazolin 20 mg/kg i.v. at induction of anesthesia	

[a]The recommendations included in this table have been extrapolated from adult data. The pediatric dosages are approximately equivalent to the adult dosages listed in Table 1. With few exceptions (aminoglycosides), pediatric dosages should not exceed the maximum dosage recommended for adults. Adult dosages should be used for children weighing more than 40–50 kg because a dosage calculated on a milligram-per-kilogram basis will exceed the maximum recommended dosage for adults.[34,35] Dosages for neonates (full-term and preterm) are not provided. The reader is referred to Neofaxfor neonatal dosing.[36]

[b]If a short-acting agent is used, it should be readministered if the operation takes more than three hours. If an operation is expected to last more than six to eight hours, it would be reasonable to administer an agent with a longer half-life and duration of action or to administer a short-acting agent at three-hour intervals during the procedure. Readministration may also be warranted if prolonged or excessive bleeding occurs or there are factors that may shorten the half-life (e.g., extensive burns). Readministration may not be warranted in patients in whom the half-life is prolonged (e.g., patients with renal insufficiency or failure).

[c]Duration is based on expert panel consensus. Prophylaxis for 24 hours or less may be appropriate.

[d]There is currently no evidence to support continuing antimicrobial prophylaxis until chest and mediastinal drainage tubes are removed.

[e]According to Hospital Infection Control Practices Advisory Committee guidelines[21] or American Heart Association recommendations for penicillin-allergic patients at high risk for endocarditis.[32] Pediatric cancer patients may require dosages greater than the standard dosage.[37,38]

[f]According to Hospital Infection Control Practices Advisory Committee guidelines.[21]

[g]The American College of Obstetricians and Gynecologists (ACOG) considers the use of prophylaxis controversial in low-risk patients.[33] ACOG does not routinely recommend prophylaxis in low-risk patients because of concerns about adverse effects, development of resistant organisms, and relaxation of standard infection-control measures and proper operative technique.

[h]According to ACOG guidelines, first-, second-, and third-generation cephalosporins can be used for vaginal, abdominal, and radical hysterectomies.[34]

[i]The necessity of continuing topical antimicrobials postoperatively has not been established by data.

[j]Laminectomy and knee, hand, and foot surgeries. The evaluated studies did not include arthroscopy procedures and did not identify specific procedures, like carpal tunnel release; however, arthroscopy and other procedures not involving implantation are similar enough to be included with clean orthopedic procedures not involving implantation.

[k]Procedures involving internal fixation devices (e.g., nails, screws, plates, wires).

[l]High risk is defined as prolonged postoperative catheterization, positive urine cultures, or hospital infection rate of greater than 20%.

[m]Prophylaxis is not indicated for brachiocephalic procedures. Although there are no data, patients undergoing brachiocephalic procedures involving vascular prosthesis or patch implantation (e.g., carotid endarterectomy) may benefit from prophylaxis.

[n]Patients undergoing lung transplantation with negative pretransplant cultures should receive antimicrobial prophylaxis as appropriate for other types of cardiothoracic surgeries.

[o]Patients undergoing lung transplantation for cystic fibrosis should receive 7–14 days of prophylaxis with antimicrobials selected according to pretransplant isolates and susceptibilities. This may include additional antibacterial or antifungal agents.

The only situations in which vancomycin is appropriate for surgical prophylaxis are major surgical procedures involving the implantation of prosthetic materials or devices at institutions that have a high rate of infections caused by MRSA or MRSE or in patients who have a life-threatening allergy to β-lactam antimicrobials.[21] A high rate of infection caused by MRSA is defined as >20% by our expert panel consensus. However, some institutions consider >10% to be a high MRSA infection rate and 20% to be a low infection rate for MRSE. Each institution is encouraged to develop guidelines for the proper use of vancomycin, as applicable to the institution. Consistent with the HICPAC recommendations, a single dose of vancomycin administered immediately before surgery is sufficient unless the procedure lasts more than six hours or major blood loss occurs, in which case the dose should be repeated.[21] Prophylaxis should be discontinued after a maximum of two doses.

The use of antimicrobials for prophylaxis in surgery contributes to changes in individuals' and institutions' bacterial flora. Studies have demonstrated that the use of antimicrobials prophylactically can alter bacterial flora, leading to colonization or resistance[5,40–45] although another study, which involved patients undergoing colorectal surgery, showed no effect on the emergence of resistant bacteria.[6] The bacterial flora affected include, but are not limited to, *Clostridium difficile*, enterococci, *Pseudomonas* species, and *Serratia* species.

Colonization with *C. difficile* has been demonstrated with prophylaxis of more than 24 hours' duration[40] and single-dose prophylaxis.[41] Colonization with *C. difficile* may lead to complications such as colitis. A retrospective review demonstrated that 55% of the *C. difficile*-associated colitis cases were associated with surgical patients receiving preoperative cephalosporins.[42]

Surgical prophylaxis may be a contributing factor to the development of VRE. An increase in VRE infection has been demonstrated in solid-organ transplant patients.[43,44] Although transplant patients receive multiple courses of antimicrobials, including vancomycin, throughout their hospital course, the use of prophylactic antimicrobials may contribute to the development of resistance. A descriptive report demonstrated higher VRE infection rates among patients on the organ transplantation service (13.2 infections per 1000 admissions) and the surgical intensive care unit (5.6 infections per 1000 admissions) compared with the medical intensive care unit (4.8 infections per 1000 admissions) and the internal medicine service (1.8 infections per 1000 admissions).[43] In a hospital surveillance study, 32 (10.4%) of the 307 patients in whom VRE were cultured were transplant recipients[44]; 24 (75%) of 32 patients developed VRE within 30 days (mean time) of transplantation. In an infant–toddler surgical ward, colorectal prophylaxis was an independent risk factor for colonization with a β-lactamase-producing, gentamicin-resistant strain of *Enterococcus faecalis*.[45]

The development of resistance to *Pseudomonas* species and *Serratia* species from the use of surgical prophylaxis has also been demonstrated.[5] An increased rate of *Pseudomonas* and *Serratia* resistance to gentamicin was detected, with a subsequent decrease in resistance after gentamicin was removed from the prophylactic regimen for open-heart surgery.

Timing. Prophylaxis implies delivery of the drug to the operative site before contamination occurs. Thus, the anti-infective drug should be given before the initial incision to ensure its presence in an adequate concentration in the targeted tissues. A landmark study demonstrated that, in a guinea pig model, antimicrobials administered before or around the time of *S. aureus* inoculation reduced the rate of infection, whereas administration after *S. aureus* exposure was less effective.[46] The effect of administering an antimicrobial in the fourth postoperative hour was no different from that seen in a control group. This was confirmed in a prospective clinical study that demonstrated that giving antimicrobials more than two hours before surgery was no more effective than giving no antimicrobials or postoperative antimicrobials alone.[47] By consensus, the ideal time of administration is within 30 minutes to one hour before the incision. For most procedures, scheduling administration at the time of induction of anesthesia ensures adequate concentrations during the period of potential contamination.[30] The exceptions are cesarean procedures, in which the antimicrobial should be administered after crossclamping of the umbilical cord,[48,49] and colonic procedures, in which oral antimicrobials should be administered starting 19 hours before the scheduled time of surgery.[50–56]

Duration. The shortest effective duration of antimicrobial administration for preventing postoperative infection is not known; however, postoperative antimicrobial administration is not necessary for most procedures.[57] For most procedures, the duration of antimicrobial prophylaxis should be 24 hours or less, with the exception of cardiothoracic procedures (up to 72 hours' duration) and ophthalmic procedures (duration not clearly established). The duration of cardiothoracic prophylaxis is based on expert panel consensus because the data do not delineate the optimal duration of prophylaxis. Prophylaxis for 24 hours or less may be appropriate for cardiothoracic procedures. At a minimum, antimicrobial coverage must be provided from the time of incision to closure of the incision. If a short-acting agent is used, it should be readministered if the operation extends beyond three hours in duration.[58] Readministration may also be warranted if prolonged or excessive bleeding occurs or there are factors that may shorten the half-life of the antimicrobial (e.g., extensive burns). Readministration may not be warranted in patients for whom the half-life is prolonged (e.g., patients with renal insufficiency or failure). If an operation is expected to last more than six to eight hours, it would be reasonable to administer an agent with a longer half-life and duration of action or to consider administering a short-acting agent at three-hour intervals during the procedure.

Route of Administration

Antimicrobials used for prophylaxis in surgery may be administered intravenously, orally, or topically. The preferred route of administration varies with the type of surgery, but, for a majority of procedures, intravenous administration is ideal because it produces reliable and predictable serum and tissue concentrations. Oral antimicrobials are often used for gut decontamination in elective colorectal operations and are an option in urologic procedures.

The use of topical antimicrobial agents, paste, and irrigations is beyond the scope of these guidelines. Intravenous and oral administration are the main focus of the guidelines, with the exception of ophthalmic procedures, for which topical administration is the primary route of administration.

Cardiothoracic Surgery

Background. Approximately 4 million cardiothoracic surgeries are performed annually in the United States.[59] Of

these, approximately 500,000 are coronary-artery bypass graft (CABG) procedures and approximately 600,000 are open-heart procedures. A relatively small number involve heart or heart–lung transplants and repair of congenital heart defects in children.

Patients who have cardiac conditions such as prosthetic cardiac valves, previous bacterial endocarditis, acquired valvular dysfunction, hypertrophic cardiomyopathy, and mitral valve prolapse with valvular regurgitation are at risk for developing bacterial endocarditis when undergoing open-heart surgery. Few controlled trials have demonstrated a benefit of prophylaxis. However, because of the morbidity and mortality associated with bacterial endocarditis, the AHA recommends antimicrobial prophylaxis.[32]

Mediastinitis and sternal wound infection are rare but serious complications of cardiothoracic surgery. The frequency of these infections with or without associated sternal dehiscence is 0.7% to 1.5%; however, the associated mortality rate is 13% to 33%.[60] Risk factors for these complications include chronic obstructive pulmonary disease, prolonged stay in the intensive care unit, respiratory failure, connective tissue disease, and male sex. Advanced age, lengthy surgery, and diabetes mellitus have also been identified as risk factors.[61]

Organisms. The primary intent of early antimicrobial prophylaxis in open-heart surgery was to reduce the frequency of postoperative endocarditis after valve repair. Early studies showed that coagulase-positive and coagulase-negative staphylococci were the primary pathogens infecting prosthetic valves.[62–64] As a result, most early prophylactic regimens were directed against staphylococci, with semisynthetic penicillins and first-generation cephalosporins emerging as the drugs of choice. With the advent of the CABG procedure and an expansion in the number of cardiothoracic procedures performed in the United States, prophylaxis must cover a broader spectrum of aerobic gram-negative pathogens that cause wound infections postoperatively at the sternal incision and the saphenous vein harvest sites.[64–67]

Efficacy. The postoperative infection rate in clean cardiothoracic surgeries is intrinsically low, and the extent of superiority of one regimen over another is relatively small. Antimicrobial prophylaxis in cardiothoracic surgery is associated with a fivefold lower rate of postoperative wound infection compared with placebo (approximately 5% versus 20% to 25%)[68]. Early placebo-controlled studies using a semisynthetic penicillin[69] or cephradine[70] were terminated early because of high infection rates in the placebo groups. Postoperative wound infection rates ranged from 9.1% to 54% in the placebo groups, compared with 0% to 6.7% in groups receiving antimicrobials. Since the routine administration of prophylactic antimicrobials for cardiothoracic surgeries, postoperative wound infection rates have ranged from 0.8% to 25%.

Choice. Cephalosporins were compared with antistaphylococcal penicillins as prophylactic agents for cardio-thoracic surgery in five studies. The antistaphylococcal penicillins were used in combination with another penicillin, an aminoglycoside, or both in four of these studies.[71–75] In four of the five studies, there were fewer total wound infections in the cephalosporin-treated patients; however, none of the differences were significant.

Published trials comparing cefazolin, cefamandole, and cefuroxime as prophylactic antimicrobials for cardiothoracic

surgery have revealed fewer total infections in the second-generation cephalosporin-treated patients; however, none of the differences were significant.[76–82] Both sternal and total wound infection rates (sternal plus leg wound infection) ranged from 2.5% to 18.8% in cefazolin-treated patients and from 0% to 13.5% in cefamandole- or cefuroxime-treated patients. Total wound infection rates were lower in patients receiving the second-generation cephalosporin in seven of the eight comparison groups. Leg wound infection rates were lower in five of the eight second-generation cephalosporin treatment groups. Meta-analysis of these results did not yield significant differences between agents when sternal and leg wounds were analyzed separately.[68] In another study, in which cefazolin and cefamandole, both with the addition of gentamicin, were compared, there was a significantly lower rate of sternal and total wound infection in the cefamandole–gentamicin group.[77] Three randomized, prospective, double-blind studies did not favor the second-generation cephalosporins: One study demonstrated no clinically or statistically significant difference between cefazolin and cefuroxime prophylaxis in 702 patients undergoing heart surgery,[83] a second study showed that cefuroxime-treated patients developed more sternal wound infections than cefazolin-treated patients,[84] and a third study showed no difference in rates of postsurgical site wound infection among cefamandole, cefazolin, and cefuroxime.[82]

In a study that compared second-generation cephalosporins, cefamandole was found to be superior to cefonicid in preventing perioperative infections.[85] No differences in total wound infection rates were found in another study in which cefuroxime was compared with ceftriaxone in 512 patients.[78] Vancomycin was superior to penicillin G in preventing total wound infections.[86]

In summary, cefamandole and cefuroxime were each associated with a lower frequency of wound infection than cefazolin, although significant differences were not consistently demonstrated. There were no differences in wound infection rates in a study that compared cefazolin with ceftriaxone. In addition, no differences in outcome were seen in studies in which cefamandole was compared with cefuroxime. No differences were found between antistaphylococcal penicillin regimens (often used in combination with aminoglycosides or other penicillins) and single-agent first- or second-generation cephalosporin regimens. These results are further supported by the results of a 30-year meta-analysis.[68]

Cephalosporins, as single agents, are at least as effective as combination regimens of antistaphylococcal penicillins and aminoglycosides and are much easier to administer. Cefazolin has been the traditional cephalosporin of choice. Further trials in a large number of patients would be required in order to demonstrate the superiority of cefamandole or cefuroxime.

There are limited data regarding the choice of an antimicrobial for penicillin-allergic patients undergoing cardiovascular procedures. Although vancomycin offers coverage against potential gram-positive pathogens, the addition of an aminoglycoside may be prudent when colonization and infection with gram-negative organisms are expected (such as a saphenous vein site).

Duration. The optimal duration of antimicrobial prophylaxis for cardiothoracic surgery was addressed by five studies, all using cephalothin as the prophylactic antimicrobial.[66,87–90] Dosages and durations in the short-duration groups ranged from a single 1-g dose of cephalothin

(as the sodium) to 2 g every six hours for two days. Long treatment regimens ranged from 2 g of cephalothin preoperatively followed by 1 g every six hours for three days to 2 g every six hours for six days. Total wound infection rates were lower in the short-duration treatment groups in two of four studies, although the differences were not significant. In another randomized study, there was no significant difference between single-dose ceftriaxone and cefuroxime three times daily until the end of the second postoperative day.[90] The researchers concluded that a single dose of ceftriaxone was a viable alternative to cefuroxime for 48 hours as prophylaxis in cardiothoracic surgical procedures. A European randomized, prospective study in 844 evaluable patients demonstrated that a single dose of cefuroxime 20 mg/kg (as the sodium) at induction of anesthesia was as effective as the same dose at induction of anesthesia followed by 750 mg three times daily for three consecutive days.[91]

Pediatric Efficacy. No well-controlled studies have evaluated the efficacy of antimicrobial prophylaxis in pediatric patients undergoing cardiovascular procedures. A survey indicated that the predominant practice in pediatric cardiovascular surgery is to use cefazolin for two days or less or until transthoracic medical devices are removed.[92]

Recommendations. For patients undergoing cardiothoracic procedures, the recommended regimen is cefazolin 1 g (as the sodium) intravenously at induction of anesthesia and every 8 hours for up to 72 hours. This duration is based on consensus of the expert panel because the data do not delineate the optimal duration of prophylaxis. Prophylaxis for 24 hours or less may be appropriate for cardiothoracic procedures. Currently there is no evidence to support continuing prophylaxis until chest and mediastinal drainage tubes are removed. Cefuroxime 1.5 g (as the sodium) intravenously at induction of anesthesia and every 12 hours for up to 72 hours or cefamandole 1 g (as the nafate) at induction of anesthesia and every six hours for up to 72 hours are suitable alternatives. Further studies are needed to demonstrate the efficacy of single-dose prophylaxis. Vancomycin 1 g (as the hydrochloride) intravenously over one hour, with or without gentamicin 2 mg/kg (as the sulfate) intravenously, should be reserved as an alternative on the basis of guidelines from HICPAC and AHA.[21,32] (Strength of evidence for prophylaxis = A.)

Pediatric Dosage. The recommended regimen for pediatric patients undergoing cardiothoracic procedures is cefazolin 20–30 mg/kg (as the sodium) intravenously at induction of anesthesia and every 8 hours for up to 72 hours. Cefuroxime 50 mg/kg (as the sodium) intravenously at induction of anesthesia and every 8 hours for up to 72 hours is an acceptable alternative. Vancomycin 15 mg/kg (as the hydrochloride) intravenously over one hour, with or without gentamicin 2 mg/kg (as the sulfate) intravenously, should be reserved as an alternative on the basis of guidelines from HICPAC and AHA.[21,32]

Gastroduodenal Surgery

Background. The gastroduodenal procedures considered in this document include resection with or without vagotomy for gastric or duodenal ulcers, resection for gastric carcinoma, revision required in order to repair strictures of the gastric outlet, and gastric bypass. Studies addressing antimicrobial prophylaxis for gastroesophageal reflux disease procedures (Nissen's fundoplication), pancreatoduodenectomy (Whipple's procedure), or highly selective vagotomy for ulcers could not be identified.

The stomach is an effective barrier to bacterial colonization; this is at least partially related to its acidity. The stomach and the duodenum typically contain small numbers of organisms ($<10^4$ CFU/mL), the most common of which are streptococci, lactobacilli, diphtheroids, and fungi.[93,94] Treatment with agents that increase gastric pH significantly increases the concentration of gastric organisms.[95–97] Alterations in gastric and duodenal bacterial flora as a result of increases in gastric pH have the potential to increase the postoperative infection rate.[98,99]

The risk of postoperative infection in gastroduodenal surgery depends on a number of factors. Patients who are at highest risk include those with achlorhydria, decreased gastric motility, gastric outlet obstruction, morbid obesity, gastric bleeding, or cancer.[100]

Organisms. The most common organisms cultured from wound infections after gastroduodenal surgery are coliforms (*Escherichia coli*, *Proteus* species, *Klebsiella* species), staphylococci, streptococci, enterococci, and, occasionally, *Bacteroides* species.[101–108]

Efficacy. In one large study, wound infection rates in patients not receiving antimicrobial prophylaxis were 6% after vagotomy and drainage, 13% after gastric ulcer surgery, 17% after surgery for gastric cancer, and 25% in patients with gastroduodenal bleeding.[109] Results of randomized, controlled trials clearly indicate that prophylactic antimicrobials are effective in decreasing postoperative infection rates in gastroduodenal surgery. Relative to other types of GI tract surgery, the number of clinical trials evaluating antimicrobial prophylaxis for gastroduodenal surgery is limited. The most common definition of wound infection used in those studies was the presence of purulent discharge. In placebo-controlled trials, infection rates ranged from 0% to 7% for patients receiving cephalosporins and from 21% to 44% for patients receiving placebo.[102,103,105–107,110–12] The difference was significant in most studies.

No efficacy data are available on highly selective vagotomy, Nissen's fundoplication, or Whipple's procedure. despite the lack of data, the expert panel supports the use of a single dose of cefazolin 1 g (as the sodium) intravenously for prophylaxis of these procedures.

Choice. No differences between first- and second-generation cephalosporins were found. The most frequently used agents were first-generation[103,105,108,110–113] and second-generation[101,102,104,106,107,113] cephalosporins. Ticarcillin,[108] amoxicillin–clavulanate,[114] mezlocillin,[104] and ciprofloxacin[101,115] were also evaluated. Relatively few studies have compared the efficacy of different agents in reducing postoperative infection rates. In comparative studies, ticarcillin (intravenous) and cephalothin (intravenous) were similarly effective,[108] as were ciprofloxacin (intravenous and oral) and cefuroxime (intravenous).[101]

Duration. Available data indicate that single-dose and multidose regimens are similarly effective. Two studies compared single- and multidose regimens of either cefamandole[113] or amoxicillin–clavulanate.[114] There was no significant difference in wound infection rates. No studies have evaluated the use of a single dose of a first-generation cephalosporin.

Pediatric Efficacy. No well-controlled studies have evaluated the efficacy of antimicrobial prophylaxis in pediatric patients undergoing gastroduodenal surgery.

Recommendation. Antimicrobial prophylaxis in gastroduodenal surgery should be considered for patients at highest risk for postoperative infections, such as patients with increased gastric pH (e.g., patients receiving histamine H_2-receptor antagonists), decreased gastric motility, gastric outlet obstruction, gastric bleeding, or cancer. Antimicrobials are not needed when the lumen of the intestinal tract is not entered.

A single dose of cefazolin 1 g (as the sodium) given intravenously at induction of anesthesia is recommended in procedures during which the lumen of the intestinal tract is entered. A single dose of cefazolin 1 g given intravenously at induction of anesthesia is recommended for highly selective vagotomy, Nissen's fundoplication, and Whipple's procedure. (Strength of evidence for prophylaxis = A when the lumen of the intestinal tract is entered.) (Strength of evidence for prophylaxis = C for highly selective vagotomy, Nissen's fundoplication, and Whipple's procedure.)

Pediatric Dosage. The recommended regimen for pediatric patients undergoing gastroduodenal surgery during which the lumen of the intestinal tract is entered, highly selective vagotomy, Nissen's fundoplication, and Whipple's procedure is a single dose of cefazolin 20–30 mg/kg (as the sodium) intravenously at induction of anesthesia.

Biliary Tract Surgery

Background. Biliary tract surgeries include cholecystectomy, exploration of the common bile duct, and choledochoenterostomy. The overall risk of postoperative infection in biliary tract surgery is approximately 5% to 20%.[116] The biliary tract is usually sterile; therefore, the risk of infection is low. However, it is generally accepted that patients with bacteria in the bile at the time of surgery are at higher risk of postoperative infection.[117,118] Factors that place patients at a higher risk of infection include obesity, age greater than 70 years, an acute episode of cholecystitis or cholelithiasis within the previous six months, diabetes mellitus, or a history of obstructive jaundice or bile duct obstruction.[116,119]

Organisms. The organisms most commonly associated with infection after biliary tract surgery include *E. coli, Klebsiella* species, and enterococci; less frequently, other gram-negative organisms, streptococci, or staphylococci are isolated. Anaerobes are occasionally reported, most commonly *Clostridium* species.[117,119–128]

Efficacy. Data from randomized, controlled trials support the use of prophylactic antimicrobials in all patients undergoing biliary tract surgery. Significantly lower rates of postoperative wound infection have been demonstrated, even in patients at low risk.

Numerous studies have evaluated the use of prophylactic antimicrobials during biliary tract surgery. Although the definition of wound infection varied between studies, the presence of purulent discharge was the most common definition. First-generation[121,127,129,138] second-generation,[118–120, 122,123,126,133,135,136,138–143] and third-generation[123,124,132,141] cephalosporins have been studied more extensively than other

antimicrobials. Limited data are available for ampicillin–gentamicin,[144] mezlocillin,[142] piperacillin,[137] amoxicillin–clavulanate,[143] and ciprofloxacin.[124,145]

Although many studies had an insufficient sample size to demonstrate a significant benefit of antimicrobial prophylaxis, a meta-analysis of 42 clinical trials that compared prophylactic antimicrobials with placebo demonstrated that active treatment significantly reduced the risk of wound infection.[116] In that analysis, the overall wound infection rate was 15% in the control group. Wound infection rates were 9% lower in the antimicrobial treatment group than the control group. When patients were stratified by low or high risk and by early or late wound inspection (early in hospital or late at follow-up), antimicrobial prophylaxis was still effective in preventing wound infections in all groups, although the largest benefit was in high-risk patients with a later wound inspection.

Laparoscopic cholecystectomy has replaced open cholecystectomy as the standard of practice because of a reduction in recovery time and a shorter hospital stay. There have been few studies of antimicrobial prophylaxis for laparoscopic cholecystectomy. The studies that have addressed this procedure were not randomized, controlled studies. In one study at the Mayo Clinic, 95% of 195 patients received a preoperative dose of an antimicrobial, usually a first-generation cephalosporin. Erythema at the trocar site was noted in 6% of patients, and wound separation was noted in 5% of patients; however, no treatment was necessary.[146] A nonrandomized study showed 14 infections in 228 patients who received antimicrobial prophylaxis and no infections in 188 patients who received only a chlorhexidine scrub before surgery.[147] The patients in this study were assigned to treatment groups according to the attending physician's treatment preference. In a study in the United Kingdom, cefuroxime 1.5 g (as the sodium) was administered at induction of anesthesia to 253 consecutive patients. At two weeks, 0.8% of patients had wound infections, 0.8% had chest infections, and 0.4% had an intra-abdominal abscess. No complications were noted at 12 months.[148] Current data do not support antimicrobial prophylaxis for laparoscopic cholecystectomies.

Choice. The data do not indicate a significant difference among first-, second-, and third-generation cephalosporins. Several studies have compared first-generation cephalosporins with second- or third-generation agents.[127,132–136,138] With one exception,[136] there was no significant difference among agents. This was confirmed by a meta-analysis that found no significant difference among first-, second-, and third-generation cephalosporins.[116] Other studies found no significant differences between ampicillin and cefamandole,[126] ciprofloxacin and ceftriaxone,[124] cefonicid and mezlocillin,[142] cefuroxime with or without metronidazole and mezlocillin,[149] amoxicillin–clavulanate and mezlocillin,[150] amoxicillin–clavulanate and cefamandole,[143] and oral and intravenous ciprofloxacin and intravenous cefuroxime.[145]

Duration. The effect of treatment duration on outcome has been evaluated. A single dose of a cephalosporin was compared with multiple doses in several studies; no significant differences were found.[118,120,121,132,139–141,151] The largest study compared one dose of cefuroxime with three doses in 1004 patients with risk factors for infection who were undergoing biliary tract surgery.[118] There was no significant difference in the rates of minor or major wound infection between the single- and multiple-dose groups.

Pediatric Efficacy. No well-controlled studies have evaluated the efficacy of antimicrobial prophylaxis in pediatric patients undergoing biliary tract surgery.

Recommendation. A single dose of cefazolin 1 g (as the sodium) administered intravenously at induction of anesthesia is recommended for open procedures in the biliary tract. (Strength of evidence for prophylaxis = A.) Antimicrobial prophylaxis is not recommended in laparoscopic cholecystectomies. (Strength of evidence against prophylaxis = B.)

Pediatric Dosage. The recommended regimen for pediatric patients undergoing open procedures in the biliary tract is a single dose of cefazolin 20–30 mg/kg (as the sodium) intravenously at induction of anesthesia.

Appendectomy

Background. Cases of appendicitis can be described as complicated or uncomplicated on the basis of the pathology. Patients with uncomplicated appendicitis have an acutely inflamed appendix. Complicated appendicitis usually includes perforated or gangrenous appendicitis, including peritonitis or abscess formation. However, in some studies patients with gangrenous appendicitis are considered to have uncomplicated disease because these patients generally have a lower infectious complication rate than patients with perforation. Because complicated appendicitis is treated as a presumed infection, it has not been addressed in these guidelines.

Approximately 80% of patients with appendicitis have uncomplicated disease.[24] Postoperative infection has been reported in 9–30% of patients with uncomplicated appendicitis who do not receive prophylactic antimicrobials.[152–156] Postoperative infection was usually defined as purulent wound discharge with or without positive cultures. Laparoscopic appendectomy has been reported to produce similar or lower rates of infection as open appendectomy when antimicrobials are used; however, there have been no randomized, controlled studies.[157]

Organisms. The most common microorganisms isolated from wound infections after appendectomy are anaerobic and aerobic gram-negative enteric organisms. *Bacteroides fragilis* is the most commonly cultured anaerobe, and *E. coli* is the most frequent aerobe, indicating that the bowel flora constitute a major source for pathogens.[24,158,159] Aerobic and anaerobic streptococci, *Staphylococcus* species, and *Enterococcus* species also have been reported. *Pseudomonas aeruginosa* has been reported infrequently.

Efficacy. As a single agent, metronidazole was no more effective in appendectomy than placebo.[152,155] cefazolin was generally less effective than placebo, with postoperative infection rates above 10%.[153] This is likely due to its limited activity against anaerobes. Clindamycin was more effective than placebo, although the postoperative infection rate tended to be relatively high (17%).[153]

Choice. Randomized, controlled trials have failed to identify an agent that is clearly superior to other agents in the prophylaxis of postappendectomy infectious complications. The second- and third-generation cephalosporins appear to have similar efficacy and are the recommended agents on the basis of cost and tolerability. Given the relatively equivalent efficacy between agents, a cost-minimization approach

is reasonable; the choice of agents should be based on local drug acquisition costs.

A wide range of antimicrobials have been evaluated for prophylaxis in uncomplicated appendicitis. The most commonly used agents were cephalosporins. In general, second-generation cephalosporins (cefoxitin, cefotetan) and third-generation cephalosporins (cefoperazone, cefotaxime) were effective, with postoperative infection rates of <5% in most studies.[156,160–166] However, one study[165] showed that single-dose cefotetan was significantly more effective than single-dose cefoxitin, perhaps because of the longer half-life of cefotetan.

Piperacillin 2 g (as the sodium) was comparable to cefoxitin 2 g (as the sodium) in a well-controlled study.[166] Metronidazole was less effective than cefotaxime, with infection rates above 10%.[160] However, when metronidazole was combined with ampicillin[167] or gentamicin,[162,168] the postoperative infection rates were 3% to 6%. Clindamycin was more effective than cefazolin, although the postoperative infection rate tended to be relatively high (17%).[153]

Duration. In most of the studies of second- or third-generation cephalosporins or metronidazole combinations, a single dose[160–162,165,166,168] or two or three doses[156,163,167] were given. Although direct comparisons were not done, there was no discernible difference in postoperative infection rates between single-dose and multidose administration in most studies.

Pediatric Efficacy. Two pediatric studies demonstrated no difference in infection rates between placebo and antimicrobials: metronidazole, penicillin plus tobramycin, and piperacillin[169] and single-dose metronidazole and single-dose metronidazole plus cefuroxime.[170] As a single agent, metronidazole was no more effective than placebo in two double-blind studies that included children 10 years of age and older[152] and 15 years of age and older.[155] In a randomized study that included pediatric patients, ceftizoxime and cefamandole demonstrated significantly lower infection rates and duration of hospitalization than placebo.[171] Both cefoxitin and a combination of gentamicin and metronidazole were associated with a lower rate of postoperative infection in a randomized study that included pediatric patients less than 16 years of age.[162] Second-generation cephalosporins (cefoxitin) and third-generation cephalosporins (cefoperazone, cefotaxime) were effective, with postoperative infection rates of <5% in two studies that included pediatric patients less than 12 years of age.[156,162,163]

Recommendation. For uncomplicated appendicitis, the recommended regimen is a cephalosporin with anaerobic and aerobic activity (cefoxitin, cefotetan, cefmetazole) 1–2 g intravenously at induction of anesthesia. An alternative is piperacillin 2 g (as the sodium) intravenously. For penicillin-allergic patients, an alternative is metronidazole 500 mg plus gentamicin 2 mg/kg (as the sulfate) intravenously at the induction of anesthesia. (Strength of evidence for prophylaxis = A.)

Pediatric Dosage. The recommended regimen for pediatric patients undergoing procedures for uncomplicated appendicitis is a single intravenous dose of cefoxitin 20–40 mg/kg (as the sodium), cefotetan 20–40 mg/kg (as the disodium), or cefotaxime or ceftizoxime 25–50 mg/kg (as the sodium) at induction of anesthesia. An alternative is piperacillin 50 mg/kg (as the sodium) intravenously at induction of anesthesia. For penicillin-allergic patients, an alternative is metronidazole 10 mg/kg plus gentamicin 2 mg/kg (as the sulfate) intravenously at induction of anesthesia.

Colorectal Surgery

Background. Wound infections are a frequent complication of surgery of the colon or rectum. Other septic complications, such as fecal fistula, intra-abdominal abscesses, peritonitis, and septicemia, are serious concerns but much less common.[172] Infectious complication rates range from 30% to 60% when antimicrobial prophylaxis is not used.[24,173] Patients receiving appropriate antimicrobial prophylaxis have infection rates of <10%. A pooled analysis of clinical trials of antimicrobial prophylaxis in colon surgery also demonstrated that the use of antimicrobials significantly reduces mortality (11.2% for control versus 4.5% for treatment).[174] The type and duration of surgery can affect the risk of infection. Rectal resection is associated with a higher risk of infection than intraperitoneal colon resection.[175,176] Surgeries lasting 3.5 hours or more are associated with a higher risk of infection than shorter procedures.[24] Other risk factors include impaired host defenses, age of >60 years, hypoalbuminemia, poor preoperative bowel preparation, bacterial contamination of the surgical wound,[177] corticosteroid therapy, and malignancy.[178]

The removal of feces and intestinal fluid by mechanical preparation is considered a prerequisite for colorectal surgery. Mechanical preparation also reduces the high concentrations of bacteria in the bowel. Traditional three- to four-day regimens of clear liquids, cathartics, and enemas have been replaced by single-day lavage techniques.[179–186]

The choice of antimicrobials for prophylaxis in colorectal surgery should be guided by the spectrum of activity of the agent. Agents should have activity against the anaerobic and aerobic flora of the bowel. There have been three main approaches to the prophylaxis of infections after colorectal surgery: oral agents, intravenous agents (usually cephalosporins), and combinations of oral and intravenous agents. Although numerous clinical trials have been conducted, the central issues of determining the most appropriate regimen (oral versus intravenous versus an oral–intravenous combination) and the optimal choice of antimicrobial have yet to be fully resolved.

Organisms. The infecting organisms in colorectal surgery are derived from the bowel lumen, where there are high concentrations of organisms. *B. fragilis* and other obligate anaerobes are the most frequently isolated organisms from the bowel, with concentrations 1,000 to 10,000 times higher than those of aerobes.[187] *E. coli* is the most common aerobe. *B. fragilis* and *E. coli* make up approximately 20% to 30% of the fecal mass. They are the most frequently isolated pathogens from infected wounds after colon surgery.[187]

Efficacy. Results from randomized, controlled trials unequivocally support the use of prophylactic antimicrobials in all patients undergoing colorectal surgery. Postoperative infection rates tend to be lower when oral antimicrobials are used for prophylaxis than after the use of intravenous agents; therefore, oral antimicrobials are preferred.

Oral regimens. A variety of oral agents administered after mechanical bowel preparation have been evaluated for prophylaxis for colorectal surgery. The most common combinations have been an aminoglycoside (neomycin and, less often, kanamycin) plus an agent that will provide sufficient anaerobic activity, usually erythromycin[50–56,188] or metronidazole.[56,182,188–192] In placebo-controlled studies,[6,50,188,192,193] the oral combination was significantly more effective than

placebo in reducing wound infections. Postoperative wound infection rates ranged from 0% to 11% with neomycin plus erythromycin[50–56] and from 2% to 13% with neomycin and metronidazole.[189–191] Combinations of neomycin and tetracycline,[6,193] and neomycin and clindamycin[189] have also been used successfully, with postoperative wound infection rates of <10%. The use of metronidazole as a single agent appears to be less effective, with reported wound infection rates of 12% to 15%.[194,195]

Oral antimicrobials have been compared with intravenous agents in a few studies. Oral neomycin plus oral erythromycin was significantly more effective than intravenous gentamicin and intravenous metronidazole[54] but was similarly effective as intravenous cefoxitin,[52] intravenous cefamandole,[53] and intravenous ceftriaxone plus intravenous metronidazole.[55]

Intravenous regimens. A wide range of intravenous antimicrobials have been evaluated for prophylaxis in colorectal surgery. Cephalosporins are the most common agents, usually administered as a single agent. First-generation cephalosporins produced inconsistent results.[196–200] With one exception,[199] single-agent first-generation cephalosporins were generally ineffective, with postoperative wound infection rates ranging from 12% to 39%.[196,197] This is not surprising given the lack of *B. fragilis* activity of these agents. Second-generation cephalosporins have been widely evaluated. In single-agent therapy, wound infection rates ranged from 0% to 17%[176,198,201–209]; however, more than half of the studies found rates of >10%. Third-generation agents have been evaluated in a few trials; postoperative wound infection rates were 8% to 19% with single-agent use.[205,210,211] In some studies, second- or third-generation cephalosporins were combined with other intravenous agents, most commonly metronidazole.[201,209–212] However, in three of four studies, a combination of a second- or third-generation cephalosporin plus metronidazole was no more effective than the cephalosporin alone.[201,209–211] Other intravenous agents that have been evaluated either alone or in combination include aminoglycosides,[54,101,213–217] clindamycin,[213] ampicillin,[214,218,219] ampicillin plus a β-lactamase inhibitor,[216,220] doxycycline,[218,221–223] ticarcillin plus a β-lactamase inhibitor,[215,224] piperacillin,[206,225] piperacillin plus a β-lactamase inhibitor,[225] imipenem,[212] and ciprofloxacin.[115]

Combination oral and intravenous regimens. Combinations of oral and intravenous antimicrobials have been used in an attempt to further reduce postoperative infection rates. Regimens include oral neomycin and erythromycin plus intravenous administration of a cephalosporin,[52,175,176,197,198,226,227] metronidazole,[228,229] or gentamicin plus clindamycin.[213] Postoperative wound infection rates in these studies ranged from 0% to 7%. With one exception,[175] there was no significant difference between oral neomycin–erythromycin plus an intravenous antimicrobial and oral neomycin–erythromycin alone.[52,197,213,226] When combination oral and intravenous agents were compared with intravenous agents alone, combination therapy tended to be superior in four of five studies[52,176,197,198,228]; the difference was significant in two of the studies.[176,197] In one study,[176] the difference was even greater among patients undergoing rectal resection, a procedure associated with a high risk of infection. The postoperative wound infection rates after rectal resection were 23% and 11%, respectively, for patients receiving intravenous cefoxitin and cefoxitin plus oral neomycin and erythromycin.

Duration. Single and multiple doses were compared in several studies.[203–205,211,219,222] However, only two of these

studies,[219,222] compared single doses with multiple doses of
the same antimicrobial. There was no significant difference
in infection rates between single-dose and multidose admini-
stration, with only one exception. A single dose of cefo-
taxime plus metronidazole was significantly more effective
than three doses of cefotaxime alone.[211]

Pediatric Efficacy. No well-controlled studies have evalu-
ated the efficacy of antimicrobial prophylaxis in pediatric
patients undergoing colorectal surgery. The safety, efficacy,
tolerability, and cost-effectiveness of intestinal lavage have
been demonstrated in pediatric patients.[230,231]

Recommendation. Patients undergoing colorectal surgery
should receive mechanical bowel preparation. Numerous
bowel preparations are available. Lavage solutions are con-
traindicated in patients with obstruction.

Oral neomycin sulfate 1 g and erythromycin base 1
g should be given after the bowel preparation is complete at
19, 18, and 9 hours before surgery. If the oral route is contra-
indicated, a single 2-g dose of an intravenous cephalosporin
with both aerobic and anaerobic activity (e.g., cefoxitin, cefo-
tetan, cefmetazole) should be given at induction of anesthesia.
Because there is no demonstrable difference in efficacy among
these cephalosporins, the choice should be based on local drug
acquisition costs. In patients undergoing high-risk surgery,
such as rectal resection, a combination of oral neomycin–
erythromycin plus a cephalosporin administered intravenously
is recommended. (Strength of evidence for prophylaxis = A.)

Pediatric Dosage. Pediatric patients undergoing colorec-
tal surgery should undergo mechanical bowel preparation.
Numerous bowel preparations are available. Lavage solu-
tions are contraindicated in patients with obstruction. One
regimen for pediatric patients is polyethylene glycol–
electrolyte lavage solution given orally or by nasogastric tube
at a rate of 25–40 mL/kg/hr until rectal effluent is clear.[230,231]

Oral neomycin sulfate 20 mg/kg and erythromycin base
10 mg/kg should be given after the bowel preparation is com-
plete at 19, 18, and 9 hours before surgery. If the oral route
is contraindicated, a single 30–40 mg/kg intravenous dose of
cefoxitin or cefotetan should be given at induction of anesthe-
sia. In patients undergoing high-risk surgery, such as rectal re-
section, a combination of oral neomycin and erythromycin plus
a cephalosporin administered intravenously is recommended.

Head and Neck Surgery

Background. Elective surgical procedures of the head and
neck can be categorized as clean or clean-contaminated.
Clean procedures include parotidectomy, thyroidectomy,
and submandibular-gland excision. Clean-contaminated proce-
dures include all procedures involving an incision through the
oral or pharyngeal mucosa.[232] These vary considerably from
tonsillectomy, adenoidectomy, and rhinoplasty to complicated
tumor-debulking procedures requiring massive reconstruction.

In prospective, randomized, double-blind trials com-
paring placebo with antimicrobials in clean-contaminated
surgeries, patients receiving placebo had postoperative
wound infection rates of 36% to 78%.[233-235] Antimicrobials
are associated with dramatically lower rates of postopera-
tive wound infection. Infection rates below 10% may be
expected when appropriate antimicrobial prophylaxis is

given.[233,234,236-241] Postoperative wound infection rates are
affected by age, nutritional status, and the presence of con-
comitant medical conditions such as diabetes mellitus. The
hospital course, including length of hospitalization before
surgery, duration of antimicrobial use before surgery, length
of surgery, and presence of implants, can also affect postop-
erative wound infection rates. If the patient has cancer, the
stage of the malignancy before operation and preoperative
radiation therapy must also be assessed.[242-244]

Organisms. The normal flora of the mouth and the orophar-
ynx are responsible for most infections that follow clean-
contaminated head and neck procedures. The predominant
oropharyngeal organisms include various streptococci (aero-
bic and anaerobic species), *S. epidermidis, Peptococcus,
Peptostreptococcus,* and numerous anaerobic gram-negative
bacteria, including *Bacteroides* species (but almost never *B.
fragilis*) and *Veillonella.* Nasal flora include *Staphylococcus*
species and *Streptococcus* species. Anaerobic bacteria are ap-
proximately 10 times more common than aerobic bacteria in the
oropharynx. As a result, postoperative wound infections are pri-
marily polymicrobial. Both aerobic and anaerobic bacteria are
cultured from infected wounds in more than 90% of cases.[245-248]
It has been suggested that aerobic gram-negative bacteria are
colonizers rather than pathogens in most patients.[237,246]

Efficacy for Clean Procedures. Systemic administration of
prophylactic antimicrobials has not proven effective in reduc-
ing wound infection rates in patients undergoing clean pro-
cedures of the head and neck; however, randomized, blinded
studies have not been performed for clean procedures. A
retrospective review of 438 patients undergoing clean pro-
cedures (parotidectomy, thyroidectomy, or submandibular
gland excision) demonstrated that 80% of the patients had
not received prophylactic antimicrobials; the associated
wound infection rate was 0.7%. Patients receiving antimi-
crobials had a similar wound infection rate.[249] Another retro-
spective cohort study of 192 patients who underwent surgery
between 1976 and 1989 did not demonstrate any difference
in infection rates between patients who did and patients who
did not receive perioperative antimicrobials.[250] However, the
authors calculated that the excess cost due to patients who
developed a postoperative wound infection was in excess
of $36,000 and that the cost of administering prophylaxis
to 100 patients is less than this amount. These retrospective
data alone do not justify prophylaxis. Other factors besides
cost need to be considered, including the potential for resis-
tance, adverse events, and prosthetic placement.

Pediatric Efficacy for Clean Procedures. No well-controlled
studies have evaluated the effect of antimicrobial prophylaxis
in the pediatric population undergoing clean surgical proce-
dures of the head and neck.

Efficacy for Clean-Contaminated Procedures. Three double-
blind, placebo-controlled trials established superiority of
antimicrobials over placebo in clean-contaminated proce-
dures.[233,234,238] In one trial, 101 patients were randomly as-
signed to receive placebo every eight hours for four doses,
cefazolin 500 mg (as the sodium) every eight hours for four
doses, cefotaxime 2 g (as the sodium) every eight hours
for four doses, or cefoperazone 2 g (as the sodium) every
eight hours for four doses.[234] Infection rates were 78% in

the placebo group, 33% in the cefazolin group, 10% in the cefotaxime group, and 9% in the cefoperazone group. The difference between each antimicrobial group and the placebo group was significant. The length of hospital stay for infected patients was twice that of noninfected patients. The second study demonstrated a wound infection rate of 12% with ampicillin plus cloxacillin, compared with 28% with placebo.[238] Although the wound infection rate (27%) for cefamandole 2 g (as the nafate) followed by 1 g every eight hours for a total of three doses was relatively high compared with the previous studies, cefamandole did demonstrate superiority over placebo (wound infection rate of 55%).[233] Another study involving cefoperazone, cefotaxime, and placebo demonstrated similar results.[235]

Choice. Various studies of prophylaxis for clean-contaminated procedures have demonstrated wound infection rates of less than 10% with clindamycin plus gentamicin,[236,251] clindamycin plus amikacin,[252] cefazolin plus metronidazole,[241] cefuroxime alone,[253] and cefuroxime plus metronidazole.[253] A prospective, randomized, double-blind study compared clindamycin 600 mg (as the hydrochloride) intravenously for a total of four doses with clindamycin 600 mg plus gentamicin 1.7 mg/kg (as the sulfate) intravenously for a total of four doses in 104 patients undergoing clean-contaminated oncological head and neck surgery.[237] The combination of gentamicin plus clindamycin demonstrated no significant advantage over clindamycin alone. The postoperative infection rate was 3.8% in both groups. The authors concluded that clindamycin alone appears effective as a prophylactic agent and that broad-spectrum antimicrobials such as cefoxitin may be unnecessary. Because clindamycin is not active against aerobic gram-negative bacteria, the authors concluded that these bacteria are probably colonizers rather than pathogens. This study suggests that aerobic gram-negative coverage (as provided by gentamicin) may be unnecessary. However, the study lacked sufficient power to show a difference among groups.

Cefazolin offers coverage against potential aerobic and anaerobic organisms, except *B. fragilis,* in clean-contaminated procedures of the head and neck. Although the need for coverage against *B. fragilis* has not been substantiated by the literature, some people consider the addition of metronidazole to cefazolin acceptable when colonization with *B. fragilis* is expected.

Dosage. Cefazolin 500 mg (as the sodium) three times daily for a total of one and five days demonstrated high infection rates (35% and 18%, respectively).[251] Another study showed similar results with cefazolin.[236] Two major flaws with these studies were the dose (500 mg) and the administration time (three hours preoperatively).

In a randomized trial, cefazolin 2 g (as the sodium) was compared with moxalactam 2 g (as the disodium), each given one hour before surgery and three more times, for a total of four doses.[254] Infection rates were not significantly different: 8.5% in the cefazolin group and 3.4% in the moxalactam group. A prospective, randomized multicenter trial compared the effectiveness of clindamycin 900 mg (as the hydrochloride) with that of cefazolin 2 g (as the sodium) before surgery and continued every 8 hours for a total of 24 hours in patients undergoing major procedures (pectoralis major myocutaneous flap reconstruction).[255] Wound infections developed in 19.6% of patients in the clindamycin group and 21.6% of patients in the cefazolin group. This difference was not significant. These two trials demonstrated that, when administered at the appropriate time, cefazolin 2 g is effective.

In a prospective, double-blind trial, 159 patients were randomly assigned to receive amoxicillin 1750 mg (as the trihydrate) with clavulanic acid 250 mg (as clavulanate potassium), clindamycin 600 mg (as the hydrochloride) plus gentamicin 80 mg (as the sulfate), or cefazolin 2 g (as the sodium).[256] All groups received a total of three intravenous doses (the cefazolin group received one 2-g dose followed by two doses of 1 g each). There was no significant difference in wound infection rates among these regimens.

Duration. There was no difference in efficacy between one day and five days of clindamycin plus gentamicin prophylaxis in a randomized, unblinded study.[236] Other studies involving prophylaxis for a total duration of one day or less also demonstrated wound infection rates of 10% or less.[235,237,239,240,2 51,253,254] Single-dose prophylaxis has not been studied.

Pediatric Efficacy for Clean-Contaminated Procedures. No well-controlled studies have evaluated the efficacy of antimicrobial prophylaxis in pediatric patients undergoing clean-contaminated surgery of the head and neck.

Recommendation. *Clean procedures.* Infection rates in clean head and neck surgical procedures are generally less than 2%. Antimicrobial prophylaxis is not justified in patients undergoing clean surgical procedures of the head and neck. If there is prosthetic placement, cefazolin 1 g (as the sodium) intravenously at induction of anesthesia is appropriate. (Strength of evidence against prophylaxis = B.) (Strength of evidence for prophylaxis with prosthesis placement = C.)

Clean-contaminated procedures. The preferred regimens for patients undergoing clean-contaminated head and neck procedures are cefazolin 2 g (as the sodium) intravenously at induction of anesthesia and every 8 hours for 24 hours or clindamycin 600 mg (as the hydrochloride) intravenously at induction of anesthesia and every 8 hours for 24 hours. The necessity of giving gentamicin with clindamycin or metronidazole with cefazolin remains controversial; if these combinations are selected, the dosages are gentamicin 1.7 mg/kg (as the sulfate) intravenously and metronidazole 500 mg intravenously every eight hours. Agents should be administered at induction of anesthesia. Prophylaxis should not exceed 24 hours. Single-dose regimens may be preferable, particularly when cost and the possibility of resistance are considered; however, this approach remains controversial. (Strength of evidence for prophylaxis = A.)

Pediatric Dosage. *Clean procedures.* Antimicrobial prophylaxis is not recommended in pediatric patients undergoing clean head and neck procedures unless there is prosthetic placement. In these cases, cefazolin 20–30 mg/kg (as the sodium) administered intravenously at induction of anesthesia is appropriate.

Clean-contaminated procedures. The recommended regimen for pediatric patients undergoing clean-contaminated head and neck procedures is cefazolin 30–40 mg/kg (as the sodium) intravenously at induction of anesthesia and every 8 hours for 24 hours or clindamycin 15 mg/kg (as the hydrochloride) intravenously, at induction of anesthesia and every 8 hours for 24 hours. The addition of gentamicin 2.5 mg/kg (as the sulfate) intravenously to clindamycin remains controversial, as does the addition of metronidazole 10 mg/kg intravenously every eight hours to cefazolin. Agents should be administered at induction of anesthesia. Single-dose regimens may be preferable, particularly when cost and the possibility of resistance are considered; however, this approach remains controversial.

Neurosurgery

Background. Clean neurosurgical procedures are those during which there is no break in surgical technique and no entry into the respiratory or GI tract. Clean procedures usually carry a risk of postoperative wound infection of less than 5%. In many hospitals the risk is 1% to 2%. It is therefore understandable that the use of injectable antimicrobials for such procedures is controversial. In addition, it is difficult to design clinical trials that could enable a distinction between infection rates of 2% and 5%. Clean-contaminated neurosurgical procedures (e.g., surgical approach through the nasopharynx or transphenoid sinus) are not addressed in these guidelines because there is a lack of data and there are no sufficiently similar procedures from which to extrapolate data.

Examples of clean neurosurgical procedures include elective craniotomy for the repair of aneurysms, correction of arteriovenous malformations, and removal of various types of brain tumors. There can be major differences (e.g., immune status, nutrition) between a person who undergoes elective surgery for a nonmalignant condition and a patient with cancer. These variables make clinical trial results difficult to interpret. Some craniotomies for ruptured aneurysms must be done on an emergency basis, and meticulous preparation of the skin cannot be ensured. Neurosurgical procedures after trauma occurring outside the hospital should never be included in comparative trials and would be considered contaminated surgery. Laminectomies (with or without the use of the operating microscope) are performed by orthopedic surgeons and neurosurgeons. Many studies include laminectomies and elective craniotomies in trials of clean neurosurgical procedures. The microscope introduces an additional source of potential contamination that should be considered. Laminectomies are addressed in this section and the orthopedic section.

Ventricular fluid-shunting procedures (ventriculo–peritoneal shunts), performed to control increased intracranial pressure in patients with hydrocephalus, have also been included in some clinical trials of clean neurosurgical procedures. Because this procedure involves the placement of a foreign body (pressure-release valve and tubing) in the cranium, another variable is introduced. Most infectious disease consultants believe that such shunting operations should be studied as a separate entity.[258] Ventricular fluid-shunting procedures are also performed after serious head trauma and in some elective craniotomy procedures to drain cerebrospinal fluid (CSF) and lower intracranial pressure. The drains are left in place for varying lengths of time, ranging from 48 hours to seven days.

Postoperative central nervous system (CNS) shunt infections are associated with serious morbidity and mortality. The rate of infection is generally reported as 5% to 20%.[259–261] Infections after surgery include meningitis, ventriculitis (most common infection), and, less frequently, wound infection.[258] In most cases, antimicrobial therapy without shunt removal is not effective in eradicating the infecting organism.[262–267] Therefore, shunt removal or replacement, in addition to intravenous antimicrobial therapy, is common practice.

Organisms. Data from most published clinical trials indicate that wound infections are primarily associated with gram-positive bacteria. *S. aureus* and coagulase-negative staphylococci are responsible for more than 85% of such infections and are isolated in mixed cultures with other gram-positive bacteria in an additional 5% to 10% of cases. Gram-negative bacteria are isolated as the sole cause of postoperative neurosurgical wound infections in only 5% to 8% of cases.[268–273] Therefore, most clinical trials of antimicrobial prophylaxis use a drug with primary activity against staphylococci: clindamycin, erythromycin, penicillinase-stable penicillins (oxacillin, nafcillin, and methicillin), first-generation cephalosporins, and vancomycin.

Staphylococci account for 75% to 80% of CNS and wound infections after shunting procedures. Gram-negative bacteria are responsible for only 10% to 20% of such infections.[261,274–281]

Efficacy for Clean Neurosurgical Procedures. Although the efficacy of antimicrobials in lowering postoperative wound infection rates after elective craniotomy and laminectomy has not been demonstrated in a pivotal clinical trial, a single dose of an antimicrobial effective against *S. aureus* can be recommended. The strongest evidence supporting prophylaxis is a meta-analysis of eight prospective, randomized, placebo-controlled trials in craniotomy patients.[282] The following data also support prophylaxis.

Studies, mostly published before 1980, of prophylactic antimicrobials in clean neurosurgery cases were uncontrolled, nonrandomized, and retrospective.[268,269,283–287] These studies seemed to favor some type of prophylactic regimen. In 1980, an excellent review of most of these studies concluded that a final recommendation regarding antimicrobial prophylaxis in clean neurosurgical procedures must await the results of controlled clinical trials.[288] A randomized, nonblinded, clinical trial involving 402 cases (including craniotomy and spinal operations) demonstrated the superiority of antimicrobial prophylaxis (vancomycin and gentamicin with a streptomycin irrigation during the surgical procedure) in preventing infections compared with controls.[271]

Prospective studies involving large numbers of patients have also demonstrated lower neurosurgical postoperative infection rates when antimicrobial prophylaxis is used.[270,289–291] One such study in craniotomy, spinal surgery, and shunting procedures was stopped early because of an excessive number of wound infections in the placebo group.[273]

Choice. In a blinded study, 826 patients undergoing clean neurological procedures were randomly assigned to receive either a single dose of ceftizoxime 2 g (as the sodium) or a combination of a single dose of vancomycin 1 g (as the hydrochloride) and gentamicin 80 mg (as the sulfate).[292] Patients undergoing cranial, spinal, or transphenoidal neurosurgical procedures who were not undergoing placement of a shunt or another foreign body were included. The rate of primary and secondary wound infections was not different between the treatment groups. Ceftizoxime was better tolerated than the vancomycin–gentamicin combination. CSF and blood samples were obtained from 19 craniotomy patients. Ceftizoxime and gentamicin were detectable in all samples. Vancomycin was detectable in the serum in all cases but was undetectable in some CSF samples. The researchers concluded that ceftizoxime is as effective as the combination of gentamicin and vancomycin but is less toxic and has better CSF penetration.

A meta-analysis also did not demonstrate a significant difference between antimicrobial regimens.[282]

Duration. A meta-analysis did not demonstrate a significant difference between single-dose and multi-dose regimens for clean neurosurgical procedures.[282]

Pediatric Efficacy for Clean Neurosurgical Procedures. A randomized, placebo-controlled, double-blind trial that included pediatric patients undergoing clean neurosurgical procedures was stopped prematurely because of an excessive number of wound infections in the placebo group.[273] The overall rate of infection was 2.8% in the antimicrobial group and 11.7% in the placebo group.

Efficacy for CSF-Shunting Procedures. Because CNS infections after shunting procedures are responsible for substantial mortality and morbidity, especially in children, the possible role of prophylactic antimicrobials in such procedures has been the subject of numerous small, but well-conducted, randomized, controlled trials.[293–300] Meticulous surgical and aseptic technique and short operation time were determined to be important factors in lowering infection rates after shunt placement. Although the number of patients studied in each trial was small, two meta-analyses of the data demonstrated that the use of antimicrobial prophylaxis in CSF-shunting procedures reduces the risk of infection by approximately 50%.[301,302]

Choice. Because no antimicrobial has been demonstrated to have greater efficacy over the others for CSF-shunting procedures, a single dose of cefazolin appears to be the best choice.

Duration. In most studies, prophylaxis was continued for 24 to 48 hours postoperatively, but regimens of different durations were not compared for efficacy. There is a lack of data evaluating the continuation of extraventricular drains with and without antimicrobial prophylaxis.

Pediatric Efficacy for CSF-Shunting Procedures. A retrospective pediatric study of 1201 CSF-shunting procedures failed to demonstrate a significant difference in infection rates between patients who received antimicrobials (2.1%) and those who did not receive antimicrobials (5.6%). Two randomized, prospective studies that included pediatric patients did not demonstrate a significant difference in infection rates between the control group and the groups that received cefotiam[300] or methicillin.[297] A randomized, double-blind, placebo-controlled study that included pediatric patients undergoing ventriculoperitoneal shunt surgeries failed to demonstrate that the use of perioperative sulfamethoxazole–trimethoprim reduced the frequency of shunt infection.[293]

Other studies have demonstrated efficacy for prophylactic antimicrobials.[295,303] A single-center, randomized, double-blind, placebo-controlled trial of perioperative rifampin plus trimethoprim was performed in pediatric patients.[303] Among patients receiving rifampin plus trimethoprim, the infection rate was 12%, compared with 19% in patients receiving placebo. The study was ended (because of the high infection rates) before significance could be achieved. Infection rates at the study institution had been 7.5% in the years before the study. An open randomized study institution that included pediatric patients demonstrated a lower infection rate in a group receiving oxacillin (3.3%) than in a control group (20%).[295]

Recommendation. A single dose of cefazolin 1 g (as the sodium) intravenously at induction of anesthesia is recommended for patients undergoing clean neurosurgical procedures or CSF-shunting procedures. Alternatively, a single intravenous dose of one of the β-lactamase-stable penicillins might be used (oxacillin 1 g [as the sodium] or nafcillin 1 g [as the sodium]). Vancomycin 1 g (as the hydrochloride) intravenously over one hour should be reserved as an alternative on the basis of previously outlined guidelines from HICPAC.[21] (Strength of evidence for prophylaxis for clean neurosurgical procedures = A.) (Strength of evidence for prophylaxis for CSF-shunting procedures = A.)

Pediatric Dosage. The recommended regimen for pediatric patients undergoing clean neurosurgical procedures or CSF-shunting procedures is a single dose of cefazolin 20–30 mg/kg (as the sodium) intravenously at induction of anesthesia. Vancomycin 15 mg/kg (as the hydrochloride) intravenously should be reserved as an alternative on the basis of previously outlined guidelines from HICPAC.[21,32]

Cesarean Delivery

Background. Approximately 1 million infants are born by cesarean delivery in the United States annually.[304] The rate of cesarean delivery has risen from 5% to 25% over the past two decades.[305] Postpartum infectious complications are common after cesarean delivery. Endometritis (infection of the uterine lining) is usually identified by uterine tenderness and sometimes abnormal or foul-smelling lochia. Wound infection is usually defined as the presence of pus at the incision site. Although febrile morbidity, or temperature elevation in an asymptomatic patient, is often considered in evaluations of antimicrobial prophylaxis, it appears that this temperature elevation is often not associated with an identifiable infectious source or with symptoms specific for infection. It may occur in women with normal physical examination results and sometimes disappears without treatment. In controlled trials, increased temperature occurred with equal frequency in placebo and treatment groups.[306,307] Moreover, women with febrile morbidity appear not to be those who later develop clinical infection. The presence or absence of febrile morbidity is not an appropriate indication of the efficacy of antimicrobial prophylaxis and therefore will not be considered in these guidelines.

Endometritis has been reported to occur in up to 85% of patients in high-risk populations.[308] High-risk patients are defined as women who have not received prenatal care; who are poorly nourished; who have prolonged labor, especially in the presence of ruptured membranes; or who have undergone multiple vaginal examinations or frequent invasive monitoring. A majority of these women are of lower socioeconomic status. In contrast, women in upper or middle socioeconomic populations, who tend to be better nourished and to have received appropriate prenatal care, are at lower risk; the postpartum rate of endometritis in these patients ranges from 5% to 15%.

The factor most frequently associated with infectious morbidity in postcesarean delivery is prolonged labor in the presence of ruptured membranes. Intact chorioamniotic membranes serve as a protective barrier against bacterial infection. Rupture of the membrane exposes the uterine surface to bacteria from the birth canal. The vaginal fluid with its bacterial flora is drawn up into the uterus when it relaxes between contractions during labor. Women undergoing labor for six to eight hours or longer in the presence of ruptured membranes should be considered at high risk for developing endometritis.[306] Other risk factors include systemic illness, poor hygiene, obesity, and anemia.

Organisms. The natural microflora of the vaginal tract are often involved in endometritis and include various aerobic and anaerobic streptococci, enterococci, staphylococci, enteric gram-negative bacilli, and anaerobic gram-negative bacteria such as *Bacteroides bivius, B. fragilis,* and *Fusobacterium* species.[306] In contrast, the organisms causing wound infections after delivery most often are *S. aureus* and other staphylococci, streptococci, and Enterobacteriaceae. Anaerobes are also present but less commonly than with endometritis.[309]

Efficacy. Most investigations of the efficacy of prophylactic antimicrobials in cesarean delivery have been conducted in high-risk patients. There has been considerable controversy about the necessity for prophylaxis in low-risk women undergoing cesarean delivery.

Despite multiple clinical trials assessing the efficacy of broad-spectrum antimicrobials or multiple doses of antimicrobials for prophylaxis in cesarean delivery, the data support the use of narrow-spectrum agents, such as first-generation cephalosporins, administered as a single dose intravenously immediately after clamping of the umbilical cord.[310,311]

Low-risk patients. Two early investigations showed significantly lower rates of postcesarean endometritis in low-risk patients with the use of prophylactic antimicrobials.[312,313] Some authorities have dismissed these benefits, arguing that limited morbidity, theoretical risks, and excessive costs do not justify prophylaxis in these patients.[314]

A randomized, prospective study compared the use of a 1-g dose of cefazolin (as the sodium) with no prophylaxis in 307 low-risk patients undergoing cesarean delivery.[315] The outcomes investigated were endometritis, wound infection, febrile morbidity, and use of antimicrobials for presumed or confirmed infection. The study showed significantly lower febrile morbidity and therapeutic antimicrobial use in the treatment group, although the sample was not large enough to enable a significant reduction in endometritis and wound infection to be detected.

A large-scale prospective study in more than 1800 low-risk women who underwent cesarean delivery was conducted from 1980 to 1982.[316] Although prophylaxis was uncontrolled for, endometritis and wound infection rates were significantly lower (0.7% and 0.2%, respectively in the group receiving prophylaxis than the group not receiving prophylaxis (2.1% and 2%, respectively). A case–control study, including the prospective data and women at high risk, determined that patients undergoing a first-time cesarean delivery were five times more likely to develop endometritis than those who had had a cesarean delivery in the past. On the basis of certain assumptions, the investigators calculated that more than $9 million could be saved annually by administering prophylaxis to low-risk patients. The cost of adverse effects was considered negligible. Thus, antimicrobial prophylaxis may be appropriate for low-risk cesarean deliveries.

However, ACOG considers the use of prophylaxis to be controversial in low-risk patients.[33] ACOG does not routinely recommend prophylaxis in low-risk patients because of concerns about adverse effects, development of resistant organisms, and relaxation of standard infection-control measures and proper operative technique.

High-risk patients. There have been more than 40 placebo-controlled, prospective trials evaluating the efficacy of prophylactic antimicrobials in cesarean delivery, most of which have been carried out in high-risk populations. A meta-analysis of these data, which combined high- and low-risk patients undergoing both emergency and elective cesarean deliveries, suggests that the rate of serious infections and endometritis is 75% lower and the rate of wound infections 65% lower among antimicrobial-treated patients than control patients.[317]

Choice. Although more than 20 different drugs have been used alone or in combination for antimicrobial prophylaxis during cesarean delivery, most obstetricians currently use either a penicillin or a cephalosporin.[318] ACOG recommends a first-generation cephalosporin, with extended-spectrum agents reserved for treatment rather than prophylaxis.[33]

In a large-scale study involving more than 1600 high-risk patients, several single-dose regimens, including cefazolin 2 g (as the sodium) or piperacillin 4 g (as the sodium), were comparably effective.[319] This provides two disparate choices, with drugs that offer differing spectra of activity with roughly equivalent efficacy. Two large-scale, randomized, double-blind trials offer a potential solution to this dilemma.[320,321] Both studies involved hundreds of high-risk patients and compared cefazolin, which has poor *Bacteroides* coverage, with cefoxitin or moxalactam, which has excellent *Bacteroids* coverage. In both studies, cefoxitin and moxalactam were slightly less effective than cefazolin in preventing endometritis, although the differences did not reach significance.

In another study of nearly 350 high-risk women undergoing cesarean delivery, a two-dose regimen of cefoxitin or piperacillin was given starting immediately after the cord was clamped.[322] Despite its superior in vitro activity against enterococci, *P. aeruginosa,* and several enteric gram-negative bacillary species, piperacillin was found to be no more effective than cefoxitin.

Timing. Unlike other surgical procedures for which antimicrobials are ideally administered just before incision, administration of antimicrobials in cesarean delivery is usually delayed until after cord clamping. This is done principally to avoid suppression of the infant's normal bacterial flora. Although toxicity in the infant is of potential concern, a majority of drugs used for this procedure (primarily β-lactams) have a documented record of safety in the treatment of infections during pregnancy, and many are used in the treatment of neonatal sepsis. ACOG and the American Academy of Pediatrics recommend administration of prophylactic antimicrobials after cord clamping.[33,34]

The issue of timing was addressed in three controlled trials. A large, randomized trial in 642 women undergoing cesarean delivery[49] and a smaller randomized, placebo-controlled study[48] demonstrated no difference in infectious complications, regardless of whether the antimicrobials were given preoperatively or after the cord was clamped. In the larger study, infants who were not exposed to antimicrobial agents in utero required significantly fewer evaluations for neonatal sepsis. A third case–control study demonstrated that a second- or third-generation cephalosporin given before incision was superior to cefazolin given as three 1-g doses starting immediately after cord clamping.[323] Thus, antimicrobials provide effective prophylaxis, even when given after clamping of the umbilical cord.[49]

Duration. Most recent trials of antimicrobial prophylaxis for cesarean delivery have assessed the efficacy of a single dose versus multiple doses (usually up to 24 hours). Early studies used regimens that lasted as long as five or six days. Two prospective, randomized studies found that a five-day course of a cephalosporin was no more efficacious than a 24-hour

course.[324,325] A third study, by contrast, found that a three-day course of ampicillin was significantly more effective than three doses of ampicillin.[326] The explanation for this difference is unclear. The efficacy of several types of β-lactam antimicrobials given in various regimens to nearly 1600 patients was assessed in an open, randomized, comparative study.[319] One group of patients was given three doses of cefazolin, and the two other groups received a single dose of cefazolin, either 1 or 2 g (as the sodium). One dose of cefazolin 2 g was superior to three doses of cefazolin 1 g. One dose of cefazolin 1 g was no different than three doses of cefazolin 1 g. It does not seem necessary to extend prophylaxis beyond a single dose. These data also suggest that cefazolin 2 g is more efficacious than cefazolin 1 g.

Pediatric Efficacy. No well-controlled studies have evaluated the effect of antimicrobial prophylaxis for low- or high-risk adolescents undergoing cesarean delivery.

Recommendation. The recommended regimen for all women (low and high risk) undergoing cesarean delivery is a single dose of cefazolin 2 g (as the sodium) intravenously immediately after clamping of the umbilical cord. (Strength of evidence for prophylaxis for low-risk women = B.) (Strength of evidence for prophylaxis for high-risk women = A.)

Pediatric Dosage. The recommended regimen for low- and high-risk adolescents undergoing cesarean delivery is a single dose of cefazolin 2 g (as the sodium) intravenously immediately after clamping of the umbilical cord.

Hysterectomy

Background. Hysterectomy is second only to cesarean delivery as the most frequently performed major gynecologic operation in the United States, with approximately 590,000 hysterectomies being performed annually. Although there appears to be a downward trend in the rate since the mid-1980s, it is not yet known whether a true decline has occurred because of recent changes in the National Hospital Discharge Survey sampling method.[327]

Uterine fibroid tumors account for 30% of all presurgical diagnoses leading to hysterectomy; other common diagnoses are dysfunctional uterine bleeding, genital prolapse, endometriosis, chronic pelvic pain, pelvic inflammatory disease, endometrial hyperplasia, and cancer.[327] The proportion of patients undergoing concurrent unilateral or bilateral oophorectomy increases with age; this procedure is performed in approximately two thirds of women over the age of 60 years who undergo hysterectomy.[309]

Hysterectomy may be performed by a transvaginal or transabdominal approach. During a vaginal hysterectomy, the uterus and, occasionally, one or two fallopian tubes, the ovaries, or a combination of ovaries and fallopian tubes are removed through the vagina. No abdominal incision is made. Because the procedure is performed in an organ that is normally colonized with bacteria, it is associated with a high risk of postoperative infection. Abdominal hysterectomy involves removal of the uterus and, in some cases, one or both fallopian tubes, the ovaries, or a combination of ovaries and fallopian tubes. Because bacterial contamination associated with this procedure is minimal, postoperative infection rates in women receiving no antimicrobial prophylaxis have often been lower than those in women undergoing vaginal hysterectomy.[328–333] Radical hysterectomy, which entails removal of the uterus, fallopian tubes, and ovaries and extensive

stripping of the pelvic lymph nodes, is performed in patients with extension of cervical cancer. Many factors increase the risk of postoperative infection. Nonetheless, because of the low rate of contamination associated with this procedure, the need for prophylaxis has not been established.

Infections after hysterectomy include operative site infections: vaginal cuff infection, pelvic cellulitis, and pelvic abscess. Wound infections are usually diagnosed by the presence of pus or a purulent discharge.[307]

Risk factors for infection after vaginal or abdominal hysterectomy include longer duration of surgery, young age, diabetes, obesity, peripheral vascular disease, collagen disease, anemia, poor nutritional status, and previous history of postsurgical infection.[309,328,334,335] The depth of subcutaneous tissue is also a significant risk factor for transabdominal hysterectomy.[336] Factors that increase the risk of postoperative infection in women undergoing radical hysterectomy for cervical cancer include extended length of surgery, blood loss and replacement, presence of malignancy, prior radiation therapy, obesity, and presence of indwelling drainage catheters.[337,338]

Organisms. The vagina is normally colonized with a wide variety of bacteria, including gram-positive and gram-negative aerobes and anaerobes. The normal flora of the vagina include staphylococci, streptococci, enterococci, lactobacilli, diphtheroids, *E. coli*, anaerobic streptococci, *Bacteroides* species, and *Fusobacterium* species.[307,339] Postoperative vaginal flora differ from preoperative flora; enterococci, gram-negative bacilli, and *Bacteroides* species increase postoperatively. Postoperative changes in flora may occur independently of prophylactic antimicrobial administration and are not by themselves predictive of postoperative infection.[307,340,341] Postoperative infections associated with vaginal hysterectomy are frequently polymicrobial; enterococci, aerobic gram-negative bacilli, and *Bacteroides* species are isolated most frequently. Postoperative wound infections after abdominal and radical hysterectomy are also polymicrobial; gram-positive cocci and enteric gram-negative bacilli predominate, and anaerobes are also frequently isolated.[341,342]

Efficacy for Vaginal Hysterectomy. The rate of postoperative infection (wound and pelvic sites) in women administered placebo or no prophylactic antimicrobials ranges from 14% to 57%.[328–333,335,340,343–354] A number of antimicrobial agents, including clindamycin,[355] metronidazole,[331,354,356,357] penicillins,[307,345,353,355,357–360] ampicillin,[345,361,362] tetracycline derivatives,[333,352,363] streptomycin,[345] and first-generation,[328–330,344,347,351,353,356,358,360,361,364–367] second-generation,[307,349,350,357–359,363] and third-generation[355,367] cephalosporins have been studied as perioperative prophylaxis for vaginal hysterectomy. Overall, the use of antimicrobials markedly reduces the frequency of postoperative infection after vaginal hysterectomy to a generally acceptable rate of less than 10%.

Choice. Cephalosporins are the most frequently used antimicrobials for prophylaxis in vaginal hysterectomy. Cefazolin is the drug of choice. Cefazolin has been associated with postoperative infection rates ranging from 0% to 12%.[346,347,351,368–370] Postoperative infection rates with various second- and third-generation cephalosporins have ranged between 0% and 16%.[349,350,355,357–359,363,371] Studies directly comparing different cephalosporins have shown no significant differences in rates of infection.[372–381] Studies directly comparing the first-generation cephalosporins with second- or third-generation cephalosporins indicate that

first-generation cephalosporins (primarily cefazolin) are equivalent to second- and third-generation agents.[367-370,382]

In light of the organisms encountered in the vaginal canal and comparative studies conducted among different classes of cephalosporins, the expert panel considers cefazolin and cefotetan appropriate first-line choices for prophylaxis during vaginal hysterectomy and cefoxitin a suitable alternative. The ACOG guidelines support the use of a first-, second-, or third-generation cephalosporin for prophylaxis.[383]

Duration. The trend in recent years has been toward use of single-dose regimens of antimicrobials, administered immediately before surgery. Studies comparing single doses of one antimicrobial with multidose regimens of a different antimicrobial have shown the two regimens to be equally effective.[346,356,363,368-371,373-379,384-392] Although there have been few comparative trials involving single-dose cefazolin,[346,370] clinical experience indicates that this regimen is effective for most women. In addition, the drug's relatively long serum half-life (1.8 hours) suggests that a single dose would be sufficient. The exception is when the procedure lasts three hours or longer or if blood loss exceeds 1500 mL, in which case a second dose is warranted.

Efficacy for Abdominal Hysterectomy. At least 25 placebo-controlled or nonantimicrobial-controlled studies involving abdominal hysterectomy have been performed.[328-333,342,347, 348,351-354,360,393-403] First- and second-generation cephalosporins and metronidazole have been studied more widely than any other agents. A meta-analysis of 25 controlled, randomized trials demonstrated the efficacy of antimicrobial prophylaxis with any of these agents in the prevention of postoperative infections.[404] The infection rate was 21.1% with placebo or no prophylaxis and 9.0% with any antimicrobial. Cefazolin was significantly more effective than placebo or no prophylaxis, with an infection rate of 11.4%.

Choice. Studies comparing second-generation cephalosporins and comparing second- and third-generation cephalosporin regimens have not shown significant differences in rates of serious infections.[376,387-392,405-407] Few comparisons have been made between second-generation cephalosporins and cefazolin. Cefazolin has been at least as effective in preventing infectious complications as third-generation cephalosporins.[369,384,399,408] However, in one double-blind, controlled study, the risk of major operative site infection requiring antimicrobial therapy was significantly higher with cefazolin (11.6%; relative risk, 1.84; 95% confidence interval, 1.03–3.29) than with cefotetan (6.3%).[334] A total of 511 women undergoing abdominal hysterectomy participated in this study and received a single dose of cefazolin 1 g (as the sodium) or cefotetan 1 g (as the disodium).

In light of the organisms involved in infectious complications from abdominal hysterectomy and the lack of superior efficacy demonstrated in comparative trials, the expert panel considers cefazolin or cefotetan an appropriate choice for prophylaxis and cefoxitin a suitable alternative. The ACOG guidelines state that first-, second-, and third-generation cephalosporins can be used for prophylaxis.[383]

Duration. A 24-hour antimicrobial regimen has been shown to be as effective as longer courses of prophylaxis for abdominal hysterectomy,[400,409] and many single-dose prophylaxis regimens have proved as effective as multidose regimens.[369,371,376,385,387-392,410] Single doses of cefotetan, ceftizoxime, or cefotaxime appear to be as effective as multiple doses of cefoxitin.[380,387,388,390-392,406]

Efficacy for Radical Hysterectomy. Six small prospective, placebo-controlled trials evaluated the impact of antimicrobial prophylaxis on wound infection rates after radical hysterectomy.[337,411-414] Rates of infection in the placebo groups ranged from 17% to 87%. In all six trials, the frequency of postoperative infection was lower with antimicrobial prophylaxis. Infection rates in antimicrobial-treated patients ranged from 0% to 64% (but generally from 0% to 15%). The antimicrobial agents used were cefoxitin, cefamandole, mezlocillin, and doxycycline. In one study in which cefamandole was given by injection and by intraperitoneal irrigation, postoperative infection rates were less than 4%.[411]

Choice. There is a lack of data comparing first- and second-generation cephalosporins. The optimal choice for prophylaxis has not been determined, but second-generation cephalosporins have demonstrated efficacy.[337,411,413] Because similar approaches are used in abdominal and radical hysterectomy and in light of the results of a recent study (described in Efficacy for abdominal hysterectomy),[334] a single dose of cefotetan may be applicable to radical hysterectomy procedures.

Appropriate cephalosporins identified by the expert panel members are cefazolin and cefotetan; an alternative is cefoxitin. The ACOG guidelines state that first-, second-, and third-generation cephalosporins can be used for prophylaxis.[383]

Duration. The optimal duration of antimicrobial prophylaxis for radical hysterectomy has not been established. The duration of prophylaxis ranged from one dose[414] to four days.[337,413] A 24-hour regimen of mezlocillin appears to be as effective as other antimicrobial regimens of longer duration.[412] A prospective, randomized study demonstrated no difference between a single dose of piperacillin plus tinidazole and a multidose (three-dose) regimen of the two drugs.[415]

Pediatric Efficacy. No well-controlled studies have evaluated the efficacy of antimicrobial prophylaxis in adolescents undergoing vaginal, abdominal, or radical hysterectomy.

Recommendation. The recommended regimen for women undergoing vaginal hysterectomy, abdominal hysterectomy, or radical hysterectomy is a single intravenous dose of cefazolin 1 g (as the sodium) or cefotetan 1 g (as the di-sodium) at induction of anesthesia. An alternative is cefoxitin 1 g (as the sodium) intravenously at induction of anesthesia. (Strength of evidence for prophylaxis for vaginal hysterectomy = A.) (Strength of evidence for prophylaxis for abdominal hysterectomy = A.) (Strength of evidence for prophylaxis for radical hysterectomy = A.)

Pediatric Dosage. The recommended regimen for adolescent women undergoing vaginal hysterectomy, abdominal hysterectomy, or radical hysterectomy is a single dose of cefazolin 1 g (as the sodium) or cefotetan 1 g (as the disodium) intravenously at induction of anesthesia. An alternative is cefoxitin 1 g (as the sodium) intravenously at induction of anesthesia.

Ophthalmic Surgeries

Background. Ophthalmic procedures include cataract extractions, vitrectomies, keratoplasties, implants, glaucoma operations, strabotomies, and retinal detachment repair. Most of the available studies involve cataract procedures.[416-427]

There is a low rate of postoperative ophthalmic infection (bacterial endophthalmitis),[417,418,424,428] but this is a devastating complication that may lead to an early loss of light sense and eventual loss of the eye if the infection is not eradicated.[420,424,425] Possible risk factors for developing postoperative ophthalmic infections include poor surgical technique, "weak ocular tissue" (not defined by the author), and multiple ophthalmic operations.[420] The duration of follow-up in studies that determined the postoperative endophthalmitis rate ranged from less than one week to 12 days[416,421,424,429]; 97% of cases of postoperative endophthalmitis occurred within the first 7 days of the 12-day follow-up period.[416] However, the appropriate duration of follow-up is not established.

Organisms. Approximately 90% of postoperative ophthalmic infections are caused by *S. aureus* or *S. epidermidis.*[420,425,430] The other organisms identified are *Streptococcus pneumoniae, Acinetobacter* species, and *P. aeruginosa.*[430] Virulent pathogens such as *P. aeruginosa, Bacillus cereus,* and *S. aureus* can cause eye destruction within 24 hours.[431]

Efficacy. Numerous studies have evaluated the effectiveness of prophylactic regimens in eradicating bacteria and reducing bacterial count on the conjunctivas, lower eyelid, eyelashes, and inner canthus (corner of the eye) preoperatively and postoperatively. There is a lack of controlled trials in the literature. The following studies had many flaws, including retrospective or uncontrolled design, inadequate follow-up, lack of confirmation of infection with cultures, difficulties in distinguishing between bacterial endophthalmitis and aseptic postoperative inflammation, inadequate aseptic surgical techniques, and inadequate preoperative and postoperative care.

Studies have shown that topical antimicrobials reduce ocular flora.[419,421,422,425,427] The studies evaluating bacteria eradication do not provide definitive antimicrobial choices, dosages, or duration of treatment because elimination of ophthalmic flora does not equate with a lower rate of infections. Although up to 95% of eye cultures are positive, few develop into infections.[420–422,425] Ciprofloxacin, norfloxacin, and ofloxacin have demonstrated antibacterial activity against organisms (staphylococcal and gram-negative organisms, in particular *Pseudomonas* species) that cause postoperative endophthalmitis,[432–435] but they cannot be recommended because of a lack of trials using fluoroquinolones prophylactically.

Choice. There have been no controlled efficacy studies supporting a particular choice of antimicrobial prophylaxis for ophthalmic surgeries. Because of the very low rate of infections (0.05% to 0.82%),[416–418,424,428,436] an enormous patient population would be required to allow determination of the most effective antimicrobial. The most efficacious antimicrobial cannot be determined from the available data because of study flaws.

A series of 16,000 cataract-extraction procedures demonstrated an infection rate of 0.6% (6 infections per 1,000 cases) with the use of an ointment containing neomycin 0.5% (as the sulfate), polymyxin B 0.1% (as the sulfate), and erythromycin 0.5% compared with 0.02% (3 infections per 15,000 cases) with the use of an ointment containing chloramphenicol 0.4%, polymyxin B 0.1% (as the sulfate), and erythromycin 0.5%.[417] Although these infection rates appear to favor chloramphenicol over neomycin, the superiority of chloramphenicol cannot be concluded because of limitations in the study design.

An open-label, nonrandomized, parallel trial demonstrated a lower rate of culture-proven endophthalmitis (0.06%) in a suite of operating rooms that used povidone-iodine preparation than in a similar suite that used topical silver protein solution (0.24%).[436] The intraocular procedures included vitrectomy, extracapsular cataract extraction, phacoemulsifications, secondary intraocular lens procedure, trabeculectomy, and penetrating keratoplasty. Recommendations cannot be made for the use of povidone-iodine as a single agent because of limitations of the study design (open-label, nonrandomized, without placebo control) and the surgeon's continued use of "customary" prophylactic antimicrobials (not identified) before, during, and after the procedure.

Prophylactic antimicrobials were administered during alternating cases in a series of 974 patients undergoing cataract extraction, glaucoma operations, corneal transplant, and pupillary membrane needling.[424] The prophylactic antimicrobial regimen was a subconjunctival combination of penicillin G 100,000 units and 3.3% streptomycin. There were seven postoperative infections (1.4%) among patients who had not received antimicrobials, compared with one infection (0.2%) among patients who received subconjunctival antimicrobials. In a follow-up series in which antimicrobials were used routinely in 1480 consecutive cases, the rate of infection was 0.14%. Organisms causing the postoperative infections in patients who received prophylactic antimicrobials were penicillin- and streptomycin-resistant *Proteus vulgaris* and *P. aeruginosa* and penicillin-sensitive *S. aureus* in a penicillin-allergic patient who received subconjunctival streptomycin only.

Route. The most often studied routes of administration are preoperative topical application and perioperative subconjunctival injection. Human data directly comparing administration routes have not been reported. Animal data demonstrated that topical application was highly effective in eliminating *Staphylococcus* and *Pseudomonas* species from the cornea but that antimicrobials administered periocularly or by intravenous injection did not significantly reduce the number of *Staphylococcus* or *Pseudomonas* organisms in the cornea.[437] Local reactions during the early postoperative period have been reported more frequently in eyes receiving subconjunctival antimicrobials than those in which no antimicrobials were used. These reactions, consisting of conjunctival hyperemia and chemosis (chemical action transmitted through a membrane) at the site of injection, usually subsided within two to four days. No systemic or serious local effects from the injections were reported.[424] Subconjunctival injections have been administered perioperatively or postoperatively because of the practicality of administering ophthalmic injections in a sedated and anesthetized patient. The ideal circumstance would be subconjunctival administration preoperatively once anesthesia is induced.

A concurrent series of 6618 patients undergoing cataract extraction were randomly assigned to receive periocular penicillin G 500,000 units or no periocular injection.[429] All patients were administered topical antimicrobials: chloramphenicol 0.5% and sulfamethazine 10% 15 to 20 hours before surgery, an unidentified ophthalmic antimicrobial ointment the day before surgery, polymyxin B 5000 units/mL (as the sulfate) and neomycin 2.5 mg/mL (as the sulfate) at the end of the procedure, an unidentified ophthalmic antimicrobial ointment the first day postoperatively, and sulfamethazine 5% solution for approximately another six days postoperatively starting the second postoperative day. The infection

rate was 0.15% with the combination of topical antimicrobials and periocular penicillin, compared with 0.45% with only topical antimicrobials. Other routes, including intraocular antimicrobials and antimicrobial-soaked collagen shields,[438] are not widely accepted at this time because of the lack of safety and efficacy data. Topical only is the most common route of administration because of ease of administration, lack of complications, high efficacy in eliminating bacterial flora, and low cost.

Duration and timing. The available data do not specifically address duration and timing of antimicrobial administration. In studies to determine infection rates, the duration of preoperative antimicrobials ranged from one to five days. Postoperative topical antimicrobial regimens ranged from no postoperative antimicrobials to administration of antimicrobials until the time of patient discharge (approximately seven days).[416,424,429] The following data may provide some guidance. A series of 2508 cataract extraction procedures demonstrated that penicillin ophthalmic ointment had to be applied every two to three hours for three to eight days to eliminate pathogenic staphylococci from the conjunctiva and the eyelids.[425] Two consecutive patient groups undergoing open lacrimal surgery were retrospectively reviewed.[439] Both groups received topical antimicrobial drops (not further defined). The infection rate was 1.6% (2 of 128 patients) in the group that received postoperative antimicrobials and 7.9% (12 of 152 patients) in the group that did not receive postoperative antimicrobials. The study was not designed to determine the best postoperative antimicrobial, but, in a majority of cases, cephalexin 250 mg orally four times daily for five days was used. Although this study demonstrated a fivefold lower rate of infection with postoperative antimicrobials, recommendations for postoperative antimicrobial prophylaxis cannot be made until controlled studies are performed. Duration and timing cannot be extrapolated from general surgery (nonophthalmic) data because of the lack of data on antimicrobial pharmacokinetics in the eye (e.g., duration, distribution, and elimination from the aqueous humor). Recommendations on timing and duration are based solely on expert opinion.

Despite the lack of well-controlled trials, the consequences of bacterial endophthalmitis support the use of prophylactic antimicrobials. No definitive studies have delineated superiority of antimicrobial route, timing, or duration. The suggested antimicrobials are relatively similar in cost.

Pediatric Efficacy. No well-controlled studies have evaluated the efficacy of antimicrobial prophylaxis in pediatric patients undergoing ophthalmic surgery.

Recommendation. The prophylactic antimicrobials used in ophthalmic procedures should provide coverage against *Staphylococcus* species and gram-negative organisms, in particular *Pseudomonas* species. The necessity of continuing topical antimicrobials postoperatively has not been established. The frequency of administration is based on usual treatment regimens.

Antimicrobials that are appropriate include commercially available neomycin–polymyxin B–gramicidin solution one or two drops topically and tobramycin 0.3% or gentamicin 0.3% solution two drops topically before the procedure. Continuation of antimicrobials postoperatively is not supported by data. Addition of a subconjunctival antimicrobial, tobramycin 20 mg (as the sulfate), is optional. (Strength of evidence for prophylaxis = C.)

Pediatric Dosage. The recommendations for the use of topical antimicrobials in pediatric patients undergoing ophthalmic procedures are the same as for adults. Subconjunctival tobramycin cannot be recommended because there is a lack of pediatric data and dosages cannot be extrapolated from the insufficient adult data.

Orthopedics

Background. Antimicrobial prophylaxis will be discussed for total joint-replacement surgery, repair of hip fractures, implantation of internal fixation devices (screws, nails, plates, and pins), and clean orthopedic procedures (not involving replacement or implantations). Open (compound) fractures are often associated with extensive wound contamination and are virtually always managed with empirical antimicrobial therapy and surgical debridement. This practice is viewed as treatment rather than prophylaxis.[440] Although antimicrobials are given to patients with prosthetic joints who undergo dental procedures to reduce the likelihood of prosthesis infection,[441] this practice has not been sufficiently studied and is beyond the scope of these guidelines.

Postoperative wound infection is one of the more frequent complications of orthopedic surgery, and it often has devastating results,[442] frequently requiring removal of the implanted hardware and a prolonged course of antimicrobials for cure. Although early studies did not support the routine use of prophylactic antimicrobials,[443,444] these studies were flawed by an improper choice of agent(s), inappropriate dosage or route of administration, or failure to institute therapy until well beyond the time of the initial surgical incision. Later work has established that antimicrobial prophylaxis is indicated in some types of orthopedic procedures.[442,445–452]

Organisms. Organisms that make up the skin flora are the most frequent causes of postoperative infections in orthopedic surgery. The pathogens involved in total joint replacement are *S. epidermidis* (40% of infected patients), *S. aureus* (35%), gram-negative bacilli (15%), anaerobes (5%), and others (5%).[24]

Clean Orthopedic Procedures Not Involving Implantation of Foreign Materials

Background. The need for antimicrobial prophylaxis in clean orthopedic procedures is not well established.[452,453] Included in this category are knee, hand, and foot surgeries and laminectomy with and without fusion. These procedures do not normally involve the implantation of foreign materials. The evaluated data do not include arthroscopy procedures and do not identify specific procedures, like carpal tunnel release; however, arthroscopy and other procedures not involving implantation are similar enough to be included with clean orthopedic procedures not involving implantation. The risks of wound infection and long-term sequelae are quite low for procedures not involving implantation. The duration of procedures may be a risk factor, with longer procedures having higher infection rates; the difference was significant in one study[453] but not in another.[452] Neither study formally evaluated procedures performed on the feet of patients with diabetes. Diabetic patients are at a higher risk for infection, and their infections are typically polymicrobial;

therefore, recommendations for procedures performed on the feet of patients with diabetes cannot be extrapolated from the following efficacy data.

Efficacy. The most extensive investigation of the efficacy of antimicrobial prophylaxis in clean orthopedic procedures was performed in the early 1970s.[452] In a randomized, double-blind, prospective study, the efficacy of cephaloridine was compared with that of placebo in reducing postoperative wound infection in more than 1500 patients undergoing clean orthopedic procedures (internal fixation device involvement was not identified). Infection rates for the two groups differed significantly: 5% with placebo and 2.8% with perioperative cephaloridine. Drug fever (loosely defined as fever occurring on the day the study drug was administered) was noted in 34 antimicrobial-treated patients and 14 placebo recipients.

Given the small difference in infection rates between groups and the lack of serious long-term sequelae from postoperative infections associated with these procedures, many authorities have questioned the need for antimicrobial prophylaxis. Attempts to correlate infection rate with the type of clean orthopedic procedure or with certain patient characteristics (e.g., age, disease) have been unsuccessful. Although one study demonstrated that prophylaxis with cefamandole was more effective than placebo when procedures were longer than two hours, prophylaxis was not more effective than placebo in procedures shorter than two hours.[453] These results were not consistent with those of the previously discussed study,[452] whose series was much larger and failed to demonstrate a difference in infection rates with procedures lasting longer than two hours.

The low rate of infection, coupled with the absence of serious morbidity as a consequence of postoperative infection, does not justify the expense or potential for toxicity and resistance associated with routine use of antimicrobial prophylaxis in this setting.

Pediatric Efficacy. No well-controlled studies have evaluated the efficacy of antimicrobial prophylaxis in pediatric patients undergoing clean orthopedic procedures.

Recommendation. Antimicrobial prophylaxis is not recommended for patients undergoing clean orthopedic procedures not involving implantation of foreign materials. (Strength of evidence against prophylaxis = C.)

Pediatric Dosage. Antimicrobial prophylaxis is not recommended for pediatric patients undergoing clean orthopedic procedures not involving implantation of foreign materials.

Hip Fracture Repair and Other Orthopedic Procedures Involving the Implantation of Internal Fixation Devices

Background. Data support the use of antimicrobial prophylaxis for hip fracture repairs. In contrast, there is a lack of data to support the use of prophylaxis for procedures other than hip fracture repairs that involve the implantation of internal fixation devices (e.g., high tibial osteotomy and ligament reconstruction). When internal fixation procedures involve the implantation of foreign bodies such as nails, screws, plates, and wires, postoperative infection can produce extensive morbidity—prolonged and repeated hospitalization, sepsis, persistent pain, and device replacement[442,454]—and possible

death. No cost analysis is available to support the use of prophylaxis for any orthopedic procedure; however, the assumed costs for the associated morbidity may be adequate to justify prophylaxis. Consequently, antimicrobial prophylaxis is frequently used, even though the infection rate is low. For example, the frequency of infection after hip fracture repair with or without prophylaxis is generally less than 5%.[442,450]

Efficacy. Hip fracture repair. The efficacy of antimicrobial prophylaxis in hip fracture repair was studied in three double-blind, randomized, placebo-controlled trials.[442,450,455] One study demonstrated a significant difference in postoperative wound infections after hip fracture repair in patients receiving placebo (4.8%, or 7 of 145 patients) and patients given nafcillin 0.5 g (as the sodium) intramuscularly every six hours for two days (0.8%, or 1 of 135 patients).[442] Some prostheses were used, but a majority of patients had pin or plate implantation. The duration of follow-up was one year. There was no difference in the frequency of infected wound hematomas between the two groups.

In another study involving 307 patients with hip fractures, a significant difference was demonstrated for major postoperative wound infection rates: 4.7% in the placebo group compared with 0.7% in patients given preoperative cephalothin 1 g (as the sodium) intravenously and every 4 hours thereafter for 72 hours.[450] The duration of follow-up was not identified. Patients who received cephalothin for prophylaxis tended to be colonized with cephalothin-resistant organisms (in urine, sputum, and blood).

Despite having a small sample size (127 patients) and an unusually high rate of wound infection in the control group, one study showed prophylaxis to be beneficial in preventing postoperative wound infection compared with no prophylaxis.[451] In contrast to the previously described studies, a randomized, double-blind, single-hospital study involving 352 patients undergoing hip fracture fixation failed to show a significant difference between four doses of cefazolin, one dose of cefazolin, and placebo.[455] These regimens did not differ in efficacy even when both treatment groups were combined and compared with the placebo group. Although hip fracture repairs are associated with low infection rates, results from these three studies[442,450,451] and the morbidity and costs associated with infectious complications in hip fracture repair support the use of short-term prophylactic antimicrobials. The long-term benefits of prophylaxis have not been determined.

Procedures other than hip surgery involving implantation of internal fixation devices. The evidence supporting antimicrobial prophylaxis for the implantation of internal fixation devices is not as strong for nonhip surgeries as for hip replacement or repair. In a randomized, double-blind study of 122 patients undergoing open reduction and internal fixation of closed ankle fractures, no difference was demonstrated between cephalothin 1 g (as the sodium) intravenously every six hours for a total of four doses and placebo.[456] However, the sample was too small. Despite the lack of studies evaluating prophylaxis for procedures involving the implantation of internal fixation devices, consideration of antimicrobial use is warranted, especially in complicated procedures, because of the associated morbidity and assumed costs of infections involving implanted devices.

Choice. Sudies comparing antimicrobials are lacking. The antimicrobials that have been studied most often for prophylaxis in orthopedic surgery are first-generation

cephalosporins. First-generation cephalosporins (particularly cefazolin) are the most suitable agents for orthopedic prophylaxis because their spectrum of activity includes *Staphylococcus* species and gram-negative bacilli (such as *E. coli*), they have desirable pharmacokinetic characteristics (adequate bone penetration),[457] and they are easy to administer, low in cost, and safe. Second- and third-generation cephalosporins offer no major advantages over first-generation agents. Second- and third-generation cephalosporins are more expensive; furthermore, indiscriminate use is likely to promote resistance, particularly among nosocomial gram-negative bacilli. Therefore, the use of a second- or third-generation cephalosporin as orthopedic surgical prophylaxis should be avoided. The increasing prevalence of MRSA warrants discriminate use of alternative antimicrobials. No studies have evaluated vancomycin as a prophylactic agent in orthopedic procedures. However, vancomycin has adequate activity against the most common pathogens involved and would be an acceptable alternative under certain circumstances.[21] Only patients with a serious β-lactam allergy or patients in institutions with a high rate of infection due to MRSA or MRSE should be administered vancomycin.

Duration. One study evaluated the duration of therapy in patients undergoing orthopedic surgery. A double-blind, randomized study compared one day of cefuroxime alone with one day of cefuroxime followed by oral cephalexin for a total of six days in 121 evaluable patients undergoing implantation surgery for intertrochanteric hip fracture repair.[458] This study, combined with the total joint-replacement studies, supports a duration of 24 hours or less.

Pediatric Efficacy. No well-controlled studies have evaluated the efficacy of antimicrobial prophylaxis in pediatric patients undergoing hip fracture repair or implantation of internal fixation devices.

Recommendation. Despite the lack of substantial data, the use of antimicrobial prophylaxis in hip fracture repair and in other orthopedic procedures involving the implantation of internal fixation devices may be substantiated by the morbidity (possible removal of an infected internal fixation device) and costs associated with infectious events. The recommended regimen is cefazolin 1 g (as the sodium) intravenously at induction of anesthesia and continued every 8 hours for 24 hours. Vancomycin 1 g (as the hydrochloride) intravenously over one hour should be reserved as an alternative agent on the basis of previously outlined guidelines from HICPAC.[21] (Strength of evidence for prophylaxis for hip fracture repair = A.) (Strength of evidence for prophylaxis for implantation procedures = C.)

Pediatric Dosage. Despite the lack of substantial data, the use of antimicrobial prophylaxis in hip fracture repair and in other orthopedic procedures involving the implantation of internal fixation devices may be substantiated by the morbidity (possible removal of an infected internal fixation device) and costs associated with infectious events. The recommended regimen for pediatric patients is cefazolin 20–30 mg/kg (as the sodium) intravenously at the induction of anesthesia and every 8 hours for 24 hours. Vancomycin 15 mg/kg (as the hydrochloride) intravenously should be reserved as an alternative on the basis of previously outlined guidelines from HICPAC.[21,32]

Total Joint Replacement

Background. It is estimated that more than 200,000 hip or knee replacements are performed each year in North America.[459] The frequency of infections complicating hip, knee, elbow, or shoulder replacement is low, ranging from 0.6% to 11%.[454] With the introduction of antimicrobial prophylaxis and the use of "ultraclean" operating rooms, the infection rate has declined substantially, generally to less than 1%.[447,448,454] The two main types of infectious complications of total joint arthroplasty are superficial and deep infections of the prosthesis. Infections of the joint prosthesis may occur early (less than one year after the procedure) or late (occurring after the first year). Infection after joint arthroplasty can be disastrous, frequently requiring removal of the prosthesis and a prolonged course of antimicrobials for cure. An analysis of the costs associated with operations in Europe demonstrated that 90% of the total expense was associated with keeping the patient in a hospital bed.[460] The stay for joint revision was much longer than the stay for primary joint replacement.

A 1992 survey documented low use of antimicrobial-impregnated bone cement and cement beads in the United States (for fewer than one procedure per month); a majority of the antimicrobial-impregnated cement was used in community hospitals.[461] Total hip arthroplasty, total knee arthroplasty, and chronic osteomyelitis were the most common indications for use. A wide variety of antimicrobials are used in these products, a majority of which have not been adequately studied in the clinical setting. Inadequate quality control during mixing and use has been identified. Prophylaxis with antimicrobial-impregnated bone cement and cement beads is not recommended. Readers are referred to a review of this topic for additional information about tissue penetration, clinical application, and safety.[462]

Efficacy. A majority of studies that have evaluated prophylactic antimicrobials in joint-replacement surgery have been conducted in patients undergoing total hip arthroplasty. There is a lack of data involving elbow and shoulder arthroplasty; however, these procedures are similar enough to justify inclusion with total hip arthroplasty.

A double-blind, randomized, placebo-controlled trial involving 2137 hip replacements in 2097 patients evaluated the efficacy of prophylactic cefazolin.[447] Cefazolin 1 g (as the sodium) was given before surgery and continued every six hours for a total of five days. After a two-year follow-up period, a significant difference in the rate of "hip infection" was found between the placebo group and the cefazolin group (3.3% and 0.9%, respectively). When these results were further analyzed for the type of operating-room environment, a significant difference was observed only when surgery was carried out in a conventional operating room. Antimicrobial prophylaxis did not significantly reduce infection when hip replacement surgery was performed in a "hypersterile" (laminar airflow) operating room (1.3% with placebo versus 0.8% with cefazolin). This study was well designed in that sufficient numbers of patients were enrolled to reduce the probability of Type I and Type II errors in terms of the efficacy of prophylaxis.

Choice. (Readers are also referred to Procedures other than hip surgery involving implantation of internal fixation devices.) Cefazolin has been compared with cefuroxime[463] and cefonicid.[464] A double-blind multicenter study of 1354 patients undergoing total joint (hip or knee) arthroplasty compared

intravenous cefuroxime 1.5 g (as the sodium) preoperatively followed by 750 mg every eight hours for a total of three doses with intravenous cefazolin 1 g (as the sodium) preoperatively followed by 1 g every eight hours for a total of nine doses.[463] The preoperative doses were administered 50 to 60 minutes before incision. Follow-up assessments were performed at two to three months and one year after the procedure. An intention-to-treat analysis demonstrated no significant difference in the wound infection rate between cefuroxime (3%) and cefazolin (3%). All three late wound infections (identified at one-year follow-up) developed in the cefazolin group. The second trial was a double-blind, randomized, controlled trial that compared three doses of cefazolin with three doses of cefonicid in 102 patients undergoing joint replacement or insertion of a metallic device for fixation.[464] The median duration of follow-up was 106 to 109 days. There were six postoperative infections among 52 patients in the cefazolin group and no infections among the 50 patients in the cefonicid group. This difference was significant. However, three of the six infections in the cefazolin group were urinary tract infections.

Antimicrobials incorporated in bone cement is a viable method for prophylaxis. However, there are limited clinical data on the use of this method. One prospective, randomized clinical trial performed in two centers involved 401 patients undergoing total joint arthroplasty. Intravenous cefuroxime was compared with cefuroxime in bone cement.[465] All patients were followed for two years. The overall rate of deep infection (infection extending to the deep fascia, with persistent wound discharge or joint pain, positive or negative cultures from deep tissues, and delay in wound healing) was 1%. No significant difference was demonstrated between the two groups. There were no late deep infections (deep infection present for at least three months and occurring up to two years after the operation). Another prospective, randomized, controlled study that compared gentamicin-impregnated bone cement with systemic antimicrobials (cloxacillin, dicloxacillin, cephalexin, or penicillin) had similar results.[466] Antimicrobial bone cement has not been shown to be superior to intravenous antimicrobials.

The impact of ultraclean operating rooms on deep infection after joint-replacement surgery was evaluated in more than 8000 hip or knee operations.[448] A significantly lower rate of deep infection was observed with the use of ultraclean operating rooms than with conventional rooms (0.6% versus 1.5%, respectively). Although not strictly controlled in this study, the use of prophylactic antimicrobials (primarily flucloxacillin) was associated with an even lower rate of deep infection of the prosthesis.

Taken together, studies reported in the medical literature suggest that a short course of antimicrobial prophylaxis can significantly reduce the rate of postoperative infection, particularly late, deep-seated infection, in joint-replacement surgery. Although infectious complications are infrequent, the consequences of an infected joint prosthesis can be devastating. The use of ultraclean operating rooms significantly reduces the rate of deep infection after joint-replacement surgery, regardless of whether antimicrobials are given.[447,448] Because such operating environments are not widely available, antimicrobial prophylaxis using agents with activity primarily against *S. aureus* is indicated in patients undergoing joint-replacement surgery.

Duration. Two studies demonstrate that prophylactic antimicrobials are essential in total joint replacement, but the studies are not particularly helpful in guiding duration of use.[446,447] Studies involving total hip replacement have used

antimicrobials for 12 hours to 14 days postoperatively.[442,445–451,467] A duration of 24 hours was supported in a randomized trial of 358 patients undergoing total hip arthroplasty, total knee arthroplasty, or hip fracture repair that compared one day with seven days of either nafcillin or cefazolin.[467] The difference in infection rates between groups was not significant. The timing and duration of prophylaxis for total joint replacement have not been established, although there is general agreement that the first dose should be given about 30 minutes before the initial incision and the second dose given intraoperatively if the procedure takes more than three hours. The duration of prophylaxis remains controversial,[24] although the available data do not support prophylaxis beyond 24 hours.

A discussion of whether prophylaxis should be continued until postoperative surgical drainage tubes are removed is outside the scope of these guidelines; however, drainage tubes carry the risk of infection and thus are a variable in postoperative infections. There is a lack of data evaluating the risk of infection with and without continued antimicrobial prophylaxis in patients with surgical drainage tubes still in place. Continuation of antimicrobials may be warranted until the tubes are removed; however, there are no available data to support continuing prophylaxis.

Pediatric Efficacy. No well-controlled studies have evaluated the efficacy of antimicrobial prophylaxis in pediatric patients undergoing total joint replacement.

Recommendation. The recommended regimen for patients undergoing total hip, elbow, knee, or shoulder replacement is cefazolin 1 g (as the sodium) intravenously at induction of anesthesia and every 8 hours for 24 hours. Although continuing prophylaxis until drainage tubes are removed may be warranted, there is currently no evidence to support this practice. Vancomycin 1 g (as the hydrochloride) intravenously over one hour should be reserved as an alternative agent on the basis of previously outlined guidelines from HICPAC.[21] (Strength of evidence for prophylaxis = A.)

Pediatric Dosage. The recommended regimen for pediatric patients undergoing total hip, elbow, knee, or shoulder replacement is cefazolin 20–30 mg/kg (as the sodium) intravenously at induction of anesthesia and every 8 hours for 24 hours. Vancomycin 15 mg/kg (as the hydrochloride) intravenously should be reserved as an alternative on the basis of previously outlined guidelines from HICPAC.[21,32]

Urologic Surgery

Background. The efficacy of antimicrobial prophylaxis in urologic surgery has been investigated in many clinical trials, particularly in patients undergoing prostatectomy through the urethra, more commonly known as transurethral resection of the prostate (TURP).[385,468–488] Many patients undergoing resection of bladder tumors have also been studied.[470,489] Non-TURP transurethral procedures, like urethral dilatation and stone extraction, involve the same organisms and risk factors as TURP. Therefore, any transurethral procedure is similar enough to be included with TURP. Prostatectomy can also be performed through the perineum (perineal) and into the bladder (suprapubic). However, perineal procedures may involve different organisms on the basis of the proximity to the anus. There is a lack of studies addressing perineal prostatectomy;

therefore, the following recommendations do not include perineal prostatectomy. *S. aureus* may be the only organism causing infection after suprapubic procedures. However, there is a lack of studies, so the following recommendations do not include suprapubic procedures.

The most common infectious complication after urologic surgery is bacteriuria, the frequency of which has varied from 0% to 54% in reported studies. More serious infections, including bacteremia, are rare after TURP. Risk factors for infection after urologic surgery include age over 60 years, prolonged preoperative hospital stay, and wound contamination.[490] Bacteriuria before open prostatectomy has also been identified as a risk factor for postoperative wound infection in patients with or without an indwelling catheter.[491] Other factors that contribute to postoperative complications are the length of postoperative catheterization and the mode of irrigation (closed versus open). No significant correlation between infection rate and diagnosis of benign prostate hyperplasia or prostate carcinoma has been identified.[480] Therefore, neither of these diagnoses is considered a risk factor. The major objective of prophylaxis is the prevention of bacteremia and surgical wound infection and secondarily the prevention of postoperative bacteriuria.[24] The benefits of preventing postoperative bacteriuria are unknown; however, a majority of studies have regarded postoperative bacteriuria, regardless of the presence or absence of infectious signs and symptoms, as a postoperative complication. Therapeutic antimicrobials directed at the appropriate pathogens and for the appropriate duration should be used in patients with preoperative urinary tract infection.

Organisms. *E. coli* is the most common isolate in patients with postoperative bacteriuria; however, other gram-negative bacilli and enterococci also cause infection.

Efficacy. A wide range of antimicrobial regimens, including cephalosporins,[385,469,471,473,475,477,479,480,483,484,486–489] aminoglycosides,[468,474,481,482] carbenicillin,[470,472] piperacillin–tazobactam,[487] trimethoprim–sulfamethoxazole,[473,476,486] nitrofurantoin,[478] and fluoroquinolones,[485,488,492–494] have been evaluated.

Four studies did not demonstrate a difference in the frequency of postoperative bacteriuria when prophylactic antimicrobials were compared with controls.[469–472] The postoperative bacteriuria rate was 10% or less for the control groups and 6% or less for the prophylactic antimicrobial groups. In eight studies, the rate of postoperative bacteriuria was 25% in the control groups and 5% or less in the antimicrobial groups.[474–476,478,482] These studies included only patients with sterile urine preoperatively. Postoperative bacteriuria was defined as greater than 10^5 CFU/mL. In most of the studies, patients who received antimicrobial prophylaxis did not have fewer febrile episodes or shorter hospital stays than control patients.

Choice. No single antimicrobial regimen appears superior. Broad-spectrum antimicrobials, such as aminoglycosides or second- and third-generation cephalosporins, are no more effective than first-generation cephalosporins or oral agents (trimethoprim–sulfamethoxazole or nitrofurantoin). One prospective, randomized study demonstrated that norfloxacin is effective in preventing stricture formation after TURP.[485] This study is relevant in that bacterial infection is believed to be the partial cause of stricture formation. Other trials have demonstrated the efficacy of lomefloxacin, another fluoroquinolone, for antimicrobial prophylaxis in urologic surgical procedures. One open-label, randomized trial showed that oral lomefloxacin is effective in preventing

postsurgical bacteriuria after visual laser ablation of the prostate.[494] Additional studies indicated that oral lomefloxacin is as effective as intravenous cefotaxime or cefuroxime in the prevention of infections after transurethral surgical procedures.[488,492,493] Other fluoroquinolones may provide the same benefit as lomefloxacin; however, there are no efficacy data at this time to support recommendation of these agents.

Duration. In a large number of the trials, prophylaxis was continued for up to three weeks postoperatively.[468,470,472, 474–476,478,480] The most recent studies suggest that continuation of prophylaxis after the preoperative dose is unnecessary.[385,479,481–486,495] However, one study suggests that giving one dose of cefotaxime one hour before catheter removal instead of at the induction of anesthesia may be beneficial.[496]

Pediatric Efficacy. Most urologic studies evaluated prophylaxis for TURP or resection of bladder tumors, and pediatric patients therefore would be unlikely to have been included.

Recommendation. Considering the low risk of serious infection after urologic surgery, antimicrobial prophylaxis should be considered only in patients at high risk of postoperative bacteriuria (patients likely to require prolonged postoperative catheterization and patients with a positive urine culture) or in hospitals with infection rates of greater than 20%. Low-risk patients do not appear to benefit from the use of perioperative antimicrobials. If oral antimicrobials are used, a single dose of trimethoprim 160 mg with sulfamethoxazole 800 mg or lomefloxacin 400 mg (as the hydrochloride) should be administered two hours before surgery. If an injectable agent is preferred, cefazolin 1 g (as the sodium) intravenously at induction of anesthesia is recommended. Continuation of antimicrobial prophylaxis postoperatively is not recommended. (Strength of evidence for prophylaxis = A.)

Pediatric Dosage. Prophylaxis for urologic surgery in pediatric patients should be considered only in patients at high risk of postoperative bacteriuria (e.g., patients likely to require prolonged postoperative catheterization and patients with a positive urine culture) or in hospitals with infection rates of greater than 20%. If oral antimicrobials are used, a single dose of trimethoprim 6–10 mg/kg with sulfamethoxazole 30–50 mg/kg two hours before surgery is recommended. If an injectable agent is preferred, a single dose of cefazolin 20–30 mg/kg (as the sodium) intravenously at induction of anesthesia is recommended. Fluoroquinolones are not recommended in pediatric patients.

Vascular Surgery

Background. Infection after vascular surgery often is associated with extensive morbidity and mortality. postoperative infection is particularly devastating if it involves the vascular graft material. As a result, antimicrobial prophylaxis is widely used with surgical revascularization.[497] Patients undergoing brachiocephalic procedures do not appear to benefit from antimicrobial prophylaxis. Although there are no data, patients undergoing brachiocephalic procedures (e.g., carotid endarterectomy) involving vascular prosthesis or patch implantation may benefit from prophylaxis. Risk factors for postoperative surgical wound infection in patients undergoing vascular surgery include lower-extremity surgery, delayed surgery after hospitalization, diabetes mellitus, and a history of vascular surgery.[498] Another risk factor is short duration of antimicrobial prophylaxis, which was

defined as a 1.5-g dose of intravenous cefamandole (as the nafate) at induction of anesthesia and 750 mg of cefamandole four and eight hours after the first dose.[498]

Organisms. The predominant organisms involved include *S. aureus, S. epidermidis,* and enteric gram-negative bacilli. At some institutions, MRSA could be an organism of concern.

Efficacy. Prophylactic antimicrobials decrease the rate of infection after procedures involving the lower abdominal vasculature and procedures required for dialysis access. The duration of follow-up for late wound complications was at least once after hospital discharge (not further defined) for most studies,[490-501] one month,[498,502,503] six months,[504] and up to three years.[505]

In the first randomized, prospective, double-blind placebo-controlled study in patients undergoing peripheral vascular surgery (*n* = 462), the infection rate was significantly lower with cefazolin than placebo (0.9% and 6.8%, respectively).[499] Four deep graft infections were observed in the placebo group; none occurred in the patients who received cefazolin. No infections were observed in patients who underwent brachiocephalic (*n* = 103), femoral artery (*n*=56), or popliteal (*n*=14) procedures. Cefazolin-susceptible *S. aureus* was the predominant pathogen; however, gram-negative aerobic bacilli, coagulase-negative staphylococci, and enterococci were also isolated.

In a subsequent controlled trial, intravenous cephradine, topical cephradine, or both were evaluated in patients undergoing peripheral vascular surgery.[505] The infection rate was significantly different between the cephradine groups (less than 6%) and the control group (25%). There were no significant differences in the infection rate among the groups that received cephradine, regardless of route. Ten of 16 infected patients grew *S. aureus; E. coli* and other gram-negative bacilli were infrequently associated with infection.

Patients undergoing vascular-access surgery for hemodialysis also benefit from the administration of antistaphylococcal antimicrobials.[504] Two of 19 cefamandole-treated patients and 8 of 19 placebo recipients developed an infection after undergoing polytetra-fluoroethylene vascular-access grafts.

Choice. More recent studies have demonstrated that cefazolin remains the preferred cephalosporin for use in vascular surgery.[500,501] There was no significant difference in infection rates between cefazolin and cefuroxime in patients undergoing abdominal aortic and lower-extremity peripheral vascular surgery[500] or between cefazolin and cefamandole in patients undergoing aortic or infrainguinal arterial surgery.[501]

There are limited data regarding the choice of an antimicrobial for penicillin-allergic patients undergoing vascular procedures. Although vancomycin offers coverage against potential gram-positive pathogens, the addition of an aminoglycoside may be prudent when colonization and infection with gram-negative organisms are expected. Given the lack of data regarding vancomycin as a single agent, definitive conclusions are not possible.

Duration. A prospective, randomized, double-blind study compared infection rates of a one-day and a three-day course of cefuroxime with placebo in patients undergoing peripheral vascular surgery.[502] The infection rates were 16.7%, 3.8%, and 4.3% in the placebo, one-day, and three-day groups, respectively. The difference in the infection rates between the one-day and three-day groups was not

significant. A prospective study that analyzed risk factors for surgical wound infection after vascular surgery found that patients randomly assigned to receive a short course of antimicrobial prophylaxis, defined as 1.5 g of cefamandole (as the nafate) at induction of anesthesia followed by 750 mg of cefamandole four and eight hours after the first dose, were more likely to develop surgical wound infection than patients randomly assigned to receive a longer course of antimicrobial prophylaxis, defined as 1.5 g of cefamandole (as the nafate) at induction of anesthesia and 750 mg every 6 hours for 48 hours after surgery.[498]

Route. The question of oral versus intravenous treatment was addressed in a multicenter, randomized, double-blind, prospective trial in 580 patients undergoing arterial surgery involving the groin.[503] Patients received two doses of ciprofloxacin 750 mg orally or three doses of cefuroxime 1.5 g intravenously on the day of surgery. The wound infection rate within 30 days of surgery was 9.2% (27 patients) in the ciprofloxacin group and 9.1% (26 patients) in the cefuroxime group. Although oral ciprofloxacin was shown to be as effective as intravenous cefuroxime in one study, this study did not address the well-founded concern about resistance developing with routine use of fluoroquinolones[506]; therefore, intravenous cefazolin remains the first-line agent for this indication. The study did, however, demonstrate the need for more studies regarding efficacy of oral agents for postoperative prophylaxis.

Pediatric Efficacy. No well-controlled studies have evaluated the efficacy of surgical prophylaxis in pediatric patients undergoing vascular surgery.

Recommendation. The recommendation for patients undergoing vascular surgery is cefazolin 1 g (as the sulfate) intravenously at induction of anesthesia and every 8 hours for 24 hours. Vancomycin 1 g (as the hydrochloride) intravenously over one hour, with or without gentamicin 2 mg/kg (as the sulfate) intravenously, should be reserved as an alternative on the basis of previously outlined guidelines from HICPAC.[21] Although there are no data, patients undergoing brachiocephalic procedures involving vascular prosthesis or patch implantation (e.g., carotid endarterectomy) may benefit from prophylaxis. (Strength of evidence for prophylaxis = A.)

Pediatric Dosage. The recommended regimen for pediatric patients undergoing vascular surgery is cefazolin 20–30 mg/kg (as the sodium) intravenously at induction of anesthesia and every 8 hours for 24 hours. Vancomycin 15 mg/kg (as the hydrochloride) intravenously over one hour, with or without gentamicin 2 mg/kg (as the sulfate) intravenously, should be reserved as an alternative on the basis of previously outlined guidelines from HICPAC.[21] Although there are no data, patients undergoing brachiocephalic procedures involving vascular prosthesis or patch implantation (e.g., carotid endarterectomy) may benefit from prophylaxis.

Solid Organ Transplantation

Few well-designed, prospective, comparative studies of antimicrobial prophylaxis have been conducted in patients undergoing solid organ transplantation, and no formal recommendations are available from professional organizations or expert consensus panels. As a result, multiple regimens are in use at different

transplant centers. A recent survey of four major U.S. centers performing combined pancreas–kidney transplantation identified four different prophylactic regimens using from one to four different drugs for two to seven days postoperatively.[507]

The recommendations given for each of the solid organ transplant procedures represent an attempt to provide guidelines for safe and effective surgical prophylaxis based on the best available literature. These recommendations will undoubtedly vary considerably from protocols in use at various transplantation centers around the United States.

Heart Transplantation

Background. Heart transplantation has emerged as a standard therapeutic option for selected patients with end-stage cardiac disease. Approximately 4000 heart transplants are performed worldwide each year, including approximately 100 in children less than 16 years of age.[508] Survival rates after heart transplantation are approximately 79% at one year and 65% at five years, illustrating the tremendous progress that has been made over the past two decades. Infection continues to be an important cause of morbidity and mortality after heart transplantation and is the major cause of death in approximately 15%, 40%, and 10% of patients at <1 month, 1–12 months, and >12 months posttransplant, respectively.

Despite the large number of heart transplantation surgeries performed, few studies have specifically examined postoperative infection rates in this population. General cardiothoracic surgery has been associated with surgical wound infection rates of 9% to 55% in the absence of antimicrobial prophylaxis.[69,70,88] Because heart transplantation is similar to other cardiothoracic surgeries, similar considerations regarding the need for antimicrobial prophylaxis apply (see Cardiothoracic surgery).[509]

Organisms. Similar to other types of cardiothoracic surgery, coagulase-positive and coagulase-negative staphylococci are the primary pathogens that cause surgical wound infection after heart transplantation. *S. aureus* was the cause of all wound infections in one study involving heart transplantation.[510]

Efficacy. In an open-label, noncomparative study, the wound infection rate was 4.5% among 96 patients administered cefotaxime plus flucloxacillin preoperatively and for 72 hours after surgery.[510] This rate of infection was similar to that seen in other cardiothoracic, non-heart-transplantation procedures in which antimicrobial prophylaxis was used. Although antimicrobial prophylaxis appears to be effective in significantly reducing infection rates, no randomized, controlled trials have specifically addressed the use of antimicrobial prophylaxis in heart transplantation.

Choice. Antimicrobial prophylaxis for heart transplantation is similar to that used for other types of cardiothoracic procedures.[509] First- and second-generation cephalosporins are considered to be equally efficacious and are the preferred agents. There appear to be no significant differences in efficacy among prophylactic regimens using agents such as cefazolin, cephalothin, cefuroxime, and cefamandole.[511] The use of antistaphylococcal penicillins, either alone or in combination with aminoglycosides or cephalosporins, has not been demonstrated to provide efficacy superior to that of cephalosporin monotherapy (see Cardiothoracic surgery).

Duration. On the basis of data concerning other cardiothoracic procedures, prophylactic regimens of 48 to 72 hours' duration appear similar in efficacy to longer regimens.

Pediatric Efficacy. There are no data specifically addressing antimicrobial prophylaxis for heart transplantation in pediatric patients. Pediatric patients should be treated according to recommendations for other types of cardiothoracic procedures.

Recommendation. On the basis of data for other types of cardiothoracic surgery, antimicrobial prophylaxis is indicated for all patients undergoing heart transplantation. The recommended regimen is cefazolin 1 g (as the sodium) intravenously at induction of anesthesia and every 8 hours for 48 to 72 hours. Currently there is no evidence to support continuing prophylaxis until chest and mediastinal drainage tubes are removed. Cefuroxime 1.5 g (as the sodium) intravenously at induction of anesthesia and every 12 hours for 48 to 72 hours and cefamandole 1 g (as the nafate) intravenously at induction of anesthesia and every 6 hours for 48 to 72 hours are acceptable alternatives. Further studies are needed to demonstrate the efficacy of single-dose prophylaxis. Vancomycin 1 g (as the hydrochloride) intravenously with or without gentamicin 2 mg/kg (as the sulfate) should be reserved as an alternative agent on the basis of previously outlined guidelines from HICPAC and AHA.[21,32] (Strength of evidence for prophylaxis = A.)

Pediatric Dosage. The recommended regimen for pediatric patients undergoing heart transplantation is cefazolin 20–30 mg/kg (as the sodium) intravenously at induction of anesthesia and every 8 hours for 48 to 72 hours. Cefuroxime 50 mg/kg (as the sodium) at induction of anesthesia and every 8 hours for 48 to 72 hours is an acceptable alternative. Vancomycin 15 mg/kg (as the hydrochloride) intravenously with or without gentamicin 2 mg/kg (as the sulfate) should be reserved as an alternative on the basis of previously outlined guidelines from HICPAC and AHA.[21,32]

Lung and Heart–Lung Transplantation

Background. Lung transplantation has become an accepted mode of therapy for a variety of end-stage, irreversible lung diseases. The most common diseases for which lung transplantation is performed are chronic obstructive pulmonary disease, emphysema associated with α_1-antitrypsin deficiency, cystic fibrosis, idiopathic pulmonary fibrosis, and primary pulmonary hypertension.[512] Approximately 1000 single-lung, bilateral-lung, and heart–lung transplants are performed in the United States every year.[508,512] National survival rates after lung transplantation are approximately 70% at one year and 50% at five years; differences in rates between single-lung and double-lung transplants are not significant.[508] Survival rates after heart–lung transplants are somewhat lower: approximately 60% at one year and 40% at five years.

Bacterial, fungal, and viral infections are the most common complications and causes of death within the first 90 days after lung or heart–lung transplantation.[512–514] Bacterial infections, particularly surgical wound infections and pneumonia, are common in the immediate postoperative period. The frequent occurrence of bacterial pneumonias is directly related to the procedure being performed. Thus antimicrobial prophylaxis is routinely administered to patients undergoing lung or

heart–lung transplantation with the aim of preventing bacterial pneumonia as well as wound infection. Although much has been published about general infectious complications associated with lung transplantation, there are no data specifically addressing the optimal prophylactic antimicrobial regimens. Fungal and viral infections are late complications not directly associated with the surgical procedure. Prophylaxis of these infections is beyond the scope of this document.

Organisms. Similar to other cardiothoracic surgeries, coagulase-positive and coagulase-negative staphylococci are the primary pathogens that cause wound infection after lung transplantation. Patients undergoing lung transplantation are also at risk for bacterial pneumonia due to colonization or infection of the lower and upper airways of the donor, the recipient, or both.[512] The donor lung appears to be a major route of transmission of pathogens; 75% to 90% of bronchial washings from donor organs are positive for at least one bacterial organism.[515,516]

Organ recipients may also be the source of infection of the transplanted organ. This is particularly true in patients with cystic fibrosis because of the frequent presence of *P. aeruginosa* in the upper airways and sinuses before transplantation.[514] These pathogens are often highly resistant to antimicrobials because of the frequent administration of broad-spectrum agents during the previous course of the disease. Multiresistant strains of *Burkholderia (Pseudomonas) cepacia* and *Stenotrophomonas maltophilia* may be a problem in cystic fibrosis patients in some transplant centers.[514,517]

Infections with *Candida* and *Aspergillus* species are also common after lung transplantation. The occurrence of early *Candida* infections has been associated with colonization of the donor lung before transplantation.[516,518]

Efficacy. No randomized, controlled trials regarding antimicrobial prophylaxis for lung transplantation have been conducted. The rate of bacterial pneumonia within the first two weeks after surgery has reportedly been decreased from 35% to approximately 10% by routine antimicrobial prophylaxis.[519–521] Improvements in surgical technique and postoperative patient care may also be important factors in the apparently lower rates of pneumonia after lung transplantation.

Choice. No formal studies have addressed optimal prophylaxis for patients undergoing lung transplantation. Antimicrobial prophylaxis for lung and heart–lung transplantation should generally be similar to that for other cardiothoracic procedures (see Cardiothoracic surgery). First- and second-generation cephalosporins are considered to be equally efficacious and are the preferred agents for these procedures. However, prophylactic regimens should be modified to include coverage for any potential bacterial pathogens that have been isolated from the recipient's airways or the donor lung.[512] Patients with end-stage cystic fibrosis should receive antimicrobials on the basis of the known susceptibilities of pretransplant isolates, particularly *P. aeruginosa.*

It has been suggested that antifungal prophylaxis should be considered when pretransplant cultures reveal fungi in the donor lung.[512] Because of the serious nature of fungal infections in the early posttransplant period and the availability of relatively nontoxic antifungal agents, prophylaxis with fluconazole should be considered when *Candida* is isolated from the donor lung and itraconazole should be considered when *Aspergillus* is isolated.[512] Amphotericin B may also be

considered.[522] No antifungal prophylaxis is necessary in the absence of positive fungal cultures from the donor lung.

Duration. No well-conducted studies have addressed the optimal duration of antimicrobial prophylaxis for lung transplantation. In the absence of positive cultures from the donor or the recipient, prophylactic regimens of 48 to 72 hours' duration are probably similar in efficacy to longer regimens.[522] In patients with positive pretransplant cultures from donor or recipient organs or patients with positive cultures posttransplant, prophylaxis should be continued for longer. Antimicrobial prophylaxis should be appropriately modified according to the specific organisms isolated and antimicrobial susceptibilities. It has been recommended that prophylactic regimens be continued for 7 to 14 days postoperatively in transplant recipients with positive cultures, particularly patients with cystic fibrosis and previous *P. aeruginosa* infection.[512,514,522]

Pediatric Efficacy. There are few data specifically concerning antimicrobial prophylaxis for lung transplantation in pediatric patients. Pediatric patients should be treated according to recommendations for other types of cardiothoracic procedures and as previously discussed for adult lung transplantation.[522]

Recommendation. On the basis of data from other types of cardiothoracic surgery, all patients undergoing lung transplantation should receive antimicrobial prophylaxis because of the high risk of infection. Patients with negative pretransplant cultures should receive antimicrobial prophylaxis as appropriate for other types of cardiothoracic surgeries. The recommended regimen is cefazolin 1 g (as the sodium) intravenously at induction of anesthesia and every 8 hours for 48 to 72 hours. There is no evidence to support continuing prophylaxis until chest and mediastinal drainage tubes are removed. Cefuroxime 1.5 g (as the sodium) intravenously at induction of anesthesia and every 12 hours for 48 to 72 hours and cefamandole 1 g (as the nafate) intravenously at induction of anesthesia and every 6 hours for 48 to 72 hours are acceptable alternatives. Further studies are needed to demonstrate the efficacy of single-dose prophylaxis. Vancomycin 1 g (as the hydrochloride) intravenously should be reserved as an alternative on the basis of previously outlined guidelines from HICPAC.[21]

The prophylactic regimen should be modified to provide coverage against any potential pathogens (e.g., *P. aeruginosa*) isolated from the donor lung or the recipient. Prophylactic regimens directed against *P. aeruginosa* may include one or two drugs with activity against this pathogen, although two-drug therapy is recommended for prophylaxis and is mandatory should prophylaxis fail and an actual infection develop. The regimen may also include antifungal agents such as fluconazole if donor lung cultures are positive for *Candida* and itraconazole if cultures are positive for *Aspergillus*. The following doses would be appropriate: fluconazole 200–400 mg intravenously or orally, or itraconazole 200 mg orally as tablet or suspension. If the use of amphotericin B is desired, doses of 0.1–0.25 mg/kg intravenously may be used. Patients undergoing lung transplantation for cystic fibrosis should receive 7 to 14 days of prophylaxis with antimicrobials selected according to pretransplant culture and susceptibility results. (Strength of evidence for prophylaxis = B.)

Pediatric Dosage. As used for other cardiothoracic procedures, the recommended regimen for pediatric patients

undergoing lung or heart–lung transplantation is cefazolin 20–30 mg/kg (as the sodium) intravenously at induction of anesthesia and every 8 hours for 48 to 72 hours. Cefuroxime 50 mg/kg (as the sodium) intravenously at induction of anesthesia and every 8 hours for 48 to 72 hours is an acceptable alternative. Vancomycin 15 mg/kg (as the hydrochloride) intravenously should be reserved as an alternative on the basis of previously outlined guidelines from HICPAC.[21] If these regimens require modification for potential pathogens isolated from the donor or the recipient, the dosages are as appropriate for the specific agent(s) chosen. Patients undergoing lung transplantation for cystic fibrosis should receive 7 to 14 days of prophylaxis with antimicrobials selected according to pretransplant isolates and susceptibilities. These antimicrobials may be antibacterial or antifungal agents.

Liver Transplantation

Background. Liver transplantation is a life-saving procedure for many patients with end-stage hepatic disease for whom there are no other medical or surgical options. Approximately 6000 liver transplants are performed worldwide each year, with one- and five-year survival rates of 76% and 65%, respectively.[523,524] Infection remains a major cause of morbidity and mortality in liver transplant recipients. Infections may occur in 42% to 83% of patients within three months of transplantation and are the cause of death in 4% to 23% of patients; these rates are highly variable and do not seem to have substantially changed in spite of advances in surgical technique and medical management.[523–529]

Liver transplantation is often considered to be the most technically difficult of the solid organ transplant procedures. Surgical procedures longer than 8 to 12 hours have been consistently identified as one of the most important risk factors for early infectious complications, including wound infections, intra-abdominal infections, and biliary tract infections.[523,527,529] Other important risk factors for infectious complications include previous hepatobiliary surgery, high pretransplantation serum bilirubin concentration, and surgical complications such as anastomotic leakage. In spite of the high rate of infections directly related to the transplantation procedure, there are few well-controlled studies concerning optimal antimicrobial prophylaxis in this setting.

Organisms. The pathogens most commonly associated with early wound and intra-abdominal infections are those derived from the normal flora of the intestinal lumen and the skin. Aerobic gram-negative bacilli, including *E. coli, Klebsiella* species, *Enterobacter* species, and *Citrobacter* species, are common causes of wound and intra-abdominal infections and account for up to 65% of all bacterial pathogens.[523,524,527,529–531] Infections due to *P. aeruginosa* may also occur but are much less frequent in the early postoperative period. *P. aeruginosa* is most commonly associated with late pneumonias, vascular infections, and secondary bacteremias.[523,524,527,529]

Enterococci are particularly common pathogens and may be responsible for 20% to 46% of wound and intra-abdominal infections. *S. aureus* and coagulase-negative staphylococci are also common causes of postoperative wound infections.[524,525,527–529] Although *Candida* species commonly cause late infections, they are less frequent causes of early postoperative infections.

Efficacy. In evaluating the efficacy of prophylactic regimens, it is important to differentiate between early infections (variously defined as those occurring within 14 to 30 days after surgery) and late infections (those occurring >30 days after surgery). Infections occurring in the early postoperative period are most commonly associated with biliary, vascular, and abdominal surgeries involved in the transplantation procedure itself and are thus most preventable with prophylactic antimicrobial regimens.[523–525,527] The frequency of these infections varies from 10% to 55% despite antimicrobial prophylaxis.[523–525,527,532] It is difficult to assess the efficacy of prophylactic regimens in reducing the rate of infection because prophylaxis has been routinely used in light of the complexity of the surgical procedure; therefore, reliable rates of infection in the absence of prophylaxis are not available. No controlled studies have compared prophylaxis with no prophylaxis.

Choice. Antimicrobial prophylaxis should be directed against the pathogens most commonly isolated from early infections (i.e., gram-negative aerobic bacilli, staphylococci, enterococci). Traditional prophylactic regimens have thus consisted of a third-generation cephalosporin (usually cefotaxime because of relatively greater staphylococcal activity) plus ampicillin.[525,526,528–530,532] The use of cefoxitin and of ampicillin–sulbactam has also been reported; the efficacy of these regimens compared with that of cefotaxime plus ampicillin cannot be assessed because of different definitions of infection used in the various studies. No randomized, controlled studies have been conducted to compare the efficacy of other antimicrobial prophylactic regimens in the prevention of early postoperative infections.

At least one study used mechanical bowel preparation in conjunction with oral erythromycin base and neomycin sulfate, followed by systemic administration of cefotaxime plus ampicillin.[526] Infection rates in that study did not appear to be different from those in studies that did not use preoperative gut sterilization.

Several studies have examined the use of selective bowel decontamination in order to eliminate aerobic gram-negative bacilli and yeast from the bowel before surgery.[525,530–534] These studies used combinations of nonabsorbable antibacterials (aminoglycosides, polymyxin E) and antifungals (nystatin or amphotericin B) administered orally and applied to the oropharyngeal cavity, in combination with systemically administered antimicrobials. The results of these studies are conflicting and do not currently support the routine use of selective bowel decontamination in patients undergoing liver transplantation.[523]

Duration. No studies have assessed the optimal duration of antimicrobial prophylaxis in liver transplantation. Although antimicrobials were administered for five days in older studies,[526,529] more recent studies have limited the duration of prophylaxis to 48 hours, with no apparent difference in early infection rates.[525,527,530,532]

Pediatric Efficacy. There are few data specifically concerning antimicrobial prophylaxis in liver transplantation in pediatric patients. The combination of cefotaxime plus ampicillin has been reportedly used in children undergoing living-related-donor liver transplantation; the efficacy of this regimen appeared to be favorable.[528]

Recommendation. All patients undergoing liver transplantation should receive antimicrobial prophylaxis because of the

high risk of infectious morbidity and mortality associated with these procedures. Cefotaxime 1 g (as the sodium) plus ampicillin 1 g (as the sodium) should be administered intravenously at induction of anesthesia, repeated every 6 hours during the procedure, and given every 6 hours for 48 hours beyond final surgical closure. Other antimicrobial regimens that provide adequate coverage against gram-negative aerobic bacilli, staphylococci, and enterococci may be appropriate, but no randomized, comparative clinical trials have been conducted. (Strength of evidence for prophylaxis = B.)

Pediatric Dosage. The recommended regimen for pediatric patients undergoing liver transplantation is cefotaxime 50 mg/kg (as the sodium) plus ampicillin 50 mg/kg (as the sodium) intravenously at induction of anesthesia and repeated every 6 hours for 48 hours beyond final surgical closure. Other antimicrobial regimens that provide adequate coverage against gram-negative aerobic bacilli, staphylococci, and enterococci may be appropriate, but no randomized, comparative clinical trials have been conducted.

Pancreas and Pancreas–Kidney Transplantation

Background. Pancreas transplantation is an accepted therapeutic intervention for type 1 diabetes mellitus; it is the only therapy that consistently achieves euglycemia without dependence on exogenous insulin. Simultaneous pancreas–kidney transplantation is an accepted procedure for patients with type 1 diabetes and severe diabetic nephropathy. Infectious complications are a major source of morbidity and mortality in patients undergoing pancreas or pancreas–kidney transplantation; the frequency of wound infection is reportedly 7% to 50%.[535–539] These patients may be at increased risk of wound and other infections because of the combined immunosuppressive effects of diabetes and the immunosuppressive drugs used to prevent graft rejection.[537] Other factors associated with increased wound infection rates include prolonged (more than four hours) operating time, organ donor of >55 years of age, and enteric rather than bladder drainage of pancreatic duct secretions.[537]

Organisms. A majority of superficial wound infections after pancreas or pancreas–kidney transplantation are caused by staphylococci (both coagulase-positive and coagulase-negative) and gram-negative aerobic bacilli (particularly *E. coli* and *Klebsiella* species). Deep wound infections also are frequently associated with gram-positive and gram-negative aerobes, as well as *Candida* species.[535–541]

Efficacy. Although no placebo-controlled studies have been conducted, several open-label, noncomparative studies have suggested that antimicrobial prophylaxis substantially decreases the rate of superficial and deep wound infections after pancreas or pancreas–kidney transplantation. Wound infection rates were 2.4% to 5% with various prophylactic regimens, compared with 7% to 50% for historical controls in the absence of prophylaxis.[507,540] However, even with antimicrobial prophylaxis, wound infection rates as high as 33% have been reported[537]; the reason for the wide disparity in infection rates observed with prophylaxis is not readily apparent.

Choice. Because of the broad range of potential pathogens, several studies have used multidrug prophylactic regimens, including imipenem–cilastatin plus vancomycin[537];

tobramycin, vancomycin, and fluconazole[540]; and cefotaxime, metronidazole, and vancomycin.[542] These three regimens resulted in overall wound infection rates of 33%, 2.4%, and 30%, respectively. A recent study evaluated wound infection rates in pancreas–kidney transplantation after single-agent, single-dose prophylaxis with cefazolin.[507] Only two patients (5%) developed superficial wound infections, defined as the presence of erythema and purulent drainage. Although four additional patients (11%) developed deep wound infections, all infections were associated with bladder anastomotic leaks or transplant pancreatitis. On the basis of limited studies, it appears that multidrug regimens offer no distinct advantage over cefazolin.

Duration. Recent studies have evaluated the use of prophylactic regimens ranging from a single preoperative dose of cefazolin to multidrug regimens of two to five days' duration.[507,537,540,542] Although longer durations of antimicrobial prophylaxis have been recommended,[543] these appear to offer no clear advantages over the single-dose regimen.

Pediatric Efficacy. There are no data concerning antimicrobial prophylaxis for pancreas or pancreas–kidney transplantation in pediatric patients.

Recommendation. The recommended regimen for patients undergoing pancreas or pancreas–kidney transplantation is cefazolin 1 g (as the sodium) intravenously at induction of anesthesia. (Strength of evidence for prophylaxis = B.)

Pediatric Dosage. The recommended regimen for pediatric patients undergoing pancreas or pancreas–kidney transplantation is cefazolin 20 mg/kg (as the sodium) intravenously administered at induction of anesthesia.

Kidney Transplantation

Background. Approximately 10,000 kidney transplants are performed in the United States each year.[544] The rate of postoperative infection after this procedure has been reported to range from 10% to 56%.[545–552] Graft loss due to infection occurs in up to 33% of cases.[548] Mortality associated with postoperative infections is substantial and ranges from approximately 5% to 30%.[546,548,550,553,554]

Well-defined risk factors for wound infection after renal transplantation include contamination of organ perfusate; factors related to the procedure, such as ureteral leakage and hematoma formation; immunosuppressive therapy; and obesity.[554] In one study, the frequency of wound infection was 12% in patients receiving immunosuppression with azathioprine plus prednisone but only 1.7% in patients receiving cyclosporine plus prednisone.[555]

Organisms. Postoperative wound infections are typically caused by flora of the skin (particularly *S. aureus* and *S. epidermidis*) and of the urinary tract (most frequently *E. coli*). Enterococci and other gram-negative aerobic pathogens are less frequent causes of postoperative infections after kidney transplantation.[545–552,555,556]

Efficacy. A number of studies have clearly demonstrated that antimicrobial prophylaxis significantly decreases postoperative infection rates in patients undergoing kidney transplantation. These have included at least one randomized controlled trial[545] and many prospective and retrospective studies comparing

infection rates with prophylaxis and historical infection rates at specific transplant centers.[546–549,552,555–557] A recent study evaluated wound infection rates in the absence of systemic prophylaxis and found only a 2% rate among 102 patients undergoing renal transplantation.[558] Possible explanations given for the very low infection rate included local wound irrigation with cefazolin, improved organ procurement techniques, and careful surgical technique employed by a single, very experienced surgical team. This study emphasizes the importance of good surgical technique during the transplant procedure as an effective means of reducing infectious complications. However, on the basis of available literature, the routine use of systemic antimicrobial prophylaxis is justified in patients undergoing renal transplantation.

Three studies using a triple-drug regimen consisting of an aminoglycoside, an antistaphylococcal penicillin, and ampicillin demonstrated infection rates of less than 2%, compared with 10% to 25% with no antimicrobial prophylaxis.[549,552] Piperacillin plus cefuroxime was also shown to be efficacious; infection rates were 3.7%, compared with 19% in patients not receiving prophylaxis.[545] Several studies have shown that single-agent prophylaxis with an antistaphylo-coccal penicillin,[556] a first-generation cephalosporin,[547,548] a second-generation cephalosporin,[557] or a third-generation cephalosporin such as cefoperazone or ceftriaxone[555,559] can reduce postoperative infection rates to between 0% and 8.4%. Antimicrobial prophylaxis with agents providing good coverage against gram-positive cocci and gram-negative enteric pathogens is very effective in reducing infection rates in patients undergoing kidney transplantation.

Choice. The data do not indicate a significant difference between single-agent regimens and regimens using two or more drugs.[545,549,552] Also, there appear to be no significant differences between single-agent regimens employing antistaphylococcal penicillins or first-, second-, or third-generation cephalosporins.[547,548,555–557,559] Studies have directly compared antimicrobial regimens in a prospective, controlled fashion. Single-agent prophylaxis with both cefazolin and ceftriaxone has been reported to result in infection rates of 0%.[547,559]

Duration. Studies have used various prophylactic regimens ranging from a single preoperative dose of cefazolin or ceftriaxone to multidrug regimens of two to five days' duration.[545–549,552,555–557] There appear to be no significant differences in wound infection rates between single-dose and multidose regimens.

Pediatric Efficacy. Although pediatric patients were included in studies demonstrating the efficacy of antimicrobial prophylaxis, there are few data specific to pediatric patients.

Recommendation. The recommended regimen for patients undergoing kidney transplantation is cefazolin 1 g (as the sodium) intravenously at induction of anesthesia. (Strength of evidence for prophylaxis = A.)

Pediatric Dosage. The recommended regimen for pediatric patients undergoing kidney transplantation is cefazolin 20 mg/kg (as the sodium) intravenously at induction of anesthesia.

References

1. ASHP Commission on Therapeutics. ASHP therapeutic guidelines on antimicrobial prophylaxis in surgery. *Clin Pharm.* 1992; 11:483–513.
2. Dotson LR, Witmer DR. Development of ASHP therapeutic guidelines. *Am J Health-Syst Pharm.* 1995; 52:254–5.
3. Taketomo CK, Hodding JH, Kraus DM. Pediatric dosage handbook. Hudson, OH: Lexi-Comp; 1996.
4. Koren G, Prober CG, Gold R, eds. Antimicrobial therapy in infants and children. New York: Marcel Dekker; 1988.
5. Roberts NJ, Douglas RG. Gentamicin use and *Pseudomonas* and *Serratia* resistance: effect of a surgical prophylaxis regimen. *Antimicrob Agents Chemother.* 1978; 13:214–20.
6. Bartlett J, Condon R, Gorbach S et al. Veterans Administration Cooperative Study on bowel preparation for elective colorectal operations: impact of oral antibiotic regimen on colonic flora, wound irrigation cultures and bacteriology of septic complications. *Ann Surg.* 1978; 188:249–54.
7. Rozenberg-Arska M, Dekker AW, Verhoef J. Ciprofloxacin for selective decontamination of the alimentary tract in patients with acute leukemia during remission induction treatment: the effect on fecal flora. *J Infect Dis.* 1985; 152:104–7.
8. Harrison GA, Stross WP, Rubin MP et al. Resistance in oral streptococci after repeated three-dose erythromycin prophylaxis. *J Antimicrob Chemother.* 1985; 15:471–9.
9. Murray BE, Rensimer ER, DuPont HL. Emergence of high-level trimethoprim resistance in fecal *Escherichia coli* during oral administration of trimethoprim or trimethoprim-sulfamethoxazole. *N Engl J Med.* 1982; 306:130–5.
10. Kern WV, Andriof E, Oethinger M et al. Emergence of fluoroquinolone-resistant *Escherichia coli* at a cancer center. *Antimicrob Agents Chemother.* 1994; 38:681–7.
11. Dupeyron C, Mangeney N, Sedrati L et al. Rapid emergence of quinolone resistance in cirrhotic patients treated with norfloxacin to prevent spontaneous bacterial peritonitis. *Antimicrob Agents Chemother.* 1994; 38:340–4.
12. Tetteroo GWM, Wagenvoort JHT, Bruining HA. Bacteriology of selective decontamination: efficacy and rebound colonization. *J Antimicrob Chemother.* 1994; 34:139–48.
13. Kotilainen P, Nikoskelainen J, Huovinen P. Emergence of ciprofloxacin-resistant coagulase-negative staphylococcal skin flora in immunocompromised patients receiving ciprofloxacin. *J Infect Dis.* 1990; 161:41–4.
14. Kauffman CA, Liepman MK, Bergman AG et al. Trimethoprim/sulfamethoxazole prophylaxis in neutropenic patients. Reduction of infections and effect on bacterial and fungal flora. *Am J Med.* 1983; 74:599–607.
15. Weinstein JW, Roe M, Towns M et al. Resistant enterococci: a prospective study of prevalence, incidence, and factors associated with colonization in a university hospital. *Infect Control Hosp Epidemiol.* 1996; 17:36–41.
16. Kunova A, Trupl J, Kremery V Jr. Low incidence of quinolone resistance in gram-negative bacteria after five-years use of ofloxacin in prophylaxis during afebrile neutropenia. *J Hosp Infect.* 1996; 32:155–6. Letter.

17. Preheim L, Rimland D, Bittner M. Methicillin-resistant *Staphylococcus aureus* in Veterans Administration Medical Centers. *Infect Control.* 1987; 8:191–4.

18. Thornsberry C. Methicillin-resistant staphylococci. *Clin Lab Med.* 1989; 9:255–67.

19. Panlilio AL, Culver DH, Gaynes RP et al. Methicillin-resistant *Staphylococcus aureus* in US hospitals, 1975–1991. *Infect Control Hosp Epidemiol.* 1992; 13:582–6.

20. Centers for Disease Control and Prevention. Nosocomial enterococci resistant to vancomycin—United States, 1989–1993. *MMWR.* 1993; 42:597–9.

21. Centers for Disease Control and Prevention. Recommendations for preventing the spread of vancomycin resistance: recommendations of the Hospital Infection Control Practices Advisory Committee (HICPAC). *MMWR.* 1994; 44:1–13.

22. Boyce J, Potter-Bynoe G, Dziobek L. Hospital reimbursement patterns among patients with surgical wound infections following open heart surgery. *Infect Control Hosp Epidemiol.* 1990; 11:89–93.

23. Roach A, Kernodle D, Kaiser A. Selecting cost-effective antimicrobial prophylaxis in surgery: are we getting what we pay for? *DICP Ann Pharmacother.* 1990; 24:183–5.

24. Gorbach SL, Condon RE, Conte JE Jr et al. Evaluation of new anti-infective drugs for surgical prophylaxis. Infectious Diseases Society of America and the Food and Drug Administration. *Clin Infect Dis.* 1992; 15(suppl 1):S313–38.

25. Antimicrobial prophylaxis in surgery. *Med Lett Drugs Ther.* 1997; 39:97–102.

26. Page CP, Bohnen JM, Fletcher R et al. Antimicrobial prophylaxis for surgical wounds. Guidelines for clinical care. *Arch Surg.* 1993; 128:79–88.

27. Platt R, Zaleznik DF, Hopkins CC et al. Perioperative antibiotic prophylaxis for herniorrhaphy and breast surgery. *N Engl J Med.* 1990; 322:153–60.

28. Platt R, Zucker JR, Zaleznik DF et al. Perioperative antibiotic prophylaxis and wound infection following breast surgery. *J Antimicrob Chemother.* 1993; 31:43–8.

29. National Academy of Sciences–National Research Council. Postoperative wound infections: the influence of ultraviolet irradiation of the operating room and of various other factors. *Ann Surg.* 1964; 160:1–195.

30. Kernodle DS, Kaiser AB. Surgical and trauma-related infections. In: Mandell GL, Bennett JE, Dolin R, eds. Principles and practice of infectious diseases. 4th ed. New York: Churchill Livingstone; 1995:2742–55.

31. Freiman JA, Chalmers TC, Smith H et al. The importance of beta, the type II error and sample size in the design and interpretation of the randomized control trial. *N Engl J Med.* 1978; 299:690–4.

32. Dajani AS, Taubert KA, Wilson W et al. Prevention of bacterial endocarditis. Recommendations by the American Heart Association. *JAMA.* 1997; 277:1794–801.

33. American College of Obstetricians and Gynecologists (ACOG). Antimicrobial therapy for obstetric patients. *ACOG Ed Bull.* 1998; 245:1–10.

34. Guidelines for perinatal care. 4th ed. Elk Grove Village, IL: American Academy of Pediatrics and American College of Obstetricians and Gynecologists; 1997.

35. Peter G, ed. 1997 Red book: report of the Committee on Infectious Diseases. 24th ed. Elk Grove Village, IL: American Academy of Pediatrics; 1997.

36. Young TE, Mangum OB. Neofax: a manual of drugs used in neonatal care. 10th ed. Columbus, NC: Ross Laboratories; 1997.

37. Chang D. Influence of malignancy on the pharmacokinetics of vancomycin in infants and children. *Pediatr Infect Dis J.* 1995; 14:667–73.

38. Chang D, Liem L, Malogolowkin M. A prospective study of vancomycin pharmacokinetics and dosage requirements in pediatric cancer patients. *Pediatr Infect Dis J.* 1994; 13:969–74.

39. Kernodle DS, Classen DC, Burke JP et al. Failure of cephalosporins to prevent *Staphylococcus aureus* surgical wound infection. *JAMA.* 1990; 263:961–6.

40. Kriesel D, Savel TG, Silver AL et al. Surgical antibiotic prophylaxis and *Clostridium difficile* toxin positivity. *Arch Surg.* 1995; 130:989–93.

41. Privitera G, Scarpellini P, Ortisi G et al. Prospective study of *Clostridium difficile* intestinal colonization and disease following single-dose antibiotic prophylaxis surgery. *Antimicrob Agents Chemother.* 1991; 35:208–10.

42. Jobe BA, Grasley A, Deveney KE et al. *Clostridium difficile* colitis: an increasing hospital-acquired illness. *Am J Surg.* 1995; 169:480–3.

43. Morris JG, Shay DK, Hebden JN. Enterococci resistant to multiple antimicrobial agents, including vancomycin: establishment of endemicity in a university medical center. *Ann Intern Med.* 1995; 123:250–9.

44. Sastry V, Brennan PJ, Levy MM. Vancomycin-resistant enterococci: an emerging problem in immunosuppressed transplant recipients. *Transplant Proc.* 1995; 27:954–5.

45. Rhinehart E, Smith NE, Wennersten C. Rapid dissemination of beta-lactamase producing aminoglycoside resistant *Enterococcus faecium* among patients and staff on an infant-toddler surgical ward. *N Engl J Med.* 1990; 323:1814–8.

46. Burke JF. The effective period of preventive antibiotic action in experimental incisions and dermal lesions. *Surgery.* 1961; 50:161–8.

47. Classen DC, Evans RS, Pestotnik SL et al. The timing of prophylactic administration of antibiotics and the risk of surgical-wound infection. *N Engl J Med.* 1992; 326:281–6.

48. Gordon HP, Phelps D, Blanchard K. Prophylactic cesarean section antibiotics: maternal and neonatal morbidity before and after cord clamping. *Obstet Gynecol.* 1979; 53:151–6.

49. Cunningham FG, Leveno KJ, DePalma RT et al. Perioperative antimicrobials for cesarean delivery: before or after cord clamping. *Obstet Gynecol.* 1983; 62:151–4.

50. Clarke J, Condon R, Bartlett J et al. Preoperative oral antibiotics reduce septic complications of colon operations: results of a prospective randomized, double-blind clinical study. *Ann Surg.* 1977; 186:251–9.

51. Nichols R, Broldo P, Condon P et al. Effect of preoperative neomycin-erythromycin intestinal preparation on the incidence of infectious complications following colon surgery. *Ann Surg.* 1973; 178:453–62.

52. Stellato T, Danziger L, Gordon N et al. Antibiotics in elective colon surgery: a randomized trial of oral, systemic, and oral/systemic antibiotics for prophylaxis. *Am Surg.* 1990; 56:251–4.

53. Petrelli N, Contre DC, Herrera L et al. A prospective randomized trial of perioperative prophylactic cefamandole in elective colorectal surgery for malignancy. *Dis Colon Rectum.* 1988; 31:427–9.

54. Felip JF, Bonet EB, Eisman FI et al. Oral is superior to systemic antibiotic prophylaxis in operations upon the colon and rectum. *Surg Gynecol Obstet.* 1984; 158:359–62.

55. Kling PA, Dahlgren S. Oral prophylaxis with neomycin and erythromycin in colorectal surgery; more proof for efficacy than failure. *Arch Surg.* 1989; 124:705–7.

56. Lewis RT, Goodall RG, Marien B et al. Is neomycin necessary for bowel preparation in surgery of the colon? Oral neomycin plus erythromycin versus erythromycin-metronidazole. *Dis Colon Rectum.* 1989; 32:265–70.

57. DiPiro JT, Cheung RP, Bowden TA et al. Single-dose systemic antibiotic prophylaxis of surgical wound infections. *Am J Surg.* 1986; 152:552–9.

58. Scher KS. Studies on the duration of antibiotic administration for surgical prophylaxis. *Am Surg.* 1997; 63:59–62.

59. American Heart Association. 1996 statistical supplement. Dallas: Heart and stroke facts.

60. Demmy TL, Sang BP, Liebler GA et al. Recent experience with major sternal wound complications. *Ann Thorac Surg.* 1990; 49:458–62.

61. Kutsal A, Ibrisim E, Catav Z et al. Mediastinitis after open heart surgery. Analysis of risk factors and management. *J Cardiovasc Surg.* 1991; 32:38–41.

62. Kittle C, Reed W. Antibiotics and extracorporeal circulation. *J Thorac Cardiovasc Surg.* 1961; 41:34–48.

63. Slonim R, Litwak R, Gadboys H et al. Antibiotic prophylaxis of infection complicating open-heart operations. *Antimicrob Agents Chemother.* 1963; 3:731–5.

64. Goodman J, Schaffner W, Collins H et al. Infection after cardiovascular surgery. *N Engl J Med.* 1968; 278:117–23.

65. Fekety F, Cluff L, Sabiston D et al. A study of antibiotic prophylaxis in cardiac surgery. *J Thorac Cardiovasc Surg.* 1969; 57:757–63.

66. Conte J, Cohen S, Roe B et al. Antibiotic prophylaxis and cardiac surgery: a prospective double-blind comparison of single-dose versus multi-dose regimens. *Ann Intern Med.* 1972; 76:943–9.

67. Firor W. Infection following open-heart surgery, with special reference to the role of prophylactic antibiotics. *J Thorac Cardiovasc Surg.* 1967; 53:371–8.

68. Kreter B, Woods M. Antibiotic prophylaxis for cardiothoracic operations. Meta-analysis of thirty years of clinical trials. *J Thorac Cardiovasc Surg.* 1992; 104:590–9.

69. Fong I, Baker C, McKee D. The value of prophylactic antibiotics in aorta-coronary bypass operations. *J Thorac Cardiovasc Surg.* 1979; 78:908–13.

70. Penketh A, Wansbrough-Jones M, Wright E et al. Antibiotic prophylaxis for coronary artery bypass graft surgery. *Lancet.* 1985; 1:1500. Letter.

71. Hill D, Yates A. Prophylactic antibiotics in open heart surgery. *Aust N Z J Med.* 1975; 81:414–7.

72. Myerowitz P, Caswell K, Lindsay W et al. Antibiotic prophylaxis for open-heart surgery. *J Thorac Cardiovasc Surg.* 1977; 73:625–9.

73. Cooper D, Norton R, Mobin M et al. A comparison of two prophylactic antibiotic regimens for open-heart surgery. *J Cardiovasc Surg (Torino).* 1980; 21:279–86.

74. Bailey J, Perciva H. Cefamandole as a prophylactic in cardiac surgery. *Scand J Infect Dis.* 1980(suppl 25):112–7.

75. Ghoneim A, Tandon A, Ionescu M. Comparative study of cefamandole versus ampicillin plus cloxacillin: prophylactic antibiotics in cardiac surgery. *Ann Thorac Surg.* 1982; 33:152–8.

76. Slama T, Sklar S, Misinski J et al. Randomized comparison of cefamandole, cefazolin and cefuroxime prophylaxis in open-heart surgery. *Antimicrob Agents Chemother.* 1986; 29:744–7.

77. Kaiser A, Petracek M, Lea J et al. Efficacy of cefazolin, cefamandole, and gentamicin as prophylactic agents in cardiac surgery. *Ann Surg.* 1987; 206:791–7.

78. Geroulanos S, Oxelbark S, Donfried B et al. Antimicrobial prophylaxis in cardiovascular surgery. *Thorac Cardiovasc Surg.* 1987; 35:199–205.

79. Conklin C, Gray R, Neilson D et al. Determinants of wound infection incidence after isolated coronary artery bypass surgery in patients randomized to receive prophylactic cefuroxime or cefazolin. *Ann Thorac Surg.* 1988; 46:172–7.

80. Wellens F, Pirlet M, Larbuisson R et al. Prophylaxis in cardiac surgery: a controlled, randomized comparison between cefazolin and cefuroxime. *Eur J Cardiothorac Surg.* 1995; 9:325–9.

81. Galbraith U, Schilling J, von Segesser LK et al. Antibiotic prophylaxis in cardiovascular surgery: a prospective, randomized, comparative trial of one-day cefazolin vs single-dose cefuroxime. *Drugs Exp Clin Res.* 1993; 19:229–34.

82. Townsend TR, Reitz BA, Bilker WB et al. Clinical trial of cefamandole, cefazolin, and cefuroxime for antibiotic prophylaxis in cardiac operations. *J Thorac Cardiovasc Surg.* 1993; 106:664–70.

83. Curtis JJ, Boley TM, Walls JT et al. Randomized, prospective comparison of first- and second-generation cephalosporins as infection prophylaxis for cardiac surgery. *Am J Surg.* 1993; 166:734–7.

84. Doebbeling B, Pfaller M, Kuhns K et al. Cardiovascular surgery prophylaxis: a randomized, controlled comparison of cefazolin and cefuroxime. *J Thorac Cardiovasc Surg.* 1990; 99:981–9.

85. Gelfand MS, Simmons BP, Schoettle P et al. Cefamandole versus cefonicid prophylaxis in cardiovascular surgery: a prospective study. *Ann Thorac Surg.* 1990; 49:435–9.

86. Joyce F, Szczepanski K. A double-blind comparative study of prophylactic antibiotic therapy in open heart surgery: penicillin G versus vancomycin. *Thorac Cardiovasc Surg.* 1986; 34:100–3.

87. Goldman D, Hopkins C, Karchmer A et al. Cephalothin prophylaxis in cardiac valve surgery; a prospective, double-blind comparison of two-day and six-day regimens. *J Thorac Cardiovasc Surg.* 1977; 73:470–9.

88. Austin T, Coles J, McKenzie P et al. Cephalothin prophylaxis and valve replacement. *Ann Thorac Surg.* 1977; 23:333–6.

89. Hillis D, Rosenfeldt F, Spicer W et al. Antibiotic prophylaxis for coronary bypass grafting. *J Thorac Cardiovasc Surg.* 1983; 86:217–21.

90. Sisto T, Laurikka J, Tarkka MR. Ceftriaxone vs cefuroxime for infection prophylaxis in coronary bypass surgery. *Scand J Thorac Cardiovasc Surg.* 1994; 28:143–8.

91. Nooyen SMH, Overbeek BP, Brutel de la Riviere A et al. Prospective randomised comparison of single-dose versus multiple-dose cefuroxime for prophylaxis in coronary artery bypass grafting. *Eur J Clin Microbiol Infect Dis.* 1994; 13:1033–7.

92. Lee KR, Ring JC, Leggiadro RJ. Prophylactic antibiotic use in pediatric cardiovascular surgery: a surgery of current practice. *Pediatr Infect Dis J.* 1995; 14:267–9.

93. Gorbach SL, Plaut AG, Nahas L et al. Studies of intestinal microflora: II. Microorganisms of the small intestine and their relations to oral fecal flora. *Gastroenterology.* 1967; 53:856–67.

94. Gorbach SL. Intestinal microflora. *Gastroenterology.* 1971; 60:1110–29.

95. Ruddell WSJ, Axon ATR, Findlay JM et al. Effect of cimetidine on the gastric bacterial flora. *Lancet.* 1980; 1:672–4.

96. Driks MR, Craven DE, Bartolome RC et al. Nosocomial pneumonia in intubated patients given sucralfate as compared with antacids or histamine type 2 blockers. *N Engl J Med.* 1987; 317:1376–82.

97. Long J, Desantis S, State D et al. The effect of antisecretagogues on gastric microflora. *Arch Surg.* 1983; 118:1413–5.

98. Sjostedt S, Levin P, Malmborg AS et al. Septic complications in relation to factors influencing the gastric microflora in patients undergoing gastric surgery. *J Hosp Infect.* 1989; 12:191–7.

99. Feretis CB, Contou CT, Papoutsis GG et al. The effect of preoperative treatment with cimetidine on postoperative wound sepsis. *Am Surg.* 1984; 50:594–8.

100. LoCiero J, Nichols RL. Sepsis after gastroduodenal operations; relationship to gastric acid, motility, and endogenous microflora. *South Med J.* 1980; 73:878–80.

101. McArdle CS, Morran CG, Pettit L et al. Value of oral antibiotic prophylaxis in colorectal surgery. *Br J Surg.* 1995; 82:1046–8.

102. Nichols RL, Webb WR, Jones JW et al. Efficacy of antibiotic prophylaxis in high risk gastroduodenal operations. *Am J Surg.* 1982; 143:94–8.

103. Stone HH. Gastric surgery. *South Med J.* 1977; 70(suppl 1):35–7.

104. Morris DL, Yound D, Burdon DW et al. Prospective randomized trial of single-dose cefuroxime against mezlocillin elective gastric surgery. *J Hosp Infect.* 1984; 5:200–4.

105. Lewis RT, Allan CM, Goodall RG et al. Discriminate use of antibiotic prophylaxis in gastroduodenal surgery. *Am J Surg.* 1979; 138:640–3.

106. Lewis RT, Allan CM, Goodall RG et al. Cefamandole in gastroduodenal surgery: a controlled prospective, randomized, double-blind study. *Can J Surg.* 1982; 25:561–3.

107. Mitchell NJ, Evans DS, Pollock D. Pre-operative, single-dose cefuroxime antimicrobial prophylaxis with and without metronidazole in elective gastrointestinal surgery. *J Antimicrob Chemother.* 1980; 6:393–9.

108. Brown J, Mutton TP, Wasilauskas BL et al. Prospective, randomized, controlled trial of ticarcillin and cephalothin as prophylactic antibiotics for gastrointestinal operations. *Am J Surg.* 1982; 143:343–8.

109. Cruse PJ, Foord R. The epidemiology of wound infection: a ten-year prospective study of 62,939 wounds. *Surg Clin North Am.* 1980; 60:27–40.

110. Pories WJ, Van Rij AM, Burlingham BT et al. Prophylactic cefazolin in gastric bypass surgery. *Surgery.* 1981; 90:426–32.

111. Polk H, Lopez-Meyer J. Postoperative wound infection: a prospective study of determinant factors and prevention. *Surgery.* 1969; 66:97–103.

112. Evans C, Pollock AV. The reduction of surgical wound infections by prophylactic parenteral cephaloridine. *Br J Surg.* 1973; 60:434–7.

113. Stone HH, Haney BH, Kolb LD et al. Prophylactic and preventive antibiotic therapy. Timing, duration and economics. *Ann Surg.* 1979; 189:691–9.

114. Bates T, Roberts JV, Smith K et al. A randomized trial of one versus three doses of Augmentin as wound prophylaxis in at-risk abdominal surgery. *Postgrad Med J.* 1992; 68:811–6.

115. McArdle CS, Morran CG, Anderson JR et al. Oral ciprofloxacin as prophylaxis in gastroduodenal surgery. *J Hosp Infect.* 1995; 30:211–6.

116. Meijer WS, Schmitz PIM, Jeeke J. Meta-analysis of randomized, controlled clinical trials of antibiotic prophylaxis in biliary tract surgery. *Br J Surg.* 1990; 77:282–90.

117. Cainzos M, Potel J, Puente JL. Prospective, randomized, controlled study of prophylaxis with cefamandole in high-risk patients undergoing operations upon the biliary tract. *Surg Gynecol Obstet.* 1985; 160:27–32.

118. Meijer WS, Schmitz PI. Prophylactic use of cefuroxime in biliary tract surgery: randomized, controlled trial of single versus multiple dose in high-risk patients. Galant Trial Study Group. *Br J Surg.* 1993; 80:917–21.

119. Grant MD, Jones RC, Wilson SE et al. Single-dose cephalosporin prophylaxis in high-risk patients undergoing surgical treatment of the biliary tract. *Surg Gynecol Obstet.* 1992; 174:347–54.

120. Lapointe RW, Roy AF, Turgeon PL et al. Comparison of single-dose cefotetan and multidose cefoxitin as intravenous prophylaxis in elective, open biliary tract surgery: a multicentre, double-blind, randomized study. *Can J Surg.* 1994; 37:313–8.

121. Strachan CJL, Black J, Powis SJA et al. Prophylactic use of cephazolin against wound sepsis after cholecystectomy. *Br Med J.* 1977; 1:1254–6.

122. Berne TV, Yellin AE, Appleman MD et al. Controlled comparison of cefmetazole with cefoxitin for prophylaxis in elective cholecystectomy. *Surg Gynecol Obstet.* 1990; 170:137–40.

123. Wilson SE, Hopkins JA, Williams RA. A comparison of cefotaxime versus cefamandole in prophylaxis for surgical treatment of the biliary tract. *Surg Gynecol Obstet.* 1987; 164:207–12.

124. Kujath P. Brief report: antibiotic prophylaxis in biliary tract surgery. *Am J Med.* 1989; 87(suppl 5A):255–7.

125. Garibaldi RA, Skolnck D, Maglio S et al. Postcholecystectomy wound infection. *Ann Surg.* 1986; 204:650–4.

126. Levi JU, Martinez OV, Hutson DG et al. Ampicillin versus cefamandole in biliary tract surgery. *Am Surg.* 1984; 50:412–7.

127. Kellum JM, Duma RJ, Gorbach SL et al. Single-dose antibiotic prophylaxis for biliary surgery. *Arch Surg.* 1987; 122:918–22.

128. Muller EL, Pitt HA, Thompson JE et al. Antibiotics in infections of the biliary tract. *Surg Gynecol Obstet.* 1987; 165:285–92.

129. Stone HH, Hooper CA, Kolb LD et al. Antibiotic prophylaxis in gastric, biliary and colonic surgery. *Ann Surg.* 1976; 184:443–52.

130. Elliot DW. Biliary tract surgery. *South Med J.* 1977; 70(suppl 1):31–4.

131. Chetlin SH, Elliot DW. Preoperative antibiotics in biliary surgery. *Arch Surg.* 1973; 107:319–23.

132. Kellum JM, Gargano S, Gorbach SL et al. Antibiotic prophylaxis in high-risk biliary operations: multicenter trial of single preoperative ceftriaxone versus multidose cefazolin. *Am J Surg.* 1984; 148:15–21.

133. Drumm J, Donovan IA, Wise R. A comparison of cefotetan and cefazolin for prophylaxis against wound infection after elective cholecystectomy. *J Hosp Infect.* 1985; 6:227–80.

134. Plouffe JF, Perkins RL, Fass RJ et al. Comparison of the effectiveness of moxalactam and cefazolin in the prevention of infection in patients undergoing abdominal operations. *Diagn Microbiol Infect Dis.* 1985; 3:25–31.

135. Crenshaw CA, Glanges E, Webber CE et al. A prospective, randomized, double-blind study of preventive cefamandole therapy in patients at high risk for undergoing cholecystectomy. *Surg Gynecol Obstet.* 1981; 153:546–52.

136. Leaper DJ, Cooper MJ, Turner A. A comparison trial between cefotetan and cephazolin for wound sepsis prophylaxis during elective upper gastrointestinal surgery with an investigation of cefotetan penetration into the obstructed biliary tree. *J Hosp Infect.* 1986; 7:269–76.

137. Krajden S, Yaman M, Fuksa M et al. Piperacillin versus cefazolin given perioperatively to high-risk patients who undergo open cholecystectomy: a double-blind, randomized trial. *Can J Surg.* 1993; 36:245–50.

138. Sirinek KR, Schauer PR, Yellin AE et al. Single-dose cefuroxime versus multiple-dose cefazolin as prophylactic therapy for high-risk cholecystectomy. *J Am Coll Surg.* 1994; 178:321–5.

139. Maki DG, Lammers JL, Aughey DR. Comparative studies of multiple-dose cefoxitin vs. single-dose cefonicid for surgical prophylaxis in patients undergoing biliary tract operations or hysterectomy. *Rev Infect Dis.* 1984; 6(suppl 4):887–95.

140. Fabian TC, Zellner SR, Gazzaniga A et al. Multicenter open trial of cefotetan in elective biliary surgery. *Am J Surg.* 1988; 155:77–80.

141. Garcia-Rodriquez JA, Puig-LaCalle J, Arnau C et al. Antibiotic prophylaxis with cefotaxime in gastroduodenal and biliary surgery. *Am J Surg.* 1989; 158:428–32.

142. Targarona EM, Garau J, Munoz-Ramos C et al. Single-dose antibiotic prophylaxis in patients at high risk for infection in biliary surgery: a prospective and randomized study comparing cefonicid with mezlocillin. *Surgery.* 1990; 107:327–34.

143. Krige JE, Isaacs S, Stapleton GN et al. Prospective, randomized study comparing amoxicillin-clavulanic acid and cefamandole for the prevention of wound infection in high-risk patients undergoing elective biliary surgery. *J Hosp Infect.* 1992; 22(suppl A):33–41.

144. McLeish AR, Keighley MRB, Bishop HM. Selecting patients requiring antibiotics in biliary surgery by immediate gram stains of bile at surgery. *Surgery.* 1977; 81:473–7.

145. McArdle CS. Oral prophylaxis in biliary tract surgery. *J Antimicrob Chemother.* 1994; 33:200–2.

146. Donohue JH, Farnell MB, Grant CS et al. Laparoscopic cholecystectomy: early Mayo Clinic experience. *Mayo Clin Proc.* 1992; 67:449–55.

147. Frantzides CT, Sykes A. A reevaluation of antibiotic prophylaxis in laparoscopic cholecystectomy. *J Laparoendosc Surg.* 1994; 4:375–8.

148. Watkin DS, Wainwright AM, Thompson MH et al. Infection after laparoscopic cholecystectomy: are antibiotics really necessary? *Eur J Surg.* 1995; 161:509–11.

149. Cann KJ, Watkins RM, George C et al. A trial of mezlocillin versus cefuroxime with or without metronidazole for the prevention of wound sepsis after biliary and gastrointestinal surgery. *J Hosp Infect.* 1988; 12:207–14.

150. Menzies D, Gilbert JM, Shepherd MJ et al. A comparison between amoxycillin/clavulanate and mezlocillin in abdominal surgical prophylaxis. *J Antimicrob Chemother.* 1989; 24:203–8B.

151. Katz S, Glicksman A, Levy Y et al. Cefuroxime prophylaxis in biliary surgery: single versus triple dose. *Israel J Med Sci.* 1993; 29:673–6.

152. Ahmed ME, Ibrahim SZ, Arabi YE et al. Metronidazole prophylaxis in acute mural appendicitis: failure of a single intra-operative infusion to reduce wound infection. *J Hosp Infect.* 1987; 10:260–4.

153. Donovan IA, Ellis D, Gatehouse D et al. One-dose antibiotic prophylaxis against wound infection after appendectomy: a randomized trial of clindamycin, cefazolin sodium and a placebo. *Br J Surg.* 1979; 66:193–6.

154. Gilmore OJ, Martin TD. Aetiology and prevention of wound infection in appendectomy. *Br J Surg.* 1974; 62:567–72.

155. Keiser TA, Mackenzie RL, Feld LN. Prophylactic metronidazole in appendectomy: a double-blind controlled trial. *Surgery.* 1983; 93:201–3.

156. Winslow RE, Rem D, Harley JW. Acute nonperforating appendicitis: efficacy of brief antibiotic prophylaxis. *Arch Surg.* 1983; 118:651–5.

157. Wilson AP. Antibiotic prophylaxis and infection control measures in minimally invasive surgery. *J Antimicrob Chemother.* 1995; 36:1–5.

158. Stone HH. Bacterial flora of appendicitis in children. *J Pediatr Surg.* 1976; 11:37–42.

159. Keighley MR. Infection: prophylaxis. *Br Med Bull.* 1988; 44:374–402.

160. Lau WY, Fan ST, Yiu TF et al. Prophylaxis of post-appendectomy sepsis by metronidazole and cefotaxime: a randomized, prospective and double-blind trial. *Br J Surg.* 1983; 70:670–2.

161. Lau WY, Fan ST, Chu KW et al. Randomized, prospective, and double-blind trial of new beta-lactams in the treatment of appendicitis. *Antimicrob Agents Chemother.* 1985; 28:639–42.

162. Lau WY, Fan ST, Chu KW et al. Cefoxitin versus gentamicin and metronidazole in prevention of post-appendectomy sepsis: a randomized, prospective trial. *J Antimicrob Chemother.* 1986; 18:613–9.

163. O'Rourke MGE, Wynne MJ, Morahan RJ et al. Prophylactic antibiotics in appendectomy: a prospective, double-blind, randomized study. *Aust N Z J Surg.* 1984; 54:535–41.

164. Panichi G, Pantosi AL, Marsiglio F. Cephalothin or cefoxitin in appendectomy? *J Antimicrob Chemother.* 1980; 6:801–4. Letter.

165. Liberman MA, Greason KL, Frame S et al. Single-dose cefotetan or cefoxitin versus multiple-dose cefoxitin as prophylaxis in patients undergoing appendectomy for acute nonperforated appendicitis. *J Am Coll Surg.* 1995; 180:77–80.

166. Salam IM, Abu Galala KH, el Ashaal YI et al. A randomized prospective study of cefoxitin versus piperacillin in appendicectomy. *J Hosp Infect.* 1994; 26:133–6.

167. Lau WY, Fan ST, Yiu TF et al. Prophylaxis of postappendectomy sepsis by metronidazole and ampicillin; a randomized, prospective and double-blind trial. *Br J Surg.* 1983; 70:155–7.

168. Al-Dhohayan A, al-Sebayl M, Shibl A et al. Comparative study of augmentin versus metronidazole/gentamicin in the prevention of infections after appendectomy. *Eur Surg Res.* 1993; 25:60–4.

169. Kizilcan F, Tanyel FC, Buyukpamukcu N et al. The necessity of prophylactic antibiotics in uncomplicated appendicitis during childhood. *J Pediatr Surg.* 1992; 27:586–8.

170. Soderquist-Elinder C, Hirsch K, Bergdahl S et al. Prophylactic antibiotics in uncomplicated appendicitis during childhood—a prospective randomized study. *Eur J Pediatr Surg.* 1995; 5:282–5.

171. Browder W, Smith JW, Vivoda LM et al. Nonperforative appendicitis: a continuing surgical dilemma. *J Infect Dis.* 1989; 159:1088–94.

172. Bartlett S, Burton R. Effects of prophylactic antibiotics on wound infection after elective colon and rectal surgery. *Am J Surg.* 1983; 145:300–9.

173. Burton RC. Postoperative wound infection in colon and rectal surgery. *Br J Surg.* 1973; 60:363–8.

174. Baum M, Anish D, Chalmers T et al. A survey of clinical trials of antibiotic prophylaxis in colon surgery: evidence against further use of no treatment controls. *N Engl J Med.* 1981; 305:795–9.

175. Coppa G, Eng K, Gouge T et al. Parenteral and oral antibiotics in elective colorectal surgery: a prospective randomized trial. *Am J Surg.* 1983; 145:62–5.

176. Coppa G, Eng K. Factors involved in antibiotic selection in elective colon and rectal surgery. *Surgery.* 1988; 104:853–8.

177. Svensson LG. Prophylactic antibiotic administration. *S Afr J Surg.* 1985; 23:55–62.

178. Singh JJ, Wexner SD. Laparoscopy for colorectal cancer. In: Keighley MRB, Williams N, eds. Surgery of the anus, rectum and colon. 2nd ed. London: Saunders; 1999.

179. Davis G, Santa Ana C, Morawiski S et al. Development of a lavage solution associated with minimal water and electrolyte absorption or secretion. *Gastroenterology.* 1980; 78:991–5.

180. Beck D, Harford F, DiPalma JA. Comparison of cleansing methods in preparation for colon surgery. *Dis Colon Rectum.* 1985; 28:491–5.

181. Jagelman D, Fazio V, Lavery I et al. Single-dose piperacillin versus cefoxitin combined with 10 percent mannitol bowel preparation as prophylaxis in elective colorectal operations. *Am J Surg.* 1987; 154:478–81.

182. Wolff B, Beart R, Dozios R et al. A new bowel preparation for elective colon and rectal surgery: a prospective, randomized clinical trial. *Arch Surg.* 1988; 123:895–900.

183. Cohen SM, Wexner SD, Binderow SR et al. Prospective, randomized, endoscopic-blinded trial comparing precolonoscopy bowel cleansing methods. *Dis Colon Rectum.* 1994; 37:689–96.

184. Smith LE, Solla JA, Rothenberger DA. Current status. Preoperative bowel preparation. A survey of colon and rectal surgeons. *Dis Colon Rectum.* 1990; 33:154–9.

185. DiPalma JA, Marshall JB. Comparison of a new sulfate-free polyethylene glycol electrolyte lavage solution versus a standard solution for colonoscopy cleansing. *Gastrointest Endosc.* 1990; 36:285–9.

186. Oliveira L, Wexner SD, Daniel N et al. Mechanical bowel preparation for elective colorectal surgery. A prospective, randomized, surgeon-blinded trial comparing sodium phosphate and polyethylene glycol-based oral lavage solutions. *Dis Colon Rectum.* 1997; 40:585–91.

187. Nichols RL. Prophylaxis for intraabdominal surgery. *Rev Infect Dis.* 1984; 6(suppl 1):276–82.

188. Wapnick S, Gunito R, Leveen HH et al. Reduction of postoperative infection in elective colorectal surgery with preoperative administration of kanamycin and erythromycin. *Surgery.* 1979; 85:317–21.

189. Gahhos FN, Richards GK, Hinchey EJ et al. Elective colon surgery: clindamycin versus metronidazole prophylaxis. *Can J Surg.* 1982; 25:613–6.

190. Dion YM, Richards GK, Prentis JJ et al. The influence of oral metronidazole versus parenteral preoperative metronidazole on sepsis following colon surgery. *Ann Surg.* 1980; 192:221–6.

191. Beggs FD, Jobanputra RS, Holmes JT. A comparison of intravenous and oral metronidazole as prophylactic in colorectal surgery. *Br J Surg.* 1982; 69:226–7.

192. Goldring J, McNaught W, Scott A et al. Prophylactic oral antimicrobial agents in elective colonic surgery: a controlled trial. *Lancet.* 1975; 2:997–9.

193. Washington J, Dearing W, Judd E et al. Effect of preoperative antibiotic regimen on development of infection after intestinal surgery. *Ann Surg.* 1974; 180:567–72.

194. Willis A, Fergunson I, Jones P et al. Metronidazole in prevention and treatment of *Bacteroides* infections in elective colonic surgery. *Br Med J.* 1977; 1:607–10.

195. Hagen TB, Bergan T, Liavag I. Prophylactic metronidazole in elective colorectal surgery. *Acta Chir Scand.* 1980; 146:71–5.

196. Lewis RT, Allan CM, Goodall RG et al. Are first-generation cephalosporins effective for antibiotic prophylaxis in elective surgery of the colon? *Can J Surg.* 1983; 26:504–7.

197. Condon RE, Bartlett JG, Nichols RL et al. Preoperative prophylactic cephalothin fails to control septic complications of colorectal operations: results of a controlled clinical trial. *Am J Surg.* 1979; 137:68–74.

198. Kaiser A, Herrington J, Jacobs J et al. Cefoxitin vs erythromycin, neomycin and cefazolin in colorectal surgery: importance of the duration of the operative procedure. *Ann Surg.* 1983; 198:525–30.

199. McDermott F, Polyglase A, Johnson W et al. Prevention of wound infection in colorectal resections by preoperative cephazolin with and without metronidazole. *Aust N Z J Surg.* 1981; 51:351–3.

200. Jones RN, Wojeski W, Bakke J et al. Antibiotic prophylaxis to 1,036 patients undergoing elective surgical procedures. A prospective randomized comparative trial of cefazolin, cefoxitin, and cefotaxime in a prepaid medical practice. *Am J Surg.* 1987; 153:341–6.

201. Morton A, Taylor E, Wells G. A multicenter study to compare cefotetan alone with cefotetan and metronidazole as prophylaxis against infection in elective colorectal operations. *Surg Gynecol Obstet.* 1989; 169:4–45.

202. Hoffman C, McDonald P, Watts J. Use of perioperative cefoxitin to prevent infection after colonic and rectal surgery. *Ann Surg.* 1981; 193:353–6.

203. Periti P, Mazzei T, Tonelli F. Single-dose cefotetan vs multiple dose cefoxitin—antimicrobial prophylaxis in colorectal surgery: results of a prospective, multicenter, randomized study. *Dis Colon Rectum.* 1989; 32:121–7.

204. Jagelman D, Fabian T, Nichols R et al. Single-dose cefotetan versus multiple dose cefoxitin as prophylaxis in colorectal surgery. *Am J Surg.* 1988; 155:71–6.

205. Shatney CH. Antibiotic prophylaxis in elective gastrointestinal tract surgery: a comparison of single-dose preoperative cefotaxime and multiple-dose cefoxitin. *J Antimicrob Chemother.* 1984; 14(suppl B):241–5.

206. Galandiuk S, Polk HC, Jagelman DG et al. Reemphasis of priorities in surgical antibiotic prophylaxis. *Surg Gynecol Obstet.* 1989; 169:219–22.

207. Arnaud JP, Bellissant E, Boissel P et al. Single-dose amoxycillin-clavulanic acid vs cefotetan for prophylaxis in elective colorectal surgery: a multicentre, prospective, randomized study. The PRODIGE Group. *J Hosp Infect.* 1992; 22(suppl A):23–32.

208. Periti P, Tonelli F, Mazzei T et al. Antimicrobial chemoimmunoprophylaxis in colorectal surgery with cefotetan and thymostimulin: prospective, controlled, multicenter study. Italian Study Group on Antimicrobial Prophylaxis in Abdominal Surgery. *J Chemother.* 1993; 5:37–42.

209. Skipper D, Karran SJ. A randomized, prospective study to compare cefotetan with cefuroxime plus metronidazole as prophylaxis in elective colorectal surgery. *J Hosp Infect.* 1992; 21:73–7.

210. Lumley JW, Siu SK, Pillay SP et al. Single-dose ceftriaxone as prophylaxis for sepsis in colorectal surgery. *Aust N Z J Surg.* 1992; 62:292–6.

211. Hakansson T, Raahave D, Hansen OH et al. Effectiveness of single-dose prophylaxis with cefotaxime and metronidazole compared with three doses of cefotaxime alone in elective colorectal surgery. *Eur J Surg.* 1993; 159:177–80.

212. Karran SJ, Sutton G, Gartell P et al. Imipenem prophylaxis in elective colorectal surgery. *Br J Surg.* 1993; 80:1196–8.

213. Barbar MS, Hirxberg BC, Rice C et al. Parenteral antibiotics in elective colon surgery? A prospective, controlled clinical study. *Surgery.* 1979; 86:23–9.

214. Madsen M, Toftgaard C, Gaversen H et al. Cefoxitin for one day vs ampicillin and metronidazole for three days in elective colorectal surgery: a prospective, randomized, multicenter study. *Dis Colon Rectum.* 1988; 31:774–7.

215. Blair J, McLeod R, Cohen Z et al. Ticarcillin/clavulanic acid (Timentin) compared to metronidazole/netilmicin in preventing postoperative infection after elective colorectal surgery. *Can J Surg.* 1987; 30:120–2.

216. AhChong K, Yip AW, Lee FC et al. Comparison of prophylactic ampicillin/sulbactam with gentamicin and metronidazole in elective colorectal surgery: a randomized clinical study. *J Hosp Infect.* 1994; 27:149–54.

217. Mendes da Costa P, Kaufman L. Amikacin once daily plus metronidazole versus amikacin twice daily plus metronidazole in colorectal surgery. *Hepatogastroenterology.* 1992; 39:350–4.

218. Roland M. Prophylactic regimens in colorectal surgery: an open randomized consecutive trial of metronidazole used alone or in combination with ampicillin or doxycycline. *World J Surg.* 1986; 10:1003–8.

219. Juul PZ, Klaaborg KE, Kronborg O. Single or multiple doses of metronidazole and ampicillin in elective colorectal surgery: a randomized trial. *Dis Colon Rectum.* 1987; 30:526–8.

220. Kwok SP, Lau WY, Leung KL et al. Amoxicillin and clavulanic acid versus cefotaxime and metronidazole as antibiotic prophylaxis in elective colorectal resectional surgery. *Chemotherapy.* 1993; 39:135–9.

221. Bergman L, Solhaug JH. Single-dose chemoprophylaxis in elective colorectal surgery. *Ann Surg.* 1987; 205:77–81.

222. Goransson G, Nilsson-Ehle I, Olsson S et al. Single-versus multiple-dose doxycycline prophylaxis in elective colorectal surgery. *Acta Chir Scand.* 1984; 150:245–9.

223. Andaker L, Burman LG, Eklund A et al. Fosfomycin/metronidazole compared with doxycycline/metronidazole for the prophylaxis of infection after elective colorectal surgery: a randomized, double-blind, multicentre trial in 517 patients. *Eur J Surg.* 1992; 158:181–5.

224. University of Melbourne Colorectal Group. A comparison of single-dose Timentin with mezlocillin for prophylaxis of wound infection in elective colorectal surgery. *Dis Colon Rectum.* 1989; 32:940–3.

225. Stewart M, Taylor EW, Lindsay G. Infection after colorectal surgery: a randomized trial of prophylaxis with piperacillin versus sulbactam/piperacillin. West of Scotland Surgical Infection Study Group. *J Hosp Infect.* 1995; 29:135–42.

226. Condon RE, Bartlett J, Greenlee H et al. Efficacy of oral and systemic antibiotic prophylaxis in colorectal operations. *Arch Surg.* 1983; 118:496–502.

227. Condon RE. Preoperative antibiotic bowel preparation. *Drug Ther.* 1983; Jan:29–37.

228. Hinchey E, Richards G, Lewis R et al. Moxalactam as single agent prophylaxis in the prevention of wound infection following colon surgery. *Surgery.* 1987; 101:15–9.

229. Jagelman DG, Fazio VW, Lavery IC et al. A prospective, randomized, double-blind study of 10% mannitol mechanical bowel preparation combined with oral neomycin and short-term, perioperative, intravenous Flagyl as prophylaxis in elective colorectal resections. *Surgery.* 1985; 98:861–5.

230. Sondheimer JM, Sokol RJ, Taylor S et al. Safety, efficacy, and tolerance of intestinal lavage in pediatric patients undergoing diagnostic colonoscopy. *J Pediatr.* 1991; 119:148–52.

231. Tuggle DW, Hoelzer DJ, Tunell WP et al. The safety and cost-effectiveness of polyethylene glycol electrolyte solution bowel preparation in infants and children. *J Pediatr Surg.* 1987; 22:513–5.

232. Weber RS, Callender DL. Antibiotic prophylaxis in clean-contaminated head and neck oncologic surgery. *Ann Otol Rhinol Laryngol.* 1992; 101:16–20.

233. Saginur R, Odell PF, Poliquin JF. Antibiotic prophylaxis in head and neck cancer surgery. *J Otolaryngol.* 1988; 17:78–80.

234. Mandell-Brown M, Johnson JT, Wagner RL. Cost-effectiveness of prophylactic antibiotics in head and neck surgery. *Otolaryngol Head Neck Surg.* 1984; 92:520–3.

235. Johnson JT, Yu VL, Myers EN et al. Efficacy of two third-generation cephalosporins in prophylaxis for head and neck surgery. *Arch Otolaryngol.* 1984; 110:224–7.

236. Johnson JT, Myers EN, Thearle PB et al. Antimicrobial prophylaxis for contaminated head and neck surgery. *Laryngoscope.* 1984; 94:46–51.

237. Johnson JT, Yu VL, Myers EN et al. An assessment of the need for gram-negative bacterial coverage in antibiotic prophylaxis for oncological head and neck surgery. *J Infect Dis.* 1987; 155:331–3.

238. Dor P, Klastersky J. Prophylactic antibiotics in oral pharyngeal and laryngeal surgery for cancer: a double-blind study. *Laryngoscope.* 1973; 83:1992–8.

239. Mombelli G, Coppens L, Dor P et al. Antibiotic prophylaxis in surgery for head and neck cancer. Comparative study of short and prolonged administration of carbenicillin. *J Antimicrob Chemother.* 1981; 7:665–7.

240. Myers EN, Thearle PB, Sigler BA et al. Antimicrobial prophylaxis for contaminated head and neck surgery. *Laryngoscope.* 1984; 94:46–51.

241. Robbins KT, Byers RM, Fainstein V et al. Wound prophylaxis with metronidazole in head and neck surgical oncology. *Laryngoscope.* 1988; 98:803–6.

242. Robbins KT, Favrot S, Hanna D et al. Risk of wound infection in patients with head and neck cancer. *Head Neck.* 1990; 12(2):143–8.

243. Tabet JC, Johnson JT. Wound infection in head and neck surgery: prophylaxis, etiology and management. *J Otolaryngol.* 1990; 3:143–8.

244. Girod DA, McCulloch TM, Tsue TT et al. Risk factors for complications in clean-contaminated head and neck surgical procedures. *Head Neck.* 1995; 17(1):7–13.

245. Becker GD, Welch WD. Quantitative bacteriology of closed-suction wound drainage in contaminated surgery. *Laryngoscope.* 1990; 100:403–6.

246. Johnson JT, Yu VL. Role of aerobic gram-negative rods, anaerobes, and fungi in wound infection after head and neck surgery: implications for antibiotic prophylaxis. *Head Neck.* 1989; 11(1):27–9.

247. Rubin J, Johnson JT, Wagner RL et al. Bacteriologic analysis of wound infection following major head and neck surgery. *Arch Otolaryngol Head Neck Surg.* 1988; 114:969–72.

248. Brown BM, Johnson JT, Wagner RL. Etiologic factors in head and neck wound infections. *Laryngoscope.* 1987; 97:587–90.

249. Johnson JT, Wagner RL. Infection following uncontaminated head and neck surgery. *Arch Otolaryngol Head Neck Surg.* 1987; 113:368–9.

250. Blair EA, Johnson JT, Wagner RL et al. Cost-analysis of antibiotic prophylaxis in clean head and neck surgery. *Arch Otolaryngol Head Neck Surg.* 1995; 121:269–71.

251. Brand B, Johnson JT, Myers EN et al. Prophylactic perioperative antibiotics in contaminated head and neck surgery. *Otolaryngol Head Neck Surg.* 1982; 990:315–8.

252. Gerard M, Meunier F, Dor P et al. Antimicrobial prophylaxis for major head and neck surgery in cancer patients. *Antimicrob Agents Chemother.* 1988; 32:1557–9.

253. Sharpe DAC, Renuich P, Mathews KHN et al. Antibiotic prophylaxis in oesophageal surgery. *Eur J Cardiothorac Surg.* 1992; 6:561–4.

254. Johnson JT, Yu VL, Myers EN et al. Cefazolin vs moxalactam? A double-blind, randomized trial of cephalosporins in head and neck surgery. *Arch Otolaryngol Head Neck Surg.* 1986; 112:151–3.

255. Johnson JT, Wagner RL, Schuller DE et al. Prophylactic antibiotics for head and neck surgery with flap reconstruction. *Arch Otolaryngol Head Neck Surg.* 1992; 118:488–90.

256. Rodrigo JP, Alvarez JC, Gomez JR et al. Comparison of three prophylactic antibiotic regimens in clean-contaminated head and neck surgery. *Head Neck.* 1997; 19:188–93.

257. Ehrenkranz NJ. Surgical wound infection occurrence in clean operations. Risk stratification for interhospital comparisons. *Am J Med.* 1981; 50:909–14.

258. Fan-Havard P, Nahata MC. Treatment and prevention of infections of cerebrospinal fluid shunts. *Clin Pharm.* 1987; 6:866–80.

259. Keucher TR, Mealey J. Long-term results after ventriculoatrial and ventriculoperitoneal shunting for infantile hydrocephalus. *J Neurosurg.* 1979; 50:179–86.

260. Yogev R, Davis T. Neurosurgical shunt infections—a review. *Childs Brain.* 1980; 6:74–80.

261. Renier D, Lacombe J, Pierre-Kahn A et al. Factors causing acute shunt infection—computer analysis of 1174 patients. *J Neurosurg.* 1984; 61:1072–8.

262. O'Brien M, Parent A, Davis B. Management of ventricular shunt infections. *Childs Brain.* 1979; 5:304–9.

263. Schoenbaum SC, Gardner P, Shillito J. Infection of cerebrospinal fluid shunts: epidemiology, clinical manifestations and therapy. *J Infect Dis.* 1975; 131:534–52.

264. Walters BC, Hoffman HJ, Hendrick EB et al. Cerebrospinal fluid shunt infection. Influences on initial management and subsequent outcome. *J Neurosurg.* 1984; 60:1014–21.

265. Wilson HD, Bean JR, James HE et al. Cerebrospinal fluid antibiotic concentrations in ventricular shunt infections. *Childs Brain.* 1978; 4:74–82.

266. James HE, Walsh JW, Wilson HD et al. The management of cerebrospinal fluid shunt infections. A clinical experience. *Acta Neurochir.* 1981; 59:157–66.

267. Mates S, Glaser J, Shapiro K. Treatment of cerebrospinal fluid shunt infections with medical therapy alone. *Neurosurgery.* 1982; 11:781–3.

268. Horwitz NH, Curtin JA. Prophylactic antibiotics and wound infections following laminectomy for lumbar disc disease. A retrospective study. *J Neurosurg.* 1975; 43:727–31.

269. Savitz MH, Malis LI. Prophylactic clindamycin for neurosurgical patients. *N Y State J Med.* 1976; 76:64–7.

270. Haines SJ, Goodman ML. Antibiotic prophylaxis of postoperative neurosurgical wound infection. *J Neurosurg.* 1982; 56:103–5.

271. Geraghty J, Feely M. Antibiotic prophylaxis in neurosurgery. A randomized, controlled trial. *J Neurosurg.* 1984; 60:724–6.

272. Mollman HD, Haines SJ. Risk factors for postoperative neurosurgical wound infection. A case-control study. *J Neurosurg.* 1986; 64:902–6.

273. Shapiro M, Wald U, Simchen E et al. Randomized clinical trial of intra-operative antimicrobial prophylaxis of infection after neurosurgical procedures. *J Hosp Infect.* 1986; 8:283–95.

274. George R, Leibrock L, Epstein M. Long-term analysis of cerebrospinal fluid shunt infections—a 25-year experience. *J Neurosurg.* 1979; 51:804–11.

275. Bayston R. Hydrocephalus shunt infections and their treatment. *J Antimicrob Chemother.* 1985; 15:259–61.

276. Forrest DM, Cooper DG. Complications of ventriculoatrial shunts. A review of 455 cases. *J Neurosurg.* 1968; 29:506–12.

277. Odio C, McCracken JC, Nelson JD. CSF shunt infections in pediatrics—a seven-year experience. *Am J Dis Child.* 1984; 138:1103–8.

278. Petrak RM, Pottage JC, Harris AA et al. *Haemophilus influenzae* meningitis in the presence of a cerebrospinal fluid shunt. *Neurosurgery.* 1986; 18:79–81.

279. Sells CJ, Shurtleff DB, Coeser JD. Gram-negative cerebrospinal fluid shunt-associated infections. *Pediatrics.* 1977; 59:614–8.

280. Shapiro S, Boaz J, Kleiman M et al. Origins of organisms infecting ventricular shunts. *Neurosurgery.* 1988; 22:868–72.

281. Gardner P, Leipzig TJ, Sadigh M. Infections of mechanical cerebrospinal fluid shunts. *Curr Clin Top Infect Dis.* 1988; 9:185–214.

282. Barker FG II. Efficacy of prophylactic antibiotics for craniotomy: a meta-analysis. *Neurosurgery.* 1994; 35:484–90.

283. Wright RL. Septic complication of neurosurgical spinal procedures. Springfield, IL: Thomas; 1970:26–39.

284. Wright RL. Postoperative craniotomy infections. Springfield, IL: Thomas; 1966:26–31.

285. Tenney JH, Vlahov D, Daleman M et al. Wide variation in risk of wound infection following clean neurosurgery. Implication for perioperative antibiotic prophylaxis. *J Meirpsirg.* 1986; 62:243–7.

286. Savitz MH, Malis LI, Meyers BR. Prophylactic antibiotics in neurosurgery. *Surg Neurol.* 1974; 2:95–100.

287. Malis LI. Prevention of neurosurgical infection by intraoperative antibiotics. *Neurosurgery.* 1979; 5:339–43.

288. Haines SJ. Systemic antibiotic prophylaxis in neurological surgery. *Neurosurgery.* 1980; 6:355–61.

289. Quartey GRC, Polyzoidis K. Intraoperative antibiotic prophylaxis in neurosurgery: a clinical study. *Neurosurgery.* 1981; 8:669–71.

290. Savitz MH, Katz SS. Prevention of primary wound infection in neurosurgical patients: a 10-year study. *Neurosurgery.* 1986; 18:685–8.

291. Blomstedt GC, Kytta J. Results of a randomized trial of vancomycin prophylaxis in craniotomy. *J Neurosurg.* 1988; 69:216–20.

292. Pons VG, Denlinger SL, Guglielmo BJ et al. Ceftizoxime versus vancomycin and gentamicin in neurosurgical prophylaxis: a randomized, prospective, blinded clinical study. *Neurosurgery.* 1993; 33:416–22.

293. Wang EL, Prober CG, Hendrick BE. Prophylactic sulfamethoxazole and trimethoprim in ventriculoperitoneal shunt surgery. A double-blind, randomized, placebo-controlled trial. *JAMA.* 1984; 251:1174–7.

294. Blomstedt GC. Results in trimethoprim-sulfamethoxazole prophylaxis in ventriculostomy and shunting procedures. *J Neurosurg.* 1985; 62:694–7.

295. Djindjian M, Fevrier MJ, Ottervbein G et al. Oxacillin prophylaxis in cerebrospinal fluid shunt procedures: results of a randomized, open study in 60 hydrocephalic patients. *Surg Neurol.* 1986; 24:178–80.

296. Blum J, Schwarz M, Voth D. Antibiotic single-dose prophylaxis of shunt infections. *Neurosurg Rev.* 1989; 12:239–44.

297. Schmidt K, Gjerris F, Osgaard O et al. Antibiotic prophylaxis in cerebrospinal fluid shunting: a prospective randomized trial in 152 hydrocephalic patients. *Neurosurgery.* 1985; 17:1–5.

298. Griebel R, Khan M, Tan L. CSF shunt complications: an analysis of contributory factors. *Childs Nerv Syst.* 1985; 1:77–80.

299. Lambert M, MacKinnon AE, Vaishnav A. Comparison of two methods of prophylaxis against CSF shunt infection. *Z Kinderchir.* 1984; 39(suppl):109–10.

300. Zentner J, Gilsbach J, Felder T. Antibiotic prophylaxis in cerebrospinal fluid shunting: a prospective randomized trial in 129 patients. *Neurosurg Rev.* 1995; 18:169–72.

301. Haines SJ, Walters BC. Antibiotic prophylaxis for cerebrospinal fluid shunts: a metanalysis. *Neurosurgery.* 1994; 34:87–92.

302. Langley JM, LeBlanc JC, Drake J et al. Efficacy of antimicrobial prophylaxis in placement of cerebrospinal fluid shunts: meta-analysis. *Clin Infect Dis.* 1993; 17:98–103.

303. Walters BC, Goumnerova L, Hoffman HJ et al. A randomized, controlled trial of perioperative rifampin/trimethoprim in cerebrospinal fluid shunt surgery. *Childs Nerv Syst.* 1992; 8:253–7.

304. Taffel SM, Placek PJ, Meien M. 1988 U.S. C-section rate at 24.7 per 100 births—a plateau? *New Engl J Med.* 1990; 323:199–200.

305. Lopez-Zeno JA, Peaceman AM, Adashek JA et al. A controlled trial of a program for the active management of labor. *New Engl J Med.* 1992; 326:450–4.

306. Faro S. Infectious disease relations to cesarean section. *Obstet Gynecol Clin North Am.* 1989; 16:363–71.

307. Hemsell DL. Infections after gynecologic surgery. *Obstet Gynecol Clin North Am.* 1989; 16:381–400.

308. Amstey MT, Sheldon GW, Blyth JF. Infectious morbidity after primary cesarean section in a private institution. *Am J Obstet Gynecol.* 1980; 136:205–10.

309. Faro S. Antibiotic prophylaxis. *Obstet Gynecol Clin North Am.* 1989; 16:279–89.

310. Crombleholme WR. Use of prophylactic antibiotics in obstetrics and gynecology. *Clin Obstet Gynecol.* 1988; 31:466–72.

311. Jakobi P, Weissmann A, Zimmer EZ et al. Single dose cefazolin prophylaxis for cesarean section. *Am J Obstet Gynecol.* 1988; 158:1049–52.

312. Duff P, Smith PN, Keiser JF. Antibiotic prophylaxis in low-risk cesarean section. *J Reprod Med.* 1982; 27:133–8.

313. Apuzzio JJ, Reyelt C, Pelosi MA et al. Prophylactic antibiotics for cesarean section: comparison of high- and low-risk patients for endometritis. *Obstet Gynecol.* 1982; 59:693–8.

314. Duff P. Prophylactic antibiotics for cesarean delivery: a simple cost-effective strategy for prevention of

postoperative morbidity. *Am J Obstet Gynecol.* 1987; 157:794–8.

315. Jakobi P, Weissman A, Sigler E et al. Post-Cesarean section febrile morbidity. Antibiotic prophylaxis in low-risk patients. *J Reprod Med.* 1994; 39:707–10.

316. Ehrenkranz NJ, Blackwelder WC, Pfaff SJ et al. Infections complicating low-risk cesarean sections in community hospitals: efficacy of antimicrobial prophylaxis. *Am J Obstet Gynecol.* 1990; 162:337–43.

317. Enkin M, Enkin E, Chalmers I et al. Prophylactic antibiotics in association with cesarean section. In: Chalmers I, Enkin M, Keiser MJNC, eds. Effective care in pregnancy and childbirth. Vol 1. London: Oxford University; 1989:1246–69.

318. Galask R. Changing concepts in obstetric antibiotic prophylaxis. *Am J Obstet Gynecol.* 1987; 157:491–5.

319. Faro S, Martens MG, Hammill HA et al. Antibiotic prophylaxis: is there a difference? *Am J Obstet Gynecol.* 1990; 162:900–9.

320. Stiver HG, Forward KR, Livingstone RA et al. Multicenter comparison of cefoxitin vs cefazolin for prevention of infectious morbidity after nonelective cesarean section. *Am J Obstet Gynecol.* 1985; 145:158–63.

321. Rayburn W, Varner M, Galask R et al. Comparison of moxalactam and cefazolin as prophylactic antibiotics during cesarean section. *Antimicrob Agents Chemother.* 1985; 27:337–9.

322. Benigno BB, Ford LC, Lawrence WD et al. A double-blind, controlled comparison of piperacillin and cefoxitin in the prevention of post-operative infection in patients undergoing cesarean section. *Surg Gynecol Obstet.* 1986; 162:1–7.

323. Fejgin MD, Markov S, Goshen S et al. Antibiotic for cesarean section: the case for 'true' prophylaxis. *Int J Gynecol Obstet.* 1993; 42:257–61.

324. D'Angelo LJ, Sokol RJ. Short-versus long-course prophylactic antibiotic treatment in cesarean section patients. *Obstet Gynecol.* 1980; 55:583–6.

325. Scarpignato C, Caltabiano M, Condemi V et al. Short-term vs long-term cefuroxime prophylaxis in patients undergoing emergency cesarean section. *Clin Ther.* 1982; 5:186–91.

326. Elliott JP, Freeman RK, Dorchester W. Short- versus long-course of prophylactic antibiotics in cesarean section. *Am J Obstet Gynecol.* 1982; 143:740–4.

327. Carlson KJ, Nichols DH, Schiff I. Indications for hysterectomy. *N Engl J Med.* 1993; 328:856–60.

328. Jennings RH. Prophylactic antibiotics in vaginal and abdominal hysterectomy. *South Med J.* 1978; 71:251–4.

329. Allen J, Rampone J, Wheeless C. Use of a prophylactic antibiotic in elective major gynecologic operations. *Obstet Gynecol.* 1972; 39:218–24.

330. Stage AH, Glover DD, Vaughan JE. Low-dose cephradine prophylaxis in obstetric and gynecologic surgery. *J Reprod Med.* 1982; 27:113–9.

331. Vincelette J, Finkelstein F, Aoki FY et al. Double-blind trial of perioperative intravenous metronidazole prophylaxis for abdominal and vaginal hysterectomy. *Surgery.* 1983; 93:185–9.

332. Mayer W, Gordon M, Rothbard MJ. Prophylactic antibiotics. Use in hysterectomy. *N Y State J Med.* 1976; 76:2144–7.

333. Wheeless CR Jr, Dorsey JH, Wharton LR Jr. An evaluation of prophylactic doxycycline in hysterectomy patients. *J Reprod Med.* 1978; 21:146–50.

334. Hemsell D, Johnson ER, Hemsell PG et al. Cefazolin is inferior to cefotetan as single-dose prophylaxis for women undergoing elective total abdominal hysterectomy. *Clin Infect Dis.* 1995; 20:677–84.

335. Goosenberg J, Emich JP Jr, Schwarz RH. Prophylactic antibiotics in vaginal hysterectomy. *Am J Obstet Gynecol.* 1969; 105:503–6.

336. Soper DE, Bump RC, Hurt GW. Wound infection after abdominal hysterectomy: effect of the depth of subcutaneous tissue. *Am J Obstet Gynecol.* 1995; 173:465–71.

337. Marsden DE, Cavanagh D, Wisniewski BJ et al. Factors affecting the incidence of infectious morbidity after radical hysterectomy. *Am J Obstet Gynecol.* 1985; 152:817–21.

338. Mann W, Orr J, Shingleton H et al. Perioperative influences on infectious morbidity in radical hysterectomy. *Gynecol Oncol.* 1981; 11:207–12.

339. Rein MF. Vulvovaginitis and cervicitis. Mandell GL, Bennett JE, Dolin R, eds. Principles and practice of infectious diseases. 4th ed. New York: Churchill Livingstone; 1995:1070–5.

340. Ohm MJ, Galask RP. The effect of antibiotic prophylaxis on patients undergoing vaginal operations. II. Alterations of microbial flora. *Am J Obstet Gynecol.* 1975; 123:597–604.

341. Ohm MJ, Galask RP. The effect of antibiotic prophylaxis on patients undergoing total abdominal hysterectomy. II. Alterations of microbial flora. *Am J Obstet Gynecol.* 1976; 125:448–54.

342. Appelbaum P, Moodley J, Chatterton S et al. Metronidazole in the prophylaxis and treatment of anaerobic infection. *S Afr Med J.* 1978; 1:703–6.

343. Ledger WJ, Sweet RL, Headington JT. Prophylactic cephaloridine in the prevention of postoperative pelvic infections in premenopausal women undergoing vaginal hysterectomy. *Am J Obstet Gynecol.* 1972; 115:766–74.

344. Breeden JT, Mayo JE. Low-dose prophylactic antibiotics in vaginal hysterectomy. *Obstet Gynecol.* 1974; 43:379–85.

345. Glover MW, Van Nagell JR Jr. The effect of prophylactic ampicillin on pelvic infection following vaginal hysterectomy. *Am J Obstet Gynecol.* 1976; 126:385–8.

346. Lett WJ, Ansbacher R, Davison BL et al. Prophylactic antibiotics for women undergoing vaginal hysterectomy. *J Reprod Med.* 1977; 19:51–4.

347. Holman J, McGowan J, Thompson J. Perioperative antibiotics in major elective gynecologic surgery. *South Med J.* 1978; 71:417–20.

348. Roberts JM, Homesley HD. Low-dose carbenicillin prophylaxis for vaginal and abdominal hysterectomy. *Obstet Gynecol.* 1978; 52:83–7.

349. Mickal A, Curole D, Lewis C. Cefoxitin sodium: double-blind vaginal hysterectomy prophylaxis in premenopausal patients. *Obstet Gynecol.* 1980; 56:222–5.

350. Hemsell DL, Cunningham FG, Kappus S et al. Cefoxitin for prophylaxis in premenopausal women undergoing vaginal hysterectomy. *Obstet Gynecol.* 1980; 56:629–34.

351. Polk B, Tager I, Shapiro M et al. Randomized clinical trial of perioperative cefazolin in preventing infection after hysterectomy. *Lancet.* 1980; 1:437–40.

352. Savage EW, Thadepalli H, Rambhatla K et al. Minocycline prophylaxis in elective hysterectomy. *J Reprod Med.* 1984; 29:81–7.

353. Davey PG, Duncan ID, Edward D et al. Cost-benefit analysis of cephradine and mezlocillin prophylaxis for abdominal and vaginal hysterectomy. *Br J Obstet Gynaecol.* 1988; 95:1170–7.

354. Willis A, Bullen C, Ferguson I et al. Metronidazole in the prevention and treatment of *Bacteroides* infection in gynaecological patients. *Lancet.* 1974; 2:1540–3.

355. Mozzillo N, Diongi R, Ventriglia L. Multicenter study of aztreonam in the prophylaxis of colorectal, gynecologic and urologic surgery. *Chemotherapy.* 1989; 35(suppl 1):58–71.

356. Hamod KA, Spence MR, Roshenshein NB et al. Single and multidose prophylaxis in vaginal hysterectomy: a comparison of sodium cephalothin and metronidazole. *Am J Obstet Gynecol.* 1980; 136:976–9.

357. Friese S, Willems FTC, Loriaux SM et al. Prophylaxis in gynaecological surgery: a prospective, randomized comparison between single-dose prophylaxis with amoxicillin/clavulanate and the combination of cefuroxime and metronidazole. *J Antimicrob Chemother.* 1989; 24(suppl B):213–6.

358. Benigno BB, Evard J, Faro S et al. A comparison of piperacillin, cephalothin, and cefoxitin in the prevention of postoperative infections in patients undergoing vaginal hysterectomy. *Surg Gynecol Obstet.* 1986; 163:421–7.

359. Faro S, Pastorek JG, Aldridge KE et al. Randomized, double-blind comparison of mezlocillin versus cefoxitin prophylaxis for vaginal hysterectomy. *Surg Gynecol Obstet.* 1988; 166:431–5.

360. Grossman J, Greco T, Minkin MJ et al. Prophylactic antibiotics in gynecologic surgery. *Obstet Gynecol.* 1979; 53:537–44.

361. Rapp RP, Van Nagell JR, Donaldson ES et al. A double-blind, randomized study of prophylactic antibiotics in vaginal hysterectomy. *Hosp Formul.* 1982; 1:524–9.

362. Benson WL, Brown RL, Schmidt PM. Comparison of short and long courses of ampicillin for vaginal hysterectomy. *J Reprod Med.* 1985; 30:874–6.

363. Hemsell DI, Hemsell PG, Nobles BJ. Doxycycline and cefamandole prophylaxis for premenopausal women undergoing vaginal hysterectomy. *Surg Gynecol Obstet.* 1985; 161:462–4.

364. Forney JP, Morrow CP, Townsend DE et al. Impact of cephalosporin prophylaxis on colonization: vaginal hysterectomy morbidity. *Am J Obstet Gynecol.* 1976; 125:100–5.

365. Ledger WJ, Child MA. The hospital care of patients undergoing hysterectomy: an analysis of 12,026 patients from the Professional Activity Study. *Am J Obstet Gynecol.* 1973; 117:423–30.

366. Ohm MJ, Galask RP. The effect of antibiotic prophylaxis on patients undergoing vaginal operations. I. The effect of morbidity. *Am J Obstet Gynecol.* 1975; 123:590–6.

367. Hemsell D, Hemsell PG, Nobles BJ et al. Moxalactam versus cefazolin prophylaxis for vaginal hysterectomy. *Am J Obstet Gynecol.* 1983; 147:379–85.

368. Hemsell D, Menon M, Friedman A. Ceftriaxone or cefazolin prophylaxis for the prevention of infection after vaginal hysterectomy. *Am J Surg.* 1984; 148:22–6.

369. Hemsell DL, Johnson ER, Bawdon RE et al. Ceftriaxone and cefazolin prophylaxis for hysterectomy. *Surg Gynecol Obstet.* 1985; 161:197–203.

370. Soper D, Yarwood R. Single-dose antibiotic prophylaxis in women undergoing vaginal hysterectomy. *Obstet Gynecol.* 1987; 53:879–82.

371. Hemsell DL, Johnson ER, Heard MC et al. Single dose piperacillin versus triple dose cefoxitin prophylaxis at vaginal and abdominal hysterectomy. *South Med J.* 1989; 82:438–42.

372. Blanco JD, Lipscomb KA. Single-dose prophylaxis in vaginal hysterectomy: a double-blind, randomized comparison of ceftazidime versus cefotaxime. *Curr Ther Res.* 1984; 36:389–93.

373. Rapp RP, Connors E, Hager WD et al. Comparison of single-dose moxalactam and a three-dose regimen of cefoxitin for prophylaxis in vaginal hysterectomy. *Clin Pharm.* 1986; 5:988–93.

374. Roy S, Wilkins J. Single-dose cefotaxime versus 3- to 5-dose cefoxitin for prophylaxis of vaginal or abdominal hysterectomy. *J Antimicrob Chemother.* 1984; 14(suppl B):217–21.

375. Roy S, Wilkins J, Hemsell DL et al. Efficacy and safety of single-dose ceftizoxime vs. multiple-dose cefoxitin in preventing infection after vaginal hysterectomy. *J Reprod Med.* 1988; 33(suppl 1):149–53.

376. Roy S, Wilkins J, Galaif E et al. Comparative efficacy and safety of cefmetazole or cefoxitin in the prevention of postoperative infection following vaginal and abdominal hysterectomy. *J Antimicrob Chemother.* 1989; 23(suppl D):109–17.

377. Mercer LJ, Murphy HJ, Ismail MA et al. A comparison of cefonicid and cefoxitin for preventing infections after vaginal hysterectomy. *J Reprod Med.* 1988; 33:223–6.

378. Hemsell DL, Heard ML, Nobles BJ et al. Single-dose cefoxitin prophylaxis for premenopausal women undergoing vaginal hysterectomy. *Obstet Gynecol.* 1984; 63:285–90.

379. Mendelson J, Portnoy J, De Saint Victor JR et al. Effect of single and multidose cephradine prophylaxis on infectious morbidity of vaginal hysterectomy. *Obstet Gynecol.* 1979; 53:31–5.

380. McGregor JA, Phillips LE, Dunne JT et al. Results of a double-blind, placebo-controlled clinical trial program of single-dose ceftizoxime versus multiple-dose cefoxitin as prophylaxis for patients undergoing vaginal and abdominal hysterectomy. *J Am Coll Surg.* 1994; 178:123–31.

381. Multicenter Study Group. Single-dose prophylaxis in patients undergoing vaginal hysterectomy: cefamandole versus cefotaxime. *Am J Obstet Gynecol.* 1989; 160:1198–201.

382. Jacobson JA, Hebertson R, Kasworm E. Comparison of ceforanide and cephalothin prophylaxis for vaginal hysterectomies. *Antimicrob Agents Chemother.* 1982; 22:643–6.

383. American College of Obstetricians and Gynecologists (ACOG). Antibiotics and gynecologic infections. *ACOG Educ Bull.* 1997; 237:1–8.

384. Campillo F, Rubio JM. Comparative study of single-dose cefotaxime and multiple doses of cefoxitin and cefazolin as prophylaxis in gynecologic surgery. *Am J Surg.* 1992; 164:12S–15S.

385. Turano A. New clinical data on the prophylaxis of infections in abdominal, gynecologic, and urologic surgery. Multicenter Study Group. *Am J Surg.* 1992; 164(4A suppl):16S–20S.

386. D'Addato F, Canestrelli M, Repinto A et al. Perioperative prophylaxis in abdominal and vaginal hysterectomy. *Clin Exp Obstet Gynecol.* 1993; 20:95–101.

387. Orr JW Jr, Varner RE, Kilgore LC et al. Cefotetan versus cefoxitin as prophylaxis in hysterectomy. *Am J Obstet Gynecol.* 1986; 154:960–3.

388. Orr JW Jr, Sisson PF, Barrett JM et al. Single center study results of cefotetan and cefoxitin prophylaxis for abdominal or vaginal hysterectomy. *Am J Obstet Gynecol.* 1988; 158:714–6.

389. Eron LJ, Gordon SF, Harvey LK et al. A trial using early preoperative administration of cefonicid for antimicrobial prophylaxis with hysterectomies. *DICP Ann Pharmacother.* 1989; 23:655–8.

390. Berkeley AS, Orr JW, Cavanagh D et al. Comparative effectiveness and safety of cefotetan and cefoxitin as prophylactic agents in patients undergoing abdominal or vaginal hysterectomy. *Am J Surg.* 1988; 155:81–5.

391. Berkeley AS, Freedman KS, Ledger WJ et al. Comparison of cefotetan and cefoxitin prophylaxis for abdominal and vaginal hysterectomy. *Am J Obstet Gynecol.* 1988; 158:706–9.

392. Gordon SF. Results of a single center study of cefotetan prophylaxis in abdominal or vaginal hysterectomy. *Am J Obstet Gynecol.* 1988; 158:710–4. (Erratum published in *Am J Obstet Gynecol.* 1989; 160:1025.)

393. Mathews D, Ross H. Randomized, controlled trial of a short course of cephaloridine in the prevention of infection after abdominal hysterectomy. *Br J Obstet Gynecol.* 1978; 85:381–5.

394. Duff P. Antibiotic prophylaxis for abdominal hysterectomy. *Obstet Gynecol.* 1982; 60:25–9.

395. Walker EM, Gordon AJ, Warren RE et al. Prophylactic single-dose metronidazole before abdominal hysterectomy. *Br J Obstet Gynaecol.* 1982; 89:957–61.

396. Manthorpe T, Justesen T. Metronidazole prophylaxis in abdominal hysterectomy. A double-blind, controlled trial. *Acta Obstet Gynecol Scand.* 1982; 61:243–6.

397. Ohm MJ, Galask RP. The effect of antibiotic prophylaxis on patients undergoing total abdominal hysterectomy. I. Effect on morbidity. *Am J Obstet Gynecol.* 1976; 125:442–7.

398. Hemsell DL, Reisch J, Nobles B et al. Prevention of major infection after elective abdominal hysterectomy. Individual determination required. *Am J Obstet Gynecol.* 1983; 147:520–3.

399. Berkeley AS, Haywork SD, Hirsch JC et al. Controlled, comparative study of moxalactam and cefazolin for prophylaxis of abdominal hysterectomy. *Surg Gynecol Obstet.* 1985; 161:457–61.

400. Gonen R, Hakin M, Samberg I et al. Short-term prophylactic antibiotic for elective abdominal hysterectomy: how short? *Eur J Obstet Gynecol Reprod Biol.* 1985; 20:229–34.

401. Senior C, Steirad J. Are preoperative antibiotics helpful in abdominal hysterectomy? *Am J Obstet Gynecol.* 1986; 154:1004–8.

402. McDonald PJ, Sanders T, Higgins G et al. Antibiotic prophylaxis in hysterectomy: cefotaxime compared to ampicillin-tinidazole. *J Antimicrob Chemother.* 1985; 14(suppl B):223–30.

403. Mamsen A, Hansen V, Moller BR. A prospective randomized double-blind trial of ceftriaxone versus no treatment for abdominal hysterectomy. *Eur J Obstet Gynecol Reprod Biol.* 1992; 47:235–8.

404. Mittendorf R, Aronson MP, Berry RE et al. Avoiding serious infections associated with abdominal hysterectomy: a meta-analysis of antibiotic prophylaxis. *Am J Obstet Gynecol.* 1993; 169:1119–24.

405. Hemsell DL, Johnson ER, Bawdon RE et al. Cefoperazone and cefoxitin prophylaxis for abdominal hysterectomy. *Obstet Gynecol.* 1984; 63:467–72.

406. Tchabo JG, Cutting ME, Butler C. Prophylactic antibiotics in patients undergoing total vaginal or abdominal hysterectomy. *Int Surg.* 1985; 70:349–52.

407. Hemsell DL, Martin NJ Jr, Pastorek JG II et al. Single-dose antimicrobial prophylaxis at abdominal hysterectomy. Cefamandole vs cefotaxime. *J Reprod Med.* 1988; 33:939–44.

408. Tuomala RE, Fischer SG, Munoz A et al. A comparative trial of cefazolin and moxalactam as prophylaxis for preventing infection after abdominal hysterectomy. *Obstet Gynecol.* 1985; 66:372–6.

409. Scarpignato C, Labruna C, Condemi V et al. Comparative efficacy of two different regimens of antibiotic prophylaxis in total abdominal hysterectomy. *Pharmatherapeutica.* 1980; 2:450–5.

410. Hemsell DL, Hemsell PG, Heard ML et al. Preoperative cefoxitin prophylaxis for elective abdominal hysterectomy. *Am J Obstet Gynecol.* 1985; 153:225–6.

411. Miyazawa K, Hernandez E, Dillon MB. Prophylactic topical cefamandole in radical hysterectomy. *Int J Gynaecol Obstet.* 1987; 25:133–8.

412. Micha JP, Kucera PR, Birkett JP et al. Prophylactic mezlocillin in radical hysterectomy. *Obstet Gynecol.* 1987; 69:251–4.

413. Sevin B, Ramos R, Lichtinger M et al. Antibiotic prevention of infection complicating radical abdominal hysterectomy. *Obstet Gynecol.* 1984; 64:539–45.

414. Rosenshein NB, Ruth JC, Villar J et al. A prospective randomized study of doxycycline as a prophylactic antibiotic in patients undergoing radical hysterectomy. *Gynecol Oncol.* 1983; 15:201–6.

415. Mayer HO, Petru E, Haas J et al. Perioperative antibiotic prophylaxis in patients undergoing radical surgery for gynecologic cancer: single dose versus multiple dose administration. *Eur J Gynaecol Oncol.* 1993; 14:177–81.

416. Christy NE, Lall P. Postoperative endophthalmitis following cataract surgery. *Arch Ophthalmol.* 1973; 90:361–6.

417. Allen HF, Mangiaracine AB. Bacterial endophthalmitis after cataract extraction. *Arch Ophthalmol.* 1974; 91:3–7.

418. Allen HF, Mangiaracine AB. Bacterial endophthalmitis after cataract extraction: a study of 22 infections in 20,000 operations. *Arch Ophthalmol.* 1964; 57:454–62.

419. Fahmy JA. Bacterial flora in relation to cataract extraction: effects of topical antibiotics on the preoperative conjunctival flora. *Acta Ophthalmol.* 1980; 58:567–75.

420. Burns RP. Postoperative infections in an ophthalmologic hospital. *Am J Ophthalmol.* 1959; 48:519–26.

421. Burns RP, Hansen T, Fraunfelder FT et al. An experimental model for evaluation of human conjunctivitis

and topical antibiotic therapy: comparison of gentamicin and neomycin. *Can J Ophthalmol.* 1968; 3:132–7.

422. Burns RP, Oden M. Antibiotic prophylaxis in cataract surgery. *Trans Am Ophthalmol Soc.* 1972; 70:43–57.

423. Ormerod LD, Becker LE, Cruise RJ et al. Endophthalmitis caused by the coagulase-negative staphylococci factors influencing presentation after cataract surgery. *Ophthalmology.* 1993; 100:724–9.

424. Kolker AE, Freeman MI, Pettit TH. Prophylactic antibiotics and postoperative endophthalmitis. *Am J Ophthalmol.* 1967; 63:434–9.

425. Dunnington JH, Locatcher-Khorazo D. Value of cultures before operation for cataract. *Arch Ophthalmol.* 1945; 34:215–9.

426. Dallison IW, Simpson AJ, Keenan JI et al. Topical antibiotic prophylaxis for cataract surgery: a controlled trial of fusidic acid and chloramphenicol. *Aust N Z J Ophthalmol.* 1989; 17:289–93.

427. Apt L, Isenberg SJ, Yoshimori R et al. The effect of povidone-iodine solution applied at the conclusion of ophthalmic surgery. *Am J Ophthalmol.* 1995; 119:701–5.

428. Kattan HM, Flynn HW Jr, Pflugfelder SC et al. Nosocomial endophthalmitis survey: current incidence of infection after intraocular surgery. *Surv Ophthalmol.* 1991; 98:227–38.

429. Christy NE, Sommer A. Antibiotic prophylaxis of postoperative endophthalmitis. *Ann Ophthalmol.* 1979; 11:1261–5.

430. Mahajan VM. Acute bacterial infections of the eye: their aetiology and treatment. *Br J Ophthalmol.* 1983; 67:191–4.

431. O'Brien TP, Green RW. Endophthalmitis. Mandell GL, Bennett JE, Dolin R, eds. Principles and practice of infectious diseases. 4th ed. New York: Churchill Livingstone; 1995:1120–9.

432. Neu HC. Microbiologic aspects of fluoroquinolones. *Am J Ophthalmol.* 1991; 112:15S–24S.

433. Shungu DL, Tutlane VK, Weinberg E et al. In vitro antibacterial activity of norfloxacin and other agents against ocular pathogens. *Chemotherapy.* 1985; 31:112–8.

434. Osato MS, Jensen HG, Trousdale MD et al. The comparative in vitro activity of ofloxacin and selected ophthalmic antimicrobial agents against ocular bacterial isolates. *Am J Ophthalmol.* 1989; 108:380–6.

435. Miller IM, Vogel R, Cook TJ et al., and The Worldwide Norfloxacin Ophthalmic Study Group. Topically administered norfloxacin compared with topically administered gentamicin for the treatment of external ocular bacterial infections. *Am J Ophthalmol.* 1992; 113:638–44.

436. Speaker MG, Menikoff JA. Prophylaxis of endophthalmitis with topical povidone-iodine. *Ophthalmology.* 1991; 98:1769–75.

437. Leibowitz HM, Ryan WJ Jr. Kupferman A. Route of antibiotic administration in bacterial keratitis. *Arch Ophthalmol.* 1981; 99:1420.

438. Starr MB, Lally JM. Antimicrobial prophylaxis for ophthalmic surgery. *Surv Ophthalmol.* 1995; 36:485–501.

439. Walland MJ, Rose GE. Soft tissue infections after open lacrimal surgery. *Ophthalmology.* 1994; 101:608–11.

440. Eron LJ. Prevention of infection following orthopedic surgery. *Antibiot Chemother.* 1985; 33:140–64.

441. Nguyen TT, Garibaldi JA. Cephalosporin vs penicillin. *J Calif Dent Assoc.* 1994; 22:46–55.

442. Boyd RJ, Burke JF, Colton T. A double-blind clinical trial of prophylactic antibiotics in hip fractures. *J Bone Joint Surg.* 1973; 55A:1251–8.

443. Olix ML, Klug TJ, Coleman CR et al. Prophylactic penicillin and streptomycin in elective operations on bones, joints, and tendons. *Surg Forum.* 1960; 10:818–9.

444. Schonholtz GJ, Borgia CA, Blair JD. Wound sepsis in orthopedic surgery. *J Bone Joint Surg.* 1962; 44A:1548–52.

445. Ericson C, Lidgren L, Lindberg L. Cloxacillin in the prophylaxis of postoperative infections of the hip. *J Bone Joint Surg.* 1973; 55A:808–13.

446. Carlsson AS, Lidgren L, Lindberg L. Prophylactic antibiotics against early and late deep infections after total hip replacements. *Acta Orthop Scand.* 1977; 48:405–10.

447. Hill C, Mazas F, Flamant R et al. Prophylactic cefazolin versus placebo in total hip replacement. *Lancet.* 1981; 1:795–7.

448. Lidwell OM, Lowbury EJL, White W et al. Effect of ultraclean air in operating room on deep sepsis in the joint after total hip or knee replacement: a randomized study. *Br Med J.* 1982; 285:10–4.

449. Pollard JP, Hughes SPF, Scott JE et al. Antibiotic prophylaxis in total hip replacement. *Br Med J.* 1979; 1:707–9.

450. Burnett JW, Gustilo RB, Williams DN et al. Prophylactic antibiotics in hip fractures. *J Bone Joint Surg.* 1980; 62A:457–62.

451. Tengve B, Kjellander J. Antibiotic prophylaxis in operations on trochanteric femoral fractures. *J Bone Joint Surg.* 1978; 60A:97–9.

452. Pavel A, Smith RL, Ballard A et al. Prophylactic antibiotics in clean orthopedic surgery. *J Bone Joint Surg.* 1974; 56A:777–82.

453. Henley MB, Jones RE, Wyatt RWB et al. Prophylaxis with cefamandole nafate in elective orthopedic surgery. *Clin Orthop.* 1986; 209:249–54.

454. Fitzgerald RH. Infections of hip prosthesis and artificial joints. *Infect Dis Clin North Am.* 1989; 3:329–38.

455. Buckley R, Hughes G, Snodgrass T et al. Perioperative cefazolin prophylaxis in hip fracture surgery. *Can J Surg.* 1990; 33:122–7.

456. Paiement GD, Renaud E, Dagenais G et al. Double-blind, randomized prospective study of the efficacy of antibiotic prophylaxis for open reduction and internal fixation of closed ankle fractures. *J Orthop Trauma.* 1994; 8:64–6.

457. Cunha BA, Gossling HR, Pasternak HS et al. The penetration characteristics of cefazolin, cephalothin, and cephradine into bone in patients undergoing total hip replacement. *J Bone Joint Surg.* 1977; 59A:856–9.

458. Hedstrom SA, Lidgren L, Sernbo I et al. Cefuroxime prophylaxis in trochanteric hip fracture operations. *Acta Orthop Scand.* 1987; 58:361–4.

459. Harris WH, Sledge CV. Total hip and total knee replacement. *New Engl J Med.* 1990; 323:725.

460. Dreghorn CR, Roughneen P, Graham J et al. The real cost of joint replacement. *Br Med J.* 1986; 292:1636–7.

461. Fish DN, Hoffman HM, Danziger LH. Antibiotic-impregnated cement use in U.S. hospitals. *Am J Hosp Pharm.* 1992; 49:2469–74.

462. Wininger DA, Fass RJ. Antibiotic-impregnated cement and beads for orthopedic infections. *Antimicrob Chemother.* 1996; 40:2675–9.

463. Mauerhan DR, Nelson CL, Smith DL et al. Prophylaxis against infection in total joint arthroplasty. *J Bone Joint Surg.* 1994; 76A:39–45.

464. Liebergall M, Mosheiff R, Rand N et al. A double-blinded, randomized, controlled clinical trial to compare cefazolin and cefonicid for antimicrobial prophylaxis in clean orthopedic surgery. *Israel J Med Sci.* 1995; 31:62–4.

465. McQueen MM, Hughes SPF, May P et al. Cefuroxime in total joint arthroplasty. Intravenous or in bone cement. *J Arthroplasty.* 1990; 5:169–72.

466. Josefsson G, Kolmert L. Prophylaxis with systematic antibiotics versus gentamicin bone cement in total hip arthroplasty. A ten-year survey of 1,688 hips. *Clin Orthop.* 1993; 292:210–4.

467. Nelson CL, Green TG, Porter RA et al. One day versus seven days of preventive antibiotic therapy in orthopedic surgery. *Clin Orthop.* 1983; 176:258–63.

468. Gibbons RP, Stark RA, Gorrea RJ et al. The prophylactic use—or misuse—of antibiotics in transurethral prostatectomy. *J Urol.* 1978; 119:381–3.

469. Ferrie B, Scott R. Prophylactic cefuroxime in transurethral resection. *Urol Res.* 1984; 12:279–81.

470. Upton JD, Das S. Prophylactic antibiotics in transurethral resection of bladder tumors: are they necessary? *Urology.* 1986; 27:421–3.

471. Houle AM, Mokhless I, Sarto N et al. Perioperative antibiotic prophylaxis for transurethral resection of the prostate: is it justified? *J Urol.* 1989; 142:317–9.

472. Fair WR. Perioperative use of carbenicillin in transurethral resection of the prostate. *Urology.* 1986; 27(suppl 2):15–8.

473. Shah P, Williams G, Chaudary M et al. Short-term antibiotic prophylaxis and prostatectomy. *Br J Urol.* 1981; 53:339–43.

474. Morris MJ, Golovsky D, Guinness MDG et al. The value of prophylactic antibiotics in transurethral prostatic resection: a controlled trial, with observations on the origin of postoperative infection. *Br J Urol.* 1976; 48:479–84.

475. Gonzalez R, Wright R, Blackard CE. Prophylactic antibiotics in transurethral prostatectomy. *J Urol.* 1976; 116:203–5.

476. Hills NH, Bultitude MI, Eykyn S. Cotrimoxazole in prevention of bacteriuria after prostatectomy. *Br Med J.* 1976; 2:498–9.

477. Dorflinger T, Madsen PO. Antibiotics prophylaxis in transurethral surgery. *Urology.* 1984; 24:643–6.

478. Matthew AD, Gonzales R, Jeffords D et al. Prevention of bacteriuria after transurethral prostatectomy with nitrofurantoin macrocrystals. *J Urol.* 1978; 120:442–3.

479. Childs SJ, Wells WB, Mirelman S. Antibiotic prophylaxis for genitourinary surgery in community hospitals. *J Urol.* 1983; 130:305–8.

480. Nielsen OS, Maigaard S, Frimφdt-Mφller N et al. Prophylactic antibiotics in transurethral prostatectomy. *J Urol.* 1981; 126:60–2.

481. Charton M, Vallancien G, Veillon B et al. Antibiotic prophylaxis or urinary tract infection after transurethral resection of the prostate: a randomized study. *J Urol.* 1987; 138:87–9.

482. Ramsey E, Sheth NK. Antibiotic prophylaxis in patients undergoing prostatectomy. *Urology.* 1983; 21:376–8.

483. Slavis SA, Miller JB, Golji H et al. Comparison of single-dose antibiotic prophylaxis in uncomplicated transurethral resection of the prostate. *J Urol.* 1992; 147:1301–6.

484. Raz R, Almog D, Elhanan G et al. The use of ceftriaxone in the prevention of urinary tract infection in patients undergoing transurethral resection of the prostate (TURP). *Infection.* 1994; 22:347–9.

485. Hammarsten J, Lindqvist K. Norfloxacin as prophylaxis against urethral strictures following transurethral resection of the prostate: an open, prospective, randomized study. *J Urol.* 1993; 150:1722–4.

486. Viitanen J, Talja M, Jussila E et al. Randomized controlled study of chemoprophylaxis in transurethral prostatectomy. *J Urol.* 1993; 150:1715–7.

487. Brewster SF, MacGowan AP, Gingell JC. Antimicrobial prophylaxis for transrectal prostatic biopsy: a prospective, randomized trial of cefuroxime versus piperacillin/tazobactam. *Br J Urol.* 1995; 76:351–4.

488. Crawford ED, Berger NS, Davis MA et al. Prevention of urinary tract infection and bacteremia following transurethral surgery: oral lomefloxacin compared to parenteral cefotaxime. *J Urol.* 1992; 147:1053–5.

489. DeBessonet DA, Merlin AS. Antibiotic prophylaxis in elective genitourinary tract surgery: a comparison of single-dose preoperative cefotaxime and multiple-dose cefoxitin. *J Antimicrob Chemother.* 1984; 14(suppl B):271–5.

490. Taha SA, Sayed AAK, Grant C et al. Risk factors in wound infection following urologic operations: a prospective study. *Int Surg.* 1992; 77:128–30.

491. Richter S, Lang R, Zur F et al. Infected urine as a risk factor for postprostatectomy wound infection. *Infect Control Hosp Epidemiol.* 1991; 12:147–9.

492. Klimberg IW, Childs SJ, Madore RJ et al. A multicenter comparison of oral lomefloxacin versus parenteral cefotaxime as prophylactic agents in transurethral surgery. *Am J Med.* 1992; 92(suppl 4):121–5.

493. Charton M, Mombet A, Gattegno B. Urinary tract infection prophylaxis in transurethral surgery: oral lomefloxacin versus parenteral cefuroxime. *Am J Med.* 1992; 92(suppl 4A):4A–118S.

494. Costa FJ. Lomefloxacin prophylaxis in visual laser ablation of the prostate. *Urology.* 1994; 44:933–6.

495. Hall JC, Christiansen KJ, England P et al. Antibiotic prophylaxis for patients undergoing transurethral resection of the prostate. *Urology.* 1996; 47:852–6.

496. Duclos JM, Larrouturou P, Sarkis P. Timing of antibiotic prophylaxis with cefotaxime for prostatic resection: better in the operative period or at urethral catheter removal? *Am J Surg.* 1992; 164(4A suppl): 21S–23S.

497. Burnakis TG. Surgical antimicrobial prophylaxis: principles and guidelines. *Pharmacotherapy.* 1984; 4:248–71.

498. Richet S, Chidiac C, Prat A et al. Analysis of risk factors for surgical wound infections following vascular surgery. *Am J Med.* 1991; 91:171S–172S.

499. Kaiser A, Clayton KR, Mulherin JL et al. Antibiotic prophylaxis in vascular surgery. *Ann Surg.* 1978; 188:283–9.

500. Edwards WH, Kaiser AB, Kernodle DS et al. cefuroxime versus cefazolin as prophylaxis in vascular surgery. *J Vasc Surg.* 1992; 15:35–42.

501. Edwards WH Jr, Kaiser AB, Tapper S et al. Cefamandole versus cefazolin in vascular surgical wound infection prophylaxis: cost-effectiveness and risk factors. *J Vasc Surg.* 1993; 18:470–5.

502. Hasselgren P-O, Ivarson L, Risberg B et al. Effects of prophylactic antibiotics in vascular surgery. A prospective, randomized, double-blind study. *Ann Surg.* 1984; 200:86–92.

503. Risberg B, Drott C, Dalman P et al. Oral ciprofloxacin versus intavenous cefuroxime as prophylaxis against postoperative infection in vascular surgery: a randomized double-blind, prospective multicentre study. *Eur J Endovasc Surg.* 1995; 10:346–51.

504. Bennion RS, Hiatt JR, Williams RA et al. A randomized, prospective study of perioperative antimicrobial prophylaxis for vascular access surgery. *J Cardiovasc Surg.* 1985; 26:270–4.

505. Pitt HA, Postier RG, Mcgowan WA et al. Prophylactic antibiotics in vascular surgery. Topical, systemic, or both. *Ann Surg.* 1980; 192:356–64.

506. Murray BE. Problems and dilemmas of antimicrobial resistance. *Pharmacotherapy.* 1992; 12:86–93.

507. Barone GW, Hudec WA, Sailors DM et al. Prophylactic wound antibiotics for combined kidney and pancreas transplants. *Clin Transplant.* 1996; 10:386–8.

508. Hosenpud JD, Novick RJ, Bennett LE et al. The registry of the International Society for Heart and Lung Transplantation: thirteenth official report—1996. *J Heart Lung Transplant.* 1996; 15:655–74.

509. Kaiser AB. Use of antibiotics in cardiac and thoracic surgery. In: Sabiston DC Jr, Spencer FC, eds. Surgery of the chest. 6th ed. Philadelphia: W. B. Saunders; 1995:98–116.

510. Khaghani A, Martin M, Fitzgerald M et al. Cefotaxime and flucloxacillin as antibiotic prophylaxis in cardiac transplantation. *Drugs.* 1988; 35(suppl 2):124–6.

511. Petri WA Jr. Infections in heart transplant recipients. *Clin Infect Dis.* 1994; 18:141–8.

512. Trulock EP. Lung transplantation. *Am J Respir Crit Care Med.* 1997; 155:789–818.

513. Davis RD Jr, Pasque MK. Pulmonary transplantation. *Ann Surg.* 1995; 221:14–28.

514. Kotloff RM, Zuckerman JB. Lung transplantation for cystic fibrosis. Special considerations. *Chest.* 1996; 109:787–98.

515. Dowling RD, Zenati M, Yousem S et al. Donor-transmitted pneumonia in experimental lung allografts. *J Thorac Cardiovasc Surg.* 1992; 103:767–72.

516. Low DE, Kaiser LR, Haydock DA et al. The donor lung: infectious and pathologic factors affecting outcome in lung transplantation. *J Thorac Cardiovasc Surg.* 1993; 106:614–21.

517. Steinbach S, Sun L, Jiang R-Z et al. Transmissibility of Pseudomonas cepacia infection in clinic patients and lung-transplant recipients with cystic fibrosis. *New Engl J Med.* 1994; 331:981–7.

518. Zenati M, Dowling RD, Dummer JS et al. Influence of the donor lung on development of early infections in lung transplant recipients. *J Heart Transplant.* 1990; 9:502–9.

519. Dauber JH, Paradis IL, Dummer JS. Infectious complications in pulmonary allograft recipients. *Clin Chest Med.* 1990; 11:291–308.

520. Deusch E, End A, Grimm M et al. Early bacterial infections in lung transplant recipients. *Chest.* 1993; 104:1412–6.

521. Paradis IL, Williams P. Infection after lung transplantation. *Semin Respir Infect.* 1993; 8:207–15.

522. Noyes BE, Kurland G, Orenstein DM. Lung and heart-lung transplantation in children. *Pediatr Pulmonol.* 1997; 23:39–48.

523. Kibbler CC. Infections in liver transplantation: risk factors and strategies for prevention. *J Hosp Infect.* 1995; 30(suppl):209–17.

524. Wade JJ, Rolando N, Hayllar K et al. Bacterial and fungal infections after liver transplantation: an analysis of 284 patients. *Hepatology.* 1995; 21:1328–36.

525. Arnow PM, Carandang GC, Zabner R et al. Randomized controlled trial of selective bowel decontamination for prevention of infections following liver transplantation. *Clin Infect Dis.* 1996; 22:997–1003.

526. Colonna JO II, Drew WJ, Brill JE et al. Infectious complications in liver transplantation. *Arch Surg.* 1988; 123:360–4.

527. George DL, Arnow PM, Fox AS et al. Bacterial infection as a complication of liver transplantation: epidemiology and risk factors. *Rev Infect Dis.* 1991; 13:387–96.

528. Uemoto S, Tanaka K, Fujita S et al. Infectious complications in living related liver transplantation. *J Pediatr Surg.* 1994; 29:514–7.

529. Kusne S, Dummer JS, Singh N et al. Infections after liver transplantation. An analysis of 101 consecutive cases. *Medicine.* 1988; 67:132–43.

530. Arnow PM, Furmaga K, Flaherty JP et al. Microbiological efficacy and pharmacokinetics of prophylactic antibiotics in liver transplant patients. *Antimicrob Agents Chemother.* 1992; 36:2125–30.

531. Gorensek MJ, Carey WD, Washington JA II et al. Selective bowel decontamination with quinolones and nystatin reduces gram-negative and fungal infections in orthotopic liver transplant recipients. *Cleve Clin J Med.* 1993; 60:139–44.

532. Bion JF, Badger I, Crosby HA et al. Selective decontamination of the digestive tract reduces gram-negative pulmonary colonization but not systemic endotoxemia in patients undergoing elective liver transplantation. *Crit Care Med.* 1994; 22:40–9.

533. Raakow R, Steffen R, Lefebre B et al. Selective bowel decontamination effectively prevents gram-negative bacterial infections after liver transplantations. *Transplant Proc.* 1990; 22:1556–7.

534. Weisner RH, Hermans PE, Rakela J et al. Selective bowel decontamination to decrease gram-negative aerobic bacterial and candidal colonization and prevent infection after orthotopic liver transplantation. *Transplantation.* 1988; 45:570–4.

535. Barker RJ, Mayes JT, Schulak JA. Wound abscesses following retroperitoneal pancreas transplantation. *Clin Transplant.* 1991; 5:403–7.

536. Douzdjian V, Abecassis MM, Cooper JL et al. Incidence, management, and significance of surgical complications after pancreas-kidney transplantation. *Surg Gynecol Obstet.* 1993; 177:451–6.

537. Everett JE, Wahoff DC, Statz C et al. Characterization and impact of wound infection after pancreas transplantation. *Arch Surg.* 1994; 129:1310–7.

538. Ozaki CF, Stratta RJ, Taylor RJ et al. Surgical complications in solitary pancreas and combined pancreas-kidney transplantations. *Am J Surg.* 1992; 164:546–51.

539. Sollinger HW, Ploeg RJ, Eckhoff DE et al. Two hundred consecutive simultaneous pancreas-kidney transplants with bladder drainage. *Surgery.* 1993; 114:736–44.

540. Freise CE, Stock PG, Roberts JP et al. Low postoperative wound infection rates are possible following simultaneous pancreas-kidney transplantation. *Transplant Proc.* 1995; 27:3069–70.

541. Smets YFC, van der Pijl JW, van Dissel JT et al. Major bacterial and fungal infections after 50 simultaneous pancreas-kidney transplantations. *Transplant Proc.* 1995; 27:3089–90.

542. Douzdjian V, Gugliuzza KK. Wound complications after simultaneous pancreas-kidney transplants: midline versus transverse incision. *Transplant Proc.* 1995; 27:3130–2.

543. Stratta RJ, Taylor RJ, Gill IS. Pancreas transplantation: a managed cure approach to diabetes. *Curr Probl Surg.* 1996; 33:709–816.

544. U.S. Renal Data System. 1995 annual report. *Am J Kidney Dis.* 1995; 26:S1–186.

545. Cohen J, Rees AJ, Williams G. A prospective randomized controlled trial of perioperative antibiotic prophylaxis in renal transplantation. *J Hosp Infect.* 1988; 11:357–63.

546. Hoy WE, May AG, Freeman RB. Primary renal transplant wound infections. *N Y State J Med.* 1981; 81:1469–73.

547. Kohlberg WI, Tellis VA, Bhat DJ et al. Wound infections after transplant nephrectomy. *Arch Surg.* 1980; 115:645–6.

548. Muakkassa WF, Goldman MH, Mendez-Picon G et al. Wound infections in renal transplant patients. *J Urol.* 1983; 130:17–9.

549. Novick AC. The value of intraoperative antibiotics in preventing renal transplant wound infections. *J Urol.* 1981; 125:151–2.

550. Ramos E, Karmi S, Alongi SV et al. Infectious complications in renal transplant recipients. *South Med J.* 1980; 73:752–4.

551. Rubin RH, Wolfson JS, Cosimi AB et al. Infection in the renal transplant recipient. *Am J Med.* 1981; 70:405–11.

552. Tilney NL, Strom TB, Vineyard GC et al. Factors contributing to the declining mortality rate in renal transplantation. *New Engl J Med.* 1978; 299:1321–5.

553. Lai M-K, Huang C-C, Chu S-H et al. Surgical complications in renal transplantation. *Transplant Proc.* 1994; 26:2165–6.

554. Schmaldienst S, Hoerl WH. Bacterial infections after renal transplantation. *Nephron.* 1997; 75:140–53.

555. Koyle MA, Glasscock RJ, Ward HJ et al. Declining incidence of wound infection in cadaveric renal transplant recipient. *Urology.* 1988; 31:103–6.

556. Judson RT. Wound infection following renal transplantation. *Aust N Z J Surg.* 1984; 54:223–4.

557. Del Rio G, Dalet F, Chechile G. Antimicrobial prophylaxis in urologic surgery: does it give some benefit? *Eur Urol.* 1993; 24:305–12.

558. Stephan RN, Munschauer CE, Kumar MSA. Surgical wound infection in renal transplantation. Outcome data in 102 consecutive patients without perioperative systemic antibiotic coverage. *Arch Surg.* 1997; 132:1315–9.

559. Capocasale E, Mazzoni MP, Tondo S et al. Antimicrobial prophylaxis with ceftriaxone in renal transplantation. Prospective study of 170 patients. *Chemotherapy.* 1994; 40:435–40.

Developed through the ASHP Commission on Therapeutics and approved by the ASHP Board of Directors on April 21, 1999. Supersedes an earlier version dated April 22, 1992.

Members of the 1998–1999 ASHP Commission on Therapeutics are Austin J. Lee, Pharm.D., BCPS, FASHP, Chair; C. Wayne Weart, Pharm.D., FASHP, Vice Chair; G. Dennis Clifton, Pharm. D.; Matthew A. Fuller, Pharm.D., BCPS, BCPP; Kent M. Nelson, Pharm.D., BCPS; William L. Green, Pharm.D., BCPS, FASHP; Mary Beth Gross, Pharm.D.; Michael D. Katz, Pharm.D.; Shirley J. Reitz, Pharm.D.; Jane E. DeWitt, Student Member; Donald T. Kishi, Pharm.D., Board Liaison; and Leslie Dotson Jaggers, Pharm. D., BCPS, Secretary.

Project Coordinator: Debbie Denzel, Pharm.D.[a] Clinical Information Specialist, Rocky Mountain Poison and Drug Center, Denver, CO.

Expert Panel: John A. Bosso, Pharm.D., BCPS, Professor of Pharmacy Practice and Administration, College of Pharmacy, Professor of Pediatrics, College of Medicine, Medical University of South Carolina, Charleston; Steven C. Ebert, Pharm.D., FCCP, Clinical Associate Professor of Pharmacy, University of Wisconsin, Clinical Specialist in Infectious Diseases, Department of Pharmacy, Meriter Hospital, Madison; John F. Flaherty, Jr., Pharm.D., FCCP[b], Clinical Sciences Liaison, Gilead Sciences Inc., Foster City, CA; B. Joseph Guglielmo, Jr., Pharm.D., Professor and Vice Chairman, Department of Clinical Pharmacy, School of Pharmacy, University of California, San Francisco; David P. Nicolau, Pharm.D., Coordinator for Research, Department of Medicine, Division of Infectious Diseases, Department of Pharmacy, Hartford Hospital, Hartford, CT; Karen Plaisance, Pharm.D., BCPS, Associate Professor, School of Pharmacy, University of Maryland, Baltimore; Joseph T. DiPiro, Pharm.D., Professor, College of Pharmacy, University of Georgia and Medical College of Georgia, Augusta; Larry H. Danziger, Pharm.D., Professor of Pharmacy Practice, College of Pharmacy, University of Illinois at Chicago.

Major Contributor: Doug Fish, Pharm.D., Assistant Professor, Department of Pharmacy Practice, School of Pharmacy, University of Colorado Health Sciences Center, Denver.

Contributors: Richard Dart, M.D., Ph.D., Lada Kokan, M.D., Edwin Kuffner, M.D., Jodi Schonbok, Luke Yip, M.D., Rocky Mountain Poison and Drug Consultation Center, Denver, CO; Bret Fulton, Louisville, CO.

ASHP Staff Liaison: Leslie Dotson Jaggers, Pharm.D., BCPS,[c] Cardiovascular Pharmacist, Fuqua Heart Center of Atlanta, Piedmont Hospital, Atlanta, GA.

[a]During the development of these guidelines, Dr. Denzel was Clinical Information Specialist, Rocky Mountain Poison and Drug Center, Denver. She is presently Medical Editor, MicroMedex, Englewood, CO.

[b]During the development of these guidelines, Dr. Flaherty was Associate Professor of Clinical Pharmacy, Division of Clinical Pharmacy, School of Pharmacy, University of California, San Francisco, CA.

[c]During the development of these guidelines, Dr. Dotson Jaggers was a Clinical Affairs Associate, ASHP.

The recommendations in this document do not indicate an exclusive course of treatment to be followed. Variations, taking into account individual circumstances, may be appropriate.

The bibliographic citation for this document is as follows: American Society of Health-System Pharmacists. ASHP therapeutic guidelines on antimicrobial prophylaxis in surgery. *Am J Health-Syst Pharm.* 1999; 56:1839–88.

Sedation, Analgesia, and Neuromuscular Blockade of the Critically Ill Adult: Revised Clinical Practice Guidelines for 2002

The critically ill and injured patient is invariably anxious, confused, uncomfortable, and in pain from immobility, wounds, and indwelling tubes and is generally distressed by the adverse environs of the intensive care unit. The restlessness associated with critical illness must nearly always, by necessity, be quelled with sedation and analgesia. Clinicians must sometimes use neuromuscular blockade as a last resort. The knowledge and practice of using sedatives, analgesics, and neuromuscular receptor blocking agents originated in and migrated out of the operating theater and postanesthesia recovery units. However, critical care clinicians have discovered that the sustained use of these agents in intentive care units has consequences that are different from those seen in the immediate perioperative period.

The Society of Critical Care Medicine (SCCM) and the American College of Critical Care Medicine (ACCM) systematically reviewed, developed, and, in 1995, published clinical practice guidelines (CPGs) for sedation, analgesia, and neuromuscular blockade in the critically ill patient.[1,2] These CPGs are the most popular and requested of the SCCM and ACCM documents because of the complexities involved in achieving appropriate levels of sedation and analgesia without inducing complications. Recommendations stemming from the 1995 CPGs, although evidence based, were limited because of the lack of prospective randomized trials comparing agents. Since that time, new evidence has emerged and ACCM believes that the CPGs require updating. ACCM and SCCM have joined forces with the American Society of Health-System Pharmacists (ASHP) to develop new CPGs on the sustained use of sedatives, analgesics, and neuromuscular blocking agents in the critically ill adult.[3,4] The quality of care can be improved by implementing the best known and tested standards, measuring the consequences of what we do, and reducing variability found in practice through the use of protocols. CPGs, in tandem with protocol development, can serve as educational tools, improve outcomes, and reduce costs.[5,6] Evidence suggests that, in real practice, recommendations such as these are often not followed.[7]

"Clinical practice guidelines" are defined by the Institute of Medicine as "systematically developed statements to assist the practitioner and patient in decisions about appropriate health care for specific clinical circumstances."[8] Clinicians need to differentiate CPGs from a summary or review article.[9–11] CPGs are vitally different from review articles and greatly valued for several reasons. Ideally, CPGs are created by a multidisciplinary task force of clinicians, including physicians, nurses, and pharmacists, as well as other health care professionals, under the auspices of

the recommendations developed by critical evaluation of the graded scientific literature. CPGs are typically more comprehensive and far-reaching in scope than review articles and serve as virtual guiding lights by providing a useful construct of available evidence and expert decision-making against which individual decisions by clinicians and programs can be evaluated.[12]

A comprehensive literature search was performed to develop the CPGs. Published studies identified through a MEDLINE search (Sedation and Analgesia 1994–2001; Neuromuscular blocking agents 1994–2001) were reviewed, as were the reference lists of the retrieved documents and abstracts from meetings of professional associations. The literature was critically evaluated for research design, patient selection, medication dose, administration route, combination treatment, test measures, statistics, and results.

The medical literature ranged in quality from prospective randomized trials and retrospective observations to expert opinions (Table 1). Pertinent references were assigned a score to account for variance in quality. The recommendations of SCCM, ACCM, and ASHP (Joint Task Force) were graded according to the strength and quality of the scientific evidence (Table 2). A substantial effort was made by the Joint Task Force to adhere to the methodology for developing scientifically sound CPGs as prescribed by the American Medical Association, the Institute of Medicine, and the Canadian Medical Association.[13–17] The 2002 clinical practice guidelines state the rationale, benefits, and harms of the recommendations, describe the expected health outcomes, and cite and rank the evidence. These CPGs will be reviewed and updated in three to five years.

Table 1.
Categories of Literature Evaluation[a]

Level	Type of Evidence
1	Results from a single PRCT[b] or from a meta-analysis of PRCTs
2	Results from a single PRCT or from a meta-analysis of PRCTs, in which the confidence interval for the treatment effect overlaps the minimal clinically important benefit
3	Results from nonrandomized, concurrent, cohort studies
4	Results from nonrandomized, historical, cohort studies
5	Results from case series
6	Recommendation based on expert opinion

[a]After the authors have identified and classified their respective studies, they grade the articles on the basis of the results of the review.
[b]PRCT = prospective, randomized, controlled trial.

Table 2.
Grades of Recommendations

Grade	Type of Evidence
A	Methods strong, results consistent, PRCTs[a], no heterogeneity
B	Methods strong, results inconsistent, PRCTs, heterogeneity present
C	Methods weak, observational studies

[a]PRCT = prospective, randomized, controlled trial.

There are major additions, besides the updating of the science, to the 2001 CPGs being issued by the Joint Task Force,[3,4] compared with the 1995 guidelines. These guidelines are the most comprehensive documents in the fields of sedation, analgesia, and neuromuscular blockade of the critically ill patient. Graded recommendations are provided and summarized in list form for efficient review at the end of each document. Clear one-page algorithms are also included in each document for sedation, analgesia, and neuromuscular blockade. There is a special focus on appropriate goals for treatment and an absolute insistence on monitoring the level of sedation, pain relief, and the degree of neuromuscular blockade or weakness to better titrate pharmacologic therapy. Moreover, tapering high-dose opioids or sedatives after prolonged treatment (more than a week) is now formally recommended to avoid withdrawal symptoms. Sleep deprivation, its contribution to states of agitation and delirium, and therapeutic approaches to relieve insomnia in critically ill patients are given new and special attention. *Use of neuromuscular blockade remains a last resort* and should always be preceded by adequate sedation. It should always be discontinued as soon as possible to avoid complications. Both documents address cost-effectiveness for their respective modalities.[3,4]

The CPGs issued for 2002 are comprehensive and based on available evidence. This field is still constrained by a dearth of high-quality, randomized, prospective trials comparing agents, monitoring techniques, and scoring scales. Critical care clinicians have a clarion mandate to understand these CPGs, to integrate this information in a manner that is appropriate for their practice setting, and to establish protocols to reduce practice variability and the complications that usually accompany variation. Once this information is applied at the bedside, there is a final obligation to measure the effects of its implementation and the ensuing consequences. The recommendations in these documents may not be appropriate for use in all clinical situations. Decisions to follow these recommendations must be based on professional judgment, level of care, individual patient circumstances, and available resources.

References

1. Shapiro BA, Warren J, Egol AB, et al. Practice parameters for intravenous analgesia and sedation for adult patients in the intensive care unit: an executive summary. *Crit Care Med.* 1995; 23:1596–600.
2. Shapiro BA, Warren J, Egol AB, et al. Practice parameters for sustained neuromuscular blockade in the adult critically ill patient: an executive summary. *Crit Care Med.* 1995; 23:1601–5.
3. Society of Critical Care Medicine and American Society of Health-System Pharmacists. Clinical practice guidelines for the sustained use of sedatives and analgesics in the critically ill adult. *Am J Health-Syst Pharm.* 2002; 59:150–78.
4. Society of Critical Care Medicine and American Society of Health-System Pharmacists. Clinical practice guidelines for sustained neuromuscular blockade in the adult critically ill patient. *Am J Health-Syst Pharm.* 2002; 59:179–95.
5. Price J, Ekleberry A, Grover A, et al. Evaluation of clinical practice guidelines on outcome of infection in patients in the surgical intensive care unit. *Crit Care Med.* 1999; 27:2118–24.
6. Luce J. Reducing the use of mechanical ventilation. *N Engl J Med.* 1996; 335:1916–7.
7. Rhoney DH, Murry KR. A national survey of the use of sedating and neuromuscular blocking agents in the intensive care unit. *Crit Care Med.* 1998; 26:A24. Abstract.
8. Institute of Medicine. Clinical practice guidelines: directions for a new program. Washington, DC: National Academy Press, 1990; 38.
9. Ostermann ME, Keenan SP, Seiferling RA, et al. Sedation in the intensive care unit: a systematic review. *JAMA.* 2000; 283:1451–9.
10. Lerch C, Park GR. Sedation and analgesia. *Br Med Bull.* 1999; 55:76–95.
11. Elliot JM, Bion JF. The use of neuromuscular blocking drugs in intensive care practice. *Acta Anaesthesiol Scand Suppl.* 1995; 106:70–82.
12. Wright J, Bibby J, Hughes J. Evidence-based practice. Guiding lights. *Health Serv J.* 1999; 109:30–1.
13. Institute of Medicine Committee to Advise the Public Health Service on Clinical Practice Guidelines. Clinical practice guidelines: directions of a new program. Washington, DC: National Academy Press; 1990.
14. Attributes to guide the development and evaluation of practice parameters. Chicago, IL: American Medical Association; 1990.
15. Quality of care program: the guidelines for Canadian clinical practice guidelines. Ottawa, Ontario: Canadian Medical Association; 1993.
16. Shaneyfelt TM, Mayo-Smith MF, Rothwangl J. Are guidelines following guidelines? The methodological quality of clinical practice guidelines in the peer-reviewed medical literature. *JAMA.* 1999; 281:1900–5.
17. Cook D, Giacomini M. The trials and tribulations of clinical practice guidelines. *JAMA.* 1999; 281:1950–1.

Developed through the Task Force of the American College of Critical Care Medicine (ACCM) of the Society of Critical Care Medicine (SCCM), in collaboration with the American Society of Health-System Pharmacists (ASHP), and in alliance with the American College of Chest Physicians. No external funding was provided.

The bibliographic citation for this document is as follows: Society of Critical Care Medicine and American Society of Health-System Pharmacists. Sedation, analgesia, and neuromuscular blockade of the critically ill adult: revised clinical practice guidelines for 2002. *Am J Health-Syst Pharm.* 2002; 59:147–9.

Clinical Practice Guidelines for Sustained Neuromuscular Blockade in the Adult Critically Ill Patient

The decision to treat a patient in the intensive care unit (ICU) with neuromuscular blocking agents (NMBAs) (for reasons other than the placement of an endotracheal tube) is a difficult one that is guided more commonly by individual practitioner preference than by standards based on evidence-based medicine. Commonly cited reasons for the use of NMBAs in the ICU are to facilitate mechanical ventilation or different modes of mechanical ventilation and to manage patients with head trauma or tetanus. Independent of the reasons for using NMBAs, we emphasize that all other modalities to improve the clinical situation must be tried, using NMBAs only as a last resort.

In 1995 the American College of Critical Care Medicine (ACCM) of the Society of Critical Care Medicine (SCCM) published guidelines for the use of NMBAs in the ICU. The present document is the result of an attempt to reevaluate the literature that has appeared since the last guidelines were published and, based on that review, to update the recommendations for the use of NMBAs in the ICU. Appendix A summarizes our recommendations. Using methods previously described to evaluate the literature and grade the evidence, the task force reviewed the physiology of the neuromuscular receptor, the pharmacology of the NMBAs currently used in the ICU, the means to monitor the degree of blockade, the complications associated with NMBAs, and the economic factors to consider when choosing a drug.

Neuromuscular Junction in Health and Disease

The neuromuscular junction consists of a motor nerve terminus, the neurotransmitter acetylcholine, and the postsynaptic muscle endplate (Figure 1). The impulse of an action potential causes the release of acetylcholine from synaptic vesicles (each containing about 10,000 molecules of acetylcholine) diffusing across the 20-nm gap to the postsynaptic endplate. The motor endplate contains specialized ligand-gated, nicotinic acetylcholine receptors (nAChRs), which convert the chemical signal (i.e., binding of two acetylcholine molecules) into electrical signals (i.e., a transient permeability change and depolarization in the postsynaptic membrane of striated muscle).

There are depolarizing and nondepolarizing NMBAs. Depolarizing NMBAs physically resemble acetylcholine and, therefore, bind and activate acetylcholine receptors. Succinylcholine is currently the only available depolarizing NMBA and is not used for long-term use in ICUs.

Nondepolarizing NMBAs also bind acetylcholine receptors but do not activate them—they are competitive antagonists. The difference in the mechanism of action also accounts for different effects in certain diseases. If there is a long-term decrease in acetylcholine release, the number of acetylcholine receptors within the muscle increases. This upregulation causes an increased response to depolarizing NMBAs but a resistance to nondepolarizing NMBAs (i.e., more receptors must be blocked). Conditions in which there are fewer acetylcholine receptors (e.g., myasthenia gravis) lead to an increase in sensitivity to nondepolarizing NMBAs.

Adult skeletal muscle retains an ability to synthesize both the mature adult nAChR as well as an immature nAChR variant in which a gamma subunit is substituted for the normal epsilon subunit. Synthesis of immature (fetal) receptors may be triggered in the presence of certain diseases (e.g., Guillain-Barré syndrome, stroke) and other conditions producing loss of nerve function. These immature nAChRs are distinguished by three features. First, immature receptors are not localized to the muscle endplate but migrate across the entire membrane surface.[2] Second, the immature receptors are metabolically short-lived (<24 hours) and more ionically active, having a 2- to 10-fold longer channel "open time." Lastly, these immature receptors are more sensitive to the depolarizing effects of such drugs as succinylcholine and more resistant to the effects of competitive antagonists, such as pancuronium. This increase in the number of immature acetylcholine receptors may account for the tachyphylaxis seen with NMBAs and some of the complications associated with their use. For the remainder of this document, only nondepolarizing NMBAs will be discussed.

Pharmacology of Neuromuscular-Receptor Blockers

Aminosteroidal Compounds. The aminosteroidal compounds include pancuronium, pipecuronium, vecuronium, and rocuronium (Tables 1 and 2).[3–11]

Pancuronium. Pancuronium, one of the original NMBAs used in ICUs, is a long-acting, nondepolarizing compound that is effective after an intravenous bolus dose of 0.06–0.1 mg/kg for up to 90 minutes. Though it is commonly given as an i.v. bolus, it can be used as a continuous infusion[12] by adjusting the dose to the degree of neuromuscular blockade that is desired (Table 1). Pancuronium is vagolytic (more than 90% of ICU patients will have an increase in heart rate of ≥10 beats/min), which limits its use in patients who cannot tolerate an increase in heart rate.[12] In patients with renal failure or cirrhosis, pancuronium's neuromuscular blocking effects are prolonged because of its increased elimination half-life and the decreased clearance of its 3-hydroxypancuronium metabolite that has one-third to one-half the activity of pancuronium.

Pipecuronium. Pipecuronium is another long-acting NMBA with an elimination half-life of about two hours, similar to pancuronium's. Khuenl-Brady and colleagues[13] conducted an open-label evaluation of pipecuronium compared with pancuronium in 60 critically ill patients to determine the minimum doses required for ventilatory management. The administration of 8 mg of either drug followed by intermittent boluses of 4–6 mg when needed resulted in optimal paralysis. Patients were paralyzed for a mean duration of 62.6 hours (45–240 hours) and 61.5 hours (46–136 hours) with pancuronium and pipecuronium, respectively. No adverse effects were attributed to either drug. Perhaps because of this lack of difference and because there are no recent studies examining pipecuronium's use in the ICU, most clinicians continue to use the more familiar drug, pancuronium.

Figure 1. Neuromuscular Junction. Schematic model of the organization and structure of the neuromuscular junction, with focus and enlargement on the postsynaptic membrane. Agrin is the nerve-derived protein that triggers receptor clustering during synapse formation. Receptor aggregation appears to occur in distinct steps, however, initiated with acetylcholine receptors (AChR) localized together by rapsyn. Meanwhile, D-dystroglycan, the extracellular component of dystrophin-associated glycoprotein complex (DGC), is the agrin receptor which transduces final AChR clustering. This process utilizes the structural organization of additional proteins like utrophin, which stabilize the mature, immobile domains by interaction with the underlying cytoskeleton (actin). When completed, this process concentrates AChR density 1000-fold compared to typical muscle membrane. ACh = acetylcholine, MuSK = muscle-specific-receptor kirase, MASC = MuSK-accessory specificity component. (Reprinted with permission, from Wall MH, Prielipp RC. Monitoring the neuromuscular junction. In: Lake C, Blitt CD, Hines RL, eds. Clinical Monitoring: Practical Applications for Anesthesia and Critical Care. Philadelphia: W.B. Saunders, 2000, Figure 10-3.)

Vecuronium. Vecuronium is an intermediate-acting NMBA that is a structural analogue of pancuronium and is not vagolytic. An i.v. bolus dose of vecuronium 0.08–0.1 mg/kg, produces blockade within 60–90 seconds that typically lasts 25–30 minutes. After an i.v. bolus dose, vecuronium is given as a 0.8–1.2-µg/kg/min continuous infusion, adjusting the rate to the degree of blockade desired. Because up to 35% of a dose is renally excreted, patients with renal failure will have decreased drug requirements. Similarly, because up to 50% of an injected dose is excreted in bile, patients with hepatic insufficiency will also have decreased drug requirements to maintain adequate blockade. The 3-desacetylvecuronium metabolite has 50% of the pharmacologic activity of the parent compound, so patients with organ dysfunction may have increased plasma concentrations of both the parent compound and the active metabolite, which contributes to the prolongation of blockade if the dose is not adjusted. Vecuronium has been reported to be more commonly associated with prolonged blockade once discontinued, compared with other NMBAs[a]. Members of the task force believe that vecuronium is being used with decreased frequency in the ICU.

Vecuronium has been studied in open-label prospective trials.[14,15] In one of these studies, the mean infusion rate for vecuronium was 0.9 ± 0.1 µg/kg/min for a mean duration of 80 ± 7 hours. Recovery of a train-of-four (TOF) ratio of ≥0.7 was significantly longer than with cisatracurium.[15] Recovery time averaged 1–2 hours but ranged from ≤30 minutes to more than 48 hours.

Although Rudis et al.[14] observed no difference in the incidence of prolonged blockade between patients receiving vecuronium with and without concomitant administration of corticosteroids, the opinion of the task force was that patients receiving vecuronium and corticosteroids were at increased risk of prolonged weakness once the drug was discontinued.

Rocuronium. Rocuronium is a newer nondepolarizing NMBA with a monoquaternary steroidal chemistry that has an intermediate duration of action and a very rapid onset. When given as a bolus dose of 0.6–1 mg/kg, blockade is almost always achieved within two minutes, with maximum blockade occurring within three minutes. Continuous infusions are begun at 10 µg/kg/min.[8] Rocuronium's metabolite, 17-des-acetylrocuronium, has only 5–10% activity compared with the parent compound.

Sparr, Khuenl-Brady, and colleagues[8,9] studied the dose requirements, recovery times, and pharmacokinetics of rocuronium in 32 critically ill patients, 27 of whom were given intermittent bolus doses, and 5 received a continuous infusion. The median duration of drug administration was 29 hours and 63.4 hours in the bolus dose and infusion groups, respectively. The mean dose of rocuronium required to maintain 80% blockade was 0.34 mg/kg, and the median infusion rate required to maintain one twitch of the TOF was 0.54 mg/kg/hr. The median time from the last bolus dose to the appearance of TOF response was 100 minutes; in the infusion group, the TOF response returned 60 minutes after the infusion was stopped.

Rapacuronium. Rapacuronium, a propionate analogue of vecuronium, was marketed as a nondepolarizing NMBA as an alternative to succinylcholine. It was withdrawn from the market on March 27, 2001, because of reports of morbidity (bronchospasm) and mortality associated with its use.

Table 1.
Selected Neuromuscular Blocking Agents[a] for ICU Use

Variable	Benzylisoquinolinium Drugs				
	D-Turbocurarine (Curare)	Cisatracurium (Nimbex)	Atracurium (Tracrium)	Doxacurium (Nuromax)	Mivacurium (Mivacron)
Introduced (yr)	1942	1995	1983	1991	1992
ED_{95}[b] dose (mg/kg)	0.51	0.05	0.25	0.025–0.03	0.075
Initial dose (mg/kg)	0.1–0.2	0.1–0.2	0.4–0.5	0.025–0.05	0.15–0.25
Duration (min)	80	45–60	25–35	120–150	10–20
Infusion described	. . .	Yes	Yes	Yes	Yes
Infusion dose (µg/kg/min)	. . .	2.5–3	4–12	0.3–0.5	9–10
Recovery (min)	80–180	90	40–60	120–180	10–20
% Renal excretion	40-45	Hofmann elimination	5–10 (uses Hofmann elimination)	70	Inactive metabolites
Renal failure	Increased duration	No change	No change	Increased duration	Increased duration
% Biliary excretion	10–40	Hofmann elimination	Minimal (uses Hofmann elimination)	Insufficient data	. . .
Hepatic failure	Minimal change to mild increased effect	Minimal to no change	Minimal to no change	. . .	Increased duration
Active metabolites	No	No	No, but can accumulate laudanosine	. . .	No
Histamine release hypotension	Marked	No	Minimal but dose dependent	No	Minimal but dose dependent
Vagal block tachycardia	Minimal	No	No	No	No
Ganglionic blockade hypotension	Marked	No	Minimal to none	No	No
Prolonged ICU block	. . .	Rare	Rare	Insufficient data	Insufficient data

	Aminosteroidal Drugs			
	Pancuronium (Pavulon)	Vecuronium (Norcuron)	Pipecuronium (Arduan)	Rocuronium (Zemuron) Introduced (yr)
1972	1984	1991	1994	ED_{95}[b] dose
(mg/kg)	0.05	0.05	0.05	0.3
Initial dose (mg/kg)	0.06–0.1	0.08–0.1	0.085–0.1	0.6–1
Duration (min)	90–100	35–45	90–100	30
Infusion described	Yes	Yes	No	Yes
Infusion dose (µg/kg/min)	1–2	0.8–1.2	0.5–2	10–12
Recovery (min)	120–180	45–60	55–160	20–30
% Renal excretion	45–70	50	50+	33
Renal failure	Increased effect	Increased effect, especially metabolites	Increased duration	Minimal
% Biliary excretion	10–15	35–50	Minimal	<75
Hepatic failure	Mild increased effect	Variable, mild	Minimal	Moderate
Active metabolites	Yes, 3-OH and 17-OH-pancuronium	Yes, 3-desacetyl–vecuronium	Insufficient data	No
Histamine release hypotension	No	No	No	No
Vagal block tachycardia	Modest to marked	No	No	Some at higher doses
Ganglionic blockade hypotension	No	No	No	No
Prolonged ICU block	Yes	Yes	Insufficient data	Insufficient data

[a]Based on drugs for use in a 70-kg man. Modified with permission from Prielipp and Coursin. Reference 3.
[b]ED_{95} = effective dose for 95% of patients studied.

Benzylisoquinolinium Compounds. The benzylisoquinolinium compounds include D-tubocuranine, atracurium, cisatracurium, doxacurium, and mivacurium (Tables 1 and 3).[12,15,16,31]

D-Tubocurarine. Tubocurarine was the first nondepolarizing NMBA to gain acceptance and usage in the ICU. This long-acting benzylisoquinolinium agent is rarely used in ICUs because it induces histamine release and autonomic

Table 2.
ICU Studies of Aminosteroidal Drugs[a]

Reference	Type of Study	Patients	Results	Level of Evidence
4	Prospective, observational, cohort	**30**	Median time to recovery with pancuronium was 3.5 hr in infusion group vs. 6.3 hr in the bolus dose group.	3
5	Prospective, open-label	25 PICU	Increased infusion requirements for pancuronium with anticonvulsants.	3
6	Prospective, open-label	6	Vecuronium clearance increased in 3 and decreased in 2 patients. V_D did not change.	3
7	Survey	. . .	Neuromuscular blockade monitored clinically with only 8.3% using TOF. All respondents indicated concomitant use of sedatives and/or opioids (75%).	5
8	Prospective, open-label	30 SICU	25 trauma patients received rocuronium 50-mg i.v. bolus dose followed by maintenance doses of 25 mg whenever TOF = 2, five patients were on continuous infusion at 25 mg/hr. Duration 1–5 days, recovery approximately 3 hr, and plasma clearance similar between groups.	3
9	Prospective, open-label	32	An initial dose of rocuronium 50 mg followed by maintenance doses of 25 mg with TOF = 2 ($n = 27$) or by continuous infusion to maintain TOF ($n = 5$). Pharmacokinetic data tabulated. Crossover with patients reported by Khuenl-Brady et al.[8]	3
10	Prospective, randomized, controlled	20 CABG	Pancuronium ($n = 10$) was compared to rocuronium ($n = 10$). Incidence of residual block higher with pancuronium than rocuronium. No effect on time to extubation.	2
11	Prospective, open-label	12 ICU	12 patients, 4 with MODS. Patients given 0.6-mg/kg bolus dose of rocuronium followed by repeated bolus ($n = 2$) or continuous infusion ($n = 10$) started at 10–12 µg/kg/min and adjusted to TOF = 1–4. No evidence of prolonged blockade.	**3**

[a]PICU = pediatric intensive care unit, SICU = surgical intensive care unit, CABG = coronary artery bypass grafting, ICU = intensive care unit, TOF = train-of-four, V_D = volume of distribution, MODS = multiple organ dysfunction syndrome.

Table 3.
ICU Studies of Benzylisoquinolinium Drugs[a]

Reference	Type of Study	Patients	Dose	Results	Level of Evidence
16	Review	. . .	. . .	Review of pharmacokinetics	5
17	Prospective, open-label, controlled	14 with hepatic failure vs. 11 controls	Cisatracurium 0.1-mg/kg i.v. bolus dose	V_D greater in liver patients but no differences in elimination $t_{1/2}$ or in duration of action	5
18	Prospective, randomized, single-blind	20 ICU	Cisatracurium ($n = 12$) 0.25 mg/kg/hr Atracurium ($n = 8$) 0.62 mg/kg/hr	Similar mean recovery time	2
19	Prospective, randomized	12 ICU	Cisatracurium 0.1-mg/kg bolus dose + 0.18-mg/kg/hr infusion Atracurium: 0.5 mg/kg + 0.6-mg/kg/hr infusion	Measured V_D, Cl, $T_{1/2}$. Laudanosine concentration was lower in patients on cisatracurium	2
20	Randomized, open-label	61 ICU	Cisatracurium ($n = 26$) 0.1-mg/kg bolus, followed by an infusion of 3 µg/kg/min; 14 pts infusion only	118 ± 19 min recovery no change in HR, BP, and ICP with bolus	3
			Atracurium ($n = 18$) 0.5 mg/kg bolus followed by an infusion of 10 µg/kg/min; 3 pts infusion only		
			Infusion adjusted to one twitch		

(Continued on Next Page)

Table 3 *(continued)*

Reference	Type of Study	Patients	Dose	Results	Level of Evidence
15	Prospective, randomized, double-blind, multicenter	58 ICU	Cisatracurium 2.5-µg/kg/min Vecuronium 1-µg/kg/min	Recovery profiles were significantly different with more prolonged recovery noted for vecuronium. TOF monitoring could not eliminate prolonged recovery and myopathy	1
21	Prospective, blinded, cross-over	14 with brain injury	Cisatracurium 0.15 mg/kg bolus Atracurium 0.75 mg/kg bolus	No change in ICP, CPP, CBF, MAP, ETCO$_2$, and HR and no histamine-related symptoms, with 3×ED$_{95}$ cisatracurium. With 3×ED$_{95}$ tracurium, ICP, CPP, CBF, and MAP decreased within 2–4 min. Five patients had typical histamine reaction; excluding these five patients, there was no difference in any variable compared with cisatracurium	2
22	Observational, prospective, open-label	24 with brain injury	0.1 or 0.2-mg/kg cisatracurium bolus dose	No change from baseline in ICP, CPP, MAP, ETCO$_2$, HR, and CBF velocity in both groups	5
23	Case	. . .	. . .	. . .	4
24	Case	. . .	. . .	. . .	4
25	Review	. . .	. . .	. . .	4
26	Editorial	. . .	. . .	. . .	4
27	Review	. . .	. . .	. . .	5
28	Review	. . .	. . .	. . .	5
12	Multicenter, prospective, double-blind, randomized	40 critically ill	Doxacurium 0.04-mg/kg bolus dose, 0.025-mg/kg maintenance; pancuronium: 0.07 mg/kg bolus dose, 0.05-mg/kg maintenance	No difference in adverse reactions or onset of blockade; pancuronium had a more prolonged and variable recovery time	1
29	Prospective, open-label	8 mechanical ventilated ICU with HD monitoring and pHi <7.35	Doxacurium: 0.03-mg/kg load; 0.03-mg/kg/hr infusion	DO$_2$ + VO$_2$ decreased, pHi increased; VO$_2$ is decreased and pHi increased. NMBA causes redistribution of blood flow to splanchnic beds	5
30	Prospective, open-label study	8 ICU with traumatic head injury	Doxacurium 0.05 mg/kg then 0.25 µg/kg/min	No significant effect in HR, BP, ICP. No adverse effects	5
31	Case report	4 with atracurium tachyphylaxis	Doxacurium 0.25–0.75 µg/kg/min	No tachyphylaxis noted	5

aICU = intensive care unit, TOF = train-of-four, V_D = volume of distribution, HR = heart rate, BP = blood pressure, ICP = intracranial pressure, CPP = cerebral perfusion pressure, CBF = cerebral blood flow, MAP = mean arterial pressure, NMBA = neuromuscular blocking agent, ETCO$_2$ = end tidal carbon dioxide, ED$_{95}$ = effective dose for 95% of patients studied, HD = hemodynamic flow, pHi = gastric mucosal pH, DO$_2$ = oxygen delivery, VO$_2$ = oxygen consumption, CBF = cerebral blood flow.

ganglionic blockade. Hypotension is rare, however, when the agent is administered slowly in appropriate dosages (e.g., 0.1–0.2 mg/kg). Metabolism and elimination are affected by both renal and hepatic dysfunction.

Atracurium. Atracurium is an intermediate-acting NMBA with minimal cardiovascular adverse effects and is associated with histamine release at higher doses. It is inactivated in plasma by ester hydrolysis and Hofmann elimination so that renal or hepatic dysfunction does not affect the duration of blockade.

Laudanosine is a breakdown product of Hofmann elimination of atracurium and has been associated with central nervous system excitation. This has led to concern about the possibility of precipitating seizures in patients who have received extremely high doses of atracurium or who are in hepatic failure (laudanosine is metabolized by the liver). There has been only one report of a surgical patient who had a seizure while receiving atracurium.[32]

Atracurium has been administered to various critically ill patient populations, including those with liver failure,[17] brain injury,[21] or multiple organ dysfunction syndrome (MODS), to facilitate mechanical ventilation. In these reports, atracurium infusion rates varied widely, but they typically ranged from 10 to 20 µg/kg/min with doses adjusted to clinical endpoints or by TOF monitoring. Infusion durations ranged from ≤24 hours to >200 hours. Recovery of normal neuromuscular activity usually occurred within one to two hours after stopping the infusions and was independent of organ function. Long–term infusions have been associated with the development of tolerance, necessitating significant dose increases or conversion to other NMBAs.[31,33] Atracurium has been associated with persistent neuromuscular weakness as have other NMBAs.[34–38]

Cisatracurium. Cisatracurium, an isomer of atracurium, is an intermediate-acting benzyliso-quinolinium NMBA that is increasingly used in lieu of atracurium. It produces few, if any, cardiovascular effects and has a lesser tendency to produce mast cell degranulation than atracurium. Bolus doses of 0.1–0.2 mg/kg result in paralysis in an average of 2.5 minutes, and recovery begins at approximately 25 minutes; maintenance infusions should be started at 2.5–3 µg/kg/min. Cisatracurium is also metabolized by ester hydrolysis and Hofmann elimination, so the duration of blockade should not be affected by renal or hepatic dysfunction. Prolonged weakness has been reported following the use of cisatracurium.[38]

Cisatracurium has been compared with atracurium and vecuronium for facilitating mechanical ventilation in several open-label prospective trials.[15,18–21] Cisatracurium infusion rates ranged from 2 to 8 µg/kg/min and were adjusted to clinical endpoints or to TOF count. Infusion durations varied from 4 to 145 hours. Recovery of a TOF ratio >0.7 occurred within 34–85 minutes after drug discontinuation and was independent of organ function. These recovery times are similar to those seen with atracurium[18,21] and less than those observed with vecuronium.[15]

Doxacurium. Doxacurium, a long-acting benzylisoquinolinium agent, is the most potent NMBA currently available. Doxacurium is essentially free of hemodynamic adverse effects. Initial doses of doxacurium 0.05–0.1 mg/kg may be given with maintenance infusions of 0.3–0.5 µg/kg/min and adjusted to the degree of blockade desired. An initial bolus dose lasts an average of 60–80 minutes. Doxacurium is primarily eliminated by renal excretion. In elderly patients and patients with renal dysfunction, a significant prolongation of effect may occur.

Murray and colleagues[12] conducted a prospective, randomized, controlled, multicenter comparison of intermittent doses of doxacurium and pancuronium in 40 critically ill patients requiring neuromuscular blockade to optimize mechanical ventilation or to lower intracranial pressure (ICP). Patients were given another bolus dose based on TOF monitoring and were paralyzed for a mean duration of 2.6 days with doxacurium or 2.2 days with pancuronium. There was a clinically significant increase in heart rate after the initial bolus dose of pancuronium compared with baseline (120 ± 23 versus 109 ± 22 beats/min, respectively) without any differences after the initial dose of doxacurium (107 ± 21 versus 109 ± 21 beats/min, respectively). Once the drugs were discontinued, the pancuronium group had a more prolonged and variable recovery time (279 ± 229 min) than the doxacurium group (135 ± 46 min).

Mivacurium. Mivacurium is one of the shortest-acting NMBAs currently available. It consists of multiple stereoisomers and has a half-life of approximately two minutes, allowing for rapid reversal of the blockade. There are little data to support its use as a continuous infusion in the ICU.

Indications

NMBAs are indicated in a variety of situations (Table 4).[8,9,12–15,17–21,30,39,42] There have been no studies randomizing patients who are considered candidates for NMBAs to a placebo versus an NMBA. We therefore reviewed many studies comparing one NMBA to another to assess the clinical indications for enrolling patients in these studies. The most common indications for long-term administration of NMBAs included facilitation of mechanical ventilation, control of ICP, ablation of muscle spasms associated with tetanus, and decreasing oxygen consumption (Figure 2). NMBAs are often used to facilitate ventilation and ablate muscular activity in patients with elevated ICP or seizures but have no direct effect on either condition. Patients who are being treated for seizures who also take NMBAs should have electroencephalographic monitoring to ensure that they are not actively seizing while paralyzed.

With the exception of atracurium and cisatracurium, which need to be given continuously because of their short half-lives, bolus administration of NMBAs offers potential advantages for controlling tachyphylaxis; monitoring for

accumulation, analgesia, and amnesia; and limiting complications related to prolonged or excessive blockade; and improving economics. However, in many ICUs, NMBAs are administered continuously, achieving adequate paralysis and faster recovery with TOF monitoring.

Facilitate Mechanical Ventilation. Numerous reports have described the use of NMBAs to facilitate mechanical ventilation. Most of the reports are limited to case studies, small prospective open-label trials, and small randomized open-label and double-blind trials enrolling a wide variety of critically ill patients to whom NMBAs were given to prevent respiratory dysynchrony, stop spontaneous respiratory efforts and muscle movement, improve gas exchange, and facilitate inverse ratio ventilation. However, none of these reports compared NMBAs to placebos.

Manage Increased ICP. The data supporting the use of NMBAs to control ICP are limited to a case report and an open-label trial. Prielipp[30] evaluated doxacurium use in eight patients with severe head injury in an open-label prospective study. NMBAs were given to facilitate ventilation or to manage brain injuries. Patients received an initial bolus injection of doxacurium 0.05 mg/kg followed by a continuous infusion of 0.25 µg/kg/min adjusted to maintain one twitch of the TOF. Doxacurium had no effect on ICP, heart rate, or blood pressure. Infusion rates were similar at the beginning (1 ± 0.1 mg/hr) and at the end (1.3 ± 0.2 mg/hr) of the study. TOF responses returned at 118 minutes; a TOF ratio of 0.7 was measured at 259 ± 24 minutes. No adverse events were reported.

McClelland et al.[40] treated three patients with atracurium for four to six days to manage increased ICP. patients could undergo a neurologic examination within minutes after discontinuing atracurium. No adverse events were reported. There have been no controlled studies evaluating the role of NMBAs in the routine management of increased ICP.

Treat Muscle Spasms. Case studies describe the use of NMBAs in the treatment of muscle contractures associated with tetanus, drug overdoses, and seizures; many were published before 1994.

Anandaciva and Koay[41] administered a continuous rocuronium infusion to control muscle tone in patients with tetanus. Muscle spasms recurred at an infusion rate of 8 µg/kg/min, and neither administering a bolus dose of 0.9 mg/kg nor increasing the infusion rate to 10 µg/kg/min controlled the muscle contractures but did increase heart rate. Switching to a different NMBA could control the spasms.

Decrease Oxygen Consumption. Freebairn et al.[42] evaluated the effects of vecuronium on oxygen delivery, oxygen consumption, oxygen extraction ratios, and gastric intramucosal pH in a randomized, placebo-controlled crossover trial in 18 critically ill patients with severe sepsis. Although the infusion of vecuronium achieved an adequate level of paralysis and improved respiratory compliance, it did not alter intramucosal pH, oxygen consumption, oxygen delivery, or oxygen extraction ratios.

Recommended Indications

There are no prospective, randomized, controlled trials assigning patients to an NMBA versus a placebo with a goal

Table 4.
Indications for the Long-Term Use of Neuromuscular Blocking Agents in Critically Ill Patients[a]

Indication	Agents (n)	Study Design	Underlying Diseases	Reference	Level of Evidence
Facilitate Mechanical Ventilation					
Facilitate management	Cisatracurium (40), atracurium (21)	Randomized, open-label	Hepatic failure, sepsis, cardiogenic shock, ARDS	20	2
Beneficial to management	Cisatracurium (12), atracurium (8)	Randomized, single-blind	Cardiac arrest, respiratory failure, postneurosurgery, trauma, multiorgan failure, asthma, cardiogenic shock	18	2
Facilitate management	Cisatracurium (6), atracurium (6)	Randomized, open-label	Multiple	19	2
Facilitate management	Cisatracurium (28), vecuronium (30)	Randomized, double-blind	Head trauma, intracranial hemorrhage, trauma, ARDS, sepsis, hepatic or renal failure, tetanus	15	2
Optimize mechanical ventilation, increase ICP	Doxacurium (19), pancuronium (21)	Prospective, randomized, double-blind	Not reported	12	2
Facilitate mechanical ventilation	Pipecuronium (30), pancuronium (30)	Prospective, open-label	Head injury, multiple trauma, sepsis, multiorgan failure	13	3
Facilitate mechanical ventilation: dose-finding pharmacokinetic study	Rocuronium (32)	Prospective, open-label	Respiratory failure, multiple trauma, blunt brain trauma	9	3
Facilitate mechanical ventilation; dose-finding pharmacokinetic study	Rocuronium (30)	Prospective, open-label	Multiple trauma and/or blunt brain trauma	8	3
Deterioration in gas exchange	Vecuronium and atracurium (1)	Case report	Respiratory failure in a kidney/pancreas transplant patient	39	5
Control ICP					
Facilitate mechanical ventilation and/or management of traumatic brain injury	Doxacurium (8)	Prospective, open-label	Severe head injury	30	3
Control ICP	Atracurium (4)	Case report	Severe head injury	40	5
Control Muscle Spasms					
Control tetanospasms	Rocuronium (1)	Case report	Tetanus	41	5
Decrease Oxygen Consumption					
Determine effect on oxygen delivery, consumption, and gastric intramucosal pH	Vecuronium (18)	Prospective, randomized, controlled, cross-over	Severe sepsis and septic shock	42	2

[a]ARDS = acute respiratory distress syndrome, ICP = intracranial pressure.

Figure 2. Use of neuromuscular blocking agents (NMBAs) in the ICU.

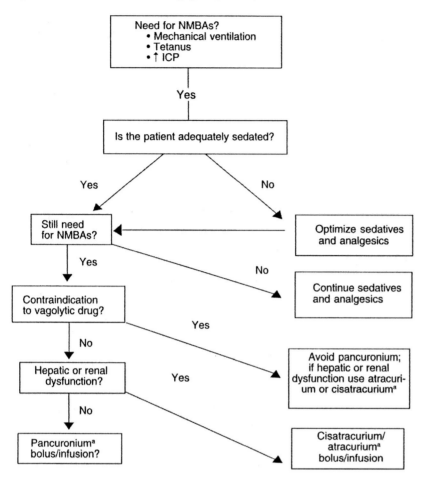

^aMonitor train-of-four ratio, protect eyes, position patient to protect pressure points, and address deep venous thrombosis prophylaxis. Reassess every 12–24 hours for continued NMBA indication.

of documenting if such patients could be managed by means other than NMBA therapy.

Recommendation: NMBAs should be used for an adult patient in an ICU to manage ventilation, manage increased ICP, treat muscle spasms, and decrease oxygen consumption only when all other means have been tried without success. (Grade of recommendation = C)

Recommended Drugs

There has, in essence, been no study since the last guidelines were published that questions the use of pancuronium for the majority of patients in an ICU. Those prospective, randomized, controlled trials (PRCTs) that have been conducted do not clearly show the benefits of using newer agents or any other agents instead of pancuronium.

There are no well-designed studies with sufficient power to make this a level A recommendation, but there is evidence in the literature that patients on pancuronium fare as well as or better than patients receiving any other NMBA.

The two adverse effects of pancuronium that are commented on frequently are vagolysis and an increase in heart rate. Therefore, patients who would not tolerate an increase in heart rate, i.e., those with cardiovascular disease, should probably receive an NMBA other than pancuronium. The indications for the use of an NMBA must outweigh the risk of tachycardia, and

that is based on interpretation of the severity of the patient's underlying cardiovascular disease. For example, a patient with a history of atrial fibrillation now in sinus rhythm and otherwise hemodynamically stable might better tolerate pancuronium than a patient who is hospitalized with cardiogenic pulmonary edema and managed with mechanical ventilation. The clinician should choose an NMBA on the basis of other patient characteristics. Any benzylisoquinolinium compound or aminosteroidal compound could be substituted for pancuronium in these circumstances.

There are no ideal PRCTs that support this recommendation, but there are data suggesting that patients recover more quickly following administration of cisatracurium or atracurium compared with patients receiving other NMBAs if they have evidence of hepatic or renal disease.

Recommendations: The majority of patients in an ICU who are prescribed an NMBA can be managed effectively with pancuronium. (Grade of recommendation = B)

For patients for whom vagolysis is contraindicated (e.g., those with cardiovascular disease), NMBAs other than pancuronium may be used. (Grade of recommendation = C)

Because of their unique metabolism, cisatracurium or atracurium is recommended for patients with significant hepatic or renal disease. (Grade of recommendation = B)

Monitoring

Monitoring neuromuscular blockade is recommended (Table 5).[12,14,43–55] Monitoring the depth of neuromuscular blockade may allow use of the lowest NMBA dose and may minimize adverse events. No PRCT has reported that reducing the dose of an NMBA can prevent persistent weakness. Despite this lack of evidence and the lack of a standardized method of monitoring, assessment of the depth of neuromuscular blockade in ICU patients is recommended.[43]

Visual, tactile, or electronic assessment of the patient's muscle tone or some combination of these three is commonly used to monitor the depth of neuromuscular blockade. Observation of skeletal muscle movement and respiratory effort forms the foundation of clinical assessment; electronic methods include the use of ventilator software allowing plethysmographic recording of pulmonary function to detect spontaneous ventilatory efforts and "twitch monitoring," i.e., the assessment of the muscular response by visual, tactile, or electronic means to a transcutaneous delivery of electric current meant to induce peripheral nerve stimulation (PNS).

Table 5.
Monitoring the Degree of Neuromuscular Blockade[a]

Monitoring Method	Study Design	Reference	Level of Evidence
TOF vs. clinical assessment to guide dosing	Prospective, randomized, single-blind	14	2
TOF vs. clinical assessment to compare depth of neuromuscular blockade	Prospective, nonrandomized	43	4
Complications with various monitoring methods	Retrospective, nonrandomized cohort	44	4
Use of TOF in comparing NMBAs	Multicenter, double-blind, PRCT	12	2
Methods of monitoring NMBAs	Editorial	45	6
Methods of monitoring NMBAs	Review	46	6
Comparison of common NMBAs/pharmacology	Review	25	6
Frequency of NMBA monitoring methods	Nonrandomized, historic, descriptive	47	4
Comparison of NMBA monitoring methods	Editorial	48	6
Comparison of NMBA monitoring methods	Expert opinion	49	6
Comparison of NMBA monitoring methods	Expert opinion	50	6
Technical aspects and problems in NMBA monitoring	Review	51	6
Technical problems with NMBAs monitoring	Review	52	6
Technical problems with NMBA monitoring	Review	53	5
Methods of assessing depth of NMBA	Prospective, randomized, blinded	54	2
Patient assessment during NMBA use	Review	55	6

[a]TOF = train-of-four, NMBA = neuromuscular blocking agent, PRCT = prospective, randomized, controlled trial.

Since the last practice guidelines were published, only two studies have examined the best method of monitoring the depth of neuromuscular blockade, and none have compared the efficacy or accuracy of specific techniques. The first study was a prospective, randomized, single-blinded trial of 77 patients in a medical ICU who were administered vecuronium based on either clinical parameters (patient breathed above the preset ventilatory rate) or TOF monitoring, with a goal of one of four twitches.[44] PNS resulted in a significantly lower total dose and lower mean infusion rate of NMBA as well as a faster time to recovery of neuromuscular function and spontaneous ventilation.

A second study sought to compare the depth of blockade induced by atracurium either by "best clinical assessment" (i.e., maintenance of patient-ventilator synchrony and prevention of patient movement) or TOF monitoring (with a goal of three of four twitches). Analysis of the 36 medical ICU patients in this prospective, nonrandomized trial revealed no difference in the total dose, mean dose, or the mean time to clinical recovery.[43] This may have been due to sample size or study design.

An additional study examining the results of the implementation of a protocol using PNS to monitor the level of blockade in patients receiving a variety of NMBAs found a reduction in the incidence of persistent neuromuscular weakness.[49]

Other methods of electronic monitoring of the depth of blockade are fraught with difficulties; TOF monitoring of PNS remains the easiest and most reliable method available,[43,44,46-50] despite its shortcomings and technical pitfalls.[51-53] Currently, there is no universal standard for twitch monitoring. The choice of the number of twitches necessary for "optimal" blockade is influenced by the patient's overall condition and level of sedation. The choice of the "best" nerve for monitoring may be influenced by site accessibility, risk of false positives, considerations for the effect of stimulation on patient visitors, and whether faint twitches should be included in the assessment of blockade.[54-56] Despite these gaps in research-generated knowledge, evidence-based practice appears to be influencing the increasing frequency with which PNS is utilized.[47] The low correlation of blockade measured peripherally compared with that of the phrenic nerve and diaphragm underscores the importance of three issues: (1) more than one method of monitoring should be utilized, (2) poor technique in using any device will invariably produce inaccurate results, and (3) more clinical studies are necessary to determine the best techniques.

Recommendations for Monitoring Degree of Blockade

Even though the patient may appear quiet and "comfortable," experienced clinicians understand the indications and therapeutic limits of NMBAs. Despite multiple admonitions that NMBAs have no analgesic or amnestic effects, it is not uncommon to find a patient's degree of sedation or comfort significantly overestimated or even ignored. It is difficult to assess pain and sedation in the patient receiving NMBAs, but patients must be medicated for pain and anxiety, despite the lack of obvious symptoms or signs. In common practice, sedative and analgesic drugs are adjusted until the patient does not appear to be conscious and then NMBAs are administered. There have been no studies of the use of electrophysiologic monitoring in assessing adequacy of sedation or analgesia.

In a phenomenological study of 11 critically ill adult trauma patients who required therapeutic NMBA, patients compared their feelings of vagueness to dreaming.[56] Few patients recalled pain or painful procedures. Family members understood the rationale for the use of the drugs and remembered being encouraged to touch and talk with patients. The use of effective pain and sedation protocols and a liberalized visiting policy may have affected the findings.

Recommendations: Patients receiving NMBAs should be assessed both clinically and by TOF monitoring (Grade of recommendation = B), with a goal of adjusting the degree of neuromuscular blockade to achieve one or two twitches. (Grade of recommendation = C)

Before initiating neuromuscular blockade, patients should be medicated with sedative and analgesic drugs to provide adequate sedation and analgesia in accordance with the physician's clinical judgment to optimize therapy. (Grade of recommendation = C)

Complications

Skeletal muscle weakness in ICU patients is multifactorial, producing a confusing list of names and syndromes, including acute quadriplegic myopathy syndrome (AQMS), floppy man syndrome, critical illness polyneuropathy (CIP), acute myopathy of intensive care, rapidly evolving myopathy, acute myopathy with selective lysis of myosin filaments, acute steroid myopathy, and prolonged neurogenic weakness (Table 6).[57,58]

There are probably two adverse events related to prolonged paralysis following discontinuation of NMBAs. We define the first, "prolonged recovery from NMBAs," as an increase (after cessation of NMBA therapy) in the time to recovery of 50–100% longer than predicted by pharmacologic parameters. This is primarily due to the accumulation of NMBAs or metabolites. By comparison, the second, AQMS, presents with a clinical triad of acute paresis, myonecrosis with increased creatine phosphokinase (CPK) concentration, and abnormal electromyography (EMG). The latter is characterized by severely reduced compound motor action potential (CMAP) amplitudes and evidence of acute denervation. In the beginning, these syndromes are characterized by neuronal dysfunction; later (days or weeks), muscle atrophy and necrosis may develop.[59]

Prolonged Recovery from NMBAs. The steroid-based NMBAs are associated with reports of prolonged recovery and myopathy.[57,60] This association may reflect an increased risk inferred by these NMBAs or may reflect past practice patterns in which these drugs may have been more commonly used.[61] Steroid-based NMBAs undergo extensive hepatic metabolism, producing active drug metabolites. For instance, vecuronium produces three metabolites: 3-des-, 17-des-, and 3,17-desacetyl vecuronium.[62] The 3-desacetyl

Table 6.
Weakness in ICU Patients: Etiologies and Syndromes[a]

1. Prolonged recovery from NMBAs (secondary to parent drug, drug metabolite, or drug–drug interaction)
2. Myasthenia gravis
3. Lambert-Eaton syndrome
4. Muscular dystrophy
5. Guillain-Barré syndrome
6. Central nervous system injury or lesion
7. Spinal cord injury
8. Steroid myopathy
9. Mitochondrial myopathy
10. HIV-related myopathy
11. Acute myopathy of intensive care
12. Disuse atrophy
13. Critical illness polyneuropathy
14. Severe electrolyte toxicity (e.g., hypermagnesemia)
15. Severe electrolyte deficiency (e.g., hypophosphatemia)

[a]ICU = intensive care unit, NMBAs = neuromuscular blocking agents, HIV = human immunodeficiency virus.

metabolite is estimated to be 80% as potent as the parent compound. The 3-desacetyl vecuronium metabolite is poorly dialyzed, minimally ultrafiltrated, and accumulates in patients with renal failure because hepatic elimination is decreased in patients with uremia. Thus, the accumulation of both 3–desacetyl vecuronium and its parent compound, vecuronium, in patients with renal failure contributes to a prolonged recovery by this ICU subpopulation. Other explanations have been proposed. One suggests that the basement membrane of the neuromuscular junction acts as a reservoir of NMBAs, maintaining NMBAs at the nAChRs long after the drug has disappeared from the plasma.[63]

Drug–drug interactions that potentiate the depth of motor blockade (Table 7) may also prolong recovery. The specific interaction of NMBAs and exogenous corticosteroids is discussed later.[57,62–65]

Physiologic changes of the nAChRs are enhanced when patients are immobilized or denervated secondary to spinal cord injury, and perhaps during prolonged NMBA drug-induced paralysis. The nAChRs may be triggered to revert to a fetal–variant structure (Figure 3), characterized by an increase in total number, frequent extrajunctional proliferation, and resistance to nondepolarizing NMBAs. The proliferation and distribution of these altered receptors across the myomembrane may account for tachyphylaxis and the neuromuscular blocking effects of these drugs.

AQMS. AQMS, also referred to as postparalytic quadriparesis, is one of the most devastating complications of NMBA therapy and one of the reasons that indiscriminate use of NMBAs is discouraged (Table 8).[65,66] This entity must be differentiated from other neuromuscular pathologies (Table 6) seen in an ICU and requires extensive testing. Reports of AQMS in patients receiving NMBAs alone are quite limited; no experimental model has been able to produce the histopathology of this syndrome by administering NMBAs. Afflicted patients demonstrate diffuse weakness that persists long after the NMBA is discontinued and the drug and its active metabolites are eliminated. Neurologic examination reveals a global motor deficit affecting muscles in both the upper and lower extremities and decreased motor reflexes. However, extraocular muscle function is usually preserved. This myopathy is characterized by low-amplitude CMAPs, and muscle fibrillations but normal (or nearly normal) sensory nerve conduction studies.[63,67] Muscle biopsy shows prominent vacuolization of muscle fibers without inflammatory infiltrate, patchy type 2 muscle fiber atrophy, and sporadic myofiber necrosis.[64] Modest CPK increases (0 to 15-fold above normal range) are noted in approximately 50% of patients and are probably dependent on the timing of enzyme measurements and the initiation of the myopathic process. Thus, there may be some justification in screening patients with serial CPK determinations during infusion of NMBAs, particularly if the patients are concurrently treated with corticosteroids. Also, since AQMS develops after prolonged exposure to NMBAs, there may be some rationale to daily "drug holidays" (i.e., stopping the drugs for a few to several hours and restarting them only when necessary). However, no one has demonstrated that drug holidays decrease the frequency of AQMS. Other factors that may contribute to the development of the syndrome include nutritional deficiencies, concurrent drug administration with aminoglycosides or cyclosporine, hyperglycemia, renal and hepatic dysfunction, fever, and severe metabolic or electrolyte disorders.

Evidence supports, but occasionally refutes,[14] the association of concurrent administration of NMBAs and cor-

Table 7.
Drug–Drug Interactions of Neuromuscular Blocking Agents (NMBAs)

Drugs that potentiate the action of nondepolarizing NMBAs	Drugs that antagonize the actions of nondepolarizing NMBAs
Local anesthetics	Phenytoin
Lidocaine	Carbamazepine
Antimicrobials (aminoglycosides, polymyxin B, clindamycin, tetracycline)	Theophylline
Antiarrhythmics (procainamide, quinidine)	Ranitidine
Magnesium	
Calcium channel blockers	
β-Adrenergic blockers	
Immunosuppresive agents (cyclophosphamide, cyclosporine)	
Dantrolene	
Diuretics	
Lithium carbonate	

Figure 3. Acetylcholine Receptor. The mature nicotinic acetylcholine receptor (AChR) (left) with its glycoprotein subunits arranged around the central cation core. Two molecules of acetylcholine bind simultaneously to the two alpha subunits to convert the channel to an open state. The immature, or fetal-variant, receptor is shown on the right, with a single subunit substitution which follows major stress such as burns or denervation. These immature receptors are characterized by 10-fold greater ionic activity, rapid metabolic turnover, and extrajunctional proliferation. (Reprinted, with permission, from Martyn JAJ, White DA, Gronert GA et al. Up-and-down regulation of skeletal muscle acetylcholine receptors. *Anesthesiology.* 1992; 76:825.)

ticosteroids with AQMS.[59,63,68,69] The incidence of myopathy may be as high as 30% in patients who receive corticosteroids and NMBAs. While no period of paralysis is risk free, NMBA administration beyond one or two days increases the risk of myopathy in this setting.[63] Similarly, there is an inconsistent correlation with the dose of corticosteroids, but total doses in excess of 1 g of methylprednisolone (or equivalent) probably increase the risk. Afflicted patients manifest an acute, diffuse, flaccid weakness and an inability to wean from mechanical ventilation. Sensory function is generally preserved.[63] Muscle biopsy shows extensive type 2 fiber atrophy, myonecrosis, disarray of sarcomere architecture, and an extensive, selective loss of myosin. Experimental evidence in animals shows that denervation for ≥24 hours induces profound negative nitrogen balance and increases expression of steroid receptors in muscle. Such denervation sensitizes muscle to even normal corticosteroid concentrations, and evidence suggests that the combination of denervation and high-dose corticosteroids precipitates myosinolysis.

Acute myopathy in ICU patients is also reported after administration of the benzylisoquinolinium NMBAs (i.e., atracurium, cisatracurium, doxacurium).[24,34,69] Common to all these reports is the coadministration of benzyliso-quinolinium NMBAs and large doses of corticosteroids, aminoglycosides, or other drugs that affect neuromuscular transmission.

Recommendations: For patients receiving NMBAs and corticosteroids, every effort should be made to discontinue NMBAs as soon as possible. (Grade of recommendation = C)

Drug holidays (i.e., stopping NMBAs daily until forced to restart them based on the patient's condition) may decrease the incidence of AQMS. (Grade of recommendation = C)

Other nerve and muscle disorders have been recognized in the last decade in ICU patients (Table 6). For instance, CIP is a sensory and motor polyneuropathy identified in elderly, septic patients or those with MODS.[58,66,70] EMG testing reveals decreased CMAP, fibrillation potentials, and positive sharp waves.[60,63,64] CIP is primarily an axonopathy and may be related to microvascular ischemia of the nerve but is not directly related to the use of NMBAs. Recovery from ICU myopathy requires a protracted (weeks or months) hospitalization. One economic analysis of 10 patients who developed AQMS showed the median additional hospital charge to be $66,000 per patient.[65] As for any critically ill patient, particularly immobilized patients, deep venous thrombosis (DVT) prophylaxis and physical therapy to maintain joint mobility are important.

Patients receiving NMBAs are also at risk of developing keratitis and corneal abrasion. Prophylactic eye care is highly variable and recommendations may include methylcellulose drops, ophthalmic ointment, taping the eyelids shut to ensure complete closure, or eye patches. In a study of 69 paralyzed or heavily sedated patients by Lenart and Garrity,[71] there was strong evidence that the use of an artificial tear ointment prevented corneal exposure. In this randomized study, patients served as their own controls.

Myositis Ossificans (Heterotopic Ossification). Myositis ossificans can develop in patients who are paralyzed for long periods of time, but inflammation is not characteristic of the ailment. The name is misleading because the process involves connective tissue (not muscle). The name originates from the ossification that occurs within the connective tissue of muscle but may also be seen in ligaments, tendons, fascia, aponeuroses,

Table 8.
Potential Complications of Neuromuscular Blockade Use in the ICU[a]

Complications and contraindications of succinylcholine in the ICU	General complications associated with NMBAs in the ICU
Loss of airway	Awake, paralyzed patient–anxiety and panic
Hyperkalemia	Risk of ventilator disconnect or airway mishap
Plasma pseudocholinesterase deficiency	Autonomic and cardiovascular effects (i.e., vagolytic)
	Decreased lymphatic flow
	Risk of generalized deconditioning
	Skin breakdown
	Peripheral nerve injury
	Corneal abrasion, conjunctivitis
	Myositis ossificans
	Risk of prolonged muscle weakness, AQMS
	Potential central nervous system toxicity

[a]NMBA = neuromuscular blocking agent, AQMS = acute quadriplegic myopathy syndrome.

and joint capsules. The acquired form of the disease may occur at any age in either sex, especially around the elbows, thighs, and buttocks. The basic defect is the inappropriate differentiation of fibroblasts into osteoblasts and is usually triggered by trauma and muscle injury, paraplegia or quadriplegia, tetanus, and burns. Treatment consists of promoting an active range of motion around the affected joint and surgery when necessary.

Tachyphylaxis. For reasons mentioned earlier, tachyphylaxis to NMBAs can and does develop.

Coursin and colleagues[31] administered doxacurium to four patients who developed tolerance to atracurium infusions (range, 16 to 40 µg/kg/min). Patients were successfully blocked with infusion rates of doxacurium 0.25–0.75 µg/kg/min.

Tschida et al.[72] described a patient whose atracurium requirement escalated from 5 to 30 µg/kg/min over 10 days. The patient was successfully blocked with a pancuronium infusion of 10–50 µg/kg/min for a period of five days.

Fish and Singletary[33] describe a patient who was inadequately blocked with a 60-µg/kg/min infusion of atracurium but adequately paralyzed for seven days with 2.3-mg/kg/hr infusion of vecuronium. Tachyphylaxis then developed to vecuronium which prompted discontinuation of NMBAs. Two days later, 50–µg/kg/min atracurium infusions were required with high-dose midazolam and fentanyl infusions to achieve adequate oxygenation and acceptable airway pressures.

> *Recommendations: Patients receiving NMBAs should have prophylactic eye care (Grade of recommendation = B), physical therapy (Grade of recommendation = C), and DVT prophylaxis. (Grade of recommendation = C)*

> *Patients who develop tachyphylaxis to one NMBA should try another drug if neuromuscular blockade is still required. (Grade of recommendation = C)*

Economics

There have been few formal pharmacoeconomic evaluations of NMBAs. In one of these economic evaluations, medication-related cost savings were found when voluntary prescribing guidelines for NMBAs were initiated in the operating room of a university hospital.[73] In another study that involved randomization to one of three NMBAs, there were no significant cost differences between atracurium, vecuronium, and rocuronium for surgeries lasting two hours or less, but vecuronium and rocuronium were economically advantageous if the duration of surgery was two to four hours.[74] In a third retrospective study, long-acting NMBAs (e.g., D-tubocurarine and pancuronium) were associated with prolonged postoperative recovery compared with shorter-acting agents (e.g., atracurium, mivacurium, and vecuronium). The authors noted in the discussion section of the paper that based on intrainstitutional recovery room costs, delays in recovery times seen with the longer-acting agents offset the expected savings in drug costs.[75] For patients transferred to the ICU, this may not be a major problem.

Two pharmacoeconomic investigations involving NMBAs in the ICU evaluated the costs associated with prolonged recovery following discontinuation of nondepolarizing NMBAs. In one study, overall costs were lower when TOF monitoring was employed.[76] In another study, patients who had prolonged motor weakness after discontinuing NMBAs were compared with a control group[77]; ICU and hospital costs were substantially higher in the patients with prolonged weakness.

A study involving 40 academic medical centers with patients undergoing coronary artery bypass graft surgery found no significant differences in duration of intubation or duration of ICU or hospital stay among patients who received pancuronium ($n = 732$), vecuronium ($n = 130$), or both ($n = 242$) agents.[78] It is unknown if these results pertain to subgroups of patients, such as those with renal or hepatic dysfunction. If the results of this study are confirmed, the choice of agent could be based solely on cost minimization using medication purchase cost information and equipotent dosage regimens.

A prospective, randomized trial comparing TOF to standard clinical assessment showed decreased NMBA usage and faster return of spontaneous ventilation with TOF monitoring.[14] TOF has the potential to decrease costs associated with NMBA use in ICUs.

Appendix B describes the basic steps involved in conducting a cost-effectiveness analysis of the NMBAs. Consequently, intrainstitutional data and assumptions can be used to perform the analysis along with local value judgments involved in selecting the appropriate agent(s).

> *Recommendations: Institutions should perform an economic analysis using their own data when choosing NMBAs for use in an ICU. (Grade of recommendation = C)*

References

1. Society of Critical Care Medicine and American Society of Health–System Pharmacists. Sedation, analgesia, and neuromuscular blockade of the critically ill adult: revised clinical practice guidelines for 2002. *Am J Health-Syst Pharm.* 2002; 59:147–9.

2. Coakley JH, Nagendran K, Yarwood GD, et al. Patterns of neurophysiological abnormality in prolonged critical illness. *Intensive Care Med.* 1998; 24:801–7.

3. Prielipp RC, Coursin DB. Applied pharmacology of common neuromuscular blocking agents in critical care. *New Horizons.* 1994; 2:34–47.

4. De Lemos JM, Carr RR, Shalansky KF, et al. Paralysis in the critically ill: intermittent bolus pancuronium compared with continuous infusion. *Crit Care Med.* 1999; 27:2648–55.

5. Tobias JD, Lynch A, McDuffee A, et al. Pancuronium infusion for neuromuscular block in children in the pediatric intensive care unit. *Anesth Analg.* 1995; 81:13–6.

6. Segredo V, Caldwell JE, Wright PM, et al. Do the pharmacokinetics of vecuronium change during prolonged administration in critically ill patients? *Br J Anaesth.* 1998; 80:715–9.

7. Appadu BL, Greiff JM, Thompson JP. Postal survey on the long–term use of neuromuscular block in the intensive care unit. *Intensive Care Med.* 1996; 22:862–6.

8. Khuenl-Brady KS, Sparr H, Pühringer F, et al. Rocuronium bromide in the ICU: dose finding and pharmacokinetics. *Eur J Anaesthesiol Suppl.* 1995; 11:79–80.

9. Sparr HJ, Wierda JMKH, Proost JH, et al. Pharmacodynamics and pharmacokinetics of rocuronium in intensive care patients. *Br J Anaesth.* 1997; 78:267–73.

10. McEwin L, Merrick PM, Bevan DR. Residual neuromuscular blockade after cardiac surgery: pancuronium vs rocuronium. *Can J Anaesth.* 1997; 44:891–5.

11. Stene J, Murray M, de Ruyter M, et al. Selective rocuronium pharmacodynamics and kinetics during ICU infusion. *Anesthesiology.* 1998; 89:A477. Abstract.

12. Murray MJ, Coursin DB, Scuderi PE, et al. Double-blind, randomized, multicenter study of doxacurium vs. pancuronium in intensive care unit patients who require neuromuscular–blocking agents. *Crit Care Med.* 1995; 23:450–8.

13. Khuenl-Brady KS, Reitstatter B, Schlager A, et al. Long-term administration of pancuronium and pipecuronium in the intensive care unit. *Anesth Analg.* 1994; 78:1082–6.

14. Rudis MI, Sikora CP, Angus E, et al. A prospective, randomized, controlled evaluation of peripheral nerve stimulation versus standard clinical dosing of neuromuscular blocking agents in critically ill patients. *Crit Care Med.* 1997; 25:575–83.

15. Prielipp RC, Coursin DB, Scuderi PB, et al. Comparison of the infusion requirements and recovery profiles of vecuronium and cisatracurium 51W89 in intensive care unit patients. *Anesth Analg.* 1995; 81:3–12.

16. Hull CJ. Pharmacokinetics and pharmacodynamics of the benzylisoquinolinium muscle relaxants. *Acta Anaesthesiol Scand Suppl.* 1995; 106:13–7.

17. De Wolf AM, Freeman JA, Scott VL, et al. Pharmacokinetics and pharmacodynamics of cisatracurium in patients with end-stage liver disease undergoing liver transplantation. *Br J Anaesth.* 1996; 76:624–8.

18. Pearson AJ, Harper NJ, Pollard BJ. The infusion requirements and recovery characteristics of cisatracurium or atracurium in intensive care patients. *Intensive Care Med.* 1996; 22:694–8.

19. Boyd AH, Eastwood NB, Parker CJ, et al. Comparison of the pharmacodynamics and pharmacokinetics of an infusion of cisatracurium (51W89) or atracurium in critically ill patients undergoing mechanical ventilation in an intensive therapy unit. *Br J Anaesth.* 1996; 76:382–8.

20. Newman PJ, Quinn AC, Grounds RM, et al. A comparison of cisatracurium (51W89) and atracurium by infusion in critically ill patients. *Crit Care Med.* 1997; 25:1139–42.

21. Schramm WM, Papousek A, Michalek-Sauberer A, et al. The cerebral and cardiovascular effects of cisatracurium and atracurium in neurosurgical patients. *Anesth Analg.* 1998; 86:123–7.

22. Schramm WM, Jesenko R, Bartuneka A, et al. Effects of cisatracurium on cerebral and cardiovascular hemodynamics in patients with severe brain injury. *Acta Anaesthesiol Scand.* 1997; 41:1319–23.

23. Grigore AM, Brusco LJr, Kuroda M, et al. Laudanosine and atracurium concentrations in a patient receiving long-term atracurium infusion. *Crit Care Med.* 1998; 26:180–3.

24. Davis NA, Rodgers JE, Gonzalez ER, et al. Prolonged weakness after cisatracurium infusion: a case report. *Crit Care Med.* 1998; 26:1290–2.

25. Reeves ST, Turcasso NM. Nondepolarizing neuromuscular blocking drugs in the intensive care unit: a clinical review. *South Med J.* 1997; 90:769–74.

26. Miller RD. Use of neuromuscular blocking drugs in intensive care unit patients. *Anesth Analg.* 1995; 81:1–2.

27. Bion J, Prielipp RC, Bihari D, et al. Cisatracurium in intensive care. *Curr Opin Anesthesiol.* 1996; 9:S47–51.

28. Werba A, Schultz AM, Hetz H, et al. Benzylisochinoline muscle relaxants in clinical practice. *Acta Anaesthesiol Scan Suppl.* 1997; 111:109–10.

29. Marik PE, Kaufman D. The effects of neuromuscular paralysis on systemic and splanchnic oxygen utilization in mechanically ventilated patients. *Chest.* 1996; 109:1038–42.

30. Prielipp RC, Robinson JC, Wilson JA, et al. Dose response, recovery, and cost of doxacurium as a continuous infusion in neurosurgical intensive care unit patients. *Crit Care Med.* 1997; 25:1236–41.

31. Coursin DB, Meyer DA, Prielipp RC. Doxacurium infusion in critically ill patients with atracurium tachyphylaxis. *Am J Health Syst-Pharm.* 1995; 52:635–9.

32. Manthous CA, Chatila W. Atracurium and status epilepticus. *Crit Care Med.* 1995; 23:1440–2.

33. Fish DN, Singletary TJ. Cross-resistance to both atracurium- and vecuronium-induced neuromuscular blockade in a critically ill patient. *Pharmacotherapy.* 1997; 17:1322–7.

34. Meyer KC, Prielipp RC, Grossman JE, et al. Prolonged weakness after infusion of atracurium in two intensive care unit patients. *Anesth Analg.* 1994; 78:772–4.

35. Manthous CA, Chatila W. Prolonged weakness after the withdrawal of atracurium. *Am J Resp Crit Care Med.* 1994; 150:1441–3.

36. Branney SW, Haenal JB, Moore FA, et al. Prolonged paralysis with atracurium infusion: a case report. *Crit Care Med.* 1994; 22:1699–701.

37. Rubjo ER, Seelig CB. Persistent paralysis after prolonged use of atracurium in the absence of corticosteroids. *South Med J.* 1996; 89:624–6.

38. Hoey LL, Joslin SM, Nahum A, et al. Prolonged neuromuscular blockade in two critically ill patients treated with atracurium. *Pharmacotherapy.* 1995; 15:254–9.

39. Prielipp RC, Jackson MJ, Coursin DB. Comparison of neuromuscular recovery after paralysis with atracurium versus vecuronium in an ICU patient with renal insufficiency. *Anesth Analg.* 1994; 78:775–8.

40. McClelland M, Woster P, Sweasey T, et al. Continuous midazolam/atracurium infusions for the management of increased intracranial pressure. *J Neurosci Nurs.* 1995; 27:96–101.

41. Anandaciva S, Koay CW. Tetanus and rocuronium in the intensive care unit. *Anaesthesia.* 1996; 51:505–6.

42. Freebairn RC, Derrick J, Gomersall CD, et al. Oxygen delivery, oxygen consumption, and gastric intramucosal pH are not improved by a computer-controlled, closed-loop, vecuronium infusion in severe sepsis. *Crit Care Med.* 1997; 25:72–7.

43. Strange C, Vaughan L, Franklin C, et al. Comparison of train–of–four and best clinical assessment during continuous paralysis. *Am J Resp Crit Care Med.* 1997; 156:1556–61.

44. Frankel H, Jeng J, Tilly E, et al. The impact of implementation of neuromuscular blockade monitoring standards in a surgical intensive care unit. *Am Surg.* 1996; 62:503–6.

45. Sladen RN. Neuromuscular blocking agents in the intensive care unit: a two-edged sword. *Crit Care Med.* 1995; 23:423–8.

46. Ford EV. Monitoring neuromuscular blockade in the adult ICU. *Am J Crit Care.* 1995; 4:122–30.

47. Kleinpell R, Bedrosian C, McCormick L. Use of peripheral nerve stimulators to monitor patients with neuromuscular blockade in the ICU. *Am J Crit Care.* 1996; 5:449–54.

48. Murray MJ. Monitoring of peripheral nerve stimulation versus standard clinical assessment for dosing of neuromuscular blocking agents. *Crit Care Med.* 1997; 25:561–2.

49. Tavernier B, Rannou JJ, Vallet B. Peripheral nerve stimulation and clinical assessment for dosing of neuromuscular blocking agents in critically ill patients. *Crit Care Med.* 1998; 26:804–5.

50. Barnette RE, Fish DJ. Monitoring neuromuscular blockade in the critically ill. *Crit Care Med.* 1995; 23:1790–1.

51. Rudis M, Guslits B, Zarowitz B. Technical and interpretative problems of peripheral nerve stimulation in monitoring neuromuscular blockade in the intensive care unit. *Ann Pharmacother.* 1996; 30:165–72.

52. Tschida SJ, Loey LL, Bryan KV. Inconsistency with train-of-four monitoring in a critically ill paralyzed patient. *Pharmacotherapy.* 1995; 15:540–5.

53. Tschida SJ, Loey LL, Mather D. Train-of-four: to use or not to use. *Pharmacotherapy.* 1995; 15:546–50.

54. Martin R, Bourdua I, Theriault S, et al. Neuromuscular monitoring: does it make a difference? *Can J Anesth.* 1996; 43:585–8.

55. Luer JM. Sedation and chemical relaxation in critical pulmonary illness: suggestions for patient assessment and drug monitoring. *AACN Clin Issues.* 1995; 6:333–43.

56. Johnson KL, Cheung RB, Johnson SB, et al. Therapeutic paralysis of critically ill trauma patients: perceptions of patients and their family members. *Am J Crit Care.* 1999; 8:490–8.

57. Watling SM, Dasta JF. Prolonged paralysis in intensive care unit patients after the use of neuromuscular blocking agents: a review of the literature. *Crit Care Med.* 1994; 22:884–93.

58. Nates J, Cooper D, Day B, et al. Acute weakness syndromes in critically ill patients—a reappraisal. *Anaesth Intensive Care.* 1997; 25:502–13.

59. Road J, Mackie G, Jiang T, et al. Reversible paralysis with status asthmaticus, steroids, and pancuronium: clinical electrophysiological correlates. *Muscle Nerve.* 1997; 20:1587–90.

60. Lacomis D, Giuliani MJ, Van Cott A, et al. Acute myopathy of intensive care: clinical, electromyographic, and pathological aspects. *Ann Neurol.* 1996; 40:645–54.

61. Elliot J, Bion J. The use of neuromuscular blocking drugs in intensive care practice. *Acta Anaesthesiol Scand Suppl.* 1995; 106:70–82.

62. Leatherman J, Fluegel W, David W, et al. Muscle weakness in mechanically ventilated patients with severe asthma. *Am J Resp Crit Care Med.* 1996; 153:1686–90.

63. David W, Roehr C, Leatherman J. EMG findings in acute myopathy with status asthmaticus, steroids and paralytics: clinical and electrophysiologic correlation. *Electromyogr Clin Neurophysiol.* 1998; 38:371–6.

64. Faragher MW, Day BJ, Dennett X. Critical care myopathy: an electrophysiological and histological study. *Muscle Nerve.* 1996; 19:516–8.

65. Latronico N, Fenzi F, Recupero D, et al. Critical illness myopathy and neuropathy. *Lancet.* 1996; 347:1579–82.

66. Bolton CF. Muscle weakness and difficulty in weaning from the ventilator in the critical care unit. *Chest.* 1994; 106:1–2.

67. Barohn RJ, Jackson CE, Rogers SJ, et al. Prolonged paralysis due to nondepolarizing neuromuscular blocking agents and corticosteroids. *Muscle Nerve.* 1994; 17:647–54.

68. Zochodne DW, Ramsay DA, Shelley S. Acute necrotizing myopathy of intensive care: electrophysiologic studies. *Muscle Nerve.* 1994; 17:285–92.

69. Marik PE. Doxacurium-corticosteroid acute myopathy: another piece to the puzzle. *Crit Care Med.* 1996; 24:1266–7.

70. Hund E, Fogel W, Krieger D, et al. Critical illness polyneuropathy: clinical findings and outcomes of a frequent cause of neuromuscular weaning failure. *Crit Care Med.* 1996; 24:1328–33.

71. Lenart SG, Garrity J. Eye care for the mechanically ventilated patient receiving neuromuscular blockade or propofol. *Mayo Clin Proc.* In press.

72. Tschida SJ, Hoey LL, Nahum A, et al. Atracurium resistance in a critically ill patient. *Pharmacotherapy.* 1995; 15:533–9.

73. Gora-Harper ML, Hessel E, Shadick D. Effect of prescribing guidelines on the use of neuromuscular blocking agents. *Am J Health-Syst Pharm.* 1995; 52:1900–4.

74. Loughlin KA, Weingarten CM, Nagelhout J, et al. A pharmacoeconomic analysis of neuromuscular blocking agents in the operating room. *Pharmacotherapy.* 1996; 16:942–50.

75. Ballantyne JC, Chang Y. The impact of choice of muscle relaxant on postoperative recovery time: a retrospective study. *Anesth Analg.* 1997; 85:476–82.

76. Zarowitz BJ, Rudis MI, Lai K, et al. Retrospective pharmacoeconomic evaluation of dosing vecuronium by peripheral nerve stimulation versus standard clinical assessment in critically ill patients. *Pharmacotherapy.* 1997; 17:327–32.

77. Rudis MI, Guslits BJ, Peterson EL, et al. Economic impact of prolonged motor weakness complicating neuromuscular blockade in the intensive care unit. *Crit Care Med.* 1996; 24:1749–56.

78. Butterworth J, James R, Prielipp RC, et al. Do shorter-acting neuromuscular blocking drugs or opioids associate with reduced intensive care unit or hospital length of stay after coronary artery bypass grafting? *Anesthesiology.* 1998; 88:1437–46.

Appendix A—Summary of Recommendations

1. NMBAs should be used for an adult patient in an ICU to manage ventilation, manage increased ICP, treat muscle spasms, and decrease oxygen consumption only when all other means have been tried without success.[1] (Grade of recommendation = C)

2. The majority of patients in an ICU who are prescribed an NMBA can be managed effectively with pancuronium. (Grade of recommendation = B)

3. For patients for whom vagolysis is contraindicated (e.g., those with cardiovascular disease), NMBAs other than pancuronium may be used. (Grade of recommendation = C)

4. Because of their unique metabolism, cisatracurium or atracurium is recommended for patients with significant hepatic or renal disease. (Grade of recommendation = B)

5. Patients receiving NMBAs should be assessed both clinically and by TOF monitoring (Grade of recommendation = B), with a goal of adjusting the degree of neuromuscular blockade to achieve one or two twitches. (Grade of recommendation = C)

6. Before initiating neuromuscular blockade, patients should be medicated with sedative and analgesic drugs to provide adequate sedation and analgesia in accordance with the physician's clinical judgment to optimize therapy. (Grade of recommendation = C)

7. For patients receiving NMBAs and corticosteroids, every effort should be made to discontinue NMBAs as soon as possible. (Grade of recommendation = C)

8. Drug holidays (i.e., stopping NMBAs daily until forced to restart them based on the patient's condition) may decrease the incidence of AQMS. (Grade of recommendation = C)

9. Patients receiving NMBAs should have prophylactic eye care (Grade of recommendation = B), physical therapy (Grade of recommendation = C), and DVT prophylaxis. (Grade of recommendation = C)

10. Patients who develop tachyphylaxis to one NMBA should try another drug if neuromuscular blockade is still required. (Grade of recommendation = C)

11. Institutions should perform an economic analysis using their own data when choosing NMBAs for use in an ICU. (Grade of recommendation = C)

Appendix B—Determination of Cost Effectiveness Using Intrainstitutional Data[a]

1. For each adverse effect (e.g., prolonged recovery) of any given neuromuscular blocking agent (NMBA), add all associated costs together and multiply this figure by the probability of the occurrence of the adverse effect. If adverse effects A, B, and C are associated with an NMBA, then

 (Drug cost + cost A1) (probability of occurrence expressed as a decimal) = $U
 (Drug cost + cost B1) (probability of occurrence expressed as a decimal) = $V
 (Drug cost + cost C1) (probability of occurrence expressed as a decimal) = $W

2. Calculate the product of the drug cost multiplied by the probability of occurrence of no adverse effects expressed as a decimal; add this product to the cost multiplied by the probability factor for each adverse effect calculated in step 1.

 (Drug cost) (probability of occurrence of no adverse effects) + $U + $V + $W = average cost of all pathways for agent
 Note: The probabilities of all adverse effects plus the probability of no adverse effects associated with the NMBA must add up to 1.

3. Determine the cost effectiveness of the agent by dividing the total costs associated with the agent by the probability of occurrence of no adverse effects expressed as a decimal.
 Example using pancuronium:

 a. [$224 (drug cost for 4 days of therapy) + $1000 (estimated cost of 1 extra day of ICU stay due to prolonged paralysis
 resulting from renal dysfunction)] [0.07 (estimated probability of renal dysfunction)] = $85.68
 [$224 (drug cost for 4 days of therapy) + $1000 (estimated cost of 1 extra day of ICU (intensive care unit) stay due to prolonged paralysis
 resulting from hepatic dysfunction)] [0.04 (estimated probability of hepatic dysfunction)] = $48.96
 b. [$224 (drug cost for 4 days of therapy, assuming no adverse effects) × 0.89 (estimated probability of no adverse effects)]
 + $85.68 + $48.96 = $334.00
 c. Cost effectiveness of pancuronium = 334.00/0.89 (probability of no adverse effects) = $375.28

[a]Note that the term "adverse effects" includes problems such as prolonged paralysis resulting from decreased medication elimination due to impaired organ function. If a neuromuscular blocking agent is eliminated by more than one organ (e.g., kidney and liver), prolonged paralysis may result from impaired elimination due to a combination of organ problems. For example, one adverse effect

may be prolonged paralysis associated with renal dysfunction, while another adverse effect may be prolonged paralysis associated with hepatic dysfunction, while a third adverse effect may be prolonged paralysis associated with combined renal and hepatic dysfunction.

Developed through the Task Force of the American College of Critical Care Medicine (ACCM) of the Society of Critical Care Medicine (SCCM), in collaboration with the American Society of Health-System Pharmacists (ASHP), and in alliance with the American College of Chest Physicians; and approved by the Board of Regents of ACCM and the Council of SCCM on November 15, 2001 and the ASHP Board of Directors on November 17, 2001.

The recommendations in this document do not indicate an exclusive course of treatment to be followed. Variations, taking into account individual circumstances, may be appropriate.

The bibliographic citation is as follows: Society of Critical Care Medicine and American Society of Health-System Pharmacists. Clinical practice guidelines for sustained neuromuscular blockade in the adult critically ill patient. *Am J Health Syst Pharm.* 2002; 59:179–95.

Clinical Practice Guidelines for the Sustained Use of Sedatives and Analgesics in the Critically Ill Adult

Maintaining an optimal level of comfort and safety for critically ill patients is a universal goal for critical care practitioners. The American College of Critical Care Medicine (ACCM) of the Society of Critical Care Medicine's (SCCM's) practice parameters for the optimal use of sedatives and analgesics was published in 1995 and recommended a tiered approach to the use of sedatives and analgesics, largely on the basis of expert opinion.[1] These clinical practice guidelines replace the previously published parameters and include an evaluation of the literature published since 1994 comparing the use of these agents. The reader should refer to the accompanying introduction for a description of the methodology used to develop these guidelines.[2]

This document is limited to a discussion of prolonged sedation and analgesia. Consistent with the previous practice guidelines, this document pertains to patients older than 12 years. The majority of the discussion focuses on the care of patients during mechanical ventilation. A discussion of regional techniques is not included. Appendix A summarizes the recommendations made herein.

Analgesia

In these guidelines, "analgesia" is defined as the blunting or absence of sensation of pain or noxious stimuli. Intensive care unit (ICU) patients commonly have pain and physical discomfort from obvious factors, such as preexisting diseases, invasive procedures, or trauma. Patient pain and discomfort can also be caused by monitoring and therapeutic devices (such as catheters, drains, noninvasive ventilating devices, and endotracheal tubes), routine nursing care (such as airway suctioning, physical therapy, dressing changes, and patient mobilization), and prolonged immobility.[3,4] Unrelieved pain may contribute to inadequate sleep, possibly causing exhaustion and disorientation. Agitation in an ICU patient may result from inadequate pain relief. Unrelieved pain evokes a stress response characterized by tachycardia, increased myocardial oxygen consumption, hypercoagulability, immunosuppression, and persistent catabolism.[5,6] The combined use of analgesics and sedatives may ameliorate the stress response in critically ill patients.[7,8] Pain may also contribute to pulmonary dysfunction through localized guarding of muscles around the area of pain and a generalized muscle rigidity or spasm that restricts movement of the chest wall and diaphragm.[9] Effective analgesia may diminish pulmonary complications in postoperative patients.[10]

Some patients recall unrelieved pain when interviewed about their ICU stays.[3,11,12] The perception of pain can be influenced by several factors, such as the expectation of pain, prior pain experiences, a patient's emotional state, and the cognitive processes of the patient.[11] Patients should be educated about the potential for pain and instructed to communicate their needs in an appropriate manner (such as using an assessment tool or other communication techniques). The goals of therapy should also be communicated to the patient and family. In many cases, pain will be managed but not completely eliminated. Fear of potent analgesics and mis-

conceptions about pain and analgesics should be addressed. Similarly, practitioner bias against the adequate use of opioids or misplaced fears of adverse effects or addiction may produce inadequate prescribing or administration.[13,14] Educating practitioners and assessing the quality of a pain management program may improve analgesia therapy, but such programs have not been universally successful.[4,15] The importance of appropriate pain management programs has been reinforced by the Joint Commission on Accreditation of Healthcare Organizations's (JCAHO's) establishment of standards on pain assessment and management.

> *Recommendation: All critically ill patients have the right to adequate analgesia and management of their pain. (Grade of recommendation = C)*

Pain Assessment. There is a limited amount of literature that directly addresses pain assessment in the critical care unit. The articles reviewed in this report include descriptions of pain assessment tools used for critically ill patients, even if these tools were not validated in this population. Studies of pain in the critically ill indicate the importance of systematic and consistent assessment and documentation.[16] The most reliable and valid indicator of pain is the patient's self-report.[17] The location, characteristics, aggravating and alleviating factors, and intensity of pain should be evaluated. Assessment of pain intensity may be performed with unidimensional tools, such as a verbal rating scale (VRS), visual analogue scale (VAS), and numeric rating scale (NRS). VAS comprises a 10-cm horizontal line with descriptive phrases at either end, from "no pain" to "severe pain" or "worst pain ever." Variations include vertical divisions or numeric markings. VAS is reliable and valid for many patient populations.[18] Though not specifically tested in the ICU, VAS is frequently used there[19-22] Elderly patients may have difficulty with VAS.[20] NRS is a zero to ten point scale and patients choose a number that describes the pain, with ten representing the worst pain. NRS is also valid, correlates with VAS, and has been used to assess pain in cardiac surgical patients.[21] Because patients can complete the NRS by writing or speaking, and because it is applicable to patients in many age groups, NRS may be preferable to VAS in critically ill patients.

Multidimensional tools, such as the McGill Pain Questionnaire (MPQ) and the Wisconsin Brief Pain Questionnaire (BPQ), measure pain intensity and the sensory, affective, and behavioral components of that pain but take longer to administer and may not be practical for the ICU environment.[18,22] The MPQ and BPQ are reliable and valid tools but have not been tested or used in the ICU.

Although the most reliable indicator of pain intensity is what the patient reports, critically ill patients are often unable to communicate their level of pain if sedated, anesthetized, or receiving neuromuscular blockade. Neither the VAS nor the NRS will resolve this problem as they rely on the patient's ability to communicate with the care provider. Behavioral–physiological scales may be useful in assessing pain in these patients. Moderate agreement was found

between the VAS and the observer-reported Faces scale for all observations, but less agreement was noted as the pain intensity increased.[19] The verbal descriptive scale (VDS) used in another trial showed moderate correlation (r> 0.60) with a behavioral pain scale in assessing pain in postanesthesia patients.[23] A behavioral–physiological scale was compared with an NRS and a moderate-to-strong correlation was observed between the scales.[24] The behavioral–physiological scale also assessed pain-related behaviors (movement, facial expression, and posturing) and physiological indicators (heart rate, blood pressure, and respiratory rate). However, such nonspecific parameters might be misinterpreted or affected by observer bias, leading to an underestimation of the degree of pain experienced by the patient.[12,24–27]

Family members or other surrogates have been evaluated for their ability to assess the amount of pain experienced by noncommunicative ICU patients. While surrogates could estimate the presence or absence of pain in 73.5% of patients, they less accurately described the degree of pain (53%).[28]

The most appropriate pain assessment tool will depend on the patient involved, his/her ability to communicate, and the caregiver's skill in interpreting pain behaviors or physiological indicators.

Recommendations: Pain assessment and response to therapy should be performed regularly by using a scale appropriate to the patient population and systematically documented. (Grade of recommendation = C)

The level of pain reported by the patient must be considered the current standard for assessment of pain and response to analgesia whenever possible. Use of the NRS is recommended to assess pain. (Grade of recommendation = B)

Patients who cannot communicate should be assessed through subjective observation of pain-related behaviors (movement, facial expression, and posturing) and physiological indicators (heart rate, blood pressure, and respiratory rate) and the change in these parameters following analgesic therapy. (Grade of recommendation = B)

Analgesia Therapy. Nonpharmacologic interventions including attention to proper positioning of patients, stabilization of fractures, and elimination of irritating physical stimulation (e.g., proper positioning of ventilator tubing to avoid traction on the endotracheal tube) are important to maintain patient comfort. Application of heat or cold therapy may be useful. Other nonpharmacologic techniques to promote patient comfort are discussed later in this document.

Pharmacologic therapies include opioids, nonsteroidal anti-inflammatory drugs (NSAIDs), and acetaminophen. Opioids mediate analgesia by interacting with a variety of central and peripheral opioid receptors. The opioids currently available have activity at a variety of these receptors, although the μ- and κ-receptors are most important for analgesia. Interaction at other receptors may contribute to adverse effects. The analgesic agents most commonly used in ICU patients (fentanyl, morphine, and hydromorphone) are addressed later.[29] Although alfentanil has previously been reported as an analgesic with sedative effects, it will not be extensively discussed because it is not commonly used in North America.[29]

Comparative trials of opioids have not been performed in critically ill patients. The selection of an agent depends on its pharmacology and potential for adverse effects. The characteristics of commonly used opioids and nonopioids are reviewed in Table 1.[30–32] Desirable attributes of an opioid include rapid onset, ease of titration, lack of accumulation of the parent drug or its metabolites, and low cost. Fentanyl has the most rapid onset and shortest duration, but repeated dosing may cause accumulation and prolonged effects. Morphine has a longer duration of action, so intermittent doses may be given. However, hypotension may result from vasodilation and an active metabolite may cause prolonged sedation in the presence of renal insufficiency. Hydromorphone's duration of action is similar to morphine's, but hydromorphone lacks a clinically significant active metabolite or histamine release. Meperidine has an active metabolite that causes neuroexcitation (apprehension, tremors, delirium, and seizures) and may interact with antidepressants (contraindicated with monoamine oxidase inhibitors and best avoided with selective serotonin-reuptake inhibitors), so it is not recommended for repetitive use.[17,33,34] Because codeine lacks analgesic potency, it is not useful for most patients. Remifentanil has not been widely studied in ICU patients and requires the use of a continuous infusion because of its very short duration of action.[35] The short duration of action could be beneficial in selected patients requiring interruptions for neurologic examination.[35]

Disease states, such as renal or hepatic insufficiency may alter opioid and metabolite elimination. Titration to the desired response and assessment of the drug's prolonged effect are necessary in all patients. The elderly may have reduced opioid requirements.[30,31,36–39]

Adverse effects of opioid analgesics are common and occur frequently in ICU patients. Of greatest concern are respiratory, hemodynamic, central nervous system, and gastrointestinal effects. Respiratory depression is a concern in spontaneously breathing patients or those receiving partial ventilatory support. Hypotension can occur in hemodynamically unstable patients, hypovolemic patients, or those with elevated sympathetic tone.[40] Opioid-mediated hypotension in euvolemic patients is a result of the combination of sympatholysis, vagally mediated bradycardia, and histamine release (when using codeine, morphine, or meperidine).[41,42] Opioid-induced depression of the level of consciousness may cloud the clinical assessment of critically ill patients, and hallucinations may increase agitation in some patients. Gastric retention and ileus are common in critically ill patients, and intestinal hypomotility is enhanced by opioids.[43,44] Routine prophylactic use of a stimulant laxative may minimize constipation. Small-bowel intubation may be needed for enteral nutrition because of gastric hypomotility.[45] Opioids may increase intra-cranial pressure with traumatic brain injury, although the data are inconsistent and the clinical significance is unknown.[46–48]

Opioid administration techniques. Preventing pain is more effective than treating established pain. When patients are administered drugs on an "as needed" basis, they may receive less than the prescribed dose and encounter significant delays in treatment, although the impact on patient outcome has not been well documented.[49] Analgesics should be administered on a continuous or scheduled intermittent basis, with supplemental bolus doses as required.[17] Intravenous administration usually requires lower and more frequent doses than intramuscular administration to titrate to patient comfort. Intramuscular administration is not recommended in hemodynamically unstable

Table 1.
Pharmacology of Selected Analgesics[1,17,30–32]

Agent	Equianalgesic Dose (i.v.)	Half-life	Metabolic Pathway	Active Metabolites (Effect)	Adverse Effects	Intermittent Dose[a]	Infusion Dose Range (Usual)	Infusion Cost per day 70 kg[b]
Fentanyl	200 µg	1.5–6 hr	Oxidation	No metabolite, parent accumulates	Rigidity with high doses	0.35–1.5 µg/kg i.v. q 0.5–1 hr	0.7–10 µg/kg/hr	100 µg/hr: $26.00
Hydromorphone	1.5 mg	2–3 hr	Glucuronidation	None	...	10–30 µg/kg i.v. q 1–2 hr	7–15 µg/kg/hr	0.75 mg/hr: $5.00–11.00
Morphine	10 mg	3–7 hr	Glucuronidation	Yes (sedation, especially in renal insufficiency)	Histamine release	0.01–0.15 mg/kg i.v. q 1–2 hr	0.07–0.5 mg/kg/hr	5 mg/hr: $3.50–12.00
Meperidine	75–100 mg	3–4 hr	Demethylation and hydroxylation	Yes (neuroexcitation, especially in renal insufficiency or high doses)	Avoid with MAOIs[c] and SSRIs[d]	Not recommended	Not recommended	...
Codeine	120 mg	3 hr	Demethylation and glucuronidation	Yes (analgesia, sedation)	Lacks potency, histamine release	Not recommended	Not recommended	...
Remifentanil	...	3–10 min	Plasma esterase	None	...	...	0.6–15 µg/kg/hr	10 µg/kg/hr: $170.00
Ketorolac	...	2.4–8.6 hr	Renal	None	Risk of bleeding, GI and renal adverse effects	15–30 mg i.v. q 6h, decrease if age > 65 yr or wt < 50 kg or renal impairment, avoid > 5 days use	...	...
Ibuprofen	...	1.8–2.5 hr	Oxidation	None	Risk of bleeding, GI and renal adverse effects	400 mg p.o. q 4–6 hr	...	...
Acetaminophen	...	2 hr	Conjugation	...	...	325–650 mg p.o. q 4–6 hr, avoid > 4 g/day	...	...

[a]More frequent doses may be needed for acute pain management in mechanically ventilated patients.
[b]Cost based on 2001 average wholesale price.
[c]MAOIs = monoamine oxidase inhibitors.
[d]SSRIs = selective serotonin-reuptake inhibitors.

Figure 1. Algorithm for the sedation and analgesia of mechanically ventilated patients. This algorithm is a general guideline for the use of analgesics and sedatives. Refer to the text for clinical and pharmacologic issues that dictate optimal drug selection, recommended assessment scales, and precautions for patient monitoring. Doses are approximate for a 70-kg adult. IVP = intravenous push.

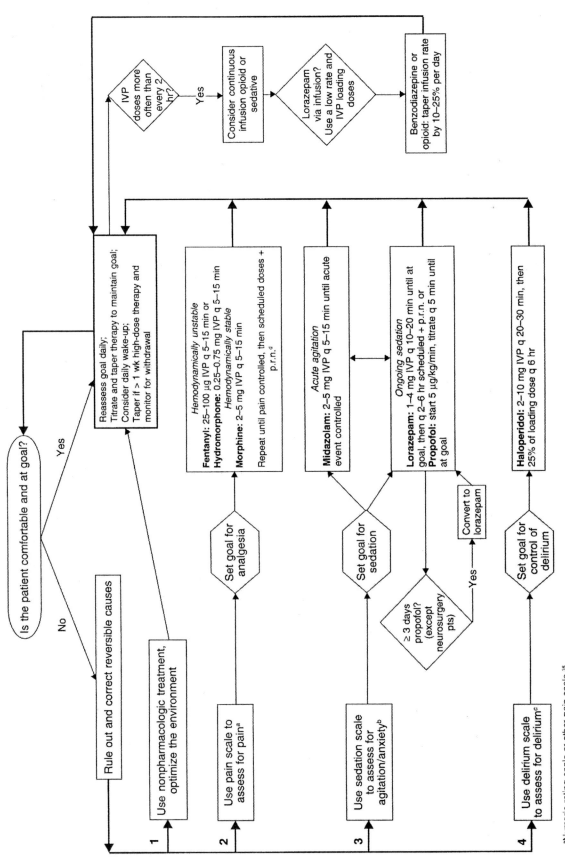

[a]Numeric rating scale or other pain scale.[18]
[b]Riker Sedation-Agitation Scale or other sedation scale.[82]
[c]Confusion Assessment Method for the ICU.[185]
[d]See Table 1 for intermittent dosing for specific agents.

patients because of altered perfusion and variable absorption. When a continuous infusion was used, a protocol incorporating daily awakening from analgesia and sedation allowed more effective analgesic titration and a lower total dose of morphine.[50] Daily awakening was associated with a shorter duration of ventilation and ICU stay.[50] A pain management plan and therapy goal should be established for each patient and reevaluated as the clinical condition changes. An algorithm that illustrates the potential use of opioid analgesics for mechanically ventilated patients is shown in Figure 1. Analgesic orders should be written to allow titration to achieve the analgesic goal and to balance the potential impact of adverse effects.

In noncritically ill patients, patient-controlled analgesia (PCA) has been reported to result in stable drug concentrations, a good quality of analgesia, less sedation, less opioid consumption, and potentially fewer adverse effects, including respiratory complications.[10,51] In addition, a basal rate or continuous infusion mode can be used for consistent analgesia during sleep. Patient selection is important when PCA is used, and particular attention should be paid to the patient's cognition, hemodynamic reserve, and previous opioid exposure. PCA devices can also be used for nurse-controlled analgesia. The elimination of paperwork can improve the timeliness of analgesic administration.

Fentanyl may also be administered via a transdermal patch in hemodynamically stable patients with more chronic analgesic needs. The patch provides consistent drug delivery, but the extent of absorption varies depending on the permeability, temperature, perfusion, and thickness of the skin. There is a large interpatient variability in peak plasma concentrations. Fentanyl patches are not a recommended modality for acute analgesia because of their 12–24-hour delay to peak effect and similar lag time to complete offset once the patch is removed. Breakthrough pain should be treated with rapid-acting agents.

The use of a reversal agent, such as naloxone, is not recommended after prolonged analgesia, because it can induce withdrawal and may cause nausea, cardiac stress, and arrhythmias. Analgesics with agonist–antagonist action, such as nalbuphine, butorphanol, and buprenorphine, can also elicit withdrawal symptoms and should be avoided during prolonged opioid use.

Recommendations: A therapeutic plan and goal of analgesia should be established for each patient and communicated to all caregivers to ensure consistent analgesic therapy. (Grade of recommendation = C)

If intravenous doses of an opioid analgesic are required, fentanyl, hydromorphone, and morphine are the recommended agents. (Grade of recommendation = C)

Scheduled opioid doses or a continuous infusion is preferred over an "as needed" regimen to ensure consistent analgesia. A PCA device may be utilized to deliver opioids if the patient is able to understand and operate the device. (Grade of recommendation = B)

Fentanyl is preferred for a rapid onset of analgesia in acutely distressed patients. (Grade of recommendation = C)

Fentanyl or hydromorphone are preferred for patients with hemodynamic instability or renal insufficiency. (Grade of recommendation = C)

Morphine and hydromorphone are preferred for intermittent therapy because of their longer duration of effect. (Grade of recommendation = C)

Nonopioid analgesics. NSAIDs provide analgesia via the nonselective, competitive inhibition of cyclooxygenase (COX), a critical enzyme in the inflammatory cascade. NSAIDs have the potential to cause significant adverse effects, including gastrointestinal bleeding, bleeding secondary to platelet inhibition, and the development of renal insufficiency. Patients with hypovolemia or hypoperfusion, the elderly, and those with preexisting renal impairment may be more susceptible to NSAID-induced renal injury.[52,53] Prolonged use (more than five days) of ketorolac has been associated with a twofold increase in the risk of renal failure and an increased risk of gastrointestinal and operative-site bleeding.[54,55] NSAIDs should not be administered to patients with asthma and aspirin sensitivity.

Administration of NSAIDs may reduce opioid requirements, although the analgesic benefit of NSAIDs has not been systematically studied in critically ill patients. Many oral agents are available, and ibuprofen and naproxen are available in liquid form. Ketorolac is currently the only parenteral NSAID. The safety of ketorolac administration in patients with severe renal insufficiency or those undergoing dialysis has not been determined.

The role, if any, of the more selective COX-2 inhibitors in the critically ill remains unknown. Selective COX-2 inhibiting agents cause less gastrointestinal irritation with long-term use than traditional NSAIDs.[56] The slow onset of action of some agents may decrease their utility for acute pain management.

Acetaminophen is an analgesic used to treat mild to moderate pain. In combination with an opioid, acetaminophen produces a greater analgesic effect than higher doses of the opioid alone.[57] The role of acetaminophen in critical care is limited to relieving mild pain or discomfort, such as that associated with prolonged bed rest or use as an antipyretic. Care must be taken to avoid excessive and potentially hepatotoxic doses, especially in patients with depleted glutathione stores resulting from hepatic dysfunction or malnutrition. Acetaminophen should be maintained at less than 2 g per day for patients with a significant history of alcohol intake or poor nutritional status and less than 4 g per day for others (Table 1).[58]

Recommendations: NSAIDs or acetaminophen may be used as adjuncts to opioids in selected patients. (Grade of recommendation = B)

Ketorolac therapy should be limited to a maximum of five days, with close monitoring for the development of renal insufficiency or gastrointestinal bleeding. Other NSAIDs may be used via the enteral route in appropriate patients. (Grade of recommendation = B)

Sedation

The indications for sedative agents are not well defined. Sedatives are common adjuncts for the treatment of anxiety

and agitation. The causes of anxiety in critically ill patients are multifactorial and are likely secondary to an inability to communicate amid continuous noise (alarms, personnel, and equipment), continuous ambient lighting, and excessive stimulation (inadequate analgesia, frequent vital signs, repositioning, lack of mobility, and room temperature). Sleep deprivation and the circumstances that led to an ICU admission may increase patient anxiety, affecting up to 50% of ICU patients.[38,59] Efforts to reduce anxiety, including frequent reorientation, maintenance of patient comfort, provision of adequate analgesia, and optimization of the environment, may be supplemented with sedatives. Some patients with respiratory failure require sedation to facilitate mechanical ventilation, although sedation should not be used in lieu of appropriate ventilation strategies.

Agitation is common in ICU patients of all ages, occurring at least once in 71% of patients in a medical–surgical ICU.[38] Agitation can be caused by multiple factors, such as extreme anxiety, delirium, adverse drug effects, and pain.[38] However, not all patients with anxiety will exhibit agitation; some patients may be fearful, anxious, and withdrawn. When patients exhibit signs of anxiety or agitation, the first priority is to identify and treat any underlying physiological disturbances, such as hypoxemia, hypoglycemia, hypotension, pain, and withdrawal from alcohol and other drugs. The prevalence of drug and alcohol abuse in the general population is high, and these substances are commonly associated with traumatic injury.[60–62] Patients in the ICU should be assessed for symptoms of intoxication or withdrawal upon admission and for several weeks thereafter.[60–62] When possible, patients should be questioned about the use of herbal medicines because these products may contribute to significant drug interactions and adverse effects.[63]

Recent studies have confirmed that agitation may have a deleterious effect on patients by contributing to ventilator dysynchrony, an increase in oxygen consumption, and inadvertent removal of devices and catheters.[38,64–67] Sedatives reduce the stress response and improve the tolerance of routine ICU procedures.[68] The use of sedatives to maintain patient safety and comfort is often essential to the ICU therapeutic care plan. The sedation of mechanically ventilated patients is often medically necessary and should be based on an individualized assessment and the patient's needs. Sedatives should be administered intermittently or on an "as needed" basis to determine the dose that will achieve the sedation goal. Sedatives, as outlined in this guideline, are not intended to be used as a method of restraint and are not to be "used as a means of coercion, discipline, convenience, or retaliation by staff" (Federal regulation 42 CFR 482.13). It is important to consider this principle in order to follow the intent of the Centers for Medicare and Medicaid Services regulation regarding restraints.

An analgesic may be the appropriate initial therapy when pain is the suspected cause of acute agitation. Although opioids may produce sedating effects, they do not diminish awareness or provide amnesia for stressful events. Sedative–amnestic therapy is required to reliably attain amnesia.[69–72] Without amnesia, many patients who recall their ICU stay report unpleasant or frightening memories, which may contribute to post-traumatic stress disorder (PTSD) symptoms.[21,73] However, some patients have vivid hypnogagic hallucinations (dreams just before loss of consciousness) with sedative–amnestic therapy.[74] As sedation blunts explicit memory, these hallucinations may be patients' only memory of the ICU experience.[75] Recalling

delusions, without memory of real events, may also contribute to acute PTSD-related symptoms.[75] Other data suggest that PTSD may be experienced by 4–15% of ICU survivors.[76,77] Amnestic sedatives may paradoxically contribute to agitation and disorientation because patients may not remember where they are or why they are in the ICU.

Recommendation: Sedation of agitated critically ill patients should be started only after providing adequate analgesia and treating reversible physiological causes. (Grade of recommendation = C)

Sedation Assessment. *Subjective assessment of sedation and agitation.* Frequent assessment of the degree of sedation or agitation may facilitate the titration of sedatives to predetermined endpoints.[78–80] An ideal sedation scale should provide data that are simple to compute and record, accurately describe the degree of sedation or agitation within well-defined categories, guide the titration of therapy, and have validity and reliability in ICU patients. Many scales are available, but a true gold-standard scale has not been established.[79] Several scales have construct validity with good correlation between the scales' measures and other measures of sedation. None of the scales have been tested for their ability to detect a patient's response to changes in sedative therapy, dosage, or withdrawal. However, a defined sedation goal, using the Ramsay scale and a protocol-driven sedation plan, was shown to reduce the duration of mechanical ventilation and length of stay.[80] The authors did not report other patient outcome measures relative to the adequacy of analgesia or sedation.

The Riker Sedation–Agitation Scale (SAS) was the first scale proven to be reliable and valid in critically ill adults.[81,82] SAS scores a patient's level of consciousness and agitation from a seven-item list describing patient behavior (Table 2). Excellent inter-rater reliability has been demonstrated and validity has been shown with two other scales. The Motor Activity Assessment Scale (MAAS), adapted from the SAS, has also been validated and shown reliable for use in critically ill patients.[83] The MAAS has seven categories to describe patient behaviors in response to stimulation (Table 2). The Ramsay scale measures three levels of awake states and three levels of asleep states (Table 2).[84] It has been shown to have an acceptable interrater reliability compared with the SAS, but has been criticized for its lack of clear discrimination and specific descriptors to differentiate between the various levels.[82,85] Nevertheless, the Ramsay scale has been used in many comparative sedation trials and is widely used clinically. The Vancouver Interaction and Calmness Scale (VICS) has also been validated for the assessment of sedation in adult critically ill patients.[86] With the VICS scoring system, patients are assessed independently for the ability to interact and communicate and for their level of activity or restlessness. The VICS has not been tested to identify optimal sedation endpoints. Another scale, the Observer's Assessment of Alertness/Sedation Scale, is often used in the operating room but lacks the ability to assess agitation and has never been tested in the ICU.[87] The COMFORT scale has been extensively tested and applied in the ICU environment, but only in children.[88]

The appropriate target level of sedation will primarily depend on a patient's acute disease process and any therapeutic and supportive interventions required. A common target level of sedation in the ICU is a calm patient that can be easily aroused with maintenance of the normal

Table 2.
Scales Used to Measure Sedation and Agitation

Score	Description	Definition
Riker Sedation–Agitation Scale (SAS)[82]		
7	Dangerous agitation	Pulling at endotracheal tube (ETT), trying to remove catheters, climbing over bedrail, striking at staff, thrashing side-to-side
6	Very agitated	Does not calm despite frequent verbal reminding of limits, requires physical restraints, biting ETT
5	Agitated	Anxious or mildly agitated, attempting to sit up, calms down to verbal instructions
4	Calm and cooperative	Calm, awakens easily, follows commands
3	Sedated	Difficult to arouse, awakens to verbal stimuli or gentle shaking but drifts off again, follows simple commands
2	Very sedated	Arouses to physical stimuli but does not communicate or follow commands, may move spontaneously
1	Unarousable	Minimal or no response to noxious stimuli, does not communicate or follow commands
Motor Activity Assessment Scale (MAAS)[83]		
6	Dangerously agitated	No external stimulus is required to elicit movement and patient is uncooperative pulling at tubes or catheters or thrashing side to side or striking at staff or trying to climb out of bed and does not calm down when asked
5	Agitated	No external stimulus is required to elicit movement and attempting to sit up or moves limbs out of bed and does not consistently follow commands (e.g., will lie down when asked but soon reverts back to attempts to sit up or move limbs out of bed)
4	Restless and cooperative	No external stimulus is required to elicit movement and patient is picking at sheets or tubes or uncovering self and follows commands
3	Calm and cooperative	No external stimulus is required to elicit movement and patient is adjusting sheets or clothes purposefully and follows commands
2	Responsive to touch or name	Opens eyes or raises eyebrows or turns head toward stimulus or moves limbs when touched or name is loudly spoken
1	Responsive only to noxious stimulus[a]	Opens eyes or raises eyebrows or turns head toward stimulus or moves limbs with noxious stimulus
0	Unresponsive	Does not move with noxious stimulus
Ramsay Scale[84]		
1	Awake	Patient anxious and agitated or restless or both
2		Patient cooperative, oriented and tranquil
3		Patient responds to commands only
4	Asleep	A brisk response to a light glabellar tap or loud auditory stimulus
5		A sluggish response to a light glabellar tap or loud auditory stimulus
6		No response to a light glabellar tap or loud auditory stimulus

[a]Noxious stimulus = suctioning or 5 seconds of vigorous orbital, sternal, or nail bed pressure.

sleep–wake cycle, but some may require deep levels of sedation to facilitate mechanical ventilation. The desired level of sedation should be defined at the start of therapy and reevaluated on a regular basis as the clinical condition of the patient changes. Regimens should be written with the appropriate flexibility to allow titration to the desired endpoint, anticipating fluctuations in sedation requirements throughout the day.

Objective assessment of sedation. Objective testing of a patient's level of sedation may be helpful during very deep sedation or when therapeutic neuromuscular blockade masks observable behavior. Vital signs, such as blood pressure and heart rate, are not specific or sensitive markers of the level of sedation among critically ill patients. Tools utilized in objective assessment include heart rate variability and lower-esophageal contractility, but most are based on a patient's electroencephalogram (EEG). The raw EEG signal has been manipulated in several devices to simplify bedside interpretation and improve reliability. For example, the bispectral index (BIS) uses a digital scale from 100 (completely awake) to 0 (isoelectric EEG).[89] Most of the literature about the use of BIS in the operating room supports strong agreement between BIS and patient recall or level of hypnosis.[90] Elective

surgery patients receiving sedatives have shown a strong inverse correlation between hypnotic drug effect and BIS.[91,92]

Although the BIS may be a promising tool for the objective assessment of sedation or hypnotic drug effect, it has limitations in the ICU environment.[93–95] BIS scores may vary between patients at the same subjective level of sedation, and subjective scales may be more reproducible during light sedation.[93,94] Muscle-based electrical activity may artificially elevate BIS scores if the patient has not received neuromuscular blockade.[94] A new version of BIS software is being tested for improved applicability in measuring ICU sedation. BIS has not been tested in patients with metabolic impairments or structural abnormalities of the brain. Studies have not compared the patient outcomes of using BIS versus subjective scales. Although BIS is likely to be useful when patients are deeply comatose or under neuromuscular blockade, routine use of this device cannot be recommended until the value and validity are confirmed.

Recommendations: A sedation goal or endpoint should be established and regularly redefined for each patient. Regular assessment and response to therapy should be systematically documented. (Grade of recommendation = C)

The use of a validated sedation assessment scale (SAS, MAAS, or VICS) is recommended. (Grade of recommendation = B)

Objective measures of sedation, such as BIS, have not been completely evaluated and are not yet proven useful in the ICU. (Grade of recommendation = C)

Sedation Therapy. *Benzodiazepines.* Benzodiazepines are sedatives and hypnotics that block the acquisition and encoding of new information and potentially unpleasant experiences (anterograde amnesia) but do not induce retrograde amnesia. Although they lack any analgesic properties, they have an opioid-sparing effect by moderating the anticipatory pain response.[96,97] Benzodiazepines vary in their potency, onset and duration of action, uptake, distribution, metabolism, and presence or absence of active metabolites (Table 3). Patient-specific factors, such as age, concurrent pathology, prior alcohol abuse, and concurrent drug therapy, affect the intensity and duration of activity of benzodiazepines, requiring individualized titration. Elderly patients exhibit slower clearance of benzodiazepines or their active metabolites and have a larger volume of drug distribution, contributing to a marked prolongation of elimination.[111] Compromised hepatic or renal function may slow the clearance of benzodiazepines or their active metabolites. Induction or inhibition of hepatic or intestinal enzyme activity can alter the oxidative metabolism of most benzodiazepines.[112]

Benzodiazepine therapy should be titrated to a predefined endpoint, often requiring a series of loading doses. Hemodynamically unstable patients may experience hypotension with the initiation of sedation. Maintenance of sedation with intermittent or "as needed" doses of diazepam, lorazepam, or midazolam may be adequate to accomplish the goal of sedation.[78] However, patients requiring frequent doses to maintain the desired effect may benefit from a continuous infusion by using the lowest effective infusion dose. Continuous infusions must be used cautiously, as accumulation of the parent drug or its active metabolites may produce inadvertent oversedation. Frequent reassessment of a patient's sedation requirements and active tapering of the infusion rate can prevent prolonged sedative effects.[80] However, awakening times after several days of sedation may be quite unpredictable in clinical use. In contrast, tolerance to benzodiazepines may occur within hours to several days of therapy, and escalating doses of midazolam have been reported.[113,114] While not well described in the literature, paradoxical agitation has also been observed during light sedation and may be the result of drug-induced amnesia or disorientation.

Diazepam has been shown to provide rapid onset and awakening after single doses (Table 3).[78,115] Because of its long-acting metabolites, a prolonged duration of sedative effect may occur with repeated doses, but this may be acceptable for long-term sedation.[78] Lorazepam has a slower onset but fewer potential drug interactions because of its metabolism via glucuronidation (Table 3).[98,112] The slow onset makes lorazepam less useful for the treatment of acute agitation. Maintenance of sedation can be accomplished with intermittent or continuous intravenous administration. Lorazepam has an elimination half-life of 12–15 hours, so an infusion is not readily titratable. Loading doses given by i.v. push should be used initially with relatively fixed infu-

Table 3.
Pharmacology of Selected Sedatives[1,30–32,98–110]

Agent	Onset After i.v. Dose	Half-life of Parent Compound	Metabolic Pathway	Active Metabolite	Unique Adverse Effects	Intermittent i.v. Dose[a]	Infusion Dose Range (Usual)	Cost per day 70 kg patient[b]
Diazepam	2–5 min	20–120 hr	Desmethylation and hydroxylation	Yes (prolonged sedation)	Phlebitis	0.03–0.1 mg/kg q 0.5–6 hr	...	20 mg q 4 hr: $5.00–20.50
Lorazepam	5–20 min	8–15 hr	Glucuronidation	None	Solvent-related acidosis/renal failure in high doses	0.02–0.06 mg/kg q 2–6 hr	0.01–0.1 mg/kg/hr	48 mg/day: $55.00
Midazolam	2–5 min	3–11 hr	Oxidation	Yes (prolonged sedation, especially with renal failure)	...	0.02–0.08 mg/kg q 0.5–2 hr	0.04–0.2 mg/kg/hr	6 mg/hr: $65.00–309.00
Propofol	1–2 min	26–32 hr	Oxidation	None	Elevated triglycerides, pain on injection	...	5–80 µg/kg/min	50 µg/kg/min: $235.00–375.00
Haloperidol	3–20 min	18–54 hr	Oxidation	Yes (EPS)[c]	QT interval prolongation	0.03–0.15 mg/kg q 0.5–6 hr	0.04–0.15 mg/kg/hr	10 mg q 6 h: $62.00–65.00

[a]More frequent doses may be needed for management of acute agitation in mechanically ventilated patients.
[b]Cost based on 2001 average wholesale price.
[c]EPS = extrapyramidal symptoms.

sion rates. Lorazepam infusions should be prepared using the 2 mg/mL injection and diluted to a concentration of 1 mg/mL or less and mixed in a glass bottle.[116,117] Despite these precautions, precipitation may develop.[118] An alternative is to administer undiluted lorazepam as an infusion using a PCA device.[78] The lorazepam solvents polyethylene glycol (PEG) and propylene glycol (PG) have been implicated as the cause of reversible acute tubular necrosis, lactic acidosis, and hyperosmolar states after prolonged high-dose infusions. The dosing threshold for this effect has not been prospectively defined, but these case reports described doses that exceeded 18 mg/hr and continued for longer than four weeks and higher doses (>25 mg/hr) continuing for hours to days.[119–121] It seems prudent to avoid doses of this magnitude. Alternatively, lorazepam and diazepam may be administered via the enteral route in tablet or liquid form.[122] Large doses of liquid lorazepam (i.e., 60 mg of 2 mg/mL every six hours) may lead to diarrhea because of the high PEG and PG content.[123]

Midazolam has a rapid onset and short duration with single doses, similar to diazepam (Table 3).[115] The rapid onset of midazolam makes it preferable for treating acutely agitated patients. Accumulation and prolonged sedative effects have been reported in critically ill patients using midazolam who are obese or have a low albumin level or renal failure.[99–103] Prolonged sedative effects may also be caused by the accumulation of an active metabolite, alpha-hydroxymidazolam, or its conjugated salt, especially in patients with renal insufficiency.[101–105] Significant inhibition of midazolam metabolism has been reported with propofol, diltiazem, macrolide antibiotics, and other inhibitors of cytochrome P450 isoenzyme 3A4, which could influence the duration of effect.[107,108,112] Daily discontinuation of midazolam infusions (wake up) with retitration to a Ramsay scale endpoint reduced midazolam requirements and was associated with a reduction in the duration of mechanical ventilation and length of ICU stay.[50] However, the patients in this trial were off of midazolam for an average of 5.3 hours per day, so this research technique may be difficult to implement. Patients should be closely monitored for self-extubation or the removal of other monitoring devices during the daily awakening sessions.

The routine use of a benzodiazepine antagonist, such as flumazenil, is not recommended after prolonged benzodiazepine therapy because of the risks of inducing withdrawal symptoms and increasing myocardial oxygen consumption with as little as 0.5 mg of flumazenil.[124] An i.v. dose of flumazenil 0.15 mg is associated with few withdrawal symptoms when administered to patients receiving midazolam infusions.[125] If flumazenil is used to test for prolonged sedation after several days of benzodiazepine therapy, a single low dose is recommended.

Propofol. Propofol is an intravenous, general anesthetic agent. However, sedative and hypnotic properties can be demonstrated at lower doses. Compared with benzodiazepines, propofol produces a similar degree of amnesia at equisedative doses in volunteers.[69] In a clinical trial of ICU patients, propofol did not produce amnesia as often as midazolam.[70] Like the benzodiazepines, propofol has no analgesic properties.

Propofol has a rapid onset and short duration of sedation once discontinued (Table 3). While most of the early literature documents the comparatively rapid resolution of sedation after propofol infusions, a slightly longer recovery has been reported after more than 12 hours of infusion.[110,126]

No changes in kinetic parameters have been reported in patients with renal or hepatic dysfunction.

Propofol is available as an emulsion in a phospholipid vehicle, which provides 1.1 kcal/mL from fat and should be counted as a caloric source. Long-term or high-dose infusions may result in hypertriglyceridemia.[127–129] Other adverse effects most commonly seen with propofol include hypotension, bradycardia, and pain upon peripheral venous injection. The hypotension is dose related and more frequent after bolus dose administration. Elevation of pancreatic enzymes has been reported during prolonged infusions of propofol.[130,131] Pancreatitis has been reported following anesthesia with propofol, although a causal relationship has not been established.[132] Prolonged use (>48 hours) of high doses of propofol (>66 μg/kg/min infusion) has been associated with lactic acidosis, bradycardia, and lipidemia in pediatric patients and doses >83 μg/kg/min have been associated with an increased risk of cardiac arrest in adults.[133,134] The adults at highest risk for cardiac complications received > 100 μg/kg/min infusion of a 2% propofol solution to achieve deep sedation after neurologic injury.[134] FDA has specifically recommended against the use of propofol for the prolonged sedation of pediatric patients. Patients receiving propofol should be monitored for unexplained metabolic acidosis or arrhythmias.

Alternative sedative agents should be considered for patients with escalating vasopressor or inotrope requirements or cardiac failure during high-dose propofol infusions.

Propofol requires a dedicated i.v. catheter when administered as a continuous infusion because of the potential for drug incompatibility and infection. Improper aseptic technique with propofol in the operating room has led to nosocomial postoperative infection.[135] However, a clinically relevant incidence of infectious complications has not been reported with ICU use.[136] The manufacturers suggest that propofol infusion bottles and tubing should hang no more than 12 hours and solutions transferred from the original container should be discarded every 6 hours. A preservative has been added to propofol to decrease the potential for bacterial overgrowth in case the vial would become contaminated. One of the propofol formulations contains edetic acid (Diprivan, AstraZeneca) and the manufacturer recommends a drug holiday after more than seven days of infusion to minimize the risk of trace element abnormalities. Another product (propofol, Gensia Sicor) contains sodium metabisulfite, which may produce allergic reactions in susceptible patients. Sulfite sensitivity occurs more frequently in patients with asthma.

While propofol appears to possess anticonvulsant activity, excitatory phenomena, such as myoclonus, have been observed. There are several case reports and small, uncontrolled studies describing the efficacy of propofol in refractory status epilepticus (after traditional treatment regimens have failed or are not tolerated) and electroconvulsive shock therapy.[137,138] Case reports have also described roles for propofol in delirium tremens refractory to high-dose benzodiazepine therapy.[139]

Propofol has been used to sedate neurosurgical patients to reduce elevated intracranial pressure (ICP).[140,141] The rapid awakening from propofol allows interruption of the infusion for neurologic assessment. Propofol may also decrease cerebral blood flow and metabolism. Propofol and morphine produced improved control of ICP compared with morphine alone in the treatment of severe traumatic brain injury (TBI).[141] Propofol reduced elevated ICP more effectively than fentanyl following severe TBI.[142] High doses of propofol should be used cautiously in this setting.[134]

Propofol infusions used to reduce elevated ICP may need to be continued longer than usually recommended for routine sedation.[141]

Central α-agonists. Clonidine has been used to augment the effects of general anesthetics and narcotics and to treat drug withdrawal syndromes in the ICU.[143–148] The more selective α-2 agonist, dexmedetomidine, was recently approved for use as a sedative with analgesic-sparing activity for short-term use (<24 hours) in patients who are initially receiving mechanical ventilation. Patients remain sedated when undisturbed, but arouse readily with gentle stimulation. Dexmedetomidine reduces concurrent analgesic and sedative requirements and produces anxiolytic effects comparable to benzodiazepines.[145–148] Rapid administration of dexmedetomidine may produce transient elevations in blood pressure. Patients maintained on dexmedetomidine may develop bradycardia and hypotension, especially in the presence of intravascular volume depletion or high sympathetic tone. The role of this new agent in the sedation of ICU patients remains to be determined.

Sedative Selection. Acute agitation arises from a variety of etiologies, including pain. A short-acting opioid analgesic, such as fentanyl, may provide immediate sedation and patient comfort; however, fentanyl has not been compared with other sedatives in a controlled trial. Midazolam and diazepam also have a rapid onset of sedation.[115] Propofol has a rapid onset, but hypotension and infusion-site pain can result from bolus dose administration. Cautious use of sedatives is recommended for patients not yet intubated because of the risk of respiratory depression.

Comparative trials of prolonged sedation have been performed in a variety of critical care settings. Many were supported by pharmaceutical industry research grants; as a result, newer products have been evaluated more frequently. Outcome is usually described in terms of the speed of onset, ability to maintain the target level of sedation, adverse effects, time required for awakening, and ability to wean from mechanical ventilation. Most of the prospective, randomized trials are experimentally flawed because they are unblinded, use uncontrolled amounts of opioids, and exclude patients with obesity or renal or hepatic insufficiency. This limits their general applicability. There is a need for more large, high-quality, randomized trials of the effectiveness of different sedative agents.[149] Most of the trials used a Ramsay scale for assessment, so the depth of sedation can generally be compared among the trials. The trials are summarized in Tables 4–6.

Duration of therapy. Short-term (<24 hours), randomized, open-label trials of sedation have compared propofol and midazolam most often (eight of nine trials) (Table 4). An opioid was available to all patients. Awakening times for patients taking propofol ranged from 1 to 105 minutes versus 1 to 405 minutes for patients receiving midazolam.[128,150–157] Time to extubation has also been compared, but other variables may influence this outcome measure. Clinically, these agents produced similar outcomes following <24 hours of infusion (Table 4).

An intermediate duration of sedation (one to three days) was reported in three randomized open-label trials (Table 5). Propofol and midazolam were compared for sedation of medical ICU patients and a mixed medical-surgical ICU population with respiratory failure.[157,158] Patients receiving propofol had statistically more predictable awakening times than patients receiving midazolam in both trials. Clinically, this time difference was not as significant and did not produce more

rapid discharge from the ICU.[157] In a three-way comparison of midazolam, lorazepam, and propofol infusions for sedation of surgical ICU patients, the authors concluded that lorazepam was the preferred agent in this population.[118] Overall, these agents were similar in the levels of sedation provided, the time required to achieve adequate sedation, and the number of dose adjustments per day. However, midazolam produced adequate sedation during a greater percentage of time while propofol was associated with more undersedation and lorazepam with more oversedation. Morphine was provided on an as needed basis and the average dose was similar in all three groups. Awakening times were not reported. Precipitation of lorazepam infusions was reported.[118]

Nine open-label, randomized trials comparing long-term sedation (more than three days) were reviewed in these guidelines (Table 6).[70,127–129,157,159–163] Most of the trials compared propofol with midazolam. All trials included opioid therapy, although administration was not controlled. Most studies used a Ramsay scale for patient assessment. In these trials, propofol consistently produced more rapid awakening than midazolam with a statistical and, probably, a clinical difference.[70,127–129,160,161] Propofol patients awakened and were extubated in 0.25–4 hours while midazolam patients required 2.8–10 hours to awaken and up to 49 hours for extubation (Table 6).[157] The greatest difference in time to awakening was seen when a deep level of sedation was the goal of therapy (Ramsay level 4–5). Patients receiving propofol awakened from deep sedation significantly faster than those receiving midazolam.[127–129] Lorazepam and midazolam were also compared for long-term sedation.[159,162] One of these studies used a double-blind study design.[162] There was no statistically significant difference in awakening time between these agents when titrated to similar levels of sedation, although the awakening times associated with lorazepam appeared to be more predictable.

Sedative comparison. Four trials compared lorazepam with midazolam.[118,154,159,162] Intermittent lorazepam doses produced sedation comparable to a midazolam infusion during an eight-hour observation period.[154] Both lorazepam and midazolam have the potential to cause accumulation and prolonged drug effects or oversedation if administered excessively via continuous infusion, especially when deep levels of sedation are attempted.[118,159] However, a rigorous protocol of assessment and titration of lorazepam infusions to moderate levels of sedation produced a less variable awakening time with lorazepam than with midazolam, although the absolute difference in awakening time was not statistically significant.[159] A nurse-managed sedation protocol, which included the active titration of lorazepam infusions to a defined endpoint, avoided a prolonged sedative effect compared with physician management of infusion rates.[80] A blinded trial of lorazepam versus midazolam found that the lorazepam infusions were easier to manage than midazolam infusions because fewer dose adjustments were required to maintain the desired level of sedation.[162] In this trial, wide inter- and intrapatient variability was noted between sedative plasma concentrations and the Ramsay score. No difference was noted in patient recovery when patients were evaluated for 24 hours after the end of the infusion. Awakening times were not reported in two of the other trials.[118,154]

When titrated to a standard endpoint, midazolam and propofol provide comparable levels of sedation with a similar onset of effect.[128,150–153,155–157] As shown in Table

Table 4.
Clinical Trials with Less Than 24 Hours of Sedation[a]

Level of Evidence (Reference)	Population Type (No. Patients)	Exclusion Criteria	Trial Design	Drugs	Mean Dosage	Actual Duration	Sedation Endpoint or Goal	Outcome Measure	Significance or Conclusion
1 (150)	MICU/SICU (100)	Obese, head injury, NMBA use	Multicenter, open-label	Propofol Midazolam Morphine: to all patients	Propofol: 1.77 mg/kg/hr Midazolam: 0.1 mg/kg/hr	Propofol: 20.2 hr Midazolam: 21.3 hr	Ramsay level 2–4	Awakening time: most awake at end of infusion, longest: Propofol: 105 min, Midazolam: 405 min	No statistical analysis reported
2 (128)	MICU/SICU (88 total, 40 short-term sedation)	Neurologic injury, ongoing NMBA use	Open-label	Propofol Midazolam Morphine: to all patients	Propofol: 2.3 mg/kg/hr Midazolam: 0.17 mg/kg/hr	Propofol: 11.9 hr Midazolam: 11.9 hr	Ramsay level 2–5 and modified GCS	Time to extubation: Propofol: 0.3 hr Midazolam: 2.5 ± 0.9 hr	$p < 0.05$, Propofol more rapid extubation
2 (151)	CABG (30)	Obese, renal or hepatic insufficiency	Open-label	Propofol Midazolam Sufentanil: to all patients	Propofol: 2.71 ± 1.13 mg/kg/hr Midazolam: 0.09 ± 0.03 mg/kg/hr	Propofol: 9.5 hr Midazolam: 9.8 hr	Ramsay level 5	Time to extubation: Propofol: 250 ± 135 min Midazolam: 391 ± 128 min	$p < 0.01$, Propofol more rapid extubation
1 (152)	CABG (84)	Renal or hepatic insufficiency	Open-label	Propofol Midazolam Morphine: p.r.n.	Propofol: 0.7 ± 0.09 mg/kg/hr Midazolam: 0.018 ± 0.001 mg/kg/hr	Propofol: 9.2 hr Midazolam: 9.4 hr	Ramsay level 3	Time to extubation: Propofol: 4.3 hr Midazolam: 3.5 hr	Not statistically significant
1 (153)	SICU (60)	None	Open-label, consecutive patients	Propofol Midazolam Morphine: p.r.n.	Propofol: 114.8 mg/hr (80.1 ± 21.1 kg) Midazolam: 2.1 ± 1.3 mg/hr (74.2 ± 24 kg)	16 hr observation, total sedation duration not defined	Ramsay level 3 and response to stimulation	Postsedation score at 5, 30, 60, and 90 min: Propofol scores lower at 5 and 30 min	$p < 0.05$, Midazolam more heavily sedated
1 (154)	MICU/SICU (61% trauma)	Cardiac insufficiency, neurosurgical or unstable	Multicenter, open-label	Lorazepam Midazolam Morphine: p.r.n.	Lorazepam: 1.6 ± 0.1 mg i.v. push Midazolam: 14.4 ± 1.2 mg infusion over 8 hr	8 hr	Multiple scales: anxiety, amnesia, pain, GCS, Ramsay level 3	Adequacy of sedation	Comparable sedation scores

(Continued on next page)

Table 4. (Continued)

Level of Evidence (Reference)	Population Type (No. Patients)	Exclusion Criteria	Trial Design	Drugs	Mean Dosage	Actual Duration	Sedation Endpoint or Goal	Outcome Measure	Significance or Conclusion
1 (155)	Cardiac surgery (41)	Renal, hepatic, or cardiac failure	Double-blind	Propofol Midazolam Morphine: p.r.n.	Propofol: 0.64 ± 0.17 mg/kg/hr Midazolam: 0.015 ± 0.001 mg/kg/hr	Propofol: 4 hr Midazolam: 4 hr	Ramsay level 2–4	Awakening time: Propofol: 88.6 ± 51 min Midazolam: 93.8 ± 59.4 min	Not statistically significant
1 (156)	CABG (75)	Renal failure, neurologic history, hepatic failure, cardiovascular dysfunction	Double-blind	Propofol Midazolam Both Propofol and Midazolam Morphine: to all patients	Propofol: 1.2 ± 0.03 mg/kg/hr Midazolam: 0.08 ± 0.01 mg/kg/hr Propofol and Midazolam: Propofol: 0.22 ± 0.33 mg/kg/hr, Midazolam: 0.02 mg/kg/hr	Propofol: 14.4 hr Midazolam: 14.1 hr Propofol and Midazolam: 14.7 hr	Modified GCS	Time to extubation: Propofol: 0.9 ± 0.3 hr Midazolam: 2.3 ± 0.8 hr Propofol and Midazolam: 1.2 ± 0.6 hr	$p = 0.01$, Midazolam vs. Propofol or Propofol and Midazolam
2 (157)	MICU/SICU (99)	Neurosurgery, coma, seizures	Multicenter, open-label, intention-to-treat analysis	Propofol Midazolam Opiates: p.r.n.	Actual doses not specified	≤24 hr - post hoc stratum Propofol: n = 21 Midazolam: n = 26	Ramsay scale, level was specified daily	Time to extubation: Propofol: 5.6 hr Midazolam: 11.9 hr	$p = 0.029$ Overall: Propofol: 60.2% of time at target Ramsay score Midazolam: 44% of time at target Ramsay score, $p < 0.05$

aMICU = medical intensive care unit, SICU = surgical intensive care unit, NMBA = neuromuscular blocking agent, GCS = Glasgow Coma Score, CABG = coronary artery bypass graft.

4, there is generally no statistical or clinical difference in awakening times between propofol and midazolam when used for short-term sedation. Data from longer trials of sedation (more than 72 hours) suggest that propofol is associated with more reliable and rapid awakening, both statistically and clinically, than midazolam.[106,127,128,156,158,160] Following long-term sedation, propofol awakening times ranged from 0.25 to 2.5 hours and midazolam awakening times ranged from 2.8 to 30 hours (Table 6). One center's comparison of two concentrations of propofol (1% and 2%) versus midazolam used in trauma patients has shown that midazolam provides deep levels of sedation more reliably than propofol, but the awakening times were much longer with midazolam.[127,163] More patients receiving 1% propofol experienced failure because of elevated triglycerides, but the 2% propofol group experienced failure because of inadequate sedation. Failure of propofol to provide adequate sedation of trauma patients was reported elsewhere, although an explanation was not apparent.[118]

Economic comparison. Several of these studies presented limited pharmacoeconomic data. In most reports, the sedative costs were the only costs considered (cost minimization).[118,154–156,162] Some studies included a portion of the costs for ICU patient care.[128,161] A sedative with a low acquisition cost may be cited as the least expensive agent for prolonged sedation (e.g., lorazepam).[1,32,118] A complete economic analysis should consider costs associated with the evaluation and treatment of sedation-induced adverse effects (e.g., prolonged sedation, infection, and hypertriglyceridemia), therapy failures (additional agents or high doses required), and drug preparation and administration costs (precipitation and tubing changes) to determine the total cost of therapy. The cost of sedation-induced prolongation of ventilation or length of ICU stay is likely to reduce the potential difference in acquisition costs between benzodiazepines and propofol.[164] Institutional variables (bed

Table 5.
Clinical Trials with One to Three Days of Sedation[a]

Level of Evidence (Reference)	Population (No. Patients)	Exclusion Criteria	Design	Drugs	Mean Dosage	Actual Duration	Sedation Endpoint/Goal	Outcome Measure	Significance/ Conclusion
1 (158)	MICU with respiratory failure (73)	. . .	Open-label	Propofol Midazolam Morphine: p.r.n.	Propofol: 1.25 ± 0.87 mg/kg/hr Midazolam: 3.1 ± 3.2 mg/hr	Up to 3 days	Behavior scale	Awakening: defined by eye opening ability to follow with eyes, hand grasp, and tongue protrusion	Many awake during infusion, Propofol: smaller range of awakening times. Used daily wake-up to reassess patients
2 (118)	Surgical or Trauma ICU(31)	Alcohol abuse, head injury, dialysis	Open-label	Propofol Midazolam Lorazepam Morphine: p.r.n.	Propofol: 2 ±1.5 mg/kg/hr Midazolam: 0.04 ± 0.03 mg/kg/hr Lorazepam: 0.02 ± 0.01 mg/kg/hr	Propofol: 86.4 ±72hr Midazolam: 60 ± 72 hr Lorazepam: 72±52.8 hr	Ramsay level 2–4	Time with adequate sedation: Midazolam: 79% Propofol: 62% Lorazepam: 68%	Lorazepam vs. midazolam p = 0.03 Midazolam vs. Propofol p = 0.01 Propofol: more undersedation 31% Lorazepam: more over-sedation 14% and precipitation 18%
2 (157)	MICU or SICU (99)	Neurosurgery, coma, seizures	Multicenter, Open-label, intention-to-treat analysis	Propofol Midazolam Opioids: p.r.n.	Actual doses not specified	24–72 hr = post hoc stratum Propofol: n = 21 Midazolam: n = 17	Ramsay scale, level was specified daily	Time to extubation Propofol: 7.4 hr Midazolam: 31.3 hr	p = 0.068, Enrollment ended early, insufficient power. Overall: Propofol: 60.2% of time at target Ramsay score Midazolam: 44% of time at target Ramsay score, $p < 0.05$

[a]MICU = medical intensive care unit, ICU = intensive care unit, SICU = surgical intensive care unit.

Table 6.
Clinical Trials of More Than Three Days of Sedation

Level of Evidence (Reference)	Population (No. Patients)	Exclusion Criteria	Design	Drugs	Mean Dosage	Actual Duration	Sedation Endpoint/Goal	Outcome Measure	Significance/Conclusion
2 (128)	MICU/SICU[a] (88 total, 28 medium-term, 20 long-term sedation)	Neurologic injury, ongoing NMBA use	Open-label	Propofol Midazolam Morphine: to all patients	Propofol 2.3 mg/kg/hr Midazolam 0.17 mg/kg/hr	Medium: Propofol: 116 hr Midazolam: 113 hr Long Propofol: 312 hr Midazolam: 342 hr	Ramsay level 2–5 and modified GCS	Time to extubation: Medium: Propofol: 0.4 ± 0.1 hr Midazolam: 13.5 ± 4 hr Long: Propofol: 0.8 ± 0.3 hr Midazolam: 36.6 ± 6.8 hr	Medium: $p < 0.05$ Long: $p < 0.05$
1 (159)	MICU (20)	CNS abnormal	Open-label	Lorazepam Midazolam Morphine: to all patients	Lorazepam: 0.06 ± 0.04 mg/kg/hr Midazolam: 0.24 ± 0.16 mg/kg/hr	Lorazepam: 77 hr Midazolam: 108 hr	Ramsay level 2–3	Return to baseline mental status: Lorazepam: 261 ± 189 min, Midazolam: 1815 ± 2322 min	Not statistically significant
1 (160)	MICU/SICU (98)	Renal, hepatic, or cardiac failure, ongoing NMBA use	Open-label, multicenter	Propofol Midazolam Morphine: p.r.n.	Propofol: 2.8 ± 1.1 mg/kg/hr Midazolam: 0.14 ± 0.1 mg/kg/hr	Propofol: 81 hr Midazolam: 88 hr	Own sedation scale	Awakening lightly sedated: Propofol: 14 ± 0.8 min Midazolam: 64 ± 20 min Deep sedation: Propofol: 27 ± 16 min Midazolam: 237 ± 222 min	Light: $p < 0.05$ Heavy: $p < 0.01$
1 (129)	MICU/SICU (108 consecutive)	Chronic liver disease, head injury, ongoing NMBA use	Open-label	Propofol Midazolam Morphine: to all patients	Propofol: 3.07–5.7 0.04 mg/kg/hr Midazolam: 14 ± 0.1 mg/kg/hr	Propofol: 139 hr Midazolam: 141 hr	Ramsay level 4–5	Time to t-tube Propofol: 4 ± 3.9hr Midazolam: 48.9 ± 47.2 hr	$p = 0.0001$ Propofol: high triglycerides 12% men, 50% women

(Continued on next page)

Table 6 (continued)

Level of Evidence (Reference)	Population (No. Patients)	Exclusion Criteria	Design	Drugs	Mean Dosage	Actual Duration	Sedation Endpoint/Goal	Outcome Measure	Significance/ Conclusion
2 (70)	MICU/SICU (68 consecutive)	None	Open-label	Propofol Midazolam Morphine: p.r.n.	Propofol: 1.8 ± 0.08 mg/kg/hr Midazolam: 0.07 ± 0.003 mg/kg/hr	Propofol: 99 hr Midazolam: 141 hr	Ramsay level 2–3 also rated amnesia	Awakening: Propofol: 1.8 ± 0.4hr Midazolam: 2.8 ± 0.4hr Amnesia: Propofol: 29% Midazolam: 100%	$p < 0.02$ More propofol patients with agitation upon awakening
2 (161)	MICU/SICU (26)	Hepatic or renal insufficiency, head injury, ongoing NMBA use	Open-label	Propofol + alfentanil Midazolam + morphine	Alfentanil: 0.5–2 ug/kg/hr Propofol: 1–4 mg/kg/hr Morphine: 17–70 µg/kg/hr Midazolam: 0.03–0.2 mg/ kg/hr	…	Own scale, goal: moderate-heavy sedation	Time to extubation: Propofol: 3 hr (1–13 hr) Midazolam: 50 hr (1–121 hr)	$p = 0.006$
1 (127)	Trauma ICU (100 consecutive)	Renal or hepatic failure	Open-label	Propofol Midazolam Propofol + midazolam Morphine: p.r.n.	Propofol: 2.12 ± 1.2 mg/kg/hr Midazolam: 0.19 ± 0.09 mg/kg/hr Propofol and Midazolam: Propofol: 1.6 ± 0.05 mg/kg/hr, Midazolam: 0.14 ± 0.08 mg/kg/hr	Propofol: 5.2 days Midazolam: 6.6 days Propofol and Midazolam: 7.2 days	Own scale, goal: moderate to heavy sedation	Awakening (excluding head trauma): Propofol: 110 ± 50 min Midazolam: 660 ± 400 min Propofol and Midazolam: 190 ± 200 min	Midazolam vs Propofol or Propofol and Midazolam: $p < 0.01$; Propofol: high triglyceride levels
1 (162)	MICU (64)	Head injury, ongoing NMBA use	Blinded	Lorazepam Midazolam Fentanyl p.r.n.	Lorazepam: 23.1 ± 14.4 mg/day Midazolam: 372 ± 256 mg/day	Lorazepam: 141 hr Midazolam: 141 hr	Addenbrooke sedation scale, initial moderate to heavy sedation, tapering to	Awakening similar, times not reported	Satisfactory sedation: Lorazepam: 87 ± 10.5%, Midazolam: 66.2 ± 23.1%

Table 6 (continued)

2 (163)	Trauma ICU (63 consecutive)	Renal or hepatic failure	Open-label	Propofol 2% Midazolam Morphine: to all patients	Propofol: 6400 ± 1797 mg/day Midazolam: 297.8 ± 103.8 mg/day	Propofol: 6.5 hr Midazolam 11.1 hr	Own scale, goal: moderate to heavy sedation	Awakening (no head trauma) Propofol: 145 ± 50 min Midazolam: 372 ± 491 min	Awakening: not statistically significant Less triglyceride elevation that historical control (reference 117)
2 (157)	MICU/SICU (99)	Neurosurgery, coma, seizures	Multicenter, open-label, intention-to-treat analysis	Propofol Midazolam Opioids: p.r.n.	Actual doses not specified	24–72 hr - post hoc stratum Propofol: $n = 4$ Midazolam: $n = 10$	Ramsay scale, level was specified daily	Time to extubation: Propofol: 8.4 hr Midazolam: 46.8 hr	$p = 0.03$, enrollment ended early, insufficient power limits conclusion Overall: Propofol: 60.2% of time at target Ramsay score Midazolam: 44% of time at target Ramsay score, $p < 0.05$

aMICU = medical intensive care unit, ICU = intensive care unit, NMBA = neuromuscular blocking agent, GCS = Glasgow Coma Score, SICU = surgical intensive care unit.

availability) or patient-specific factors (other injuries and the need for observation) may impact a patient's length of stay more than the sedation regimen. More rapid extubation with propofol was not associated with a shorter length of stay in a multicenter Canadian trial.[157] Research that considers all of these cost factors is needed to estimate the overall cost of sedative regimens. Since the frequency of sedation-induced adverse effects has not been well described, there are insufficient data to create pharmacoeconomic models comparing the potential costs of sedative regimens. The acquisition costs of sedatives vary widely among institutions, and costs may decline with the availability of generic products (Table 3).

Multidisciplinary development and implementation of sedation guidelines have been shown to reduce direct drug costs (from $81.54 to $18.12 per patient per day), ventilator time (317 to 167 hours), and the lengths of ICU stay (19.1 to 9.9 days) and total stay without a change in mortality.[165] Although an economic analysis was not performed, a nursing-implemented sedation protocol using lorazepam reduced the duration of sedation and mechanical ventilation and the tracheostomy rate.[80] A systematic multi-disciplinary team approach to sedation and analgesia will produce clinical and economic benefits.

An algorithm was developed to incorporate many of the assessment issues with the therapy options in this document (Figure 1). When using this algorithm, the pharmacology, potential adverse effects, and therapeutic issues discussed in this document should be considered.

Recommendations: Midazolam or diazepam should be used for rapid sedation of acutely agitated patients. (Grade of recommendation = C)

Propofol is the preferred sedative when rapid awakening (e.g., for neurologic assessment or extubation) is important. (Grade of recommendation = B)

Midazolam is recommended for short-term use only, as it produces unpredictable awakening and time to extubation when infusions continue longer than 48–72 hours. (Grade of recommendation = A)

Lorazepam is recommended for the sedation of most patients via intermittent i.v. administration or continuous infusion. (Grade of recommendation = B)

The titration of the sedative dose to a defined endpoint is recommended with systematic tapering of the dose or daily interruption with retitration to minimize prolonged sedative effects. (Grade of recommendation = A)

Triglyceride concentrations should be monitored after two days of propofol infusion, and total caloric intake from lipids should be included in the nutrition support prescription. (Grade of recommendation = B)

The use of sedation guidelines, an algorithm, or a protocol is recommended. (Grade of recommendation = B)

Sedative and Analgesic Withdrawal

Patients exposed to more than one week of high-dose opioid or sedative therapy may develop neuroadaptation or physiological dependence. Rapid discontinuation of these agents could lead to withdrawal symptoms. Opioid withdrawal signs and symptoms include dilation of the pupils, sweating, lacrimation, rhinorrhea, piloerection, tachycardia, vomiting, diarrhea, hypertension, yawning, fever, tachypnea, restlessness, irritability, increased sensitivity to pain, cramps, muscle aches, and anxiety. Benzodiazepine withdrawal signs and symptoms include dysphoria, tremor, headache, nausea, sweating, fatigue, anxiety, agitation, increased sensitivity to light and sound, paresthesias, muscle cramps, myoclonus, sleep disturbances, delirium, and seizures. Propofol withdrawal has not been well described but appears to resemble benzodiazepine withdrawal.

The occurrence of sedative and analgesic withdrawal has been described in both adult and pediatric ICU populations.[166-168] In adults, withdrawal is associated with the length of stay, mechanical ventilation, and the dose and duration of analgesic and sedative therapy. Patients at highest risk include those who stay greater than seven days in the ICU, receive greater than 35 mg/day of lorazepam, or greater than 5 mg/day of fentanyl.[166]

Studies of pediatric patients have found that the rate of medication weaning may be very important in the development of withdrawal syndromes.[167,169] Although not tested prospectively, it has been recommended that daily dose decrements of opioids not exceed 5–10% in high-risk patients.[170] If the drug is administered intermittently, changing the therapy to longer-acting agents may also attenuate withdrawal symptoms.[171] Another recommendation for opioid weaning is to decrease a continuous infusion rate by 20–40% initially and make additional reductions of 10% every 12–24 hours, depending on the patient's response.[172] Conversion to a continuous subcutaneous infusion has also been used for gradual fentanyl and midazolam weaning in children.[173] Patient care costs may be increased unnecessarily if sedatives and analgesics are withdrawn too slowly.

Recommendation: The potential for opioid, benzodiazepine, and propofol withdrawal should be considered after high doses or more than approximately seven days of continuous therapy. Doses should be tapered systematically to prevent withdrawal symptoms. (Grade of recommendation = B)

Delirium

As many as 80% of ICU patients have delirium, characterized by an acutely changing or fluctuating mental status, inattention,

disorganized thinking, and an altered level of consciousness that may or may not be accompanied by agitation. Placing severely ill patients in a stressful environment for prolonged periods exacerbates the clinical symptoms of delirium.[174-177] Delirium is usually characterized by fluctuating levels of arousal throughout the day, associated with sleep–wake cycle disruption, and hastened by reversed day–night cycles.[178] Delirium may be associated with confusion and different motoric subtypes: hypoactive, hyperactive, or mixed.[179,180] Hypoactive delirium, which is associated with the worst prognosis, is characterized by psychomotor retardation manifested by a calm appearance, inattention, decreased mobility, and obtundation in extreme cases. Hyperactive delirium is easily recognized by agitation, combative behaviors, lack of orientation, and progressive confusion following sedative therapy.

Assessment of Delirium. The gold standard criteria used to diagnose delirium is the clinical history and examination as guided by the *Diagnostic and Statistical Manual of Mental Disorders, 4th edition (DSM-IV).*[177] Although many scales and diagnostic instruments have been developed to facilitate the recognition and diagnosis of delirium, these scales routinely exclude ICU patients because it is often difficult to communicate with them.[178,181] Several groups of delirium investigators have recently collaborated to develop and validate a rapid bedside instrument to accurately diagnose delirium in ICU patients, who are often nonverbal because they are on mechanical ventilation. This instrument is called the Confusion Assessment Method for the ICU (CAM-ICU).[181,182] The work was begun by Hart and colleagues with their publication of the Cognitive Test for Delirium and a later version called the Abbreviated Cognitive Test for Delirium.[183,184] These two investigations were limited because they included approximately 20 patients each and excluded some of the most severely ill patients who are often cared for in the ICU. These factors led the authors to recommend that additional research with delirium assessment tools be conducted before routine application in mechanically ventilated patients.[184]

Collaboration among specialists in pulmonary and critical care, neurology, psychiatry, neuropsychology, and geriatrics has led to the development of a useful assessment tool.[182,185] It is based on the Confusion Assessment Method (CAM), which was designed specifically for use by health care professionals without formal psychiatric training, and incorporates *DSM-IV* criteria for the diagnosis of delirium.[186] CAM, which is the most widely used Delirium assessment instrument for non-psychiatrists, is easy to use and has demonstrated utility in important clinical investigations.[187,188]

Critical care nurses can complete delirium assessments with the CAMICU in an average of 2 minutes with an accuracy of 98%, compared with a full *DSM-IV* assessment by a geriatric psychiatric expert, which usually requires at least 30 minutes to complete. The CAM-ICU assessments have a likelihood ratio of over 50 for diagnosing delirium and high inter-rater reliability (kappa = 0.96).[185] In the two subgroups expected to present the greatest challenge to the CAM-ICU (i.e., those over 65 years and those with suspected dementia), the instrument retained excellent interrater reliability, sensitivity, and specificity. To complete the CAM-ICU, patients are observed for the presence of an acute onset of mental status change or a fluctuating mental status, inattention, disorganized thinking, or an altered level of consciousness (Table 7). With the CAM-ICU, delirium was diagnosed in

Table 7.
The Confusion Assessment Method for the Diagnosis of Delirium in the ICU (CAM-ICU)[182,185]

Feature	Assessment Variables
1. Acute Onset of mental status changes or Fluctuating Course	Is there evidence of an acute change in mental status from the baseline?
	Did the (abnormal) behavior fluctuate during the past 24 hours, i.e., tend to come and go or increase and decrease in severity?
	Did the sedation scale (e.g., SAS or MAAS) or coma scale (GCS) fluctuate in the past 24 hours?[a]
	Did the patient have difficulty focusing attention?
2. Inattention	Is there a reduced ability to maintain and shift attention?
	How does the patient score on the Attention Screening Examination (ASE)? (i.e., Visual Component ASE tests the patient's ability to pay attention via recall of 10 pictures; auditory component ASE tests attention via having patient squeeze hands or nod whenever the letter "A" is called in a random letter sequence)
3. Disorganized thinking	If the patient is already extubated from the ventilator, determine whether or not the patient's thinking is disorganized or incoherent, such as rambling or irrelevant conversation, unclear or illogical flow of ideas, or unpredictable switching from subject to subject.
	For those still on the ventilator, can the patient answer the following 4 questions correctly?
	1. Will a stone float on water?
	2. Are there fish in the sea?
	3. Does one pound weigh more than two pounds?
	4. Can you use a hammer to pound a nail?
	Was the patient able to follow questions and commands throughout the assessment?
	1 "Are you having any unclear thinking?"
	2. "Hold up this many fingers." (examiner holds two fingers in front of patient)?
	3. "Now do the same thing with the other hand." (not repeating the number of fingers)
4. Altered level of consciousness (any level of consciousness other than alert (e.g., vigilant, lethargic, stupor, or coma))	Alert: normal, spontaneously fully aware of environment, interacts appropriately
	Vigilant: hyperalert
	Lethargic: drowsy but easily aroused, unaware of some elements in the environment, or not spontaneously interacting appropriately with the interviewer; becomes fully aware and appropriately interactive when prodded minimally
	Stupor: difficult to arouse, unaware of some or all elements in the environment, or not spontaneously interacting with the interviewer; becomes incompletely aware and inappropriately interactive when prodded strongly; can be aroused only by vigorous and repeated stimuli and as soon as the stimulus ceases, stuporous subjects lapse back into the unresponsive state.
	Coma: unarousable, unaware of all elements in the environment, with no spontaneous interaction or awareness of the interviewer, so that the interview is impossible even with maximal prodding

PATIENTS ARE DIAGNOSED WITH DELIRIUM IF THEY HAVE BOTH FEATURES 1 AND 2 AND EITHER FEATURE 3 OR 4.

[a]SAS = Sedation–Analgesia Scale, MAAS = Motor Activity Assessment Scale, GCS = Glasgow Coma Scale.

87% of the ICU patients with an average onset on the second day and a mean duration of 4.2 ± 1.7 days.[185] Ongoing research will assist in understanding the etiology of delirium and the effects of therapeutic interventions.

Another instrument for delirium screening was validated in ICU patients by comparison with a psychiatric evaluation.[189] The use of these tools in prospective trials will delineate the long–term ramifications of delirium on the clinical outcomes of ICU patients. The study of delirium and other forms of cognitive impairment in mechanically ventilated patients and other risk factors for neuropsychological sequelae after ICU care may be an important advancement in the monitoring and treatment of critically ill patients.

Recommendation: Routine assessment for the presence of delirium is recommended. (The CAM-ICU is a promising tool for the assessment of delirium in ICU patients.) (Grade of recommendation = B)

Treatment of Delirium. Inappropriate drug regimens for sedation or analgesia may exacerbate delirium symptoms. Psychotic or delirious patients may become more obtunded and confused when treated with sedatives, causing a paradoxical increase in agitation.[190]

Neuroleptic agents (chlorpromazine and haloperidol) are the most common drugs used to treat patients with delirium.

They are thought to exert a stabilizing effect on cerebral function by antagonizing dopamine-mediated neurotransmission at the cerebral synapses and basal ganglia. This effect can also enhance extrapyramidal symptoms (EPS). Abnormal symptomatology, such as hallucinations, delusions, and unstructured thought patterns, is inhibited, but the patient's interest in the environment is diminished, producing a characteristic flat cerebral affect. These agents also exert a sedative effect.

Chlorpromazine is not routinely used in critically ill patients because of its strong anticholinergic, sedative, and α-adrenergic antagonist effects. Haloperidol has a lesser sedative effect and a lower risk of inducing hypotension than chlorpromazine. Droperidol, a chemical congener of haloperidol, is reported to be more potent than haloperidol but has been associated with frightening dreams and may have a higher risk of inducing hypotension because of its direct vasodilating and antiadrenergic effects.[191,192] Droperidol has not been studied in ICU patients as extensively as haloperidol.

Haloperidol is commonly given via intermittent i.v. injection.[193] The optimal dose and regimen of haloperidol have not been well defined. Haloperidol has a long half-life (18–54 hours) and loading regimens are used to achieve a rapid response in acutely delirious patients. A loading regimen starting with a 2-mg dose, followed by repeated doses (double the previous dose) every 15–20 minutes while agitation persists, has been described.[193,194] High doses of haloperi-

dol (>400 mg per day) have been reported, but QT prolongation may result. However, the safety of this regimen has been questioned.[192, 195–200] Once the delirium is controlled, regularly scheduled doses (every four to six hours) may be continued for a few days; then therapy should be tapered over several days. A continuous infusion of haloperidol (3–25 mg/hr) has been used to achieve more consistent serum concentrations.[81,201] The pharmacokinetics of haloperidol may be affected by other drugs.[202]

Neuroleptic agents can cause a dose-dependent QT-interval prolongation of the electrocardiogram, leading to an increased risk of ventricular dysrhythmias, including torsades de pointes.[195–200] Significant QT prolongation has been reported with cumulative haloperidol doses as low as 35 mg, and dysrhythmias have been reported within minutes of administering i.v. doses of 20 mg or more.[199] A history of cardiac disease appears to predispose patients to this adverse event.[200] The actual incidence of torsades de pointes associated with halperidol use is unknown, although a historical case-controlled study suggests it may be 3.6%.[199]

EPS can occur with these agents. A slowly eliminated active metabolite of haloperidol appears to cause EPS.[203–208] EPS has been reported less frequently after i.v. versus oral haloperidol administration, but concurrent benzodiazepine use may mask EPS appearance. Self-limited movement disorders can be seen several days after tapering or discontinuing haloperidol and may last for up to two weeks.[209] Treatment of EPS includes discontinuing the neuroleptic agent and a clinical trial of diphenhydramine or benztropine mesylate.

Other adverse effects have also been described. Haloperidol therapy for the control of agitation after a traumatic brain injury may prolong the duration of posttraumatic amnesia, but the effect on functional recovery has not been well demonstrated in humans.[210] Although haloperidol is the most common antipsychotic agent associated with neuroleptic malignant syndrome and has been implicated in approximately 50% of reported episodes (only three cases were reported in critically ill patients receiving intravenous haloperidol), its adverse effects may be underreported.[211–214]

Haloperidol therapy for acutely agitated or delirious patients has not been studied prospectively in agitated ICU patients, but its utility has been suggested in case series.[81,193,201]

> Recommendations: Haloperidol is the preferred agent for the treatment of delirium in critically ill patients. (Grade of recommendation = C)

> Patients should be monitored for electrocardiographic changes (QT interval prolongation and arrhythmias) when receiving haloperidol. (Grade of recommendation = B)

Sleep

Sleep is believed to be important to recover from an illness. Sleep deprivation may impair tissue repair and overall cellular immune function.[215] Sleeplessness induces additional stress in critical care patients.[3,216] Allowing a patient to obtain an adequate amount of sleep may be difficult in a critical care unit. Sleep in the ICU has been characterized by few complete sleep cycles, numerous awakenings, and infrequent rapid-eye-movement (REM) sleep.[217] Atypical sleep patterns were demonstrated in critically ill patients receiving high doses of sedatives.[218]

Sleep Assessment. Similar to pain assessment, the patient's own report is the best measure of sleep adequacy, since polysomnography is not a clinically feasible tool in the critical care setting. If self-report is not possible, systematic observation of a patient's sleep time by nurses has been shown to be a valid measure.[219] A VAS or questionnaire can be used to assess sleep for specific patients.[220]

Nonpharmacologic Strategies. Titrating environmental stimulation. Nonpharmacologic interventions to promote sleep and increase overall patient comfort may include environment modification, relaxation, back massage, and music therapy. Noise in critical care settings is an environmental hazard that disrupts sleep.[221–223] Sources of noise include equipment, alarms, telephones, ventilators, and staff conversations. Noise levels above 80 decibels cause arousal from sleep. Sleep occurs best below 35 decibels.[222] Earplugs effectively decreased noise and increased REM sleep in healthy volunteers in a study that simulated noise heard in an ICU.[224] A creative unit design with single rooms may ameliorate noise and provide lighting that better reflects a day–night orientation.[225] Lighting mimicking the 24-hour day helps patients achieve normal sleep patterns, so bright lights should be avoided at night. In addition, care should be coordinated to minimize frequent interruptions during the night.

Relaxation. Head-to-toe relaxation may benefit anxious critically ill patients who can follow directions. Relaxation will lead to a parasympathetic response and a decrease in respiratory rate, heart rate, jaw tension, and blood pressure. Relaxation techniques include deep breathing followed by the sequential relaxation of each muscle group.[226] Relaxation, in combination with music therapy, is effective in patients with myocardial infarction.[227]

Music therapy. Music therapy relaxes patients and decreases their pain. Music intervention with cardiac surgery patients, during the first postoperative day, decreased noise annoyance, heart rate, and systolic blood pressure.[228] In mechanically ventilated patients, music therapy decreased anxiety and promoted relaxation.[229] Music therapy is a proven intervention for anxious patients in other critical care settings.[229–231] Music can decrease heart rate, respiratory rate, myocardial oxygen demand, and anxiety scores and improve sleep.[232,233] When selecting music, a patient's personal preference should be considered.

Massage. Back massage is an alternative or adjunct to pharmacologic therapy in critically ill patients. Approximately 5–10 minutes of massage initiates the relaxation response and increases a patient's amount of sleep.[234,235]

Pharmacologic Therapy to Promote Sleep. Patients may remain sleep-deprived despite nonpharmacologic interventions. Most patients need a combination of analgesics, sedatives, and relaxation techniques to decrease pain and anxiety and promote sleep. Sedative-hypnotics can induce sleep in healthy individuals, but little is known of their use in the critically ill. There was no difference in sleep quality between two groups of nonintubated ICU patients receiving midazolam or propofol.[59] Oral hypnotics, such as benzodiazepines or zolpidem, are used in nonintubated patients to decrease sleep latency while increasing total sleep time without affecting sleep architecture in stages three and four and REM sleep.[215]

Recommendation: Sleep promotion should include optimization of the environment and nonpharmacologic methods to promote relaxation with adjunctive use of hypnotics. (Grade of recommendation = B)

References

1. Shapiro BA, Warren J, Egol AB, et al. Practice parameters for intravenous analgesia and sedation for adult patients in the intensive care unit: an executive summary. *Crit Care Med.* 1995; 23:1596–600.
2. Society of Critical Care Medicine and American Society of Health-System Pharmacists. Sedation, analgesia, and neuromuscular blockade of the critically ill adult: revised clinical practice guidelines for 2002. *Am J Health-Syst Pharm.* 2002; 59:147–9.
3. Novaes MA, Knobel E, Bork AM, et al. Stressors in ICU: perception of the patient, relatives and healthcare team. *Intensive Care Med.* 1999; 25:1421–6.
4. Desbiens NA, Wu AW, Broste SK, et al. Pain and satisfaction with pain control in seriously ill hospitalized adults: findings from the SUPPORT research investigators. *Crit Care Med.* 1996; 24:1953–61.
5. Epstein J, Breslow MJ. The stress response of critical illness. *Crit Care Clin.* 1999; 15:17–33.
6. Lewis KS, Whipple JK, Michael KA, et al. Effect of analgesic treatment on the physiological consequences of acute pain. *Am J Hosp Pharm.* 1994; 51:1539–54.
7. Mangano DT, Silician D, Hollenberg M, et al. Postoperative myocardial ischemia; therapeutic trials using intensive analgesia following surgery. *Anesthesiology.* 1992; 76:342–53.
8. Parker SD, Breslow MJ, Frank SM, et al. Catecholamine and cortisol responses to lower extremity revascularization: correlation with outcome variables. *Crit Care Med.* 1995; 23:1954–61.
9. Desai PM. Pain management and pulmonary dysfunction. *Crit Care Clin.* 1999; 15:151–66.
10. Gust R, Pecher S, Gust A, et al. Effect of patient-controlled analgesia on pulmonary complications after coronary artery-bypass grafting. *Crit Care Med.* 1999; 27:2218–23.
11. Carroll KC, Atkins PJ, Herold GR, et al. Pain assessment and management in critically ill postoperative and trauma patients: a multisite study. *Am J Crit Care.* 1999; 8:105–17.
12. Ferguson J, Gilroy D, Puntillo K. Dimensions of pain and analgesic administration associated with coronary artery bypass in an Australian intensive care unit. *J Adv Nurs.* 1997; 26:1065–72.
13. Whipple JK, Lewis KS, Quebbeman EJ, et al. Analysis of pain management in critically ill patients. *Pharmacotherapy.* 1995; 15:592–9.
14. Sun X, Weissman C. The use of analgesics and sedatives in critically ill patients: Physicians'; orders versus medications administered. *Heart Lung.* 1994; 23:169–76.
15. Caswell DR, Williams JP, Vallejo M, et al. Improving pain management in critical care. *Jt Comm J Qual Improvement.* 1996; 22:702–12.
16. Hamill-Ruth RJ, Marohn ML. Evaluation of pain in the critically ill patient. *Crit Care Clin.* 1999; 15:35–54.
17. Acute Pain Management Guideline Panel. Acute pain management: operative or medical procedures and trauma. Clinical practice guideline. Rockville, MD: Agency for Health Care Policy and Research, 1992 AHCPR publication no. 92–0032.
18. Ho K, Spence J, Murphy MF. Review of pain management tools. *Ann Emerg Med.* 1996; 27:427–32.
19. Terai T, Yukioka H, Asada A. Pain evaluation in the intensive care unit: observer-reported faces scale compared with self-reported visual analog scale. *Reg Anesth Pain Med.* 1998; 23:147–51.
20. Puntillo KA. Dimensions of procedural pain and its analgesic management in critically ill surgical patients. *Am J Crit Care.* 1994; 3:116–28.
21. Meehan DA, McRae ME, Rourke DA, et al. Analgesia administration, pain intensity, and patient satisfaction in cardiac surgical patients. *Am J Crit Care.* 1995; 4:435–42.
22. Melzack R, Katz J. Pain measurement in persons in pain. In: Wall PD, Melzack R, eds. Textbook of pain. Edinburgh, Scotland: Churchill Livingstone; 1994:337–51.
23. Mateo OM, Krenzischek DA. A pilot study to assess the relationship between behavioral manifestations of pain and self-report of pain in post anesthesia care unit patients. *J Post Anesth Nurs.* 1992; 7:15–21.
24. Puntillo KA, Miaskowski C, Kehrle K, et al. Relationship between behavioral and physiological indicators of pain, critical care patients' self-reports of pain, and opioid administration. *Crit Care Med.* 1997; 25:1159–66.
25. Sjostrom B, Haljamae H, Dahlgren LO, et al. Assessment of postoperative pain: impact of clinical experience and professional role. *Acta Anaesthesiol Scand.* 1997; 41:339–44.
26. Hall-Lord ML, Larsson G, Steen B. Pain and distress among elderly intensive care unit patients: comparison of patients' experiences and nurses' assessments. *Heart Lung.* 1998; 27:123–32.
27. Stannard D, Puntillo K, Miaskowski C, et al. Clinical judgement and management of postoperative pain in critical care patients. *Am J Crit Care.* 1996; 5:433–41.
28. Desbiens NA, Mueller-Rizner N. How well do surrogates assess the pain of seriously ill patients? *Crit Care Med.* 2000; 28:1347–52.
29. Watling SM, Dasta JF, Seidl EC. Sedatives, analgesics, and paralytics in the ICU. *Ann Pharmacother.* 1997; 31:148–53.
30. Wagner BKJ, O'Hara DA. Pharmacokinetics and pharmacodynamics of sedatives and analgesics in the treatment of agitated critically ill patients. *Clin Pharmacokinet.* 1997; 33:426–53.
31. Barr JB, Donner A. Optimal intravenous dosing strategies for sedatives and analgesics in the ICU. *Crit Care Clin.* 1995 11:827–47.
32. AmeriSource Corporation, ECHO software, version 3.1Q, release 00112. Accessed 2001 Feb 6.
33. Danziger LH, Martin SJ, Blum RA. Central nervous system toxicity associated with meperidine use in hepatic disease. *Pharmacotherapy.* 1994; 14:235–8.
34. Hangmeyer KO, Mauro LS, Mauro VF. Meperidine-related seizures associated with patient-controlled analgesia pumps. *Ann Pharmacother.* 1993; 27:29–32.
35. Tipps LB, Coplin WM, Murry KR, et al. Safety and feasibility of continuous infusion of remifentanil in the neurosurgical intensive care unit. *Neurosurgery.* 2000; 46:596–602.

36. Lay TD, Puntillo KA, Miaskowski MI. Analgesics prescribed and administered to intensive care cardiac surgery patients: does patient age make a difference? *Prog Cardiovasc Nurs.* 1996; 11:17–24.

37. Macintyre PE, Jarvis DA. Age is the best predictor of postoperative morphine requirements. *Pain.* 1995; 64:357–64.

38. Fraser GL, Prato S, Berthiaume D, et al. Evaluation of agitation in ICU patients: incidence, severity, and treatment in the young versus the elderly. *Pharmacotherapy.* 2000; 20:75–82.

39. Hofbauer R, Tesinsky P, Hammerschmidt V, et al. No reduction in the sufentanil requirement of elderly patients undergoing ventilatory support in the medical intensive care unit. *Eur J Anaesthesiol.* 1999; 16:702–7.

40. McArdle P. Intravenous analgesia. *Crit Care Clin.* 1999; 15:89–105.

41. Grossman M, Abiose A, Tangphao O, et al. Morphine-induced venodilation in humans. *Clin Pharmacol Ther.* 1996; 60:554–60.

42. Flacke JW, Flacke WE, Bloor BC, et al. Histamine release by four narcotics: a double-blind study in humans. *Anesth Analg.* 1987; 66:723–30.

43. Yuan C, Foss JF, O'Connor MF, et al. Effects of low-dose morphine on gastric emptying in healthy volunteers. *J Clin Pharmacol.* 1998; 38:1017–20.

44. Heyland DK, Tougas G, King D, et al. Impaired gastric emptying in mechanically ventilated, critically ill patients. *Intensive Care Med.* 1996; 22:1339–44.

45. Bosscha K, Nieuwenhuijs VB, Vos A, et al. Gastro–intestinal motility and gastric tube feeding in mechanically ventilated patients. *Crit Care Med.* 1998; 26:1510–7.

46. Albanese J, Viviand X, Potie F, et al. Sufentanil, fentanyl, and alfentanil in head trauma patients: a study on cerebral hemodynamics. *Crit Care Med.* 1999; 27:407–11.

47. Sperry RJ, Bailey PL, Reichman MV, et al. Fentanyl and sufentanil increase intracranial pressure in head trauma patients. *Anesthesiology.* 1992; 77:416–20.

48. DeNaal M, Munar F, Poca MA, et al. Cerebral hemodynamic effects of morphine and fentanyl in patients with severe head injury. *Anesthesiology.* 2000; 92:11–9.

49. Dasta JF, Fuhrman TM, McCandles C. Patterns of prescribing and administering drugs for agitation and pain in patients in a surgical intensive care unit. *Crit Care Med.* 1994; 22:974–80.

50. Kress JP, Pohlman AS, O'Connor MF, et al. Daily interruption of sedative infusions in critically ill patients undergoing mechanical ventilation. *N Engl J Med.* 2000; 342:1471–7.

51. Boldt J, Thaler E, Lehmann A, et al. Pain management in cardiac surgery patients: comparison between standard therapy and patient-controlled analgesia regimen. *J Cardiothorac Vasc Anesth.* 1998; 12:654–8.

52. Pearce CJ, Gonzalez FM, Wallin JD. Renal failure and hyperkalemia associated with ketorolac tromethamine. *Arch Intern Med.* 1993; 153:1000–2.

53. Schlondorff D. Renal complications of nonsteroidal anti-inflammatory drugs. *Kidney Int.* 1993; 44:643–53.

54. Feldman HI, Kinman JL, Berlin JA, et al. Parenteral ketorolac: the risk for acute renal failure. *Ann Intern Med.* 1997; 126:193–9.

55. Strom BL, Berlin JA, Kinman JL, et al. Parenteral ketorolac and risk of gastrointestinal and operative site bleeding. *JAMA.* 1996; 275:376–82.

56. Bombardier C, Laine L, Reicin A, et al. Comparison of upper gastrointestinal toxicity of rofecoxib and naproxen in patients with rheumatoid arthritis. *N Engl J Med.* 2000; 343:1520–8.

57. Peduta VA, Ballabio M, Stefanini S. Effiacacy of propacetamol in the treatment of postoperative pain. Morphine sparing effect in orthopedic surgery. Italian Collaborative Group on Propacetamol. *Acta Anaesthesiol Scand.* 1998; 42:293–8.

58. Zimmerman HJ, Maddrey W. Acetaminophen hepatotoxicity with regular intake of alcohol. Analysis of instances of therapeutic misadventure. *Hepatology.* 1995; 22:767–73.

59. Treggiari-Venzi M, Borgeat A, Fuchs-Buder T, et al. Overnight sedation with midazolam or propofol in the ICU: effects on sleep quality, anxiety and depression. *Intensive Care Med.* 1996; 22:1186–90.

60. Jenkins DH. Substance abuse and withdrawal in the intensive care unit: contemporary issues. *Surg Clin North Am.* 2000; 80:1033–53.

61. Cornwell EE, Belzberg H, Velmahos G, et al. The prevalence and effect of alcohol and drug abuse on cohort-matched critically injured patients. *Am Surg.* 1998; 64:461–5.

62. Spies CD, Rommelspacher H. Alcohol withdrawal in the surgical patient: prevention and treatment. *Anesth Analg.* 1999; 88:946–54.

63. Kaye AD, Clarke RC, Sabar R, et al. Herbal medicines: current trends in anesthesiology practice—a hospital survey. *J Clin Anesth.* 2000; 12:468–71.

64. Atkins PM, Mion LC, Mendelson W, et al. Characteristics and outcomes of patients who self-extubate from ventilatory support: a case-control study. *Chest.* 1997; 112:1317–23.

65. Vassal T, Anh NGD, Gabillet JM, et al. Prospective evaluation of self-extubations in a medical intensive care unit. *Intensive Care Med.* 1993; 19:340–2.

66. Fraser GL, Riker RR, Prato BS, et al. The frequency and cost of patient-initiated device removal in the ICU. *Pharmacotherapy.* 2001; 21:1–6.

67. Conti J, Smith D. Haemodynamic responses to extubation after cardiac surgery with and without continued sedation. *Br J Anaesth.* 1998; 80:834–6.

68. Cohen D, Horiuchi K, Kemper M, et al. Modulating effects of propofol on metabolic and cardiopulmonary responses to stressful intensive care unit procedures. *Crit Care Med.* 1996; 24:612–7.

69. Veselis RA, Reinsel RA, Feshchenko VA, et al. The comparative amnestic effects of midazolam, propofol, thiopental, and fentanyl at equi-sedative concentrations. *Anesthesiology.* 1997; 87:749–64.

70. Weinbroum AA, Halpern P, Rudick V, et al. Midazolam versus propofol for long-term sedation in the ICU: a randomized prospective comparison. *Intensive Care Med.* 1997; 23:1258–63.

71. Wagner BK, O'Hara DA, Hammond JS. Drugs for amnesia in the ICU. *Am J Crit Care.* 1997; 6:192–201.

72. Wagner BK, Zavotsky KE, Sweeney JB, et al. Patient recall of therapeutic paralysis in a surgical critical care unit. *Pharmacotherapy.* 1998; 18:358–63.

73. Schelling G, Stoll C, Meier M, et al. Health-related quality of life and posttraumatic stress disorder in survivors of adult respiratory distress syndrome. *Crit Care Med.* 1998; 26:651–9.

74. Jones C, Griffiths RD. Disturbed memory and amnesia related to intensive care. *Memory.* 2000; 8:79–94.

75. Jones C, Griffiths RD, Humphris G, et al. Memory, delusions, and the development of acute post-traumatic stress disorder-related symptoms after intensive care. *Crit Care Med.* 2001; 29:573–80.

76. Schnyder U, Morgeli H, Nigg C, et al. Early psychological reactions to life-threatening injuries. *Crit Care Med.* 2000; 28:86–92.

77. Scragg P, Jones A, Fauvel N. Psychological problems following ICU treatment. *Anaesthesia.* 2001 56:914.

78. Watling SM, Johnson M, Yanos J. A method to produce sedation in critically ill patients. *Ann Pharmacother.* 1996; 30:1227–31.

79. DeJonghe B, Cook D, Appere-De-Vecchi C, et al. Using and understanding sedation scoring systems: a systematic review. *Intensive Care Med.* 2000; 26:275–85.

80. Brook AD, Ahrens TS, Schaiff R, et al. Effect of a nursing-implemented sedation protocol on the duration of mechanical ventilation. *Crit Care Med.* 1999; 27:2609–15.

81. Riker RR, Fraser GL, Cox PM. Continuous infusion of haloperidol controls agitation in critically ill patients. *Crit Care Med.* 1994; 22:89–97.

82. Riker RR, Picard JT, Fraser GL. Prospective evaluation of the Sedation-Agitation Scale for adult critically ill patients. *Crit Care Med.* 1999; 27:1325–9.

83. Devlin JW, Boleski G, Mlynarek M, et al. Motor Activity Assessment Scale: a valid and reliable sedation scale for use with mechanically ventilated patients in an adult surgical intensive care unit. *Crit Care Med.* 1999; 27:1271–5.

84. Ramsay MA, Savege TM, Simpson BR, et al. Controlled sedation with alphaxalone–alphadolone. *Br Med J.* 1974; 2:656–9.

85. Hansen-Flaschen J, Cowen J, Polomano RC. Beyond the Ramsay scale: need for a validated measure of sedating drug efficacy in the intensive care unit. *Crit Care Med.* 1994; 22:732–3.

86. DeLemos J, Tweeddale M, Chittock DR. Measuring quality of sedation in adult mechanically ventilated critically ill patients: the Vancouver Interaction and Calmness Scale. *J Clin Epidemiol.* 2000; 53:908–19.

87. Chernik DA, Gillings D, Laine H, et al. Validity and reliability of the Observer's Assessment of Alertness/ Sedation Scale: study with intravenous midazolam. *J Clin Psychopharmacol.* 1990; 10:244–51.

88. Ambuel B, Hamlett KW, Marx CM, et al. Assessing distress in pediatric intensive care environments: the COMFORT scale. *J Pediatr Psychol.* 1992; 17:95109.

89. Rosow C, Manberg PJ. Bispectral index monitoring. *Anesthesiol Clin North Am.* 1998; 2:89–107.

90. Liu J, Singh H, White PF. Electroencephalographic bispectral index correlates with intraoperative recall and depth of propofol-induced sedation. *Anesth Analg.* 1997; 84:185–9.

91. Doi M, Gajraj RJ, Mantzaridis H, et al. Relationship between calculated blood concentration of propofol and electrophysiological variables during emergence from anesthesia: comparison of bispectral index, spectral edge frequency, median frequency, and auditory evoked potential index. *Br J Anaesth.* 1997; 78:180–4.

92. Liu J, Singh H, White PF. Electroencephalogram bispectral analysis predicts the depth of midazolam-induced sedation. *Anesthesiology.* 1996; 84:64–9.

93. Simmons LE, Riker RR, Prato BS, et al. Assessing sedation levels in mechanically ventilated ICU patients with the bispectral index and the sedation-agitation scale. *Crit Care Med.* 1999; 27:1499–504.

94. Riker RR, Simmons LE, Fraser GL, et al. Validating the sedation-agitation scale with the bispectral index and visual analog scale in adult ICU patients after cardiac surgery. *Intensive Care Med.* 2001; 27:853–8.

95. De Deyne C, Struys M, Decruyenaere J, et al. Use of continuous bispectral EEG monitoring to assess depth of sedation in ICU patients. *Intensive Care Med.* 1998; 24:1294–8.

96. Ghoneim MM, Mewaldt SP. Benzodiazepines and human memory: a review. *Anesthesiology.* 1990; 72:926–38.

97. Gilliland HE, Prasad BK, Mirakhur RK, et al. An investigation of the potential morphine sparing effect of midazolam. *Anaesthesia.* 1996; 51:808–11.

98. Greenblatt DJ, Ehrenberg BL, Gunderman J, et al. Kinetic and dynamic study of intravenous lorazepam: comparison with intravenous diazepam. *J Pharmacol Exp Ther.* 1989; 250:134–9.

99. Vree TB, Shimoda M, Driessen JJ, et al. Decreased plasma albumin concentration results in increased volume of distribution and decreased elimination of midazolam in intensive care patients. *Clin Pharmacol Ther.* 1989; 46:537–44.

100. Driessen JJ, Vree TB, Guelen PJ. The effects of acute changes in renal function on the pharmacokinetics of midazolam during long-term infusion in ICU patients. *Acta Anaesthesiol Belg.* 1991; 42:149–55.

101. Greenblatt DJ, Abernethy DR, Locniskar A, et al. Effect of age, gender, and obesity on midazolam kinetics. *Anesthesiology.* 1984; 61:27–35.

102. Patel IH, Soni PP, Fukuda EK, et al. The pharmacokinetics of midazolam in patients with congestive heart failure. *Br J Clin Pharmacol.* 1990; 29:565–9.

103. Macgilchrist AJ, Birnie GG, Cook A, et al. Pharmacokinetics and pharmacodynamics of intravenous midazolam in patients with severe alcoholic cirrhosis. *Gut.* 1986; 27:190–5.

104. Boulieu R, Lehmann B, Salord F, et al. Pharmacokinetics of midazolam and its main metabolite 1-hydroxy-midazolam in intensive care patients. *Eur J Drug Metab Pharmacokinet.* 1998; 23:255–8.

105. Malacrida R, Fritz ME, Suter P, et al. Pharmacokinetics of midazolam administered by continuous infusion to intensive care patients. *Crit Care Med.* 1992; 20:1123.

106. Bauer TM, Ritz R, Haberthur C, et al. Prolonged sedation due to accumulation of conjugated metabolites of midazolam. *Lancet.* 1995; 346:145–7.

107. Hamaoka N, Oda Y, Hase I, et al. Propofol decreases the clearance of midazolam by inhibiting CYP3A4: an in vivo and in vitro study. *Clin Pharmacol Ther.* 1999; 66:110–7.

108. Gorski JC, Jones DR, Haehner-Daniels BD, et al. The contribution of intestinal and hepatic CYP3A to the interaction between midazolam and clarithromycin. *Clin Pharmacol Ther.* 1998; 64:133–43.

109. Ahonen J, Olkkola KT, Salmenpera M, et al. Effect of diltiazem on midazolam and alfentanil disposition in patients undergoing coronary artery bypass grafting. *Anesthesiology.* 1996; 85:1246–52.

110. Bailie GR, Cockshott ID, Douglas EJ, et al. Pharmacokinetics of propofol during and after long-term continuous infusion for maintenance of sedation in ICU patients. *Br J Anaesth.* 1992; 68:486–91.

111. Hammerlein A, Derendorf H, Lowenthal DT. Pharmacokinetic and pharmacodynamic changes in the elderly. *Clin Pharmacokinet.* 1998; 35:49–64.

112. Michalets EL. Update: clinically significant cytochrome P-450 drug interactions. *Pharmacotherapy.* 1999; 18:84–112.

113. Shelly MP, Sultan MA, Bodenham A, et al. Midazolam infusions in critically ill patients. *Eur J Anaesthesiol.* 1991; 8:21–7.

114. Nishiyama T. Sedation during artificial ventilation by continuous intravenous infusion of midazolam: effects of hepatocellular or renal damage. *J Intensive Care Med.* 1997; 12:40–4.

115. Ariano RE, Kassum DA, Aronson KJ. Comparison of sedative recovery time after midazolam versus diazepam administration. *Crit Care Med.* 1994; 22:1492–6.

116. Newton DW, Narducci WA, Leet WA, et al. Lorazepam stability in and sorption from intravenous admixture solutions. *Am J Hosp Pharm.* 1983; 40:424–7.

117. Hoey LL, Vance-Bryan K, Clarens DM, et al. Lorazepam stability in parenteral solutions for continuous intravenous administration. *Ann Pharmacother.* 1996; 30:343–6.

118. McCollam JS, O'Neil MG, Norcross ED, et al. Continuous infusions of lorazepam, midazolam and propofol for sedation of the critically-ill surgery trauma patient: a prospective, randomized comparison. *Crit Care Med.* 1999; 27:2454–8.

119. Laine GA, Hamid Hossain SM, Solis RT, et al. Polyethylene glycol nephrotoxicity secondary to prolonged high-dose intravenous lorazepam. *Ann Pharmacother.* 1995; 29:1110–4.

120. Seay RE, Graves PJ, Wilkin MK. Comment: possible toxicity from propylene glycol in lorazepam infusion. *Ann Pharmacother.* 1997; 31:647–8.

121. Arbour RB. Propylene glycol toxicity related to high-dose lorazepam infusion: case report and discussion. *Am J Crit Care.* 1999; 8:499–506.

122. Lugo RA, Chester EA, Cash J, et al. A cost analysis of enterally administered lorazepam in the pediatric intensive care unit. *Crit Care Med.* 1999; 27:417–21.

123. Shepherd MF, Felt-Gunderson PA. Diarrhea associated with lorazepam solution in a tube-fed patient. *Nutr Clin Pract.* 1996; 11:117–20.

124. Kamijo Y, Masuda T, Nishikawa T, et al. Cardiovascular response and stress reaction to flumazenil injection in patients under infusion with midazolam. *Crit Care Med.* 2000; 28:318–23.

125. Breheny FX. Reversal of midazolam sedation with flumazenil. *Crit Care Med.* 1992; 20:736–9.

126. Kowalski SD, Rayfield CA. A post hoc descriptive study of patients receiving propofol. *Am J Crit Care.* 1999; 8:507–13.

127. Sanchez-Izquierdo-Riera JA, Caballero-Cubedo RE, Perez-Vela JL, et al. Propofol versus midazolam: safety and efficacy for sedating the severe trauma patient. *Anesth Analg.* 1998; 86:1219–24.

128. Carrasco G, Molina R, Costa J, et al. Propofol versus midazolam in short-, medium-, and long-term sedation of critically ill patients. *Chest.* 1993; 103:557–64.

129. Barrientos-Vega R, Sanchez–Soria MM, Morales-Garcia C, et al. Prolonged sedation of critically ill patients with midazolam or propofol: impact on weaning and costs. *Crit Care Med.* 1997; 25:33–40.

130. Kumar AN, Achwartz DE, Lim KG. Propofol-induced pancreatitis: recurrence of pancreatitis after rechallenge. *Chest.* 1999; 115:1198–9.

131. Possidente CJ, Rogers FB, Osler TM, et al. Elevated pancreatic enzymes after extended propofol therapy. *Pharmacotherapy.* 1998; 18:653–5.

132. Leisure GS, O'Flaherty J, Green L, et al. Propofol and postoperative pancreatitis. *Anesthesiology.* 1996; 84:224–7.

133. Bray RJ. Propofol infusion syndrome in children. *Paediatr Anaesth.* 1998; 8:491–9.

134. Cremer OL, Moons KGM, Bouman EAC, et al. Long-term propofol infusion and cardiac failure in adult head-injured patients. *Lancet.* 2001; 357:117–8.

135. Bennett SN, McNeil MM, Bland LA, et al. Postoperative infections traced to contamination of an intravenous anesthetic, propofol. *N Engl J Med.* 1995; 333:147–54.

136. Webb SA, Roberts B, Breheny FX, et al. Contamination of propofol infusions in the intensive care unit: incidence and clinical significance. *Anaesth Intensive Care.* 1998; 26:162–4.

137. Avramov MN, Husain MM, White PF. The comparative effects of methohexital, propofol, and etomidate for electroconvulsive therapy. *Anesth Analg.* 1995; 81:596–602.

138. Stecker MM, Kramer TH, Raps EC, et al. Treatment of refractory status epilepticus with propofol: clinical and pharmacokinetic findings. *Epilepsia.* 1998; 39:18–26.

139. McCowan C, Marik P. Refractory delirium tremens treated with propofol: a case series. *Crit Care Med.* 2000; 28:1781–4.

140. Herregods L, Verbeke J, Rolly G, et al. Effect of propofol on elevated intracranial pressure. Preliminary results. *Anaesthesia.* 1988; 43(suppl):107–9.

141. Kelly DF, Goodale DB, Williams J, et al. Propofol in the treatment of moderate and severe head injury: a randomized, prospective double-blinded pilot trial. *J Neurosurg.* 1999; 90:1042–52.

142. Herregods L, Mergaert C, Rolly G, et al. Comparison of the effects of 24-hour propofol or fentanyl infusions on intracranial pressure. *J Drug Dev.* 1989; 2(suppl 2):99–100.

143. Spies CD, Dubisz N, Neumann T, et al. Therapy of alcohol withdrawal syndrome in intensive care unit patients following trauma: results of a prospective, randomized trial. *Crit Care Med.* 1996; 24:414–22.

144. Ip Yam PC, Forbes A, Kox WJ. Clonidine in the treatment of alcohol withdrawal in the intensive care unit. *Br J Anaesth.* 1992; 69:328.

145. Aantaa RE, Kanto JH, Scheinin M. Dexmedetomidine pre-medication for minor gynecologic surgery. *Anesth Analg.* 1990; 4:407–13.

146. Venn RM, Bradshaw CJ, Spencer R, et al. Preliminary UK experience of dexmedetomidine, a novel agent for postoperative sedation in the intensive care unit. *Anaesthesia.* 1999; 54:1136–42.

147. Hall JE, Uhrich TD, Barnet JA, et al. Sedative, amnestic, and analgesic properties of small-dose dexmedetomidine infusions. *Anesth Analg.* 2000; 90:699–705.

148. Belleville JP, Ward DS, Bloor BC, et al. Effects of intravenous dexmedetomidine in humans. *Anesthesiology.* 1992; 77:1125–33.

149. Osterman ME, Keenan SP, Seiferling RA, et al. Sedation in the intensive care unit, a systematic review. *JAMA.* 2000; 283:1451–9.

150. Aitkenhead AR, Willatts SM, Park GR, et al. Comparison of propofol and midazolam for sedation in critically ill patients. *Lancet.* 1989; 2(8665):704–9.

151. Roekaerts PM, Huygen FJ, deLange S. Infusion of propofol versus midazolam for sedation in the intensive care unit following coronary artery surgery. *J Cardiothorac Vasc Anesth.* 1993; 7:142–7.

152. Higgins TL, Yared JP, Estafanous FG, et al. Propofol versus midazolam for intensive care unit sedation after coronary artery bypass grafting. *Crit Care Med.* 1994; 22:1415–23.

153. Ronan KP, Gallagher TJ, George B, et al. Comparison of propofol and midazolam for sedation in intensive care unit patients. *Crit Care Med.* 1995; 23:286–93.

154. Cernaianu AC, DelRossi AJ, Flum DR, et al. Lorazepam and midazolam in the intensive care unit: a randomized, prospective, multicenter study of hemodynamics, oxygen transport, efficacy, and cost. *Crit Care Med.* 1996; 24:222–8.

155. Searle NR, Taillefer J, Gagnon L, et al. Propofol or midazolam for sedation and early extubation following cardiac surgery. *Can J Anaesth.* 1997; 44:629–35.

156. Carrasco G, Cabre L, Sobrepere G, et al. Synergistic sedation with propofol and midazolam in intensive care patients after coronary artery bypass grafting. *Crit Care Med.* 1998; 26:844–51.

157. Hall RI, Sandham D, Cardinal P, et al. Propofol vs midazolam for ICU sedation. A Canadian multicenter randomized trial. *Chest.* 2001; 119:1151–9.

158. Kress JP, O'Connor MF, Pohlman AS, et al. Sedation of critically ill patients during mechanical ventilation. *Am J Resp Crit Care Med.* 1996; 153:1012–8.

159. Pohlman AS, Simpson KP, Hall JB. Continuous intravenous infusions of lorazepam versus midazolam for sedation during mechanical ventilatory support: a prospective, randomized study. *Crit Care Med.* 1994; 22:1241–7.

160. Chamorro C, DeLatorre FJ, Montero A, et al. Comparative study of propofol versus midazolam in the sedation of critically ill patients: results of a prospective, randomized, multicenter trial. *Crit Care Med.* 1996; 24:932–9.

161. Manley NM, Fitzpatrick RW, Long T, et al. A cost analysis of alfentanil + propofol vs. morphine + midazolam for the sedation of critically ill patients. *Pharmacoeconomics.* 1997; 12:247–55.

162. Swart E, van Schijndel RJM, van Loenen AC, et al. Continuous infusion of lorazepam versus midazolam in patients in the intensive care unit: sedation with lorazepam is easier to manage and is more cost effective. *Crit Care Med.* 1999; 27:1461–5.

163. Sandiumenge Camps A, Sanchez-Izquierdo Riera JA, Toral Vazquez D, et al. Midazolam and 2% propofol in long-term sedation of traumatized critically ill patients: efficacy and safety comparison. *Crit Care Med.* 2000; 28:3612–9.

164. Kollef MH, Levy NT, Ahrens TS, et al. The use of continuous i.v. sedation is associated with prolongation of mechanical ventilation. *Chest.* 1998; 114:541–8.

165. Mascia MF, Koch M, Medicis JJ. Pharmacoeconomic impact of rational use guidelines on the provision of analgesia, sedation, and neuromuscular blockade in critical care. *Crit Care Med.* 2000; 28:2300–6.

166. Cammarano WB, Pittet JF, Weitz S, et al. Acute withdrawal syndrome related to the administration of analgesic and sedative medications in adult intensive care unit patients. *Crit Care Med.* 1998; 26:676–84.

167. Katz R, Kelly HW, His A. Prospective study on the occurrence of withdrawal in critically ill children who received fentanyl by continuous infusion. *Crit Care Med.* 1994; 22:763–77.

168. Fonsmark L, Rasmussen YH, Carl P. Occurrence of withdrawal in critically ill children. *Crit Care Med.* 1999; 27:196–9.

169. Carr DB, Todres ID. Fentanyl infusion and weaning in the pediatric intensive care unit: toward science-based practice. *Crit Care Med.* 1994; 22:725–7.

170. Buck M, Blumer J. Opioids and other analgesics: adverse effects in the intensive care unit. *Crit Care Clin.* 1991; 7:615–37.

171. American Pain Society. Principles of analgesic use in the treatment of acute pain and cancer pain. 3rd ed. Skokie, IL: 1992

172. Anand KJS, Ingraham J. Tolerance, dependence, and strategies for compassionate withdrawal of analgesics and anxiolytics in the pediatric ICU. *Crit Care Nurse.* 1996; 16:87–93.

173. Tobias JD. Subcutaneous administration of fentanyl and midazolam to prevent withdrawal after prolonged sedation in children. *Crit Care Med.* 1999; 27:2262–5.

174. Koolhoven I, Tjon-A-Tsien MRS, van der Mast RC. Early diagnosis of delirium after cardiac surgery. *Gen Hosp Psychiatry.* 1996; 18:448–51.

175. Sanders KM, Stern TA, O'Gara PT, et al. Delirium during intra-aortic balloon pump therapy. *Psychosomatics.* 1992; 33:35–44.

176. Dyer CB, Ashton CM, Teasdale TA. Postoperative delirium. A review of 80 primary data collection studies. *Arch Intern Med.* 1995; 155:461–5.

177. American Psychiatric Association. DSM-IV: diagnostic and statistical manual of mental disorders. Washington, DC: American Psychiatric Press; 1994.

178. Trzepacz PT. Delirium—advances in diagnosis, pathophysiology, and treatment. *Psychiatr Clin North Am.* 1996; 19:429–49.

179. Lipowski ZJ. Delirium in the elderly patient. *N Engl J Med.* 1989; 320:578–82.

180. Meagher DJ, Trzepacz PT. Motoric subtypes of delirium. *Semin Clin Neuropsychiatry.* 2000; 5:75–85.

181. Ely EW, Siegel MD, Inouye S. Delirium in the intensive care unit: an underrecognized syndrome of organ dysfunction. *Semin Resp Crit Care Med.* 2001; 22:115–26.

182. Ely EW, Margolin R, Francis J, et al. Evaluation of delirium in critically ill patients: Validation of the confusion assessment method for the intensive care unit (CAM-ICU). *Crit Care Med.* 2001; 29:1370–9.

183. Hart RP, Levenson JL, Sessler CN, et al. Validation of a cognitive test for delirium in medical ICU patients. *Psychosomatics.* 1996; 37:533–46.

184. Hart RP, Best ALN, Sessler CN, et al. Abbreviated cognitive test for delirium. *J Psychosom Res.* 1997; 43:417–23.

185. Ely EW, Inouye SK, Bernard GR, et al. Delirium in mechanically ventilated patients: validity and reliability of the confusion assessment method for the intensive care unit (CAM-ICU). *JAMA.* 2001; 286:2703–10.

186. Inouye SK, van Dyck CH, Alessi CA, et al. Clarifying confusion: the confusion assessment method. *Ann Intern Med.* 1990; 113:941–8.

187. Smith MJ, Breitbart WS, Meredith MP. A critique of instruments and methods to detect, diagnose, and rate delirium. *J Pain Symptom Manage.* 1995; 10:35–77.

188. Inouye SK, Bogardus ST, Charpentier PA, et al. A multicomponent intervention to prevent delirium in hospitalized older patients. *N Engl J Med.* 1999; 340:669–76.

189. Bergeron N, Dubois MJ, Dumont M, et al. Intensive care delirium screening checklist: evaluation of a new screening tool. *Intensive Care Med.* 2001; 27:859–64.

190. Breitbart W, Marotta R, Platt MM, et al. A double-blind trial of haloperidol, chlorpromazine, and lorazepam in the treatment of delirium in hospitalized AIDS patients. *Am J Psychiatry.* 1996; 153:231–7.

191. Frye MA, Coudreaut MF, Hakeman SM, et al. Continuous droperidol infusion for management of agitated delirium in an intensive care unit. *Psychosomatics.* 1995; 36:301–5.

192. Faigel DO, Metz DC, Kochman ML. Torsade de pointes complicating the treatment of bleeding esophageal varices: association with neuroleptics, vasopressin, and electrolyte imbalance. *Am J Gastroenterol.* 1995; 90:822–4.

193. Tesar GE, Murray GB, Cassem NH. Use of haloperidol for acute delirium in intensive care setting. *J Clin Psychopharmacol.* 1985; 5:344–7.

194. Tesar GE, Stern TA. Rapid tranquilization of the agitated intensive care unit patient. *J Intensive Care Med.* 1988; 3:195–201.

195. DiSalvo TG, O'Gara PT. Torsade de pointes caused by high-dose intravenous haloperidol in cardiac patients. *Clin Cardiol.* 1995; 28:285–90.

196. Metzger E, Friedman R. Prolongation of the corrected QT and torsades de pointes cardiac arrhythmia associated with intravenous haloperidol in the medically ill. *J Clin Psychopharmacol.* 1993; 13:128–32.

197. Wilt JL, Minnema AM, Johnson RF, et al. Torsade de pointes associated with the use of intravenous haloperidol. *Ann Intern Med.* 1993; 119:391–4.

198. Hunt N, Stern TA. The association between intravenous haloperidol and torsades de pointes. *Psychosomatics.* 1995; 36:541–9.

199. Sharma ND, Rosman HS, Padhi D, et al. Torsades de pointes associated with intravenous haloperidol in critically ill patients. *Am J Cardiol.* 1998; 81:238–40.

200. Lawrence KR, Nasraway SA. Conduction disturbances associated with administration of butyrophenone antipsychotics in the critically ill: a review of the literature. *Pharmacotherapy.* 1997; 17:531–7.

201. Seneff MG, Mathews RA. Use of haloperidol infusions to control delirium in critically ill adults. *Ann Pharmacother.* 1995; 29:690–3.

202. Kudo S, Ishizaki T. Pharmacokinetics of haloperidol. *Clin Pharmacokinet.* 1999; 37:435–56.

203. Fang J, Baker GB, Silverstone PH, et al. Involvement of CYP3A4 and CYP2D6 in the metabolism of haloperidol. *Cell Mol Neurobiol.* 1997; 17:227–33.

204. Tsang MW, Shader RI, Greenblatt DJ. Metabolism of haloperidol: clinical implications and unanswered questions. *J Clin Psychopharmacol.* 1994; 14:159–62.

205. Avent KM, Riker RR, Fraser GL, et al. Metabolism of haloperidol to pyridinium species in patients receiving high doses intravenously: is HPTP an intermediate? *Life Sci.* 1997; 61:2383–90.

206. Eyles DW, McLennan HR, Jones A, et al. Quantitative analysis of two pyridinium metabolites of haloperidol in patients with schizophrenia. *Clin Pharmacol Ther.* 1994; 56:512–20.

207. Usuki E, Pearce R, Parkinson A, et al. Studies on the conversion of haloperidol and its tetrahydropyridine dehydration product to potentially neurotoxic pyridinium metabolites by human liver microsomes. *Chem Res Toxicol.* 1996; 9:800–6.

208. Eyles DW, McGrath JJ, Pond SM. Formation of pyridinium species of haloperidol in human liver and brain. *Psychopharmacology.* 1996; 125:214–9.

209. Riker RR, Fraser GL, Richen P. Movement disorders associated with withdrawal from high-dose intravenous haloperidol therapy in delirious ICU patients. *Chest.* 1997; 111:1778–81.

210. Rao N, Jellinek HM, Woolston DC. Agitation in closed head injury: haloperidol effects on rehabilitation outcome. *Arch Phys Med Rehabil.* 1985; 66:30–4.

211. Shalev A, Hermesh H, Munitz H. Mortality from neuroleptic malignant syndrome. *J Clin Psychiatry.* 1989; 50:18–25.

212. Still J, Friedman B, Law E, et al. Neuroleptic malignant syndrome in a burn patient. *Burns.* 1998; 24:573–5.

213. Levitt AJ, Midha R, Craven JL. Neuroleptic malignant syndrome with intravenous haloperidol. *Can J Psychiatry.* 1990; 35:789. Letter.

214. Burke C, Fulda GJ, Casellano J. Neuroleptic malignant syndrome in a trauma patient. *J Trauma.* 1995; 39:796–8.

215. Krachman SL, D'Alonzo GE, Criner GJ. Sleep in the intensive care unit. *Chest.* 1995; 107:1713–20.

216. Stein-Parbury J, McKinley S. Patients' experiences of being in an intensive care unit: a select literature review. *Am J Crit Care.* 2000; 9:20–7.

217. Redeker NS. Sleep in acute care settings: an integrative review. *J Nurs Scholarsh.* 2000; 32:31–8.

218. Cooper AB, Thornley KS, Young GB, et al. Sleep in critically ill patients requiring mechanical ventilation. *Chest.* 2000; 117:809–18.

219. Edwards GB, Schuring LM. Pilot study: validating staff nurses' observations of sleep and wake states among critically ill patients using polysomnography. *Am J Crit Care.* 1993; 2:125–31.

220. Richardson SJ. A comparison of tools for the assessment of sleep pattern disturbance in critically ill adults. *Dimens Crit Care Nurs.* 1997; 16:226–39.

221. Meyers TJ, Eveloff SE, Bauer MS, et al. Adverse environmental conditions in the respiratory and medical ICU settings. *Chest.* 1994; 105:1211–6.

222. Aaron JN, Carlisle CC, Carskadon MA, et al. Environmental noise as a cause of sleep disruption in an intermediate respiratory care unit. *Sleep.* 1996; 19:707–10.

223. Freedman NS, Kotzer N, Schwab RJ. Patient perception of sleep quality and etiology of sleep disruption in the intensive care unit. *Am J Resp Crit Care Med.* 1999; 159:1155–62.

224. Wallace CJ, Robins J, Alvord LS, et al. The effect of ear-plugs on sleep measures during exposure to simulated intensive care unit noise. *Am J Crit Care.* 1999; 8:210–9.

225. Horsburgh CR. Healing by design. *N Engl J Med.* 1995; 333:735–40.

226. Griffin JP, Myers S, Kopelke C, et al. The effects of progressive muscular relaxation on subjectively re-ported disturbance due to hospital noise. *Behav Med.* 1988; 14:37–42.

227. Guzzetta CE. Effects of relaxation and music therapy on patients in a coronary care unit with presumptive myocardial infarction. *Heart Lung.* 1989; 18:609–16.

228. Byers JF, Smyth KA. Effect of a music intervention on noise annoyance, heart rate, and blood pressure in car-diac surgery patients. *Am J Crit Care.* 1997; 6:183–91.

229. Chlan L. Effectiveness of a music therapy intervention on relaxation and anxiety for patients receiving venti-latory assistance. *Heart Lung.* 1998; 27:169–76.

230. Updike P. Music therapy results for ICU patients. *Dimens Crit Care Nurs.* 1990; 9:39–45.

231. Bolwerk CA. Effects of relaxing music on state anxi-ety in myocardial infarction patients. *Crit Care Nurs Q.* 1990; 13:63–72.

232. White JM. Effects of relaxing music on cardiac auto-nomic balance and anxiety after acute myocardial in-farction. *Am J Crit Care.* 1999; 8:220–30.

233. Zimmerman L, Nieveen J, Barnason S, et al. The ef-fects of music interventions on postoperative pain and sleep in coronary artery bypass graft (CABG) patients. *Sch Inq Nurs Pract.* 1996; 10:153–70.

234. Labyak SE, Metzger BL. The effects of effleurage backrub on the physiological components of relax-ation: a meta-analysis. *Nurs Res.* 1997; 46:59–62.

235. Richards KC. Effect of a back massage and relaxation intervention on sleep in critically ill patients. *Am J Crit Care.* 1998; 7:288–99.

Appendix A—Summary of Recommendations

1. All critically ill patients have the right to adequate analgesia and management of their pain. (Grade of recommendation = C)

2. Pain assessment and response to therapy should be performed regularly by using a scale appropriate to the patient population and systematically documented. (Grade of recommendation = C)

3. The level of pain reported by the patient must be con-sidered the current standard for assessment of pain and response to analgesia whenever possible. Use of the NRS is recommended to assess pain. (Grade of recom-mendation = B)

4. Patients who cannot communicate should be assessed through subjective observation of pain-related behaviors (movement, facial expression, and posturing) and physi-ological indicators (heart rate, blood pressure, and respi-ratory rate) and the change in these parameters following analgesic therapy. (Grade of recommendation = B)

5. A therapeutic plan and goal of analgesia should be established for each patient and communicated to all caregivers to ensure consistent analgesic therapy. (Grade of recommendation = C)

6. If intravenous doses of an opioid analgesic are required, fentanyl, hydromorphone, and morphine are the recom-mended agents. (Grade of recommendation = C)

7. Scheduled opioid doses or a continuous infusion is preferred over an "as needed" regimen to ensure con-sistent analgesia. A PCA device may be utilized to deliver opioids if the patient is able to understand and operate the device. (Grade of recommendation = B)

8. Fentanyl is preferred for a rapid onset of analgesia in acutely distressed patients. (Grade of recommendation = C)

9. Fentanyl or hydromorphone are preferred for patients with hemodynamic instability or renal insufficiency. (Grade of recommendation = C)

10. Morphine and hydromorphone are preferred for inter-mittent therapy because of their longer duration of ef-fect. (Grade of recommendation = C)

11. NSAIDs or acetaminophen may be used as adjuncts to opi-oids in selected patients. (Grade of recommendation = B)

12. Ketorolac therapy should be limited to a maximum of five days, with close monitoring for the development of renal insufficiency or gastrointestinal bleeding. Other NSAIDs may be used via the enteral route in appropriate patients. (Grade of recommendation = B)

13. Sedation of agitated critically ill patients should be started only after providing adequate analgesia and treating reversible physiological causes. (Grade of recommendation = C)

14. A sedation goal or endpoint should be established and regularly redefined for each patient. Regular assess-ment and response to therapy should be systematically documented. (Grade of recommendation = C)

15. The use of a validated sedation assessment scale (SAS, MAAS, or VICS) is recommended. (Grade of recom-mendation = B)

16. Objective measures of sedation, such as BIS, have not been completely evaluated and are not yet proven use-ful in the ICU. (Grade of recommendation = C)

17. Midazolam or diazepam should be used for rapid seda-tion of acutely agitated patients. (Grade of recommen-dation = C)

18. Propofol is the preferred sedative when rapid awaken-ing (e.g., for neurologic assessment or extubation) is important. (Grade of recommendation = B)

19. Midazolam is recommended for short-term use only, as it produces unpredictable awakening and time to extubation when infusions continue longer than 48–72 hours. (Grade of recommendation = A)

20. Lorazepam is recommended for the sedation of most patients via intermittent i.v. administration or continu-ous infusion. (Grade of recommendation = B)

21. The titration of the sedative dose to a defined endpoint is recommended with systematic tapering of the dose or daily interruption with retitration to minimize prolonged sedative effects. (Grade of recommendation = A)

22. Triglyceride concentrations should be monitored after two days of propofol infusion, and total caloric intake from lipids should be included in the nutrition support prescription. (Grade of recommendation = B)

23. The use of sedation guidelines, an algorithm, or a pro-tocol is recommended. (Grade of recommendation = B)

24. The potential for opioid, benzodiazepine, and propo-fol withdrawal should be considered after high doses or more than approximately seven days of continuous

therapy. Doses should be tapered systematically to prevent withdrawal symptoms. (Grade of recommendation = B)

25. Routine assessment for the presence of delirium is recommended. (The CAM-ICU is a promising tool for the assessment of delirium in ICU patients.) (Grade of recommendation = B)

26. Haloperidol is the preferred agent for the treatment of delirium in critically ill patients. (Grade of recommendation = C)

27. Patients should be monitored for electrocardiographic changes (QT interval prolongation and arrhythmias) when receiving haloperidol. (Grade of recommendation = B)

28. Sleep promotion should include optimization of the environment and nonpharmacologic methods to promote relaxation with adjunctive use of hypnotics. (Grade of recommendation = B)

Developed through the Task Force of the American College of Critical Care Medicine (ACCM) of the Society of Critical Care Medicine (SCCM), in collaboration with the American Society of Health-System Pharmacists (ASHP), and in alliance with the American College of Chest Physicians; and approved by the Board of Regents of ACCM and the Council of SCCM on November 15, 2001, and the ASHP Board of Directors on November 17, 2001.

The recommendations in this document do not indicate an exclusive course of treatment to be followed. Variations, taking into account individual circumstances, may be appropriate.

The bibliographic citation is as follows: Society of Critical Care Medicine and American Society of Health-System Pharmacists. Clinical practice guidelines for the sustained use of sedatives and analgesics in the critically ill adult. *Am J Health-Syst Pharm.* 2002; 59:150–78.

Index

Index

C

D

E

F

 G

H

M

Q

R

 V

 W